North Carolina Nurse Aide I

Hegner

Acello

Needham

THOMSON
DELMAR LEARNING

Australia · Canada · Mexico · Singapore · Spain · United Kingdom · United

North Carolina Nurse Aide I

Hegner / Acello / Needham

Executive Editors:
Michele Baird, Maureen Staudt & Michael Stranz

Project Development Manager:
Linda deStefano

Sr. Marketing Coordinators:
Lindsay Annett and Sara Mercurio

Production/Manufacturing Manager:
Donna M. Brown

Production Editorial Manager:
Dan Plofchan

Pre-Media Services Supervisor:
Becki Walker

Rights and Permissions Specialist:
Kalina Ingham Hintz

Cover Image
Getty Images*

Printed in the
United States of America
1 2 3 4 5 6 7 10 09 08 07

For more information, please contact Thomson Custom Solutions, 5191 Natorp Boulevard, Mason, OH 45040. Or you can visit our Internet site at www.thomsoncustom.com

The Adaptable Courseware Program consists of products and additions to existing Thomson products that are produced from camera-ready copy. Peer review, class testing, and accuracy are primarily the responsibility of the author(s).

North Carolina Nurse Aide I /
Hegner/Acello/Needham

ISBN-13: 978-1-4283-1732-1
ISBN-10: 1-4283-1732-5

International Divisions List

Asia (Including India):
Thomson Learning
(a division of Thomson Asia Pte Ltd)
5 Shenton Way #01-01
UIC Building
Singapore 068808
Tel: (65) 6410-1200
Fax: (65) 6410-1208

Australia/New Zealand:
Thomson Learning Australia
102 Dodds Street
Southbank, Victoria 3006
Australia

Latin America:
Thomson Learning
Seneca 53
Colonia Polano
11560 Mexico, D.F., Mexico
Tel (525) 281-2906
Fax (525) 281-2656

Canada:
Thomson Nelson
1120 Birchmount Road
Toronto, Ontario
Canada M1K 5G4
Tel (416) 752-9100
Fax (416) 752-8102

UK/Europe/Middle East/Africa:
Thomson Learning
High Holborn House
50-51 Bedford Row
London, WC1R 4LS
United Kingdom
Tel 44 (020) 7067-2500
Fax 44 (020) 7067-2600

Spain (Includes Portugal):
Thomson Paraninfo
Calle Magallanes 25
28015 Madrid
España
Tel 34 (0)91 446-3350
Fax 34 (0)91 445-6218

*Unless otherwise noted, all cover images used by Thomson Custom Solutions have been supplied courtesy of Getty Images with the exception of the *Earthview* cover image, which has been supplied by the National Aeronautics and Space Administration (NASA).

Acknowledgements

The publisher would like to thank Betty Rivers of Forsyth Tech Community College for her countless hours of effort in helping select the content adherent to North Carolina's Nursing Aide standards. Her expert abilities and attention to detail have been invaluable during the creation of this textbook.

Table of Contents

Acknowledgements I

Unit I—Introduction to Health Care I

Unit 2—Communication, Interpersonal Skills, Observation, Recording . . 29
Part A: Communication and Interpersonal Skills 29
Part B: Observation, Recording, and Reporting 47
Part C: Comfort, Pain, Rest, and Sleep 68
Part D: Admission, Transfer, and Discharge 80

Unit 3—Infection Control 91

Unit 4—Safety and Emergencies 131

Unit 5—Legal and Ethical Responsibilities 167

Unit 6—Nutrition and Hydration 183

Unit 7—Common Diseases & Conditions of Body Systems 211

Unit 8—The Residence Environment 341

Unit 9—Personal Care and Grooming 357

Unit 10—Basic Nursing Skills 399

Unit 11—Resident Care Procedures 433
Part A: Elimination/Specimen Collection 435
Part B: Applying Warm or Cold Applications 469
Part C: Assisting with Coughing and Deep Breathing Exercises 484
Part D: Applying Elastic Stocking (TED Hose) and Elastic Bandages . . . 486
Part E: Non-sterile Dressing and Bandages 494

Unit 12—Death and Dying 499

Unit 13—Basic Restorative Services 513
Part A: Restorative Care 513
Part B: Assisting Residents with Mobility 551
Unit 14—Prevention of Pressure Ulcers 585
Unit 15—Restraints 605
Unit 16—Psychological Effects of Aging 623
Glossary 653
Index 667

UNIT 1

Introduction to Health Care

OBJECTIVES

After reading this unit, you will be able to:

- Spell and define key terms.
- List five settings in which health care is delivered and describe the function of each.
- Differentiate care given in an acute care hospital, subacute unit, health maintenance organization, private home, and long-term care facility.
- Describe the purpose and function of the interdisciplinary team.
- Explain the chain of command and describe why using the chain of command is important.
- Describe at least five desirable qualities of the nursing assistant.
- Describe responsible behavior and list nine ways to show that you are responsible.
- List six general categories of nursing assistant responsibilities in the long-term care facility.

Welcome to the field of health care! You are on the way to becoming a respected health care worker who provides direct care to ill or injured persons in the long-term care facility. The services you provide will be under the direction and supervision of a licensed nurse.

Many titles are used to describe the person who delivers personal care to residents. These include nursing assistant, nurse assistant, nurse aide, patient care technician, patient care associate, attendant or assistant, primary caregiver, and health care technician. This caregiver is very important to resident comfort and well-being. Some health care facilities employ **multiskilled workers**. The multiskilled worker has completed a basic nursing assistant program and has taken advanced classes to be able to provide additional resident care skills. Successfully completing the nursing assistant program is the first step in the health care ladder and will provide you with a secure, rewarding career.

Health Care Delivery

Health care is provided in many settings. Many professional and nonprofessional workers provide patient care in these sites. The type of care given is determined by the types of services the sites deliver, but the basic skills you will learn in this course are used to some degree in all health care settings.

Hospitals

Hospitals are health care agencies that give care to persons with **acute illnesses** and injuries. An acute illness is one that occurs quickly and does not last very long. The person receiving care in the hospital is called a **patient**. Patients usually stay in the hospital for a short period of time. When the patient is medically stable, he or she returns home or is transferred to a facility or unit in which patients are not acutely ill and require a lower level of care. The goal is for the individual eventually to return to his or her own home.

Long-Term Care Facilities

Long-term care facilities are agencies that care for persons with **chronic illnesses** who require **rehabilitation, restorative care,** or assistance with personal care. A chronic illness is one that lasts for a long time, perhaps for life. An example of a chronic illness is heart disease. Sometimes a chronic illness can cause an acute problem. Acute problems related to chronic illnesses are usually treated in the hospital. Rehabilitation and restorative care are individualized programs designed to assist residents to attain and maintain the highest level of function possible in their individual situations. These programs help residents overcome the disabling effects of their illness or injury.

The person receiving care in the long-term care facility is called a **resident** because the facility is considered "home," either temporarily or permanently. Long-term care facilities may be called by many different names. Some of these names are nursing homes, nursing facilities, convalescent homes, rehabilitation centers, care centers, care facilities, and skilled nursing facilities.

Long-term care facilities are regulated and inspected by government agencies. Agency representatives visit the facility unannounced to inspect resident care and facility cleanliness. Facilities that are not in compliance with the law must pay penalties and fines according to the nature and severity of the problems surveyors observe. The nursing assistant has an important responsibility to follow all laws, rules, and facility policies. If you follow facility policies and do your job in the way that you were taught, you will stay in compliance with the law.

Skilled nursing units in hospitals must follow the same laws as long-term care facilities. They follow requirements listed in the OBRA legislation. Inspections in hospital skilled units are done by state or federal surveyors who use the same survey tool that is completed in long-term care facilities. The survey process is discussed in detail in Section 6.

Types of Residents in Long-Term Care Facilities

Long-term care facilities are home for many types of residents. Some will spend the rest of their lives in the facility. Others come to the facility for a short time for rehabilitation and restoration, which help residents regain strength after an acute illness or injury. These residents then return to their own homes or a less intensive care setting. Regardless of discharge plans, remember that the quality of the resident's life is as important as the length of the resident's life. As a nursing assistant, you should try to give all residents the highest quality of life possible.

All humans have **developmental tasks** that must be completed throughout each stage of life. These are intellectual, social, and emotional skills that a person must master at a certain age level. The tasks are simple in early childhood, and

TABLE 1-1 Developmental Tasks

Age	Stage of Development	Developmental Tasks
Birth to 1 Year	Infant	Learns to trust self and others
Toddler	1–3 years	Learns to differentiate self from other people
Preschool	3–5 years	Develops initiative and is able to plan and initiate tasks
School Age	6–11 years	Develops physical and mental ability; develops relationships with others
Adolescence	12–18 years	Develops a sense of identity and sexuality
Young Adulthood	19–25 years	Establishes intimate relationships with a spouse or significant other
Middle Adulthood	26–50 years	Self-realization in marriage and family, establishes a career
Late Adulthood	51–65 years	Adjusts to the aging process, helps adult children
Old Age	65+ years	Critical review of the events and circumstances of life, develops feelings of fulfillment, acceptance, and self-worth

become more complex as a person ages. Developmental tasks are described in Table 1.1. Residents in the long-term care facility, like everyone else, have developmental tasks that they must complete while living in the nursing facility.

Geriatrics. Many residents in the long-term care facility are *geriatric,* or elderly. Geriatrics refers to the care of the elderly. Some residents of long-term care facilities have a physical or mental condition, or **disability,** that prevents them from taking care of themselves in the community.

Residents who are mentally retarded. Some residents may be **mentally retarded**. These residents have lower-than-average intelligence that prevents them from caring for themselves or living independently. Most can learn new things, but learning may take a long time.

Residents with developmental disability. Some residents have a **developmental disability**. People with a developmental disability developed this condition before the age of 22. They may have a physical impairment, mental impairment, or a combination of both. Individuals with mental retardation or developmental disabilities may not be admitted to skilled nursing facilities unless their medical needs require skilled nursing care. If they do not require skilled care, they are usually admitted to special facilities that provide services to meet their highly individual needs and teach skills to make them as independent as possible.

Young and middle-aged adults. Not all residents in the long-term care facility are elderly. Some are young and middle-aged adults who have chronic diseases or have suffered severe trauma and cannot live independently. Still others have infectious diseases, such as AIDS.

Making the transition from living in the community to life in a long-term care facility may be very difficult for this population. Over the course of a lifetime, our experiences teach us flexibility. Elderly individuals gradually learn to cope with losses of friends, family, and health. They understand the vulnerability that comes with age and chronic illness, although they do not necessarily like it. Younger residents do not always have the benefit of learning to cope with losses gradually. Many are admitted into the facility as a result of sudden illness or trauma. They have not had a lifetime to adjust to their losses. They are often learning to accept and cope with their physical losses at the same time they are trying to adjust to living in a facility. They may fear what the future holds for them. This is a difficult and frustrating time for the resident. They may view staff as their peer group because they are closer in age than the geriatric residents. By empathizing with the resident and understanding the frustration he or she feels, the nursing assistant can help to make the transition easier.

Infants and children. Some specialized long-term care facilities care for infants and young children. The laws vary among the states with regard to children in nursing facilities. Some facilities are licensed strictly for children. In other facilities, children are mixed into the adult population.

Infants, Children, Young, and Middle-Aged Adults in the Long-Term Care Facility

Some long-term care facilities have a mixed population, with residents of all ages. It is very difficult for facility staff to meet the needs of all age groups at the same time. Each group has different needs. Young individuals admitted to long-term care must complete the developmental tasks for their age group while they are residents of the facility. If they fail to complete the developmental tasks because of illness or facility admission, their emotional growth slows or stops at the point where it was before their illness.

Long-term care facilities that accept younger residents find they must adapt their activity programs to the needs of the younger population. The videotapes that the geriatric residents watch are of no interest to children and younger adults. More out-of-facility shopping trips and outings are often planned. The menu must be adapted to meet the nutritional needs and preferences of younger residents. Children and young and middle-aged adults may want yogurt, pizza, tacos, or Chinese stir-fry recipes. These foods are not normally on the nursing home menu. However, younger populations want and need the same foods they would eat if they were living in the community. They may also need larger portions than the geriatric residents. This population also looks for the same social and intellectual stimulation they had in the community.

Infants and Children

Children are often admitted to the long-term care facility as a result of problems occurring at birth or in early childhood. They often have complex medical problems and needs. Children in long-term care facilities attend school, if they are able. Infants and children must be able to trust the people who care for them. They will develop a sense of autonomy from reassurance and support. Understanding what these tasks are and helping children achieve them is an important responsibility.

Young Adults

Young adults are commonly admitted to the long-term care facility because of trauma and severe injuries. They may feel a sense of great loss when they are admitted to long-term care. Their lives have been disrupted. Their relationships frequently fall apart, which is emotionally trying. Friends and loved ones go on with their lives, leaving the young adult resident behind. Behavior problems, including drug and alcohol abuse, are not uncommon in this age group. Young adult residents are in the same age group as many of the staff members. They attempt to form relationships with staff that are not always healthy. They are frequently manipulative and play staff members against each other, because their coping skills are not well developed. The manipulation often causes them to be labeled as "problem residents." Their behavior often interferes with their care. Young adult residents often feel misplaced in the long-term care facility because there are very few residents in their age group.

Middle-Aged Adults

Middle-aged adults are commonly admitted to the long-term care facility as a result of chronic illnesses, such as multiple sclerosis. Middle-aged adults often are in the prime of their lives and careers. They have great worries about their children's education and their families' security and future. They are often frustrated by the effects of their illnesses, and feel a great sense of loss. Spouses may feel guilty over placing their loved ones in a nursing facility. They may distance themselves, visiting less often and for shorter periods of time. They may have difficulty managing their homes and families alone. Some become lonely and seek other companionship. The emotional effects of the injury or illness and separation can be devastating to both the resident and the spouse.

Helping Special Resident Populations

Meeting the needs of special populations in the facility is not difficult. The most important thing to remember is that not all residents fit into one mold. All are individuals, with both physical and emotional needs. Staff must be realistic about the resident's conditions and abilities. Avoid becoming friends with residents. Viewing them as friends causes you to lose objectivity as a caregiver and may violate professional ethics.

Likewise, avoid viewing yourself as a savior of the residents. Many will not get better. They may spend their lives in a facility. Your personal goal should be to contribute to providing the highest possible quality of life for each resident in your assignment. Because we are all different, what constitutes quality of life will vary with the individual. Follow the care plan and strive to give personalized care that meets each resident's needs.

Infants and Children. The nursing assistant who provides long-term care to infants and children should strive to keep routines as normal, consistent, and secure as possible for the child. Children often fear separation from their parents. Facility staff become parent figures to the child. Staff must not get so caught up in physical caregiving that they forget about the child's emotional needs. Helping the youngest residents to live as normally as possible and master their developmental tasks are important goals.

Young and Middle-Aged Adults. Adjusting to life in a long-term care facility may be difficult for young and middle-aged adults. These residents often prefer to stay up late at night, then sleep in the morning. Many elderly residents prefer to live by the adage, "early to bed, early to rise." The movies, music, food, and television shows that young adults prefer are different from those enjoyed by the geriatric age group. Young and middle-aged residents cannot relate to residents with dementia.

The interdisciplinary team will involve residents in developing their plans of care. If the resident establishes and agrees to the goals, he or she is more likely to work toward meeting them. Give residents as much control over their daily routines as possible. Make eye contact and use good communication skills. Avoid labeling the resident as a "behavior problem" or "uncooperative." Show the resident that he or she can depend on you. If a resident will not cooperate, ask if there would be a better time. Or say, "I want to give you the care you need, but cannot do so if you call me names. I will return in five minutes." When you leave the room, inform the nurse of the problem and your actions. When you return, start fresh and forget the problems that occurred previously. Set limits on the resident's behavior. Compliment the resident for positive behavior.

Skilled Nursing Facilities

Often the name of the agency describes the type of care that the facility provides. Some hospitals have units called *skilled units*. These units are licensed as long-term care facilities. Some nursing homes are licensed to provide skilled care in all areas of the facility. Others license only specific wings or units to provide skilled care. Residents who require skilled care have illnesses or injuries that require daily services that only a licensed health care professional can provide. These services can involve one or more disciplines within the health care facility. For example, nurses must administer injections and are responsible for complex treatments. The services of a licensed nurse are also required to assess the residents' medical condition and take appropriate action if problems are noted. If the resident has many complex needs, planning and monitoring daily care is considered a skilled service. Licensed therapy personnel provide skilled therapy on a daily basis to rehabilitate the resident. Skilled nursing facilities provide care for residents who have highly specialized medical needs, but who are medically stable and not acutely ill.

Subacute Units

Care may also be given in **subacute** care centers or units. The subacute unit is a transitional step between the hospital and the skilled nursing facility. These units may be part of a hospital or long-term care facility. Residents in subacute units have complex medical needs, but are not critically ill. However, they require close monitoring by health care professionals because their conditions may change at any time. The residents are not ill enough to require the services of the acute care hospital, but still require frequent care. They usually require many services from the nursing assistant. Some facilities call the person receiving care "patient." Others use the term "resident."

Assisted Living Facilities

Assisted living facilities (ALFs) are a rapidly growing segment of the long-term care industry. Other names for assisted living facilities are residential care facilities, personal care facilities, and adult congregate care facilities. Assisted living facilities are designed to meet consumer needs for independence in a safe, homelike, residential setting. They provide housing and personal care support services to residents. Residents are encouraged to remain involved with their families and the community. Some facilities provide specialized services, such as caring for residents with Alzheimer's disease. A resident in an assisted living facility can rent one room or an entire apartment. Each unit has an emergency call system. The services vary somewhat depending on the type of services offered, and state laws. Other services provided by most assisted living facilities are:

- 24-hour security
- 24-hour staff availability
- Three meals a day in a common dining area; some units have limited cooking and refrigeration facilities residents can use to prepare meals and store food
- Assistance with eating, bathing, dressing, toileting, and walking
- Medication management
- Social and recreational activities
- Transportation
- Housekeeping services
- Personal laundry services
- Access to health and medical services; hands-on delivery of health services is not provided in most assisted living facilities
- Exercise and wellness programs

Residents of assisted living facilities may:

- Display signs of mental or emotional disturbance, but are not considered at risk of harm to self or others.
- Need some assistance with movement; residents who are immobile or totally dependent on staff are not appropriate for an ALF.
- Require assistance with bathing, dressing, and grooming.
- Need assistance with routine skin care, such as application of lotions, or treatment of minor cuts and burns.
- Need reminders to use the toilet to prevent incontinence.
- Be incontinent without pressure sores.
- Need assistance with toileting.
- Need assistance with medications, supervision of self-medication, or administration of medication.
- Need special diets.
- Need assistance with meals, or require encouragement to eat, monitoring, or prompting during meals.
- Be hearing-impaired or speech-impaired.
- Need self-help devices.

Assisted living facilities promote the concept of "aging in place," in keeping with state rules and regulations governing resident health and safety. Whenever possible, the facility provides services so the resident does not have to move his or her living space. The assisted living facility provides assistance or supervision with personal care activities, and monitors resident health and safety. The facility coordinates any services by outside health care providers and agencies needed by the resident. Rules and licensing regulations vary from state to state. Some states require special education and certification for staff members. Many nursing assistants work in assisted living facilities.

Home Care

Many health care consumers receive care in the home from qualified caregivers. The person who receives care in the home is called the **client**. Most care is provided by home health agencies. These agencies have many workers who are responsible for care and supervision of clients in the home. Commonly, the nursing assistant is the primary caregiver. In the home care setting, the assistant may be called a home care aide or home care assistant. The home care assistant provides personal care, cares for the client's environment, makes observations, and reports abnormal findings to the registered nurse supervisor (case manager). Home health care is one of the fastest growing segments of health care today.

Some clients receiving home health care are acutely ill and need 24-hour care. Many require only short visits daily or several times a week. A visit usually lasts from 45 minutes to 2 hours. Other workers, such as physical, occupational, speech, or respiratory therapists, may also visit the home to perform services for the client.

The caregiver who works in the home does so without direct supervision. A **registered nurse (RN)** is responsible for planning and supervising the care given in the home, but the RN may not be present when the care is actually given. An RN has completed two to four years of nursing education and has passed a state licensing examination. The personal care given in the home is the same as care provided in other settings. Sometimes you must improvise by using common items in the home to care for the client. Caring for the client in the home may also involve preparing meals, shopping for groceries, doing light housekeeping, and doing laundry. The nursing assistant must follow a plan of care developed by the RN case manager. Because a caregiver may not be in the home at all times, making accurate observations and reporting your findings to your nurse manager by telephone and in writing is important.

Hospice Care

Hospice care may be provided in the home and also in a health care facility. A **hospice** is an organization dedicated to caring for persons with limited life expectancy. In hospice care, the resident and family are considered a single unit. A team of workers ensures that the physical, psychological, and spiritual needs of the entire family are met. Team members provide the resident the opportunity to die with dignity, in comfortable, familiar surroundings. Emphasis is given to keeping the resident pain-free and maintaining the highest quality of life possible. Support is provided so the resident and family members are not left alone in a time of crisis.

Because people are living longer, quality of life has become an important consideration in health care delivery. Many health care decisions are made with the future quality of the individual's life in mind. Quality-of-life policies and requirements focus on creating and maintaining an environment that humanizes and individualizes each person. In some situations, preserving the quality of the resident's life is viewed as more important than the length or duration of life. In any event, assisting each individual to maintain the highest possible quality of life is very important.

Other Types of Health Care Facilities

Health care may also be delivered in many other settings. These include:

- Freestanding clinics and emergency care centers
- Mental health facilities
- Adult day care facilities
- Adult group living centers

FINANCING HEALTH CARE

Health care is paid for in many different ways. Some individuals pay for care out of their personal bank accounts. Others pay premiums to insurance companies. When these people get sick, the insurance company **reimburses,** or pays, the facility for providing medical care. **Medicaid** is a health care program funded by both the state and federal governments that pays for health care for individuals with low incomes. **Medicare** is a federally funded program for individuals who are elderly or disabled. Medicare pays for certain services in hospitals, long-term care facilities, and home health care settings. Although most hospitals accept payment from the Medicare and Medicaid programs, some home health agencies and long-term care facilities do not.

Occasionally, other sources pay for health care. The Veterans Administration has special hospitals to care for veterans with service-related illnesses and injuries. It also pays long-term care facilities for care they provide to veterans in certain circumstances. Private agencies in the community may also help pay the cost of care for certain individuals.

The **health maintenance organization (HMO)** is a group of health care providers and hospitals. An HMO may be funded by Medicare, Medicaid, or the patient's private money. HMO members are given a list of physicians, clinics, offices, and hospitals from which they may receive care. The member must see only certain doctors and go to only designated hospitals, except in certain situations and emergencies. The HMO pays the doctor (or group of doctors) a fee for each member every month. The doctor is paid the fee even if the member does not visit. The doctor or clinic is expected to deliver all care, whenever needed, for this monthly fee. There are no additional payments. Some HMOs have special outpatient clinics in which outpatient surgery, diagnostic testing, patient teaching, and preventive health care are delivered. Medical care may be provided for individuals with acute illness. Usually the patient returns home after treatment in the clinic.

Another common method of paying for health care is through a **preferred provider organization (PPO)**. The PPO consists of various doctors, hospitals, and other health care agencies that contract with insurance companies to care for their subscribers. When members are sick, they can choose a physician or agency on the preferred provider list to care for them. The member's out-of-pocket expenses are reduced as long as the patient uses the physicians and agencies on the list. The patient may go to any other service provider of his or her choosing. However, going to providers who are not on the PPO list will cost the member more.

OBRA LEGISLATION

OBRA is an abbreviation used to describe the *Omnibus Budget Reconciliation Act*. The OBRA legislation of 1987 was designed to improve the quality of life, quality of care, health, and safety of residents in long-term care facilities. Residents' rights are emphasized. Residents in long-term care facilities have the same legal rights as all other citizens. The facility must maintain a homelike environment (Figure 1.1) and maintain or improve the quality of the residents' lives.

The OBRA legislation requires that all states follow minimum standards to ensure that nursing assistants working in long-term care facilities are educated and competent to give personal care. The legislation specifies that a

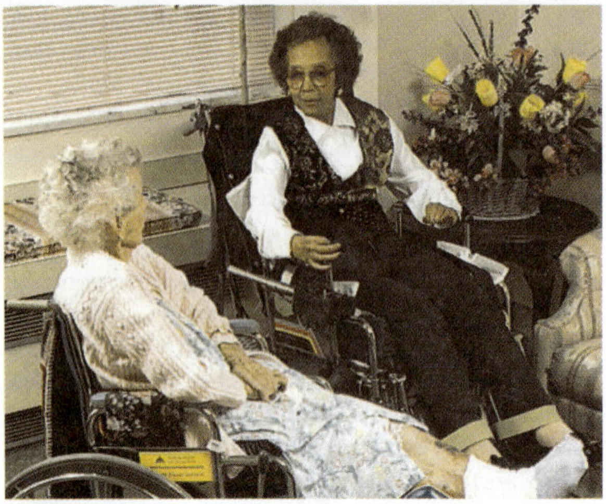

FIGURE 1-1 The long-term care facility is the residents' home. Providing a comfortable, homelike environment enhances quality of life.

nursing assistant must have a minimum of 75 hours of instruction in certain subject matter to work in long-term care. Many states require more than 75 hours of preparation. The skills learned in the nursing assistant program are the basic skills required for entry-level positions in most health care settings.

Before the OBRA legislation, each state decided whether nursing assistants should receive special preparation to work in long-term care. Some states had no education requirement. Although many states did require nursing assistant classes prior to OBRA, the content of programs varied widely from state to state. OBRA recognizes that the person receiving care, the health care facility, and the nursing assistant all benefit from the nursing assistant education program. The information learned is useful in many different health care settings and also in the assistant's personal life. The care required by the OBRA legislation translates into good care regardless of the setting. However, the OBRA legislation was specifically designed to improve the quality of care in the long-term care facility and the skilled unit of the hospital.

OBRA Requirements

The OBRA law requires facilities to maintain or improve the resident's condition. **Declines** are deteriorations in condition that are not allowed unless they are medically unavoidable. The resident's condition is assessed on admission by licensed facility staff, and a record is made of this assessment. The facility is expected to maintain or improve the resident's condition compared with how the resident was at the time of admission. For example, if the skin was free from injury on admission, the facility is expected to keep the skin free from injury. If the skin was injured at the time of admission, the facility is expected to take steps to heal the injured area. Although this is a simple example, it is important to remember that the resident should not have declines in any area of life.

The long-term care facility must help the resident function at the highest level possible for his or her individual situation. To do this, long-term care facilities use a written tool developed by the government to assess residents. This tool is called the **Minimum Data Set 2.0** (MDS), part of which is shown in Figure 1.2. **Risk factors** are conditions that could cause the resident's health to worsen. The MDS assists facility personnel in identifying risk factors in advance, so a plan of care can be developed to prevent the resident's condition from worsening. For example, a resident who is in bed all the time is at risk of skin breakdown and other problems. If the resident does not have bowel and bladder control, the risk of skin problems increases. The MDS identifies the resident's risk of skin breakdown, and the facility is expected to take steps to prevent it. The MDS is the basic assessment on which the care plan is built. However, additional assessment tools may also be used, and many factors are considered when planning resident care. When the interdisciplinary team reevaluates the resident's care plan goals, they will look for signs of decline and plan ways to avoid them. Declines will be addressed in other units of the book, but understanding what declines are and how to prevent them is important. Preventing declines is a good practice in all health care settings.

The OBRA laws require caregivers to look at the resident in the long-term care facility holistically. We are not to look at the medical problems alone. Needs in one area of life can affect the resident's entire life and well-being. For example, a resident may need help to overcome problems with sadness and depression. If this need is not met, the resident may stop eating, refuse therapy, and eventually give up on living entirely. Many people can be taught to use their own strengths to meet their needs.

Resident ________________ Numeric Identifier ________________

SECTION D. VISION PATTERNS

1.	VISION	*(Ability to see in adequate light and with glasses if used)* 0. *ADEQUATE*—sees fine detail, including regular print in newspapers/books 1. *IMPAIRED*—sees large print, but not regular print in newspapers/books 2. *MODERATELY IMPAIRED*—limited vision; not able to see newspaper headlines, but can identify objects 3. *HIGHLY IMPAIRED*—object identification in question, but eyes appear to follow objects 4. *SEVERELY IMPAIRED*—no vision or sees only light, colors, or shapes; eyes do not appear to follow objects
2.	VISUAL LIMITATIONS/ DIFFICULTIES	Side vision problems—decreased peripheral vision (e.g., leaves food on one side of tray, difficulty traveling, bumps into people and objects, misjudges placement of chair when seating self) a. Experiences any of following: sees halos or rings around lights; sees flashes of light; sees "curtains" over eyes b. *NONE OF ABOVE* c.
3.	VISUAL APPLIANCES	Glasses; contact lenses; magnifying glass 0. No 1. Yes

SECTION E. MOOD AND BEHAVIOR PATTERNS

1.	INDICATORS OF DEPRESSION, ANXIETY, SAD MOOD	***(Code for indicators observed in last 30 days, irrespective of the assumed cause)*** 0. Indicator not exhibited in last 30 days 1. Indicator of this type exhibited up to five days a week 2. Indicator of this type exhibited daily or almost daily (6, 7 days a week)

VERBAL EXPRESSIONS OF DISTRESS

a. Resident made negative statements—e.g., *"Nothing matters; Would rather be dead; What's the use; Regrets having lived so long; Let me die"*

b. Repetitive questions—e.g., *"Where do I go; What do I do?"*

c. Repetitive verbalizations—e.g., calling out for help, (*"God help me"*)

d. Persistent anger with self or others—e.g., easily annoyed, anger at placement in nursing home; anger at care received

e. Self deprecation—e.g., *"I am nothing; I am of no use to anyone"*

f. Expressions of what appear to be unrealistic fears—e.g., fear of being abandoned, left alone, being with others

g. Recurrent statements that something terrible is about to happen—e.g., believes he or she is about to die, have a heart attack

h. Repetitive health complaints—e.g., persistently seeks medical attention, obsessive concern with body functions

i. Repetitive anxious complaints/concerns (non-health related) e.g., persistently seeks attention/reassurance regarding schedules, meals, laundry, clothing, relationship issues

SLEEP-CYCLE ISSUES

j. Unpleasant mood in morning

k. Insomnia/change in usual sleep pattern

SAD, APATHETIC, ANXIOUS APPEARANCE

l. Sad, pained, worried facial expressions—e.g., furrowed brows

m. Crying, tearfulness

n. Repetitive physical movements—e.g., pacing, hand wringing, restlessness, fidgeting, picking

LOSS OF INTEREST

o. Withdrawal from activities of interest—e.g., no interest in long standing activities or being with family/friends

p. Reduced social interaction

2.	MOOD PERSISTENCE	**One or more indicators** of depressed, sad or anxious mood **were not easily altered by attempts to "cheer up", console, or reassure the resident over last 7 days** 0. No mood indicators 1. Indicators present, easily altered 2. Indicators present, not easily altered
3.	CHANGE IN MOOD	Resident's mood status has changed as compared to status of **90 days ago** (or since last assessment if less than 90 days) 0. No change 1. Improved 2. Deteriorated
4.	BEHAVIORAL SYMPTOMS	**(A) *Behavioral symptom frequency in last 7 days*** 0. Behavior not exhibited in last 7 days 1. Behavior of this type occurred 1 to 3 days in last 7 days 2. Behavior of this type occurred 4 to 6 days, but less than daily 3. Behavior of this type occurred daily **(B) *Behavioral symptom alterability in last 7 days*** 0. Behavior not present OR behavior was easily altered 1. Behavior was not easily altered

	(A)	(B)
a. WANDERING (moved with no rational purpose, seemingly oblivious to needs or safety)		
b. VERBALLY ABUSIVE BEHAVIORAL SYMPTOMS (others were threatened, screamed at, cursed at)		
c. PHYSICALLY ABUSIVE BEHAVIORAL SYMPTOMS (others were hit, shoved, scratched, sexually abused)		
d. SOCIALLY INAPPROPRIATE/DISRUPTIVE BEHAVIORAL SYMPTOMS (made disruptive sounds, noisiness, screaming, self-abusive acts, sexual behavior or disrobing in public, smeared/threw food/feces, hoarding, rummaged through others' belongings)		
e. RESISTS CARE (resisted taking medications/ injections, ADL assistance, or eating)		

5.	CHANGE IN BEHAVIORAL SYMPTOMS	Resident's behavior status has changed as compared to **status of 90 days ago** (or since last assessment if less than 90 days) 0. No change 1. Improved 2. Deteriorated

SECTION F. PSYCHOSOCIAL WELL-BEING

1.	SENSE OF INITIATIVE/ INVOLVEMENT	At ease interacting with others	a.
		At ease doing planned or structured activities	b.
		At ease doing self-initiated activities	c.
		Establishes own goals	d.
		Pursues involvement in life of facility (e.g., makes/keeps friends; involved in group activities; responds positively to new activities; assists at religious services)	e.
		Accepts invitations into most group activities	f.
		NONE OF ABOVE	g.
2.	UNSETTLED RELATIONSHIPS	Covert/open conflict with or repeated criticism of staff	a.
		Unhappy with roommate	b.
		Unhappy with residents other than roommate	c.
		Openly expresses conflict/anger with family/friends	d.
		Absence of personal contact with family/friends	e.
		Recent loss of close family member/friend	f.
		Does not adjust easily to change in routines	g.
		NONE OF ABOVE	h.
3.	PAST ROLES	Strong identification with past roles and life status	a.
		Expresses sadness/anger/empty feeling over lost roles/status	b.
		Resident perceives that daily routine (customary routine, activities) is very different from prior pattern in the community	c.
		NONE OF ABOVE	d.

SECTION G. PHYSICAL FUNCTIONING AND STRUCTURAL PROBLEMS

1. (A) ADL SELF-PERFORMANCE—***(Code for resident's PERFORMANCE OVER ALL SHIFTS during last 7 days—****Not including setup)*

0. *INDEPENDENT*—No help or oversight —OR— Help/oversight provided only 1 or 2 times during last 7 days
1. SUPERVISION—Oversight, encouragement or cueing provided 3 or more times during last7 days —OR— Supervision (3 or more times) plus physical assistance provided only 1 or 2 times during last 7 days
2. *LIMITED ASSISTANCE*—Resident highly involved in activity; received physical help in guided maneuvering of limbs or other nonweight bearing assistance 3 or more times —OR—More help provided only 1 or 2 times during last 7 days
3. *EXTENSIVE ASSISTANCE*—While resident performed part of activity, over last 7-day period, help of following type(s) provided 3 or more times:
   —Weight-bearing support
   — Full staff performance during part (but not all) of last 7 days
4. *TOTAL DEPENDENCE*—Full staff performance of activity during entire 7 days
8. *ACTIVITY DID NOT OCCUR* during entire 7 days

(B) ADL SUPPORT PROVIDED—***(Code for MOST SUPPORT PROVIDED OVER ALL SHIFTS during last 7 days; code regardless*** *of resident's self-performance classification)*

0. No setup or physical help from staff
1. Setup help only
2. One person physical assist
3. Two+ persons physical assist
8. ADL activity itself did not occur during entire 7 days

			(A) SELF-PERF	(B) SUPPORT
a.	BED MOBILITY	How resident moves to and from lying position, turns side to side, and positions body while in bed		
b.	TRANSFER	How resident moves between surfaces—to/from: bed, chair, wheelchair, standing position (EXCLUDE to/from bath/toilet)		
c.	WALK IN ROOM	How resident walks between locations in his/her room		
d.	WALK IN CORRIDOR	How resident walks in corridor on unit		
e.	LOCOMOTION ON UNIT	How resident moves between locations in his/her room and adjacent corridor on same floor. If in wheelchair, self-sufficiency once in chair		
f.	LOCOMOTION OFF UNIT	How resident moves to and returns from off unit locations (e.g., areas set aside for dining, activities, or treatments). **If facility has only one floor,** how resident moves to and from distant areas on the floor. If in wheelchair, self-sufficiency once in chair		
g.	DRESSING	How resident puts on, fastens, and takes off all items of **street clothing**, including donning/removing prosthesis		
h.	EATING	How resident eats and drinks (regardless of skill). Includes intake of nourishment by other means (e.g., tube feeding, total parenteral nutrition)		
i.	TOILET USE	How resident uses the toilet room (or commode, bedpan, urinal); transfer on/off toilet, cleanses, changes pad, manages ostomy or catheter, adjusts clothes		
j.	PERSONAL HYGIENE	How resident maintains personal hygiene, including combing hair, brushing teeth, shaving, applying makeup, washing/drying face, hands, and perineum (EXCLUDE baths and showers)		

MDS 2.0 September, 2000

FIGURE 1-2 The Minimum Data Set is an important assessment tool used to evaluate the residents' most common problems and needs. (Page 2 is shown.)

Nursing Assistant Certification

After completing the nursing assistant program, you must understand how to get and keep your certification. Some states require the employing long-term care facility to complete a criminal background check on all applicants. This background check will show if the applicant has ever been arrested. In these states, if an individual has been convicted of certain crimes, he or she cannot work in a long-term care facility.

After completing the state-approved course, the nursing assistant must take written and manual competency skills examinations given or sponsored by the state. After passing these examinations, the nursing assistant is entered into the state nursing assistant registry. To keep nursing assistant certification active, you must work in a health care agency for pay every two years. The number of hours you must work in the two-year period varies with the state. If you do not work for 24 months or longer, you must complete another nursing assistant program or refresher course and successfully complete another competency evaluation test to work as a nursing assistant again. Some states will allow you to take the test over without repeating the class. The OBRA legislation requires the nursing assistant to attend a minimum of 12 hours of continuing education each year to remain active. Some states require more than the 12-hour minimum. The facility that you work for will offer these classes. It is your responsibility to attend them to maintain your certification. Your facility is required to evaluate your skills every year to be sure that you can perform your duties in the way you were taught.

Supervision of the Nursing Assistant

In the most health care facilities, you will provide personal care to residents under the supervision of a licensed nurse. The director of nursing in the long-term care facility must be an RN. The nurse who directly supervises you is usually your charge nurse. This person may also be an RN. Some nurses are **licensed practical nurses (LPN)**. In Texas and California, these nurses are called **licensed vocational nurses (LVN)**. LPNs and LVNs have completed 1 year to 18 months of full-time nursing education and have passed a state licensing examination. The nurse will give you your assignment at the beginning of your shift. You will report your concerns and observations to this nurse.

Interdisciplinary Team

The health care team is also called the **interdisciplinary team**. The interdisciplinary team consists of many individuals who contribute to the care, health, and well-being of residents. The residents and family members that residents want to be included are also members of the team. All team members are important. We need each other, and the residents need us. To be successful, we must work together and cooperate with each other.

Members of the Interdisciplinary Team

Many individuals, both inside and outside the health care agency, are members of the interdisciplinary team. We must use whatever resources are necessary to meet the physical, mental, and emotional needs of residents. The goal of the interdisciplinary team is to assist residents to maintain the highest possible level of physical, mental, emotional, and psychosocial well-being. Team members meet shortly after a new resident admission and periodically after that to develop a **care plan** for that resident (Figure 1.3). The care plan is a mutually agreed-upon list of problems, goals, and approaches to help the resident reach his or her highest potential. A system, called **Nursing Interventions Classification (NIC)**, is being used by many facilities. This system provides specific approaches that all team members use to deliver care. The effectiveness of the approaches and all care provided is measured by **Nursing Outcomes Classification (NOC)**. Using these systems provides consistent care and a method of measuring whether the care is helping the resident meet the goals established by the interdisciplinary team.

All team members must know the information and follow the instructions on the care plan. When everyone follows the care plan, all staff members are using the same approaches and working on the same goals for the benefit of the resident. Team members that provide services to residents are listed in Table 1.2.

Chain of Command

The **chain of command** (Figure 1.4) is very important to the proper operation of all health care facilities. The chain of command is the line of authority that each department follows in reporting information. You will report your observations, problems, and concerns to the nurse. If you have a problem with another department, you will also report this information to the nurse. The nurse will contact the appropriate person in that department to solve the problem. It is your responsibility to know and follow your facility's chain of command.

MARYSVILLE CARE CENTER

CARE PLAN

09/07/20XX

FORM # 280L

PROBLEM	SHORT TERM GOAL	APPROACH
(1) DEFICIT FLUID VOLUME RELATED TO DECREASED FLUID INTAKE. ONSET 09/06/XX TARGET 12/05/XX RESOLVE 00/00/00	(1) REHYDRATE/ESTABLISH FLUID BALANCE. BEGIN 09/06/XX TARGET 12/05/XX RESOLVE 00/00/00	(1) RECORD INTAKE AND OUTPUT EVERY SHIFT. DISC: NSG (2) CHECK & RECORD B.P. AS ORDERED. DISC: NSG (3) MONITOR SKIN TURGOR. DISC: NSG (4) ENCOURAGE ADEQUATE FLUID INTAKE DAILY. DISC: NSG NA D (5) OFFER FLUIDS OF CHOICE. DISC: ALL (6) INCREASE AMOUNT OF FLUID INTAKE TO 2500CC DAILY. DISC: NSG (7) CHECK MUCOUS MEMBRANE MOISTNESS Q SHIFT DISC: NSG (8) MONITOR VITAL SIGNS Q 4 HOURS AND PRN. DISC: NSG
(2) POTENTIAL FOR IMPAIRED SKIN INTEGRITY DUE TO DECREASED MOBILITY. ONSET 09/06/XX TARGET 12/05/XX RESOLVE 00/00/00	(1) FREE FROM RED OR OPEN AREAS. BEGIN 09/06/XX TARGET 12/05/XX RESOLVE 00/00/00 (2) MAINTAIN SKIN INTEGRITY. BEGIN 09/06/XX TARGET 12/05/XX RESOLVE 00/00/00	(1) HAVE DIETITIAN CONSULT ABOUT DIET. DISC: D (2) INCREASE AMOUNT OF FLUID INTAKE DAILY. DISC: NSG (3) INCREASE MEAT/PROTEIN IN DIET. DISC: NSG D

PHYSICIAN / ALT. PHYSICIAN	PHONE NO.	ALLERGIES / NOTES
SMART, NANCY D.O. KEELEY, SHAWN D.O.	(555) 888-1212	

RESIDENT	STATION / ROOM / BED	ADMISSION NUMBER / DATE	SEX	DATE OF BIRTH	CARE PLAN DATE	PAGE #
MARTIN, FRANK	WEST-322-B	23891 09/22/XX	M	08/04/1918	09/07/XX	1

FIGURE 1-3 The care plan directs and guides resident care. It is updated for changes in condition. Your assignment will reflect care plan goals for each resident.

MARYSVILLE CARE CENTER

CARE PLAN

09/07/20XX

FORM # 280L

PROBLEM	SHORT TERM GOAL	APPROACH
		(4) KEEP BED LINEN OFF EXTREMITIES. DISC: NSG (5) KEEP EXTREMITIES IN GOOD ALIGNMENT & PROPERLY SUPPORTED. DISC: NSG (6) KEEP LEGS ELEVATED ON PILLOWS SO HEELS ARE OFF THE MATTRESS TO REDUCE PRESSURE. DISC: NSG (7) KEEP DRY AND CHANGE AFTER VOIDING. DISC: NSG (8) KEEP SKIN CLEAN, DRY AND FREE OF PRESSURE. DISC: NSG (9) TURN EVERY 2 HOURS AND PRN. MAINTAIN GOOD BODY ALIGNMENT WITH PILLOWS. DISC: NSG (10) MULTIVITAMINS WITH IRON AND VITAMIN C. DISC: NSG (11) SPENCO MATTRESS TO BED AND CHAIR. DISC: NSG
(3) CONSTIPATION. ONSET 09/06/XX TARGET 12/05/XX RESOLVE 00/00/00	(1) WILL HAVE A B.M. EVERY OTHER DAY. BEGIN 09/06/XX TARGET 12/05/XX RESOLVE 00/00/00	(1) OFFER PRUNE JUICE AT BREAKFAST. DISC: D NSG (2) MONITOR BOWEL SOUNDS DAILY. DISC: NSG (3) DO DIGITAL BOWEL CHECK IF CONSTIPATION SUSPECTED. DISC: NSG (4) INCREASE FIBER IN DIET AS ALLOWED BY DIET ORDER. DISC: NSG D

PHYSICIAN / ALT. PHYSICIAN	PHONE NO.	ALLERGIES / NOTES
SMART, NANCY D.O. KEELEY, SHAWN D.O.	(555) 888-1212	

RESIDENT	STATION / ROOM / BED	ADMISSION NUMBER / DATE	SEX	DATE OF BIRTH	CARE PLAN DATE	PAGE #
MARTIN, FRANK	WEST-322-B	23891 09/22/XX	M	08/04/1918	09/07/XX	2

FIGURE 1-3 *Continued*

MARYSVILLE CARE CENTER

CARE PLAN

09/07/19XX

FORM # 280L

PROBLEM	SHORT TERM GOAL	APPROACH
		(5) ADMINISTER MEDICATIONS AS ORDERED BY NANCY SMART D.O. DISC: NSG (6) ENCOURAGE FLUIDS. DISC: NSG (7) ACTIVITY AS TOLERATED. DISC: NSG (8) OBSERVE FOR MEDICATION EFFECTIVENESS. DISC: NSG (9) MONITOR AND RECORD BOWEL MOVEMENTS. DISC: NURSING
*** CURRENT MEDICATIONS ***		
*** WEIGHT HISTORY ***		
*** CURRENT DIAGNOSIS ***		

PHYSICIAN / ALT. PHYSICIAN	PHONE NO.	ALLERGIES / NOTES
SMART, NANCY D.O. KEELEY, SHAWN D.O.	(555) 888-1212	

RESIDENT	STATION / ROOM / BED	ADMISSION NUMBER / DATE	SEX	DATE OF BIRTH	CARE PLAN DATE	PAGE #
MARTIN, FRANK	WEST-322-B	23891 09/22/XX	M	08/04/1918	09/07/XX	3

FIGURE 1-3 *Continued*

TABLE 1-2 Interdisciplinary Health Care Team Members

Team Member	Responsibilities
Provide Most of the Direct Care Services to Residents	
Licensed Nurse (licensed nurses may be either RNs or LPN/LVNs)	Directs the care of residents, administers medications, and performs treatments. Supervises and directs nursing assistant staff.
Nursing Assistant (NA, CNA, or STNA)	Provides most of the personal care to residents under the supervision of the licensed nurse. The nursing assistant spends more time with the residents than other team members.
Medication Aide (MA) (Certified Medication Assistant [CMA]) (Medication Technician [MT])	A certified nursing assistant who has met certain criteria, taken additional classes in medication administration methods, and completed a state certification examination. Allowed to pass medications in skilled nursing facilities, assisted living facilities, and home health care in 25 states.
Restorative Nursing Assistant (RNA)	A certified nursing assistant who has additional education and experience in restorative nursing care. Delivers care designed to assist the resident to attain and maintain his or her highest level of function, and prevent physical deformities.
Dining Assistant (Feeding Assistant, Nutrition Assistant)	A single task worker with at least 8 hours education in nutrition and hydration. Assists stable residents with eating and drinking. May not assist residents with complex feeding problems.
Dietary Staff Member	Prepares meals and is responsible for ordering groceries, washing dishes, and other kitchen duties.
Registered Dietitian (RD)	Writes the menus for meals prepared by the dietary department. Responsible for seeing that residents on special diets receive the right food in the proper amounts. Assesses each resident's individual dietary needs; calculates individual calorie, fluid, and other requirements; and makes recommendations for care of chronic illnesses and complications.
Activities	Provides activities for resident enjoyment. Some activities are done to provide exercise for residents. Other types of activities are designed to provide positive **self-esteem.** Self-esteem is how you feel about yourself. Activities also provide opportunities for residents to socialize with others.
Social Service Worker (LSW or SSD)	Helps meet residents' mental and emotional needs. Coordinates functions with personnel and agencies inside and outside the facility to see that resident needs are met. When it is time for the resident to be discharged home or to another health care agency, the social worker coordinates the resources the resident will need and makes the transition as smooth as possible. An LSW is a licensed social worker. The SSD is a social services designee.

Physical Therapist (PT, LPT)	Helps residents regain strength and physical function lost because of illness or injury. The goal of the therapist is to help the resident achieve the highest possible level of physical function. The physical therapist also teaches residents and staff how to perform physical activities in a safe manner. A physical therapy assistant (PTA) may assist with physical therapy services.
Occupational Therapist (OT, OTR/L)	Helps residents regain strength and physical function lost because of illness or injury. This therapist helps residents to relearn self-care skills, such as feeding, bathing, grooming, and dressing. The goal of care is to help the resident become as independent as possible. Residents who have lost physical function may be able to use adaptive or self-help devices to be independent. The occupational therapist helps residents obtain these devices and learn how to use them. The OT may also fabricate or order splints and other equipment to prevent deformities. An occupational therapy assistant (OTA) may assist in providing occupational therapy services.
Respiratory Care Practitioner (RCP)	Works with residents who have breathing problems and those who need oxygen and other special treatments for their lungs. The goal of the treatment is to see that residents receive enough oxygen to meet their needs.
Speech Language Pathologist (SLP)	Works with residents who have diseases or injuries that have affected their ability to speak properly. This therapist also helps residents who have swallowing problems to learn to eat and drink without choking.
Physician (MD or DO)	Orders the resident's medical plan of care. Medications, diagnostic tests, and treatments must be ordered by the physician.
Clinical Nurse Specialist (CNS)	An advanced-practice registered nurse with a master's degree who focuses on a very specific resident population (e.g., medical, surgical, diabetic, cardiovascular, operating room, emergency room, critical care, geriatric, neonatal, etc.).
Nurse Practitioner (NP)	A registered nurse with advanced academic and clinical experience, which enables him or her to diagnose and manage common acute and chronic illnesses, either independently or as part of a health care team. A nurse practitioner provides some care previously offered only by physicians and in most states is legally permitted to prescribe medications.
Physician Assistant (PA)	A health care professional licensed to practice medicine with physician supervision. PAs conduct physical examinations, diagnose and treat illnesses, order and interpret tests, counsel on preventive health care, assist in surgery, and in most states are permitted to write prescriptions. Because of the close working relationship the PA has with the physician, PAs are educated in the medical model designed to complement physician training.

TABLE 1-2 *(continued)*

Team Member	Responsibilities
Provide Less Direct Resident Care	
Clergy	Members of the **clergy** are pastors of churches or other religious workers who help residents meet their spiritual needs.
Bookkeeping or Office Worker	Responsible for answering the telephone, recordkeeping, and taking care of business and financial functions.
Medical Records Worker	Keeps permanent records of residents' care and treatment. Records are an important tool for communication with other members of the health care team. They are legal documents that may be used in court.
Maintenance Worker*	Responsible for seeing that the building and equipment are safe and in good repair at all times.
Laundry Worker*	Washes facility linen and keeps the nursing units supplied with sheets, towels, and other items needed to care for residents. The laundry worker in most long-term care facilities also washes residents' personal clothing.
Housekeeping Personnel*	Keeps the facility clean and sanitary.
Beautician/Barber	Provides haircuts and other services needed to care for residents' hair.

*The departments may be combined into one environmental service department.

Responsibilities of the Nursing Assistant

The nursing assistant is an important member of the health care team. You will spend more time with residents than any other caregiver and perform many valuable services to assist residents and other team members.

Responsibilities for Providing Personal Care

You will help residents with bathing, personal hygiene, and grooming. You may need to help residents with dressing and undressing. Some residents may need assistance turning and positioning in bed or moving from one place to another. Some require help with toileting and elimination needs.

Providing Food Service and Mealtime Assistance

An important responsibility of the nursing assistant is to provide food and fluids. You are responsible for delivering food trays, special supplements, and snacks. There may be times when you will help residents eat, or even feed them. You are also responsible for passing fresh drinking water and encouraging residents to drink enough liquid.

Caring for the Resident's Unit and Belongings

The resident's room is called the **unit**. The unit consists of a bed, chair, overbed table, night-stand, dresser, wastebasket, and closet. You are responsible for keeping the unit tidy and safe. You will make beds and handle the residents' clothing and belongings. Treating personal items with care shows respect for the residents. Many residents bring only their most important possessions with them to the health care facility. It is your responsibility to see that these items are kept safe.

Observation and Reporting

A very important responsibility of the nursing assistant is to make observations of resident conditions

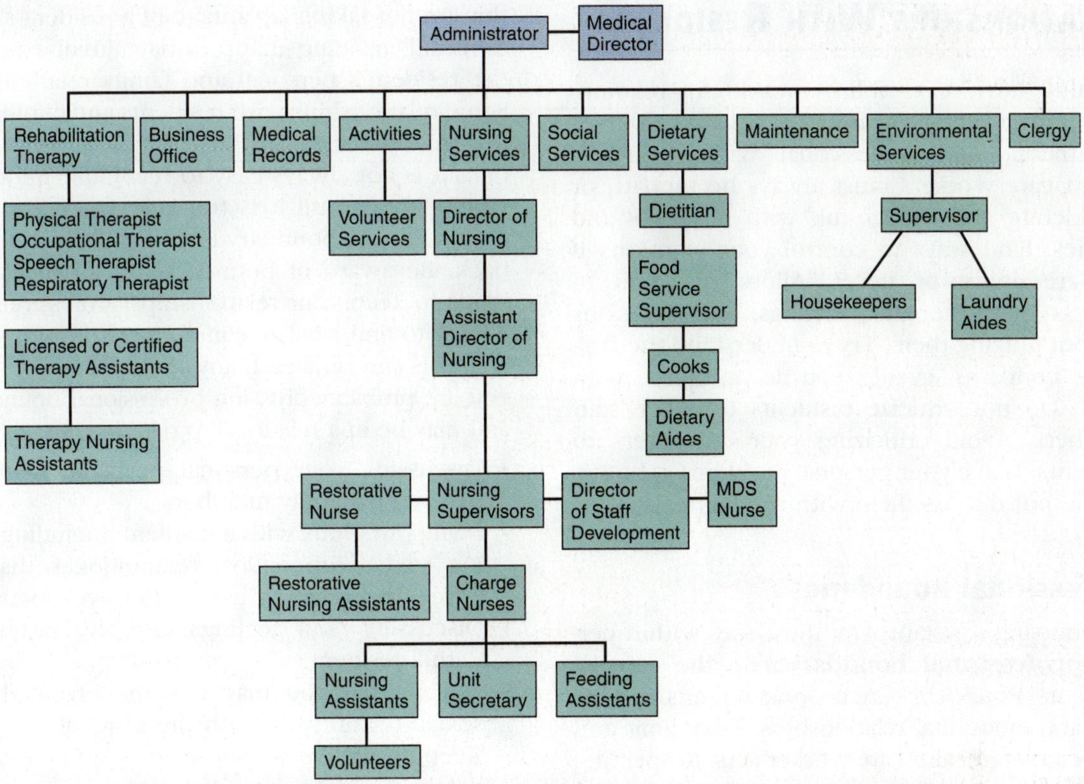

FIGURE 1-4 Following the chain of command for reporting shows respect and enhances communication in the long-term care facility.

and report changes to the nurse. The nursing assistant spends more time with the resident than any other caregiver. This puts you in an ideal position to get to know how the resident is most of the time. Because of this close contact, you may be the first person to recognize a variation from the resident's normal condition. All changes, even if they seem minor, may be important and should be reported to the nurse. Observation and reporting are discussed in detail in Unit 2.

Caring for Equipment and Supplies

Many different pieces of equipment are used in the health care facility. Some are used once and thrown away. Others are used for one resident only. Some pieces of equipment are used for many residents. They are cleaned and disinfected after each use. You will learn how to safely care for and use the equipment found in the health care facility. Take this responsibility very seriously.

Recordkeeping, Communication, and Messenger Duties

We communicate in many different ways in the health care facility. These will be discussed in more detail in Unit 2. You will be responsible for keeping accurate records in writing and for communicating information to others verbally. You will report changes in resident condition to your supervisor. There will be times when you will be asked to inform other departments and staff members of pertinent information.

LEGAL LIMITATIONS OF NURSE AIDE

a. Does not give medications
b. Does not insert or remove tubes
c. Does not take order from a physician
d. Does not do sterile procedures
e. Does not give information about diagnosis or treatment plans to residents or their family
f. Does not diagnose or prescribe treatments or medications for residents
g. Does not supervise the work of other nurse aides
h. Does not agree to do something beyond scope of practice as defined by Board of Nursing

Relationships With Residents

Learning how to establish meaningful relationships with residents is important. Always be kind, empathetic, and professional with residents. Health care workers must always be **tactful,** or considerate and thoughtful, with residents and families. Find ways to control your emotions if you are angry or upset. Allow residents to express their thoughts, feelings, and emotions without judging them. Try to understand the residents' concerns, even if you do not agree with them. Do not criticize residents to other staff members. Avoid criticizing your coworkers to residents. Leave your personal problems at home, and do not discuss them with residents.

Professional Boundaries

As a nursing assistant, you must stay within certain **professional boundaries** in the care of residents. Boundaries are unspoken limits on physical and emotional relationships. They limit and define how a health care worker acts. Respecting boundaries involves using your best behavior, ethical practices, and good judgment when caring for residents. Respecting boundaries is one way that you will act appropriately on the job.

You see boundary lines when looking at a map. However, when you drive down the road, you do not see the boundaries when you cross from one city or state to the next. Professional boundaries are the same way. They exist, but you cannot see them. You must be aware of boundaries and avoid crossing them. You may cross them inadvertently or deliberately, thinking that you are meeting a resident's need. It takes good judgment and experience to identify boundaries and keep from crossing them.

Being aware of boundaries is especially important when caring for residents with emotional stress. To avoid crossing boundaries, strive to act professionally, as you were taught in class. Avoid putting yourself in a position in which you think and act as a family member or friend. Use good judgment and determine the amount of contact and assistance that are right for the resident. Too much or too little contact can be unhealthy for both the assistant and the resident. Treat all residents professionally. Consult the nurse if you are uncertain.

Ethical behavior with residents and families. Because you are a nursing assistant, residents expect you to act in their best interests and to treat them with dignity. Ways in which you do this are not taking advantage of a resident's situation and avoiding inappropriate involvement in the resident's personal and family relationships. Some relationships with residents and families are not healthy for the resident or the nursing assistant. It is not always easy to recognize unhealthy relationships until it is too late. Once you have crossed over a boundary line, it is difficult to turn back. Be aware of boundaries at all times, and strive to keep your relationships professional.

Try to find a balance in your relationships with residents and families. If any of the following occur, you are probably crossing professional boundaries and may be in a relationship danger zone:

- Discussing your personal problems with the resident or family members.
- Being flirtatious with a resident, including making sexual innuendos, telling jokes that are sexual in nature, or using offensive language.
- Discussing your feelings of sexual attraction with a resident.
- Feeling that you may become involved in a sexual relationship with the resident.
- Keeping secrets with a resident and becoming defensive when someone questions your relationship or involvement with the resident's personal life.
- Thinking you are immune from having an unhealthy relationship with a resident.
- Believing that you are the only nursing assistant who can meet the resident's needs.
- Spending an inappropriate amount of time with the resident, including off-duty visits or trading assignments with others so you can be with the resident.
- Reporting only partial information about the resident to the nurse because you fear disclosing unfavorable information or secrets the resident has told you.
- Feeling that you must protect the resident from other health care workers and always siding with the resident's position.

If you have trouble staying objective, or think you may cross a boundary, seek help from the nurse, clergy, or another professional person whom you trust.

Desirable Qualities in the Nursing Assistant

The nursing assistant is a special person. The successful assistant likes people, takes responsibility seriously, and believes in the importance of the position.

Personal Qualities

A pleasant personality is an important quality for health care workers. You will learn how to communicate and interact with many different people. Being pleasant and polite to everyone is important, even if they have not treated you this way. Treat others with respect and dignity. Show genuine concern for your residents and coworkers. Be available to help others and accept help if you need it. Do not judge other people's feelings. You will become more aware of how to assist residents with their feelings as you learn more about emotional needs. Remember, behavior is influenced by things such as culture, personality, illness, and emotional health. Understanding why others respond as they do will help you accept and deal with people's behavior.

A positive **attitude** is an important characteristic to bring to your job. Your attitude is the outer reflection of the way you feel. Others can see your attitude by your behavior. The tone of your voice and your body language can change the message you are trying to send. Your attitude will be reflected in your work. Be positive about your job and your contribution to resident care.

You must also learn to work as a team player. This means that you depend on other people to help care for residents. It also means that other people can depend on you. Good resident care cannot be accomplished by one person or department. It takes many people and departments working together to meet the residents' needs.

Practice tact. **Tact** involves the ability to say and do things at the right time. Being tactful means you are considerate, polite, and thoughtful. Be sensitive to the problems and needs of others. Do not judge others or give advice. Treat residents and coworkers with courtesy, respect, and consideration. Do not argue, gossip, criticize your employer or others, or use abusive language.

Be proud of what you do, and feel good about yourself. It takes a special person to provide personal care to other people. The nursing assistant is a very important person to the operation of the long-term care facility. Work to do the best job you can. Others will follow your example.

Professional appearance. You should be clean, neat, and well groomed at all times (Figure 1.5). A **professional** appearance gives others confidence in you and sends a message that you feel good about yourself and the job you do. A professional is a person who is capable, competent, and efficient. Your facility will have a dress code or uniform that you must wear. Be sure to wear the clothing your facility requires. Your uniform must be clean and wrinkle-free each day. The color and design of your undergarments should not be visible beneath your uniform.

A name pin is a very important part of your uniform. The name pin identifies you by name and title. Residents have the right to know the name and position of the person caring for them. Many facilities issue name badges that are also used to electronically scan the time clock. If your facility does not issue a badge, it is your responsibility to obtain a name tag.

Because you will be standing and walking for much of the day, having comfortable, well-fitting shoes is important. Some facilities require athletic shoes or shoes with closed toes that provide good foot support. Your shoes are an important part of your uniform. Keep them clean and in good repair.

Good personal hygiene, grooming, and personal health. Staying clean is one way to maintain your personal health. Take a bath or shower every day. Use a deodorant or antiperspirant. Keep your hair clean and neat. If your hair is long, wear it up or pulled back. Your hair is like a magnet for germs. Keeping it short makes it easier to care for. Washing your hair regularly is best. Keeping long hair pulled back reduces the risk of injury from hair becoming entangled in equipment or being inadvertently pulled by a

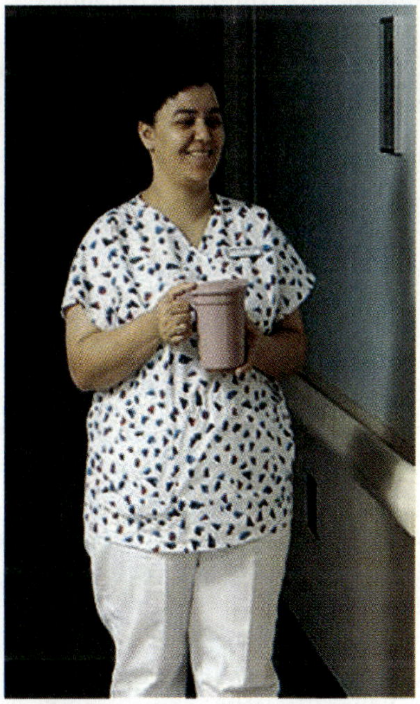

FIGURE 1-5 A professional appearance projects a positive image to residents, families, and other staff.

resident. Long fingernails, artificial nails, and chipped nail polish are also good hiding places for germs. Avoid acrylic and artificial nails. Keep your natural nails short and clean.

Jewelry should be kept to a minimum. Jewelry also harbors germs. Sharp stones and settings can injure residents and tear gloves. Only simple jewelry should be worn when on duty. Small stud-type pierced earrings also reduce your risk of injury from an earring being pulled or caught. Many facilities allow only a watch and wedding band. Cologne and aftershave should not be worn when on duty. Some residents have allergies to different fragrances. Residents who are nauseated or have other medical problems may become ill from the scent of cologne. Others with respiratory problems may have difficulty breathing with a heavy fragrance in the room.

Body piercings and tattoos. Residents in the long-term care facility are elderly, and many are offended by, do not understand, or are afraid of employees with piercings and tattoos. In communities with gang activity, residents may associate piercings and tattoos with gang membership. Most facilities do not permit employees to have conspicuous body piercings in areas of the body other than the ears. This includes the tongue. If you have piercings in other areas, cover them with clothing. Conspicuous tattoos are unacceptable in many facilities. A tattoo is considered conspicuous when it is visible. Methods of concealing tattoos, such as makeup and bandages, are usually not permitted in facilities. The only acceptable covering is clothing. Some facilities will not permit employees with visible tattoos to work in resident care positions.

Personal communication devices. Most facilities have policies prohibiting the use of non-work-related personal communication devices, such as cell phones and pagers. Safety and care of residents is paramount and communication devices distract employees from this purpose. Plan to make and return phone calls during your breaks. Personal communication devices should not be worn in resident care areas. In some facilities, employees may carry electronic pagers or cellular phones set for a silent alert that is imperceptible to others. However, staff are not permitted to respond to calls when on duty. Remember, you are being paid to work, and interrupting care even briefly to make or answer calls is not consistent with your job description. Another great concern is that some radio frequency devices will interfere with medical equipment and may jeopardize resident health and safety, as well as facility operations.

Personal Health and Safety

If you are to do your job well, you must be in good physical and emotional health. You will learn many health and safety principles and practices throughout this course that you can apply to your personal life.

Preventing physical illness. Practice the principles of proper nutrition, good health, and personal hygiene taught in this class. Eat three well-balanced meals each day. Avoid fad diets and junk foods. Avoid using alcohol, tobacco, and drugs. These substances endanger you and others.

Get adequate rest. Most people need eight hours of sleep each night. Exercise for at least 30 minutes three times each week. This is a good way to keep your body healthy, and it helps relieve stress.

See your doctor regularly for checkups and preventive health care. Treat your medical problems early. Do not wait for them to become worse.

Men should perform testicular self-examination monthly. Women should practice breast self-examination each month and have mammograms as recommended by their treating physicians.

Preventing physical illness is very important. You will learn principles of infection prevention in Unit 3. These principles will help you prevent infection and communicable disease. Avoid going to work if you have a cold, flu, diarrhea, or other illness that may be infectious. Follow your facility policy for reporting your absence. If you think you have been exposed to an illness at work, notify your supervisor and follow his or her instructions.

Immunizations. **Immunizations** involve the administration of medications to stimulate your immune system to protect you against certain communicable diseases. Some states require health care workers to be immunized against certain diseases. Immunizations will protect you from many diseases. Table 1.3 lists recommended immunizations for health care workers. The recommendations do not distinguish workers in long-term care facilities from those employed in other settings. However, the likelihood of contracting measles and mumps in a long-term care facility is minimal. Additional immunizations may be necessary in special circumstances.

Health and safety education. Attend classes on health and safety. In addition to learning how to protect residents from illness and injury, you

TABLE 1-3 Immunizations

Vaccine name	Primary booster dose schedule	Indications	Major precautions	Special considerations
Hepatitis B (recombinant vaccine)	Two doses 4 weeks apart. Third dose 5 months after second dose. No booster necessary.	Health care personnel who may be exposed to blood and body fluids.	***Warning: May cause shock in individuals allergic to baker's yeast.***	No apparent adverse effects to developing fetuses. Not contraindicated in pregnancy.
Influenza vaccine (inactivated whole or split virus vaccine)	Annual single-dose vaccine with current virus strain.	Health care personnel who have contact with high-risk residents in long-term care facilities; individuals with high-risk medical conditions.	***Warning: May cause shock in individuals allergic to eggs.***	No evidence of maternal or fetal risk when given to pregnant women with underlying medical conditions that cause high risk for serious influenza complications.
Measles (live virus vaccine)	One dose immediately, second dose 1 month later.	Health care workers born in or after 1957 without documentation of previous vaccine, physician-diagnosed measles, or laboratory evidence of immunity. Vaccine should be considered for all workers born before 1957 who have no proof of immunity.	***Do not use during pregnancy, immunocompromised state,* history of shock following gelatin ingestion, or receipt of neomycin. Do not use if recent recipient of immune globulin.***	A combined measles-mumps-rubella (MMR) vaccine is the vaccine of choice if the health care worker is also susceptible to rubella and/or mumps. Persons vaccinated between 1963 and 1967 or who were treated with a vaccine of unknown type should consider being revaccinated.
Mumps (live virus vaccine)	One dose, no booster.	Health care workers who are believed to be susceptible. Adults born before 1957 can be considered immune.	***Do not use during pregnancy, immunocompromised state,* history of shock following gelatin ingestion or receipt of neomycin.***	MMR is the vaccine of choice if the health care worker is also susceptible to rubella and/or measles.

(continues)

TABLE 1-3 *(continued)*				
Vaccine name	**Primary booster dose schedule**	**Indications**	**Major precautions**	**Special considerations**
Rubella (live virus vaccine)	One dose, no booster.	Health care personnel who lack documentation of live vaccine on or after their first birthday, or of laboratory evidence of immunity. Adults born before 1957 can be considered immune except women of childbearing age.	***Do not use during pregnancy, immunocompromised state,* history of shock following receipt of neomycin.***	Risk to fetus if pregnant when vaccinated or if woman becomes pregnant within 3 months of vaccination. MMR is the vaccine of choice if the health care worker is also susceptible to mumps and/or measles.
Varicella zoster (live virus vaccine)	Two doses, 4-8 weeks apart.	Health care workers without reliable history of chickenpox or laboratory evidence of immunity.	***Do not use during pregnancy, immunocompromised state,* history of shock following gelatin ingestion or receipt of neomycin. Salicylate use should be avoided for 6 weeks after vaccination.***	Many individuals without a history of chickenpox are immune. Serologic testing may be cost-effective.
Bacille Calmette Guerin (BCG) vaccine (tuberculosis [TB])	One dose, no booster	Should be considered only in areas where multidrug-resistant TB is prevalent, a strong likelihood of infection exists, and comprehensive TB control precautions have failed to prevent transmission in health care workers.	***Do not use during pregnancy or immunocompromised state.****	In the United States, TB control efforts are aimed at early identification, treatment, and preventive therapy.

*Persons immunocompromised because of immune deficiency diseases, HIV infection (who should normally not receive BCG, OPV, and yellow fever vaccines), leukemia, lymphoma or generalized malignancy, or who are immunosuppressed as a result of therapy with corticosteroids, alkylating drugs, antimetabolites, or radiation.

will learn how to protect yourself and family members.

Other methods of preventing illness. Follow your facility policies and procedures for prevention of infection and injury. If you identify health risks, take the proper precautions. It is your responsiblity to learn and follow these practices. Cooperate with your infection control nurse or department during audits, education, investigation of outbreaks and exposure, and review of infection control practices. Sometimes recommendations to prevent infection change. It is your responsibility to learn new techniques and make changes in the way you practice.

Preventing injuries. Safety practices taught in this class will protect both you and the residents you care for. The most common causes of employee injuries in health care facilities are slips, falls, and back injuries caused by improper lifting and moving. Wear a back support for lifting and moving if this is your preference or the policy of your employer. Lifting, moving, and using your body correctly while on duty will be discussed in detail in Unit 13. Know and follow your facility policies for reporting injuries of residents or employees, and follow them if an accident or injury occurs.

Your Emotional Health

Your feelings and behavior are your responsibility, and you must work to control them. A sign of maturity is your ability to control your emotions. Ask yourself how your behavior will affect others. If you are upset, leave the area and take time out, if necessary. If you feel angry, upset, or impatient, try to understand why you feel this way. Find acceptable ways to cope with these feelings. Do not take negative comments from residents personally. Often the resident is reacting to a situation, not to you. Try to understand why the resident is acting this way. You must respond with respect and courtesy even if the resident is not kind to you.

Stress in the workplace. **Stress** is emotional and physical tension that can be harmful to your health. Working in a health care facility can be stressful at times. Your job may be physically or emotionally demanding. Stress is sometimes unavoidable when you are helping other people with their problems. If stress goes unchecked, you may feel overwhelmed and out of control. Personal or family problems may also contribute to the stress you feel. If your physical health is not good, stress may seem to worsen. **Burnout** is complete mental and physical exhaustion that occurs as the result of a buildup of stress. Feel good about yourself and the job you are doing. Having good self-esteem helps you cope with stressful situations. Use stress-reducing techniques to help cope with stress or sadness. The goal of stress management is to prevent burnout. Try to think through a problem before you worry about it. Understand that health care is constantly changing, and that to be successful, you must change with it. If stress is caused by change, resolve to accept it. If you know of a stress-relieving technique that works for you, use it.

Ways of managing stress. Everyone has certain ways of managing stress. Learn which ways work for you and practice them regularly. Some suggestions for controlling stress are:

- Be nice to yourself. Be aware of your own needs. Leave home problems at home and work problems at work.
- Replay the good things that you have done in your mind. Dwell on these things and not on mistakes you have made.
- Do something that you enjoy and have fun.
- Exercise.
- Take a break and relax in a pleasant atmosphere (Figure 1.6).
- Sit with your feet up and your eyes closed and relax for a few minutes. Take a few deep breaths. Try to think of a pleasant scene or event. Imagine that you are there.
- Use specific relaxation techniques or audio or videotapes.
- Soak in a warm bath.
- Listen to quiet music or read a book.
- Find a hobby that you enjoy.
- Talk with a friend.
- Get in touch with nature. Contact with plants and animals has been proven to reduce stress.
- Watch a funny movie or do something that makes you laugh. Laughing is a good stress reliever.
- Sing. Singing relieves stress.
- Have someone give you a massage.
- Employ spiritual practices, such as prayer, yoga, or meditation.

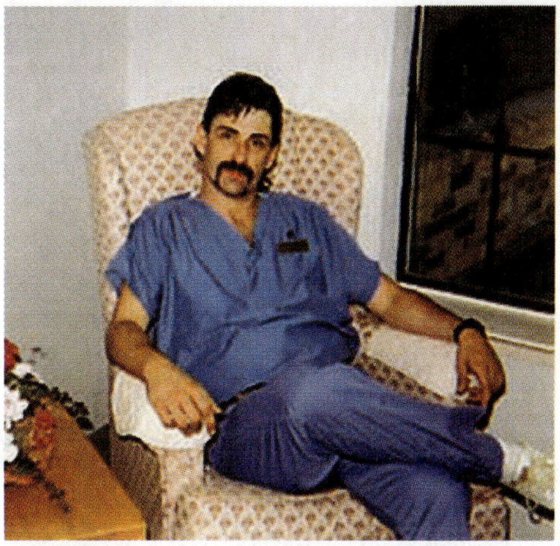

FIGURE 1-6 Taking a break and relaxing in a pleasant, comfortable atmosphere is a good stress reliever.

Proper Equipment

Health care facilities and agencies have different requirements for equipment that you will be expected to provide. By law, the health care facility is required to supply you with well-fitting gloves and other protective equipment. Gloves and personal protective equipment are used when some care is given to prevent the spread of infection. This will be explained in detail in Unit 3. In most cases you will be expected to furnish your own uniform and name pin. Some facilities expect their employees to provide a **gait belt,** also called a transfer belt. This is a canvas belt used for moving and walking residents. Some facilities also require you to have a back-support belt, blood pressure cuff and stethoscope, watch with second hand, pen, and pocket-sized note pad. Know and follow your facility policies.

Responsible Behavior

Responsible behavior is very important for workers in health care professions. Practicing responsible behavior means being dependable and trustworthy. If a member of the health care team is not responsible, residents and coworkers suffer. Because you care for the health and welfare of human beings, you must take your job duties very seriously. Think of how you would feel if a family member was a resident of a health care facility. You would want the best care possible for your loved one. To deliver the best care, all team members must demonstrate responsible behavior.

Health care facility rules must be followed even if you do not agree with them. Learn and profit from constructive criticism. Responsible behavior includes:

- Honesty in word and behavior.
- Reporting to work on time on the days that you are scheduled.
- Keeping absences to a minimum. If you must be absent, follow your facility policy for reporting your absence. Notify the facility as early as possible so that it can call in a replacement. If the facility does not know you will be absent, care will suffer and your coworkers will have to work much harder than usual.
- Keeping your promises to residents and other staff members.
- Completing tasks that are assigned to you quickly and accurately.
- Demonstrating initiative; this means doing things that you see need to be done without waiting to be told to do them.
- Cooperating with other staff members in all departments.
- Being **dependable,** so that residents and coworkers will trust you to do your job to the best of your ability. A person who is dependable is trustworthy and can be relied upon.
- Reporting safety and infection control problems.
- Reporting mistakes if you make them.
- Giving proper notice of resignation if you must resign from your position. Most facilities require a minimum of two weeks notification.

Organization of Your Work

Practice organizing your work. Organization is not something that can be taught in the classroom. The principles of organization will be taught by your instructor, but it is up to you to learn, practice, and master them. Organizing your work means learning how to set **priorities**. Prioritizing your work means performing tasks in order of importance. It also means that you will anticipate your own supply needs and residents' personal needs. Bring needed items to the room before you begin your care. This will save time and steps. If you can plan and prepare to meet these needs in advance, the quality of care you give will be better and the job will be much easier for you.

Manage your time well. Report for duty at your assigned time. Listen to the report and get your assignment (Figure 1.7) from the nurse. Set your priorities to make the most of your day. Setting priorities makes the job easier. Good organization also reduces stress.

When organizing your work, rate each assignment in order of importance. Do not become frustrated if your priorities change or must be adjusted midway through the shift. Priorities are constantly changing in health care because of resident illness and other emergencies.

After you have established your priorities, plan your work for the most efficient use of your time. Identify tasks that you can group together. For example, a well-organized worker can make the bed while the resident is sitting in a chair or washing at the bathroom sink. Plan your schedule around meal times, activities, appointments, and the residents' rehabilitation schedules. Plan for tasks that will require someone else to help you or for which you will need special equipment.

CNA ASSIGNMENT SHEET 10/12/XX														
Room	Resident Name	Bath	Position Schedule	Range of Motion	Vital Signs	Weight	Toileting	B & B	ADL Program	Ambulate	Transfer or Gait Belt	Restraint or Alternative	Safety	I & O
300A	Mary King	S	X	PROM			X					Wedge in chair	X	
300B	Susan Kowalski	WP	X	PROM			X						X	
301A	June Lee		X	PROM		X			X					
301B	Elena Hernandez	BB	X	PROM	X							Side rails	X	X
302	John Murray			AROM					X	X	X			
303A	Albert Strong	S		AROM	X					X				X
303B	Norman Jones		X	PROM			X					Lap buddy	X	
304	Hazel Urich	TB		AROM		X		X		X	X			

Nursing Assistants' Daily Assignments

DATE: 10/12/XX
UNIT: 3rd Floor

Everyone must participate in passing food trays and feeding residents so that hot food is served

Cindy	John	Mary	Susan	James	Norma
Res. group 1 300A-304	Res. group 2 305A-309B	Res. group 3 310-314B	Res. group 4 315A-320A	Res. group 5 320B-325	Res. group 6 326A-330B
Break time: 8:30	Break time: 8:45	Break time: 9:00	Break time: 8:30	Break time: 8:45	Break time: 9:00
Meal time: 10:45	Meal time: 11:15	Meal time: 12:30	Meal time: 10:45	Meal time: 11:15	Meal time: 12:30

SPECIAL ASSIGNMENTS

Fresh Water Pass (AM & PMs)
- John AM
- Norma PM

Mealtime Assignments
- James - hall tays
- Norma - feeders
- Others to main dining room

Water Pitcher Collection (PM)

Tub Room/Shower Room
- Cindy

Utility Rooms/Soiled Linen
- Mary

Deliver Nourishments
- Susan

Utensil Collection (PMs)

Fill Humidifiers

CHARGE NURSE NOTES:

Bible Study - 10:00
Current Events - 11:00
Bingo - 2:00
All beds made by 10 AM Please

RESIDENT APPOINTMENTS:

304 - Beauty shop 9:30
317B - Daughter picking up 11:00 for lunch
323A - Dentist - 2:00

TREATMENTS:

WEIGHTS:	INTAKE/OUTPUT:
301A -	301B -
321B -	303A -
329 -	312 -
VITAL SIGNS:	317B -
301B -	324B -
316A -	326B
321A -	329A -

See Routine Equipment Cleaning Assignment Form on clipboard

FIGURE 1-7 The nurse will give you an assignment each day based on the problems, goals, and needs listed on the care plan for each resident. (Two examples are shown.) Use the assignment to set priorities for your shift. If you believe you will have trouble completing your assignment, inform the nurse promptly.

Check on all of your residents before beginning your assignment. Take care of immediate needs. List special procedures that must be done and the time, such as positioning and turning residents according to an assigned schedule. Check to see if residents are scheduled for tests, appointments, or other activities during your shift. Follow your assignment sheet and the resident's care plan.

Remember that while you are at work, you are on duty. You are being paid to work the whole time. Report to the nurse when you go on break. Return from lunch and breaks on time. If you run out of things to do, help your coworkers or perform tasks that need to be done on your unit. Do these things without being told.

Other Qualities of the Successful Nursing Assistant

The successful nursing assistant delivers quality care to the residents in the long-term care facility. Always do things in the manner in which you were taught. Taking shortcuts can be dangerous. Do not perform procedures unless you have been taught to do so and your facility allows nursing assistants to perform the procedure in question. For example, giving medication is not taught in your class, so this is something that you cannot do without additional education. Some states allow specially prepared nursing assistants to pass medications, but in most states the nursing assistant cannot legally give medicine. If you are not sure how to carry out a procedure, consult the nurse or check the procedure manual. Inform the nurse if you will be unable to complete a job.

Conduct yourself as a professional at all times. Being **compassionate** and **empathetic** with residents and families shows that you care and sets a good example for others. A nursing assistant who is compassionate treats others with mercy and kindness. Empathy is the art of understanding how someone else feels.

Continue to Learn and Grow

This class is just the beginning of your career. Health care changes daily, and it is your responsibility to keep up. You can learn much from your coworkers and by reading books and journals. Attend continuing education classes offered by your employer to learn new information and maintain your certification.

There are professional organizations, support groups, and publications available for nursing assistants. Participating in a professional organization or support group will help you learn and grow.

Protect Yourself Legally

Follow your facility policies and procedures even if you do not agree with them. This protects you as an employee and ensures that you will do your job in accordance with the law. Anticipate residents' needs and meet them in a timely manner. Protect the rights of the residents in your health care facility. These rights and your legal responsibilities are discussed in detail in Unit 5.

KEY POINTS

- Hospitals provide care to patients with acute illnesses.
- Long-term care facilities provide care to residents with chronic illnesses and those who need personal care.
- Subacute care is given to residents who have complex medical or rehabilitation needs.
- Skilled nursing facilities provide care to residents who are medically stable, but require daily skilled services and intervention by licensed health care professionals.
- Home care is provided to clients in their residences by qualified caregivers.
- The OBRA legislation was designed to improve the quality of life for residents of long-term care facilities. This legislation also specifies requirements for nursing assistant education.
- The health care agency, resident, nurse, and nursing assistant all benefit from nursing assistant education and certification.
- The nursing assistant is supervised by a licensed nurse.

- The interdisciplinary team is a group of caregivers who contribute to the care, health, and well-being of residents.
- The chain of command describes the lines of authority used in the health care facility for reporting information.
- Desirable qualities include a professional appearance, good personal hygiene and grooming, good personal health, responsible behavior, dependability, and good organizational skills.

REVIEW

A. Multiple Choice

Select the one best answer.

1. People with acute illnesses are usually cared for in
   a. home care.
   b. hospitals.
   c. long-term care facilities.
   d. physicians' offices.
2. The person who receives care in the long-term care facility is the
   a. client.
   b. patient.
   c. resident.
   d. invalid.
3. The OBRA legislation
   a. is concerned with improving the quality of life for residents in home health care.
   b. describes requirements for nursing assistant education.
   c. describes requirements for professional nurse education.
   d. regulates employee saftey.
4. Benefits of nursing assistant education to the health care facility include all of the following *except*
   a. allowing the nursing assistant to give medicine to residents.
   b. improving the quality of care given to residents.
   c. lowering infection rates because the nursing assistant understands how to prevent infection.
   d. improving the image of the health care facility.
5. According to the OBRA (federal) rules, the minimum number of hours of continuing education that the nursing assistant must have every year is
   a. two.
   b. four.
   c. eight.
   d. twelve.
6. Personal care is provided to residents under the supervision of the
   a. administrator.
   b. clergy.
   c. licensed nurse.
   d. social worker.
7. Your uniform should
   a. be all white.
   b. include a stethoscope.
   c. include well-fitting, comfortable shoes.
   d. identify you as a nurse.
8. Responsible behavior includes
   a. working at least three of every five days that you are scheduled.
   b. calling your facility in advance if you are unable to come to work.
   c. doing only those tasks that you want to do.
   d. not taking breaks.
9. The interdisciplinary team always includes the:
   a. resident.
   b. resident's roommate.
   c. resident's friends.
   d. resident's children.

B. True/False

Answer each statement true (T) or false (F).

10. __________ Everyone involved with the resident's care should follow the care plan.
11. __________ The resident is a member of the interdisciplinary team.

C. Fill in the Blanks

Complete each sentence by adding the missing word.

12. A __________ illness is one that lasts for a long time.
13. A __________ employee is one whom residents and coworkers trust.
14. To maintain nursing assistant certification, you must work in a health care facility for pay for a specified period of time every __________ years.
15. The nursing assistant must be compassionate and __________ with residents and families.

16–20. List five members of the interdisciplinary team.

16. ______________________________
17. ______________________________
18. ______________________________
19. ______________________________
20. ______________________________

D. Clinical Applications

Please read the following case study, then answer the questions.

The Meadows Nursing Center has three nursing assistants on the day shift on Wing A. These assistants care for 24 residents. Mary is a 26-year-old CNA. She completed her CNA class two years ago. She works two jobs and states that she "really doesn't like this work, but needs the money." Mary's resident care is fast and thorough. When she is finished caring for her residents, she often sneaks out the back door for a quick cigarette. She frequently complains of being tired and calls in sick at least once every two to four weeks. She tells her friends that she was not really sick, but was just too tired to get up for work. Kevin is 39 years old. He has been a nursing assistant for 15 years. He is well liked by the residents and staff. He is kind to residents and his care is thorough. He does extra tasks without being asked. Kevin is satisfied with his career choice and says he does not think he would be happy doing any other type of work. Lisa is 19 years old. She says she would eventually like to become a nurse. She recently completed her nursing assistant program and has been working at The Meadows for two months. She is having trouble getting all her work done by the end of the shift.

21. Does Mary demonstrate responsible behavior? Why or why not?
22. Instead of sneaking outside to smoke, what should Mary do if her assignment is complete?
23. When Kevin does extra tasks without being asked, what positive trait is he demonstrating?
24. Lisa is frustrated because she cannot get her work done by the end of the shift. What advice can you give to help her?
25. On Saturday, Lisa is assigned to care for Mrs. Straight. Mrs. Straight's daughter will be picking her up at 9:00 a.m. and taking her out for the day. The resident finishes eating breakfast at 8:15. Lisa has seven other residents to care for in her assignment. What advice can you give to help her make sure that Mrs. Straight is ready to leave when her daughter arrives?

UNIT 2

Communication, Interpersonal Skills, Observation, Recording

A: Communication and Interpersonal Skills

OBJECTIVES

After reading this unit, you will be able to:

- Spell and define key terms.
- List five methods of communicating with others and give an example of each.
- Describe the four elements of communication.
- List eight barriers to communication and give an example of each.
- Describe goal-oriented communication.
- List six communication styles.
- Explain why listening is an important part of communication.
- Describe how to communicate with residents who have physical disabilities, vision loss, or hearing impairments, residents who are mentally confused, and those who are unable to speak.

OBSERVATIONS TO MAKE AND REPORT RELATED TO COMMUNICATION AND INTERPERSONAL SKILLS

Change in consciousness, awareness, or alertness
Changes in mood, behavior, or emotional status
Changes in orientation to person, place, time, season
Change in communication
Changes in memory
Excessive drowsiness
Changes in ability to respond verbally or non-verbally
Sleepiness for no apparent reason
Sudden onset of mental confusion
Threats of suicide or harm to self or others

Communication

Communication involves sending and receiving messages to exchange information with others. Verbal communication is the most common method, but many forms of communication are used in health care. You will communicate verbally, in writing, through gestures, and through use of your body. To be successful, you must understand and practice effective communication. You will communicate with residents, families, visitors, coworkers, and managers. The messages you send and receive must be interpreted accurately. Communication is more than saying words. It is showing honest concern and care for other people.

Factors that Influence Communication with Residents

Sickness, medication, anesthesia, pain, aging, culture, and disease can affect the resident's ability to communicate. Some residents may have trouble seeing, hearing, or speaking. Some residents have language barriers and do not speak English well or at all. When residents have difficulty communicating, the nursing assistant must always practice **empathy**. This involves putting yourself in the resident's shoes and understanding how he or she feels. Empathy is a positive quality. **Sympathy** is feeling sorry for someone because of his or her physical condition or situation. Avoid feeling sympathy for residents. Sympathy is not healthy for you or the resident. Feeling sympathetic can cause you to cross professional boundaries and enter the relationship danger zone.

Imagine how frustrating it would be if you were unable to make your needs known and communicate with others! Be patient and show empathy when communicating with residents who have physical and mental impairments. Do not assume that residents who are unable to speak are mentally confused. Residents who cannot speak often understand what is said to them. Treat all residents with dignity and respect.

Posture, appearance, and body language also affect communication. All of us use our bodies to communicate (Figure 2.1). You must become sensitive to the body language of others and monitor your own body language to be sure that it sends the correct message. Your words and body language should both say the same thing. You may be surprised to learn that whenever there is a conflict between spoken words and body language, the body language is most accurate.

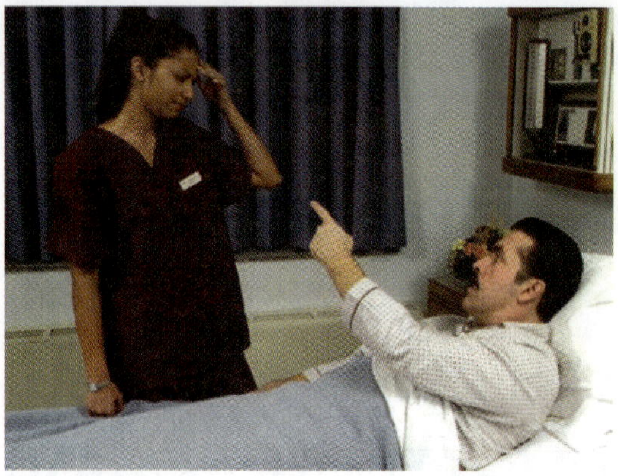

FIGURE 2-1 This resident's body language is sending a message that he is angry.

Elements of Communication

Understanding the elements of communication will help you communicate effectively. Each message has four parts:

1. *Sender*—the person who originates the communication
2. *Message*—the information the sender wants to communicate
3. *Receiver*—the person for whom the communication is intended
4. *Feedback*—confirmation that the message was received as intended

Feedback may be verbal or nonverbal. An example of verbal feedback is responding to what you say. An example of nonverbal feedback is a nod of the head indicating understanding.

Verbal Communication

We communicate with others by the words we speak. Although the words that you speak are important, your tone of voice also affects communication. In fact, one-third of the message is communicated through the tone and pitch of your voice. The tone and pitch of your voice can change the meaning of the communication. If the tone and pitch of your voice contradict the spoken words, the tone and pitch will overshadow the message. Be aware of the effect that the tone, pitch, and quality of your voice have on the way your message is interpreted. Choose your words carefully. Avoid using slang or words with more than one meaning. Use words that the receiver is likely to be familiar with. Speak slowly and clearly. Look at the receiver when speaking.

Paraphrasing. **Paraphrasing** is an effective method of showing that you understand what has been said. When using paraphrasing, restate your understanding of what was said. Listening to the message and paraphrasing provide feedback and show that you are sincerely interested in the conversation.

Nonverbal Communication

Attending behavior shows that you are alert and interested in what the other person is saying to you. Five components of attending behavior are:

1. Eye contact
2. Gestures
3. Posture
4. Physical distance from the other person
5. Paraphrasing

Good eye contact is important to communication. The eyes are very powerful messengers. Even if the body is still, a great deal can be learned about what a person is feeling or thinking by looking at the eyes. In fact, eye contact is often the most remembered part of making an impression. You can create a positive atmosphere by looking at the other person.

In North America, eye contact is very important to communication. This is not true in all cultures. Be sensitive to cultural differences of residents and coworkers. In North America, people who do not make eye contact may be considered dishonest or fearful. Making eye contact can open communication channels and create a bond between two people. During conversation, eye contact communicates interest, concern, warmth, trust, feelings, and credibility. Eye contact can send many different messages. Here are some common interpretations of the signals sent by the eyes:

- Avoiding eye contact may indicate that you wish to continue speaking.
- Looking directly at someone without speaking often indicates that you wish the other person to speak.
- Looking away while someone else is speaking may signal disinterest in the message.
- Glancing downward suggests modesty or insecurity.
- Glaring or staring suggests coldness, disgust, or anger.
- Wide eyes suggest excitement, wonder, amazement, disbelief, honesty, or fright.
- Raised eyebrows suggest disbelief, surprise, or curiosity.
- Excessive blinking suggests nervousness, insecurity, or dishonesty.

The best way to maintain eye contact is to look directly at the person you are speaking to for five to seven seconds. If you maintain eye contact for longer than this, the receiver of your message may think you are staring. Making eye contact is important as you finish speaking. Doing this invites the other person to speak. Learning how to use your eyes effectively in communication may take practice, but practicing this skill is a good investment of your time.

Gestures can be movements of your body or face. We gesture with our facial muscles, eyebrows, mouth, hands, and feet. We may shift restlessly about in a chair. Although we may not be aware of it, these movements send powerful messages to others.

Use gestures and facial expressions to reinforce what you say. Using positive gestures is very important to communication. Use gestures only when you speak. Avoid distracting movements, such as twisting your ring, clicking your pen, or playing with your hair. Doing these things when you are speaking suggests that you are nervous and may undermine your credibility. When someone else is speaking, these actions suggest that you are disinterested or impatient. Smiling is a very effective way to signal your openness. If you fail to smile, people may think you are not interested, cold, or aloof. A warm smile is like hanging out a welcome sign that invites people to relate to you.

Touch is a very powerful means of communication. Touch can communicate a calm, caring attitude. All human beings need to be touched. It sends a message of compassion, caring, and acceptance. Use touch appropriate to the resident's age. For example, holding an adult resident's hand or firmly resting your hand on the forearm or shoulder communicates caring. In a child, patting or stroking the head communicates caring.

Posture is how you hold your body when you stand or sit. When you are seated, leaning forward in the chair while another person speaks shows that you are interested. Standing with the hands on your hips suggests anger, disgust, or impatience. Shaking your finger when you speak indicates anger. Communication is most effective when your body is relaxed.

Physical distance is important for effective communication. In the United States, a comfortable physical distance from others is about 18 to 36 inches. If you are closer than this, others may be uncomfortable. If you are farther away, the receiver may be offended, or the message misinterpreted because the receiver could not see or hear you correctly. The nursing assistant must realize that comfortable physical distance for communication varies with the culture of the resident and nursing assistant.

When speaking with others, always remember the impact of nonverbal communication. Your words represent only 7% of your message. The remainder of the message is interpreted through facial expressions, gestures, and overall body language. Your tone of voice represents 38% of the meaning. Gestures, facial expressions, and other body language represent 55% of your total communication.

Barriers to Communication

A **barrier** is something that interferes with communication. It can be physical, such as trying to speak with a resident whose ears are bandaged after surgery. Eliminate barriers whenever possible. If this is not possible, as in the case of the resident with bandaged ears, find other means to communicate, such as writing. Barriers can also be mental. Mental barriers occur when you have formed a negative opinion about another person or culture. Avoid forming opinions about others based on appearances. Enter each communication with an open mind.

Sometimes other barriers are present, such as with residents with mental confusion, speech and hearing disorders, or those who do not speak English. If you are not sure of the resident's ability to communicate, ask the resident's name and speak with him or her about the season or weather. Provide orienting information if necessary and evaluate the resident's response. Keep your questions simple and ask only one question at a time. If the resident does not understand, rephrase the question. Do not make fun of the resident's lack of understanding. Laugh with the resident, if appropriate. Use the information you have obtained from your evaluation of the resident's understanding to plan your care. Other barriers to communication are:

- Teasing and kidding. Although these are not always barriers, they may be offensive, so avoid them if you do not know the resident well.
- Threatening and warning. Never threaten residents that you will withhold care because of something they have said or done. Consult the nurse if a resident does not cooperate with care.
- Preaching, moralizing, or passing judgment. Do not judge the resident for what he or she has said or done. Not expressing your opinion is better. To be successful, you must try to be neutral and objective even if you disagree.
- Directing and ordering. Your tone of voice, choice of words, and body language can turn a request into an order. This can cause the resident to deliberately do the opposite of what you want. It may also frighten the resident. Select your words carefully and monitor the tone of your voice and body language to avoid sounding like you are giving the resident no choice.
- Arguing. This may make the resident defensive, angry, or upset, and the intent of the original communication will be lost.
- Pretending to be busy, or giving the resident the impression that you are rushed. This sends a message that you do not have time for the resident, or that caring for the resident is a bother.
- Using sound-alike words, such as "haul" and "hall". This can be very confusing for elderly individuals, especially those who are confused or have difficulty hearing. Make sure the context is clear.
- Using slang or cultural terms that are not familiar to the resident, and may be misinterpreted.
- Interrupting or changing the subject. This sends a message to the resident that what he or she has to say is not worthwhile, and may inhibit the resident from future conversation.
- Giving answers such as, "Don't worry about it." This sends a message to the resident that his or her concerns are not important.
- Providing false reassurance, such as, "everything will be all right." The resident will not trust you when he or she learns you were not sincere.
- Talking to the resident about your personal problems. This is never appropriate in the long-term care setting.
- Not waiting long enough for a reply. Elderly residents may take longer to process information, especially if they have hearing problems. Allow enough time for a response.

GUIDELINES FOR COMMUNICATION

Use every contact with residents as an opportunity for communication. Show that you value the residents and respect them by calling them by their preferred names. If you do not know what they prefer to be called, use Mr. or Mrs., followed by the surname. Pet names such as "honey", "dear", and "gramps" are not appropriate. Smile and speak to residents, families, and visitors when you pass in the hallway. Speak to residents when giving care. Set aside time to talk. This shows that you like other people and are genuinely concerned for the well-being of others.

GUIDELINES FOR

Having a Conversation

- Knock on the door, introduce yourself by name and title, and address the resident by his or her preferred name.
- Approach the resident in a friendly, courteous manner.
- If you are in the room to perform a procedure, explain it before beginning. Allow time for the resident to ask questions and show understanding. This shows respect for the resident.
- If your time is limited, prepare the resident in advance by stating how much time you have and when you will need to leave.
- Speak in terms that are familiar to the resident.
- Make eye contact during the conversation.
- Be polite.
- Speak clearly and distinctly.
- Listen to what the resident says. Ask questions or make comments to show that you are interested.
- Use touch to communicate caring, if appropriate.

GUIDELINES TO

Use When Speaking

Techniques to use to make all types of communication more meaningful are:

- Maintain eye contact during the conversation.
- Sit at the resident's eye level, if possible (Figure 2.2).
- Speak clearly and distinctly.
- Use language the resident will understand. Avoid using medical terms.
- Keep your message brief and concise. This should not be difficult if you have thought about your communication and selected a goal in advance.
- Use nonverbal communication, such as touch, posture, gestures, and body language, as appropriate.
- Use open-ended questions to encourage the resident to speak.
- Be courteous and polite.
- Send positive messages by using praise, encouragement, touch, and smiles.
- Give, receive, and request feedback.

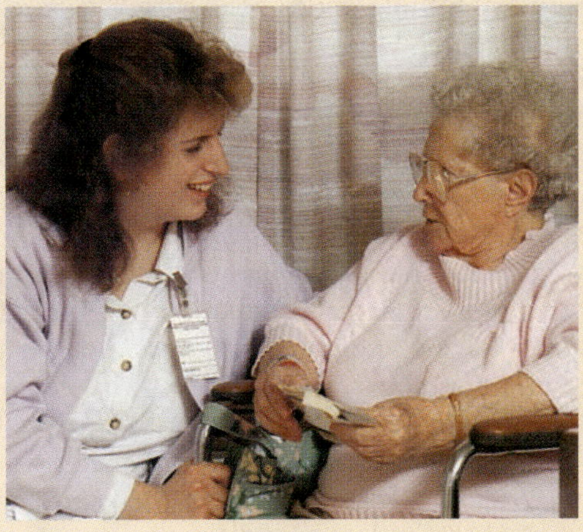

FIGURE 2-2 Sit at the resident's eye level and maintain eye contact during the conversation.

Communication should be goal-oriented. Before beginning a conversation, set a goal. Think about what you want to accomplish and focus on the topic. Arrange the main points of what you would like to say in logical order. Eliminate unrelated or unnecessary information that may confuse the message.

Communication Styles

After you have set a goal for your conversation, select the style of communication that will help you meet this goal. Six types of conversations and the goal of each are listed in Table 2.1.

TABLE 2-1 Forms of Conversation

Type of Conversation	Goal
Social conversation	To create a comfortable, relaxed atmosphere. Talk about pleasant things that the resident may be interested in. Do not discuss your problems or complaints with residents. Avoid discussing facility business or gossiping about other residents or employees.
Interviewing	To obtain information that will help you meet the resident's needs. For example, ask if the resident prefers to take a shower in the morning or evening. Interviewing helps you plan your routine and shows the resident that you are genuinely interested in his or her well-being.
Teaching	To show and tell the resident something that he or she will learn, understand, and use. All health care workers are teachers.
Reporting	To communicate accurate information. Reporting is done to the nurse. Accurate reporting involves communicating factual information.
Problem solving	To help meet the resident's needs. It is different from interviewing. In this situation, you know what the resident wants. Your objective is to find a way to do it.
Therapeutic communication	To encourage the resident to talk about feelings. This type of communication is particularly sensitive because you must be careful not to pass judgment on what the resident thinks or feels. Monitor your body language carefully.

Listening

Hearing is nothing more than being aware of sound. Listening is an active, deliberate process in which you focus and make an effort to hear and understand what the resident is saying. Listening is an important part of communication. Listening to what someone else is saying may be difficult when you have other things on your mind. Your body language may betray you by sending a message that you are not interested in what the other person is saying. Although this may not be the case, monitor your movement and expressions closely to avoid misunderstanding. Paraphrasing is a good technique to use to show that you are listening. Silence is also a good technique. Silence shows acceptance and respect. It encourages the resident to speak. You may be uncomfortable with silence. If so, work to overcome your discomfort.

Communicating with Residents who have Disabilities and Sensory Impairments

Sensory impairments can take many forms. Some forms, such as speech, hearing, or language problems, interfere directly with communication. Other problems, such as physical impairments, may make you uncomfortable and unsure of what to say without being offensive. People with disabilities are much like you are. They have the same wants and needs. They can do many of the same things you can, but may need to adapt the environment in order to do them. Although the end result is the same, people with disabilities may perform the task differently. Their bodies work differently! As a rule, people with disabilities do not want to be treated differently from anyone else. Many are self-sufficient, have led productive lives, and are valuable and equal members of society. They may be physically challenged, but many have developed other talents and qualities using nonphysical skills.

Nursing assistants have a responsibility to emphasize the uniqueness and worth of all persons, rather than the differences between people. Your efforts will do much to encourage acceptance of people with disabilities. Treat people with disabilities the way you like to be treated. You will leave the experience feeling fulfilled and richly rewarded.

Communicating with Residents Who Have Vision Loss

Vision loss can range from problems that can be corrected with glasses to complete blindness. Some people are legally blind, but still have

GUIDELINES FOR

Listening

- Use open posture. Lean toward the resident. Avoid crossing your arms in front of your body or placing your hands on your hips.
- Give the resident your full attention (Figure 2.3).
- Maintain eye contact.
- Show interest in the resident's activities, interests, and concerns.
- Monitor the resident's body language to see if it confirms or conflicts with the verbal message the resident is sending.
- Encourage the resident to talk about feelings and concerns. Allow the resident to express anger and negative feelings without passing judgment or becoming defensive.
- Use touch to communicate caring, if appropriate.
- Use silence to allow the resident to think and continue the conversation.
- Pay attention and show interest in what the resident is saying. Ask questions if necessary. Use paraphrasing to show interest and understanding. Use noncommittal responses, such as "I understand," to show that you are listening.
- Use responses such as, "I would like to hear more about that," or "Then what happened?" to show that you are interested.
- Use responses such as, "So you felt bad about that," to show empathy.
- Wait until the resident is finished speaking before responding.
- Request help from the nurse, if needed, to solve problems.

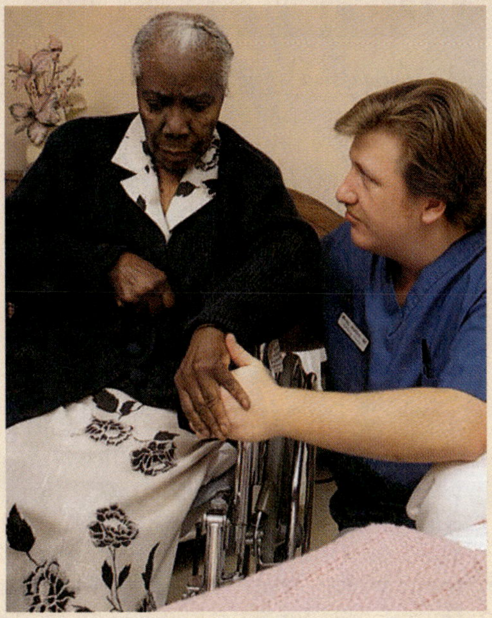

FIGURE 2-3 Pay close attention to what the resident is saying through her words and gestures.

GUIDELINES FOR

Ending a Conversation

- Inform the resident that you have to leave.
- Tell the resident what time you will be back, and be sure to return at this time.
- Tell the resident that you enjoyed the conversation.
- Ask if the resident needs anything before you leave.
- Before leaving the room, make sure that the resident is safe, comfortable, and has the call signal and needed personal items within reach.

limited vision. Do not assume that residents who are wearing glasses can see. Some residents who wear glasses are severely impaired. People who are blind are like residents with other disabilities. They may have a loss in one area of their life, but they have developed other areas. Most are self-sufficient, but may need environmental adaptations. Do not rearrange furniture, equipment, supplies, or personal items in the room without the resident's approval. People with visual impairments memorize the location of items. Moving things could result in accidents, injuries, or frustration because the resident is unable to find a needed item. When you are providing care or would like the resident

GUIDELINES FOR

Communicating with and about Residents Who Have Disabilities

- Avoid referring to the resident as a condition, such as "the **paraplegic** in 221." Say instead, "Mrs. Smith in 221." A person who is paralyzed has no feeling or movement. A paraplegic has no feeling or movement from the waist down. Always emphasize the person over the condition.
- Use common sense when talking to someone who has a disability. Talk to the person the same way you would anyone else. People with disabilities do not want to be treated differently.
- Do not assume that someone is not disabled or pretending because the disability is not visible. Some medical conditions are severely disabling, but the person may not appear disabled.
- Shaking hands is appropriate with people who have upper extremity disabilities. Residents with limited movement or a **prosthesis** are able to shake hands. A prosthesis is an artificial body part. Shake hands gently with a person who has arthritis.
- Before helping someone who has a disability, ask if you can help. It is all right to offer to help, but unless the resident is struggling, do not intervene without asking.
- It is all right to ask residents about their disabilities. Many residents are comfortable, and will talk about them, but it is also all right if they do not want to talk about it. People who are newly disabled may not have reached a point of mental acceptance and may be uncomfortable speaking about their problem.
- When caring for a resident with a disability, do not assume that the resident can or cannot do something. Assuming can be offensive. Always ask.
- Always stress the resident's ability and not the disability.
- Residents who use wheelchairs, canes, walkers, and crutches because of a disability are not always sick. Avoid making assumptions.
- Residents in wheelchairs do not like to be treated as if they are mentally impaired! Most have no mental problem. Talk to the person in the wheelchair, not to a companion.
- When talking to a resident in a wheelchair, position yourself at his or her eye level.
- Be polite. Show the same manners that you would with anyone else.
- Use good manners if you walk in front of a resident in a wheelchair by excusing yourself.
- If you are in a crowded area, such as when attending an activity, avoid standing in front of a person in a wheelchair. This blocks the resident's view.
- The wheelchair is an extension of the disabled person's body. Leaning or hanging on the chair is an invasion of the resident's personal space.
- Words such as "see," "hear," "run," and "walk" can be used when speaking with people who have disabilities.
- Choose words that are positive and nonjudgmental. Avoid using words like "cripple," "gimp," "spastic," "retard." This is demeaning and promotes negative perceptions of the physically challenged. Table 2.2 gives examples of acceptable and unacceptable terminology to use in conversation. Remember, always emphasize the person first. Emphasizing the disease is demeaning. Table 2.3 lists phrases to avoid when speaking about persons with disabilities.

TABLE 2-2 Recommended Phrases for Use in Conversation

Offensive and unacceptable Do not use in conversation	Acceptable use in conversation
Disabled person	A person with a disability
Blind person	A person who is vision impaired
Deaf person	A person who is hearing impaired
A hunchback	A person who has curvature of the spine
The disabled	People who are disabled; the disabled community
He is a cripple (gimp)	He has a disability (or mobility problem)
Dumb (or deaf and dumb)	A person who has a speech or hearing impairment
She is nuts, crazy	She has an emotional disability or mental illness
Retard	A person with mental retardation
Birth defect	A person who is disabled from birth
Fit	Seizure
Normal person as compared with a person who has a disability	A person who is not disabled as compared with a person who is
Confined to a wheelchair	A person who uses a wheelchair
Honey, sweetie, baby, or gramps	Call the person by his or her preferred name

- People who have disabilities like to laugh and have fun (Figure 2.4). Do not leave them out!
- Canine companions, such as seeing eye dogs or hearing ear dogs, are on duty. Do not feed them or pet them without the owner's permission. This distracts them and prevents them from doing their job.

TABLE 2-3 Words to Avoid

Words to avoid when speaking with or about persons who are disabled	
Abnormal	Gimp
Afflicted	Invalid
Burden	Imbecile
Cerebral palsied	Maimed
Confined to a wheelchair	Moron
Courageous	Normal
Cripple	Palsied
Crippled	Poor
Deaf and dumb	Spastic
Deaf mute	Stricken with
Defect	Sufferer
Defective	Suffers with
Deformity	Suffering
Diseased	Unfortunate
Epileptic	Victim

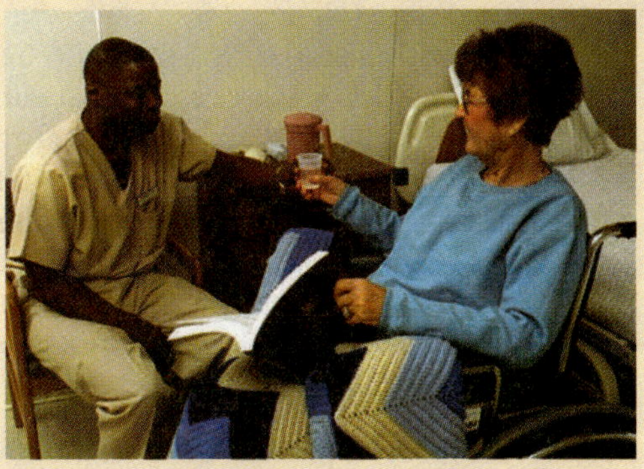

FIGURE 2-4 Residents who have disabilities like to laugh and have fun. You are privileged to share intimate moments of their lives. Enjoy the time you spend with them.

GUIDELINES FOR

Communicating with Residents Who Have Vision Loss

- Knock on the door and identify yourself by name and title before entering the room. Call the resident by the preferred name.
- Help residents clean their glasses and encourage them to wear them.
- When speaking, sit in a good light where the resident can see your face. The light source should not be behind your back, as it will shine in the resident's eyes from this position.
- Speak clearly and directly in a normal tone of voice. Blindness does not interfere with the resident's ability to hear.
- Use touch to communicate, if appropriate, but do so slowly and gently so the resident is not startled.
- When you are performing tasks in the room, tell the resident what you are doing. It is acceptable to discuss new things you see, interesting changes, and what various people are doing. This is not offensive. You are the resident's eyes!
- Always ask the resident what he or she would like to wear. Describe the color and style of the clothes.
- Tell the resident when you are finished.
- Replace everything in its original location.
- Tell the resident when you are leaving the room. Make sure the resident is comfortable and safe, with the call signal and needed personal items within reach.
- When assisting a resident who has a visual impairment to walk, have the resident hold your upper arm (Figure 2.5). Walk alongside and slightly ahead of the resident. The resident can tell a great deal from feeling your body movement. Walk naturally at the resident's pace. Tell the resident when there are steps, obstacles, when to turn left or right, if you must go through a door, and so forth. Be specific when giving directions. Pause slightly before stairs, or when making a turn. Avoid revolving doors and escalators if you are in a public place. If you are walking and are interrupted by someone, let the resident know you will be stopping.
- When using stairs, guide the resident's hand to the railing. Stop on each step before proceeding to the next step.
- When seating the resident, place the resident's hand on the back or arm of the chair.
- Do not leave a resident who is visually impaired or blind in an open area. Lead him or her to the side of a room, chair, or landmark from which he or she can obtain a direction for travel.

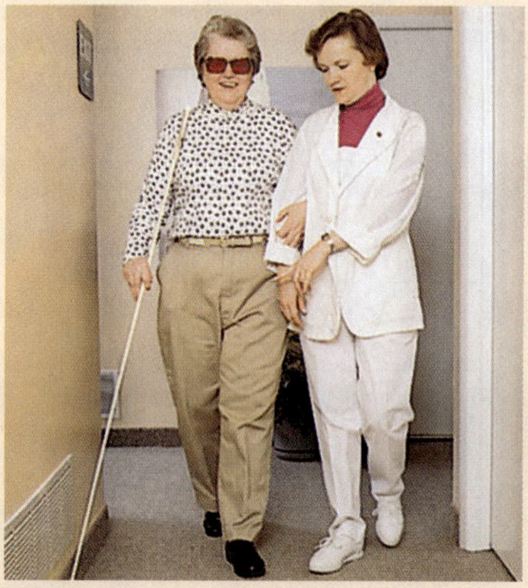

FIGURE 2-5 Have the resident hold your upper arm lightly while you walk at the resident's pace.

to assist with a procedure, provide detailed, step-by-step directions.

Communicating with Residents Who Have Hearing Loss

Hearing loss can mean that a resident has difficulty hearing or that the resident is completely deaf. There are many causes of hearing loss. Some hearing loss can be corrected with hearing aids. Other types can be corrected with surgery. Some people have uncorrected hearing loss. People who are deaf communicate in many different ways. Some use sign language. This is a combination of hand signals and facial expressions. Others

GUIDELINES FOR

Communicating with Residents Who Have Hearing Loss

- Approach the resident from the front or side. Lightly touch the resident's arm or shoulder without startling the resident.
- Eliminate as much background noise and activity as possible.
- Assist the resident to use a hearing aid, if appropriate.
- Be aware that individuals with hearing loss hear and understand less well when they are ill.
- Avoid speaking from another room, when walking away, or with your back turned to the resident.
- If the resident hears better in one ear, position yourself on that side when speaking.
- Sit in a good light where the resident can see your face. The light source should not be behind your back.
- Do not chew gum, eat, or put your hands in front of your mouth when speaking.
- Be considerate and try to make the resident feel confident in you.
- Look directly at the resident when speaking.
- Speak slowly, clearly, and distinctly. Use your lips to emphasize words.
- Choose short, simple words. Use short sentences.
- Speak in a lower pitched voice than normal. You may need to raise the loudness of your voice, but do not shout. Shouting distorts the voice and makes you sound angry.
- Tell the resident what you are going to talk about.
- Use gestures, body language, and facial expressions to convey meaning.
- Write down key words, if necessary. Use communication boards or other adaptive equipment, if available.
- If the resident with hearing impairment has difficulty with letters or numbers, say, "M as in Mary, 2 as in twins, B as in boy." Say each number separately. Say "six seven" instead of "sixty-seven."
- Some residents benefit from placing a stethoscope in their ears, which amplifies the sound when you speak into the diaphragm.
- If the resident does not understand a word, use a different word instead of repeating what you said more loudly.
- Keep conversations brief and limited to a single topic.
- Do not convey impatience by your body language.
- If you do not understand what a person who is deaf or has a speech impairment says, asking him or her to repeat is acceptable.
- If an interpreter is helping you, speak to the resident, not the interpreter.
- Tell the resident when you are leaving the room. Make sure the resident is comfortable and safe, with the call signal and needed personal items within reach.

read lips. Some people use reading and writing as their primary form of communication. Special telephone and television communication systems and amplifiers are available for people who are deaf and hearing impaired. Residents who are hearing impaired can function independently, but as with other disabilities, may need environmental adaptations. Remember that residents with vision and hearing loss will need help in an emergency, such as when the fire alarm sounds.

Caring for residents with hearing aids. Some residents use hearing aids to help them hear more clearly. The hearing aid amplifies the sound and improves communication. However, the resident may still be unable to hear normally, even with the hearing aid in place. Many types of hearing aids are available, but they all work on the same principle (Figure 2.6). The aid contains a tiny microphone that changes sound and increases the strength of electrical signals. A tiny speaker converts the signal to a sound wave and sends the message to the resident's ear.

Communicating with Residents Who Have Problems with Language and Understanding

Some residents have illnesses or injuries that affect their ability to speak and understand what is spoken to them. They may be able to understand some things, but not others. You must assume that

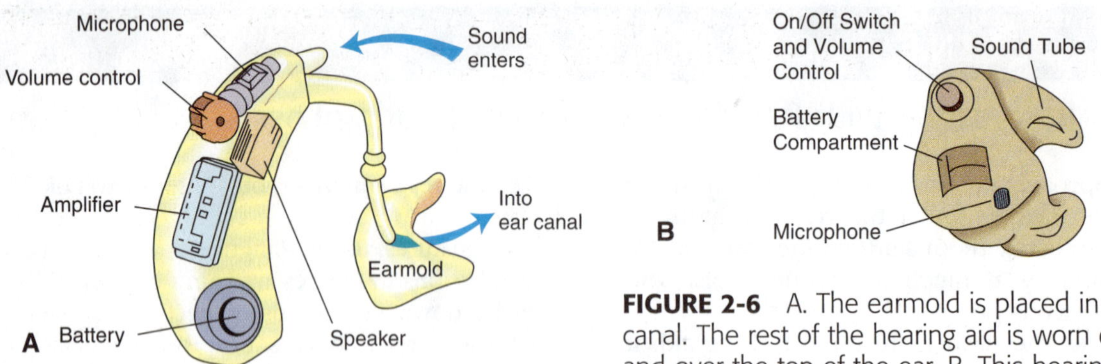

FIGURE 2-6 A. The earmold is placed in the ear canal. The rest of the hearing aid is worn outside and over the top of the ear. B. This hearing aid fits inside the outer ear canal.

GUIDELINES FOR

Caring for Hearing Aids

- The hearing aid is fragile and expensive. Avoid dropping it. Always hold the hearing aid over a soft surface or table when cleaning or caring for it.
- Keep the hearing aid clean. Remove it daily and wipe off any dust, ear wax, or body oil with a tissue. Avoid using alcohol wipes to clean the aid. Use a damp cloth.
- If the hearing aid is the cannula type, remove ear wax from the speaker opening with a pipe cleaner or special appliance cleaner. Ask the resident if he or she has a tool called a wax loop, and use this, if available. Never use a toothpick, paper clip, or other sharp object.
- When caring for a female resident, do not spray hairspray when the hearing aid is in place.
- Remove the hearing aid before using a hair dryer or blow dryer. Never apply a source of heat to the hearing aid.
- Organize your work so that male residents who shave with an electric razor can shave or be shaved before the hearing aid is applied. If this is not possible, turn the aid off or remove it before using the electric razor. The buzzing of the razor is very loud and annoying with the hearing aid in place.
- Avoid getting the hearing aid wet. If it has an outer ear mold, the ear piece may be washed with mild soap and warm water. The part of the hearing aid containing the batteries should never get wet. Allow the mold to dry thoroughly before reattaching it to the unit.
- Remove the hearing aid when bathing the resident or washing his or her hair.
- Turn the hearing aid off when it is not in the resident's ear. Opening the battery case when the aid is stored prevents unnecessary drain on the battery.
- Remove the battery at night and check it for leaks. Store the hearing aid and battery in the case. Replace worn-out or leaking batteries. Wipe the battery gently with a clean cloth before reinserting it.
- Avoid temperature extremes. Do not store the aid in a cold area, on a radiator, or in direct sunlight.
- If the hearing aid has a cord, check it for cracks or breaks.
- Insert the hearing aid properly. Sometimes the shape of the ear changes with aging and the hearing aid may need to be refitted. If the resident complains of pain or the aid is difficult to insert, this may be the problem. Advise the nurse if this occurs.
- When communicating with the resident, follow the same guidelines that you use when communicating with a resident who has a hearing impairment.
- Check the bed linen carefully before placing it in the soiled linen hamper. A hearing aid is small, expensive, and easily lost. It will not survive a trip through the washer and dryer!
- Remove the hearing aid and allow the ear to "cool" before taking a tympanic temperature.

GUIDELINES FOR

Troubleshooting Hearing Aid Problems

Never try to repair a hearing aid yourself. However, if the resident has problems with the aid, there are several things you can do that may resolve them.

- Check the hearing aid to see if it is turned on. Some models have settings marked on them. These are "M" for microphone, "T" for telephone, and "O" for off. Set the switch to the "M" setting.
- Check the volume of the hearing aid to be sure it is turned up loud enough for the resident to hear.
- Hold the hearing aid in the palm of your hand. Turn the volume up all the way. Cup the aid between your hands. You should hear a loud whistle. A weak or absent sound indicates that the battery is low.
- Before changing the battery, check the position of the old battery so you can put the new one in the same way. When inserting a new battery, place it in the unit gently. If you meet resistance, do not force it. Consult the nurse.
- Check the ear mold for wax. If wax is present, remove it.
- Ask the nurse to check the resident's ears with an otoscope for wax buildup.
- If the hearing aid is in the resident's ear and makes a loud, whistling sound, check the position. The aid should be securely in the ear. Make sure that hair, ear wax, or clothing are not interfering with the position. Check the tubing for cracks. Whistling usually indicates an air leak.
- If the hearing aid works intermittently or makes a scratchy sound, check for dirt under and around the battery. Also check the volume control and connections. If the hearing aid has a connecting wire, make sure it is plugged in tightly and is not cracked or bent.

they understand you. Try to communicate with them as you would with other residents. Do not make the mistake of being silent when you are caring for them. Your silence may be received as a negative message by the resident. These residents may be able to speak, but what they say does not make sense. They may have certain words or phrases that have meaning to them, but not to you. Sincerely try to understand what they are saying. Be empathetic and do not show frustration. If you learn what they are saying, share this information with other members of the interdisciplinary team. This will enable all team members to help meet the resident's needs. Some residents are unable to speak correctly, but they understand what is spoken to them. Do not assume that the resident with a speech problem is mentally confused. Test the resident's ability to answer yes or no questions, or to follow simple directions, to determine the resident's mental status.

Communicating with Residents Who Have Problems Speaking

Some diseases and injuries leave residents unable to speak. **Aphasia** is a condition in which the speech center in the brain has been damaged. This commonly occurs when the resident has had a stroke. Residents with **expressive aphasia** have difficulty saying what they want to say. They may also have trouble with gestures and writing. Residents with **receptive aphasia** have trouble understanding what is spoken to them. The resident may also have trouble reading and understanding gestures. **Global aphasia** involves both speaking and understanding. **Dysarthria** is a condition in which the resident has weakness or paralysis of the lips, tongue, or throat. This is often due to a head injury or stroke. The resident may be able to make noise, but not form words. However, the resident often understands what you are saying. Do not make the mistake of thinking that a resident has a mental impairment because of the inability to speak. Over time, some residents are able to regain their speech with aggressive therapy. Some develop other methods of communication. These residents are often able to make themselves understood by gestures, writing, or with other adaptive communication devices.

Communicating with Residents Who Are Mentally Retarded

Mental retardation affects about 3% of the population in the United States. A person who is

GUIDELINES FOR

Caring for Residents Who Have Problems with Language and Understanding

- Knock on the door and identify yourself by name and title before entering the room. Call the resident by the preferred name.
- Approach the resident in a friendly, courteous manner. Approach from the front to avoid startling the resident.
- Assist the resident with the use of glasses and hearing aids, if used.
- Explain what will be done.
- Use short, simple words. Pronounce them clearly and slowly.
- Focus on one topic and use short sentences.
- Use gentle touch to show that you care.
- Keep conversations short but frequent.
- Use your facial expression and gestures to convey your message.
- Allow adequate time for the resident to respond. Do not be tempted to complete a sentence for the resident.
- Listen carefully to the response. Pay close attention to what the resident is saying.
- If you think you understand what the resident is saying, use paraphrasing to give the resident feedback.
- Allow the resident time to finish speaking. Do not cut him or her off.
- Monitor your body language. Avoid communicating frustration due to your inability to understand the resident.
- Accept responsibility for being unable to understand. The resident is doing his or her best. He or she is probably more frustrated than you are. Do not discourage or blame the resident for the break-down in communication.
- Assume that the resident understands you if you are not sure and cannot get a response.
- Encourage the resident to point to things and use gestures.
- Use adaptive devices, such as picture boards (Figure 2.7), if available. The speech-language pathologist will often provide these devices and teach the resident to use them.
- Tell the resident when you are leaving the room. Make sure the resident is comfortable and safe, with the call signal and needed personal items within reach.

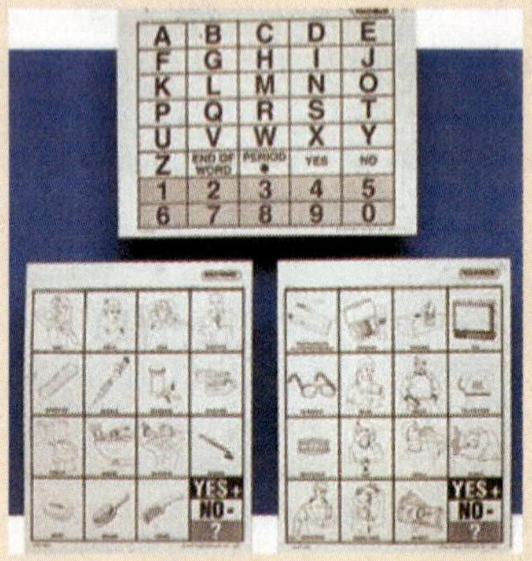

FIGURE 2-7 Picture boards are tools the resident can use to communicate wants and needs. *(Permission given for reprint/reproduction to Maddack's, Communicard Trio)*

mentally retarded has experienced difficulty learning since childhood. Mental retardation is like any other disability. The condition developed because of conditions before birth or in early childhood, and was not caused by the resident. There are many levels of retardation, ranging from profound to mild. Residents with profound retardation function at the level of an infant. People with mild retardation function at the fourth-grade level. Of all people diagnosed with mental retardation, 89% are mildly retarded. People who are mentally retarded have the same needs as you, but learn more slowly and are limited in what they can learn. Most are able to live productive lives.

Individuals who are mentally retarded need acceptance and attention. Like all other residents, they must be treated with dignity and respect. They must be able to express themselves and relieve stress. They are able to make simple choices, but may become overwhelmed if they are given too many options. If making decisions overwhelms the resident, limit choices to one of two. Residents with mental retardation respond

GUIDELINES FOR

Communicating with Residents Who Have Problems Speaking

- Knock on the door and identify yourself by name and title before entering the room. Call the resident by the preferred name.
- Approach the resident in a friendly, courteous manner.
- Assist the resident with the use of glasses and hearing aids, if used.
- Keep conversations short but frequent.
- Use questions that can be answered with yes or no answers. Tell the resident to nod his or her head in response. If the resident is unable to nod the head, tell him or her to blink the eyes once for yes and twice for no.
- Allow adequate time for the resident to respond.
- Give the resident a pen and paper to write with, if able, or use assistive communication devices such as picture or word boards.
- Listen carefully to the response.
- If you think you understand what the resident is saying, use paraphrasing to give the resident feedback.
- Do not pretend to understand the resident if you do not.
- Emphasize the positive aspects of the message, such as words and gestures that you do understand.
- Allow time to complete the conversation, to avoid sending the message that you are impatient with the resident.
- Assume that the resident understands you if you are not sure and cannot get a response.
- Use appropriate body language. Do not convey frustration at your inability to understand.
- Encourage the resident to point to things and use gestures.
- Tell the resident when you are leaving the room. Make sure the resident is comfortable and safe, with the call signal and needed personal items within reach.

GUIDELINES FOR

Communicating with Residents Who Are Mentally Retarded

- Keep your words and sentences short and simple.
- Give clear, concise instructions.
- Do not "talk down" to the resident. Treat adults as adults.
- Listen to what the resident says. Often he or she knows more than you think.
- People who are mentally retarded are very sensitive to the moods of others. If you are upset, they will be too. If you are happy and relaxed, they will be too. Ask yourself how you look to them.
- If making decisions is upsetting to the resident, limit choices to two.
- If you notice the resident becoming frustrated, slow down. Do not push.
- Praise and compliment the resident for even small accomplishments.
- Treat people who are mentally retarded with the same respect that you would give others.

well to consistent treatment and expectations. When caring for these residents, use of the care plan by all staff is very important because this ensures consistent care. It is important for people who are mentally retarded to feel worth-while. They like to help and feel like they are contributing. Most are happy and loving.

People who are mentally retarded should not be pressured to learn things or perform new tasks. They can be taught, but teaching them requires great patience. They often do not function well in high-pressure situations, and may not function well in large, loud, confusing groups unless someone is there to support them. They know if others are ridiculing them, and feel hurt and rejection.

Communicating with the Resident's Family, Friends, and Visitors

You are a representative of the health care facility to visitors. Speak and smile to visitors in the hallway. If someone looks lost, ask if you can help. Maintain an open, friendly, and supportive attitude with visitors. Show them where the lounges, vending machines, cafeteria, restrooms, and smoking areas are. Answer any questions they have about your facility's policies and procedures. However, you must protect resident confidentiality, even with family members. If they ask you questions about the resident's condition, refer them to the nurse. You may tell them something about the resident's activities, such as "He ate a good lunch."

Families may react in different ways to the resident's illness. They may show anxiety or anger. Be patient and understanding. Do not argue with them. Listen carefully and be empathetic. If family members have complaints or if you notice a resident becoming upset when visitors are in the room, report this to the nurse.

Sometimes you must perform a procedure on a resident when visitors are in the room. Ask the visitors to step out until you have completed the procedure. Show them where they can wait. When you are done with the procedure, inform them that they can return to the room.

Answering the telephone. Nursing assistants are required to answer the telephone in many long-term care facilities. If this is your responsibility, answer the phone by stating the name of your facility or unit. Identify yourself by name and title. Be courteous and polite. If a physician is on the line to give orders for a resident, you must get a nurse to take the call. Unlicensed personnel cannot legally take orders from a physician. If the caller is not a physician, determine what is requested and provide the information, if possible. However, avoid giving out personal information about residents. If the caller is not a physician, obtain the information, or transfer the caller to the proper person. If the person being called cannot come to the telephone, take a clear message. Write down the date, time of the call, name of the caller, and a brief message. Sign your name and title to the message. Inform the caller that you will deliver the message. Thank the person for calling.

KEY POINTS

- Many factors influence communication.
- Health care workers communicate with many people verbally, in writing, and through gestures, touch, and body language.
- The four elements of communication are the sender, message, receiver, and feedback.
- Using goal-oriented communication involves deciding what you want to accomplish and focusing on a topic.
- People with disabilities should be treated the way you like to be treated. Some people with disabilities have special communication needs.
- Courtesy is important when answering the telephone in the health care facility.

REVIEW

A. Multiple Choice

Select the one best answer.

1. Communication may be influenced by
   a. the season.
   b. the day of the week.
   c. acute or chronic illness.
   d. the eye color of the receiver.

2. Empathy means
   a. understanding how the resident feels.
   b. feeling sorry for the resident.

c. understanding emotional needs.
d. solving problems for the resident.

3. The sender is the person who

a. gets the message.
b. initiates a communication.
c. interprets the message.
d. relays communication to another person.

4. Feedback is

a. your interpretation of what the nurse said.
b. your interpretation of what the resident said.
c. confirmation that a message was received as intended.
d. obtaining information to meet the resident's needs.

5. Which of the following are components of attending behavior?

a. eye contact and gestures
b. thinking and feeling
c. crossing your arms and legs
d. physical appearance and dress

6. Comfortable personal space in the United States is

a. 8 inches to 10 inches.
b. 18 inches to 36 inches.
c. 28 inches.
d. 48 inches.

7. Paraphrasing is

a. repeating what the speaker says word for word.
b. interpreting the message for another person.
c. using sign language for a deaf resident.
d. restating a message in clear, simple terms.

8. Something that interferes with communication is a

a. gesture.
b. barrier.
c. suggestion.
d. symptom.

9. Thinking about what you want to accomplish in a conversation and focusing on a topic is an example of using

a. goal-oriented communication.
b. paraphrasing.
c. empathy.
d. feedback.

10. A communication style in which you want to obtain information to meet the resident's needs is

a. therapeutic communication.
b. problem solving.
c. interviewing.
d. social conversation.

11. When communicating with a resident in a wheelchair, you should avoid using the word

a. see.
b. run.
c. walk.
d. crippled.

12. When caring for residents with vision or hearing loss, you should

a. be as quiet as possible when you are in the room, so the resident is not disturbed.
b. make as much noise as possible when you are in the room, so the resident knows what you are doing.
c. announce yourself by name and title when entering the room.
d. approach the resident from the side or rear.

13. When caring for residents who have problems with speech or understanding, you should

a. explain the care you will be giving in medical terms.
b. choose short, simple words and use short sentences.
c. use sign language that the resident understands.
d. avoid speaking whenever possible.

14. When caring for a person who is mentally retarded, you should

a. treat the resident with courtesy and respect.
b. not explain procedures.
c. never smile, because this is upsetting to the resident.
d. avoid touch as this upsets the resident.

15. You answer the telephone on your unit. The caller identifies herself as Dr. Gonzales and says that she wants to give orders for Mrs. Keene. You should

a. ask the doctor to hold while you get the nurse.
b. write down the orders the doctor gives you.
c. tell the doctor to call back later.
d. inform the doctor that the nurse is not at the desk.

B. Clinical Applications

Answer the following questions.

16. You are assigned to pass trays on Wing B. You have never passed trays on this hall before. You enter Mr. Haney's room and notice that he is standing by the dresser picking up items and feeling them. You think Mr. Haney may be visually impaired. How do you find out?
17. Mrs. Stone wears a hearing aid. You served her breakfast tray in bed. She had the hearing aid in her ear at that time. After breakfast, Mrs. Stone got out of bed and you completely changed the bed linen. Her hearing aid is missing. She says the last time she remembers using it was when she was eating breakfast. She does not know what became of it. The food trays have been returned to the kitchen. The soiled linen hamper has been taken to the laundry. What should you do?
18. Mr. White recently had a stroke and has lost the ability to speak. The speech-language pathologist is working with him. Mr. White is able to write and communicates by writing notes on a magic slate. You enter the room and ask Mr. White what time he would like his shower. He throws the magic slate against the wall and glares at you angrily. Why do you think Mr. White is behaving this way? How will you handle the situation?
19. You are assigned to care for Mrs. Chacko, a 73-year-old resident who came to the United States from India. Until recently, she lived in her daughter's home. However, the daughter was unable to care for her and admitted her to the long-term care facility. Mrs. Chacko's daughter tells you that the resident previously spoke English. However, since her stroke, she has been speaking only in her native language. You are assigned to give Mrs. Chacko a shower and walk her in the hallway. How do you explain the procedures to the resident?
20. You answer the telephone on your unit. The caller identifies himself as Mr. Peterman's brother from out of state. He says he is concerned about his brother and is requesting information about Mr. Peterman's medical condition and medications. The nurse is in a room with a resident doing a treatment and cannot come to the telephone. What should you do?

B: Observation, Recording, and Reporting

OBJECTIVES

After reading this unit, you will be able to:

- Spell and define key terms.
- Differentiate between signs and symptoms and between subjective and objective observations.
- Describe how to report and record resident information.
- List 10 guidelines for documenting in the medical record.
- Demonstrate correct use of medical terminology and abbreviations.

Communicating with Other Members of the Health Care Team

You will communicate with other members of the health care team frequently throughout your shift. Some communication is written. Some is spoken (verbal). Reporting and recording your observations and care are an important part of your job. Take this responsibility very seriously. Remember the principles of goal-oriented communication.

Report

The facility will have a procedure for report at the beginning of every shift (change-of-shift report). In most facilities, the offgoing nurse gives a verbal report to the oncoming nurse. Some facilities use a tape-recorded report. The report will provide information about the residents' conditions during the previous shift. Resident illness, pain, hospitalization, and other changes in condition will be discussed. In some facilities, all nursing staff listen to this report. In other facilities, only the nurses receive report. They in turn will have a separate report for the nursing assistants after the offgoing shift leaves. Although the procedure varies from one facility to the next, it is safe to say that you will receive some type of report at the beginning of every shift.

Having a report at the beginning of the shift helps to provide **continuity of care**. This means that all staff are working on the same goals, using the same approaches 24 hours a day to benefit the residents. The report provides information that will help you to set priorities and anticipate the care you will give the residents during your shift. It will alert you to things you should be monitoring and observing. The report is objective. Baseline information is provided, such as "Mrs. Stone's temperature was 97.8 °F. She complained of feeling cold, so we gave her extra blankets." From hearing this, you know that the resident was cold, and that you should monitor her for feeling cold during your shift. The nurse may also ask you to check her temperature. If you find it is significantly different from the previous shift, this indicates a problem that must be reported immediately. Likewise, if the resident complains of feeling extremely hot for no apparent reason, this must also be reported promptly.

You will report information to the nurse throughout your shift. At the end of the shift, you will report off on all your residents. You will describe your observations, the care given, and other information. The nurse will use this as a basis for reporting off to the oncoming shift and completing her or his assessments and documentation. As you can see, your shift begins with communication. You communicate with others throughout the shift, then end the shift with more communication. Reporting and recording information on the residents' records are also forms of communication. Making observations, communicating with residents and other staff, reporting, and recording are important skills to master.

Observing the Resident

The nursing assistant is responsible for making observations about the resident and reporting them to the nurse. This is an important responsibility. Because you will spend more time with the residents than other health care workers, you are in a position to notice changes immediately. You will use your senses to make observations. Many changes that you detect will be things that you can see. You may notice changes in movement, position, facial expression, or color. These changes may indicate pain or another problem. Use your ears to observe changes you can hear. These are things such as noisy breathing or things the resident tells you. Your sense of smell is useful to detect unusual odors that may indicate a problem. You will note temperature changes or moisture on the skin with your sense of touch.

Observation of the resident is a continuous process. Important observations for which the nursing assistant is responsible are listed in Table 2.4.

Bath time gives you the perfect opportunity to make observations of the resident's entire body and note changes. If you see, feel, hear, or smell anything that seems abnormal, report your observations to the nurse. Even changes that seem insignificant may indicate a problem. For example, a red area on the skin may seem minor, but the area can quickly turn into a serious pressure sore. Report your observations to the nurse, who will decide on the course of action.

Reporting Your Observations

Signs are seen or observed by using your senses. The red area you noticed on the resident's skin during the bath is a sign. **Symptoms** are things residents notice about their conditions and tell you. They cannot be detected by using your senses. **Objective** observations are factual. They are made by seeing, hearing, feeling, touching, and smelling. **Subjective** observations may or may not be factual. Subjective observations are based on what you think or information the resident gives you that may or may not be true. Reporting that the resident did not eat lunch is an objective observation. Reporting that the resident ate a good breakfast and probably was not hungry at lunch is subjective. It reflects what you think. In fact, the resident may have felt nauseated, had pain, been upset, or had another reason for not eating. Information reported to the nurse should be objective.

Recording Your Observations

The resident's **chart** (Figure 2.8) is a notebook or binder containing the **medical record**. The medical record is a legal document. It can be subpoenaed and used in court. It is a record of the resident's true condition, progress, and care. Policies vary regarding who is responsible for recording information on the chart. You may be responsible for documenting information. A common rule in health care is, "If it is not charted, it was not done." Documentation of care given is very important and should be taken seriously. Documentation on the medical record should be objective. It should be accurate, clear, concise, and easy to read. Many facilities use flow-sheet charting (Figure 2.9). This is common for vital statistics, such as vital signs, height, and weight. Routine care, such as bathing, bowel movements, and turning/repositioning, is also commonly recorded on flow sheets. Other charting is done by narrative note. Know and follow your facility policy.

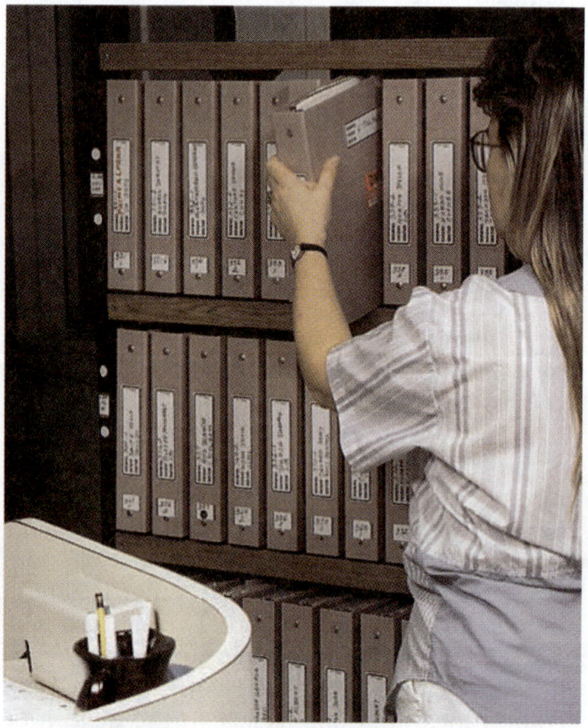

FIGURE 2-8 The resident's medical record is a confidential legal document.

TABLE 2-4 Nursing Assistant Observations

Activity	***Observations***
Activities of daily living	• What the resident can do independently • The resident's need for assistance, how much assistance, type of assistance needed • The resident's ability to tolerate activity (does he become fatigued, short of breath, etc.) • The resident's motivation, preferences, abilities
Dressing and grooming	• Overall appearance—tidy, untidy, neat, clean
Walking	• Difficulty getting up and down • Need for an assistive device, such as a cane or walker • Safety awareness • Gait steady, unsteady, shuffling, rigid, etc. • Posture • Sudden onset of falls, difficulty balancing
Position, movement	• Ability to position/reposition self • Need for staff to reposition • Special positioning aids • Ability to move unassisted • Presence of contractures • Able/unable to move • Movements shaky, jerking, tremors, muscle spasms, etc. • Presence or absence of pain upon movement • Deformity, edema • Normal or abnormal range of motion • Ability to sit, stand, move, or walk
Eating	• Food likes and dislikes, refusals • Feeding ability, need for assistance, how much assistance, type of assistance needed • Percentage of meal consumed • Difficulty chewing or swallowing, coughing, choking
Drinking	• Ability to take a drink at will without assistance • Ability to drink from straw, cup, or need for special device • Need for assistance, how much assistance, type of assistance needed • Beverage preferences • Accepts or refuses water, if offered • Fluid intake • Difficulty swallowing liquids, coughing, choking
Urinary elimination	• Frequency of elimination • Inability to urinate, or voiding frequently in small amounts • Will the resident use the bathroom if given the opportunity? • Is the resident incontinent? • Color, clarity, odor, amount of urine • Presence of mucus, sediment, or other abnormalities in urine • Pain, burning, frequency of urination • Does the resident have a urinary catheter; if so, is it draining properly, leaking, etc.?
Bowel elimination	• Frequency of elimination • Will the resident use the bathroom if given the opportunity? • Is the resident incontinent?

	• Appearance of stool, presence of blood, mucus, parasites, or foreign matter; liquid or solid stool • Abnormal color stool (black, clay color, etc.) • Small or extremely large stool • Loose, watery stool • Complaints of pain, constipation, diarrhea, bleeding • Excessive gas (flatus)
Gastrointestinal system	• Frequent belching • Fruity smell to breath • Complaints of indigestion, gas (flatus), nausea, vomiting • Choking • Abdominal pain • Abdominal distention (swelling) • Oral or rectal bleeding • Vomitus, stool, or drainage from a nasogastric tube that looks like coffee grounds • Condition of mouth and teeth; report ulcerations, pain, drainage, obvious cavities, lesions on lips or inside mouth, abscesses, cracked or broken teeth, loose teeth, abnormalities such as grinding teeth • Dentures fit properly and do not cause pain or pressure • Dentures in good repair and marked with name or initials according to facility policy • Teeth/dentures clean, breath is fresh • Moisture of lips and mucous membranes inside mouth versus dry, chapped lips or dry mucous membranes (report)
Level of consciousness	• Conscious • Unconscious • Change in consciousness, awareness, or alertness • Ability to respond verbally or nonverbally • Sleepiness for no apparent reason
Sleeping	• Ability to sleep, or can't sleep • Sleeps constantly • Awakens easily • Difficult to awaken • Moves about in sleep • Need to be awakened for toileting • Repositions self or needs to be repositioned by staff
Skin	• Skin dry, oily, normal • Redness, unusual skin color, such as blue or gray color of the skin, lips, nail beds, roof of mouth, or mucous membranes • Redness in the skin that does not go away within 30 minutes after pressure is relieved from a bony prominence or pressure area • In dark or yellow-skinned residents, spots or areas that are darker in appearance than normal skin tone • Pressure ulcers, open areas/skin breakdown, skin tears, abrasions, lacerations • Irritation, rash, bruises, skin discoloration, swelling, lumps, abnormal skin growths, change in color of a wart or mole, hives • Abnormal sweating, excessive heat or coolness to touch • Drainage • Foul odor • Complaints such as numbness, burning, tingling, itching • Signs of infection • Skin growths • Poor skin turgor/tenting of skin on forehead or over sternum • Edema, swelling • Moisture of lips and mucous membranes inside mouth

Cardiovascular system	• Pulse rate, regularity, strength • Blood pressure • Presence or absence of chest pain • Color, appearance of skin, nail beds, mucous membranes
Respiratory system	• Respiratory rate, rhythm, regularity • Respirations noisy, labored, quiet • Shortness of breath, gasping for breath, Cheyne-Stokes respirations • Wheezing • Presence or absence of coughing (dry or moist/productive) • Retractions • Skin color, color of lips, nail beds, mucous membranes
Nervous system	• Weakness • Sensation, ability to feel touch, absence of sensation • Presence or absence of pain • Numbness, tingling • Normal, abnormal or involuntary motor function, spasticity • Ability or inability to move a body part • Coordination, lack of coordination

Charting time. Entries in the chart are made in chronological order, by date and time. Some facilities color-code charting to identify the shift. For example, blue ink is used for the day shift, green for the second shift, and red for the night shift. A more common practice is for all shifts to document on the chart in black ink. When this is done, the time of the entry must be written using the 24-hour clock (Table 2.5). When this system is used, indicating times by noting a.m. or p.m. is not necessary. The day starts at midnight, or 2400 hours. This is the same as 12:00 a.m. For the first hour, only minutes are recorded. 12:25 a.m. is recorded as 0025. After the first hour, each hour increases by one until 24 hours are reached. 8:00 a.m. is recorded as 0800. 2:00 p.m. is recorded as 1400. 6:00 p.m. is recorded as 1800.

Confidentiality and privacy. The medical record is a private and confidential document. Protect the medical records from access by unauthorized persons. Likewise, you should not be reading resident charts out of curiosity. Medical records should be accessed only by those with a need to know the information.

In 1996, Congress passed the **Health Insurance Portability and Accountability Act (HIPAA).** This law has many provisions. One portion applies to resident privacy, confidentiality, and medical records. The HIPAA rules are:

- Increase residents' control over their medical records.
- Restrict the use and disclosure of resident information.
- Make facilities accountable for protecting resident data.
- Require the facility to implement and monitor its information release policies and procedures.

The HIPAA regulations protect all individually identifiable health information in any form. The rules apply to paper, verbal, and electronic documentation, billing records, and clinical records. Staff should receive only the information needed to carry out their duties. Because of this, all resident information should be used or disclosed on a need-to-know basis. For example, the dietary department would need to know if the resident was on a diabetic diet. They would not need to know that the resident has an infectious disease. The nursing assistant would need to know about both the diabetes and the infection. Facilities must monitor how and where they use resident information. Policies must protect resident charts, places where resident information is discussed, faxing resident documents, and disclosing other personal information.

The HIPAA rules ask providers to analyze how and where resident information is used, and develop procedures for protecting confidential data. This includes the areas where resident charts are stored, the places where resident information is discussed, and how residents' personal health information is distributed. The HIPAA policies and procedures for each facility are individualized to the facility.

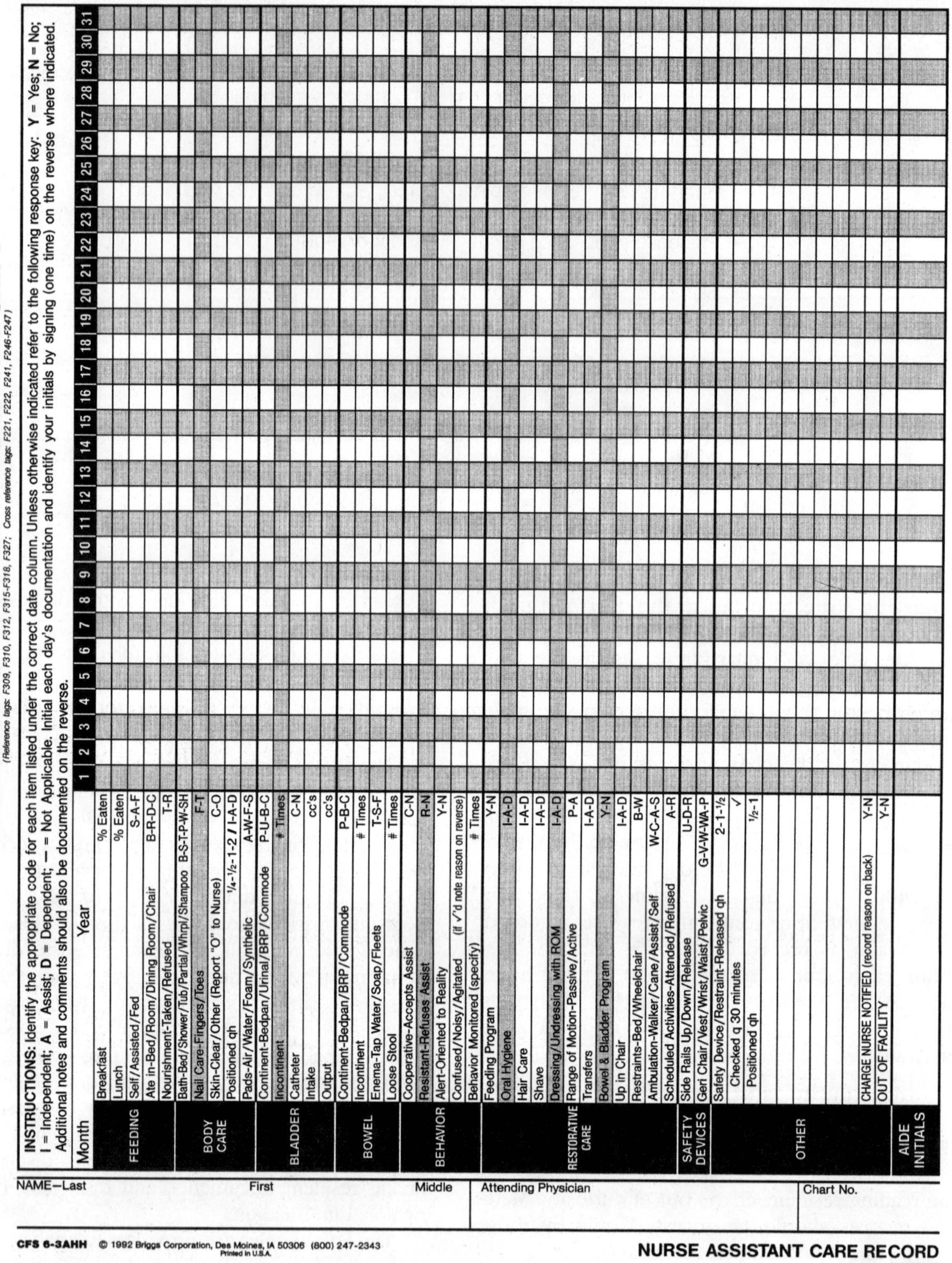

NURSE ASSISTANT CARE RECORD—A.M. SHIFT

(Reference tags: F309, F310, F312, F315-F318, F327; Cross reference tags: F221, F222, F241, F246-F247)

INSTRUCTIONS: Identify the appropriate code for each item listed under the correct date column. Unless otherwise indicated refer to the following response key: **Y** = Yes; **N** = No; **I** = Independent; **A** = Assist; **D** = Dependent; **— –** = Not Applicable. Initial each day's documentation and identify your initials by signing (one time) on the reverse where indicated. Additional notes and comments should also be documented on the reverse.

Month	Year		1	2	3	4	5	6	7	8	9	10	11	12	13	14	15	16	17	18	19	20	21	22	23	24	25	26	27	28	29	30	31
FEEDING	Breakfast	% Eaten																															
	Lunch	% Eaten																															
	Self/Assisted/Fed	S-A-F																															
	Ate in-Bed/Room/Dining Room/Chair	B-R-D-C																															
	Nourishment-Taken/Refused	T-R																															
BODY CARE	Bath-Bed/Shower/Tub/Partial/Whrpl/Shampoo	B-S-T-P-W-SH																															
	Nail Care-Fingers/Toes	F-T																															
	Skin-Clear/Other (Report "O" to Nurse)	C-O																															
	Positioned qh	¼-½-1-2 / I-A-D																															
	Pads-Air/Water/Foam/Synthetic	A-W-F-S																															
BLADDER	Continent-Bedpan/Urinal/BRP/Commode	P-U-B-C																															
	Incontinent	# Times																															
	Catheter	C-N																															
	Intake	cc's																															
	Output	cc's																															
BOWEL	Continent-Bedpan/BRP/Commode	P-B-C																															
	Incontinent	# Times																															
	Enema-Tap Water/Soap/Fleets	T-S-F																															
	Loose Stool	# Times																															
BEHAVIOR	Cooperative-Accepts Assist	C-N																															
	Resistant-Refuses Assist	R-N																															
	Alert-Oriented to Reality	Y-N																															
	Confused/Noisy/Agitated (if ✓'d note reason on reverse)																																
	Behavior Monitored (specify)	# Times																															
RESTORATIVE CARE	Feeding Program	Y-N																															
	Oral Hygiene	I-A-D																															
	Hair Care	I-A-D																															
	Shave	I-A-D																															
	Dressing/Undressing with ROM	I-A-D																															
	Range of Motion-Passive/Active	P-A																															
	Transfers	I-A-D																															
	Bowel & Bladder Program	Y-N																															
	Up in Chair	I-A-D																															
	Restraints-Bed/Wheelchair	B-W																															
	Ambulation-Walker/Cane/Assist/Self	W-C-A-S																															
	Scheduled Activities-Attended/Refused	A-R																															
SAFETY DEVICES	Side Rails Up/Down/Release	U-D-R																															
	Geri Chair/Vest/Wrist/Waist/Pelvic	G-V-W-WA-P																															
OTHER	Safety Device/Restraint-Released qh	2-1-½																															
	Checked q 30 minutes	✓																															
	Positioned qh	½-1																															
	CHARGE NURSE NOTIFIED (record reason on back)	Y-N																															
	OUT OF FACILITY	Y-N																															
AIDE INITIALS																																	

NAME—Last First Middle | Attending Physician | Chart No.

CFS 6-3AHH © 1992 Briggs Corporation, Des Moines, IA 50306 (800) 247-2343 Printed in U.S.A.

NURSE ASSISTANT CARE RECORD A.M. SHIFT

FIGURE 2-9 Most long-term care facilities use flow-sheet charting to record daily care. *(Compliments of Briggs Corporation (800) 247-2343.)*

TABLE 2-5 The 24-Hour Clock

Standard Clock	*24-Hour Clock*	*Standard Clock*	*24-Hour Clock*
12:00 midnight	2400 or 0000	12:00 noon	1200
1:00 a.m.	0100	1:00 p.m.	1300
2:00 a.m.	0200	2:00 p.m.	1400
3:00 a.m.	0300	3:00 p.m.	1500
4:00 a.m.	0400	4:00 p.m.	1600
5:00 a.m.	0500	5:00 p.m.	1700
6:00 a.m.	0600	6:00 p.m.	1800
7:00 a.m.	0700	7:00 p.m.	1900
8:00 a.m.	0800	8:00 p.m.	2000
9:00 a.m.	0900	9:00 p.m.	2100
10:00 a.m.	1000	10:00 p.m.	2200
11:00 a.m.	1100	11:00 p.m.	2300

GUIDELINES FOR
Charting

- Select the correct resident's chart.
- Document on the correct form.
- Charting must be accurate and legible. Follow your facility policy for printing or charting in script. Make sure the entry can be clearly read.
- Know the meaning and correct spelling of words before you write them on the chart.
- Chart in sequence.
- Chart the facts. Be specific and objective. Avoid making judgments or charting your personal opinion.
- Use the correct color pen with permanent ink. Never chart in pencil, erasable ink, or ink that runs when wet.
- Use short, concise phrases.
- Chart after an event occurs or care is given. Never chart in advance.
- Chart the exact time of the event.
- Use only facility-approved abbreviations. Never make up an abbreviation. Your facility will have a listing of abbreviations that are approved for documentation. Use abbreviations only if they are on this list.
- Leave no blank lines or spaces. Draw a single line through unused space at the end of a sentence.
- If you make a mistake, do not erase or use correction fluid. Do not mark through the entry so that it cannot be read. Draw a single line through the entry and write "error" and your initials.
- Sign your first initial, last name, and title immediately after your entry.
- Fill in all the boxes on flow-sheet charting. Blank spaces indicate that care was not given. Flow sheets are very important if the chart is involved in a lawsuit.
- Make sure that documentation of your care is complete and accurate, including turning and repositioning; feeding; food intake substitutes, snacks, and supplements; fluids given; safety measures and restraints; and range-of-motion exercises. Other data

GUIDELINES FOR

Charting *continued*

that may be carefully considered in a lawsuit are urine and bowel elimination, bathing and incontinent care, oral hygiene, ambulation, and use of special devices, such as hand rolls, restraints, and pressure-relieving mattresses.

- Read what you are documenting on flow sheets. It is easy to skip up or down a line. Be sure you are documenting on the correct line.
- Make sure the intake and output totals are accurate and recorded. If the fluid intake appears inadequate, notify the nurse.
- Notify the nurse if something is missing from a computerized flow sheet. The nurse will add missing information that is listed on the resident's care plan. For example, your facility routinely charts that residents are turned and repositioned every two hours. You routinely turn and reposition Mrs. Long, according to her plan of care. However, there is no place to document this important care on the flow sheet.
- Never chart for another person.
- Never chart care that you have not given.
- If you forget to chart something, follow your facility policy for making a late entry note on the chart.
- If you will be initialing a form, such as a flow sheet, make sure that you sign the initial key with your full signature and title.

Computers in Health Care Facilities

Use of computers has become common in long-term care facilities. A large amount of information can be stored, processed, and retrieved easily. Departments can communicate with each other by computer. The information is legible and easy to read. Resident information is readily available and easy to find. Using a computer to complete the Minimum Data Set saves a great deal of time. Statistics and data can be retrieved from the computer to spot problems and trends. Nursing units do not use the normal word processing programs for recording resident information. Special health care programs are available. These programs are usually simple to use, even for those with no computer experience. Some facilities print forms on which staff document routine care (Figure 2.10). Some facilities do all documentation by computer (Figure 2.11).

If you will be working with the computer, your facility will teach you about the programs you will be using. Do not be afraid of the computer. Becoming computer-literate may be frustrating at first, but it can make your job much easier! Look at it as an opportunity to learn something new that will benefit you and allow you to spend more time with the residents.

Fax Machines

Fax machines transmit printed information from one location to another over telephone lines. Long-term care facilities frequently use fax machines for laboratory and x-ray reports, physician orders, and communication with physicians and other health care agencies. You may be responsible for sending information over the fax machine. This involves placing one or more papers in the machine, dialing the telephone number of the receiving party, and pressing the start button. When sending information over the fax machine, remember that resident confidentiality laws apply. Double-check the number for accuracy before sending the documents. Your facility will teach you how to use the type of machine you will be operating.

Medical Terminology

Medicine has a language of its own. This language is used to describe the **diagnosis**, or what is wrong with the resident. Some medical terminology describes body parts, procedures, orders, measurements, treatments, activities, time, and place. Vocabulary words are listed in each chapter of your text. Learning these terms

Southaven Subacute Care — Page 1
10/03/XX Shift 2 thru 10/04/XX Shift 3

SHIFT	SIGNATURE	TITLE	INT

57Y SEX: M
ACCT: 0127601961 319-01 TYPE: I/P
PHYS: PC:
DOB: 01/17/32 ADM: 10/03/XX LOS: 1
ISO: SMK: NO
ALG: paxil levaquin zithromax centr
SGY:
DX: ACUTE RESP DIST COPD
MR#: 00015435

DEMOGRAPHIC/PRECAUTION INFORMATION
HT: 6'0.0"/182.9cm PRECAUTIONS: FALL PROTOCOL
WT: 167lbs/75.751kg
REL: CATHOLIC LANG: ENGLISH

ACTIVITIES OF DAILY LIVING		0700-1500	1500-2300	2300-0700
Date Ord	ADL Description			
10/03	BEDREST -A-* W/BRP ONLY			
10/03	ELIMINAT'N-E-TOILETING W/1			
10/03	HYGIENE -H-BATH-PARTIAL			
10/03	HYGIENE -H-HS CARE W/ASSIST			
10/03	I & O-Q8H			
10/03	LINEN CHG-UNOCCUPIED BED			
10/03	NUTRITION -N-FEED SELF W/TRAY SET			
10/03	POS/TURN-ASSIST ALL TRANSFERS			
10/03	SAFETY-S-* PATIENT ROUND Q2H			
10/03	SAFETY-S-LEVEL 2			
10/03	VS-ADULT-V-Q4H			

DIETARY ORDERS — Status Percent Consumption
Diet — Act B____% L____% S____%
REGULAR (GENERAL)

CLINICAL ORDERS	Request	Stop	Freq
Dpt Description	Date/Time	Date/Time	
LAB CULTURE, BLOOD, ARD	10/03/XX 1325	10/03/XX 0125P	ONCE
LAB CULTURE, BLOOD, ARD	10/03/XX 1325	10/03/XX 0125P	ONCE
EKG EKG-REVANA	10/03/XX 1330	10/03/XX 0130P	ONCE

THERAPY/MISC. ORDERS	
Dpt Description	Req Date/Time
RT HAND HELD NEBULIZER	10/03/XX 2138
: ALBUTEROL 0.5 UNIT DOSE Q4H	
RT OXY 02 INCL P/H	10/03/XX 2137
:	
RT STAT BLOOD GAS	10/03/XX 1329
:	

TREATMENT ORDERS	0700-1500	1500-2300	2300-0700
10/03/XX 2142 : IVPB MED: SOLUMEDROL 60MG Q6 X 3 DOSES			

FIGURE 2-10 Individual care sheets are printed daily. Staff initial care when it is completed.

will help you master medical terminology. You will use medical terms to communicate with other members of the interdisciplinary team and to document on the resident's medical record.

Word Elements

Medical terms are a combination of word elements. You cannot expect to remember every medical term. You can, however, use your

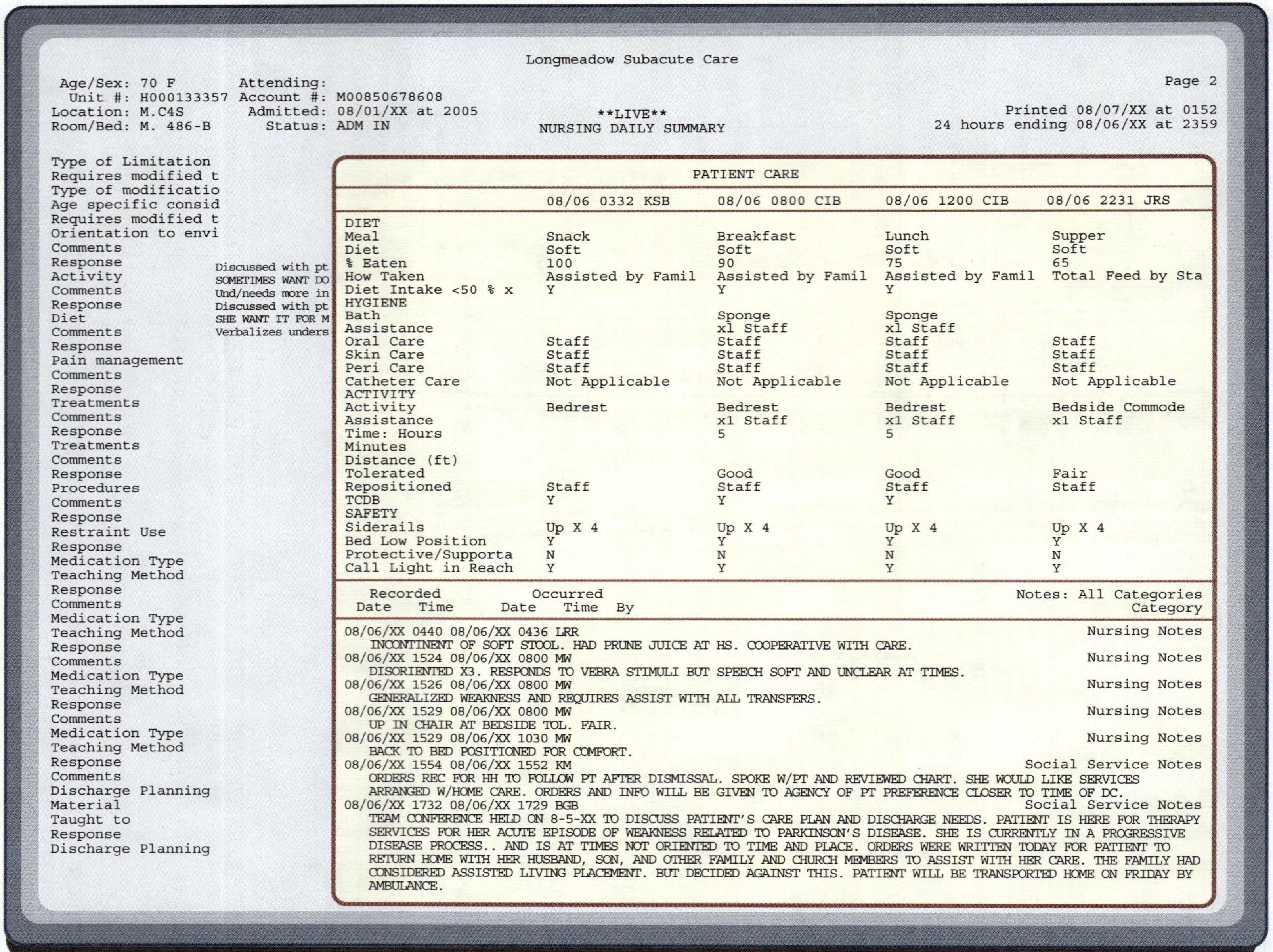

Longmeadow Subacute Care

Age/Sex: 70 F Attending:
Unit #: H000133357 Account #: M00850678608
Location: M.C4S Admitted: 08/01/XX at 2005
Room/Bed: M. 486-B Status: ADM IN

LIVE
NURSING DAILY SUMMARY

Page 2
Printed 08/07/XX at 0152
24 hours ending 08/06/XX at 2359

Type of Limitation
Requires modified t
Type of modificatio
Age specific consid
Requires modified t
Orientation to envi
Comments
Response — Discussed with pt
Activity — SOMETIMES WANT DO
Comments — Und/needs more in
Response — Discussed with pt
Diet — SHE WANT IT FOR M
Comments — Verbalizes unders
Response
Pain management
Comments
Response
Treatments
Comments
Response
Treatments
Comments
Response
Procedures
Comments
Response
Restraint Use
Response
Medication Type
Teaching Method
Response
Comments
Medication Type
Teaching Method
Response
Comments
Medication Type
Teaching Method
Response
Comments
Medication Type
Teaching Method
Response
Comments
Discharge Planning
Material
Taught to
Response
Discharge Planning

PATIENT CARE

	08/06 0332 KSB	08/06 0800 CIB	08/06 1200 CIB	08/06 2231 JRS
DIET				
Meal	Snack	Breakfast	Lunch	Supper
Diet	Soft	Soft	Soft	Soft
% Eaten	100	90	75	65
How Taken	Assisted by Famil	Assisted by Famil	Assisted by Famil	Total Feed by Sta
Diet Intake <50 % x	Y	Y	Y	
HYGIENE				
Bath		Sponge	Sponge	
Assistance		x1 Staff	x1 Staff	
Oral Care	Staff	Staff	Staff	Staff
Skin Care	Staff	Staff	Staff	Staff
Peri Care	Staff	Staff	Staff	Staff
Catheter Care	Not Applicable	Not Applicable	Not Applicable	Not Applicable
ACTIVITY				
Activity	Bedrest	Bedrest	Bedrest	Bedside Commode
Assistance		x1 Staff	x1 Staff	x1 Staff
Time: Hours		5	5	
Minutes				
Distance (ft)				
Tolerated		Good	Good	Fair
Repositioned	Staff	Staff	Staff	Staff
TCDB	Y	Y	Y	
SAFETY				
Siderails	Up X 4	Up X 4	Up X 4	Up X 4
Bed Low Position	Y	Y	Y	Y
Protective/Supporta	N	N	N	N
Call Light in Reach	Y	Y	Y	Y

Recorded Date Time — Occurred Date Time By — Notes: All Categories Category

08/06/XX 0440 08/06/XX 0436 LRR — Nursing Notes
INCONTINENT OF SOFT STOOL. HAD PRUNE JUICE AT HS. COOPERATIVE WITH CARE.
08/06/XX 1524 08/06/XX 0800 MW — Nursing Notes
DISORIENTED X3. RESPONDS TO VEBRA STIMULI BUT SPEECH SOFT AND UNCLEAR AT TIMES.
08/06/XX 1526 08/06/XX 0800 MW — Nursing Notes
GENERALIZED WEAKNESS AND REQUIRES ASSIST WITH ALL TRANSFERS.
08/06/XX 1529 08/06/XX 0800 MW — Nursing Notes
UP IN CHAIR AT BEDSIDE TOL. FAIR.
08/06/XX 1529 08/06/XX 1030 MW — Nursing Notes
BACK TO BED POSITIONED FOR COMFORT.
08/06/XX 1554 08/06/XX 1552 KM — Social Service Notes
ORDERS REC FOR HH TO FOLLOW PT AFTER DISMISSAL. SPOKE W/PT AND REVIEWED CHART. SHE WOULD LIKE SERVICES ARRANGED W/HOME CARE. ORDERS AND INFO WILL BE GIVEN TO AGENCY OF PT PREFERENCE CLOSER TO TIME OF DC.
08/06/XX 1732 08/06/XX 1729 BGB — Social Service Notes
TEAM CONFERENCE HELD ON 8-5-XX TO DISCUSS PATIENT'S CARE PLAN AND DISCHARGE NEEDS. PATIENT IS HERE FOR THERAPY SERVICES FOR HER ACUTE EPISODE OF WEAKNESS RELATED TO PARKINSON'S DISEASE. SHE IS CURRENTLY IN A PROGRESSIVE DISEASE PROCESS.. AND IS AT TIMES NOT ORIENTED TO TIME AND PLACE. ORDERS WERE WRITTEN TODAY FOR PATIENT TO RETURN HOME WITH HER HUSBAND, SON, AND OTHER FAMILY AND CHURCH MEMBERS TO ASSIST WITH HER CARE. THE FAMILY HAD CONSIDERED ASSISTED LIVING PLACEMENT. BUT DECIDED AGAINST THIS. PATIENT WILL BE TRANSPORTED HOME ON FRIDAY BY AMBULANCE.

FIGURE 2-11 Nursing assistants document all daily care on the computer.

GUIDELINES FOR

Documentation on the Computerized Medical Record

- Do not be afraid of computerized charting.
- When documenting on a specific resident, double-check to make sure you have entered the correct identification code.
- Do not give your identification code or password to others.
- Access only information that you are authorized to obtain.
- Document only in areas that you are authorized to use.
- Many computer programs place expert reminders or error codes on the screen. Read and follow the directions.
- Log off when leaving the computer.
- The procedure for late entry and addendum documentation will be different than in a narrative system. Know and follow your facility policies for this type of charting.
- Keep in mind that audit trails track the machine name, user, date, time, and exactly which medical records were accessed based on the user identification.
- If you print documents from the electronic medical record, make sure they are used correctly or discarded according to facility policy. Placing them in the wastebasket is prohibited in many facilities because of privacy laws.
- Stay current. Attend continuing education programs to learn how to maximize the use of computerized charting and information systems.

knowledge of the language of medicine to understand what unfamiliar terms mean.

The three elements of medical words are the prefix, suffix, and root. The **prefix** is the word element at the beginning of the word. A **suffix** is the word element ending the word. The **root** is the element that provides the meaning of the word. For example, the root *arth* means joint. The suffix *-algia* means pain. If you see the word arthralgia, you will know that it means pain in the joints. The letters *i* or *o* are sometimes added to the root word to make the word easier to connect and pronounce. Medical words can consist of a prefix and a suffix, a prefix and a root, a root and a suffix, or two roots.

Word roots. The word root (or root word) provides the basic meaning of the word. A list of common word roots is found in Table 2.6.

Prefixes. The prefix is found at the beginning of a medical term. It does not stand alone. It is always accompanied by a root, a suffix, or both. A list of common prefixes is found in Table 2.7.

Suffixes. The suffix is found at the end of the medical term. Like the prefix, it does not stand alone. It is combined with a root, a prefix, or both. A list of common suffixes is found in Table 2.8.

Word combinations. Table 2.9 shows some common examples of how different elements are combined to form words.

ABBREVIATIONS

An **abbreviation** is the shortened form of a word. In health care, abbreviations are used frequently to save space and time. Sometimes medical abbreviations represent Latin terms for a word. Other medical abbreviations are a combination of the letters used to form the word. For example, AIDS is the abbreviation for acquired immune deficiency syndrome. Learning common medical abbreviations is important. Abbreviations are used in conversation, in documentation, in the care plan, and on your assignment sheet. Some abbreviations are facility specific. Each facility will have a list of abbreviations approved for use in charting. Refer to this list if you do not understand the meaning of an abbreviation. Sometimes an abbreviation can mean more than one thing. For example, D/C is the abbreviation for discontinue. It can also be used to mean discharge. The context of the sentence in which it is written should give you a clue to its meaning. Table 2.10 lists common medical abbreviations.

TABLE 2-6 Word Roots

Root	Meaning	Root	Meaning	Root	Meaning
abdomin(o)	abdomen	*gloss(o)*	tongue	*ped(i)(o)*	child
aden(o)	gland	*glyc(o)*	sugar	*pharyng(o)*	throat
angi(o)	vessel	*gynec(o)*	female	*phleb(o)*	vein
arteri(o)	artery	*hem(o)*	blood	*pneum(o)*	lung, air
arth(o)	joint	*hemat(o)*	blood	*proct(o)*	rectum
bronch(i)(o)	bronchus	*hepat(o)*	liver	*psych(o)*	mind
cardi(o)	heart	*hydr(o)*	water	*pulm(o)*	lung
cephal(o)	head	*hyster(o)*	uterus	*py(o)*	pus
cerebr(o)	brain	*lapar(o)*	abdomen, flank, loin	*rect(o)*	rectum
chol(e)	bile	*laryng(o)*	larynx	*rhin(o)*	nose
col(o)	colon	*lith(o)*	stone	*splen(o)*	spleen
crani(o)	skull	*mamm(o)*	breast	*stern(o)*	sternum
cyst(o)	bladder, cyst	*mast(o)*	breast	*thorac(o)*	chest
cyt(o)	cell	*men(o)*	menstruation	*thromb(o)*	clot
dent(i)(o)	tooth	*my(o)*	muscle	*tox(o)*	poison
dermat(o)	skin	*myel(o)*	bone marrow, spinal cord	*trache(o)*	trachea
encephal(o)	brain	*nephr(o)*	kidney	*ur(o)*	urine
enter(o)	small intestine	*neur(o)*	nerve	*urethr(o)*	urethra
erythr(o)	red	*ocul(o)*	eye	*urin(o)*	urine
fibr(o)	fiber	*ophthalm(o)*	eye	*uter(i)(o)*	uterus
gastr(o)	stomach	*oste(o)*	bone	*ven(o)*	vein
geront(o)	elderly				

TABLE 2-7 Prefixes

Prefix	Meaning	Prefix	Meaning	Prefix	Meaning
a-, an-	without, not	*hemi-*	half	*per-*	by, through
ab-	away from	*hyper-*	high, above, excessive	*peri-*	around
ad-	toward	*hypo-*	low, below normal	*poly-*	many
ante-	before	*inter-*	between	*post-*	after
anti-	against	*intra-*	inside, within	*pre-*	before

bi-	double, two	*leuk-*	white	*pseud-*	false
bio-	life	*micro-*	small	*retro-*	backward
brady-	slow	*neo-*	new	*semi-*	half
circum-	around	*non-*	not	*septic-*	infection
dys-	difficult, abnormal	*pan-*	all	*sub-*	under, below
epi-	on, over			*tachy-*	fast

TABLE 2-8 Suffixes

Suffix	***Meaning***	***Suffix***	***Meaning***	***Suffix***	***Meaning***
-algia	pain	*-megaly*	enlargement	*-pnea*	breathing
-alysis	analyze	*-meter*	instrument that measures	*-ptosis*	sagging, falling
-ectomy	surgical removal	*-ostomy*	surgical opening	*-rrhagia*	excessive flow
-emia	blood	*-otomy*	surgical opening	*-rrhea*	discharge
-gram	record	*-pathy*	disease	*-scope*	instrument that examines
-itis	inflammation of	*-penia*	deficiency	*-stasis*	constant
-logy	study of	*-phasia*	speaking	*-therapy*	treatment
-lysis	destruction of	*-plegia*	paralysis	*-uria*	condition of urine

TABLE 2-9 Combining Word Parts to Form Medical Terms

Medical Term	***Prefix***	***Root***	***Suffix***	***Meaning***
antiseptic	anti-	septic		against infection
arthritis		arthr	-itis	inflammation of joints
cardiology		cardi	-ology	study of the heart
colostomy		col	-ostomy	surgical opening into the colon
dyspnea	dys-		-pnea	difficult breathing
hemiplegia	hemi-		-plegia	paralysis in one half of the body
hypoglycemia	hypo-	glyc	-emia	low blood sugar
glycosuria		glyc	-uria	sugar in urine
leukemia	leuk-		-emia	condition of white blood cells
urinalysis	urin-		-alysis	analysis of the urine

TABLE 2-10 Common Abbreviations

Abbreviation	Meaning
$\bar{a}$	before
AAROM	active assistive (assisted) range of motion
abd	abdomen
ABT, ABX	antibiotic therapy
$\overline{ac}$	before meals
ACT	active, actively, activities
AD	Activity Director
ADA	American Dietetic Association, American Diabetic Association
add.	adduction
ad lib	as desired
ADLs	activities of daily living
adm	admission
AEB	as evidenced by
AFO	ankle/foot orthosis
AIDS	acquired immune deficiency syndrome
aka	above-the-knee amputation, also known as
alt	alternate, alternating
am	morning
AMA	against medical advice
amb	ambulate
amt	amount
ant	anterior
A&P	anatomy and physiology
AROM	active range of motion
ASAP	as soon as possible
assist	assistance
as tol	as tolerated
ax	axillary (under the arm)
B, (B),Ⓑ	bilateral, both
B&B	bowel and bladder
BB	bed bath
bid	twice a day
bilat	bilateral
BKA	below-the-knee amputation
BLE	both lower extremities
BM	bowel movement
BP, B/P	blood pressure
BPM	beats per minute
BR	bed rest, bathroom
BRP	bathroom privileges
BS	blood sugar
BSC	bedside commode
BSE	breast self-examination
BUE	both upper extremities
C	Celsius, centigrade
$\bar{c}$	with
c, cm	centimeter
C1, C2, C3, etc.	first cervical vertebrae, second cervical vertebrae, third cervical vertebrae, etc.
CA	cancer
CAD	coronary artery disease
cal, kcal	calorie
cath	catheter
CBB	complete bed bath
CBC	complete blood count
CC	chief complaint
cc	cubic centimeter
CHF	congestive heart failure
ck, ✓	check
ck or ✓ freq	check frequently
cl liq	clear liquid
CMA	certified medication aide

Abbreviation	Meaning
CNA	certified nursing assistant or certified nurse administrator
c/o	complains of
COLD, COPD	chronic obstructive lung (pulmonary) disease
CP	care plan, clinical pathway, critical pathway
CPM	continuous passive motion machine
CPR	cardiopulmonary resuscitation
C & S	culture and sensitivity
cu	cubic
CVA	cerebrovascular accident, stroke
CXR	chest x-ray
d	day
D/C, DC	discontinue, discharge
DDS	Doctor of Dental Science (dentist)
dep	dependent
dept.	department
diab	diabetes, diabetic
DJD	degenerative joint disease
DNR	do not resuscitate
DO	Doctor of Osteopathy
DOA	dead on arrival
DOB	date of birth
DPM	Doctor of Podiatric Medicine
DR, D/R	dining room
Dr.	doctor
DSD	dry sterile dressing
DSM	Dietary Services Manager
DT	dietetic technician
DVT	deep vein thrombosis (blood clot)
Dx	diagnosis
E	enema

Abbreviation	Meaning
ECG, EKG	electrocardiogram
EENT	eye, ear, nose, and throat
ENT	ear, nose, and throat
ER, ED	emergency room, emergency department
ESRD	end stage renal disease
et	and
ETOH	ethanol (often used to refer to alcoholic beverages)
Eval	evaluation
ex.	exercise
exam	examination
ext.	extension, extremity, external
F	Fahrenheit
FB	foreign body
FBS	fasting blood sugar
FE	Fleet's enema
FF	force fluids
flex	flexion
freq	frequently
FS	frozen section, finger stick
FSBS	finger stick blood sugar
FU, F/U	follow up
FUO	fever of unknown origin
FWB	full weight bearing
Fx	fracture
G	good
g/c, GC	geriatric chair
GERD	gastroesophageal reflux disease
GI	gastrointestinal
G/T, GT	gastrostomy tube
gtt	drop
GU	genitourinary
Gyn	gynecology

TABLE 2-10 *(continued)*

Abbreviation	Meaning
h	hour
H	hydrogen
HAV, HBV, HCV, etc.	hepatitis A virus, hepatitis B virus, hepatitis C virus, etc.
hemi	half, hemiplegia
Hg	mercury
HIV	human immunodeficiency virus
H_2O	water
H_2O_2	hydrogen peroxide
HOB	head of bed
HOH	hard of hearing
H & P	history and physical
hr	hour
hs	bedtime (hour of sleep)
ht	height
Hx	history
Ⓘ, *ind.*	independent, independently
ID	initial dose
IDCP	interdisciplinary care plan
IDDM	insulin-dependent diabetes mellitus
IDT	interdisciplinary team
IM	intramuscular
I & O	intake and output
int.	internal
IPPB	intermittent positive pressure breathing
isol	isolation
IV	intravenous
K, K^+	potassium
L	liter, left
L1, L2, etc.	first lumbar vertebra, second lumbar vertebra, etc.
lab	laboratory

Abbreviation	Meaning
lat	lateral
lb	pound
LBP	low back pain
LE	lower extremity
lg, lge	large
liq	liquid
L/min, LPM	liters per minute
LL	left leg
LLE	left lower extremity
LLQ	left lower quadrant
LOC	loss of consciousness, level of consciousness, level of care
LPN	licensed practical nurse
lt	left
LTC	long-term care
LTCF	long-term care facility
LTG	long-term goal
LUQ	left upper quadrant
LVN	licensed vocational nurse
M	meter
MA	medication aide
max	maximum
MD	muscular dystrophy, medical doctor
MDR	main dining room
MDS	Minimum Data Set
mech soft	mechanical soft
med rec	medical records
meds	medications
MI	myocardial infarction (heart attack)
min	minimum, minimal, minute
mL or ml	milliliter

Abbreviation	Meaning
mm	millimeter
mmHg	millimeters of mercury
mod	moderate
MRSA	methicillin-resistant Staphylococcus aureus
MS	multiple sclerosis
mult.	multiple
NA, N/A	not applicable, nursing assistant (meaning determined by context)
Na^+	sodium
NACEP	Nurse Aide Competency Evaluation Program
NAR	no adverse reaction
NAS	no added salt
NATCEP	Nurse Aide Training and Competency Evaluation Program
N/C, no c/o	no complaints
neg, –, ⊖	negative
NG	nasogastric
NGT	nasogastric tube
NIDDM	non-insulin-dependent diabetes mellitus
NKA	no known allergies
NN	nurse's notes
noc	night
NPO	nothing by mouth
N/S, NSS	normal saline, normal saline solution
N & V	nausea and vomiting
NVD	nausea, vomiting, and diarrhea
NWB	nonweight-bearing
O_2	oxygen
OA	osteoarthritis
obj	objective
OBS	organic brain syndrome
obs	observations
occ	occasional
OOB	out of bed
ORIF	open reduction, internal fixation
os, o	mouth
OT	occupational therapy
oz, ℥	ounce
℥*i,* ℥*ii,* ℥*iii, etc.*	1 ounce, 2 ounces, 3 ounces, etc.
$\overline{p}$	after
P	pulse, poor
PB, PBB	partial bath, partial bed bath
$\overline{pc}$	after meals
PCT	Patient Care Technician
PE	physical examination
peds, pedi	pediatrics
per	by, through
pm	afternoon or evening
PN	progress notes, practical nurse
po	by mouth
pos, +, ⊕	positive
PPE	personal protective equipment
PPS	post polio syndrome, prospective payment system
preop	preoperative
prep	prepare
prn	as needed
prog	prognosis, progress
PROM	passive range of motion
pt or Pt	patient
PT	physical therapy
PUD	peptic ulcer disease
PVD	peripheral vascular disease
PWB	partial weight bearing

TABLE 2-10 *(continued)*

Abbreviation	Meaning
$\bar{q}$	each, every
$\bar{q}d$	every day
$\bar{q}h$	every hour
$\bar{q}2h$, $\bar{q}3h$, $\bar{q}4h$, etc.	every 2 hours, every 3 hours, every 4 hours, etc.
$\bar{q}hs$	every night at bedtime
qid	four times a day
$\bar{q}m$, $\overline{qam}$	every morning
$\overline{qod}$	every other day
$\overline{qs}$	sufficient quantity
qt	quart
quad	quadrant, quadriplegic
R	rectal, respiration, right
RA	rheumatoid arthritis, right arm
RAI	Resident Assessment Instrument
RCP	Respiratory Care Practitioner
RD	Registered Dietitian
re:	regarding
reg	regular, regulation
rehab	rehabilitation
res, Res	resident
resp, R	respirations
RL	right leg
RLE	right lower extremity
RLQ	right lower quadrant
rm	room
RN	registered nurse
RNA	restorative nursing assistant
R/O	rule out
ROM	range of motion
rot.	rotation
rt, R	right
RT	respiratory therapy
r/t	related to
RUE	right upper extremity
RUQ	right upper quadrant
Rx	prescription, therapy, treatment
$\bar{s}$	without
SBA	standby assistance
semi	half
sm	small
SNF	skilled nursing facility
SNU	skilled nursing unit
SOB	shortness of breath
spec	specimen
SS	social service
S/S, S & S	signs and symptoms
SSE	soapsuds enema
S/T	skin tear
ST	speech therapy
stat	immediately
Std prec	standard precautions
STG	short-term goal
STNA	state tested nursing assistant
supp	suppository
SW	social worker
Sx	symptoms
T, temp	temperature
T1, T2, etc.	first thoracic vertebra, second thoracic vertebra, etc.
TB	tuberculosis
TF	tube feeding
TIAN	toilet in advance of need
TID, tid	three times a day
TKO	to keep open
TLC	tender loving care
TPN	total parenteral nutrition

Abbreviation	Meaning
TPR	temperature, pulse, respiration
trach	tracheostomy
TT	therapeutic touch
TTWB	toe-touch weight bearing
TWE	tap water enema
Tx	traction, treatment
UA, U/A	urinalysis
UE	upper extremity
URI	upper respiratory infection
UTI	urinary tract infection
vag	vaginal
vc, VC	verbal cues
VRE	vancomycin-resistant Enterococcus
VS	vital signs
WA, W/A	while awake
WB	weight bearing
WBAT	weight bearing as tolerated
w/c	wheelchair
WFL	within functional limits
WNL	within normal limits
wt	weight
x, X	times
XR, X/R	x-ray

Abbreviation	Meaning
y/o	years old
yr	year
↑	up, increase
↓	down, decrease
1°	first, primary, first degree
2°	second, secondary, secondary to, second degree
3°	third, tertiary, third degree
1x, 2x, etc.	one time, one person, two times, etc.
i, ii, iii, etc.	one, two, three, four, etc.
@	at
//	parallel
=	equals, equal to
>, ≥	greater than
<, ≤	less than
±, +/−	plus or minus
△(triangle)	change, change to
°	degrees
Ø	zero, none, nothing
*	important
♀	female
♂	male

KEY POINTS

- The nursing assistant communicates with other members of the health care team verbally and in writing.
- Observations about the resident are reported to the nurse for assessment and action.
- The nursing assistant records information about the resident in the medical record in writing or by using the computer.
- The nursing assistant will use the senses of sight, hearing, smell, and touch to make valuable observations.
- Signs can be seen or observed. Symptoms are things the resident tells you.

- Objective observations are factual. Subjective observations are based on what you think or what the resident tells you.
- The medical record is a factual, permanent record of the resident's progress and care.
- The medical record is a legal document, and entries in it must be accurate and complete.
- Understanding medical terminology and medical abbreviations is important if you are to communicate well and accurately with other members of the health care team.

REVIEW

A. Multiple Choice

Select the one best answer.

1. A sign is an observation that
   a. you detect with your senses.
   b. you think.
   c. you believe.
   d. reflects your opinion.
2. A symptom is
   a. something you know to be true.
   b. what the resident tells you.
   c. what you think.
   d. what you detect with your senses.
3. Objective means
   a. something you think and feel.
   b. a complaint of pain.
   c. something you observe.
   d. what you believe is true
4. The medical record
   a. is a legal document.
   b. cannot be used in court.
   c. contains fictional information.
   d. can be read by any interested party.
5. When using the 24-hour clock, 5:15 p.m. is
   a. 0515 hours.
   b. 1515 hours.
   c. 1715 hours.
   d. 2015 hours.
6. The following is true about documenting in the resident's chart:
   a. Correction fluid should be used if you make a mistake.
   b. Factual information should be written on the chart.
   c. Charting is always done before care is given.
   d. Turning and repositioning need not be documented.
7. The prefix is found
   a. at the beginning of a word.
   b. at the end of a word.
   c. in the middle of a word.
   d. in the root of a word.
8. A suffix is found
   a. at the beginning of a word.
   b. at the end of a word.
   c. in the middle of a word.
   d. in the root of a word.
9. The root
   a. introduces the word.
   b. describes the suffix.
   c. provides depth.
   d. provides meaning.
10. The term *myalgia* means
    a. heart attack.
    b. infection of the bone.
    c. pain in the muscles.
    d. inflammation of the throat.
11. The term *colectomy* means
    a. removal of the colon.
    b. removal of a cyst.
    c. pain in the small intestine.
    d. irritation of the gallbladder.
12. The term *phlebitis* means
    a. infection of the lungs.
    b. inflammation of a vein.
    c. irritation of the throat.
    d. pus in a wound.
13. Hydrotherapy is
    a. a disease of the lungs.
    b. removal of the uterus.
    c. water therapy.

d. oxygen therapy.

14. The nurse writes on your assignment sheet, Mr. Dominguez, room 611—"B/P at H.S." You know this means:

   a. Take the blood pressure at bedtime.
   b. Give Mr. Dominguez the bedpan at his side.
   c. The resident should have big portions for his supper.
   d. Mr. Dominguez has a blood problem with his system.

15. Mrs. Shane is to ambulate in the hallway TID. You know this means to walk the resident

   a. every other day.
   b. twice a day.
   c. three times a day.
   d. ten times a day.

B. Definitions

Define the meaning of the following words based on your knowledge of medical terminology.

16. tachycardia ________________
17. bradycardia ________________
18. gastritis ________________
19. ophthalmology ________________
20. nephrectomy ________________
21. pyuria ________________
22. dyspnea ________________
23. hemolysis ________________
24. dysuria ________________
25. mastectomy ________________
26. intraabdominal ________________

C. Clinical Applications

Answer the following questions.

27. Linda Mason, CNA, is in a hurry to leave. She has an appointment as soon as she gets off work. Linda states that Mrs. Long and Mr. Thomas need to be repositioned. She completes all her other resident care, but does not get all of her charting done. She asks you to finish it for her. How should you handle this situation?
28. Your friend, John, asks if your long-term care facility has a fax machine. He asks you to fax some very important papers to another state. He said the office supply store will charge $22.00 for this and he cannot afford it. Although the fax machine is available at the nurses' station, your facility policies state that the fax is to be used for facility business only. What should you do?

C: Comfort, Pain, Rest, and Sleep

OBJECTIVES

After reading this unit, you will be able to:

- Spell and define key terms.
- Explain why nursing comfort measures are important to residents' well-being.
- List six observations to make and report for residents who have pain.
- Describe nursing assistant measures to increase comfort and relieve pain.
- List nursing comfort measures that promote rest.
- Describe the phases of the sleep cycle and the importance of each.
- List nursing measures to promote sleep.
- Define religion and spirituality and explain how they are different.
- Describe methods of supporting residents' spirituality.

OBSERVATIONS TO MAKE AND REPORT RELATED TO COMFORT, PAIN, REST, AND SLEEP

Chest pain
Pain that radiates
Pain upon movement
Pain during urination
Pain when having a bowel movement
Splinting an area upon movement
Grimacing, or facial expressions suggesting pain
Body language suggesting pain
Moaning or sighing
Pattern of behavior suggesting pain, such as screaming upon movement
Acute headache
Complaints of binding pain or sensation around forehead
"Splitting" headache
Unrelieved pain after pain medication has been given
Pain is *never* normal; *all* complaints of pain should be reported to the nurse promptly

Resident Comfort

All humans need comfort, rest, and sleep for physical and emotional well-being, health, and wellness. **Comfort** is a state of physical and emotional well-being. The resident is calm and relaxed, and is not in pain or upset. Assisting residents with their comfort needs is a major nursing assistant responsibility. In fact, assisting residents with physical or emotional comfort needs is at the very heart of nursing care. Many factors affect residents' comfort. Environmental factors that interfere with comfort are unfamiliar environment, lack of privacy, noise, odor, temperature, lighting, and ventilation. Personal and uncontrollable factors that increase or contribute to discomfort include age, activity, injury, illness, surgery, stress, and pain. As a rule, residents are uncomfortable when their physical or emotional needs are not met. Unmet needs cause tension and anxiety, and interfere with comfort and rest (Figure 2.12). Using basic nursing measures to meet residents' needs promotes comfort and relaxation, and provides a sense of well-being.

Pain

Pain (Figure 2.13) is a state of discomfort that is unpleasant for the resident. Pain is always a warning that something is wrong. It interferes with the resident's optimal level of function and self-care. Residents may limit movement when they are having pain. Unrelieved pain contributes to complications of immobility, increasing the risk of pneumonia, skin breakdown, and other problems. Pain decreases quality of life, and may cause hopelessness, anxiety, depression, and a feeling of helplessness. Pain may cause acting out, crying, and other strange, belligerent, or combative behavior. It is a major preventable public health problem that slows recovery in individuals with acute illness, complicates chronic illness, and increases health care costs. Relieving pain has always been an important nursing responsibility. Nursing staff must identify residents who are having pain, and those who are at risk for pain, then take the appropriate action to make the residents as comfortable as possible.

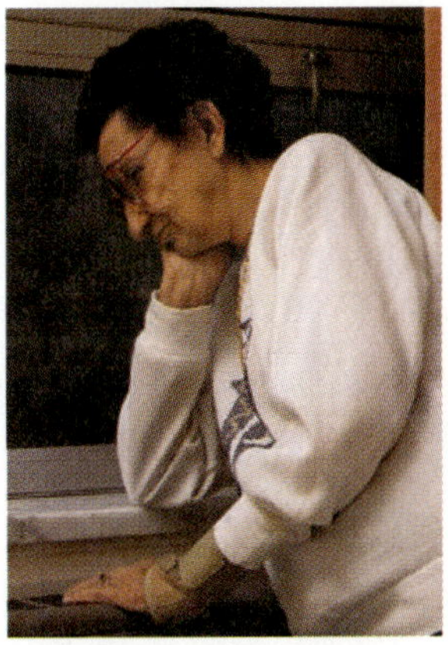

FIGURE 2-12 This resident's body language betrays the emotional distress she is feeling.

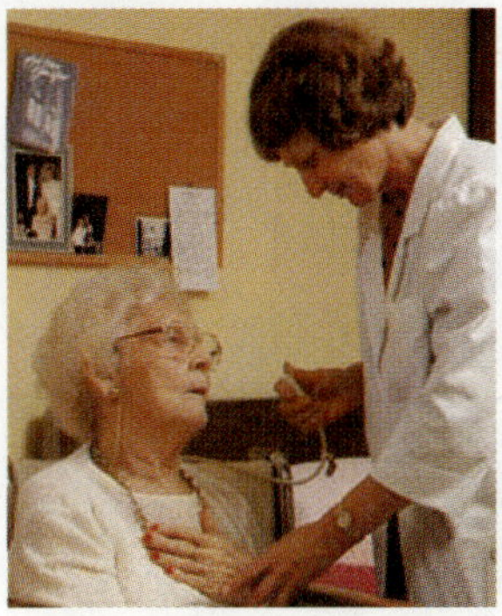

FIGURE 2-13 This resident is having severe pain.

Residents' Responses to Pain

Residents' responses to pain vary widely. Some individuals do not feel pain as acutely as others. Some try to ignore the pain. Other residents may try to deny pain because they are afraid of what it means. Ignoring or denying pain increases the risk of injury, because the normal warning that pain gives goes unrecognized or unheeded. Confused residents may display behavior problems when they are having pain. Some moan, sigh, or yell during movement. Never ignore body language or other signs of pain in residents. Always report signs and symptoms of pain to the nurse. Your observations are a valuable contribution to the nursing assessment and residents' comfort.

Residents' responses to pain may be related to culture. People from some cultures are very emotional when they are in pain. Others are very stoic. Some think that showing pain is a sign of weakness, whereas others believe that pain is a punishment from a higher power. Pain causes stress and anxiety, interfering with comfort, rest, and sleep (Figure 2.14). Rest and sleep are necessary for the body to restore strength and energy, and to repair itself. Inability to sleep, restlessness, and disturbed sleep may be caused by pain.

Identifying Residents in Pain

Pain is a serious condition that affects well-being and quality of life. Residents have the right to timely pain assessment and management. Many

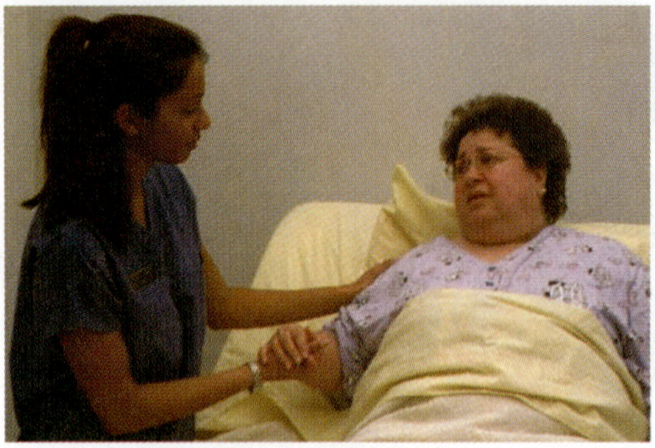

FIGURE 2-14 This resident's pain is interfering with her ability to sleep.

factors affect residents' reactions to pain. The reactions may be different from one moment to the next, and one resident to the next. Four types of pain are listed in Table 2.11. Monitor the residents' body language for signs of pain. Regularly ask residents if they are in pain. Some will not volunteer this information if not asked directly. Some residents will yell or cry out during transfers or movement. This may be interpreted as confusion instead of pain.

Body language is often the first clue that a resident is having pain. This may be the only clue in some cognitively impaired residents, those from other cultures, and residents who are comatose. Look for pain upon movement, facial expressions, crying, moaning, rigid posture, and guarded positioning. The resident may withdraw when he or she is touched or repositioned. Watch for restlessness, irregular or erratic respirations, periodic breath-holding, dilated pupils, and sweating. The resident may favor one extremity. He or she may become irritable, fatigued, or withdrawn. The resident may refuse to eat for no apparent reason. The resident may act opposite of normal. For example:

- A cognitively impaired resident who is normally very quiet becomes noisy
- A resident with garbled speech accurately describes his or her pain
- The agitated and combative resident becomes quiet and nonverbal
- A friendly and outgoing resident cries easily and withdraws
- The resident who is normally active becomes still and quiet

Always suspect pain if the resident's behavior changes. Although the resident may not display an outward appearance of pain, asking if he or she is having pain is the best way to find out. Report your observations to the nurse compared with the normal behavior for the resident. If the behavior changes back to normal after the nurse administers an **analgesic** (pain-relieving) medication, this confirms that the change in body language or behavior was caused by pain. The nurse will inform the interdisciplinary team that further evaluation is necessary to determine the best ways of managing the pain.

The resident's self-report of pain is the most accurate indicator of the existence and intensity of pain, and should be respected and believed. Avoid making assumptions about a resident's pain. Although many residents with pain display outward signs through their body language and behavior, avoid making assumptions about the presence or absence of pain if the resident is

TABLE 2-11 Types of pain

Type of Pain	Description
Acute pain	Occurs suddenly and without warning. Acute pain is usually the result of tissue damage, caused by conditions such as injury or surgery. Typically, acute pain decreases over time, as healing takes place.
Persistent (chronic) pain	Persistent pain lasts longer than six months. (Another, older term for this type of pain is *chronic pain*). It may be intermittent or constant. Persistent pain may be caused by multiple medical conditions.
Phantom pain	Phantom pain occurs as a result of an amputation. The resident has had a body part, such as a leg, removed, but complains of pain in the missing toes. The pain is real, not imaginary.
Radiating pain	Radiating pain moves from the site of origin to other areas. For example, when a resident is having a heart attack, the pain may radiate from the chest to the jaw or arm.

laughing, talking, or sleeping. For example, some health care workers assume that residents who are smiling or laughing cannot be in pain. Vital signs may be normal. These workers believe that residents who are having pain should be grimacing, frowning, or crying. This is untrue. Some residents may appear comfortable while having severe pain. Once again, avoid judging the resident. His or her self-report of pain is the most accurate and reliable indicator of pain. Notify the nurse without passing judgment.

When asking about pain, make sure the resident can see and hear you. Allow enough time for the resident to process your questions and respond. Be patient. Use language that is appropriate for the resident's age and mental status. Remember that residents may use different words for pain, such as "hurt," "sore," or "tender." Residents who are mentally confused may surprise you. Some can describe their pain accurately. Some residents will admit to having pain only if you ask them directly, so do not omit this important step. Always ask residents who are crying, those whose body language suggests pain, and those with behavior suggesting pain.

Observing and Reporting Signs and Symptoms of Pain

Pain always requires further intervention. It should never be ignored. Always report verbal complaints of pain, describing the pain in the resident's exact words. Be aware of signs and symptoms of pain in residents who have difficulty communicating, such as residents who cannot speak and residents who are cognitively impaired. Facial expressions and grimacing; moaning; refusing to move; stiff, rigid, or limited movements; and crying, yelling, or screaming may be clues that the resident is having pain. Inform the nurse promptly. Pain is always an observation that must be reported immediately. A nursing assessment of pain involves many different factors. Your observations contribute to this assessment and the resident's well-being.

Using a Pain Rating Scale. Your facility will have policies and procedures for pain management. Most facilities have adopted several different pain rating scales to evaluate the level of residents' pain. In fact, many facilities now consider pain the "fifth vital sign." In these facilities, pain is regularly and frequently evaluated.

Because pain is personal and subjective, consistent pain evaluation among health care workers is a concern. Using a pain rating (assessment) scale helps nurses assess the resident and keeps caregivers from forming their own opinions about the level of the resident's pain. Using a pain scale prevents subjective opinions, provides consistency, eliminates some barriers to pain management, and gives the resident a means of describing the pain accurately. Pain scales are important tools for communication. The resident selects the scale that helps *best describe* his or her pain. Pain rating scales can be used to evaluate pain in residents of all ages and cultures.

Although you will not be directly assessing the residents' pain, you must understand the purpose of the scales used in your facility and how they are interpreted. Many facilities use a 0 to 10 scale, with 0 meaning no pain and 10 meaning intolerable pain. If the resident tells you that she is having pain at "level 5," for example, you must know what this means and report the problem to the nurse. Likewise, if the resident complains of pain at "level 9" an hour after receiving pain medication, this suggests a potentially serious problem and must be reported immediately.

Many different pain scales are used in health care (Figure 2.15). These scales are only examples. Your facility may use similar or different tools for evaluating pain. Pain scales use pictures, words, or numbers to help the resident describe pain intensity. Most scales range from no pain to very severe pain. Picture scales use smiling faces, neutral faces, frowns, and tears.

Managing Pain

Unrelieved pain has a negative effect on the resident's health and functional status. Notify the nurse as soon as the resident complains, before pain becomes severe or out of control. Report your observations objectively. Observe the resident carefully after pain medications have been given, and report your observations to the nurse.

Sometimes the physician orders several different medications for each resident's pain. The nurse will select which drug to use based on an assessment of the resident. Your observations, the resident's self-report of pain intensity, and physical assessment findings are all considered when determining which medication to administer, when more than one is ordered. If the first drug does not relieve the pain, the nurse may have the option of administering another, so always report unrelieved pain. The quality of pain control is influenced by the education, experience, and attitude of the health care providers caring for the resident.

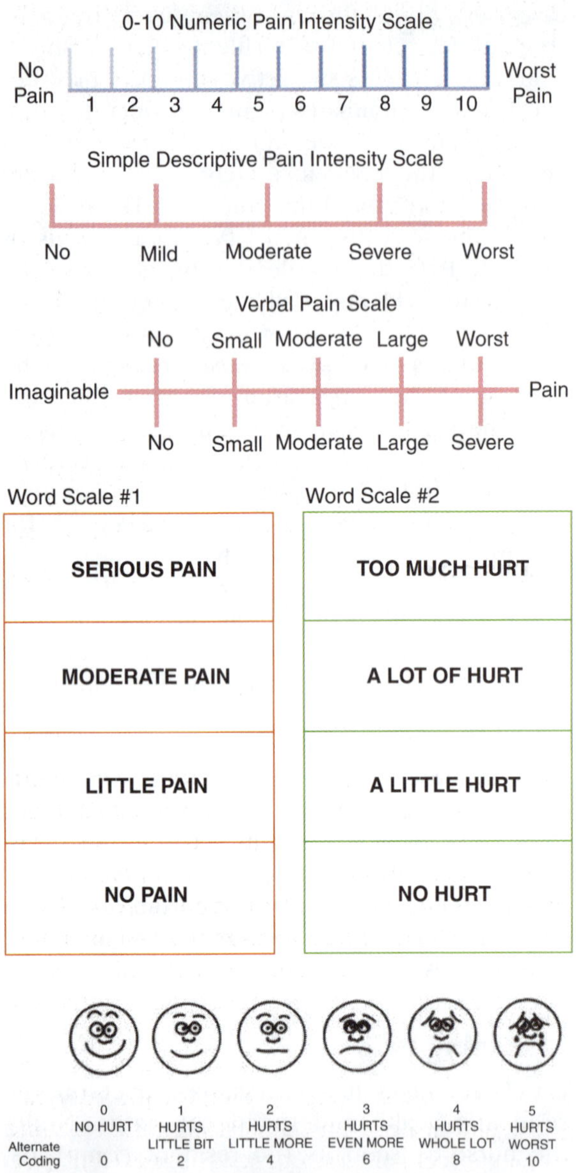

FIGURE 2-15 The resident will select the pain scale that best helps him or her communicate the level and intensity of his or her pain. **(FACES scale from Wong D. L. et al. Wong's Essentials of Pediatric Nursing, ed. 6, St. Louis: Mosby, 2001, p. 1301. Reprinted with permission.)**

Pain management is an important part of resident care. Take complaints of pain very seriously. Respect and support the residents' right to pain assessment and management without judgment or disbelief. You are responsible for promptly reporting the information to the nurse, who will assess the resident and take the appropriate action. Avoid passing judgment on residents who take narcotic medications to control their pain. Many health care workers try to discourage residents from taking these drugs because of the potential for addiction. Studies have shown that very few residents with severe pain become addicted to the drugs.

Although the nursing assistant is not directly responsible for pain management, your observations and nursing care are very important, because you work so closely and intimately with the residents. Understanding the responsibilities that health care providers have for pain relief will help you provide nursing comfort measures, monitor for signs and symptoms of pain, and report your observations to the nurse.

Nursing Assistant Comfort Measures. As a nursing assistant, you can provide many basic nursing measures to make the resident more comfortable. Relieving discomfort helps reduce pain and anxiety. These include:

- Telling residents what you plan to do and how you will do it
- Providing privacy
- Assisting the resident to get into a comfortable position (Figure 2.16)
- Repositioning the resident to relieve pain and muscle spasms
- Changing the angle of the bed to relieve tension on surgical sites or injured areas

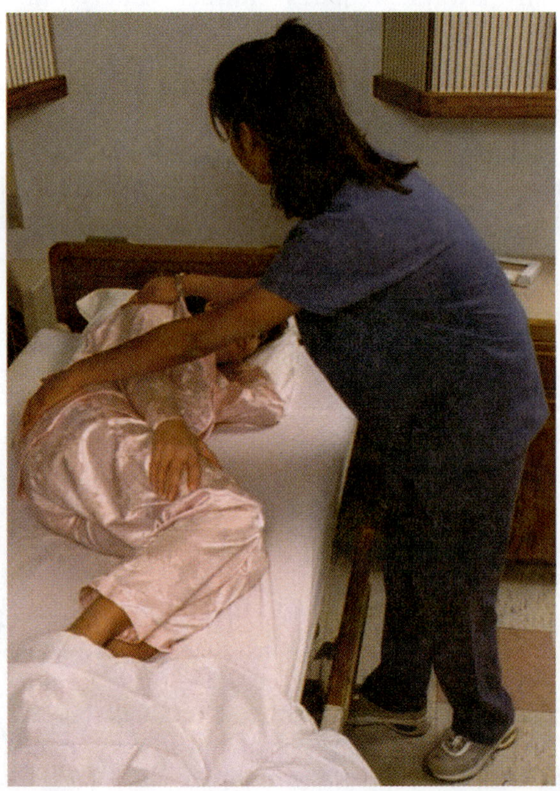

FIGURE 2-16 Help the resident find a comfortable position.

- Avoiding sudden, jerking movements when moving or positioning the resident
- Performing passive range-of-motion exercises to reduce stiffness and maintain mobility
- Using pillows to support the affected body part(s) (Figure 2.17)
- Providing extra pillows and blankets for comfort and support
- Straightening the bed and linen
- Giving a back rub
- Washing the resident's face and hands
- Providing a cool, damp washcloth on the resident's forehead
- Providing oral hygiene
- Providing fresh water, food, or beverages as permitted
- Playing soft music to distract the resident
- Listening to resident's concerns
- Providing emotional support
- Touching the resident, if appropriate
- Maintaining a comfortable environmental temperature
- Providing a quiet, dark environment
- Eliminating unpleasant sights, sounds, and odors from the environment
- Waiting at least 30 minutes after the nurse administers pain medication before moving the resident or performing procedures or activities
- Timing resident care to coincide with pain medication

Regularly incorporate these steps into your resident care. Follow the individual directions on the care plan. The nurse may also direct you to apply warm or cold applications to make the resident more comfortable.

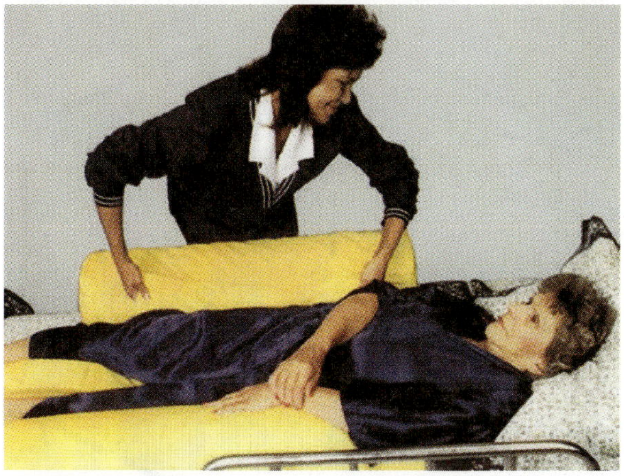

FIGURE 2-17 Use pillows, props, and supports to position body parts for comfort. *(Courtesy of Briggs Corporation, Des Moines, IA (800) 247-2343)*

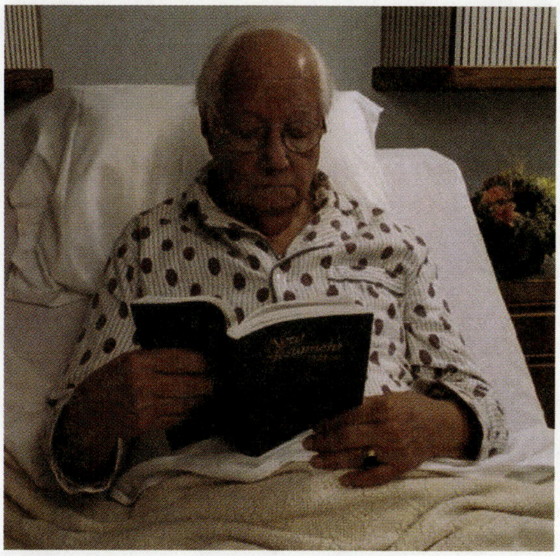

FIGURE 2-18 Reading the Bible is a pleasurable activity that helps this resident rest.

Rest

Rest is a state of mental and physical comfort, calmness, and relaxation. The resident's basic needs of hunger, thirst, elimination, and pain must be met before effective rest is possible. He or she should be dressed comfortably and feel fresh and clean. The resident may sit or lie down, or may do things that are pleasant and relaxing. Some residents have rituals, such as reading the Bible (Figure 2.18) or saying the rosary. The environment should be calm and quiet to promote rest. If basic care is tiring for the resident, allow him or her to rest before continuing. Some residents feel refreshed after 15 minutes of rest. Others need more time. Some residents must rest frequently throughout the day. Plan your schedule and activities to allow for rest periods. Providing a back rub, nursing comfort measures, or other relaxation activities may assist the resident to rest. Follow the care plan and the nurse's instructions.

Sleep

Sleep is a period of continuous or intermittent unconsciousness in which physical movements are decreased, allowing the mind and body to rest. Sleep is a basic need of all humans. Adequate sleep is necessary for the body and mind to function properly. Sleep occurs in a cycle that lasts for several hours at a time.

The body repairs itself during sleep. Because movement and activity are limited, the body's

TABLE 2-12 Sleep needs throughout the life cycle

- Newborn infants sleep in 3- to 4-hour intervals for a total of 16 to 20 hours of sleep a day
- Infants require 12 to 16 hours of sleep a day
- Toddlers require 12 to 14 hours of sleep a day, usually broken into 10 to 12 hours of sleep at night, with one or more daytime naps
- Preschool children require 10 to 12 hours per day
- Elementary school children require 10 to 12 hours a day
- Adolescents require 8 to 10 hours per day
- Young adults aged 18 to 40 require about 7 to 8 hours a day
- Middle-aged adults aged 40 to 65 require about 7 hours a day
- Elderly adults over the age of 65 require about 5 to 7 hours per day

metabolic needs are reduced. The resident may need a blanket because he or she is not moving, and may become cold. It is common for vital signs to decrease during sleep. The need for sleep decreases as a person ages. Infants and children require more sleep than adults. Elderly residents require less sleep than younger adults or middle-aged residents. Children require more sleep than adults. In fact, newborns may sleep as much as 20 hours a day. Sleep needs by age group are listed in Table 2.12. Weight loss may decrease the need for sleep, whereas weight gain often increases the need for sleep.

Many factors affect sleep. Sleep problems often result from a combination of many factors. Obvious problems that may interfere with the quality and quantity of sleep are:

- Pain
- Hunger
- Thirst
- Need to eliminate
- Illness
- Exercise
- Noise
- Temperature
- Ventilation
- Light intensity
- Physical discomfort
- Some medications
- Caffeine intake
- Alcohol, drugs
- Some foods and beverages
- Lifestyle changes
- Anxiety, stress, fear, emotional problems
- Changes in the environment, unfamiliar environment
- Treatments and therapies
- Staff providing routine care

Worry is another factor that interferes with comfort, rest, and sleep. Residents worry about many things, such as:

- What the future will bring
- How much the stay in the facility will cost
- Who is taking care of their responsibilities
- Whether they are dying

You will not have the answers to all these pressing concerns. You can listen, however. Share these concerns with the nurse. This is not gossiping. The nurse and the other members of the staff may be able to help the resident solve the problems. With worries reduced, the resident will rest easier.

The Sleep Cycle

Each person has a sleep–wake cycle. An internal biological clock tells the person when it is time to sleep and wake up. The sleep cycle includes two types of sleep (Figure 2.19).

- **Nonrapid eye movement (NREM) sleep** has four phases, progressing from light to very deep. This part of the sleep cycle begins when the resident first falls asleep. In the first two phases, the resident is easily aroused. As he or she progresses through the cycle, arousal becomes more difficult and sleep becomes deeper.
- **Rapid eye movement (REM) sleep** restores mental function. If you look closely, you will see the resident's eyes moving behind closed

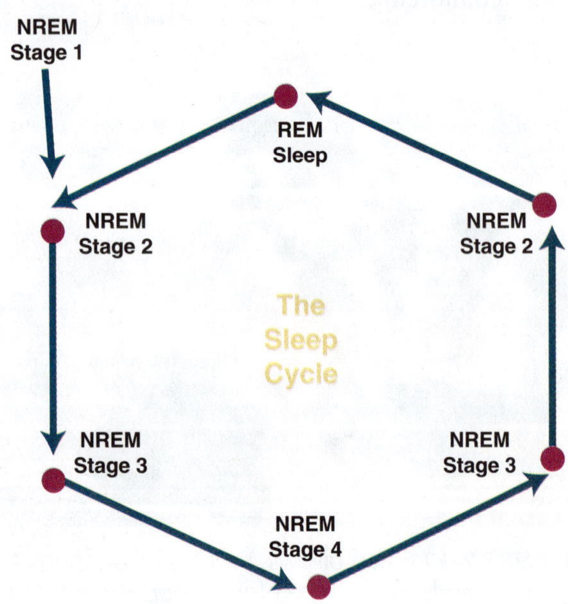

FIGURE 2-19 The sleep cycle

lids during this phase. Avoid awakening a resident who is in REM sleep, whenever possible. This is the part of the cycle in which dreams occur. The resident passes into REM sleep within approximately 60 to 90 minutes after falling asleep. Hospitalized residents may not experience prolonged periods of sleep time, so total REM time is less than normal. They awaken feeling less rested and may be more tired during the day.

Sleep is important to prevent feelings of fatigue, and for healing of medical and surgical problems. Getting enough sleep and rest allows residents to function at their highest level. Moving through the stages of the sleep cycle uninterrupted is important. Some residents become irritable if they do not have enough sleep. Elderly residents who do not sleep well may become disoriented. This correctable problem may be mistaken for confusion! It is easily solved by allowing uninterrupted sleep. Other signs and symptoms of inadequate sleep are:

- Slow mental and physical responses
- Decreased attention span
- Forgetfulness, difficulty remembering things
- Reduced reasoning and judgment
- Puffy, red, swollen eyes
- Dark circles under the eyes
- Disorientation
- Mood swings, moodiness
- Lethargy, sleepiness, fatigue
- Agitation, restlessness
- Clumsiness, incoordination
- Difficulty finding the right word(s) to say
- Slurred speech
- Hallucinations in severe **sleep deprivation**, or prolonged sleep loss (inadequate quality or quantity of REM or NREM sleep).

Nursing Assistant Measures to Promote Comfort, Rest, and Sleep

Basic nursing comfort measures, such as those used to relieve pain, are also effective in helping residents to rest and sleep. Specific measures for each resident will be listed in the care plan. Measures that promote comfort, rest, and sleep are:

- Helping the resident into loose-fitting, comfortable clothing or nightwear
- Assisting with toileting, cleanliness, oral care, and personal hygiene needs
- Providing a warm bath or shower, if permitted
- Avoiding serving beverages containing caffeine after the evening meal
- Providing a snack, if desired; snacks with protein and/or calcium, such as meat, cheese, milk, nuts, and peanut butter, promote sleep (peanut butter is not permitted in some facilities and states)
- Straightening the bed
- Assisting the resident into a comfortable position, providing pillows and props as needed for comfort
- Giving a back rub (Figure 2.20)
- Providing a comfortable environmental temperature and ventilation
- Providing an extra blanket, if desired
- Eliminating unpleasant odors
- Eliminating noise
- Adjusting the lighting to a comfortable level, darkening the room as much as possible for sleep or providing a nightlight, if desired
- Reporting pain to the nurse
- If the resident is having pain, waiting for at least 30 minutes after pain medication before performing procedures
- If the resident is anxious, listening to what he or she says and eliminating the cause of the anxiety, if possible
- Not startling the resident
- Handling the resident gently during care
- Organizing routine care to allow the resident uninterrupted sleep or rest
- Avoiding physical activity or other activities that are upsetting to the resident before bedtime
- Assisting with personal bedtime rituals, if any
- Allowing the resident to select his or her own bedtime
- Allowing the resident to read, watch television, or listen to the radio, if desired
- Reading to the resident from a favorite book
- Assisting with relaxation exercises and activities, as directed (Figure 2.21)
- If the resident receives a sleeping medication, making sure the resident is ready for sleep before the nurse administers the medication
- Closing the door to the resident's room

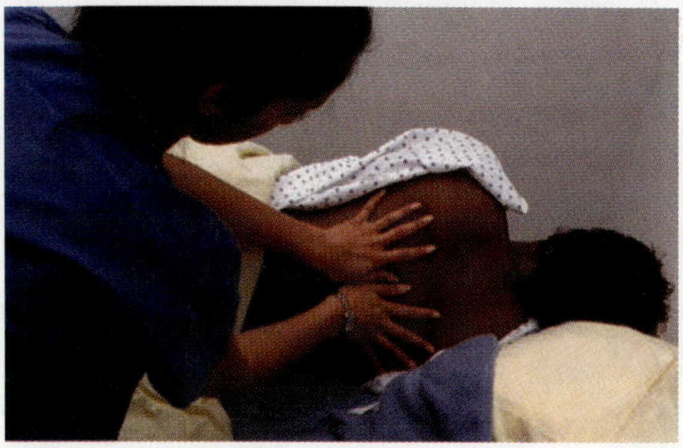

FIGURE 2-20 A back rub is relaxing and relieves muscle tension.

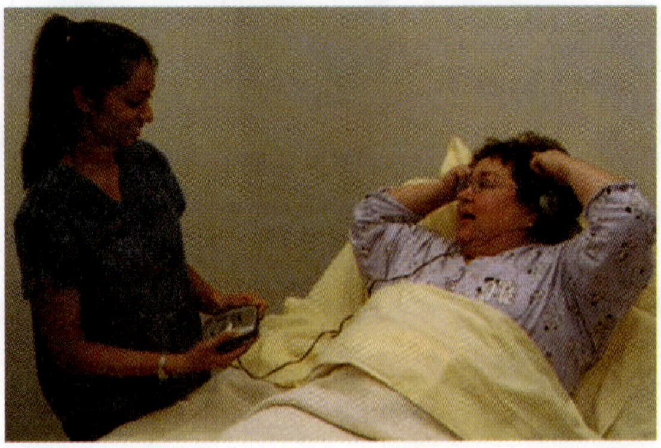

FIGURE 2-21 This resident uses music as a form of relaxation.

Spirituality

Spirituality and religion can provide great comfort and support to residents, particularly during times of illness and emotional distress. Many people believe that spirituality and religion are the same thing, but they are not. *Spirituality* is a broader term that includes:

- Our perceptions of our place in the universe (Figure 2.22)
- Belief in a higher power (if any)
- Our ideas about responsibilities to others
- Our fears and beliefs about living and dying

The need for spirituality may be fueled by experiences, relationships, and opportunities that provide the motivation for deeper healing and growth throughout life. Illness can be a powerful motivator for eliminating emotional, mental, and physical patterns that limit and restrict spiritual growth. A key to caring for residents' spiritual needs is respecting each resident as an individual, and remembering that no two people are alike.

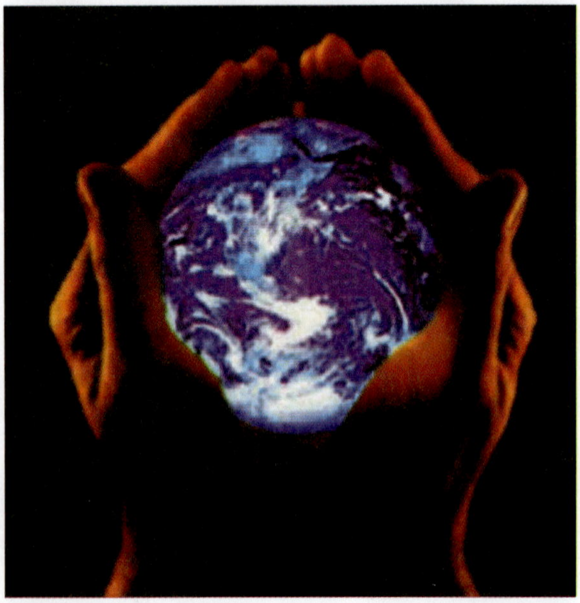

FIGURE 2-22 Spirituality involves our perceptions of our place in the universe.

When residents use spirituality for healing, they allow the power of the spirit to work more fully in their lives, leading to greater harmony and balance. It is usually a quiet time for introspection and questioning. Healing may require making changes. It involves blending of the physical, mental, emotional, and spiritual aspects of self. When a person experiences deep physical or emotional healing, all parts of the self are changed. Physical problems often involve thoughts and emotions. Residents sometimes have surprises during periods of intense spirituality. They may release a great emotional burden instead of experiencing a physical recovery. The lifting of the emotional burden often brings a great sense of inner peace.

Nursing Assistant Actions

The nursing assistant must recognize that all humans are spiritual beings, although we all choose different paths. Be sensitive to the residents' paths and choices. Avoid passing judgment about residents' religious, spiritual, ethnic, and cultural practices and choices in health care treatment. Although spiritual beliefs are usually considered a private concern, the need for spiritual caring is fundamental when serious health problems occur. The resident may question the meaning and purpose of life, the sense of hope, belief in self, belief in caregivers' ability, belief in the physician's ability, and belief in a higher power. Health care personnel are privileged to have a presence and role in these very personal times of significant stress and turmoil in residents' lives. Pay attention to what the resident is saying. Your role is to listen, to reflect, and to clarify information. Never try to interpret or define spiritual meaning or truth to the resident. Avoid imposing your beliefs on the resident. Avoid pat, uncaring answers to questions. Never give residents false hope. Never use problem-solving techniques to analyze spiritual truths for residents. Admitting that you do not know an answer is all right.

Remember that caring for residents during very private moments is a privilege. Do not be so distracted with your workload or the environment that you fail to show sensitivity when residents express spiritual concerns. Provide privacy and support while they work through challenges to their health and well-being. Inform the nurse or social worker of the resident's concerns. They may be able to provide assistance, intervention, or referrals to other sources of help.

KEY POINTS

- All humans need comfort, rest, and sleep for physical and emotional well-being, health, and wellness.
- Comfort is a state of physical and emotional well-being.
- Pain is a state of discomfort that is unpleasant for the resident; it is always a warning that something is wrong.
- Residents' responses to pain may be related to culture.
- Body language may be the first (and only) clue that a resident is having pain.
- Relieving pain is an important nursing responsibility.
- The resident's self-report of pain is the most accurate indicator of the existence and intensity of pain, and should be respected and believed.
- Residents may have pain when they are laughing, talking, or sleeping; vital signs may be normal.
- Pain rating scales are important tools for communication. They prevent subjective opinions, provide consistency, eliminate some barriers to pain management, and give the resident a means of describing the pain accurately.
- The incidence of drug addiction is very low in individuals with persistent pain who take narcotic analgesics.
- Rest is a state of mental and physical comfort, calmness, and relaxation. The basic needs of hunger, thirst, elimination, and pain must be met before effective rest is possible.
- Sleep is a period of continuous or intermittent unconsciousness in which physical movements are decreased and the mind and body rest.
- Sleep is a basic need. Adequate sleep is necessary for the body and mind to function properly.
- Less sleep is required as people age.
- Rapid eye movement sleep restores mental function.
- Spirituality and religion can provide great comfort and support during times of illness and emotional distress.
- Spirituality and religion are not the same thing.
- Spirituality includes our perceptions of our place in the universe, belief in a higher power (if any), ideas about our responsibilities to others, and our fears and beliefs about living and dying.
- Caring for residents during very private moments is a privilege. The nursing assistant should show sensitivity when residents express spiritual concerns.

REVIEW

A. Multiple Choice

Select the one best answer.

1. Pain is
   a. not the nursing assistant's responsibility.
   b. a sign of something wrong.
   c. always a sign of acute illness.
   d. a normal condition in the elderly.

2. Pain
   a. never interferes with rest and sleep.
   b. is not stressful or worrisome.
   c. negatively affects well-being.
   d. can usually be ignored.

3. If a resident expresses her problems and worries, the nursing assistant should
   a. stay out of the resident's business.
   b. avoid sharing the information with the nurse.
   c. allow her to talk about it; be a good listener.
   d. provide answers to the problems.

4. Pain assessment is considered to be the
   a. primary vital sign.
   b. frequency at which pain is evaluated.
   c. fifth vital sign.
   d. effectiveness of pain medication.

5. The resident who is having pain
   a. may be laughing or sleeping.
   b. will have abnormal vital signs.
   c. will always limit movement.
   d. always displays painful body language.
6. A state of mental calmness, comfort, and relaxation is
   a. security.
   b. sleep.
   c. leisure.
   d. rest.
7. A period of continuous or intermittent unconsciousness in which physical movements are decreased is
   a. relaxation.
   b. comfort.
   c. sleep.
   d. diversion.
8. When a resident is sleeping,
   a. vital signs may be lower than usual.
   b. temperature increases.
   c. movement increases.
   d. the pulse decreases and respirations increase.
9. During the REM sleep cycle, the resident
   a. dreams.
   b. awakens readily.
   c. progresses through four sleep phases.
   d. may feel hot to the touch.
10. Sleep deprivation is
    a. getting too much sleep.
    b. not getting enough sleep.
    c. a condition caused by snoring.
    d. a sign of mental confusion.
11. Spirituality
    a. is the same as religion.
    b. includes perceptions about one's place in the universe.
    c. is a very private matter between the resident and God.
    d. should be managed only by a qualified social worker.

B. True/False

Answer each question true (T) or false (F).

12. _________The nurse selects the pain scale for the resident to use.
13. _________Lack of privacy can affect a resident's comfort.
14. _________Unrelieved pain can lead to complications of immobility.
15. _________Persistent pain never lasts longer than one month.
16. _________Acute pain results from tissue damage.
17. _________Phantom pain is imaginary pain.
18. _________Radiating pain always encircles the area in which the pain originates.
19. _________Assume that the resident is not in pain if he or she does not complain.
20. _________Rest and sleep are necessary for the body to restore strength and energy, and to repair itself.
21. _________Pain always indicates something wrong.
22. _________Culture has no effect on residents' responses to pain.
23. _________The resident's self-report of pain is the most accurate indicator of the existence and intensity of pain.

C. Matching

Choose the correct term from Column II to match the phrases in Column I. Write the letter of that term in the blank.

Column I	Column II
24. _________state of physical and emotional well-being	a. sleep deprivation
25. _________period of unconsciousness in which movements are decreased	b. analgesic
26. _________progresses from light to very deep	c. REM sleep
27. _________restores mental function	d. rest
28. _________pain-relieving medication	e. pain
29. _________mental and physical comfort, calmness, and relaxation	f. comfort
30. _________inadequate sleep	g. NREM sleep
31. _________state of discomfort	h. sleep

D. Fill in the Blanks

32–39. Complete the statements by writing in the correct word from the following list:

acute	comfort	pain
amputation	NREM	phantom
persistent	REM	radiating

32. Full-color dreaming occurs during the_________phase of the sleep cycle.
33. _________is a state of well-being.
34. _________sleep restores mental function.
35. _________is an unpleasant state of discomfort that indicates something is wrong.
36. _________pain occurs as a result of the removal of an extremity,or _________
37. Pain that lasts longer than six months is _________or chronic pain.
38. _________pain moves from the site of origin to other areas.
39. _________pain is usually the result of tissue damage; it occurs suddenly and without warning.

E. Clinical Applications

Mr. Wong is grimacing and supporting his right side with his hands when you enter the room. He smiles and nods at you. Answer questions 40–44 regarding this resident.

40. Can Mr. Wong smile if he is having pain?
41. If Mr. Wong's right side hurts, how can you position him for comfort and support?
42. Should Mr. Wong's body language be reported to the nurse?
43. Should you ask Mr. Wong if he is having pain?
44. List six nursing assistant measures you can take to make Mr. Wong more comfortable.

Mrs. Lee is a mentally confused resident. She often cries during your shift, but despite your best efforts, you are unable to comfort her. Mrs. Lee goes to therapy several times a week for a warm paraffin wax treatment on her hands. The nurse tells you the resident has arthritis. When the resident leaves the therapy department, she is often smiling. Answer questions 45–47 regarding this resident.

45. Can pain cause crying in a cognitively impaired resident?
46. List four observations you will make of this resident's crying behavior to report to the nurse.
47. List one nursing assistant approach to use for this resident when she is crying.

D: Admission, Transfer, and Discharge

OBJECTIVES

After reading this unit, you will be able to:

- Spell and define key terms.
- Explain why first impressions are important and describe how they set the tone for the resident's stay.
- Describe family dynamics and emotions that occur when a loved one is admitted to a long-term care facility.
- List ways in which the nursing assistant can develop positive relationships with family members.
- Describe the nursing assistant's responsibilities in the admission, transfer, and discharge processes.
- Demonstrate procedures related to admission, transfer, and discharge.

OBSERVATIONS TO MAKE AND REPORT RELATED TO ADMISSION, TRANSFER, AND DISCHARGE

Pay particular attention to the patient's skin condition:

Rashes
Bruises
Pressure ulcers
Any other abnormalities

The nurse will assess the resident on admission and begin a care plan. Likewise, the nurse will assess the resident's discharge needs. Your observations and measurements of vital signs, height, and weight contribute to this assessment. Note and report:

Vision problems
Hearing problems
Communication problems, including ability to make needs known and call for help
Ability to ambulate and transfer safely
Ability to use the bathroom safely

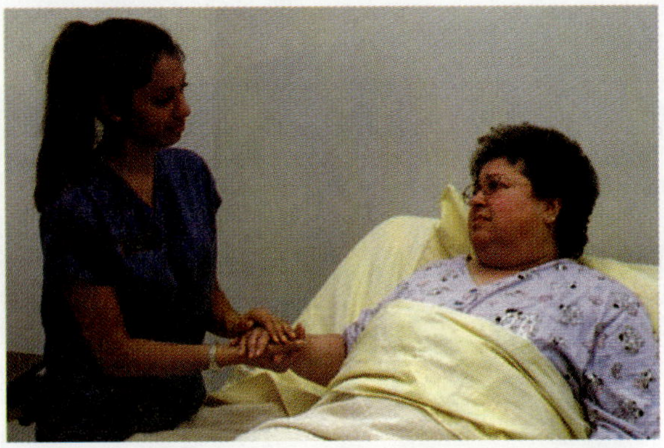

FIGURE 2-23 A positive first impression is long lasting, and will help relieve the resident's fear and anxiety.

Admitting, Transferring, and Discharging a Resident

One responsibility of the nursing assistant is to assist residents with **admission**, **transfer**, and **discharge** in the health care facility. You are expected to gather information, meet the resident's basic needs, and make the process as smooth and comfortable as possible. Your pleasant and courteous manner sets the tone for the admission process. During transfer, being calm and understanding will ease any fears the resident may have. Upon discharge, the professionalism you have shown throughout the resident's stay will be remembered and appreciated.

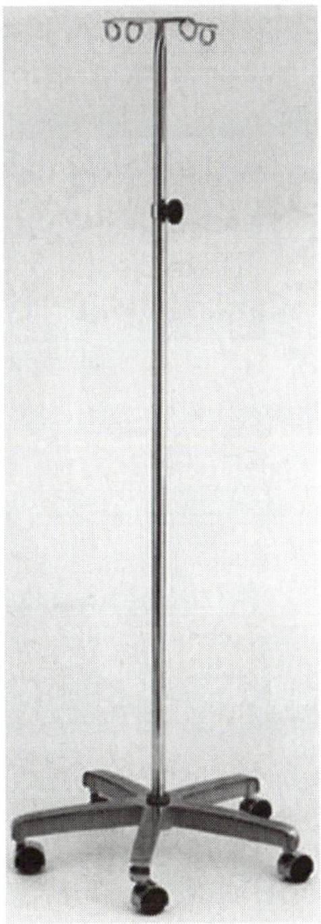

FIGURE 2-24A The intravenous standard is used for hanging IV solutions, IV pumps, tube-feeding solutions, and tube-feeding pumps. Occasionally, it is used to help elevate a resident's arm after an injury. *(Courtesy of Medline Industries, Inc. 1-800-MEDLINE)*

Admission

The nursing assistant is frequently the person who admits residents to the long-term care facility. This may be a difficult, frightening time for the resident. There is a common expression that "first impressions are usually lasting ones." The resident's perception of what is happening may be affected by illness, pain, and fear. Making a good first impression on the resident and family members is important. If the first impression of the nursing assistant is negative, it will affect the resident's impression of all health care providers, and even the long-term care facility. Think about this, remember the resident's fears during the admission process, and do your best to provide a positive, professional impression (Figure 2.23).

Each facility has policies and procedures for resident admissions. Usually, you will be aware of the admission in advance and should prepare the room. If the resident will be admitted by ambulance and put to bed, elevate the bed to the highest horizontal height and open the bed. Move furnishings if necessary, so that the stretcher can be positioned next to the bed. If the resident will require special equipment, such as an **IV standard** (Figure 2.24) or bed trapeze (Figure 2.25), the equipment should be

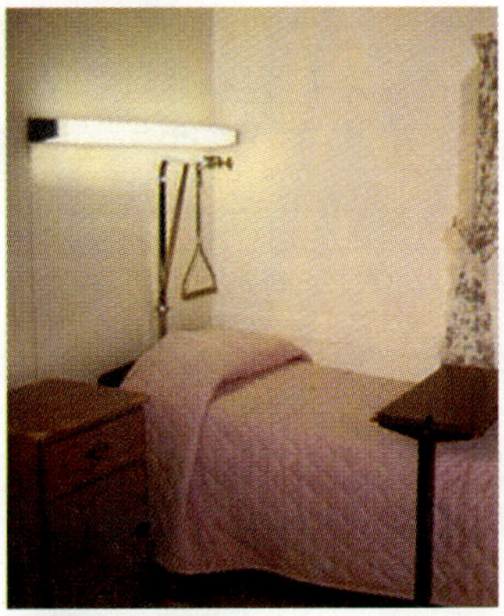

FIGURE 2-24B The trapeze is a heavy piece of equipment that should be installed on the bed before the resident arrives.

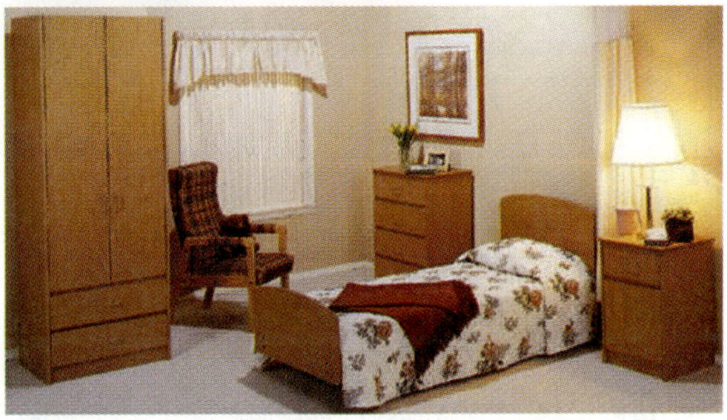

FIGURE 2-24C Arrange the room so it is comfortable and inviting. Placing the resident's personal belongings in prominent positions will make the resident feel more at home. *(Courtesy of Medline Industries, Inc. 1-800-MEDLINE)*

INVENTORY OF PERSONAL EFFECTS

(Reference tag: F252)

INSTRUCTIONS: Upon admission, identify the resident's personal belongings by indicating quantity of those items listed. Use the space allowed to write in additional items as necessary. The original copy shall be kept in the resident's chart. The copy is given to the resident or resident representative. Update as necessary throughout the resident's stay by using the space provided. Upon discharge, use the "✓" columns to indicate that all personal belongings are accounted for.

QTY.	ARTICLES	✓
	Belts	
	Blouses	
	Coats	
	Dresses	
	Gloves	
	Handkerchiefs	
	Hats	
	Housecoats/robes	
	Jackets	
	Nightgowns/pajamas	
	Purses	
	Shaving kit	
	Shoes	
	Shorts	
	Slacks	
	Slippers	
	Slips	
	Shirts	
	Socks/hose	
	Suitcases	
	Suits	
	Suspenders	
	Sweaters	
	Ties	
	Undershirts	
	Underwear	
	Hearing aid	
	Dentures: ❑ Up ❑ Low ❑ Part	
	Eyewear	
	Cane	
	Walker	
	Wheelchair	
	Brace	
	Prosthesis	

ITEMS OF SPECIFIC VALUE (JEWELRY, APPLIANCES, FURNITURE)

QTY	DESCRIPTION	VALUE		✓
		$		

ITEMS ACQUIRED AFTER ORIGINAL ENTRY

DATE	ITEM	HOW RECEIVED	INITIAL	✓

USE THIS SPACE TO RECORD MISCELLANEOUS INFORMATION (i.e. LOST, STOLEN, RETURNED/GIVEN TO FAMILY, ETC.)

DATE	DESCRIPTION / EXPLANATION	INITIAL	✓

CERTIFICATION OF RECEIPT

ON ADMISSION	ON DISCHARGE
Signed X ______ Resident or resident representative ______ Date	Signed X ______ Resident or resident representative ______ Date
Signed ______ Facility representative ______ Title ______ Date	Signed ______ Facility representative ______ Title ______ Date
If resident unable to sign, state reason:	If resident unable to sign, state reason:
Signed ______ Witness ______ Date	Signed ______ Witness ______ Date

NAME—Last	First	Middle	Attending Physician	Chart No.

CFS 1-12/2P R1098 © 1992 Briggs Corporation, Des Moines, IA 50306 (800) 247-2343 Printed in U.S.A.

INVENTORY OF PERSONAL EFFECTS

FIGURE 2-25 The nursing assistant is responsible for completing the personal effects inventory form. *Briggs Corporation, Des Moines, IA (800) 247-2343*)

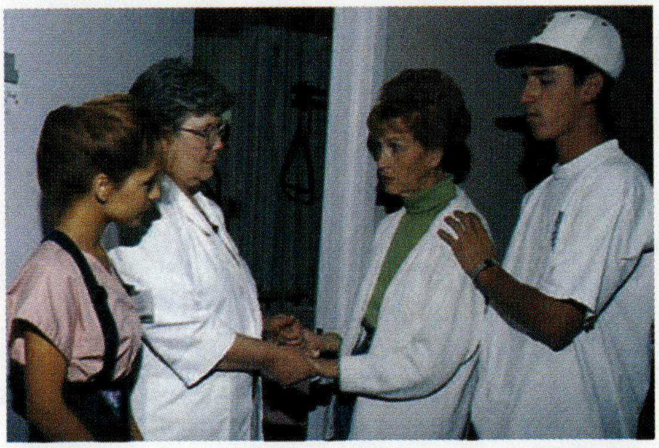

FIGURE 2-26 Families experience a wide range of emotions when a loved one is admitted to a long-term care facility. Introduce yourself and explain the nursing assistant's responsibilities in the care of the residents. Be sincere, and show that you are honestly interested in the resident's well-being.

taken to the room prior to admission. If the resident is ambulatory or will be up in a chair, prepare the room so that it looks clean, comfortable, and inviting. Leave the bed closed. If the family has dropped off personal items, arrange them in the room in an attractive manner (Figure 2.26). Having personal items from home will help the resident make the transition to facility living. Make sure that all lights, electrical items, and outlets are in working order. Check the call signals at the bed and in the bathroom to make sure they are in working order.

When you meet the resident, introduce yourself by name and title. Ask the resident what he or she prefers to be called. Avoid addressing adults by the first name without permission. Your responsibility is to make the resident feel secure and welcome. You will begin gathering information that will be used by other members of the interdisciplinary team. You may be responsible for gathering information for the admission checklist, checking and listing the resident's belongings (Figure 2.27), and obtaining vital signs, height, and weight. Provide information about the health care facility to the resident and visitors. Before you leave the room, provide fresh drinking water, if allowed, and make sure the resident knows how to use the call signal, telephone, television, and electric bed controls. Label disposable equipment such as the water pitcher, drinking glass, bedpan, urinal, emesis basin, and other personal care items with the resident's name according to facility policy. Mark resident clothing and personal items with a permanent marker, according to facility policy. When marking clothing, take care to mark the name on the inside of the garment, where it is not visible from the outside. Mark items in a location where the marker will not bleed through to the outside of the garment. If this is not possible, consult the nurse for an alternate method of labeling the garment. Ask the resident if he or she needs anything else, and do what he or she asks, if possible.

After you have completed your part of the admission, the nurse will **assess**, or evaluate, the resident. This helps identify the resident's problems and needs. Assessment is the first step of the **nursing process**. The nursing process is a four-step process that provides the structure for nursing action. The nursing assistant is an active participant in the nursing process. **Planning** is the second step. Assessment and planning involve gathering information to determine the resident's problems and needs, and then planning care to meet them. The nurse will begin to develop the care plan based on his or her assessment and the information you provide. **Implementation** is the next step. The interdisciplinary team will implement the care plan. **Evaluation** is the final step of the nursing process. The resident's response to the care plan is evaluated and the plan is revised continuously throughout the resident's stay to ensure that his or her needs are met.

Family Dynamics

The family is an extension of the resident. Like the resident, they must make many adjustments during the transition to the long-term care facility. Admitting a loved one to a long-term care facility is usually a very emotional time. Emotions range from relief in getting help with the resident's care to guilt for being unable to care for the loved one. Other common emotions family members experience are:

- Fear. Some family members feel fearful about leaving their relative in the facility. They may have preconceived or incorrect notions about long-term care based on news reports, rumors, or other sources.
- Anger. Some families become angry about the admission. They feel as if they are losing control and are being replaced. They may take their anger out on the staff.
- Uncertainty. The family may feel uncertain about placing a loved one in a facility. They worry that they have made the wrong decision. They may seem afraid, worried, nervous, and tense.
- Sadness. The family may have difficulty coping with being separated from the resident.

- Guilt. The family may feel guilty for turning the care of the resident over to complete strangers.
- Helplessness. Family members may feel helpless because the resident's physical and/or mental condition has worsened, and despite their best efforts, they cannot change the situation.
- Worry. Family members may worry about their loved one's well-being. They may worry about how to pay the bills, or what to do with the house or pets. They often feel overwhelmed with decisions and responsibilities.

Understanding the emotions that families experience should give you an appreciation of why making a good first impression is so important. In addition, you must use good communication skills and show that you care. Greet each family member with warmth, courtesy, kindness, and respect. Introduce yourself and explain your responsibilities as a nursing assistant in the care of their loved one (Figure 2.28). Introduce the resident and family to roommates and other staff members. Make them feel welcome, and show that you are sincerely interested in the resident. If appropriate, make comments such as, "I know this must be very difficult for you."

Offer to assist in unpacking and storing the resident's belongings. Mark personal items with the resident's name in an inconspicuous location, such as the labels of clothing. Make sure the marker does not bleed through to the outside of the garment. Encourage the family to bring in items from home to personalize the room and make it comfortable for the resident.

Knowing when to ask a visitor to leave the room takes tact and diplomacy. Try to schedule your care when the resident is alone, if this is possible. If not, ask visitors to leave any time the resident's body will be exposed or a procedure will be performed. If the resident requests that the visitor be allowed to stay, honor the request. However, do not ask the resident in the presence of others if he or she would like the visitor to stay. Consult the nurse if you are unsure of how to handle a visitor situation.

Admission to the long-term care facility need not be a negative experience. A competent, caring, professional staff will calm residents' and family members' fears and turn a potentially negative experience into a positive one.

GUIDELINES FOR

Family Dynamics

- Get to know family members. Greet them warmly when they come to the facility.
- Wear a name badge. Introduce yourself by name and position.
- Work to build a positive and trusting relationship with the family.
- Be available to talk to the family. Listen carefully to what they have to say and respond appropriately.
- Let the family know that you respect and support their role as their loved one's caregivers.
- Provide information about the resident's activities and daily routines, if requested.
- Familiarize the family with facility routines and services.
- Refer questions of a medical or personal nature to the nurse.
- Listen to family members' suggestions, complaints, and comments. Inform the nurse of family complaints or concerns, or refer the family to the nurse, as appropriate.
- Listen closely to family members' advice about resident care. If the family has been caring for the resident at home, they often know what works best. Pass the information on to the nurse.
- Inform the nurse if a visit is stressful or tiring to a resident.
- Avoid judging the family and decisions they make. Stay out of family disagreements.
- Avoid gossiping with the family, and do not discuss facility business with family members.
- Allow the family to participate in the resident's care, if the resident does not object. Avoid making the family feel as if they must provide care for the resident.

PROCEDURE 1

Admitting the Resident

1. Perform your beginning procedure actions.
2. Gather supplies needed: admission checklist, pen and paper, gloves, hospital gown (if needed), clothing inventory list, scale, tape measure for height, sphygmomanometer, stethoscope, thermometer, standard agency admission kit (Figure 2.27), if used.
3. Remove the contents of the admission kit, mark them with the resident's name, and put them away.
4. Bring permanent equipment to the room, if needed for resident care.
5. Upon resident arrival, introduce yourself by name and title.
6. Introduce the resident to roommates.
7. Provide privacy, and inform family members where they can wait.
8. Obtain the resident's height and weight.
9. Obtain the vital signs.

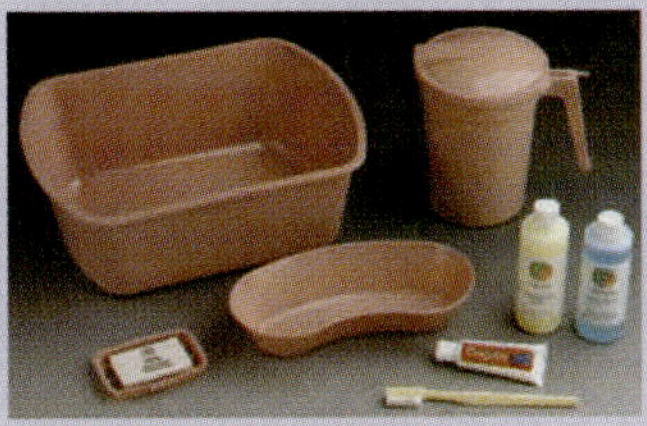

FIGURE 2-27 A standard admission kit. *Medline Industries, Inc. 1-800-MED-LINE)*

10. Complete the information on the admission checklist and personal inventory.
11. Assist the resident to put personal articles and toilet items away, if necessary. Mark items with the resident's name, if needed.
12. Familiarize the resident with his or her surroundings. Show the resident how to use the call signal, and explain the intercom system. Explain the use of the telephone, bed controls, and any other equipment in the room.
13. Provide water, if allowed (Figure 2.28).
14. Make the resident comfortable.
15. Perform your procedure completion actions. Do not leave the room until the resident is settled and has no more questions or requests.

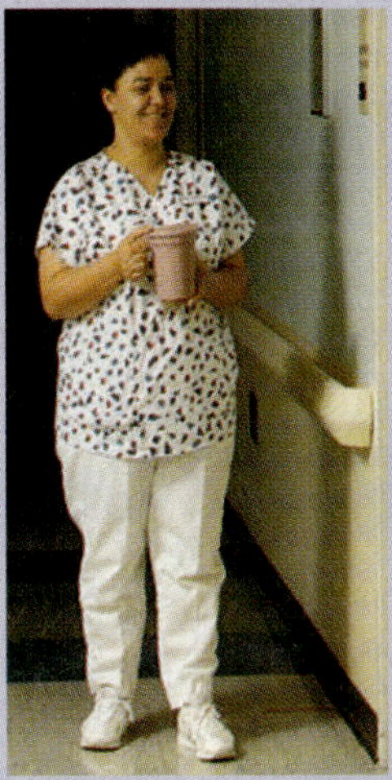

FIGURE 2-28 After admitting the resident, provide fresh water, if allowed.

TRANSFER

There are two types of health care facility transfers. The nursing assistant usually assists with both types. Performing this procedure correctly will ease the resident's fears about going to a new, unfamiliar unit or location. You are responsible for moving the resident and belongings, making the resident comfortable in the new unit, and introducing the staff who will be caring for him or her.

PROCEDURE 2

Transferring the Resident

1. Perform your beginning procedure actions.
2. Gather supplies needed: wheelchair or stretcher, cart for resident's belongings, chart, other medical supplies as instructed by the nurse.
3. Gather the resident's belongings and other items to be transferred and place them on the cart (Figure 2.29). Make sure you have the resident's dentures, glasses, and hearing aid, if used.
4. Assist the resident to transfer to the wheelchair or stretcher for transportation to the new unit. Reassure the resident that family and visitors will be given information about the new location.
5. Transport the resident and belongings to the new unit (Figure 2.30).
6. Introduce the resident to the roommate and nursing staff.
7. Put away the resident's belongings, if this is your facility policy.
8. Make the resident comfortable.
9. Before leaving the unit, make sure that the call signal is within reach and that the resident knows how to use it.
10. Return to your unit.
11. Inform the nurse that the transfer has been completed, and report the resident's reaction and any other observations.
12. Strip the resident's unit and remove any permanent equipment from the room, according to facility policy. Notify the **environmental services department** that the unit is ready to be cleaned. Environmental services is the department responsible for cleanliness and sanitation in the long-term care facility.
13. Perform your procedure completion actions.

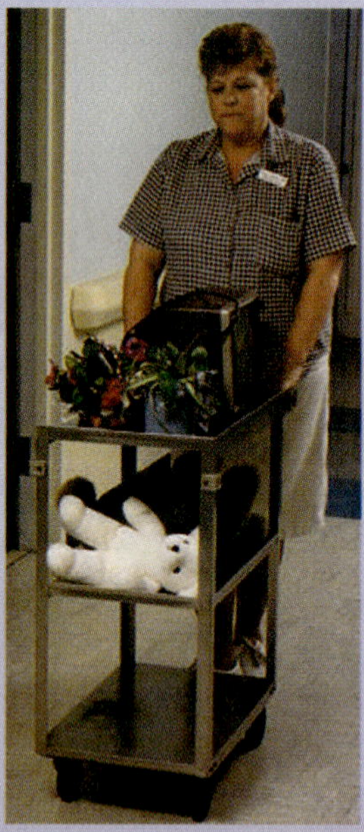

FIGURE 2-29 Use good body mechanics by moving the resident's belongings to the receiving unit on a cart.

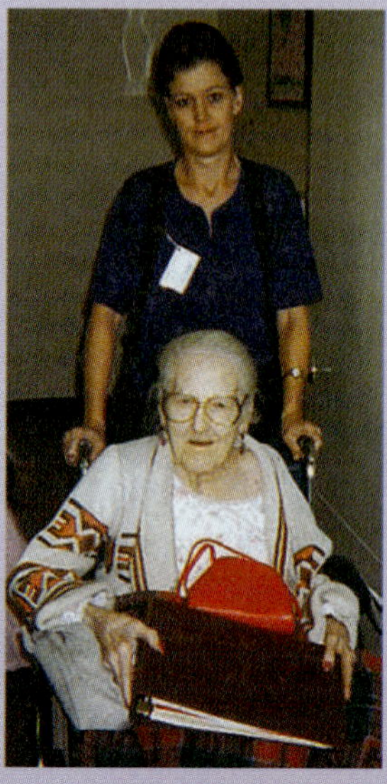

FIGURE 2-30 Transport the resident to her new room in a wheelchair and make her feel comfortable.

PROCEDURE 3

Discharging the Resident

1. Perform your beginning procedure actions.
2. Gather supplies needed: wheelchair, cart for resident's belongings, discharge slip (if used by your agency), clothing list or personal inventory, instructions and supplies provided by the nurse.
3. Collect the resident's belongings.
4. Check the belongings against the personal inventory or clothing list to ensure that the resident has all belongings.
5. Complete and have the resident sign the clothing inventory.
6. Assist with packing, if necessary.
7. Assist the resident to dress, if necessary.
8. Assist the resident to transfer to the wheelchair.
9. Check with the nurse to see if prescriptions, medications, or other supplies will be given to the resident before he or she leaves.
10. Transport the resident to the car. Assist the resident into the car.
11. Say goodbye to the resident.
12. Return to your unit.
13. Inform the nurse that the discharge has been completed, and report the resident's reaction and any other observations.
14. Strip the resident's unit and remove any permanent equipment from the room according to facility policy. Notify the environmental services department that the unit is ready to be cleaned.
15. Perform your procedure completion actions.

After the initial admission to the health care facility, the resident's needs may change. This may require a transfer to another unit within the facility. For example, the resident is admitted to a skilled nursing unit for intensive rehabilitation therapy. The resident makes good progress and is discharged from therapy. The resident is not receiving any other skilled services and does not need the high level of care provided in the skilled unit. The resident is transferred to another unit in the nursing facility.

Residents may become acutely ill and require transfer to the hospital for acute care. For example, a resident who has suffered a stroke is admitted to the acute care hospital. After the medical symptoms of the stroke have stabilized, the resident is transferred to a subacute care unit, rehabilitation center, or skilled nursing facility to complete the recovery. In this case the resident is discharged from one facility and admitted to another facility. This process is also called a "transfer," although you will be performing the procedure in the same manner as a discharge.

DISCHARGE

Discharge planning begins at the time of admission. Many members of the interdisciplinary team are involved with this process. In long-term care, the social worker also functions as a **discharge planner**. The social worker plans for discharge and is responsible for making arrangements with other community agencies, assisting with social and financial concerns, and providing continuity of care between the long-term care facility and the community. The social worker fills an important role throughout the resident's stay and during the discharge process.

When a resident is ready to leave the facility, you will perform the discharge procedure. This involves assisting the resident to gather personal belongings and escorting him or her to a waiting car or ambulance outside the facility. The nurse is responsible for resident teaching and providing discharge instructions before the resident leaves. You may be asked to assist with this process during routine care to ensure that the resident understands the instructions. For example, the resident who has a paralyzed arm will need to learn how to perform basic activities of daily living using the nonparalyzed arm. You will assist the resident to perform these procedures when you are assisting with bathing and other personal care. A correctly performed discharge will increase the resident's confidence in his or her ability to manage and adjust in the new location.

The physician must write an order for discharge. If the resident advises you that he or she is leaving without a physician order, inform the nurse immediately.

KEY POINTS

- The first impression that the resident has of the health care agency and its workers is a lasting one.
- The resident's perception of the admission process may be clouded by pain, illness, and fear.
- The nursing assistant is responsible for admitting the resident, gathering information, and making the resident comfortable.
- The nursing process involves assessment, planning, implementation, and evaluation.
- The nursing assistant makes valuable contributions to the nursing process.
- The family is an extension of the resident and will experience many emotions upon the resident's admission to a long-term care facility. A professional demeanor and good communication skills will help make the admission a positive experience.
- The nursing assistant is responsible for transferring the resident to a new unit within the health care facility and ensuring the resident's comfort before leaving the unit.
- A physician's order is required for discharge from the health care facility.
- The nursing assistant is responsible for gathering the resident's belongings and safely escorting the resident to the car.

REVIEW

A. Multiple Choice

Select the one best answer.

1. Which of the following statements is true?
   a. Sick residents do not care about first impressions.
   b. First impressions are important for family members only.
   c. First impressions are often lasting ones.
   d. Illness does not affect the resident's fear of admission.

2. An IV standard is the
   a. pump used to administer an intravenous feeding.
   b. metal pole that supports the IV pump, bottle, or bag.
   c. standard of care for administering IVs.
   d. bag that contains the intravenous fluid.

3. During the admission process, the nursing assistant is responsible for gathering the following assessment information
   a. vital signs, height, weight.
   b. food likes and dislikes.
   c. disease diagnoses.
   d. the resident's bedtime.

4. After you have admitted a resident, what should you do before leaving the room?
   a. Show the resident how to use the call signal.
   b. Call the nurse to the room.
   c. Always provide fresh water.
   d. Always put the resident to bed.

5. Which step of the nursing process involves gathering information?
   a. planning
   b. implementation

c. assessment
d. evaluation

6. Which step of the nursing process involves providing care to meet the resident's needs?

a. planning
b. implementation
c. assessment
d. evaluation

7. Which step of the nursing process involves analyzing information and developing a care plan?

a. planning
b. implementation
c. assessment
d. evaluation

8. Which step of the nursing process involves determining whether the care plan is working?

a. planning
b. implementation
c. assessment
d. evaluation

9. Discharge planning begins

a. at admission.
b. at discharge.
c. several days before discharge.
d. a month before discharge.

10. When discharging the resident, the nursing assistant is responsible for

a. taking vital signs, height, and weight.
b. safely escorting the resident to the car.
c. providing instructions on medications to use at home.
d. designing a discharge teaching plan.

11. Admitting a loved one to a long-term care facility

a. is usually an emotional time for family members.
b. is usually not an emotional experience.
c. often signifies unstable family relationships.
d. is not a significant event for stable families.

12. Which of the following is *not* an important characteristic when working with resident's families?

a. warmth and courtesy
b. having all the answers
c. kindness and respect
d. showing that you care

B. Clinical Applications

Answer the following questions.

13. Mrs. Davis has been a resident on the skilled nursing unit for three months. She has reached her maximum potential in therapy, and Medicare will no longer pay for her care. Mrs. Davis's daughter is transferring her to an assisted living facility for financial reasons. Mrs. Davis confides in you that she is nervous and scared about the transfer, because she does not know anyone at the assisted living facility. How can you assist the resident?
14. Mr. Truehart fell and fractured his hip. He has been transferred to the hospital in an ambulance. The nurse informs you that he will remain in the hospital for surgical hip repair. Mr. Truehart has a lock box containing some papers, a bank passbook, a few inexpensive rings, a watch, and $7.32. The box is unlocked on the nightstand in his room. What should you do?
15. The nurse informs you that a new resident will be admitted to room 732. The female resident will be on bed rest. She has a gastrostomy tube feeding. The nurse informs you that the resident is underweight and is at risk for pressure ulcers. How will you prepare the room for admission?
16. The new resident, Mrs. Brady, arrives in an ambulance at 1:15 p.m. Mrs. Brady is mentally confused, weak, and quiet. She is accompanied by her daughter. The EMTs transfer the resident to bed and leave the room. Mrs. Brady's daughter immediately starts complaining that she doesn't like the view out the window. She says she wanted her mother admitted to another nursing facility. However, her brother is the mother's legal guardian, and this is the facility he selected. What should the nursing assistant do?
17. Mr. Harris is being discharged from the nursing facility this afternoon. After you help him pack his clothing, he gives you a $20 bill for "being so nice" during his stay at the facility. What should you do?

UNIT 3

Infection Control

OBJECTIVES

After reading this unit, you will be able to:

- Spell and define key terms.
- Define medical asepsis and describe how it is used to prevent the spread of infection.
- List three ways that infection is spread.
- List eleven things you can do to prevent the spread of infection.
- Describe how bloodborne pathogens are spread and list measures to take to prevent the spread of bloodborne pathogens to yourself and others.
- Describe the three types of transmission-based precautions and explain when each type is used.
- Discuss infectious conditions that are seen in long-term care facilities.
- Describe how pathogens become drug resistant and explain why this is a problem.
- Describe how to recognize head lice and scabies and explain how each is treated.
- Define bioterrorism.
- Demonstrate procedures related to infection control.

OBSERVATIONS TO MAKE AND REPORT RELATED TO SIGNS AND SYMPTOMS OF INFECTION

New mental confusion or worsening mental confusion (may be the first sign of infection in elderly individuals)
Elevated temperature (elderly persons can be very ill, but have a normal or below-normal temperature; they do not always have a fever because of aging changes to the immune system)
Rapid pulse
Rapid respirations
Noisy respirations
Abnormally low blood pressure
Sweating
Chills
Skin hot or cold to touch
Skin color abnormal (flushed, red, gray, or blue)
Inflammation of skin (redness, swelling, heat, pain)
Drainage from any skin opening or body cavity
Any unusual body discharge, such as mucus or pus
Rash

Medical Asepsis

Infection is a state of illness caused by foreign organisms in the body. Preventing the spread of infection is an important responsibility. **Medical asepsis** is also called **infection control.** It involves practices that prevent the spread of infection in the long-term care facility. Infection control practices prevent the spread of infection to many people. These practices protect you and your family members, residents and their family members, other staff members, and visitors to the health care facility.

Nosocomial infection is a serious risk for health care facility workers and residents. A nosocomial infection is one that originates in the health care facility. Some infections are **localized** or confined to one area of the body. Signs of a localized infection are redness, swelling, and drainage at the site of the infection. An infection can also be **generalized.** A generalized infection is spread throughout the body. Signs of a generalized infection are fever, chills, pain, disorientation, fatigue, and nausea. Report any signs or symptoms of infection to the nurse.

The **immune system** is part of the circulatory system. It recognizes invading germs and works to eliminate them from the body. If the immune system recognizes a harmful microbe, the body's natural defenses are stimulated. The body then works to eliminate the organism and prevent infection. Some diseases weaken and destroy the immune system. **Susceptibility** is the body's ability to resist infection and is determined by age, presence of an underlying disease, health, nutritional state, and certain medications. When the immune system is weakened, the resident's body cannot defend well against invading organisms, and infection may occur. Elderly residents, those receiving cancer treatments, and others with certain diseases often have weakened immune systems.

Microorganisms are also called *microbes* (Figure 3.1). They are living organisms that cannot be seen with the eye. They are present everywhere in the environment. Some are harmless and do not cause disease. **Normal flora** are microbes that are helpful to the function of the body. For example, the normal flora in the digestive tract help break down food and turn it into waste products. However, when these organisms gain access to an area of the body where they do not belong, they may cause disease.

Pathogen are microbes that cause disease. **Bacteria** are microorganisms that can be eliminated with **antibiotics. Viruses** are tiny pathogens that cause many diseases and cannot be eliminated by antibiotics. However, many viral infections can be prevented by vaccines. We can destroy many pathogens in the environment by a process known as **disinfection.** This commonly involves scrubbing or soaking an item with a special chemical or cleaning agent. The item is then rinsed to remove all traces of the chemical. **Sterilization** eliminates all microbes and can be done by using heat, gas, or chemicals. An **antiseptic** is a product used to cleanse the skin and as a scrub to remove microorganisms before certain invasive procedures. Antiseptics should not be used on equipment or for cleaning environmental surfaces.

Spread of Infection

Infection is spread by many methods. The most common methods are by contact and in the air. The spread of infection by contact occurs in two different ways. Infections spread by **direct**

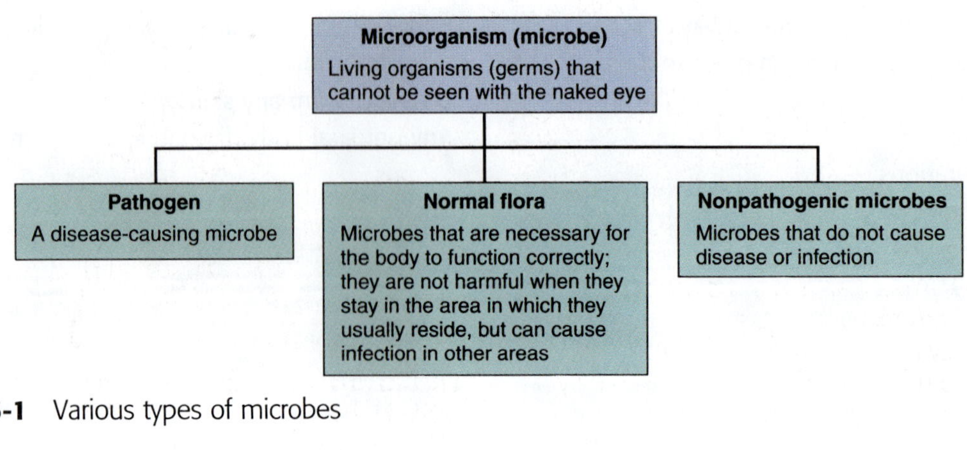

FIGURE 3-1 Various types of microbes

contact are caused by touching a resident or person who has the infection. A handshake is an example of direct contact. Your hands pick up the pathogen when you shake hands. If the pathogen can enter your body through broken skin or the mucous membranes of your eyes, nose, mouth, or genital area, an infection may develop. Pathogens may also be spread by **indirect contact.** This involves touching environmental surfaces and **fomites** such as linen, supplies, or equipment that have pathogens on them (Figure 3.2). You pick up the pathogen on your hands and spread it to the inside of your body through nonintact skin or by touching your mucous membranes.

Infection may also be spread by the **airborne** route. Pathogens spread by this method are very tiny and lightweight. They enter the air in respiratory **secretions.** Secretions are drainage from the body. In this case, mucus from the nose and mouth contains the pathogens. A cough or sneeze expels the pathogens into the air. Because they are so light, they travel long distances in the ventilation system, in dust, or on moisture particles in the air. Because of their weight, these pathogens do not drop to the ground quickly and are easily inhaled by others.

Pathogens may also enter the air and spread infection by the **droplet** method. Droplets are also respiratory secretions, such as those produced by sneezing or coughing. Pathogens spread by droplets are larger and heavier than those spread by the airborne method. Because of their size and weight, they usually do not spread beyond three feet from the **host** (Figure 3.3). Understanding the difference between the airborne and droplet methods of transmission is important so you can follow proper procedures to prevent infection from spreading.

Infections can also be spread by a **common vehicle.** Examples of common vehicles are food, water, or medication containing pathogens. The pathogens are taken into the body by eating and drinking.

Vectors (Figure 3.4) are insects and small animals that can carry pathogens.

Table 3.1 lists common ways microbes are spread.

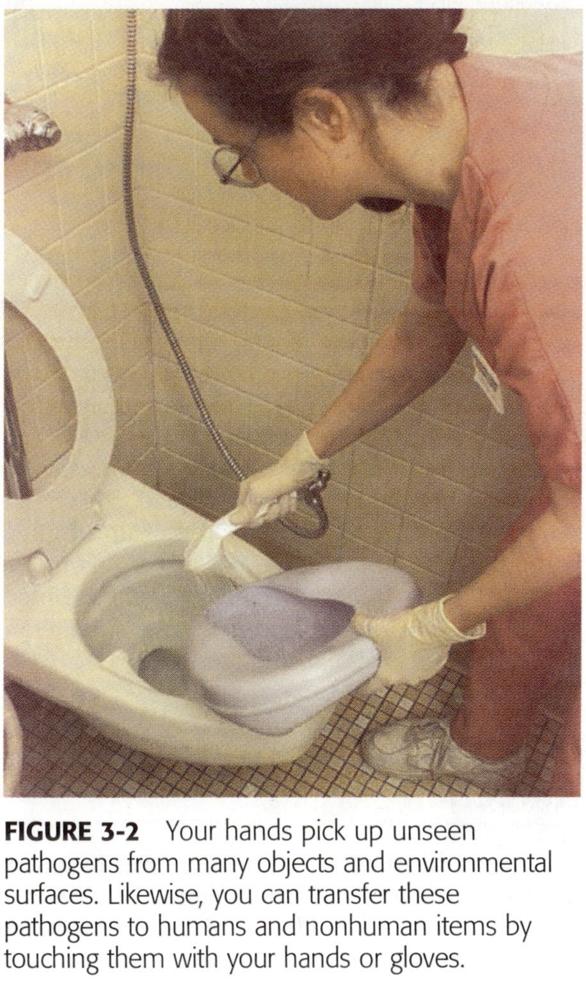

FIGURE 3-2 Your hands pick up unseen pathogens from many objects and environmental surfaces. Likewise, you can transfer these pathogens to humans and nonhuman items by touching them with your hands or gloves.

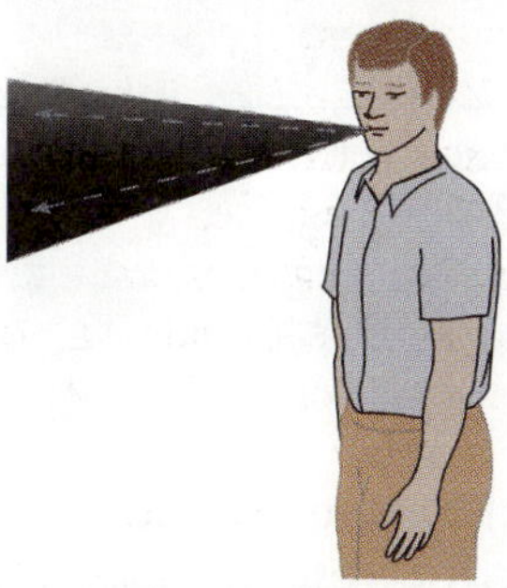

FIGURE 3-3 Droplets generated by sneezing do not usually spread more than three feet from the carrier (source of the infection).

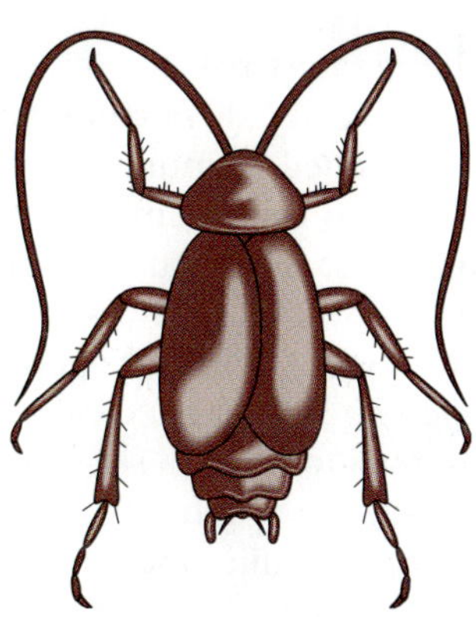

FIGURE 3-4 Vectors carry microbes from one place to another.

TABLE 3-1 Modes of Transmission of Microbes

Mode	Description
Airborne	Tiny microbes are carried by moisture or dust particles in air and are inhaled
Droplet	*Droplets spread* within approximately three feet (no personal contact). Droplets are larger and heavier than airborne microbes, so they cannot travel as far. Droplet nuclei are inhaled: • Coughing • Sneezing • Talking • Laughing • Singing
Contact	*Direct contact* of health care provider with resident: • Touching • Toileting (urine and feces) • Bathing • Secretions or excretions from patient • Rubbing • Blood, body fluid, mucous membranes, or nonintact skin
	Indirect contact of health care provider with objects used by residents: • Clothing • Bed linens • Personal belongings • Personal care equipment • Instruments and supplies used in treatments • Dressings • Diagnostic equipment • Permanent or disposable health care equipment • Environmental surfaces such as counters, faucets, and doorknobs
Common Vehicle	Spread to many people through contact with items such as: • Food • Water • Medication • Contaminated blood products
Vector-Borne	Intermediate hosts such as: • Flies • Fleas • Ticks • Rats • Mice • Roaches

Chain of Infection

The **chain of infection** (Figure 3.5) describes six factors necessary for an infection to develop. The **causative agent** is the germ that causes disease. The **mode of transmission** is the way in which the pathogen is spread. The **susceptible host** is the person who can become infected. Persons at the greatest risk for infection are the very young, the very old, persons with chronic diseases or weakened immune systems, people who are exposed to large numbers of pathogens, and individuals who do not use good hygiene or infection control practices. The **source** or **reservoir** is the place where the pathogen can grow. A **carrier** is a person who is infected with a disease that can be spread to others. The carrier may not know that he or she is infected. The **portal of entry** is where the microbe enters the body. Pathogens can enter through any opening, such as a tiny cut or crack in the skin. They can also enter through the mucous membranes of the eyes, nose, mouth, or genital area. The **portal of exit** is the way pathogens leave the body. This may be in excretions, secretions, or body fluids, such as urine, feces, saliva, tears, drainage from open wounds, blood, mucus, or respiratory fluids. If any part of the chain of infection is broken, the disease will not spread. Figure 3.5 shows breaks in each link of the chain of infection. Using one of the methods listed next to any link will break the chain and prevent an infection from developing. Table 3.2 lists some common elements in each link of the chain.

Preventing the Spread of Infection

You have learned that infective organisms are everywhere in the environment. You have an important responsibility to prevent the spread of infection. This is done in many ways.

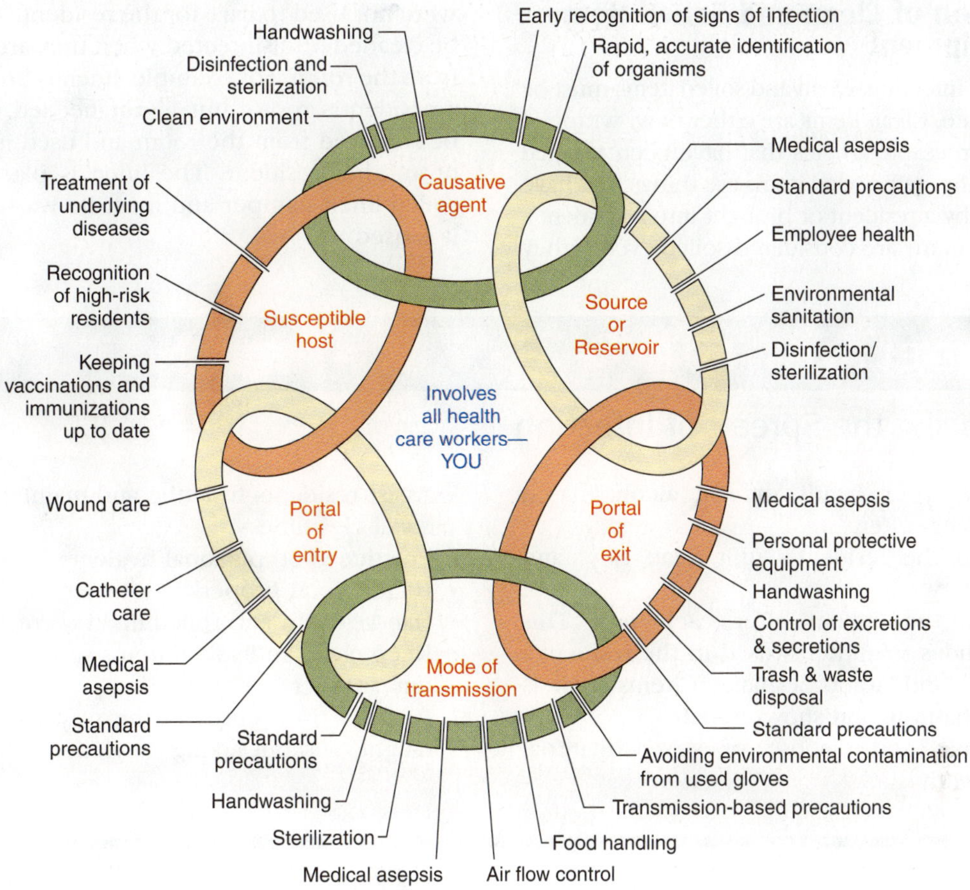

FIGURE 3-5 If one link in the chain is broken, the infection cannot be spread to others. This diagram shows the chain of infection, with examples of how health care workers can break each link of the chain.

TABLE 3-2 Elements in the Chain of Infection

Causative Agent	Source or Reservoir	Portal of Exit	Mode of Transmission	Portal of Entry	Susceptible Host
Bacteria	People	Blood	Direct contact	Mucous membranes	Chronic diseases
Fungi	Medicine	Moist body fluid	Indirect contact	Nonintact skin	Immuno-suppression
Viruses	Food	Droplets	Airborne	Urinary tract	Surgery
Parasites	Water	Secretions	Droplet	GI tract	Diabetes
	Equipment	Excretions	Fomites	Respiratory tract	Elderly residents
		Skin	Common vehicle	Blood	Burns
			Vectors	Body fluid	Cardiopulmonary disease

Separation of Clean and Soiled Items and Equipment

To prevent infection, clean and soiled items must be kept separate. Clean items are either new, wrapped articles or reusable articles that have been washed or cleaned by staff. Soiled items are things that have been used by a resident or brought into a resident's room. The items are considered soiled even if they were not used to care for the resident. They must be cleaned or disinfected when they are removed from the room. For example, linen is brought into a resident's room, but is not needed. It cannot be removed from the room and used in the care of another resident. The linen is placed in the soiled linen hamper and must be washed before it is used.

GUIDELINES FOR

Reducing the Spread of Infection

- Wash your hands or use alcohol-based cleaners often.
- Keep the resident's unit neat, tidy, and sanitary.
- Clean equipment after each use. This includes small items used in the resident's room and larger, permanent items such as the bathtub and shower chair.
- Handle and dispose of soiled material properly.
- Assist residents to bathe and maintain personal cleanliness.
- Practice good personal hygiene.
- Handle food properly.
- Handle clean and soiled linen correctly.
- Keep clean and soiled items separate from one another.
- Perform procedures in the way you were taught, without taking shortcuts.

GUIDELINES FOR

Separating Clean and Soiled Items

- Keep the food cart and clean linen cart separated from the housekeeping cart and soiled linen hamper by at least one room's width (Figure 3.6). The food cart and clean linen cart are clean items. The housekeeping cart and linen hamper are contaminated items.
- Remove the housekeeping cart from the hallway when food trays are being served. Many facilities also remove soiled linen hampers from the hallway when food is being served.
- Many long-term care facilities have pets. They should not enter areas where food is being prepared or served. Wash your hands after you touch a pet.
- Wash soiled items in the soiled utility room. After cleaning, move them to the clean utility room for storage. Be sure that items are dry before storing them.
- Bring only necessary linen and supplies into the resident's room. Avoid carrying these items next to your uniform.
- Avoid carrying trash, linen, or other contaminated items next to your uniform.

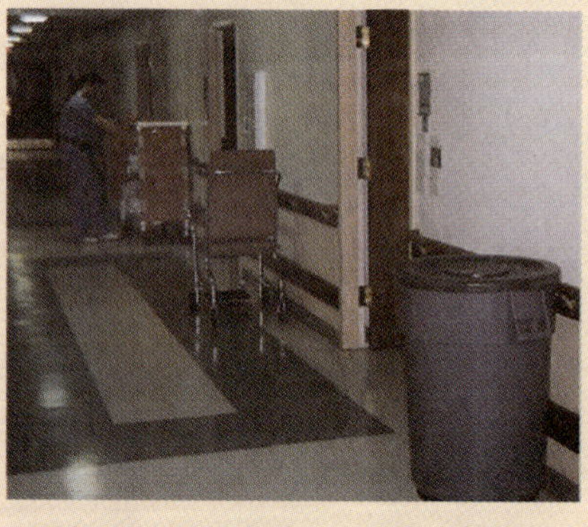

FIGURE 3-6 Keep clean and soiled items separated by at least one room's width in the hallway.

- Dispose of trash contaminated with blood or body fluid according to facility policy in covered containers in a special storage area.
- Wear gloves if needed to apply the principles of standard precautions when caring for residents. Wash your hands before applying gloves. Use gloves for the care of one resident only. After each resident, remove the gloves and wash your hands again.
- Gloves are contaminated after resident contact. Avoid contaminating clean supplies, linen, equipment, or environmental surfaces with them. You can do this by removing one glove and using your ungloved hand for touching other items or by placing a clean paper towel under one glove and contacting environmental surfaces with the towel.
- Dispose of used gloves according to facility policy. Generally they are not discarded in the open waste-basket in the resident's room. Some facilities place extra plastic bags in the bottom of the wastebasket. If you must put soiled gloves and other contaminated items into the wastebasket, remove the bag containing the contaminated items, tie it, and take it with you when you leave the room. Replace it with a new bag from the bottom of the wastebasket.
- Follow facility policy for covering soiled items in the hallway during transport. If use of gloves is necessary, remove one glove. Carry the soiled item in the gloved hand (Figure 3.7). Use the ungloved hand to turn on faucets, open doors, and touch items considered clean. Follow the same procedure when emptying bedpans and urinals in resident bathrooms. Use the ungloved hand to open the door, turn on faucets, and flush the toilet.
- Cover bedpans and urinals when you are carrying them.
- Lab specimens are never stored in the refrigerator with food or beverages. A separate, specially marked refrigerator or cooler should be used.

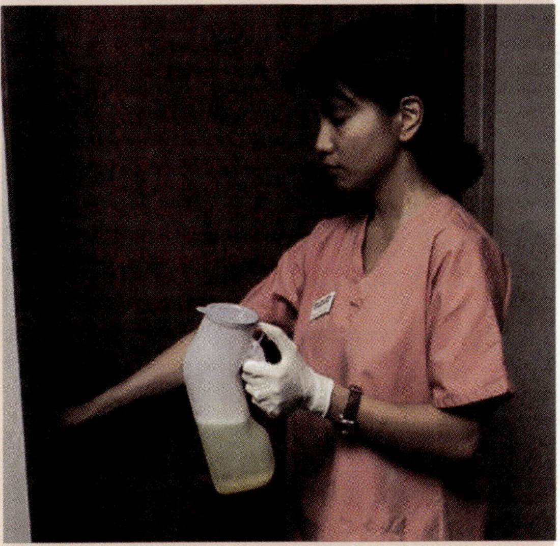

FIGURE 3-7 The one-glove technique is used for disposing of contaminated items and avoiding environmental contact with and contamination from used gloves. Remove the glove from one hand and carry it in the other hand with the soiled item. Use the ungloved hand to open doors, turn on faucets, pull up side rails, and so forth. If you cannot remove one glove, hold a paper towel under your gloved hand to contact environmental surfaces.

- Follow your assignment and facility cleaning schedule for washing and disinfecting resident care items. Special cleaners are used to disinfect reusable items. The friction created by wiping is important to remove microorganisms. Make sure supplies are completely dry before storing them. Store clean supplies in an area designated for clean items. You may be asked to date and initial items after they are cleaned.
- When working in rooms with two or more beds, clearly mark each resident's drinking glass and water pitcher, bedpan, urinal, emesis basin, and personal care items so that they are not accidentally mixed up.
- Use liquid soap whenever possible. Keep residents' individual bars of soap separated. Soap should be stored in a container that allows water to drain away from the bottom of the bar.

(continues)

GUIDELINES FOR

Separating Clean and Soiled Items, *continued*

- Cover food and beverages when you carry them in the hallway.
- Monitor resident rooms for snacks and other food items, which should be stored in a sealed package or covered container. Make sure the items can be safely stored unrefrigerated.
- Additional guidelines for handling of clean and soiled linen are listed in Unit 8.

Hand Hygiene

In the health care facility, many infections are spread on the hands (Figures 3.8A and B). Because of this, special attention is given to hand hygiene. Keep the skin on your hands in good condition. Outside of the facility, wear gloves when performing tasks, such as gardening or washing dishes, that put the hands at risk of injury. Use hand lotion in moderation to keep the skin supple and prevent drying and irritation. Many facilities do not permit caregivers to wear artificial fingernails of any type, including nail tips, overlays, silk wraps, gels, sculptured, or acrylic nails. Long nails (beyond the fingertips) are also not usually permitted. Keep natural nail tips less than 1/4-inch long. Long and artificial nails have been proven to hold microbes and increase the risk of infection. They are difficult to clean and may cause gloves to tear. Avoid chipped nail polish as well. Chips and cracks in nail polish also hide germs. Wear only simple rings, such as a plain wedding band. Rings with many stones and elaborate settings can also hold harmful pathogens, and are difficult to clean. Microbes may also hide under the rings. The stones and settings on rings may also tear gloves.

Handwashing is the most important method used to prevent the spread of infection. You can pick up microbes on your hands and introduce them to your own body. You can also transfer the microbes on your hands to residents. If your hands touch a clean object, the microbes on your hands may be transferred there. This is a potential source of indirect contact transmission.

Quickly rinsing the hands with water, then drying them on a towel, does not remove germs. Oils on your skin must be washed away, along with attached germs. This can be done only by using warm water, soap, and friction. You must spend enough time to wash the germs away. The purpose of handwashing is to clean the hands and prevent microorganisms from spreading. Handwashing should take a minimum of 15 seconds. If your hands are visibly soiled, you will need to take longer. The longer the handwashing, the more microbes are eliminated. The most important part of the handwashing procedure is the friction caused by rubbing your hands together. The friction removes the microbes from your hands.

Rules for Handwashing

Never wash your gloved hands. Handwashing damages the gloves so that they will not protect you. Remove gloves, wash your hands, and then reapply a clean pair of gloves.

1. Avoid leaning against the sink during the handwashing procedure. The inside of the sink and the faucet handles are contaminated. The outside of the sink may contaminate your uniform.
2. Avoid splashing your uniform when washing your hands.
3. Keep your fingertips pointed down during the handwashing procedure.
4. Bar soap can hold microorganisms on its surface. Use liquid soap whenever possible.
5. Turn the faucets on and off with a clean, dry paper towel.

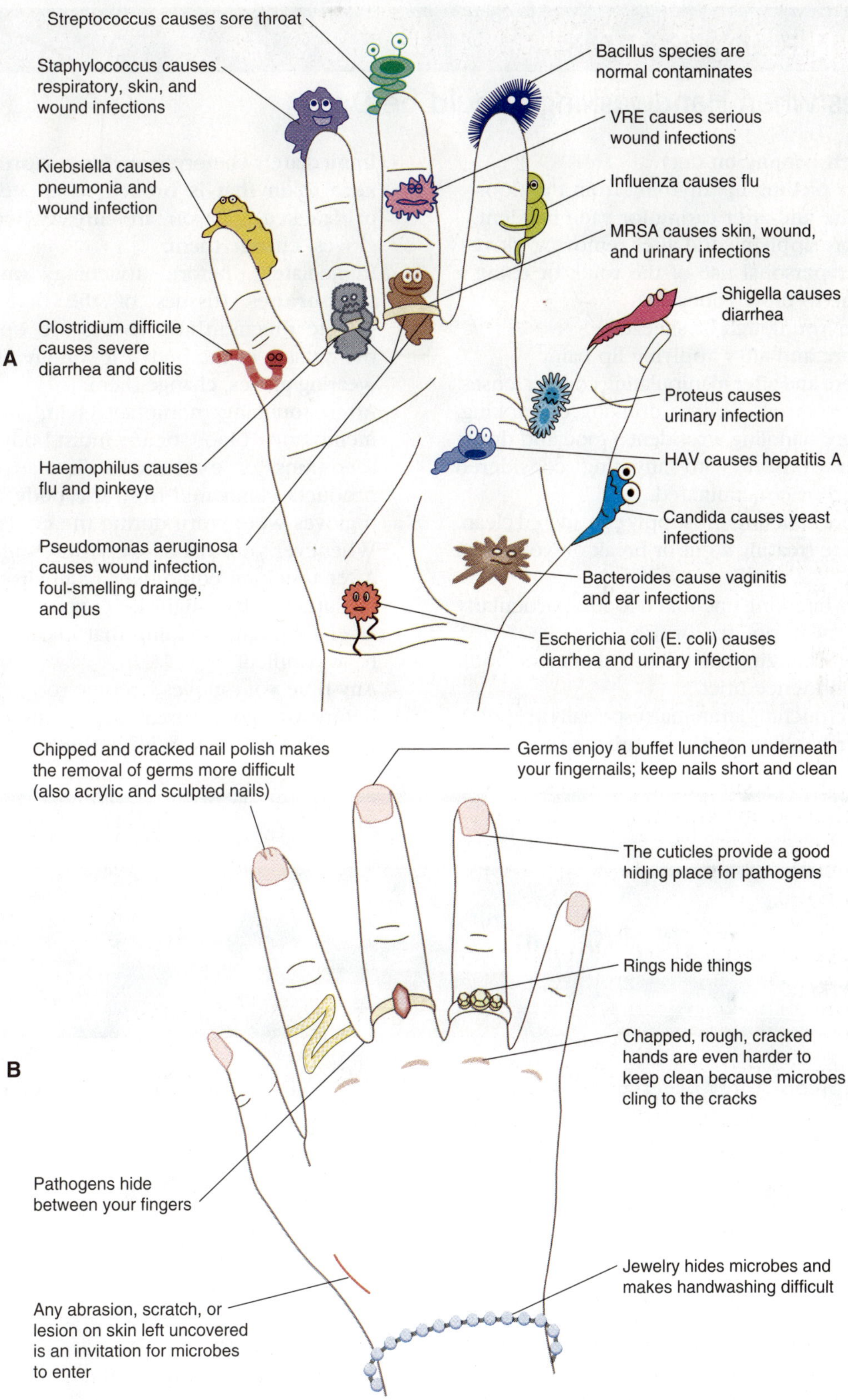

FIGURE 3-8 (A) Many infections are spread on the hands, so health care workers must pay close attention to good hand hygiene and eliminating areas where pathogens can hide. (B) Jewelry with many stones or complicated settings provides a hiding place for pathogens. Long fingernails, chipped nail polish, and acrylic nails also provide hiding places for microbes. Chapped, cut, cracked hands increase the risk of contracting an infection.

GUIDELINES FOR

Times when Handwashing Should be Done

- When coming on duty.
- After picking up anything from the floor.
- Before and after caring for each resident.
- Before applying and after removing gloves.
- After personal use of the toilet or using a tissue to blow your nose.
- After you cough or sneeze.
- Before and after applying lip balm.
- Before and after manipulating contact lenses.
- Before and after eating, drinking, or smoking.
- Before handling a resident's food and drink.
- After contact with anything considered soiled or contaminated.
- Before handling any supply considered clean.
- Before treating a cut or break on your own skin.
- After handling uncooked foods, particularly raw meat, poultry, or fish.
- After changing an infant's diaper or adult incontinence brief.
- After touching an animal (especially a reptile).
- After handling trash or garbage.
- Immediately before touching **nonintact skin** (skin that is broken, chapped, cut, or cracked); if you are already wearing gloves, change them.
- Immediately before touching **mucous membranes** (tissues of the body that secrete mucus; these tissues are open to the outside of the body); if you are already wearing gloves, change them.
- After touching nonintact skin, mucous membranes, blood, or any moist body fluid, secretions, or **excretions** (human waste products eliminated from the body), even if gloves were worn during the contact.
- Whenever your hands are visibly soiled.
- After touching equipment or environmental surfaces that might be contaminated.
- After touching anything that many people have handled.
- Any time your gloves become torn.
- Before you go on break and at the end of your shift before you leave the facility.

PROCEDURE 4

Handwashing

1. Turn on warm water using a paper towel.
2. Wet your hands. Keep your fingertips pointed down.
3. Apply soap from the dispenser.
4. Rub your hands together vigorously to create a lather. Rub the hands together in a circular motion for at least 15 seconds. Rub all surfaces of the hands. Pay particular attention to the area between your fingers. Keep your fingertips pointed down (Figure 3.9).
5. Rub the fingernails against the palm of the opposite hand. Clean the nails with a brush or an orange stick if they are soiled.

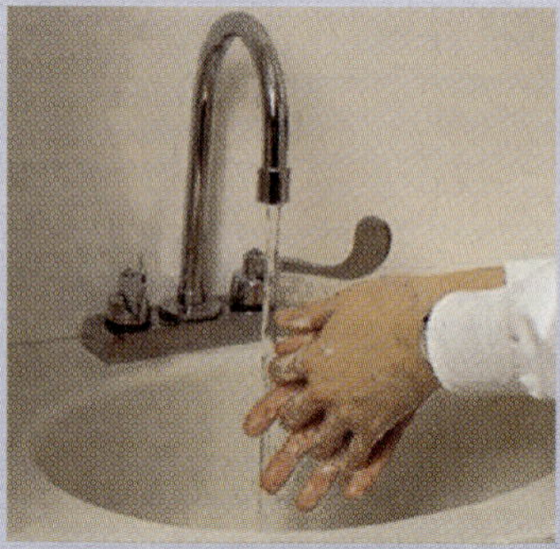

FIGURE 3-9 Keep your fingertips pointed down to prevent contaminants from rolling down your hands and arms.

6. Rinse your hands from the wrist to the fingertips. Keep the fingers pointed down.
7. Dry your hands with a paper towel.
8. Use a clean, dry paper towel to turn off the faucet (Figure 3.10). Do not touch the faucet handle with your hand.
9. Discard the paper towel.
   Note: Avoid touching the sink with your body or clothing during this procedure. Avoid splashing water onto your clothing.

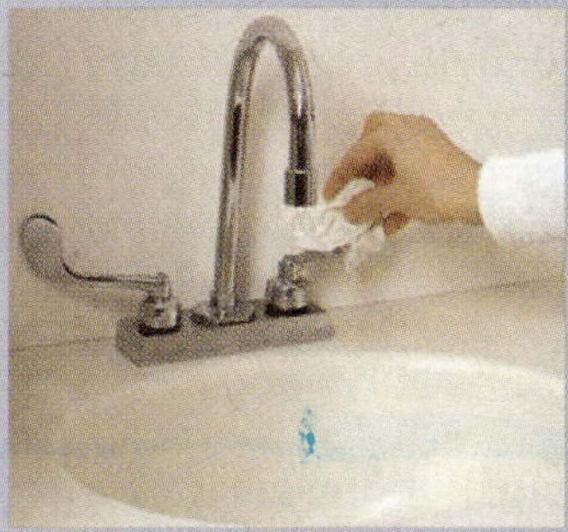

FIGURE 3-10 The faucet is contaminated with microbes deposited when people with unclean hands turned the water on. Use a paper towel to turn it off, to avoid picking up unwelcome guests on your clean hands.

Waterless Hand Cleaners

Many facilities provide dispensers containing waterless hand cleaners (Figure 3.11) in various locations in the facility. The hand cleaners contain an alcohol-based gel, lotion, or foam that is dispensed in small dime- to quarter-sized portions (approximately 2 to 3 mL). Alcohol-based products are often less irritating to the hands than washing repeatedly with soap. Most alcohol solutions contain moisturizers that prevent drying of the skin. In addition, paper towels are not necessary when alcohol products are used. Paper towels contain wood fibers that can be very irritating to sensitive skin.

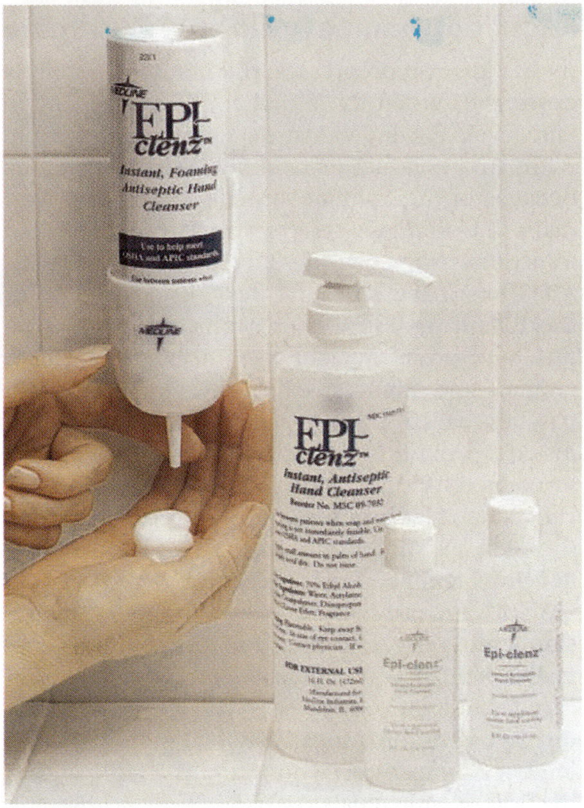

FIGURE 3-11 Alcohol-based hand cleaners may safely be used instead of washing at the sink unless your hands are contaminated with a protein substance. (*Courtesy of Medline, Industries, Inc. 1-800-MEDLINE*)

Each facility has directions for using waterless hand cleaners and policies and procedures for when the product may be used. A waterless hand cleaner may safely be used instead of handwashing during routine resident care. However, washing at the sink should be done any time the hands are visibly soiled.

To use the waterless cleaning product, dispense the proper amount into the palm of your hand. Rub the product into the hands until it dries, making sure to rub all areas and surfaces, including the nail beds and between the fingers. This should take at least 15 seconds. Become familiar with the products used by your facility and their applications. They are very effective in reducing infection and eliminating pathogens from the hands.

Bloodborne Pathogens

Bloodborne pathogens are microbes that cause disease through contact with blood, non-intact skin, mucous membranes, secretions, excretions, or any moist body fluid except sweat. Many diseases can be transmitted by contact with these substances. **Hepatitis B,hepatitis C, human immunodeficiency virus (HIV) disease,** and **acquired immune deficiency syndrome (AIDS)** are diseases that are commonly spread through contact with blood and body fluids.

Hepatitis

Hepatitis means "inflammation of the liver." It can be caused by a number of factors, including drugs, toxins, autoimmune disease, and infectious agents (viruses). Six main types of viral hepatitis are prevalent in the United States. Table 3.3 summarizes the various types of hepatitis.

Hepatitis B. Hepatitis B is a virus that causes an infection of the liver. This disease can cause liver damage, liver cancer, and death. Individuals with hepatitis B may have no symptoms at all, but may still be infectious. These people are carriers of the disease. The presence of the hepatitis B virus (HBV) can be diagnosed only by a blood test. You probably cannot tell that the carrier is sick by his or her appearance. Some people may be sick with mild symptoms that mimic the flu. Common symptoms of hepatitis B are fever, aches and pains, nausea, and fatigue. Urine may turn dark in color. The skin, mucous membranes, and white area of the eyes may appear **jaundiced,** or yellow in color. A person can transmit the disease even after recovering from the symptoms. Many people who have had hepatitis B have permanent liver damage and are disabled for life.

Hepatitis C. Hepatitis C is transmitted in the same manner as HIV and hepatitis B. There are also documented cases of transmission from unclean medical instruments. Hepatitis C is primarily a disease of the liver, but can also affect the white blood cells. At first, hepatitis C may be mistaken for the flu. Common signs and symptoms are extreme fatigue, depression, fever, mood changes, and weakness. There are many other signs and symptoms, ranging from pain to loss of appetite. Hepatitis C may cause liver cancer and liver failure. People with hepatitis C may have the disease for years and not know it. Even though the infected person is unaware of it, the disease is silently destroying the liver. The hepatitis C virus (HCV) changes constantly, so finding a treatment is difficult. Presently there is only one approved treatment for hepatitis C in the United States, and it does not work for all patients. Hepatitis C is the leading cause of the need for liver transplants in the United States. Many patients die waiting for a transplant.

Human Immunodeficiency Virus Disease

Human immunodeficiency virus is the virus that causes HIV disease and AIDS. An infected person is called "HIV-positive," or "HIV3." A newer term for this is to say that the individual has HIV disease. Most, but not all, people with HIV disease develop AIDS over time. After exposure to HIV, a person may have no symptoms at all. Sometime between one week and six months later, the exposed person may develop fever and flu-like symptoms. When this occurs, the blood converts from HIV-negative to HIV-positive. This can be very confusing, because some individuals can go for longer periods before the blood converts from negative to positive. Some people convert from negative to positive, but do not experience the flu-like symptoms. These people do not know that they are HIV-positive. The only way to know for sure is to get a blood test. Once a person converts to HIV-positive, it may take six to ten years or more for AIDS to develop. The HIV-positive person becomes a lifelong carrier and can spread the virus to others.

Acquired Immune Deficiency Syndrome

As HIV disease progresses, the immune system is destroyed. When the blood count reaches a certain level, the individual develops AIDS. People with AIDS contract many illnesses and infections because of the immune system destruction. Normally the immune system would prevent these infections from causing illness. A person with AIDS may have a chronic fever and swelling of the lymph nodes, particularly in the neck, armpits, and groin. Weight loss, diarrhea, extreme fatigue, and night sweats are common. White patches called thrush (Figure 3.12) may form inside the mouth and throat. Occasionally, Kaposi's sarcoma develops (Figure 3.13). This is a form of cancer in which raised, purple spots appear on the skin and internal organs. Many individuals develop chronic herpes (Figure 3.14). People with advanced AIDS may develop mental confusion, emotional problems, and loss of motor control. When these individuals enter the long-term care facility, they are often in the end stage of the disease. Caring for them may be emotionally trying because many are young adults. Staff may feel that these individuals are too young to die and have not had a chance at life. Some have young families and children. When caring for residents with AIDS, the staff must support each other and may need outside resources to help them deal with their feelings about the disease. AIDS was

TABLE 3-3 Types of Hepatitis

Type	Mode of Transmission	Signs & Symptoms	Vaccine	U.S. statistics	Treatment	Comments
Hepatitis A	Oral/fecal; on hands or transferred to food	Abdominal pain, loss of appetite fatigue, nausea, diarrhea, dark urine, jaundice	Vaccine available; immune globulin used for short term immunity	125,000 to 200,000 cases and approxi mately 100 deaths annually	Bed rest and limited activity for up to 30 days	usually lasts less than two months; not a chronic condition
Hepatitis B	Blood and body fluid; mother to fetus	Abdominal pain, loss of appetite, fatigue, nausea, diarrhea, dark urine, jaundice	Vaccine available	140,000 to 320,000 total infections; approximately 5,000 to 6,000 deaths annually	Most recover within 6 months; for chronic cases, interferon	More than 1 million chronically in-fected; can lead to cirrhosis or liver cancer
Hepatitis C	Blood and body fluid; mother to fetus	Most asymptomatic; abdominal pain, loss of appetite, fatigue, nausea, diarrhea, dark urine, jaundice	None	28,000 to 180,000 total infections; approximately 10,000 deaths annually	Interferon;effective in approximately 33% of patients	Approximately 4 million chronically infected; can lead to cirrhosis or liver cancer. Leading cause of liver transplant in U.S. Many carriers are asymptomatic for years before learning of infection
Hepatitis D	Blood and body fluid	Abdominal pain, loss of appetite, fatigue, nausea, diarrhea, dark urine, jaundice	Hepatitis B vaccine	Approximately 5,000 infections annually	Interferon may be effective in some patients	Develops only in the presence of hepatitis B or acquired simultaneously with HBV; few chronic cases. 70% to 80% develop cirrhosis
Hepatitis E	Oral/fecal; contaminated water	Abdominal pain, loss of appetite, fatigue, nausea, diarrhea, dark urine, jaundice	None	Rare in U.S.	Rest, limited activity for 2 weeks	Almost all U.S. cases are in travelers returning from high-risk areas (primarily Mexico, Asia, Africa); few chronic cases
Hepatitis G	Blood	Most patients are asymptomatic	None	900 to 2,000 cases annually	Rest	Serious disease rare

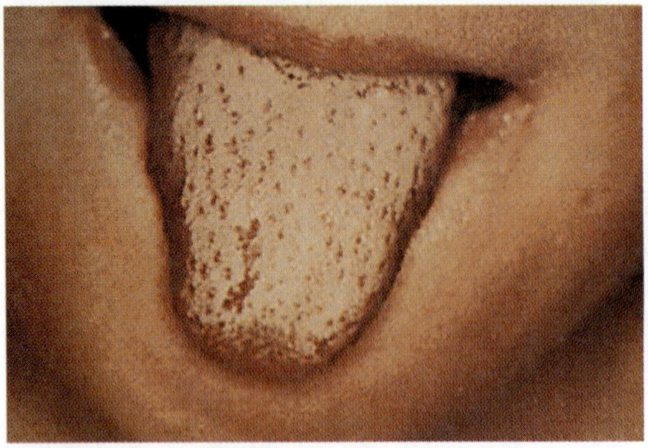

FIGURE 3-12 Oral thrush in an AIDS patient. *(Courtesy of Daniel J. Barbaro, MD, Fort Worth, Texas)*

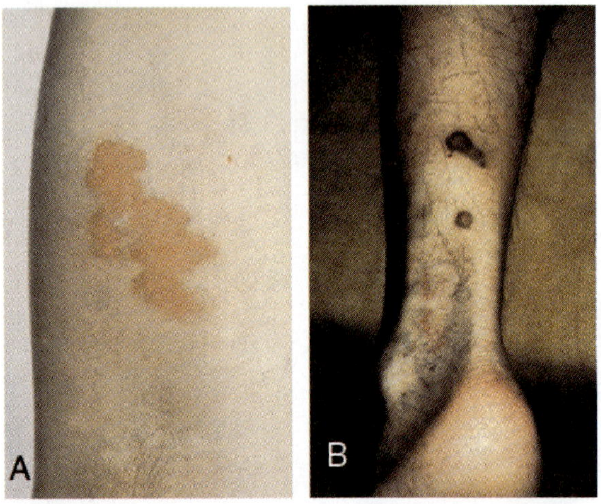

FIGURE 3-13 (A) Typical purple lesions caused by Kaposi's sarcoma. (B) Raised Kaposi's sarcoma lesions. *(Courtesy of Daniel J. Barbaro, MD, Fort Worth, Texas)*

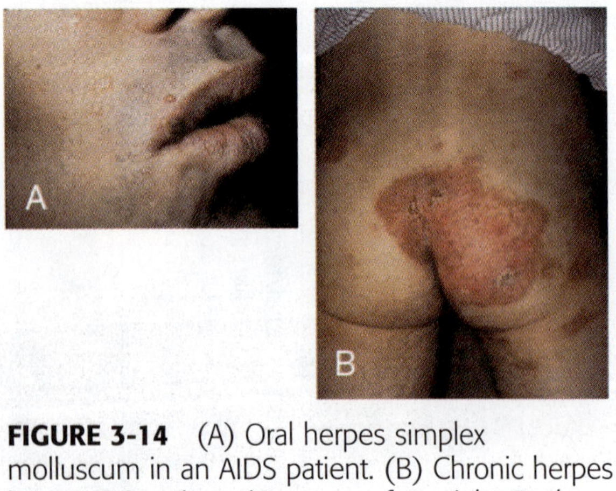

FIGURE 3-14 (A) Oral herpes simplex molluscum in an AIDS patient. (B) Chronic herpes in an AIDS patient. *(Courtesy of Daniel J. Barbaro, MD, Fort Worth, Texas)*

previously the main cause of death in males between the ages of 25 and 44. With new advances in care and treatment, it is now the second-leading cause of death in this age group. Nevertheless, AIDS continues to take a great many lives and remains a very serious public health concern.

AIDS is seen in all races and socioeconomic groups. State and federal laws prohibit discrimination against people with AIDS. Some health care workers have contracted the HIV virus at work, but the total number of work-related cases is small. Estimating the number of new AIDS cases each year is very difficult. In 2001, a total of 43,158 new cases had been reported. An estimated 344,178 persons with HIV were living in the United States. Remember that AIDS is *not the same* as HIV disease. The best way to prevent HIV disease and AIDS is to know how the disease is transmitted. Hepatitis B, hepatitis C, and HIV are transmitted in the same manner. Methods of transmission are listed in Table 3.4. Take measures to protect yourself both at work and in your personal life.

Treatment

Over the past few years, great strides have been made in treating HIV disease and AIDS. A laboratory test called the viral load is used as an indicator of when and how to medicate. By monitoring the viral load, the physician knows when to begin medications and when to change the drug regi-

TABLE 3-4 Methods of HIV, HBV and HCV Transmission
Heterosexual and homosexual sexual intercourse
Sharing needles and other paraphernalia with IV drug users
Occupational exposure through direct or indirect contact with blood and body fluids of an infected person
Transfusion with contaminated blood or blood products
Mother-to-infant transmission, prenatally or through breastfeeding
Tattooing and body piercing with unclean instruments
Sharing household items such as razors and toothbrushes with infected individuals

men. Several different types of drugs are used in combination to treat the HIV virus in the body. These drugs do not eliminate the disease. Treatment is geared to controlling symptoms. The combination drug therapy is effective in many individuals because each drug works on a different part of the HIV virus in the body. The drugs control new virus that is produced in the body each day. They do not reverse damage that was done before drug therapy was started. Taking the drugs exactly as ordered is important because the HIV virus can become drug resistant in a very short time. Following directions exactly increases the time the individual will benefit from drugs, before resistance develops. Because of progress in treating the HIV virus, HIV disease and AIDS are now viewed as chronic, manageable diseases rather than fatal illnesses.

Risk Factors for Diseases Spread by Bloodborne Pathogens

Because hepatitis B, hepatitis C, and HIV are spread by blood and body fluid contact, the diseases are seen in heterosexual, homosexual, and bisexual individuals. People who use intravenous drugs and share needles are at particularly high risk. Children born to mothers who are infected may also develop the disease. People who received blood between 1978 and 1984 may have contracted HIV from the blood transfusion. Since 1984, donor blood has been routinely tested for HIV. You cannot contract HIV by donating blood at a blood bank or hospital.

You can contract HIV, HBV, and HCV by contacting the virus through your nonintact skin. This means that cut or chapped skin touches blood, body fluid, secretions, excretions, or nonintact skin containing the virus. The virus can also be passed by contact with the mucous membranes of the eyes, nose, mouth, and genital area. You cannot contract the virus through casual contact or airborne transmission.

HBV is much more contagious than HIV. Imagine that $^{1}/_{4}$ teaspoon of HBV is mixed into a 24,000-gallon swimming pool of water. Someone draws a quarter teaspoon of that water into a syringe and injects you with it. Although the virus is extremely diluted, you will become HBV-positive. Now imagine that 10 people are in the room. Someone takes $^{1}/_{4}$ teaspoon of HIV and mixes it into a quart of water. Each person is injected with $^{1}/_{4}$ teaspoon of this solution. Only one person in the room will become HIV-positive. Hepatitis B, then, is a much greater threat to health care workers than HIV. We now know that some people do not contract HIV because of certain elements within their cells. These elements are not easy to identify, however, so everyone must assume that they can contract the disease and take the proper precautions. A vaccine is available to prevent hepatitis B. If your job involves handling blood or body fluids routinely, your employer is required to provide you with the vaccination free of charge. The vaccine is given in a series of three injections over several months. Presently, there is no vaccine to prevent hepatitis C, HIV disease, or AIDS.

Each health care facility is required to have an **exposure control plan,** which is a written program that describes what to do if you contact blood or body fluid. Immediately wash the area thoroughly. Report accidental contact with blood or body fluid to the nurse immediately. You will be treated according to the established plan, have blood samples taken, and may begin drug therapy to prevent a blood-borne disease from developing. Medical care and monitoring will continue over a long period of time.

Protecting Yourself and Others from Exposure to Bloodborne Pathogens by Using Standard Precautions

Health care workers can take measures to prevent the spread of infection to themselves and others. These measures are called **standard precautions** (Figure 3.15). The purpose of using standard precautions is to prevent the spread of infection. We cannot tell whether someone has a disease or infection by appearance, so standard precautions are used in the care of all residents regardless of their disease or diagnosis. Standard precautions are based on the assumption that all blood and body fluids are potentially infectious. Many individual infection factors are very difficult to control. Standard precautions are directed mainly at preventing the transmission of microbes. Standard precautions effectively prevent the spread of many diseases besides HIV disease, AIDS, and hepatitis B and C.

Standard precautions include the use of **personal protective equipment (PPE)** when performing certain tasks. Personal protective equipment consists of garments and apparel that protect the health care worker from contracting a disease from a resident. It also protects the resident from contracting a disease from a microbe passed from the worker's hands.

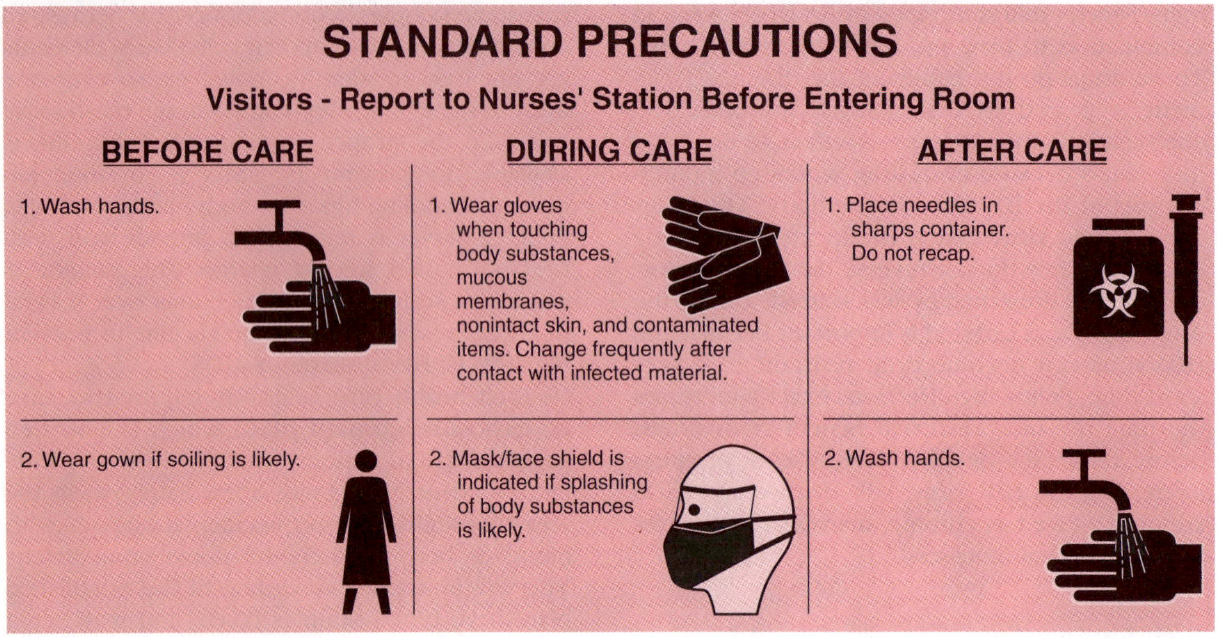

FIGURE 3-15 Standard precautions are used in the care of all residents, regardless of disease or diagnosis. (*Courtesy of Briggs Corporation, Des Moines, IA 800-247-2343*)

Selection and Use of Personal Protective Equipment

Standard precautions are used anytime the health care worker anticipates contact with blood or any moist body fluid (except sweat), secretions, or excretions. They are also used anytime you will have mucous membrane contact. Mucous membranes are found in the eyes, nose, mouth, and genital area. If either you or the resident has nonintact or broken skin, PPE is also used. There are many variables in resident care situations, so there are no absolute rules for the use of PPE. The nursing assistant must think about the situation and use good judgment. You are responsibile for applying the principles of standard precautions and selecting the PPE according to the task to be done. Equipment is worn during some direct resident care activities. Table 3.5 will guide you in selecting PPE for common tasks. Personal protective equipment is also worn during cleaning procedures when contact with blood, body fluids, secretions, or excretions is likely.

Personal protective equipment will protect you only if it fits properly, if it is free from defects, and if you use it regularly in the way you were taught. Never use equipment that is torn or has defects. You must study and learn the principles of standard precautions so you can apply them correctly. It is your responsibility to use standard precautions to protect yourself and facility residents. Always follow the infection control policies and procedures for your facility.

Rules for Standard Precautions

Certain common procedures apply to using standard precautions in resident care. You must anticipate and select the correct type of PPE and use handwashing before and after every procedure.

Handwashing. Handwashing or use of alcohol-based hand cleaners must be done before all resident care and procedures. It is also done before applying and after removing gloves. It is possible to pick up a microbe on your hands even when you are wearing gloves. Sometimes this occurs because of microscopic defects in the gloves. It is also possible to unknowingly contact microbes when your gloves are removed. Handwashing is also done immediately if your hands contact blood or any moist body fluid except sweat. Handwashing is performed at the end of each procedure, after gloves are removed.

Barrier precautions. Personal protective equipment is also called *barrier equipment.* Using barrier precautions involves wearing gloves for handling or touching blood, any moist body fluid (except sweat), secretions, excretions, mucous membranes, or nonintact skin. If your gloves

TABLE 3-5 Examples of Personal Protective Equipment in Basic Resident Care

Resident Care Task	Gloves	Gown	Goggles/ Face Sheild	Surgical Mask
Controlling bleeding when blood is squirting	Yes	Yes	Yes	Yes
Wiping a wheelchair, shower chair, or bathtub with disinfectant solution	Yes	No	No	No
Emptying a catheter bag	Yes	Yes, if facility policy	Yes, if facility policy	Yes, if facility policy
Serving a meal tray	No	No	No	No
Giving a back rub to a resident who has intact skin	No	No	No	No
Brushing a resident's teeth	Yes	No	No	No
Helping the dentist with a procedure	Yes	Yes, if facility policy	Yes	Yes
Cleaning a resident and changing the bed after an episode of diarrhea	Yes	Yes	No	No
Changing a bed in which the linen is not visibly soiled	No, or follow facility policy. if gloves are worn for removing soiled linen, remove and wash hands before handling clean linen	No	No	No
Taking an oral temperature with a glass thermometer (gloves are not necessary with an electronic thermometer)	Yes	No	No	No
Taking a rectal temperature	Yes	No	No	No
Taking a blood pressure	No	No	No	No
Cleaning soiled utensils, such as bedpans	Yes	Yes, if splashing is likely	Yes, if splashing is likely	Yes, if splashing is likely
Shaving a resident with a disposable razor	Yes, because of the high risk of this procedure for contact with blood	No	No	No
Giving eye care	Yes	No	No	No
Giving special mouth care to an unconscious resident	Yes	No, unless coughing is likely	No, unless coughing is likely	No, unless coughing is likely

(continues)

TABLE 3-5 *(continued)*

Resident Care Task	Gloves	Gown	Goggles/ Face Sheild	Surgical Mask
Washing the resident's genital area	Yes	No	No	No
Washing the resident's arms and legs when the skin is not broken	No	No	No	No

Notes: There are exceptions to every rule. Use this chart as a guideline only. Add personal protective equipment if special situations, such as possible splashing, exist. Follow your facility policies on use of PPE routine tasks.

become visibly soiled, you should remove them, wash your hands, and apply a clean pair of gloves. When using barrier precautions, you should remove your gloves, wash your hands, and reapply clean gloves *immediately* before contact with mucous membranes and nonintact skin. You may have to change your gloves and wash your hands several times during the care of one resident. Change gloves:

- Before each resident contact
- After each resident contact
- *Immediately before* touching mucous membranes
- *Immediately before* touching nonintact skin
- After you touch a resident's secretions or excretions, before moving to care for another part of the body
- After touching blood or body fluids, before moving to care for another part of the body
- After touching contaminated environmental surfaces or equipment
- Anytime your gloves become visibly soiled
- If your gloves become torn

Your facility is required to have barrier equipment available in a variety of sizes in locations where use can be reasonably anticipated. Gloves (Figure 3.16) are also worn for touching dressings, tissues, infective items, and contaminated surfaces or equipment. Do not carry glove use to extremes. Use gloves when necessary, but do not use them for all resident contact. Using gloves at all times sends a negative message. It says that the resident is untouchable. Touching is very important to all human beings. Gloves should be used only when contact with blood, body fluids, secretions, excretions, mucous membranes, or nonintact skin is likely. Gloves are also worn for resident contact if the skin on your hands is cut, cracked, or chapped. Be very careful not to contaminate clean equipment, supplies, or environmental surfaces with used gloves.

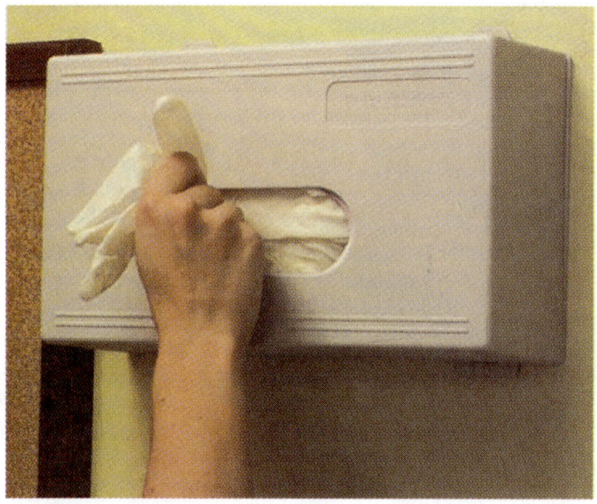

FIGURE 3-16 Gloves are stored in convenient locations near areas where they are likely to be used.

A gown (Figure 3.17) is worn anytime your clothing may contact blood or any of the body fluids mentioned. The gown may be cloth or paper, but must be fluid resistant. Many gowns are specially treated so they will resist fluid.

A face shield (Figure 3.18A) or goggles (Figure 3.18B) and a mask are worn during procedures when body fluids or secretions may splash into your face. A good rule to follow is that you can wear a mask without eye protection, but you should never wear eye protection without a mask. An alternate type of mask with a plastic eye shield attached may also be used (Figure 3.18C). The facial barriers protect the mucous membranes in your eyes, nose, and mouth. It is your responsibility to anticipate what you will need and apply

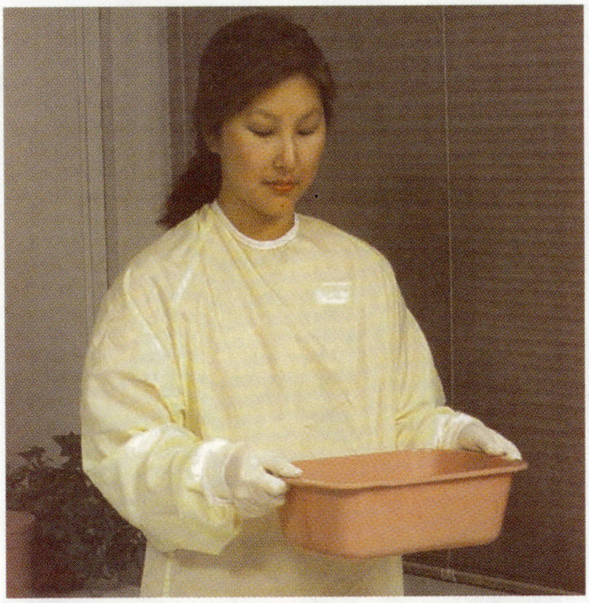

FIGURE 3-17 Gowns are specially treated to resist fluid.

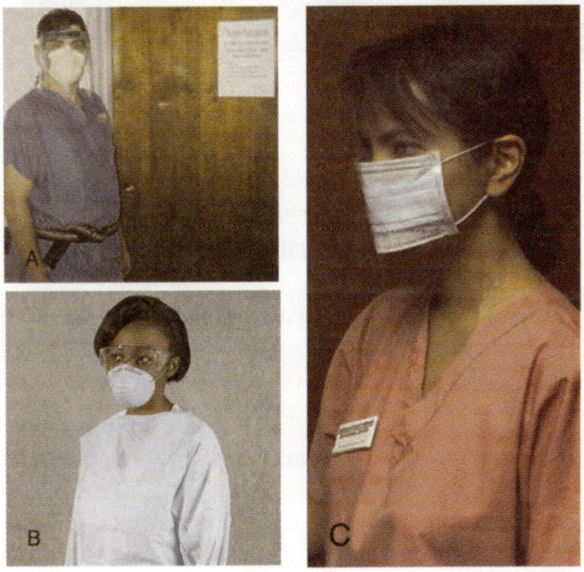

FIGURE 3-18 (A) A mask should always be worn with a regular face shield. (B) Goggles are always worn with a mask. (C) This mask has a protective eye shield attached.

it before you begin a procedure. Check the equipment before you use it. If it is cut or torn, it will not protect you and should be replaced. If you tear your gloves during a procedure, remove them as soon as possible. Wash your hands and put on a new pair of gloves before continuing.

Personal protective equipment is discarded, laundered, or decontaminated according to facility policy after use. Be sure to replace what you have used so it is available the next time it is needed. Wash protective eyewear with soap and water after each use.

Handling needles and sharps. Needle and sharp precautions are also used. Handle needles, razors, and other sharp objects with care. Needles should never be cut, bent, broken, or recapped by hand. After using a sharp object, dispose of it in a puncture-resistant "sharps" container (Figure 3.19). The sharps container should not be overfilled. The cap is placed on the container when it is three-quarters full. The cap is designed so it cannot be snapped back off after it is closed. The sealed sharps container is stored until it can be picked up with the **biohazardous waste.** The biohazardous waste disposal area is used for discarding items contaminated with blood or body fluids. Special precautions are taken to contain waste in this area.

If you must clean up broken glass, always wear gloves. Do not pick up glass with your hands. Use a broom and dustpan (Figure 3.20), forceps, or other mechanical method. Protect your hands from being cut. Dispose of the broken glass in a puncture-resistant container.

Cleaning blood and body fluid spills. Follow your facility policy for cleaning up spills of blood or body fluid. Many facilities use an absorbent powder to soak up the fluid. After the fluid has been absorbed, sweep it up (Figure 3.21). Wipe the area with a facility-approved disinfectant. If your facility uses bleach as a disinfectant, it should be mixed in a container using one part bleach to ten parts of water. Some facilities are now using a different concentration of bleach solution for cleaning blood spills. Research has shown that a much lower concentration (1:100) is needed to eliminate bloodborne pathogens. Know and follow your facility policy. The container should be labeled with the contents and the date it was mixed.

Disposing of biohazardous waste. Items that have contacted blood or body fluids are biohazardous waste. Dispose of linen and trash contaminated with blood or body fluids according to your facility policy. Contaminated trash is discarded in containers marked with the biohazardous waste emblem (Figure 3.22). The bio-hazard emblem has a red or orange background with a black biohazard symbol. Biohazardous waste requires special handling when it is removed from the facility. Having biohazardous waste removed is very expensive, so do not place nonbiohazardous

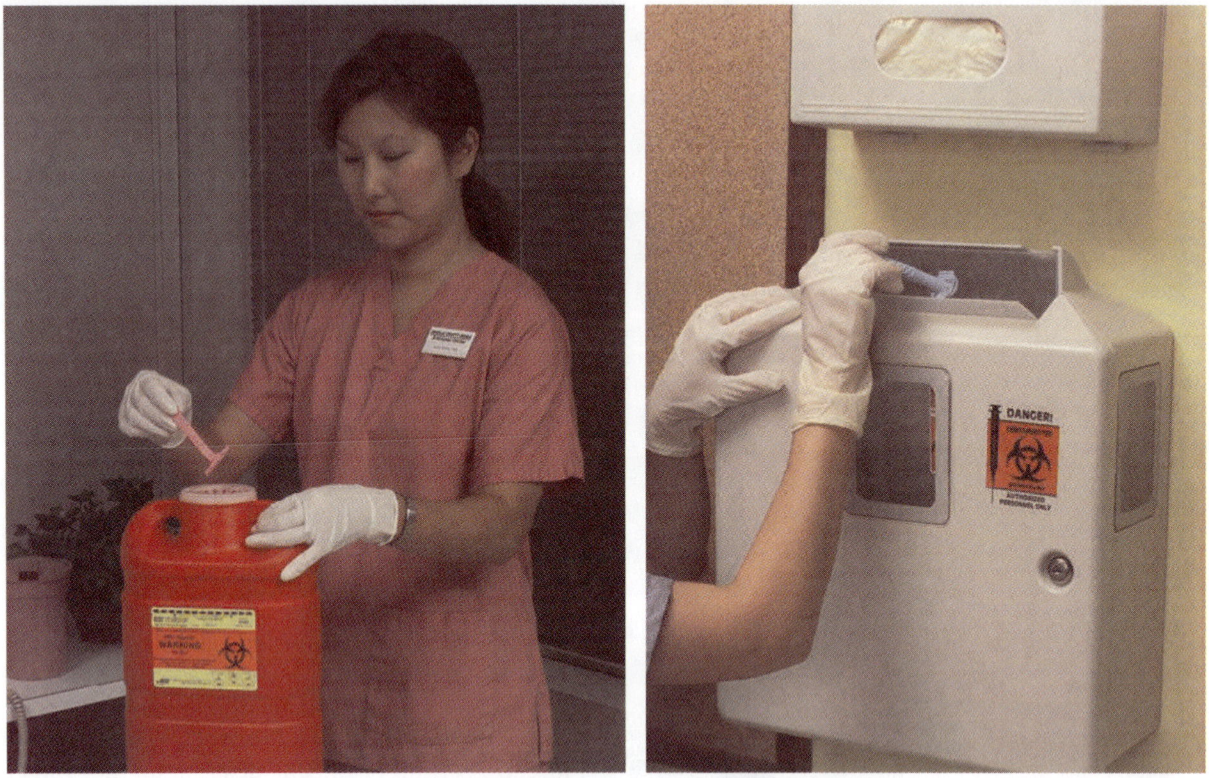

FIGURE 3-19 Razors, needles, blades, broken glass, and other potentially hazardous sharp objects are discarded promptly after use in the puncture-resistant sharps container.

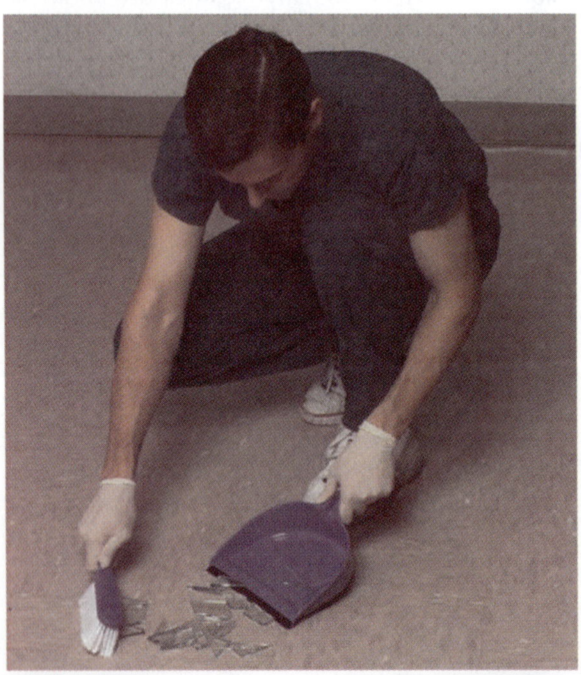

FIGURE 3-20 Never pick up broken glass with your bare hands. Always wear gloves and use an instrument to clean broken glass, even if the amount is small.

materials into this trash container. Biohazardous trash is stored in a special holding area until it can be safely removed.

Body fluids such as urine can safely be disposed of in a drain connected to a sanitary sewer. Your instructor will teach you facility policies for handling and disposing of biohazardous waste.

Laboratory specimens. Laboratory specimens are always considered potentially infectious. They are collected in covered containers. The containers are placed in sealed plastic transport bags with a biohazard emblem on them before they are transported to the lab. If a specimen must be refrigerated, it should not be stored in a refrigerator with food or beverages. A separate refrigerator or cooler, marked with a biohazard emblem, is used.

Cleaning equipment. Each facility has policies and procedures for cleaning equipment that will be reused for resident care. If the equipment may have been contaminated with blood or body fluid, always use personal protective equipment. Utility gloves are better for cleaning duties than the disposable gloves used in resident care. The chemicals used for cleaning make the pores of the disposable gloves too large. Although you probably

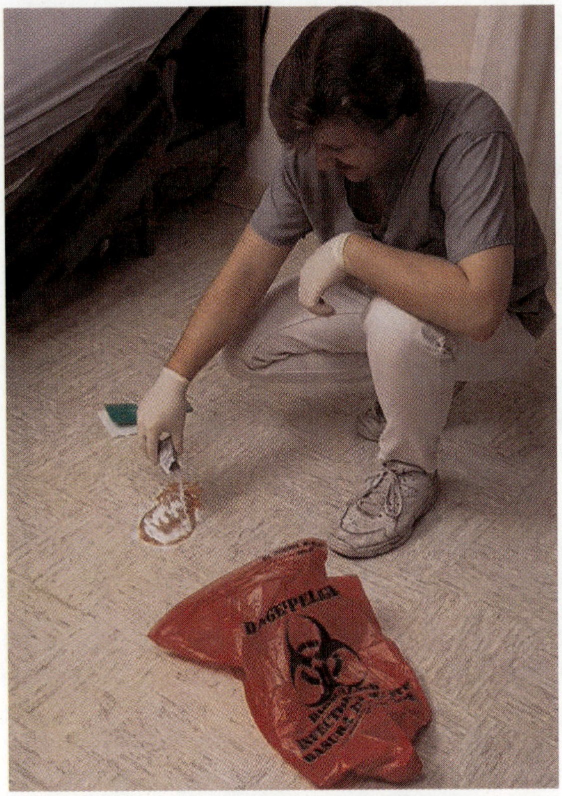

FIGURE 3-21 The absorbent powder turns the body fluid spill into a solid material for easy cleanup. The floor must be disinfected after the powder is removed.

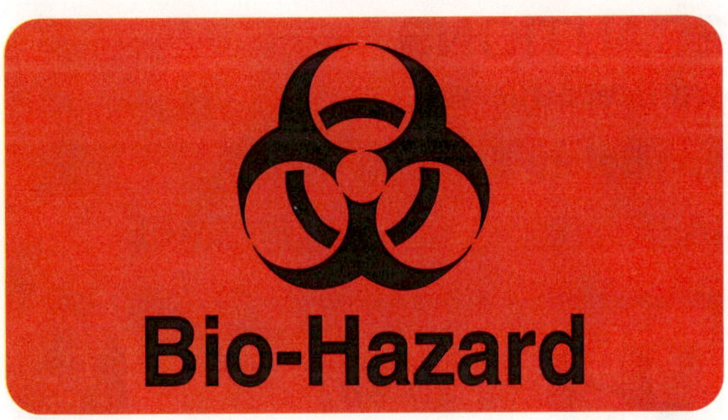

FIGURE 3-22 The biohazard emblem has a red or orange background with a black symbol.

cannot see this defect, the large pores allow microbes to pass through the gloves to your hands. Follow your facility policy for the use of gloves.

Latex allergies. Some health care workers develop allergies to latex because of repeated exposure to latex gloves and other supplies. Avoiding powdered gloves can decrease the risk of latex sensitivity. The powder in the gloves absorbs latex proteins. When the gloves are removed, the particles are inhaled, increasing sensitivity. If you are allergic to latex, your facility will provide you with another type of glove. Glove liners and topical barrier products are also available to individuals who are allergic to latex. The liner or topical product forms a barrier and prevents the latex from touching the skin.

Isolation Measures

Isolation measures are used when certain pathogens are present in a resident. Isolation is used to prevent others from becoming infected. Some facilities place residents with diseases of the immune system in **reverse** or **protective isolation.** Residents in protective isolation do not have a contagious disease. Because of their immune system disorder, they can catch diseases easily. They are isolated to prevent them from contracting pathogens from others and from the environment. Residents with other conditions, such as burns, and those receiving cancer treatment may also be placed in protective isolation. Some facilities do not use this category of isolation.

When caring for a resident in isolation, remember that you are isolating the pathogen and not the person. Isolation can be emotionally difficult for a resident. The resident may feel unclean, unwanted, and untouchable. He or she may not like being confined to a room and separated from others. Staff and visitors must wear personal protective equipment when they are in the room. Sometimes this is upsetting to the resident. A confused resident may be very frightened of staff wearing isolation garments. Because of the difficulty involved in putting on PPE, staff may not visit residents as often. This, too, can be difficult for the resident. Do everything you can to teach the resident about the purpose of the isolation. Check on residents in isolation frequently, and avoid making them feel unclean, unwanted, and unloved. The least amount of isolation possible to contain the pathogen is used. It is unnecessary to use extra precautions beyond those that are required to prevent the spread of disease.

Transmission-Based Precautions

The **Centers for Disease Control and Prevention (CDC)** is a governmental agency that studies infectious diseases and makes recommendations to prevent their spread. The CDC recommends three types of **transmission-based precautions.**

These are isolation categories designed to interrupt the mode of transmission so the pathogen cannot spread. Standard precautions are always used in addition to transmission-based precautions. The type of precautions used is selected by the nurse manager and physician according to how the disease is spread. Transmission-based precautions are used because ordinary cleanliness and standard precautions may not protect you or others from the spread of certain pathogens. Residents with the same disease may share a room. Otherwise, a private room is used to confine the pathogen to the resident's unit.

Airborne precautions. **Airborne precautions** (Figure 3.23) are used for residents whose disease is spread by the airborne method of transmission. The type of pathogen involved is very tiny and light. It can be suspended on dust and moisture in the air and travel for long distances in the ventilation system. Because of the mode of transmission, special precautions are taken to contain the microbe. A private room is necessary. This room must have a special ventilation system that prevents the pathogen from escaping into the rest of the facility. In a normal health care facility room, the air is forced downward from the ventilation system. In an airborne precautions room, the ventilation is reversed so that room air is drawn upward into the vents. This creates a **negative pressure environment.** The ventilation is either specially filtered or exhausted directly to the outside of the building. This room has six to twelve complete changes of air per hour. The door to the room is always kept closed.

Some long-term care facilities do not have the special ventilation required for airborne precautions rooms. These facilities use portable units that are placed in the room to filter the air and create a negative pressure environment. They are slightly noisier than the ventilation system, but are effective in eliminating airborne pathogens.

Staff entering the room must wear a special mask, called a **high efficiency particulate air (HEPA) respirator** (Figure 3.24). This mask has very small pores that prevent the tiny pathogen from entering. The mask must be fit-tested by a professional to be sure it fits the employee properly and does not leak. Each time you apply the mask, you must check the fit yourself. After the HEPA mask is professionally fit-tested, the employee must also have a medical exam to be sure that use of the HEPA mask is not dangerous to his or her health. The medical examination is done because some individuals have underlying diseases that make working in such a mask difficult or impossible. Men with facial hair cannot

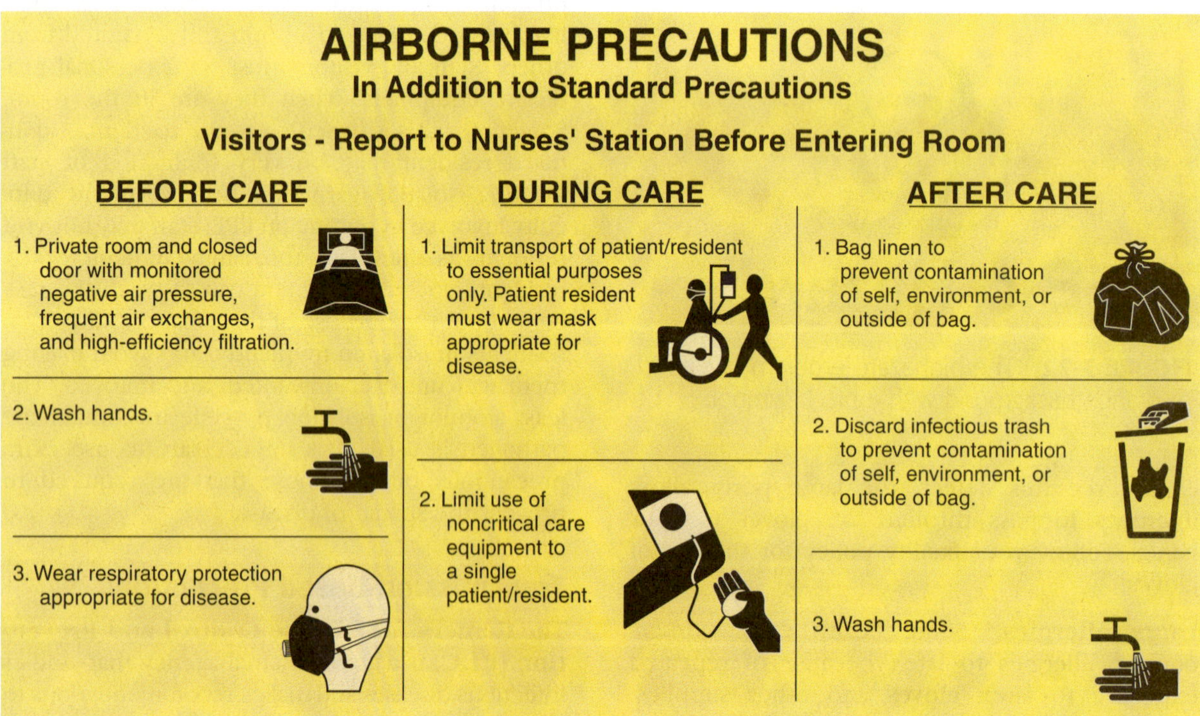

FIGURE 3-23 Airborne precautions. (*Courtesy of Briggs Corporation, Des Moines, IA 800-247-2343*)

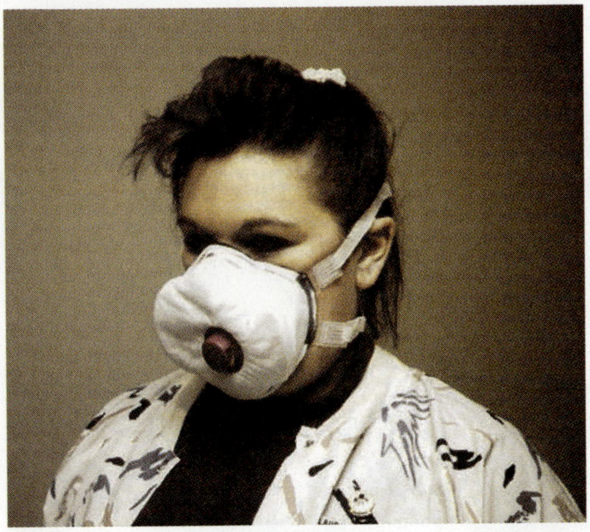

FIGURE 3-24 The HEPA respirator filter

wear the HEPA mask because the facial hair prevents a tight seal. If a man with facial hair must enter the room, a special hood is worn. Because of the fit-testing and health examination requirements, facilities may select only certain employees to work in rooms where airborne precautions are used. When working in an airborne precautions room, no other personal protective equipment is necessary unless it is needed to apply the principles of standard precautions.

A **PFR95 respirator** (Figure 3.25A) or **N95 respirator** (Figure 3.25B) may be worn instead of the HEPA mask. Some health care workers prefer these masks because they are lighter in weight and more comfortable to wear. As with the HEPA mask, there are fit-testing and health examination requirements. These masks are also fit-tested by the worker each time they are worn (Figure 3.26).

Droplet precautions. **Droplet precautions** (Figure 3.27) are used for some residents whose infections are spread in the air. An example of a disease for which droplet precautions are used is influenza. The pathogen is spread by the droplets in mucus from oral, nasal, and respiratory secretions. The droplets usually remain within three feet of the resident. The secretions containing the pathogen are too large and heavy to be carried in the air currents. A private room is necessary, but special ventilation is not used. Regular surgical masks are worn. The pathogen is too large to fit between the pores of the surgical mask. The door to the room does not have to be kept closed unless direct care is being performed, because the organism stays within three feet of the resident. No other personal protective equipment is necessary unless it is needed to apply standard precautions.

Contact precautions. **Contact precautions** (Figure 3.28) are used to contain pathogens that are spread by direct or indirect contact. The microbes that spread the disease in residents in contact precautions are usually found in infections of the skin, urine, and fecal material. Standard precautions are used in addition to contact precautions. Gloves are worn anytime you enter the

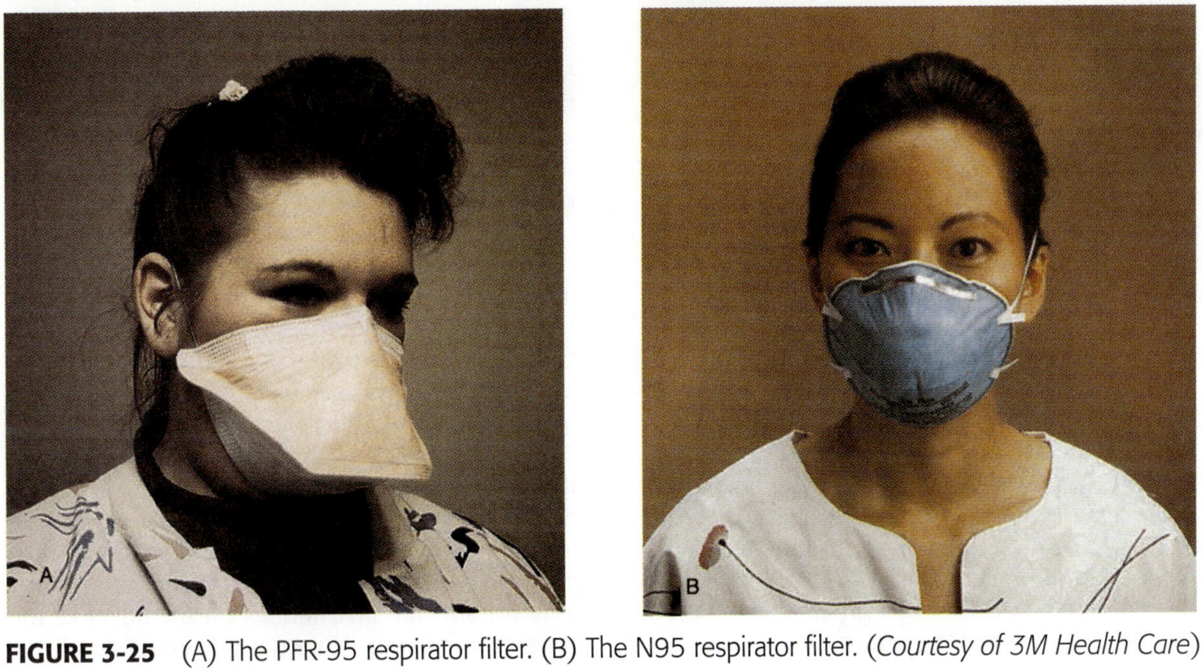

FIGURE 3-25 (A) The PFR-95 respirator filter. (B) The N95 respirator filter. (*Courtesy of 3M Health Care*)

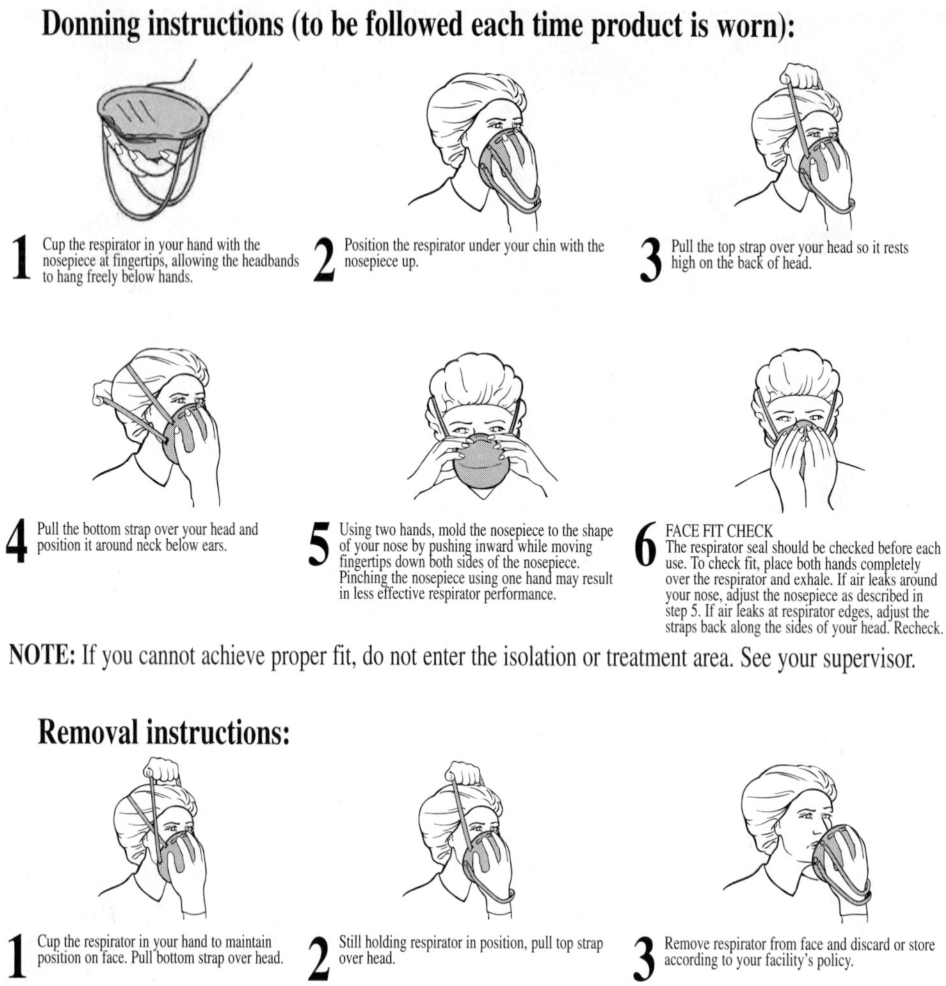

FIGURE 3-26 All respirators must be fit-tested by the employee each time he or she wears one. (*Courtesy of 3M Health Care*)

room. No other personal protective equipment is necessary unless you anticipate having direct contact with the resident or with environmental surfaces. When contact is expected, you must wear a gown to cover your uniform. Additional PPE is used only if you anticipate splashing of secretions. If you think this may happen, you will need a face shield or goggles and a surgical mask to protect the mucous membranes in your eyes, nose, and mouth. The principles of standard precautions are also used for residents in contact precautions.

Special circumstances. Residents may have infections that are transmitted by more than one method. A resident may have an infection, such as a cold, that is spread by the droplet method. The resident may also have a separate infection of the skin. Some diseases, such as chickenpox, and shingles, are spread by more than one method. In this case, two types of isolation are used in addition to standard precautions.Table 3.6 lists common diseases and the type of transmission-based precautions used for each.

Identifying residents in isolation. Most facilities post signs on the door to the room when a resident is in isolation. The sign provides directions on personal protective equipment to wear and describes precautions to take. Some facilities feel that posting signs on the door of the resident's room is an invasion of privacy. These facilities usually post a stop sign on the door that advises you to check with the nurse before entering the room. Before caring for these residents, you must get verbal directions from the nurse or look for specific instructions on the cover of the resident's chart or other designated location.

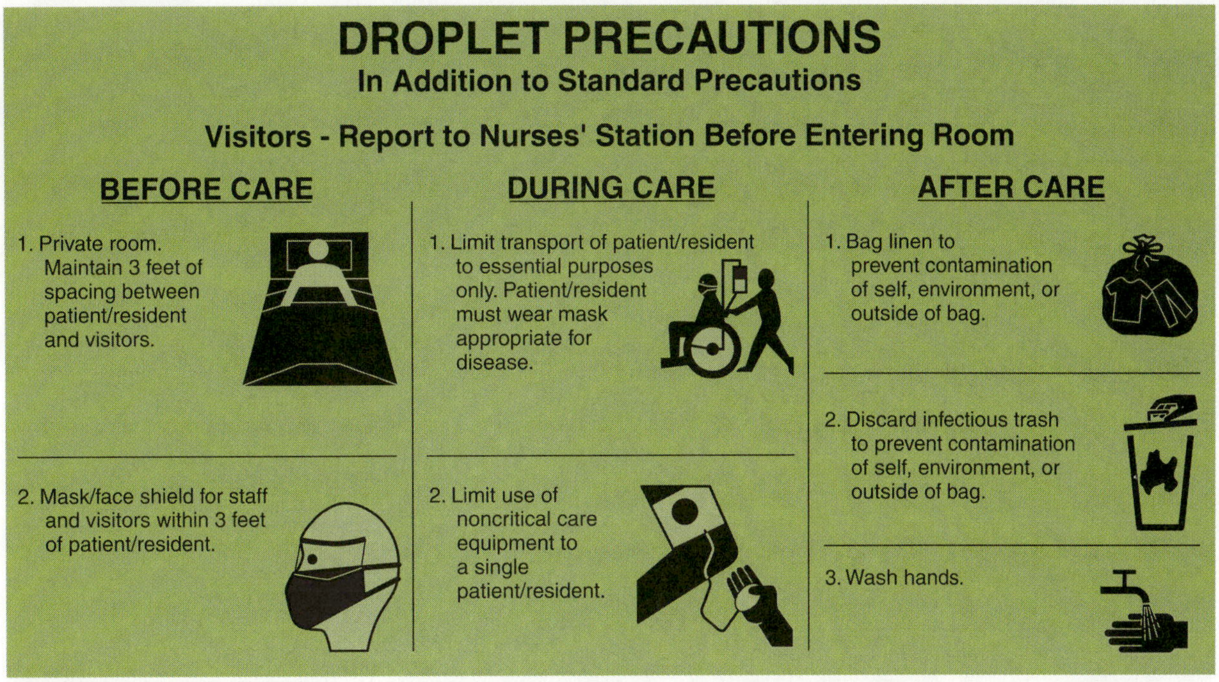

FIGURE 3-27 Droplet precautions. (*Courtesy of Briggs Corporation, Des Moines, IA 800-247-2343*)

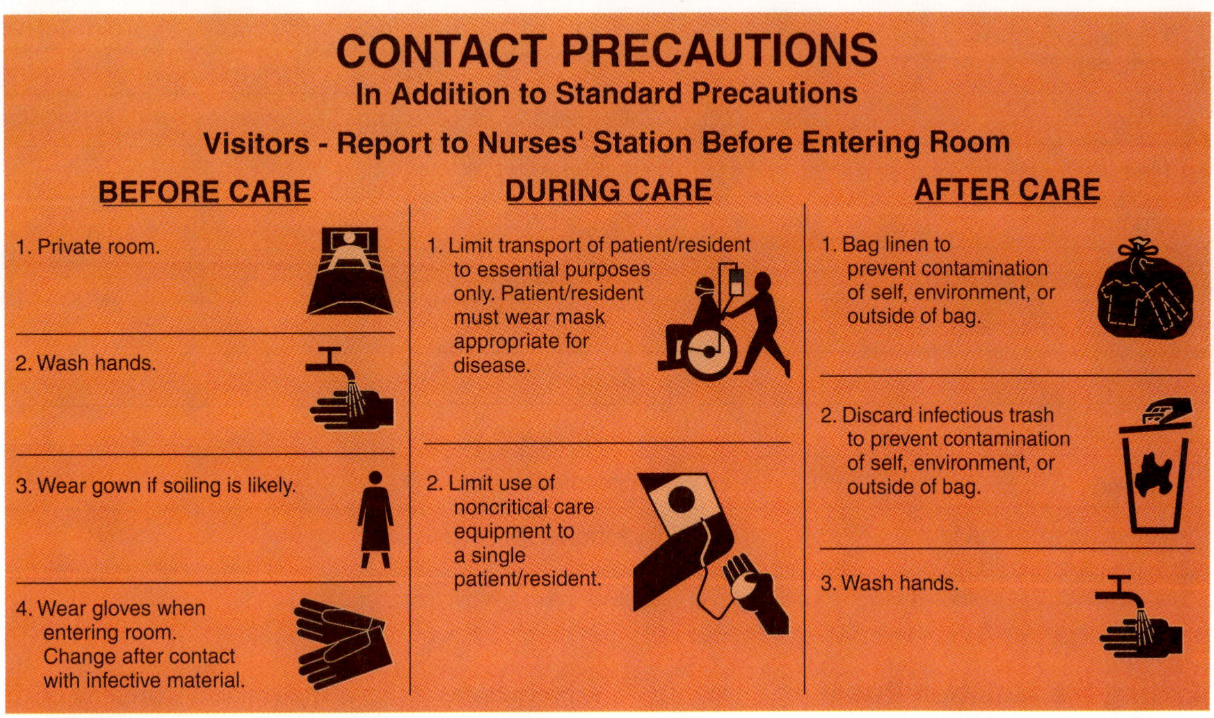

FIGURE 3-28 Contact precautions. (*Courtesy of Briggs Corporation, Des Moines, IA 800-247-2343*)

Sequence for Applying and Removing Personal Protective Equipment

There are times when you must wear full isolation garments in a resident's room. If you will be using your watch in the room, you should remove it first and place it on a clean paper towel. You will carry the watch on the towel. The sequence in which you apply and remove your personal protective equipment is important.

TABLE 3-6 Diseases Requiring Transmission-Based Precautions

Disease or Condition	Type of Precautions
AIDS	Standard
Chickenpox	Airborne and contact
Diarrhea	Standard
Drug-resistant skin infections	Contact
E. coli 0157:H7	Contact
German measles	Droplet
Head or body lice	Contact
Hepatitis, type A	Standard. Use contact if diarrhea or incontinent resident.
Hepatitis, other types	Standard
HIV disease	Standard
Impetigo	Contact
Infected pressure sore with no drainage	Standard
Infected pressure sore with heavy drainage	Contact
Infectious diarrhea caused by a known pathogen	Contact
Influenza	Droplet
Measles	Airborne
Mumps	Droplet
Oral or genital herpes	Standard
Pseudomembranous colitits	Contact
Scabies	Contact
Shingles	Airborne and contact
Syphilis	Standard
Tuberculosis of the lungs	Airborne

Note: Use standard precautions in addition to other types of precautions listed.

Exiting the Isolation Room

If you used your watch in the isolation room, pick it up after removing your personal protective equipment and put it on your wrist. Holding the clean upper side of the paper towel, pick up the towel and discard it in the trash. Obtain a clean paper towel from the dispenser and use it to open the door of the room. After the door is open, discard the towel inside the room. The door may be left open in contact and droplet precautions if this is the resident's preference. It is a good idea to wash your hands again after leaving the room.

Problematic Pathogens

Escherichia Coli

Escherichia coli (E. coli) is a type of bacteria that normally resides in the intestines. Outside of

GUIDELINES FOR

Isolation Handwashing

- Roll your sleeves up to your elbows.
- Wash your hands and forearms following the procedural guidelines for handwashing.
  - Wash your hands:
  - Before entering an isolation room.
  - After removing the isolation gown and gloves.
  - Before and after removing an isolation mask.
- Immediately before leaving the isolation room. Use a paper towel to turn the doorknob when leaving the room; discard the towel in the room.
- Any other time that handwashing is required to practice standard precautions.
- Any time your hands touch a contaminated or potentially contaminated surface.

PROCEDURE 5

Applying and Removing Personal Protective Equipment (Disposable Gloves, Gown, Surgical Mask, Protective Eyewear)

Applying Disposable Isolation Gloves

1. Wash your hands.
2. Remove clean gloves from the box.
3. Put hands into the gloves, adjusting the fingers for comfort and fit.
4. Pull the cuff of the gloves over the sleeve of the gown, if worn.

Removing Disposable Isolation Gloves

1. Grasp the outside of the glove on the nondominant hand at the cuff. Pull the glove off so that the inside of the glove faces outward (Figure 3.29A and 3.29B). Avoid touching the skin of your wrist with the fin-gers of the glove.
2. Place this glove into the palm of the hand that is still gloved.
3. Put the fingers of the ungloved hand inside the cuff of the gloved hand. Pull the glove off (Figure 3.29C) inside out. The first glove removed should be inside the second glove (Figure 3.29D).

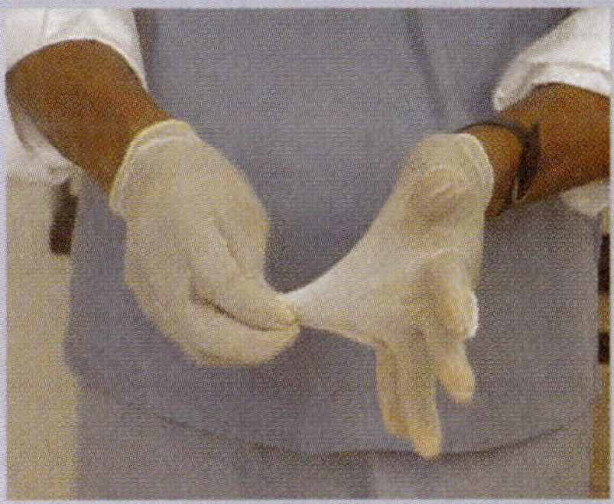

FIGURE 3-29A Grasp the outside cuff or center of the palm of the glove without touching your hand.

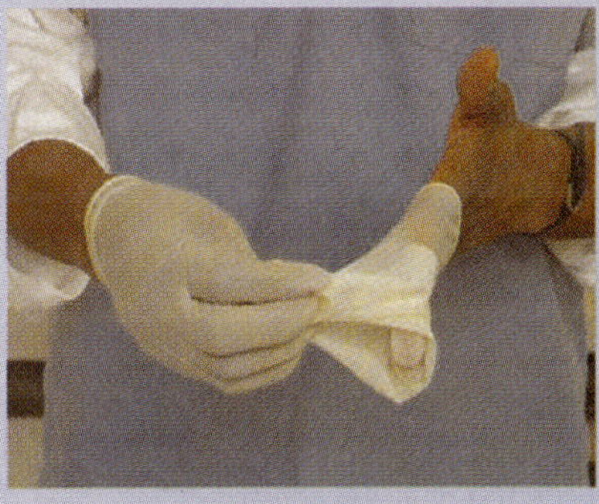

FIGURE 3-29B Pull the glove off inside out.

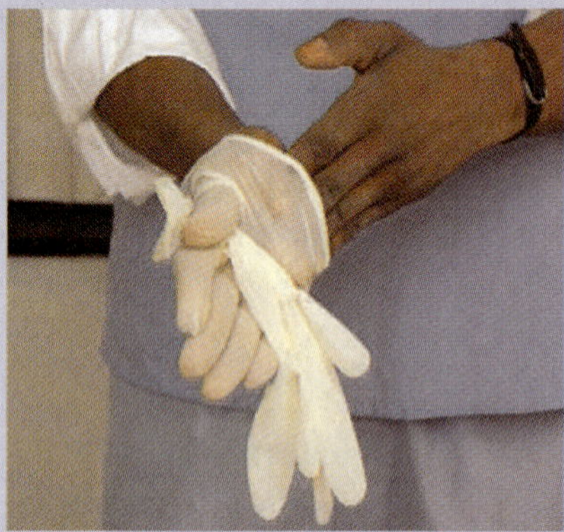

FIGURE 3-29C Hold the glove in your hand.

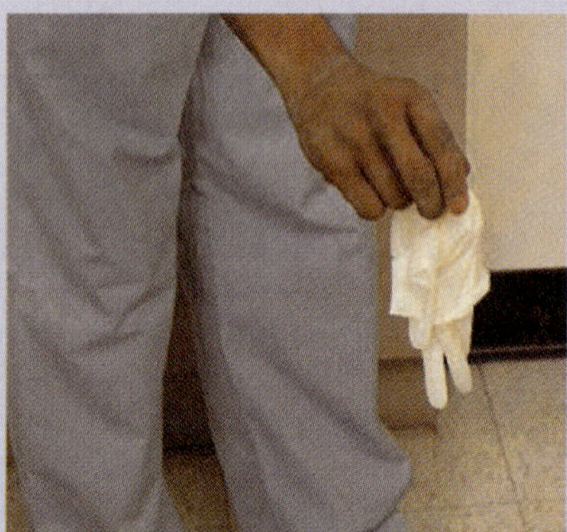

FIGURE 3-29D Remove the opposite glove inside out.

4. Discard the gloves into a covered container or isolation trash, according to facility policy.
5. Wash your hands.

Putting On an Isolation Gown

1. Wash your hands.
2. Hold the clean gown by the neck in front of you, letting it unfold. Do not let the gown touch the floor.
3. Place your arms in the sleeves and slide the gown up to your shoulders.
4. Slip your hands inside the neck band and grasp the ties. Tie them at the neck.
5. Cover your uniform at the back with the gown and tie the ties at the waist. The gown must completely cover your clothing.

Removing the Isolation Gown

1. Untie the waist ties of the gown.
2. Remove gloves.
3. Wash your hands.
4. If a mask is worn, untie the bottom ties of the mask, then the top ties.
5. Discard the mask, holding it only by the ties.
6. Untie the neck ties of the gown and loosen it at the shoulders, touching only the inside of the gown.
7. Grasp the neck ties and pull the gown off inside out.
8. Roll the gown away from your body. Touch only the inside. Discard according to facility policy.
9. Wash your hands.

Applying the Surgical Mask

1. Wash your hands. Remove a mask from the box by holding the ties.
2. Cover your nose and mouth with the mask.
3. Pinch the metal nose piece over the bridge of your nose until it fits comfortably.
4. Tie the top tie or stretch the elastic over the top of your head or ears, depending on the type of mask used.
5. Tie the bottom tie.
6. Wash your hands.

Removing the Isolation Mask

1. Remove gloves.
2. Wash your hands.
3. Untie the neck tie of the mask.
4. Untie the upper tie.
5. Remove the mask by touching only the ties.
6. Discard according to facility policy.
7. Wash your hands.

Applying Protective Eyewear

1. Wash your hands and apply the surgical or HEPA mask.
2. Apply the goggles and secure the elastic strap around the back of your head, or apply the face shield.
3. Wash your hands.

Removing Protective Eyewear

1. Remove your gloves and wash your hands.
2. Lift the protective goggles or face shield away from your face.
3. Remove your surgical or HEPA mask.
4. Wash your hands.

GUIDELINES FOR

Putting on Personal Protective Equipment

1. Wash your hands.
2. Put on the isolation gown.
3. Put on the isolation mask.
4. Apply goggles or face shield, if needed.
5. Put on the isolation gloves.

GUIDELINES FOR

Removing Personal Protective Equipment

1. Remove gloves.
2. Wash your hands.
3. Remove protective eyewear, if worn.
4. Wash your hands.
5. Untie the waist tie of the isolation gown.
6. Untie the neck tie of the gown and remove it carefully.
7. Wash your hands.
8. Remove your mask.
9. Wash your hands.

the intestines, it can cause serious problems. This bacterium sometimes causes urinary tract infections. Another strain, **E. coli 0157:H7,** has caused outbreaks resulting in serious illness and death. This is a nonhuman strain that is found in the intestines of some cattle. A small amount of this bacteria can contaminate a large amount of meat, particularly ground beef. It is transmitted in contaminated and undercooked meat, by produce that has been rinsed in water contaminated with feces, or by a person who has been handling contaminated food. It has been found on cutting boards and utensils. The bacteria have been found in unpasteurized milk and apple juice, and in pools and lakes contaminated with fecal matter. The best way to prevent its spread is to use good handwashing and food preparation practices. Ground beef (hamburger) should be cooked until it is well done in the center. The high temperature required to cook meat to well done will kill the pathogen.

Signs and Symptoms. When E. coli 0157:H7 enters the human intestinal tract, it multiplies rapidly, producing large amounts of toxins. One to two days later, the person develops watery diarrhea, nausea, vomiting, and cramping. In another day or two, the diarrhea becomes bloody. The abdomen becomes **distended** (enlarged) and very tender. The resident may show signs of dehydration, swelling, and **petechiae,** small purplish spots on the body surface, caused by minute hemorrhages. The diarrhea may subside in five to seven days, but the condition injures the mucous membranes, causing the pathogen to escape into the bloodstream.

This creates a situation in which bloodflow to the brain, kidneys, and other organs is endangered. The resident develops signs and symptoms of serious illness, such as:

- Decreased urine output that may progress to complete renal failure
- Mental confusion
- Seizures (convulsions)
- Muscle weakness
- Pain and numbness of the feet and legs

Treatment. In some conditions, the risk of transmitting infection is highest before the diagnosis is made. Because of this, many facilities place residents in contact precautions if one of these conditions is suspected. Diapered and incontinent residents remain in contact precautions for the duration of the illness. Standard precautions may safely be used for other residents. E. coli 0157:H7 can be deadly, particularly in elderly adults and persons with conditions that weaken the immune system. Care is supportive, and the resident must be carefully monitored. Unfortunately, many drugs increase the risk of kidney damage. Water intake is very important, but liquid intake must be observed closely because of the potential for kidney damage. Careful monitoring of the resident's vital signs is required.

Pseudomembranous Colitis

Many bacteria live in the bowel of a healthy person. Most of them are harmless, and some friendly bacteria help with digestion. A few of these have the potential to be troublemakers if they get out of control. Most of the time, the bad bacteria are outnumbered by the good bacteria, and no harm comes to the person. Taking antibiotics can upset the balance in the colon. Many people experience a brief bout of diarrhea because the balance is upset, but the condition resolves quickly on its own.

Pseudomembranous colitis is a very serious condition in which the diarrhea is caused by a bacterium called Clostridium difficile (C. difficile). It is often called by its nickname, "C. diff." This condition develops in residents who have been on antibiotic therapy. The friendly (good) bacteria die as a result of the antibiotic, and the harmful (bad) bacteria grow out of control. Without the other friendly bacteria to keep it in check, C. difficile breeds rapidly, producing toxins that cause serious illness.

C. difficile is very common in health care facilities. It is picked up on the hands from bedpans, bedside commodes, toilets, sinks, countertops, bed rails, doorknobs, and other surfaces that have been contaminated by stool. It spreads into the body (most commonly the mouth) by unwashed hands.

Signs and Symptoms. Pseudomembranous colitis may occur several weeks or months after the resident has completed the course of antibiotics, so it can be difficult to diagnose. C. difficile produces a toxin that causes inflammation of the intestine. This results in sudden, severe, foul-smelling, watery diarrhea. Stopping the antibiotic will not stop the diarrhea. The diarrhea may be so frequent and severe that the resident becomes dehydrated rapidly and develops other serious imbalances within the body. Other signs and symptoms are:

- Cramping and pain in the lower abdomen; sometimes this begins several days before the diarrhea starts
- Fever
- Mucus, pus, or blood in the stool
- Abdomen very tender to touch
- In severe cases, low blood pressure and signs of shock

If the condition is not promptly treated, it can cause ruptured bowel and a condition in which the bowel becomes severely distended and retains stool.

Diagnosis and Treatment. If pseudomembranous colitis is suspected, the doctor will order laboratory tests on one or more stool specimens. The laboratory will identify the bacteria that are causing the illness. The antibiotic suspected of causing the problem is stopped, if possible. Another drug is used to eliminate the harmful bacteria in the colon. The resident may be given yogurt to eat and several other medications to increase the balance of healthful flora in the bowel. Although drug therapy usually eliminates the condition, it sometimes recurs, making a second course of therapy necessary. The resident is placed in contact precautions until 72 hours after the appearance and frequency of stools return to normal, or as ordered by the physician. Use good handwashing techniques with antibacterial soap and water. Do not use alcohol-based hand cleaners. This disease is spread by spores, and alcohol will not eliminate them. The friction and running water will remove them from your hands during handwashing.

Hantavirus

In May 1993, a cluster of unexplained deaths occurred among young Native Americans in the southwestern United States. An investigation revealed a virus that was previously unknown. This situation attracted a great deal of media attention. Several additional outbreaks have been reported since 1993. This strange disease is called **hantavirus.** It is spread by contact with rodents (rats and mice) or their excretions, including urine and stool. Once disturbed, viral particles in the excretions become airborne and are inhaled by the susceptible host. Signs and symptoms appear one to five weeks later. They include high fever, chills, muscle aches, cough, nausea, vomiting, diarrhea, dizziness, and feeling very tired. As the disease progresses, the resident becomes very short of breath. When this occurs, the disease progresses rapidly, and the resident becomes seriously ill. The resident may be transferred to the hospital for respiratory support. Hantavirus is not transmitted from person to person. Spread of this condition can be reduced by taking steps to prevent rodents from entering the facility or home, and eliminating them if they are present.

Shingles

Shingles (herpes zoster) is a condition that occurs only in people who have had chickenpox. Although the person recovered from the chickenpox, the virus that caused the condition remained hidden in the nervous system. The immune system kept it in an inactive state. The immune system weakens with age. In some people, it is no longer able to contain the virus. The resident develops blister-like lesions on the torso that are often mistaken for a rash. The lesions follow the nerve pathways, and are extremely painful. Health care workers who have not had chickenpox should not enter the room, if other immune caregivers are available. Inhaling airborne viruses will cause chicken-pox in workers who are not immune. The lesions are infectious in the blister state. Airborne precautions may be used for residents if there is a widespread outbreak, and for those who are immune-compromised. Contact precautions are also used, at least until all blisters have burst and crusted over. For a minor, localized outbreak, standard precautions may be used.

Drug-Resistant Organisms

Drug-resistant organisms are pathogens that cannot be eliminated by the usual antibiotics. These microbes have become a problem because eliminating them may be difficult or impossible. If antibiotics are available to eliminate the pathogen, they are often very expensive and have toxic side effects such as kidney, liver, and hearing damage. The elderly are very vulnerable to the side effects of antibiotics. The pathogens have become drug resistant for several reasons:

1. People took antibiotics for minor conditions for which antibiotics were not necessary. Over the years, many unnecessary antibiotics have been prescribed.
2. People who were taking antibiotics stopped taking them when they felt better, but before finishing the prescription. The pathogens were still in the body and built up resistance to the antibiotic. The next time the pathogen was exposed to the antibiotic, the drug had no effect.

Methicillin-Resistant *Staphylococcus Aureus*

Methicillin-resistant Staphylococcus aureus (MRSA), is a common drug-resistant organism found in health care facilities. MRSA is very difficult to control and treat. It causes many different types of infections. Skin and urinary infections caused by this pathogen are common. Occasionally, a resident will develop respiratory MRSA. As with the other pathogens discussed earlier, you cannot always tell that the person has an infection. MRSA is spread primarily by direct and indirect contact. Use of standard precautions will prevent the spread of MRSA, particularly in urine and skin infections. Contact precautions are used if the resident is known to have MRSA in a wound or urine. Droplet precautions are used when a resident is known to have MRSA in the respiratory tract.

Vancomycin-Resistant *Enterococcus*

Vancomycin-resistant Enterococcus (VRE), is a newer drug-resistant organism. It originates in the colon, but can cause severe infections in other parts of the body. This organism is spread by contact. Standard precautions and contact precautions are used to prevent the spread of this pathogen.

Tuberculosis

Tuberculosis (TB) is a disease that has been with us for many years. The incidence of tuberculosis was steadily declining until the 1980s, when it began increasing. Many cases of tuberculosis that we see today are drug resistant. TB is spread only through the airborne method. The organism is very small and can travel long distances in the air. Tuberculosis can occur in many different sites in the body, but it is always spread by the airborne method and not through contact.

Signs and Symptoms of Tuberculosis

Signs and symptoms of tuberculosis include feeling tired and sleepy all the time, fever, night sweats, weight loss, cough, coughing up blood-tinged mucus, chest pain, and shortness of breath. When a resident has tuberculosis, airborne precautions are used. A HEPA mask is worn, and the room must have negative pressure ventilation. A resident can usually be removed from isolation after two to three weeks of antibiotics, but treatment will continue for six months to a year.

Testing for Tuberculosis

Health care facilities are required to test residents and employees periodically for the presence of the organism that causes TB. Skin testing is done. Health care facilities are using a two-step test for the initial testing. A one-step test is used thereafter. Employees are tested upon employment and every 3 to 12 months thereafter. The frequency of the testing is determined by how high the risk of infection is in your health care facility and community. If the skin test is positive, the employee is referred to a physician or public health agency for follow-up. A chest x-ray and other lab tests are done. If the tests are negative, another x-ray will be required if the employee later develops symptoms suggestive of tuberculosis. A positive skin test does not mean that an individual has TB. It indicates exposure to the pathogen that causes tuberculosis, and further testing and treatment may be indicated. Individuals over the age of 35 are not always treated because the drugs used to treat the infection could cause complications in persons of this age. The decision on whether to treat is left to the individual, the personal physician, and the local health authority.

Treating Tuberculosis

Tuberculosis is treated with a combination of antibiotics. It is very important to take the antibiotics exactly as ordered, and for as long as directed, to prevent drug resistance. If the individual is not treated, the TB germ can remain in the body for many years. It may become active sometime in the future. In some people it never becomes active.

Tuberculosis in the Long-Term Care Facility

Tuberculosis should be taken very seriously in long-term care facilities. Many elderly residents were exposed to tuberculosis years ago when the disease was common. Their skin tests are positive, indicating that the microbe is in the body and that they were not treated. The immune systems weaken with age. It is possible for the tuberculosis microbe to become active because the weakened immune system is no longer able to contain it. Fatigue is often the only sign of tuberculosis in the elderly, so a number of people can be infected before the disease is detected.

HEAD LICE

Head lice are **parasites.** Parasites are tiny animals that survive by feeding off humans or other animals. Fleas and ticks are examples of common parasites.

Head lice are spread primarily by direct contact with an infected person. You cannot contract head lice from pets and animals. They are spread by sharing personal belongings such as brushes, combs, ribbons, caps, clothing, and bedding with others. Head lice (Figure 3.30) do not hop, jump, or fly, but they can crawl very quickly. When performing hair care, check residents for **nits** (Figure 3.31A). Nits are tiny, oval shaped eggs that are yellow-white. They look like dandruff, but are firmly attached to the hair and are usually very difficult to remove. Empty nit cases are shown in Figure 3.31B. These nits have hatched into live lice. *Lice* are tiny brown insects about the size of a sesame seed. They move away from light quickly. Figure 3.31C shows how hair spray drops appear on the hair. Figure 3.31D is a magnified picture of dandruff. Figure 3.31E shows hair casts. Casts and plugs occur when oil glands in the scalp are overactive. They are easily removed. It may be difficult to differentiate

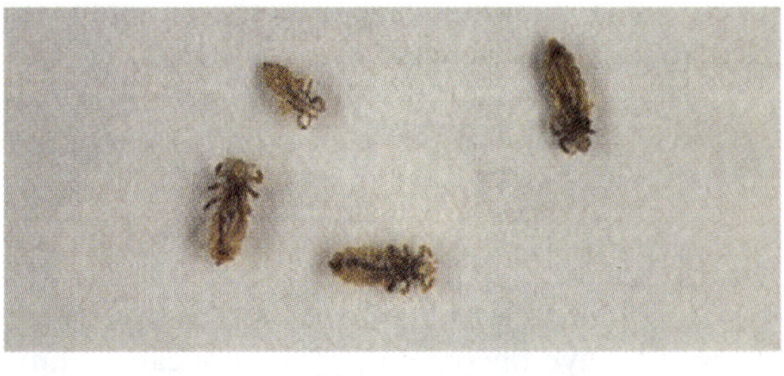

FIGURE 3-30 Head lice are tiny and run very quickly. They do not jump, hop, or fly.

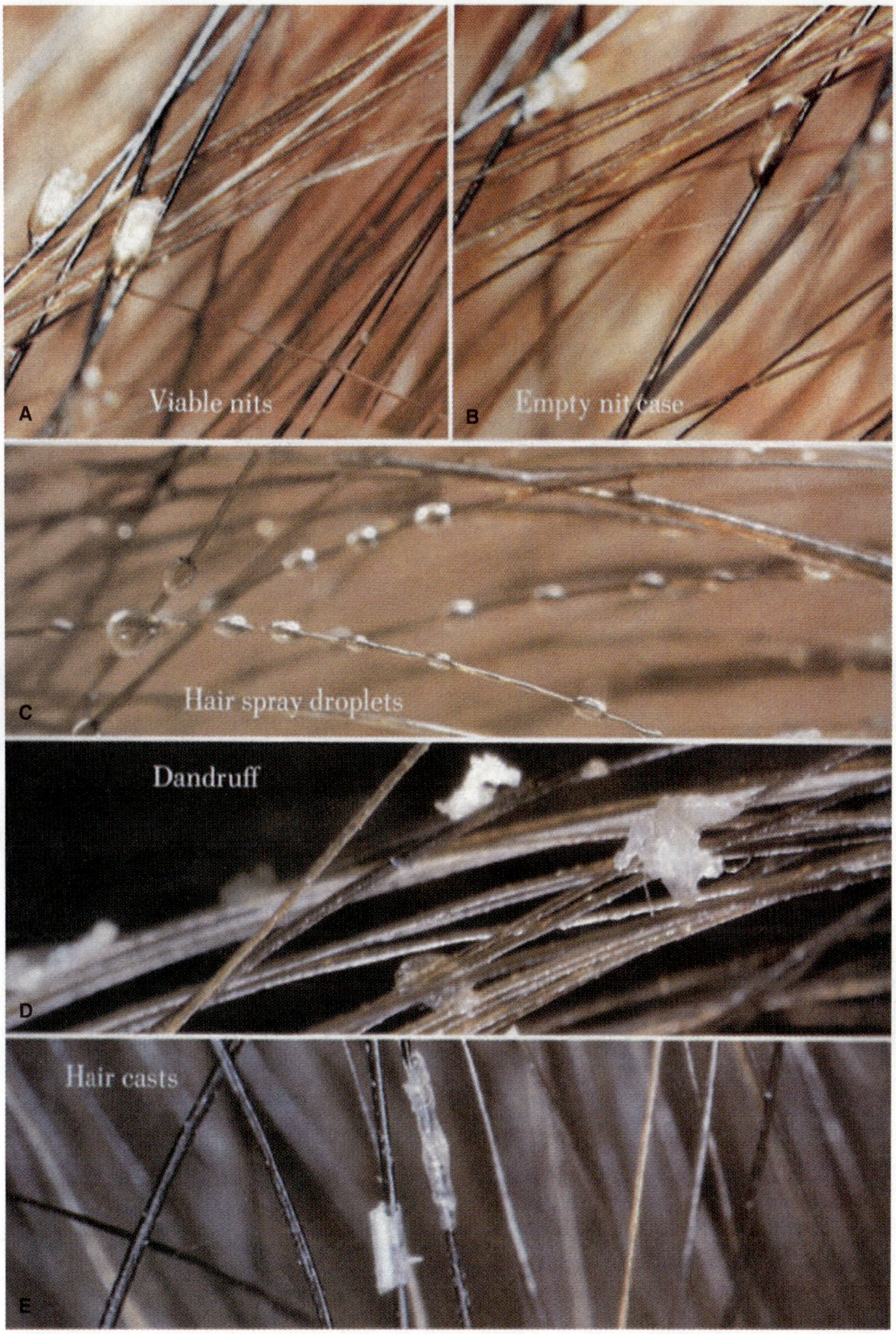

FIGURE 3-31 Nits and eggs that attach firmly to the hair shaft are very difficult to remove. Differentiating one condition from another may be difficult. *(Courtesy of Hogil Pharmaceutical)*

nits from other conditions of the scalp. Notify the nurse for further assessment if you notice any abnormalities.

Treatment for Head Lice

If you suspect that nits or lice are present, notify the nurse immediately. You will be directed to wear gloves for further resident contact. You must also wear gloves and a gown when handling the resident's clothing or linen. The physician will be contacted for an order for a special medicated shampoo to kill the parasite. The resident's hair must be washed with this shampoo. Shampoos containing the chemical lindane have proven to be toxic to some people, and are not recommended. Contact precautions will be used for 24 hours after the resident is treated. A special comb is used to remove nits from the hair. If the nits cannot be removed by combing, it may be necessary to snip the hair with eggs attached with a pair of safety scissors. The nurse will inspect the resident's scalp the day after the medicated shampoo to look for additional lice and nits. It is important to remove all of the nits, as the shampoo may not kill them. They may be difficult to remove, and this is a time-consuming task. You may be directed to check other residents for the presence of head lice, because the parasite is highly contagious.

As with other diseases, some head lice have become resistant to the medicated shampoos used to eliminate them. If the lice cannot be eliminated with a shampoo, the only way to remove them is by checking the head and eliminating them manually. Manual removal of lice and nits is done using a comb, tweezers, or double-sided tape. It may be necessary for two people to check the head simultaneously, because the lice can run very quickly. Shining a flashlight on the head may be helpful, as the lice move away from the light source. Always wear gloves when caring for the hair of a resident with known or suspected head lice.

All clothing and linen must be bagged and sent to the laundry for washing. Furniture and personal items in the room must be vacuumed to eliminate lice in the environment. Vacuuming is safer and more effective than using pesticide sprays, which leave a toxic residue. After vacuuming, wipe environmental surfaces with a facility-approved disinfectant to eliminate microbes left from the outside of the vacuum cleaner. Previously, toxic sprays were used to eliminate lice from environmental surfaces and personal belongings, but this is no longer recommended.

Scabies

Scabies is a skin condition caused by a parasite called a **mite** (Figure 3.32). A mite is a microscopic organism that cannot be seen with the eye. Scabies is highly contagious and is spread by direct and indirect contact. It causes a rash (Figure 3.33A) and severe itching of the skin. The rash may be seen in the webs of the fingers, inside the wrists, outside the elbows, in the underarm, or on the waist and nipple area. It is also sometimes seen in the genital area in men

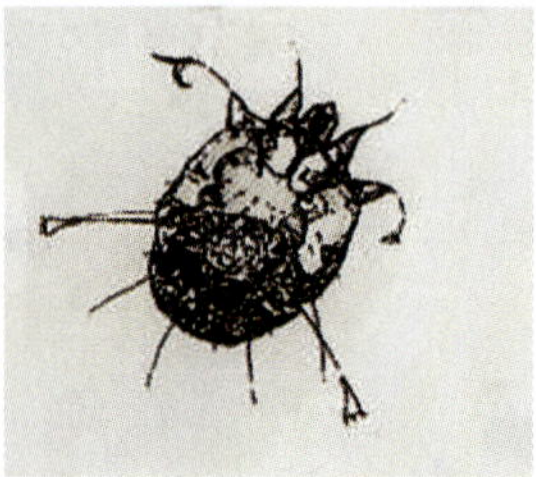

FIGURE 3-32 The scabies mite is microscopic and cannot be seen without a microscope. *(Courtesy of L.E. Morris and Donna J. Lewis, Management of Chronic, Resistive Scabies: A Case Study, Geriatric Nursing 16 [Sept/Oct 1995]: 230–37)*

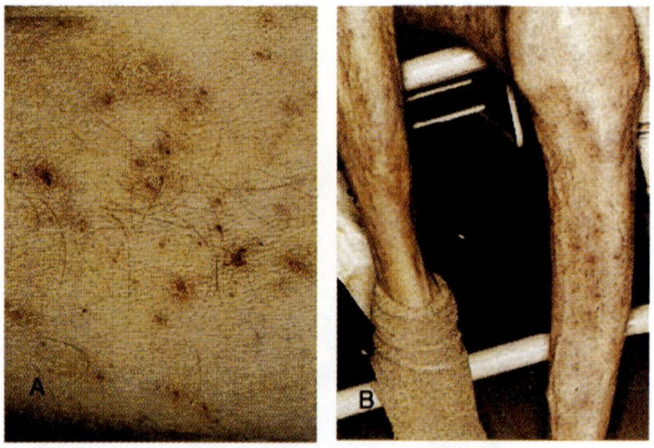

FIGURE 3-33 (A) Typical rash of scabies on the back. (B) Typical rash of scabies on the legs and knees. *(Courtesy of L.E. Morris and Donna J. Lewis, Management of Chronic, Resistive Scabies: A Case Study, Geriatric Nursing 16 [Sept/Oct 1995]: 230–37)*

and around the knees (Figure 3.33B) and lower buttocks. One type of scabies causes scaling of the skin on the palms of hands and soles of feet. If you notice a rash, notify the nurse immediately. As with head lice, you will be directed to wear a gown and gloves for further resident contact.

Treatment for Scabies

Special medicated creams and lotions are used to kill the mites. Products containing the chemical lindane are toxic and are not recommended. Some strains of scabies have become resistant to commonly used treatments. The resident's nails should be clipped before beginning the procedure. The medicated treatment is worked into and around the fingernail area with a cotton swab. The resident must not be bathed before or after the lotion is applied. You may be directed to apply the lotion to the resident's entire body, not just the rash area. It is not applied to the eyelids or lips. Wear a gown and gloves when applying this treatment. The lotion remains on the resident's skin for 12 to 24 hours, then is washed off in the tub or shower. If the resident's hands are washed during this period, reapply the lotion. Depending on the solution used, another treatment may be required several days to several weeks later. It takes about a month from the first treatment for the rash to disappear. The resident may experience itching even after the scabies are eliminated. You may be directed to check other residents for the appearance of a rash. Facility personnel who have had direct contact with the host resident may also be treated to prevent the spread of the mite.

The resident's room, clothing, and linen must also be cleaned. Wear a gown and gloves when you are assigned to this task. The room and furnishings should be vacuumed thoroughly to capture mites in the environment. Check the mattress and furniture for cracks, as the mite often crawls into the foam padding. If items cannot be vacuumed, they are bagged in a sealed plastic bag for 14 days. The mite cannot live beyond this time without food. Some facilities expose the bags to extreme heat or cold to kill the mite more quickly. The mattress is turned and vacuumed, then wiped with a facility-approved disinfectant to remove microbes left from the outside of the vacuum cleaner. Contact precautions are used for 24 hours after the resident is treated. If the resident requires a second treatment, the cleaning procedure is repeated for clothing, linen, and furnishings.

Drug resistance. As with other microbes, lice and scabies have become resistant to some of the common pesticides used in shampoos and body lotions. When treating for head lice or scabies, it is important to use the products exactly as directed. If live parasites are noted after a resident has been properly treated, it is recommended that the treatment product be changed or discontinued. Products for treating lice and scabies are pesticides and repeated use can cause toxicity and other serious complications.

BIOTERRORISM

Bioterrorism is the use of biological agents, such as pathogenic organisms or agricultural pests, for terrorist purposes. Since October 2001, state, local, and governmental public health authorities have been investigating cases of bioterrorism-related illness in the United States. Some individuals died from inhalation anthrax, a condition that was spread by a powdery substance sent through the mail. A number of other individuals developed the cutaneous (skin) version of this disease. Cutaneous anthrax is not fatal. Anthrax cannot be passed from one person to the next. It is transmitted only through contact with spores. Fortunately, the number of workplaces and individuals contaminated was small, but it raised concerns regarding future terrorist attacks. Many individuals could be infected by a biological weapon before the exposure is detected and diagnosed. Some of the diseases that can potentially be used as biological weapons have been eradicated for years and today's health care professionals have never seen or treated them. Thus, bioterrorism potentially represents a significant threat.

Many health care facilities have developed disaster plans to address bioterrorism. The plans outline the steps necessary for responding to bioterrorism with the most common agents, including smallpox, botulism, anthrax, and plague. The disaster plan covers information for residents, employees, and visitors, and lists public health precautions and protocols to follow in the event of an emergency. Unfortunatedly, health care facilities must be prepared for potential terrorist actions in the future.

KEY POINTS

- Medical asepsis refers to practices used in health care facilities to prevent the spread of infection.
- Microorganisms are everywhere. Pathogens are microorganisms that cause disease.
- The most common methods for spread of infection are airborne, droplet, direct contact, and indirect contact.
- The nursing assistant plays an important role in preventing the spread of infection.
- The nursing assistant must know which items are considered clean and which are considered soiled. These items must be separated to prevent the spread of infection.

- Handwashing is the most important method used to prevent the spread of infection.
- Bloodborne pathogens are microbes that cause disease through contact with blood, any moist body fluid except sweat, secretions, excretions, nonintact skin, and mucous membranes.
- HIV disease, hepatitis B, and hepatitis C are examples of diseases that are spread by contact with bloodborne pathogens.
- Hepatitis B is a greater threat to health care workers than HIV.
- Standard precautions are measures used in the care of all residents to prevent the spread of disease.
- The nursing assistant is responsible for selecting and using the correct personal protective equipment for the procedure being performed.
- Needles, razors, and other sharps are disposed of in puncture-resistant biohazardous waste containers.
- Trash and linen that have contacted blood or body fluids are biohazardous waste.
- Transmission-based precautions are isolation categories designed to interrupt the mode of transmission so the pathogen cannot spread.
- Isolation can be emotionally difficult for the resident.
- A HEPA mask is used when a resident is in airborne precautions. A PFR95 or N95 respirator may be worn instead.
- A surgical mask is used when a resident is in droplet precautions.
- A gown and gloves are used when a resident is in contact precautions.
- Standard precautions are used in addition to transmission-based precautions.
- Escherichia coli is a type of bacteria that normally resides in the intestines. It can cause serious illness outside the intestinal tract.
- E. coli 0157:H7 is a nonhuman strain that is found in the intestines of some cattle. It is most commonly spread in undercooked hamburger, and has caused outbreaks resulting in serious illness and death.
- Pseudomembranous colitis occurs when antibiotics destroy the normal, helpful bowel flora, except for C. difficile. Without the other friendly bacteria to keep it in check, C. difficile breeds rapidly, producing toxins that cause diarrhea and serious illness.
- Hantavirus causes serious respiratory illness. It is spread by contact with rodents or their excretions, including urine and stool.
- Shingles develop only in individuals who have had chickenpox. The resident develops painful, blister-like lesions on the torso that are often mistaken for a rash.
- Health care workers who have not had chickenpox should not enter the room of a resident who has shingles, if other immune caregivers are available.
- Drug-resistant organisms are a problem in health care facilities. Their spread can be prevented by medical asepsis and use of standard precautions.
- Tuberculosis is a growing public health problem that is detected by a skin test and treated with antibiotics.
- Head lice and scabies are highly contagious and require the use of contact precautions for 24 hours after the resident is treated.
- Bioterrorism is the use of biological agents, such as pathogenic organisms or agricultural pests, for terrorist purposes.

REVIEW

A. Multiple Choice

Select the one best answer.

1. Medical asepsis is
   a. a surgical technique.
   b. practices used to prevent the spread of infection.
   c. of concern only to licensed personnel.
   d. part of the chain of infection.

2. An infection that develops when a person is a resident in a health care facility is called a/an

   a. facility infection.
   b. acquired infection.
   c. nosocomial infection.
   d. delayed infection.

3. Some factors that affect the body's natural ability to resist disease are

   a. height.
   b. nutritional status and presence of other diseases.
   c. range of motion.
   d. a heater in the room to prevent chilling.

4. The system that detects pathogens in the body and stimulates the body's defenses to prevent disease is the

   a. immune system.
   b. nervous system.
   c. genitourinary system.
   d. respiratory system.

5. Infections can be spread by

   a. direct contact.
   b. inhaling a microbe.
   c. vectors.
   d. all of the above.

6. An example of common vehicle method of transmission is

   a. touching a contaminated object.
   b. eating contaminated food.
   c. inhaling droplets in the air.
   d. shaking hands.

7. Droplets usually are confined to a space within

   a. 3 feet of the resident.
   b. 6 feet of the resident.
   c. 12 feet of the resident.
   d. 24 feet of the resident.

8. Pathogens spread by the airborne method:

   a. are confined to a space within three feet of the resident.
   b. pose no threat to others.
   c. travel long distances in the ventilation system.
   d. are contracted in a negative-pressure room.

9. The six factors necessary for an infection to spread are called the

   a. mode of transmission.
   b. reservoir of infection.
   c. portal of exit.
   d. chain of infection.

10. _______ must be used in the care of all residents.

    a. Standard precautions
    b. Substance isolation
    c. Skin precautions
    d. Isolation precautions

11. The most important measure health care workers use to prevent the spread of infection is

    a. wearing a mask.
    b. handwashing.
    c. surgical asepsis.
    d. wearing a gown.

12. Handwashing should be performed

    a. at least three times a day.
    b. after work only.
    c. before applying and after removing gloves.
    d. before visiting with a resident.

13. Handwashing should be done for a minimum of

    a. 3 seconds.
    b. 5 seconds.
    c. 15 seconds.
    d. 60 seconds.

14. A vaccination is available to protect health care workers from

    a. AIDS.
    b. hepatitis B.
    c. herpes.
    d. MRSA.

15. Hepatitis B, hepatitis C, and AIDS are spread by

    a. blood and body fluid contact.
    b. the inhalation method.
    c. casual contact.
    d. using the same bathroom.

16. Gloves should be worn when

    a. combing a resident's hair.
    b. entering a resident's room.
    c. taking a blood pressure.
    d. brushing a resident's teeth.

17. The transmission-based precautions category in which a gown is routinely worn during close resident care is
    a. airborne precautions.
    b. contact precautions.
    c. droplet precautions.
    d. standard precautions.
18. When working in an airborne precautions room, you should wear a
    a. HEPA mask (or equivalent).
    b. surgical mask (or equivalent).
    c. gown.
    d. face shield.
19. Trash that is contaminated with blood or body fluids is identified by
    a. using a black bag.
    b. a circle with a slash through it.
    c. the biohazard emblem.
    d. a pink label.
20. Apply personal protective equipment in this order
    a. gloves, gown, mask.
    b. mask, gown, gloves.
    c. gown, mask, gloves.
    d. gloves, mask, gown.
21. Drug-resistant organisms
    a. are of no concern to the nursing assistant.
    b. can be eliminated easily with most antibiotics.
    c. are a threat to residents and health care workers.
    d. are very uncommon.
22. Tuberculosis is
    a. a growing public health concern.
    b. a disease that was eliminated in the 1960s.
    c. easily treated.
    d. a vector-borne respiratory illness.
23. Head lice and scabies are
    a. the same as nits.
    b. fomites.
    c. parasites.
    d. viruses.
24. When a resident has scabies, he or she will be placed in
    a. airborne precautions.
    b. contact precautions.
    c. droplet precautions.
    d. secretion precautions.
25. Alcohol-based hand cleansers
    a. should not be used during resident care.
    b. may be used unless hands are visibly soiled.
    c. are used only when a sink is not available.
    d. may be used only by nurses during medication pass.
26. After removing gloves
    a. wash your hands or use an alcohol-based cleanser.
    b. quickly rinse your hands with cool water and dry them.
    c. scrub your hands with disinfectant solution.
    d. handwashing is not necessary.
27. Pseudomembranous colitis
    a. occurs only in infants wearing diapers.
    b. is spread by rats and other rodents.
    c. is contracted by the airborne method.
    d. is diarrhea caused by antibiotics.
28. Shingles
    a. occurs only in residents who have had measles.
    b. does not readily spread to others.
    c. follows the nerve pathways, causing pain.
    d. is spread by vectors and fomites.
29. Petechiae are
    a. small, purple spots on the skin.
    b. swollen and painful.
    c. breaks in the skin surface.
    d. immune factors.
30. The use of biological agents for terrorist purposes is
    a. bioterrorism.
    b. chemical warfare.
    c. biology.
    d. biomedical warfare.

B. True/False

Answer each statement true (T) or false (F).

31. ______The term infection control refers to practices that reduce the spread of infection in the health care facility.

32. ______ Susceptibility is the ability of the body to resist disease.

33. _____ Hepatitis B destroys the immune system.

34. _____ A handshake is an example of the spread of infection through indirect contact.

35. ______ A microbe that is capable of causing disease is a pathogen.

36. ________ The objective of using medical asepsis is to break the chain of infection.

37. ____ Always wear gloves on both hands when carrying contaminated items in the hallway.

38. _______ It is not necessary to wash your hands after gloves are removed.

39. ______ Standard precautions are used in the care of all residents.

40. ______ Gloves should be changed immediately before contact with mucous membranes.

41. ______ Artificial fingernails may be worn when on duty, as long as they are kept short.

42. ________ Rings may hide pathogens.

43. ________ Flora are microbes that inhabit the internal and external surfaces of healthy individuals.

C. Fill in the Blanks

44–49. List six times when you should wash your hands.

44. ______________ 47. ______________
45. ______________ 48. ______________
46. ______________ 49. ______________

D. Clinical Applications

Answer the following questions.

50. David Long, a nursing assistant, has just completed caring for Mr. Brent. The resident had a loose bowel movement in a bedpan. David must carry the bedpan to the bathroom and clean it. David has BM on his gloves. How does David pull up the side rail and open the bathroom door without contaminating the environment with his soiled gloves?

51. Sam and John have been roommates for years. Both are mentally confused and walk around in the room. You are assigned to pass fresh water to the residents on Hall C. When you get to Sam and John's room, you find two water pitchers and two cups sitting side by side on the counter in the bathroom. You do not know which pitcher and cup belong to which resident. What should you do?

52. Susan Lange is a 37-year-old resident with AIDS. She has bumped her leg on the side rail and is bleeding. You accidentally get some blood on your hand. What should you do?

53. You are assigned to care for Mr. Jefferson, who is in contact precautions for an MRSA infection of a surgical wound. Mr. Jefferson is alert, oriented, and cooperative. He feeds himself. What personal protective equipment will you wear when you
    a. Serve the meal tray?
    b. Change the linen on the bed?

54. While caring for Mr. Jefferson, your gloves become soiled. You are not through with giving care. What should you do?

UNIT 4

Safety and Emergencies

OBJECTIVES

After reading this unit, you will be able to:

- Spell and define key terms.
- Describe measures to take to keep the environment safe.
- List three measures to take to prevent burns.
- Describe safety factors to consider when using heat and cold applications.
- Describe safety factors to use when caring for a resident who is using oxygen.
- List the three elements necessary to start a fire.
- Describe your responsibilities if there is a fire, tornado, hurricane, earthquake, or bomb threat.
- Describe what to do if you find a resident in an emergency situation.
- List seven guidelines to follow in an emergency.
- State the purpose of early access defibrillation.
- Demonstrate procedures related to safety and emergencies.

OBSERVATIONS TO MAKE AND REPORT RELATED TO SAFETY AND EMERGENCIES

Chest pain
Shortness of breath
Difficulty breathing
Weakness or dizziness
Headache
Pain or body language suggesting pain
Nausea or vomiting
Diarrhea (multiple loose stools; one loose stool is not diarrhea)
Cough
Cyanosis or change in color
Change in mental status
Excessive thirst
Lethargy
Unusual drainage from the skin, a wound, or a body cavity
Abnormal appearance of urine or feces
Inability to hear blood pressure or palpate pulse
Changes in vital signs
Abnormal behavior, including crying
Requests for medication for an acute problem

IMPORTANCE OF SAFETY IN THE LONG-TERM CARE FACILITY

Safety is everyone's concern. Special safety measures are described throughout this text. Every employee is responsible for keeping the environment safe and preventing **accidents**. However, because of their close and consistent contact with the residents, much of the burden for maintaining a safe environment rests with the nursing assistants.

Accidents are unexpected events that often result in injuries, which can range from minor to serious. An **incident** is an occurrence that disrupts the normal procedures and routine of the facility. It may be the result of an accident. A fall is an accident, but it is also an incident. If a confused resident wanders away, but is returned unharmed, an incident has occurred. An incident report (Figure 4.1) is completed by the charge nurse on all accidents and incidents. The incident report states what happened, describes injuries, lists witnesses, and records special notifications of the doctor and resident's family. Information written on the incident report is always **factual**. This is information that you *know* is true, not what you *think* may have happened. You may be asked to do extra monitoring of the resident until the signs of the incident are **resolved**. An incident is resolved when the charge nurse is certain that problems related to the incident are over and the resident is stable and out of danger.

Most accidents can be prevented. Accidents can occur to residents, visitors, and employees. Everyone benefits from a safe environment. The most common accidents in long-term care facilities are falls and burns.

Physical and Mental Changes in Disease and Aging that Increase the Risk of Incidents

Physical and mental changes occur with aging and with certain diseases. Many of these changes affect the resident's awareness of hazards in the environment, and thus increase the risk of incidents. Factors that influence resident safety include:

- Changes in vision affect the resident's ability to see unsafe conditions. Other changes in vision may cause residents to be unable to judge distance.
- Changes in hearing may affect the resident's ability to hear warnings, or approaching carts or equipment.
- Some diseases cause **tremors**, or shaking that the resident cannot control. Tremors affect the resident's balance and increase the risk of falls.
- Changes in the blood vessels may cause residents to become dizzy when they stand up.
- **Reflexes** are slower in the elderly and in people with certain diseases. Reflexes are automatic, involuntary reactions that cause us to pull away from danger. Because some individuals react more slowly, they cannot move away quickly. For example, if you place your hand under very hot water, you quickly pull away. If a resident with impaired reflexes placed a hand under hot water, he or she would remove it more slowly, and could be burned.
- Some residents have mental changes that cause them to be confused and forgetful. These residents may not use good judgment and may not be aware of common dangers.
- Some residents may be weak because of an illness or injury. This may cause them to fall.
- Some medications have side effects that can cause dizziness, visual disturbances, blood pressure changes, and other problems that increase the risk of injury.

Some residents may not be aware that their activities can be harmful to them. They may resent the staff's efforts to protect them. They feel that they can protect themselves. Residents may also be in **denial**. When a person is in denial, he or she is afraid to admit that something is true. Residents may be afraid that if they admit to having a need, they will no longer be independent. Speak with residents about safety. Explain what you are doing to keep the environment safe. Explain safety to residents during the procedures that you do. Always be alert to safety factors when you enter and leave a room.

Providing a Safe Environment

You can do many things to make the long-term care facility safe. If you notice an unsafe condition that you can correct, you should do so immediately. Report unsafe conditions that you cannot correct to the nurse or the proper person in your facility. Warn others of safety hazards. Follow facility policies and procedures. Set a good example for others by using safe practices. Attend classes on health and safety issues and practice what you are taught.

Safety in the hallways. Everyone is responsible for keeping the hallways safe. If you notice a spill on the floor, wipe it up immediately and place a "wet floor" sign (Figure 4.2). Keep all equipment

RESIDENT INCIDENT REPORT

IF INJURY SERIOUS, GIVE IMMEDIATE NOTICE TO THE ADMINISTRATOR AND DIRECTOR OF NURSING SERVICE

NOTE: PLEASE COMPLETE IN DETAIL

INSTRUCTIONS: Completed report to D.O.N. for review and filing in Administrator's Office. Make detailed report in Nurses Notes/Resident Records.

DATE OF OCCURRENCE 1/4/XX PLACE Room 304 TIME 4:30 AM (PM)

NAME Jane Walther TEMP 98.4 BLOOD PRESSURE 134/88 PULSE 80 RESPIRATIONS 16

ASSISTANCE NEEDED (Partial or Total)	FUNCTIONING (Partial or Total)	MENTAL STATUS*** Yes No	BEHAVIOR PROBLEMS 1-Minimum 2-Moderate 3-Maximum
P T Ambulation	P T Bedfast	(Y) N Lucid	2 Confused
P T Amb. w/Cane, Crutch, Walker	P T Fecal Incontinent	Y (N) Labile	0 Withdrawn
(P) T Transferring	P T Urinary Incontinent	(Y) N Disoriented	0 Hyperactive
(P) T Wheelchair Mobility	(P) T Blindness	Y (N) Comatose	0 Wanders
P T Bedside Chair	P T Deafness	Y (N) Semi-Comatose	0 Suspicious
(P) T Bathing	P T Aphasia	(Y) N Forgetful	0 Combative
(P) T Dressing	P T Speech Problem	Y (N) Controlled with Medication	2 Supervised for Safety
P T Grooming			0 Causes Mgt. Problems

RESTRAINTS ORDERED: ☐ YES ☑ NO ☐ NOT APPLICABLE

Complete this section ***ONLY IF mental status contributed to incident/accident

IF NOT USED, WHY?

WAS PRN MEDICATION ADMINISTERED BEFORE INCIDENT? ☐ YES ☑ NO ☐ NOT APPLICABLE

NAME OF DRUG ADMINISTERED & TIME ADMINISTERED

DESCRIPTION OF INCIDENT (include circumstances under which incident occurred): Resident attempted to transfer self from bed to w/c unassisted. No witnesses to incident. Res. was found on floor. Brakes to w/c were not locked. Footrests to w/c were in down position. Res. had socks on feet, but no shoes. States "I slipped".

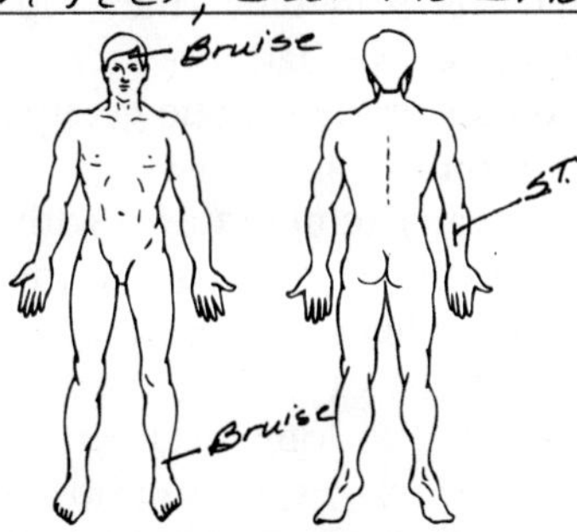

INDICATE ON FIGURES PART OF BODY AFFECTED AND DESCRIBE EXTENT OF INJURY:

Bruise (L) temple
Skin tear (R) forearm
Bruise (L) ankle

PHYSICIAN'S NAME John Dennis, D.O.

PHYSICIAN NOTIFIED: DATE 1/4/XX TIME 4:50 AM (PM)

PHYSICIAN'S ORDERS, TREATMENT OR STATEMENT: Cleanse skin tear + apply dry dressing.

HOSPITALIZED: ☐ YES ☒ NO NAME OF HOSPITAL

FIGURE 4-1 An incident report is completed on all incidents and accidents.

and supplies on the same side of the hallway. Your goal is to have one side of the hallway free so that residents can walk safely without having to go around large pieces of equipment or the wheelchairs of others. Follow your facility policy for separating items considered clean or soiled. Pick up any items, papers, or equipment dropped on the floor.

Never run in the hallways. Teach residents to use the handrails when they walk in the hallway. If you are transporting residents or equipment in the hall, watch where you are going. Approach corners slowly and look before you go around them. Take care when approaching or going through swinging doors. Avoid blocking exit doors or automatic fire doors with equipment or furnishings. Back wheelchairs and stretchers in and out of elevators, down ramps, and over thresholds in doorways.

Safety in the resident's room. Be sure there is enough light in residents' rooms. Visual changes

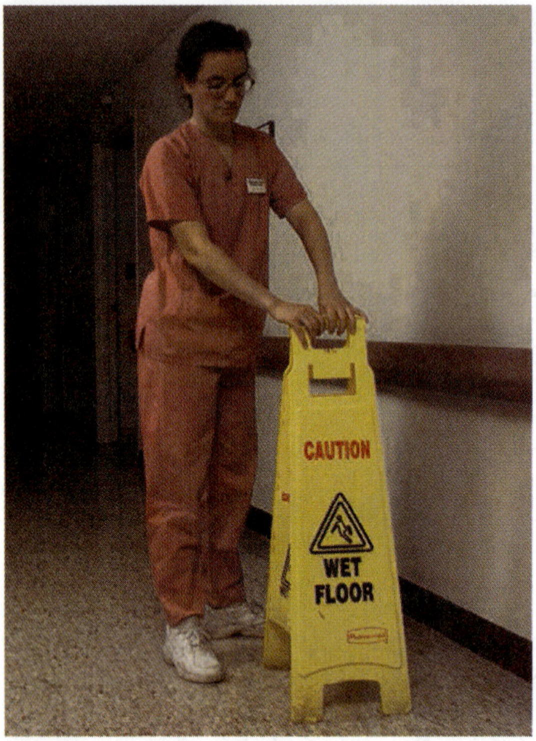

FIGURE 4-2 A wet floor sign warns others of slippery spots.

as a result of aging and disease make it difficult to see in dim lighting. However, avoid bright lights that shine directly into the residents' eyes. Remove any items that have fallen on the floor. Arrange the furniture so it is against the walls, not in the middle of the room.

Avoid dressing residents in long clothing that may cause them to trip. Avoid clothing or linen that may get caught in the wheels of a wheelchair. If residents will be walking or transferring from a bed to a wheelchair, make sure their footwear is appropriate for the floor surface. In facilities with tile floors, nonslip footwear is best. On carpeted floors, leather or plastic soles may work better. Nonslip soles may catch on carpeting, causing the resident to stumble. Residents should not walk or transfer in socks or with bare feet, because of the risk of falls.

Follow your facility policy for use of electrical appliances, such as televisions, radios, heating pads, and hair dryers in resident rooms. Most facilities require that appliances brought in from home be checked by the maintenance department for safety before they are used. Extension cords are not permitted. If you observe an electrical hazard, notify the proper person immediately. Follow your facility policy for removing it from service.

Perform procedures in the way you were taught and avoid taking shortcuts. Taking shortcuts in your work may cause injury to yourself and others.

All residents should have a call signal within reach at all times. Residents who are mentally confused must also have a call signal available. Answer all call signals as soon as possible. If residents are unable to get up from their beds or chairs, make sure that needed personal items are within reach. If residents have to bend or stretch to reach items they need, they may lose their balance and fall.

If you notice items in a room that you think are unsafe, follow your facility policy for removing them, or ask the nurse for advice. Common items, such as nail polish remover and denture cleaning tablets, can be harmful if swallowed by a confused resident.

Safety in the bathroom. Many accidents occur in the bathroom. Residents may be in a hurry to get to the bathroom. They may lose their balance, slip, trip, and fall. Sometimes they slip on a wet floor. Always check the bathroom for safety. Leave a nightlight on for residents who get up at night to use the bathroom.

Check hot water temperatures with a thermometer before bathing residents. If a thermometer is not available, check the temperature on the inside of your wrist or forearm. Water temperatures are regulated in long-term care facilities to keep the water from getting too hot. Sometimes the regulators fail. If you have to add cold water to wash your hands, the water may be too hot. Ask the proper person in your facility to check the temperature. The hottest temperature allowed by law may be too hot for some residents. Use a thermometer so that you know the exact temperature of the water. Turn hot water on last and off first. Some whirlpool and bathing units have built-in thermometers. These thermometers are checked by the maintenance department regularly. However, the thermometers sometimes fail. Use common sense. If the built-in thermometer on the whirlpool shows a low reading, but the water feels hot to touch, or is steaming, do not put the resident in the tub until you have checked the temperature with another thermometer. Follow your facility policy for using bath oil. It is not used in some facilities because it makes the tub very slippery. Use shower chairs in the shower. Do not leave residents alone in the bathtub, whirlpool, or shower.

Safe use of chemicals. Many different types of **chemicals** are used in long-term care facilities. Chemicals are substances that may be harmful if they touch the skin or mucous membranes. They are usually harmful if swallowed or inhaled. Most cleaning products are chemicals. Keep all chemicals in their original containers. All chemicals must be labeled. Never pour them into unmarked containers. Never use the contents of an unmarked container. If you think the label on a container is incorrect, do not use the product. The label on the package of cleaning products will have a warning if the chemical is dangerous. Some cosmetics, such as nail polish remover, also contain harmful chemicals. Cosmetic manufacturers are not required to provide as much information on the label as other chemical manufacturers. Use each chemical according to the directions on the package. Cleaning products should be stored in a locked area when not in use. Avoid storing them in the same area as food or beverages. If you are using a cleaning product in a resident care area, you must be able to see it at all times. Never put a bottle down and turn your back on it. If you suspect that a resident has swallowed a chemical product, take the container to the nurse immediately.

The Hazardous Communication Right to Know program is designed to make employees aware of the correct use and hazards of chemicals used in the workplace. The long-term care facility is required to keep **material safety data sheets (MSDS)** (Figure 4.3) for all chemicals used. Know the location of these information sheets in your department. The MSDS will provide information and instructions for safe use, identify health risks, and describe first aid and safety precautions.

Safety with mentally confused residents. Besides the safety practices already discussed, keep sharp objects and plants away from residents who are mentally confused. If you are not sure about the safety of an item, check with the nurse.

Equipment safety. Use equipment only according to manufacturers' directions. If you have not been taught to use electrical or mechanical equipment, do not use it. If you feel that a piece of equipment is unsafe, follow your facility policy for notifying the proper person. Many facilities use a **lockout-tagout** system. Under this program, a locking device is placed on the equipment in a way that prevents the equipment from being used. A special tag identifies the equipment as broken and warns others not to use it (Figure 4.4). Always follow your facility policy for reporting and removing unsafe or broken equipment from service.

Answering Call Signals

Your facility will have policies for staff to follow for answering call signals. The call signal may be the only way that the resident has to get help in an emergency. Remember, all residents should have a call signal available at all times.

Most facilities require all staff to answer residents' call signals, whether or not they are assigned to care for that resident. Facilities usually have two types of call signals. One type is the regular signal used in resident rooms (Figure 4.5A). The other type is an emergency signal (Figure 4.5B) used in bathrooms, tubs, and shower rooms. Become familiar with both types of signals. Regular call signals should be answered as soon as possible, usually within three minutes or less. Emergency call signals should be answered immediately.

When you answer a call signal, knock on the resident's door and wait for a response before entering. Identify yourself and ask how you can help. Turn the call signal off. Do what the resident asks, or notify the proper person of the resident's request.

Resident Identification Systems

Many types of identification systems are used by health care facilities. The most common type is the **identification band** system. The identification band is a plastic band, placed around the resident's wrist or ankle, that contains identifying information. Some facilities use color-coded identification bands for specific purposes. For example, many facilities use pink or red bands to identify residents with diabetes. Residents at risk of wandering outside may have a special color band. Some facilities use self-adhesive colored dots on the identification band. These dots have special meanings. For example, a resident who needs extra liquids may have a blue dot on the identification band. Some facilities place a dot on the identification band with the resident's "code" status. This tells staff at a glance if CPR should be performed if the resident experiences a cardiac arrest. Facilities use color-coded bands and dots for many different conditions. Find out the meaning of these systems, if used by your facility.

Many long-term care facilities place the resident's name on the door of the room. Some also place the resident's picture by the door. The resident or responsible party must give permission

Material Safety Data Sheet

PRODUCT CODE NUMBERS:
MSC5300

SECTION 1

ISSUE DATE: 9-21-96
IDENTITY: **Exuderm Hydrocolloid Ultra Dressing**

MARKETED OR DISTRIBUTED BY:
Medline Industries, Inc.
One Medline Place
Mundelein, IL 60060
1.800.MEDLINE

Emergency Telephone Number:
Contact Your Regional Poison Control Center

SECTION 2 - HAZARDOUS INGREDIENTS/IDENTITY INFORMATION

HAZARDOUS COMPONENTS (SPECIFIC CHEMICAL IDENTITY, COMMON NAME(S)	CAS#	OSHA PEL	ACGIH TLV	OTHER LIMITS RECOMMENDED	% (OPTIONAL)
None					

SECTION 3 - PHYSICAL/CHEMICAL CHARACTERISTICS

BOILING POINT: N/A	SP GRAVITY (WATER=1): N/A
VAPOR PRESSURE (MM HG): N/A	MELTING POINT: N/A
VAPOR DENSITY (AIR=1): N/A	EVAPORATION RATE(BUTYL ACETATE=1): N/A
SOLUBILITY IN WATER: N/A	
APPEARANCE AND ODOR: Light caramel in color and no odor	

SECTION 4 - FIRE AND EXPLOSION HAZARD DATA

FLASH POINT (METHOD USED): N/A		
FLAMMABLE LIMITS: N/A	LEL: N/A	UEL: N/A
EXTINGUISHING MEDIA: Water, dry chemical or foam		
SPECIAL FIRE FIGHTING PROCEDURES: None		
UNUSUAL FIRE AND EXPLOSIVE HAZARDS: None		

SECTION 5 - REACTIVITY DATA

STABILITY: Stable
CONDITIONS TO AVOID: Avoid overheating and freezing.
INCOMPATIBILITY (MATERIALS TO AVOID): N/A
HAZARDOUS DECOMPOSITION OR BYPRODUCTS: N/A
HAZARDOUS POLYMERIZATION: Will not Occur
CONDITIONS TO AVOID: N/A

SECTION 6 - HEALTH HAZARD DATA

ROUTE(S) OF ENTRY: INHALATION: N/A	SKIN: N/A		INGESTION: N/A
HEALTH HAZARDS (ACUTE AND CHRONIC): None			
CARCINOGENICITY? N/A	NTP? N/A	IARC? N/A	OSHA REGULATED? N/A
SIGNS AND SYMPTOMS OF EXPOSURE: May cause moderate irritation in eyes			
MEDICAL CONDITIONS GENERALLY AGGRAVATED BY EXPOSURE: N/A			
EMERGENCY AND FIRST AID PROCEDURES: Eye contact: Flush. Excessive Ingestion: Induce vomiting and consult physician.			

SECTION 7 - SPILL, LEAK, AND WASTE DISPOSAL PROCEDURES

STEPS TO BE TAKEN IN CASE MATERIAL IS RELEASED OR SPILLED: N/A
WASTE DISPOSAL METHOD: In accordance with all local, state and federal regulations.
PRECAUTIONS TO BE TAKEN IN HANDLING AND STORING: N/A
OTHER PRECAUTIONS: N/A

SECTION 8 - CONTROL MEASURES

RESPIRATORY PROTECTION (SPECIFY TYPE): N/A		
VENTILATION:	LOCAL EXHAUST: N.A.	SPECIAL: N/A
	MECHANICAL (GENERAL): N/A	OTHER: N/A
PROTECTIVE GLOVES: N/A		EYE PROTECTION: N/A
SPECIAL CLOTHING: N/A		
WORK/HYGIENIC PRACTICES: None		

SECTION 9 - SPECIAL PRECAUTIONS

None

SECTION 10 - ADDITIONAL INFORMATION

Exuderm Hydrocolloid Dressing has passed all testing required for medical devices as outlined in the FDA Biocompatibility Guidelines for short term devices in contact with breached or compromised skin.

The information provided in this Material Safety Data Sheet has been obtained from sources believed to be reliable.

Medline Industries, Inc. provides no warranties, either expressed or implied and assumes no responsibility for the accuracy or completeness of the data contained herein.

ISSUE DATE: 9-21-96
Revised: 10/31/01 Updated telephone information

FIGURE 4-3 Material Safety Data Sheets provide important information and instructions on chemical use, health risks, first aid, and safety precautions. (*Courtesy of Medline Industries, Inc., 1-800-MEDLNE*)

to list the resident on a roster, or to post the name by the door of the room. The facility cannot disclose the names of residents without consent. Sometimes special decorations, such as bows or decorated hats, are placed on the doors to help confused residents find their rooms. They are

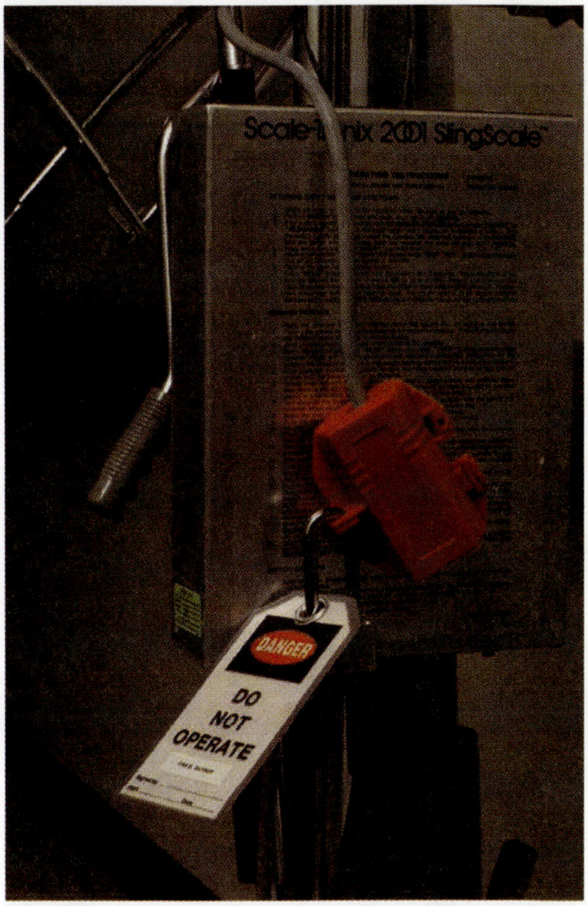

FIGURE 4-4 A tag is locked to a broken piece of electrical or mechanical equipment, to warn others not to use it.

directed to find the "blue bow" or the "straw hat" when they are looking for their rooms.

Some long-term care facilities use special identification systems for residents who may be in danger if they wander away. These devices are discussed in detail in Unit 15. However, the visual appearance of the device is distinct, so you can assume that if a resident is wearing one, he or she is at high risk of leaving the facility and will require close monitoring. Commonly, these are bracelets with magnetic sensors in them (Figure 4.6). The sensors are similar to the devices used in stores to prevent shoplifting. Use of the sensor allows the resident to move freely about the facility. If the resident tries to leave through an outside door, an alarm will sound. The bracelets are usually put on the wrist of the dominant hand to make them difficult to remove.

Always identify residents before giving care. Check the resident's identification band and call the resident by name. Some residents will answer to any name they are called, so make sure that

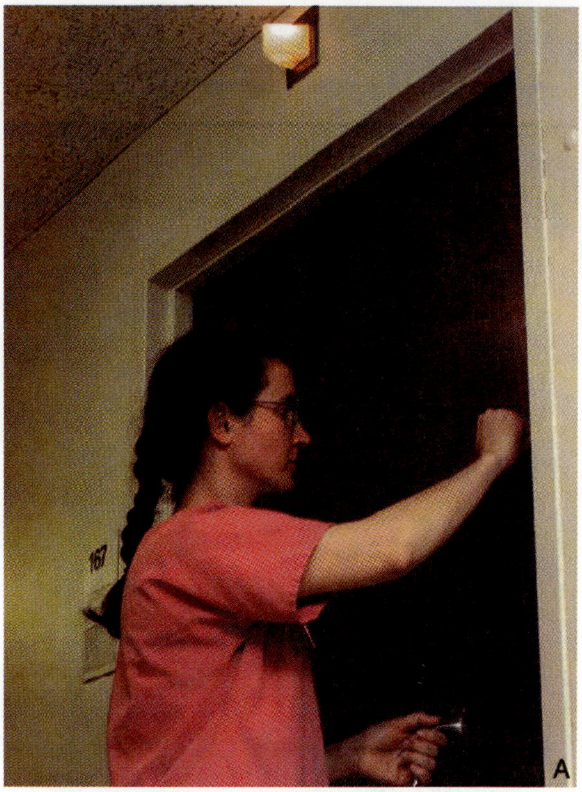

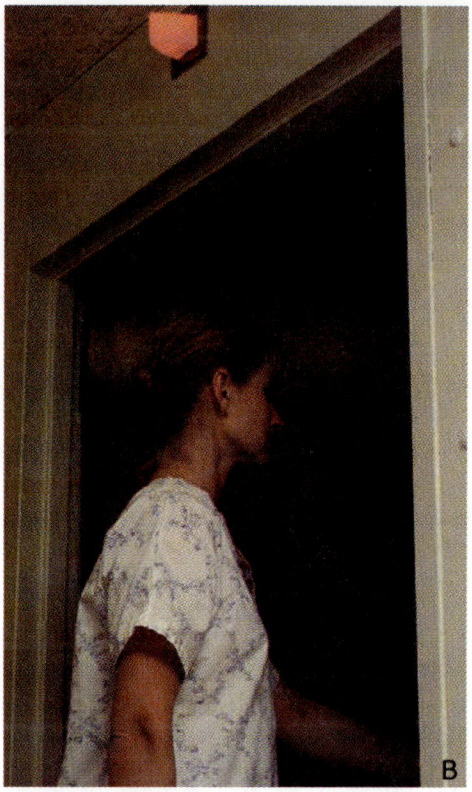

FIGURE 4-5A (A) The regular call signal is white and does not blink. (B) The emergency call signal is red and blinks, indicating that the resident needs immediate attention.

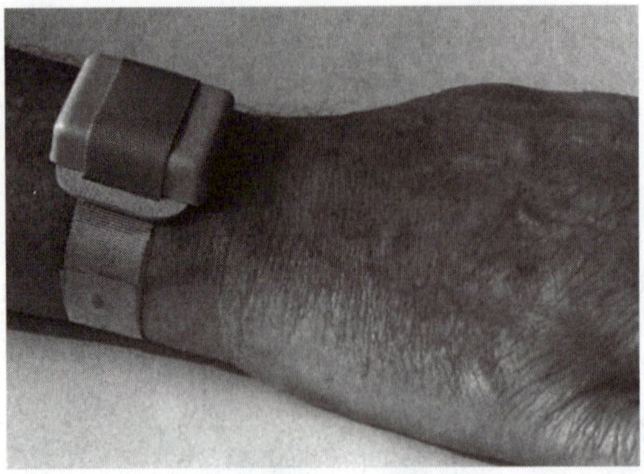

FIGURE 4-6 The magnetic sensor band is used in addition to the facility identification band. The sensor sets off an alarm if the resident tries to leave through an exit door, or enter a dangerous area, such as the stairwell. (© *1996 RF Technologies. Used by permission*)

you have the right resident before giving care. Do not be embarrassed if you have to ask a resident his or her name. It is better to ask than to provide care to the wrong resident.

Burn Prevention

Burns are a leading cause of injury. Residents with some diseases do not feel heat as acutely as healthy people. Hot water may burn them during bathing or treatments. Occasionally, hot liquids are spilled on residents, resulting in burns. Unsafe cigarette smoking is also a leading cause of burns.

Cigarette smoking. Know and follow your facility policy for cigarette smoking. If you smoke, do so only in designated areas. Some facilities allow smoking outside. Others do not allow smoking anywhere on the property. Some facilities do not allow residents to keep smoking materials. Most require that residents be supervised when they smoke. Residents are not allowed to smoke in their rooms except in special circumstances, and then only with direct supervision. Provide large, deep ashtrays for residents to use. Empty ashtrays only into metal cans with lids.

Thermal burns. **Thermal burns** are common injuries in long-term care facilities. Thermal burns are caused by contact with a hot substance or object, or an open flame. Be sure that you do not serve very hot food or liquids to residents. Help residents who are confused or who have poor hand control. Thermal burns are also caused by water that is too hot and careless smoking.

Heat and Cold Applications

Heat and cold applications are used for many different purposes. Moist applications can be hot or cold. In this type of application, water touches the skin. Dry applications are those in which no water touches the skin. Some dry applications have water inside them, such as hot water bottles. However, the outside of the application stays dry, and the skin does not get wet. Sometimes dry applications are used to maintain the temperature of moist applications.

A **localized application** is used to apply heat or cold to a specific area of the body. An example of this type of application is an ice bag applied to a swollen ankle. A **generalized application** is used to apply heat or cold to the resident's entire body. An example of this type of application is the cooling or **tepid** sponge bath to reduce a resident's temperature. Many facilities use cooling blankets for this purpose.

General Principles for Using Heat and Cold Applications

Localized heat and cold applications that touch the resident's skin should have a protective cover. Covers are usually made of flannel. Pillowcases and towels are also used. Some facilities use a thin layer of protective foam. Check with the nurse for the type of cover to use. If the device you are using, such as a hot water bottle or ice collar, has a metal cap, face the cap away from the resident. The metal in the cap can conduct heat or cold and cause injury to the resident.

Check the resident's skin under the application every 10 minutes. If the skin under a heat application appears very red, or if a dark area

GUIDELINES FOR

Using Heat and Cold Applications

Before using a heat or cold application, you should know the:

- Type of application
- Area of the resident's body to be treated
- Length of time the application is to stay in place
- Proper temperature of the application
- Safety precautions to use
- Side effects to watch for

appears, stop the application and notify the nurse. When using a cold application, stop the application and notify the nurse immediately if the resident's skin appears blue, pale, white, or bright red. If the resident is shivering and cold, remove the application, cover the resident with a blanket, and notify the nurse.

Applying Heat and Cold

Heat applications **dilate** or enlarge the blood vessels to bring oxygen and nutrients to an area. Heat may be used to relieve pain and speed healing. Local cold applications are used to relieve pain and prevent or relieve **edema**. Edema, or swelling, is common after an injury. Cold applications can also be used to stop or control bleeding. Cooling reduces the blood flow to the area and **constricts** blood vessels (makes them smaller). Generalized cooling may be used to reduce body temperature. This is done by cooling the entire body. The elderly may be very sensitive to heat and cold. When performing heat and cold treatments, assist the resident into a comfortable position that he or she can maintain for the duration of the treatment. Expose only the part of the body that you will be treating.

Follow all safety rules to prevent spills and falls. If the resident has a dressing covering the area to be treated, ask the nurse for assistance. Wear gloves if your hands will contact blood, moist body fluids (except sweat), secretions, excretions, nonintact skin, or mucous membranes. Always check the temperature of the solution to be used with a thermometer. You may need to add more liquid to the solution during the treatment to maintain the temperature. When you are done with the treatment, pat the skin dry. Make the resident comfortable. Clean and put away used equipment. Remove gloves, if worn, and dispose of them according to facility policy. Wash your hands. Report to the nurse that the procedure was completed, and also report the resident's reaction.

Oxygen Safety

Oxygen is necessary for life. We take in oxygen from the air when we breathe. Some diseases and conditions cause the resident to be unable to take in enough oxygen. In these cases, the doctor will usually order additional oxygen to be given by an oxygen delivery system. The doctor will order how much oxygen is to be used, the method of oxygen delivery, and the length of time it is to be applied. **You should not start, stop, or change the flow rate of oxygen.** However, you must know how to check the flow rate and know general safety measures to take when oxygen is in use. You must also be aware of where oxygen is stored in your facility, because the nurse may send you for the oxygen supply in an emergency. In many facilities, the nursing assistant is also responsible for cleaning oxygen equipment. Know and follow your facility policy.

Usually, the resident who is receiving oxygen will need the head of the bed elevated. Elevating the head of the bed makes breathing easier. Follow the instructions on your assignment sheet and the resident's care plan.

Oxygen Delivery Systems

Several types of oxygen delivery systems (Figure 4.7) are used in long-term care facilities. Oxygen may be piped in through the wall. Most facilities use oxygen tanks or concentrators. The oxygen concentrator converts room air to oxygen and delivers it to the resident. Oxygen also comes in a liquid canister (Figure 4.8). This canister delivers a higher concentration of oxygen than a concentrator, but is portable and convenient. It does not require electricity to operate. The canister is quiet compared with a concentrator, which has an electric motor and makes a

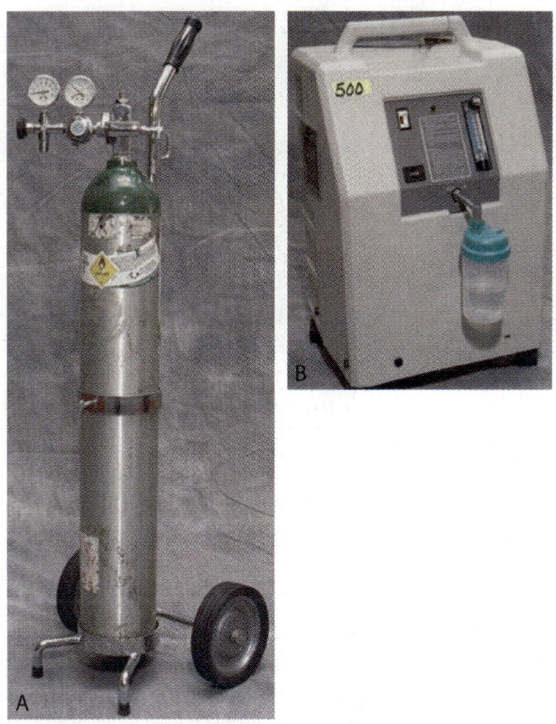

FIGURE 4-7 Most long-term care facilities use oxygen in (A) tanks and (B) concentrators.

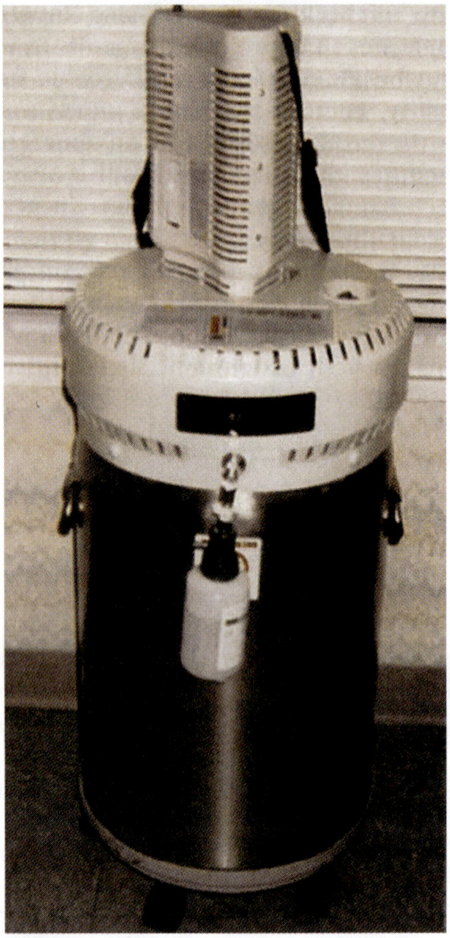

FIGURE 4-8 Liquid oxygen is portable and convenient. The small upper tank can be filled from the larger lower tank.

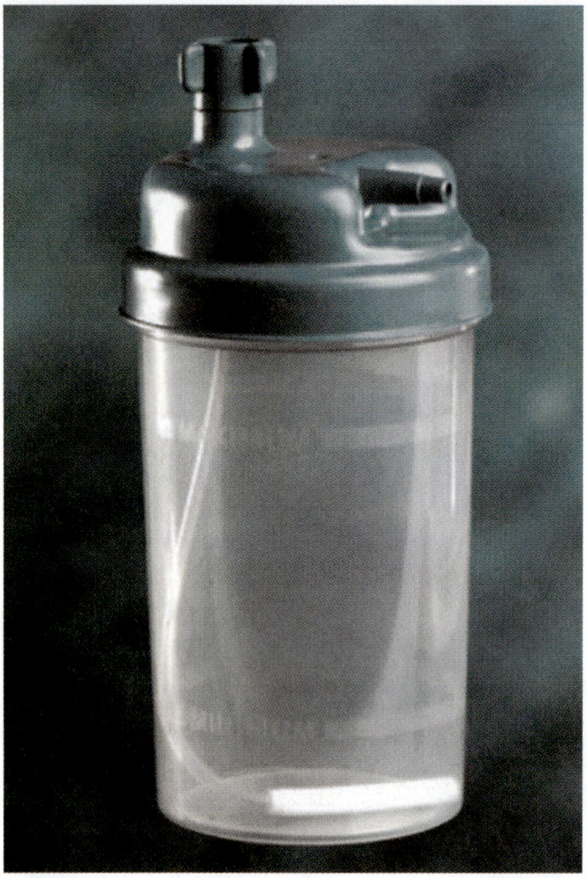

FIGURE 4-9A Humidification is not necessary for residents receiving low liter flows of oxygen, but some facilities use humidifiers to provide extra moisture and comfort. *(Courtesy of Hudson RCI, Temecula, CA, USA)*

humming noise. It is also more economical for the resident.

Oxygen can be very drying and uncomfortable for the resident. Dry oxygen thickens the respiratory secretions, making breathing more difficult. The oxygen may pass through a **humidifier** before it reaches the resident. The humidifier is a water bottle that moistens the oxygen for comfort and prevents drying of the mucous membranes in the nose, mouth, and lungs. Use of oxygen humidifiers is a controversial subject. Humidification is not necessary in liter flows below 5. Humidifiers are not used at all in some facilities.

The humidifier bottle (Figure 4.9A) screws into a male adapter on the flow meter. Oxygen passes through the water in the humidifier, picking up moisture, before it reaches the resident. The delivery device plugs into a male adapter on the side of the humidifier. Checking and changing the humidifier is a nursing assistant responsibility in some facilities. Sterile distilled water is always used. Avoid tap water. Inhalation of tap water is associated with an increased incidence of Legionnaire's disease. The water level in the humidifier should always be at or above the "minimum fill" line on the bottle. When the oxygen delivery system is functioning correctly, the water in the humidifier will bubble. Oxygen will not exit the tubing into the mask or cannula if the tubing is kinked or obstructed. If this occurs, pressure builds up in the unit and discharges through a pressure relief valve.

Two types of humidifiers are used. The *prefilled* type of humidifier is disposable. This unit is usually changed once a week, when it is empty, or according to manufacturers' directions or facility policies. Discard the bottle after replacing it with a new one. Your facility may require you to attach a sticker to the bottle listing the date and time it was changed, and your initials.

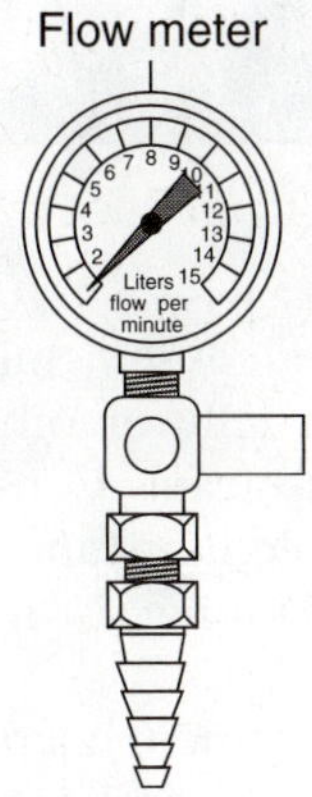

FIGURE 4-9B The flow meter shows how much oxygen the resident is receiving.

Refillable humidifiers are washed, rinsed, and sterilized every 24 to 48 hours, or according to facility infection control policies. Refill the sterile bottle with sterile distilled water. Never add water to a partially filled humidifier. A sticker may be attached to this bottle showing the date and time it was changed.

Oxygen is given through a flow meter (Figure 4.9B) that shows how many liters of oxygen are being delivered to the resident each minute. Although you will not be responsible for adjusting this meter, you should check it each time you are in the room to be sure it is set at the proper rate. If you notice a difference from the ordered rate, report this important information to the nurse. The gauge on the oxygen tank also shows how much oxygen is left in the tank (Figure 4.10). Oxygen is measured in pounds. Follow your facility policy for checking this gauge, and notify the nurse before the tank is empty. Many

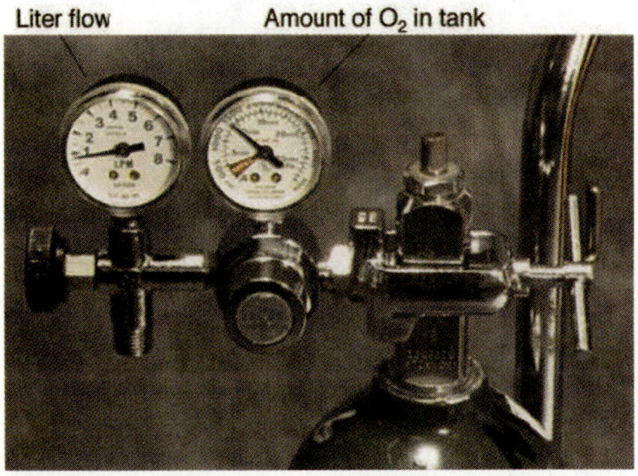

FIGURE 4-10 One gauge shows the liter flow the resident receives. The other indicates how much oxygen is in the tank.

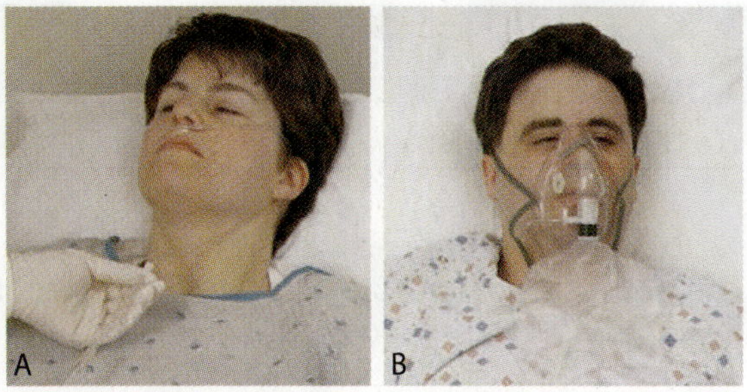

FIGURE 4-11 Oxygen is usually delivered through (A) a cannula for liter flows of five or less and (B) a mask for high liter flows.

facilities consider tanks to be empty when the pressure reaches 500 pounds. The tanks are changed when this pressure is reached.

Oxygen delivery equipment. Many different types of oxygen delivery equipment are used. The most common devices are cannulas and masks (Figure 4.11). The doctor will order the type of equipment to use. You must observe the skin under the device to be sure that it does not become red or irritated from the elastic that holds it in place. Report any skin problems to the nurse. Residents receiving oxygen may need extra liquids to drink. They will also need frequent care of the mouth and nose. Sometimes residents feel warm when receiving oxygen and will perspire heavily. Extra bathing and linen changes may be necessary. You may need to adjust the temperature in the room and help the resident change into lightweight clothes. The care plan and your assignment sheet will provide information on how and when to perform these procedures.

Being unable to breathe is very frightening. Residents who are receiving oxygen may need reassurance and emotional support. Check on the resident frequently and spend as much time in the room as possible. Difficulty in breathing makes it hard to talk, so the resident may be unable to carry on a normal conversation. Just being with the resident without talking is very reassuring.

Use of Oxygen in an Emergency

There are several differences between routine oxygen use and use of oxygen in an emergency. In an emergency, high concentrations of oxygen are necessary. Tanks, liquid oxygen, or oxygen piped in through the wall are used. Oxygen is usually delivered through a mask for emergency purposes. A mask should not be used with liter

GUIDELINES FOR

Safe Use of Oxygen

Extra oxygen in the air may cause objects to burn or explode. By itself, oxygen is not explosive. The resident's gown and linen on the bed absorb extra oxygen from the air. Special precautions should be taken when oxygen is in use.

- Before initiating oxygen therapy, check the resident's room to make sure it is safe for oxygen delivery.
- When using tank oxygen, identify the contents of the cylinder. Oxygen cylinders are always green. Read the label listing the contents as a double-check.
- Never use grease or oil on oxygen tank connections.
- Post "Oxygen in Use" signs over the bed and on the door of the room, or according to facility policy. The sign should list warnings, such as not smoking.
- Teach the resident and visitors the precautions to take.
- Do not force the flow meter into the wall or tank when assembling an oxygen unit. Forcing the flow meter may cause a valve to stick in an open position, allowing oxygen to leak out.
- Some electrical appliances can cause a spark. Check with the nurse before using a hair dryer, electric shaver, fan, radio, or television.
- Never use **flammable** liquids such as nail polish remover or adhesive tape remover. Avoid using alcohol-based aftershave, colognes, perfumes, or other products on residents receiving oxygen. Flammable liquids are combustible and will burn readily.
- Tank oxygen should be secured in a base or chained to a carrier or the wall.
- Smoking is not allowed in the room when oxygen is in use.
- Cover the resident with a cotton blanket. Avoid using wool and synthetic blankets and clothing.
- Some facilities remove the call signal and replace it with a bell that is used manually. The call signal may cause a spark.
- Avoid sparks. Static electricity can start a fire.
- Residents receiving oxygen receive frequent oral and nasal care because the oxygen dries the mucous membranes. Avoid using petroleum jelly or other petroleum products as a lubricant. Consult the nurse for a water-soluble lubricant.
- Make sure the tubing is not kinked or obstructed.
- Respond to equipment alarms, including oxygen equipment, immediately. Take corrective action or notify the appropriate person.
- If oxygen equipment makes an unusual noise, take corrective action or notify the appropriate person. If you suspect that a tank is leaking, remove the resident from the room and close the door.
- Learn how to turn off oxygen in case of a fire emergency. Piped-in oxygen may be turned off at a zone valve in the hallway. Tanks, canisters, and concentrators must be turned off at the unit.
- Learn facility policies for emergency transportation and evacuation of residents who need continuous oxygen.
- Follow infection control precautions when caring for residents receiving oxygen, such as keeping the cannula covered when not in use. Keep the oxygen cannula and tubing off the floor.
- Learn facility policies for using liquid oxygen. When liquid oxygen is used, high concentrations of oxygen build up quickly. Some materials are very flammable when saturated with oxygen. Follow all safety precautions for preventing sparks and fires.
- Liquid oxygen is nontoxic, but will cause severe burns upon direct contact. Avoid opening, touching, or spilling the container. If your skin or clothing contacts the liquid oxygen, flush the area immediately with a large amount of water. Never seal the cap or vent port on the liquid oxygen. Doing so will increase the pressure within the system, creating a potentially dangerous situation. If a bottle falls or tips, evacuate yourself and the resident from the room and close the door. Follow facility policies for getting assistance in this type of emergency.

flows of less than 5 because it has a smothering effect.

A concentrator will not deliver an adequate amount of oxygen for emergencies. Concentrators cannot deliver liter flows over 5. Most facilities use small, portable tanks for emergency purposes. In an emergency, oxygen may be delivered dry if necessary, until sterile distilled water is available. Avoid using tap water, because it increases the resident's risk of contracting Legionnaire's disease.

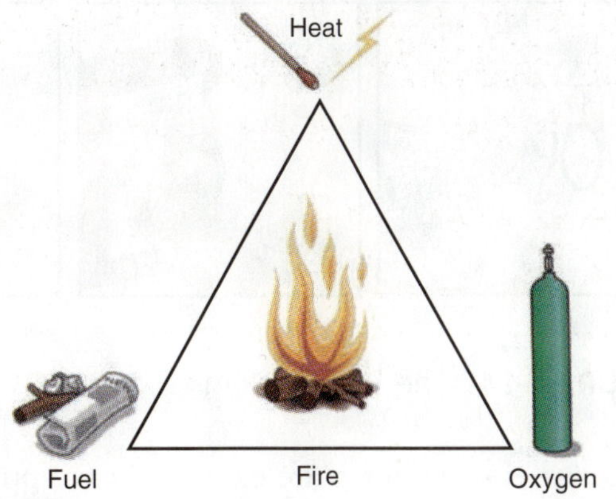

FIGURE 4-13 The three elements necessary to start a fire

Fire Safety

Long-term care facilities are built with safety features that will prevent fires from spreading. These safety features include doors that close automatically when the fire alarm sounds, an automatic sprinkler system, smoke detectors, and fire exits. Fire alarms and fire extinguishers are located on the walls in the hallways. The facility will have an evacuation plan posted (Figure 4.12). Many materials used on the floors, doors, walls, and furnishings are fire rated. This means that they will take longer to burn. Nevertheless, fire prevention is an important responsibility. Despite the built-in safety features, long-term care facilities can catch fire. Many lives can be lost.

Your facility will have periodic fire drills. Take these drills seriously and follow instructions. Your actions in a fire drill must become automatic, so that if a real fire starts you will react properly. Find the evacuation plan on your unit and become familiar with the escape routes. Know the location of fire alarms and fire extinguishers. Your facility may conduct inservices to teach you how to use the fire extinguisher.

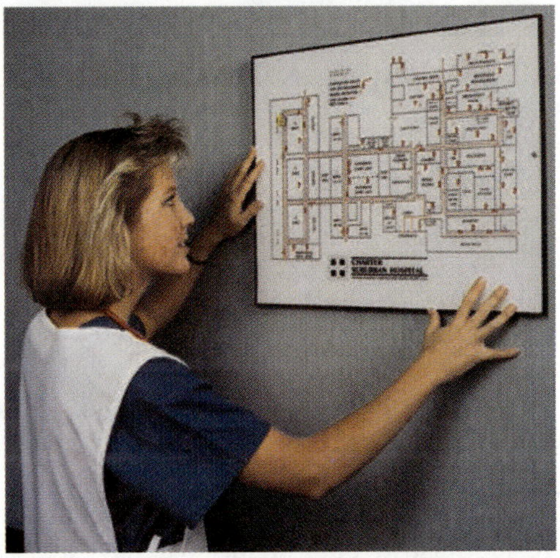

FIGURE 4-12 Become familiar with your facility evacuation plan. Commit it to memory so that you will be prepared in an emergency.

Three elements are necessary for a fire to start. These are oxygen, fuel, and a spark or source of ignition (Figure 4.13). Oxygen is in the air. Wood, paper, linens, and other materials provide fuel. Because two of the three elements necessary for fires are everywhere, the only thing missing is the spark, or source of ignition.

Careless and unsupervised smoking is a major cause of fire in long-term care facilities. Follow facility smoking policies. Check for and remove smoking materials from resident rooms, if this is your facility policy. Another common cause of fire is electrical problems. Avoid over-loading electrical outlets. Report frayed wires or other problems with electrical equipment to the proper person. Lock and tag this equipment out if this is your facility policy.

Other steps you should take to prevent fires are to store flammable materials correctly, and dispose of trash and other wastes in the proper location.

Steps to Take in a Fire Emergency

In a fire emergency, remain calm and do not panic. Most facilities use the **RACE System** (Figure 4.14). The resident is removed from immediate danger. After the alarm is sounded, the fire is contained by closing doors and windows. Residents are moved behind closed doors to keep them safe. Closing doors and windows slows the spread of fire. The hallways are cleared of residents and pieces of equipment that will burn. If the fire is large and spreading rapidly, residents may be evacuated from the building.

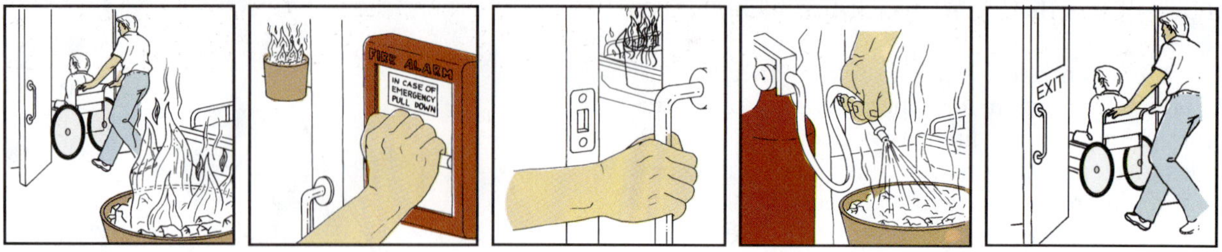

Remove Activate Contain or Extinguish or Evacuate

FIGURE 4-14 The RACE system

If the fire is small, use a fire extinguisher to put it out. Fire extinguishers are rated A, B, C, or according to the type of fire they are used on.

- A is used for trash, wood, and paper fires.
- B is used for flammable liquids, such as grease and oil.
- C is used for electrical fires.
- ABC is used on any type of fire.

Fire extinguishers are used by aiming the spray at the base of the fire. Remembering the word PASS will help you remember how to use the fire extinguisher:

P—Pull the pin out of the upper extinguisher handle.
A—Aim the extinguisher at the base of the fire.
S—Squeeze the handle to discharge the contents of the extinguisher.
S—Sweep the extinguisher from side to side while keeping it aimed at the base of the fire. Hold the hose securely when spraying.

In a fire, smoke is very dangerous. If you are in a smoke-filled area, stay as close to the floor as possible. If you can crawl to an exit, cover your mouth and stay on your knees. The floor has the most oxygen available, because smoke rises. Before entering a room, touch the door with the *back* of your hand (Figure 4.15). *If the door is hot to touch, do not open it*. If you are trapped in a room and the door is hot to touch, stay in the room and place wet blankets or towels under the door to keep the smoke out. Opening the door could cause the fire to enter explosively.

Never use the elevator in a fire emergency. If you are instructed to evacuate, you must use the stairs.

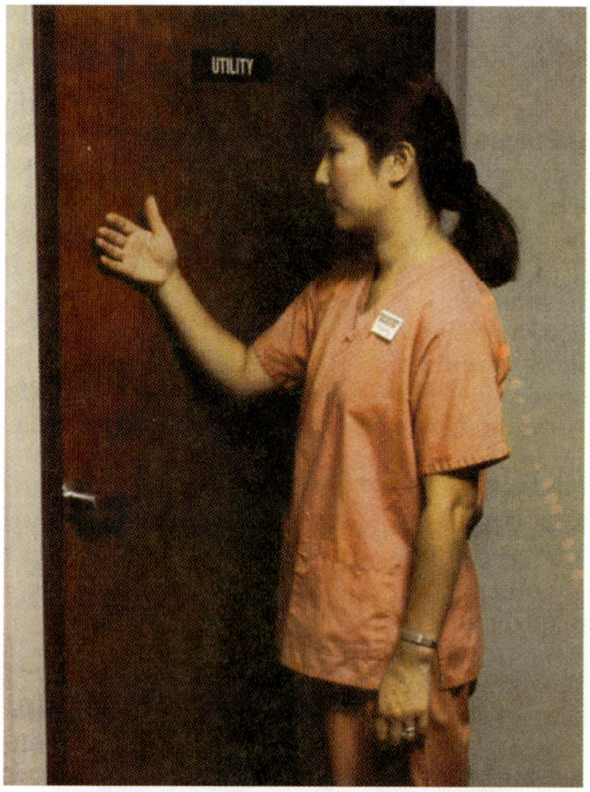

FIGURE 4-15 If you suspect a fire, touch the door with the back of your hand. Do not open the door if it feels hot.

Other Types of Emergencies

When a natural disaster occurs, many people can be injured in a short period of time. Know what natural disasters are possible in your area and find out what evacuation or safety measures are used by your facility. If evacuation is anticipated, you may be instructed to tell ambulatory residents to stay out of bed and to get bedfast residents up in wheelchairs so that they can be moved quickly. You will evacuate ambulatory residents first, followed by residents in wheelchairs. Evacuate bedfast residents last. Your facility will have a disaster plan that describes what actions to take. Regardless of the type of emergency, remaining calm is very important.

GUIDELINES FOR

Tornado Safety

Tornado Watch

The nurse will monitor the weather. During the watch, you may be instructed to:

- Remove nonessential items from hallways.
- Close windows and drapes. Remove items from window sills.
- Put sharp or heavy objects away in drawers or closets.
- Clear desks and countertops of nonessential items.
- Ask residents to return to their rooms or units.
- Remove or secure outdoor furniture or other objects.
- Turn on lights if the sky darkens.
- Locate and verify working order of flashlights and battery radios.
- Locate extra wheelchairs and small oxygen tanks and bring them to a central area in case they are needed for resident evacuation.
- Account for all residents on the unit; you may be asked to tape a list to the desk, or give it to the nurse.
- Instruct residents not to leave the building.

Tornado Warning (Severe Thunderstorm Warning)

- You may be asked to move residents before an official warning is issued.
- If a warning is announced, return to your assigned unit.
- Help move residents to the designated area(s). Move ambulatory residents first, followed by residents in wheelchairs. Evacuate bedfast residents last. Cover residents' heads with blankets. Be calm and reassuring.
- After each room is evacuated, close the door. You may be instructed to place a paper or the corner of the privacy curtain out of the door to signify that the room has been evacuated.
- If a resident refuses to move, move other residents, then return and try to persuade the resident. If he or she continues to refuse, inform the nurse. If the resident is in a potentially life-threatening situation, the nurse may instruct you to move the resident against his or her will.
- Instruct visitors and residents not to leave the building.
- If there is no time to evacuate, cover residents with blankets, push beds away from windows, and pull privacy curtains. (Window drapes should already be closed and window sills cleared.) If time allows, protect the side of the bed closest to the window by padding it with pillows or other soft materials. Begin in the area of the building where the storm is approaching.

Tornado Safety

Although rare in some parts of the country, a tornado can occur anywhere. All facilities have specific policies for natural disasters. Your community may be placed under a **tornado watch** or **tornado warning**. A tornado watch means that conditions are favorable for a tornado to develop. A tornado warning means that a tornado is actually in the area. Residents are not evacuated during a tornado watch. Someone is designated to monitor the weather in case the situation changes.

During a tornado warning, you will help with the evacuation of residents. This means that all residents will be moved to the basement, if the facility has one. In multiple-story buildings, residents are moved to the lowest level. Frequently, residents are moved to a strong area in the center of the building. Residents should not be moved to areas where there are windows, because flying glass may cause serious injuries. Evacuation must be done very quickly, because tornadoes strike with little warning. If residents cannot walk, they are moved in wheelchairs or beds. You may be instructed to cover residents with blankets to protect them from flying debris. You may also be required to close the room doors, fire doors, windows, and curtains facing the direction of the oncoming tornado. Remove items from window sills, such as plants and pictures. Put sharp or heavy objects away in drawers or closets. If there is time, check the outside of the facility. Bring lawn furniture, tools, and other objects inside the building. Locate and carry a flashlight to use in case of a power failure. Do not go near the windows during the storm. Follow the nurse's directions until the tornado has left the area.

Hurricanes

Some facilities in coastal areas are at risk for hurricanes. Hurricanes are not like other emergencies because they can be predicted in advance and there is adequate time to evacuate residents before the hurricane strikes. If a hurricane warning occurs, facility management may give the order to evacuate residents to an area farther inland. Residents, medications, and residents' charts are also moved. Follow the directions of facility management during the evacuation procedure.

If residents are not evacuated, you may be instructed to move them into interior rooms or hallways. As with a tornado, residents should be protected from flying glass and other debris. Close the doors to rooms and fire doors. Avoid blocking the emergency exits.

Earthquakes

During an earthquake, the ground shakes. It may cause building destruction and fires. Windows may break and objects may fly around. Earthquakes occur suddenly and without warning. If an earthquake strikes, remain calm. Cover or protect your head from flying debris. Take cover under a large heavy object, or in a door frame, if possible.

After the earthquake, check residents for injuries. Avoid moving injured residents unless they are in danger. Clean up spills on the floor to prevent falls. Do not smoke or use candles, matches, or open flames. Earthquakes can rupture gas lines and cause chemicals to spill, creating fire hazards. Be prepared for aftershocks. Avoid using electrical appliances. Use a flashlight for light, if needed. Listen to a battery-powered radio for emergency information.

Bomb Threats

Occasionally a long-term care facility will receive a phone call warning of a bomb. A bomb threat should be taken seriously. Facility management may order the building to be evacuated quickly. Law enforcement and fire officials will be notified. They will search the facility for a bomb, and may help with the evacuation. If you answer the telephone and the caller tells you there is a bomb in the building, stay on the line for as long as possible and obtain as much information as possible (Figure 4.16). Be polite and remain calm. Ask where the bomb is, or where it will explode and at what time. Be alert to the sound of the caller's voice, and try to determine the age, sex, and other identifying factors such as an accent. Listen for any background noise such as music, church bells, or machinery. This information will be useful to the police later in trying to identify the caller. Follow the nurse's directions in evacuating the facility. Law enforcement authorities will advise facility management when it is safe to return.

Other Types of Emergencies

Facilities have many policies and procedures for disasters. If your facility is in a flood plain, you will have a policy and procedure to be used in the event of high water. There may also be policies and procedures for other types of disasters, such as interruptions in food and water supplies, loss of gas and electricity, ice and snow emergencies, and chemical spills. Your facility will teach you how to respond to the appropriate disasters in your community.

OTHER SAFETY REQUIREMENTS

Many governmental agencies regulate safety in health care facilities. These agencies routinely inspect health care agencies and respond to complaints about unsafe conditions. Some laws pertain to the nursing assistant. Facilities receive citations and fines if unsafe conditions exist, or if workers are not following safe practices, so take your responsibilities for safe practices very seriously.

Occupational Safety and Health Administration

The **Occupational Safety and Health Administration (OSHA)** is an agency of the federal government that is responsible for overseeing employee safety in the workplace. Government statistics show that long-term care facilities have the third highest rate of injuries of all workplaces. In 2002, nursing assistants and truck drivers had more back injuries than any other workers. OSHA's role is to see that the workers are protected. Other agencies deal with resident safety. For years, OSHA inspected other types of businesses regularly, but did not inspect health

Bomb Threat Checklist

Questions to ask the caller:

- Where is the bomb right now? ______________________________
- Did you place the bomb? ______________________________
- Why did you place the bomb? ______________________________
- When is the bomb going to explode? ______________________________
- What will cause the bomb to explode? ______________________________
- What kind of bomb is it? ______________________________
- Where are you? ______________________________
- What is your name? ______________________________

Exact wording of the call:

____

____

____

Date and time of the call: ______________________________

Length of the call: ______________________________

Caller's gender (sex): ____________ Approximate age: __________ Accent: ________________

Caller's Voice; Circle all that apply

calm	nasal	loud	distinct	lisp	clearing throat
angry	slow	laughing	slurred	raspy	coughing
agitated	rapid	crying	ethnic	deep	deep breathing
excited	soft	normal	stutter	ragged	cracking
disguised	foreign	accent	familiar		

If the voice sounded familiar, whose voice did it sound like? ______________________________

Language; Circle all that apply

Well-spoken (educated)	Irrational	Message read by caller
Foul	Incoherent	Accent or dialect (specify) __________
	Taped message	

Background Sounds

Street (cars, buses, etc.)	Motor (fan, air conditioning)	Local call	Other (specify)
Airplanes	Church bells	Phone booth	__________
PA system	Animal noises	Office machinery	__________
Music	Clear	Video games, pinball, bowling, etc.	
House (dishes, TV, radio)	Static	Factory machinery	
Construction			

FIGURE 4-16 A bomb threat information checklist is available in some facilities. Using the checklist helps obtain essential information.

care facilities. This has changed, however, and in recent years, OSHA has become one of the agencies that actively inspects and has regulatory authority over health care facilities.

OSHA inspects facilities to see if they are following governmental safety requirements. Facilities must have an eyewash station and total body wash station within a reasonable distance of areas where chemicals are used. This is to protect employees in case chemicals are splashed into their eyes or spilled on their bodies. Most facilities designate the shower or tub rooms for this

GUIDELINES FOR

Violence Prevention

The nursing assistant should follow all facility policies and procedures involving safety and security. Other things you can do to prevent potential incidents are:

- Report suspicious individuals or other potential safety hazards to the nurse.
- If you are responsible for a secured area, control access to the area and keep it locked.
- Follow facility policy for locking all entrance doors at a designated time each evening. If your facility has a doorbell, respond to it quickly so oncoming workers are not outside alone in the dark.
- Participate in continuing education programs to learn how to recognize and manage escalating agitation, assaultive behavior, or criminal intent.
- Attend classes on cultural diversity that teach sensitivity on racial and ethnic issues and differences.
- Report assaults or threats of assaults to the nurse immediately.
- Avoid wearing scarves, necklaces, earrings, and other jewelry that could cause injury if a resident or other individual attacks you.
- Avoid remote, dark areas when you are alone.
- Exercise caution in elevators, stairwells, and unfamiliar areas. Immediately leave the area if you believe a hazard exists.
- If your facility has security personnel, request that they escort you in dark or potentially dangerous areas. If no security personnel are on duty, ask other staff members to accompany you.
- Use the "buddy system" if personal safety may be threatened.
- If a resident or other person is "acting out," or you believe you may be assaulted, do not let the person come between you and the exit.

purpose. OSHA also monitors the MSDS. The inspectors monitor the use of infection control precautions and isolation procedures and check to see that the facility is following guidelines to prevent the spread of tuberculosis and other infectious diseases. Your facility will teach you the OSHA requirements. It is your responsibility to attend class, learn the material, and apply it to the job you do in the long-term care facility.

Take safety very seriously. This will keep your facility in compliance with the various agencies that inspect it, and protect employees and residents from illness and injury.

Safe Medical Devices Act

The Safe Medical Devices Act of 1991 requires the health care facility to notify the United States Food and Drug Administration of death or serious injury caused by any medical device or equipment. This federal agency investigates all reports of serious injury and death. Using medical equipment according to manufacturers' directions is important to prevent injury. Do not use electrical or mechanical equipment unless you have been taught how to use it safely.

Concealed Handgun Laws

Some states allow citizens to carry concealed weapons. In these states guns *may not* be carried into a health care facility. Law enforcement personnel are exempt from this requirement. If a visitor is carrying a concealed handgun, he or she must leave it in the trunk of the car before entering the facility. If you notice any individual carrying a gun, notify the nurse immediately.

Violence in the Health Care Facility

Episodes of violence in the workplace are increasing in our society. Long-term care facilities are not exempt from violence. Serious episodes have occurred in both rural and urban communities. Many facilities have violence prevention education programs. The goal is to eliminate or reduce worker exposure to conditions that can lead to injury. OSHA has developed guidelines for preventing violence in the health care facility, and many employers use these guidelines to implement safety programs and teach their employees.

Potential reasons for violence in the health care facility include:

GUIDELINES FOR

Dealing with a Violent Individual

- Remain calm and avoid raising your voice, which may agitate the perpetrator.
- Speak slowly, softly, and clearly.
- Call for help, if possible, or send someone to get help. Pull the call light from the wall to activate the emergency signal.
- Move away from heavy or sharp objects that might be used as weapons.
- Monitor your body language and avoid movements that could be challenging, such as placing your hands on your hips, moving toward the perpetrator, pointing your finger, or staring directly at the person. However, focus your attention on the person so you know what he or she is doing at all times.
- Position yourself at right angles to the perpetrator. Avoid standing directly in front of him or her.
- Maintain a distance of three to six feet from the perpetrator.
- Position yourself so that an exit is accessible.
- Avoid making sudden movements.
- Listen to what the person is saying. Encourage the person to talk, and communicate that you care and will genuinely try to help. Acknowledge that you understand he or she is upset. Break big problems into smaller, manageable ones.
- Avoid arguing and defensive statements. Accept criticism in a positive way. If you sincerely feel that criticism is unwarranted, ask clarifying questions.
- Ask the person to leave and return when more calm.
- Ask questions to help regain control of the conversation.
- Avoid challenging, bargaining, or making promises you cannot keep.
- Describe the consequences of abusive behavior.
- Avoid touching an angry person.
- If a weapon is involved, ask the person to place it in a neutral location while you continue talking. Avoid trying to disarm the person, which may put you in danger.
- Follow facility policies for subduing or restraining the individual.

- The prevalence of handguns and other weapons
- Acute and chronically mentally ill residents
- Individuals, including coworkers, who abuse alcohol and drugs
- Overwhelming personal or financial stress
- The availability of drugs in the facility, making it a likely robbery target
- The increasing number of gangs and gang members in many communities
- Unrestricted movement of the public in health care facilities
- Distraught family members and other individuals who become angry and frustrated
- Low staffing levels during meals and at other times when staff is busy caring for residents and unable to observe activity in the hallways
- Poorly lighted parking lots, garages, and ramps
- Lack of staff awareness of risk factors, such as locking doors and reporting suspicious individuals
- Residents with dementia
- Residents who are incontinent and nonverbal

EMERGENCY PROCEDURES

When an emergency occurs in a long-term care facility, the licensed nurse is responsible for treatment of the resident. Follow the nurse's directions. Sometimes, however, you must act before the nurse arrives, to keep the resident from serious harm.

Caring for a Resident Who Has Fainted

Syncope, or fainting, occurs when the blood supply to the brain is not adequate. This sometimes occurs as a result of medical problems when residents sit or stand too quickly. The medical condition causes a temporary decrease in the blood flow to the brain, and the resident may lose consciousness. The purpose of emergency treatment for this condition is to restore the blood supply to the resident's brain and prevent injury. During this procedure, you will be required to take the resident's **vital signs**, or temperature, pulse, respiration, and blood pressure.

GUIDELINES TO Follow in All Emergencies

- If you discover a resident who is ill or injured, stay with the resident and call for help. Your facility will teach you the procedure for getting help. Some facilities instruct employees to call out. Others instruct you to pull the call signal or bathroom emergency signal.
- Do not move residents who have fallen to the floor unless they are in immediate danger. Moving the resident may worsen an injury. The nurse will check the resident and give permission for the move.
- Stay calm and do not panic.
- Start emergency measures that are permitted to do while you are waiting for help to arrive.
- Once the nurse arrives, do as he or she directs.
- Know facility procedures and phone numbers for reporting emergencies and completing incident reports.
- Know the location of emergency equipment and supplies on your unit. You may be instructed to get emergency supplies.
- Many emergencies involve bleeding. Remember that the potential for contact with blood, body fluid secretions (except sweat), excretions, mucous membranes, and non-intact skin still exists. Always remember and apply the principles of standard precautions. Know where personal protective equipment is kept.

PROCEDURE 6 Emergency Care for the Resident Who Has Fainted

1. Stay with the resident and call for help.
2. Lowering the resident's head will increase the blood supply to the brain.
   - If the resident is standing, help him or her sit or lie down.
   - If the resident is sitting, have him or her lean forward and place the head between his or her knees.
   - Once the resident is lying down, elevate his or her legs. Elevate them on pillows, if possible to increase blood flow to the brain. Keep the resident's head flat.
3. If the resident is nauseated, or is vomiting, position him or her on the side. If this is not possible, turn the resident's head to the side.
4. Loosen any tight or restrictive clothing.
5. Apply a cool, wet towel to the forehead.
6. Check the vital signs as directed by the nurse. You may be asked to monitor them at 5- to 15-minute intervals until the resident's condition is stable.
7. Keep the resident quiet, with the head lowered, until directed by the nurse.
8. Help the resident sit up gradually. Be prepared to act if the resident faints again.
9. Leave the resident in a position of comfort and safety. Usually, the resident is returned to bed with the side rails up until he or she has recovered. Leave the call signal and needed personal items within reach.
10. Wash your hands.
11. Report to the nurse:
    - The time the resident fainted, and how long he or she was unconscious.

- A description of the resident's appearance when the incident occurred.
- Any measures that you took to assist the resident and the results.
- Visual problems, change in color, or excessive perspiration.
- Presence of nausea, vomiting, changes in color or temperature of the skin, and changes in the resident's **level of consciousness**, which is determined by how responsive and alert the resident is. The level of consciousness is the resident's degree of awareness, which ranges from fully awake and alert to confusion or unconsciousness.
- Vital signs.

Caring for a Resident Who Is Having a Seizure

A **seizure** or convulsion is caused by a disturbance of the impulses in the brain. It is seen in epilepsy and other diseases. It is usually characterized by jerking and shaking of the body. Injuries, medication, fever, and infection can also cause seizures. Residents have different types of seizures. Some appear mild, whereas others appear severe. The most common types of seizures are related to epilepsy. These are described in Table 4.1. A seizure is a serious medical emergency. The goal of seizure care is to prevent injury. Some residents have a sensation called an **aura** immediately before a seizure. An aura is a sensation, smell, taste, or a bright light that precedes the onset of a seizure.

TABLE 4-1 Characteristics of Common Types of Seizures

Type of Seizure	Signs of Seizure Activity	Comment
Generalized tonic-clonic seizure (Grand mal seizure)	May be proceded by an aura. Loss of consciousness, convulsive activity, characterized by rigid stiffening of muscles and jerking movement of the arms and legs. Saliva runs from the mouth. Resident's color may change because of lack of oxygen. Incontinence of bowel and bladder.	Usually lasts three to four minutes. The resident may be very tired after the seizure and may have a headache. The resident may be mentally confused, have slurred speech, and be very weak. The resident will not remember the seizure.
Absence seizure (Petit mal seizure)	Staring, blinking, or stopping what the resident is doing. The resident may stare blankly. One muscle group may twitch or jerk.	Petit mal seizures usually last less than a minute, but may occur many times a day.
Simple-Partial (Jacksonian)	Muscle spasms of the face, hands, or feet. Starts at one extremity, such as an arm or leg, and progressively moves upward on that side of the body.	May spread to other areas in the brain, resulting in a grand mal seizure.
Complex-Partial (Psychomotor)	Abnormal acts, irrational behavior, or loss of judgment due to a temporary change in consciousness. Automatic behavior, such as typing or eating, may continue normally. The resident may uncontrollably smack his or her lips, wander aimlessly, or uncontrollably twitch part of his or her body.	Usually lasts only a few seconds. The resident usually does not remember the seizure.

(continues)

		=x(12)x(13)
Myoclonic	Consists of one or more myoclonic jerks. The resident remains conscious but cannot control the muscle movement.	The resident is aware that an extremity is jerking but is unable to stop it. The resident remains conscious throughout and can remember the seizure activity.
Status epilepticus	Multiple seizures occurring simultaneously with no break between seizures.	Status epilepticus may be precipitated by sudden withdrawal of antiseizure medications, fever, and infection. This type of seizure is dangerous and can lead to decreased mental function, neurological impairment, and death.

PROCEDURE 7 Emergency Care for the Resident Who Is Having a Seizure

1. Stay with the resident and call for help.
2. Use standard precautions if contact with blood, moist body fluids (except sweat), mucous membranes, secretions, excretions, or nonintact skin is likely.
3. If the resident is in bed, remove the pillow and raise the side rails.
4. If the resident is not in bed, gently lower the resident to the floor, protecting the head. Pad the head with a soft, flat object, such as a towel.
5. Turn the resident on the side. If this is not possible, turn the head to the side. This allows secretions to drain from the resident's mouth.
6. Move any hard objects, or pad objects that may injure the resident with pillows, blankets, or other available items, such as chair cushions.
7. Loosen tight and restrictive clothing.
8. Provide privacy by asking onlookers to leave, closing the door to the resident's room, and pulling the privacy curtain.
9. Avoid restraining the resident in any way.
10. Do not try to place any object in the resident's mouth. Doing this could break teeth and cause injury to the resident and yourself.
11. Check the resident's vital signs as requested by the nurse. You may be instructed to check vital signs frequently until the resident is stable.
12. Assist the nurse as directed. The nurse may need to suction the resident, administer oxygen, or give medication to stop the seizure.
13. When the seizure stops, tell the resident where he or she is and what happened. Assist the resident to bed. The resident will be very tired. Allow him or her to sleep.
14. Leave the resident in a position of comfort and safety. Leave the call signal and needed personal items within reach.
15. Remove gloves, if worn, and dispose of them according to facility policy.
16. Wash your hands.
17. Report to the nurse:
    - Any change in the resident before the seizure, such as an aura, confusion, or change in behavior
    - Loss of control of bowel or bladder, eyes rolling upward, rapid blinking, biting tongue

- Time the seizure started and stopped
- A description of the way the seizure looked, including the body parts involved
- Condition of the resident after the seizure
- Vital signs

PROCEDURE

8

Emergency Care for Falls and Suspected Fractures

If you are walking with a resident who starts to fall, you should:

1. Keep your back straight, your feet about 12 inches apart, and your knees bent.
2. If the resident is wearing a gait belt (Figure 4.17), hold the center back of the belt firmly with an underhand grasp. Ease the resident down your legs to the floor. Protect the head from hitting the floor. Guide the resident so that he or she does not hit hard objects in the area.

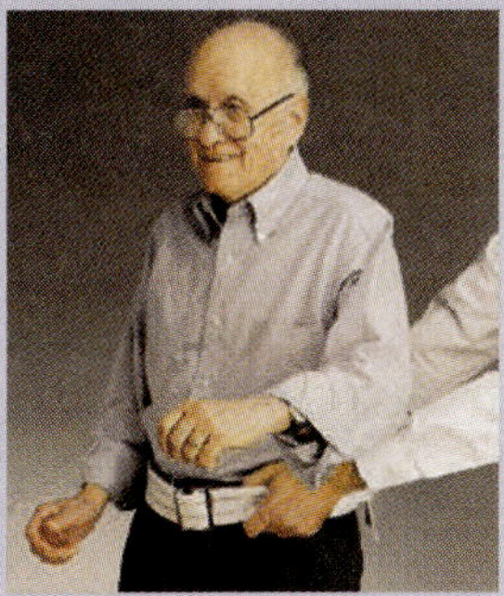

FIGURE 4-17 A gait belt is a safety device used for transfers and ambulation. *(Courtesy of Skil-Care Corporation, Yonkers, NY, 1-800-431-2972)*

3. If the resident is not wearing a gait belt, move close to the resident and wrap your arms around the resident's waist.
4. Pull the resident close to your body, sliding him or her down your leg and easing him or her to the floor. Protect the resident from hitting the head. Guide the resident so that he or she does not hit any hard objects.

Assisting the Resident after a Fall

1. Stay with the resident and call for help. Reassure the resident.
2. Use standard precautions if contact with blood or moist body fluids (except sweat) is likely.
3. Do not move the resident until the nurse has examined him or her and gives approval.
4. Check the resident's vital signs, and assist him or her to bed as instructed by the nurse.
5. Leave the resident in a position of comfort and safety. Place the call signal and needed personal items within reach.
6. Wash your hands.
7. The nurse may direct you to monitor the resident's vital signs frequently until the resident is stable.

Assisting the Resident with a Suspected Fracture

1. Stay with the resident and call for help. Reassure the resident.
2. Use standard precautions if contact with blood or moist body fluids (except sweat) is likely.

(continues)

PROCEDURE 8 Emergency Care for Falls and Suspected Fractures, *continued*

3. Do not move the resident until the nurse has examined him or her and gives approval.
4. Keep the resident as quiet as possible.
5. Immobilize the injured area by supporting it to prevent movement. If the area appears out of shape, bent, or deformed, do not attempt to straighten it.
6. Check the resident's vital signs, and assist him or her to bed as instructed by the nurse.
7. If a fracture is suspected, several staff members must assist the resident to bed. One staff member is assigned to move the injured extremity. If possible, splint it with a rigid object, such as a rolled magazine. Other staff members will move the rest of the resident's body. A sheet or other lifting device may be used to move the resident.
8. Leave the resident in a position of comfort and safety. Leave the call signal and needed personal items within reach.
9. Wash your hands.
10. The nurse may direct you to monitor the resident's vital signs frequently until he or she is stable.
11. You may also be directed to apply a cold treatment to the injured area.
12. Observe for and report:
    - The time of the fall
    - The cause of the fall, if known; avoid guessing and report only what you know to be true
    - Measures taken to break the fall
    - Measures taken to assist the resident
    - Known injuries, such as bleeding, deformities, bruises, or changes in the resident's level of consciousness
    - Circulatory problems and abnormal color of the injured extremity
    - Appearance of the injured area and steps taken to immobilize it
    - Witnesses to the fall
    - Vital signs
    - Any additional information needed to fill out the incident report

PROCEDURE 9 Application of Cold Packs to Strains and Bruises

1. Notify the nurse of the injury.
2. If the resident is on the floor, stay with him or her and call for help.
3. Do not move the resident until the nurse examines him or her.
4. Wash your hands.
5. Position the resident in a comfortable position.
6. Use standard precautions if contact with blood or moist body fluids (except sweat) is likely.

7. Prepare the cold pack as directed by the nurse and according to facility policy:
   - Place a cloth or flannel cover over the cold pack.
   - Apply the cold pack above or on top of the injured area, as directed. If the resident complains that the cold pack increases the pain, remove it and consult the nurse.
   - Secure the cold pack in place if necessary. You may need to prop it or tie it in place with a gauze bandage.
   - Check the area under the cold pack every 10 minutes and remove it if numbness or discoloration of the skin occurs.
   - Remove the cold pack after 20 minutes.
   - Reapply the cold pack as directed.
8. Wash your hands.
9. Leave the resident in a position of comfort and safety. Leave the call signal and needed personal items within reach.
10. Observe for and report:
    - The time and description of the injured area
    - Edema, deformities, or other injuries
    - Cause of the injury, if known
    - The type of cold pack applied and time
    - Response to the cold pack

PROCEDURE 10 Emergency Care for a Resident with Burns

1. Stay with the resident and call for help. Reassure the resident.
2. Use standard precautions, because contact with body fluids and nonintact skin is likely.
3. Keep the resident's airway open, if necessary, by tilting the head back with one hand while gently lifting the chin with the other hand. Make sure that the resident is breathing.
4. Remove the source of heat, if present.
5. If the burn is minor and the skin is not broken:
   - Remove the resident's clothing from the burned area. Do not remove clothing stuck to the skin.
   - Immerse the burned area in cool water. Do not use ice or ice water.
6. If the burn is very large or deep, do not get the area wet. Do not try to remove clothing stuck to the skin.
7. Cover the burned area with a clean pad, gauze, or cloth.
8. Keep the resident as quiet as possible.
9. Cover the resident to maintain body temperature.
10. Check the resident's vital signs as directed. You may be instructed to check the vital signs frequently until the resident is stable. If the resident's upper arms are burned, do not take the blood pressure. Check with the nurse for further instructions.
11. Do not give the resident food or fluids.
12. Remove gloves, if worn, and dispose of them according to facility policy.

(continues)

PROCEDURE 10 Emergency Care for a Resident with Burns, *continued*

13. Wash your hands.
14. Leave the resident in a position of comfort and safety. Leave the call signal and needed personal items within reach.
15. Observe for and report:
    - Time the resident was discovered
    - Cause of the burn, if known
    - Appearance of the burned area
    - Emergency measures taken
    - Other observations or resident response
    - Witnesses to the incident
    - Vital signs
    - Any additional information needed by the nurse to complete the incident report

Caring for a Resident Who Has Fallen and Has a Suspected Fracture

Falls are common emergencies in health care facilities. Bones become more brittle and lose calcium during the aging process. Joints are not as flexible as they were when the resident was younger. Because of these aging changes, **fractures**, or broken bones, occur more readily in the elderly. Sometimes fractures are obvious right away. An area of the body may appear swollen or deformed. If the fracture occurs in a hip, the leg on the affected side may appear shorter than the other and rotate outward. Injuries may bleed. The purpose of emergency treatment for falls is to prevent injuries and to assist residents who have suspected fractures.

Head Injury

A resident with a known or suspected head injury always requires close observation and monitoring. Bleeding inside the skull commonly occurs when the head strikes a broad, hard object, such as the floor. Some serious complications of head injuries may not be apparent until 72 hours or longer after a head injury. This is particularly true in the elderly. As people age, the brain shrinks. This does not affect the resident mentally. The space between the brain and the skull allows extra room for swelling and bleeding. Signs and symptoms of an acute bleeding problem may not be apparent for several days until the problem progresses to a point where it increases pressure on the brain. A very tiny bleed can take up to six weeks to show symptoms. This may be long after the original injury has been forgotten. Signs and symptoms of head injury are:

- Change in the resident's alertness or consciousness
- Change in orientation (ability to recognize time, place, person)
- Memory loss
- Unequal pupils
- Visual disturbances
- Blood or clear fluid leaking from ears or nose
- Change in ability to speak or make self understood
- Change in ability to follow directions
- No response to verbal stimulation
- Weakness of arms or legs, difficulty maintaining balance
- Complaint of headache
- Nausea and/or vomiting

Remember that signs and symptoms of a problem may not occur for several days. If you notice any of these, you should:

- Stay with the resident and call for help.
- Monitor the pulse and respirations while waiting for the nurse to arrive.
- If you suspect a spinal cord injury, instruct the resident not to move. Immobilize the head, neck, and trunk as much as possible.
- Keep the environment quiet and calm.
- Avoid giving the resident anything to drink.

- Reassure and orient the resident.
- Elevate the head on a pillow.
- Avoid moving the resident if he or she is on the floor; wait for the nurse's instructions.
- Cover the resident with a blanket to maintain body temperature.
- Monitor vital signs regularly after the injury, as instructed.

Caring for a Resident with Strains and Bruises

Strains are injuries that occur from overstretching or overusing a muscle. **Bruises** are injuries to the skin caused by hitting, bumping, or striking. The bruised area usually turns black and blue in color. The medical term for a bruise is **ecchymosis**. These injuries are painful, and edema may occur. Cold packs are commonly used to decrease pain and swelling. You should apply cold packs only if you are instructed to do so by the nurse. Cold packs are usually left in place for 20 minutes and then removed to avoid tissue damage.

Caring for a Resident with Burns

Burns are commonly caused by hot water or other hot liquids and careless cigarette smoking. *Thermal burns* are caused by flame and hot objects. *Chemical burns* are caused by harmful chemicals contacting the skin, eyes, or mucous membranes. Burns can range from minor to severe. Severe burns can lead to loss of skin, damage to the muscle, infection, and death. Even small burns can be very painful. The purpose of burn care is to relieve pain, prevent infection and other complications, and promote healing.

Caring for a Resident Who Is Hemorrhaging

Hemorrhage, or severe bleeding, can occur inside or outside the body. Bleeding inside the body cannot be seen or treated by the nursing assistant. This section discusses bleeding on the outside of the body. Many different injuries can cause bleeding. If bleeding is not controlled quickly, serious complications can result. One serious complication is **shock**. Shock is the result of blood loss and causes inadequate blood flow to the heart and brain. If shock is untreated, it can lead to death. The purpose of these guidelines is to control bleeding and prevent shock.

Caring for a Resident with Vomiting and Aspiration

Food and air are both taken into the body through the mouth. The passageway by which food and air enter is shared (Figure 4.18). The passage branches into two divisions in the throat. Food goes into the esophagus, then to the stomach. Air goes into the trachea, then the lungs. A small flap, called the **epiglottis**, covers the trachea when you swallow. This flap prevents food and liquid from running into the lungs. The ability to swallow is less efficient in people with some diseases and in the elderly. Occasionally food, water, or other objects accidentally go down the trachea and into the lungs. This is called **aspiration**, and can occur when a resident is vomiting, bleeding, eating, or drinking. Sometimes thick secretions from the mouth enter the lungs. Aspiration can cause serious complications. It can be prevented by turning the resident's body to the side if he or she is vomiting while lying down. If turning the resident's body is not possible, turn the head to the side. Fluid cannot enter the lungs in this position. The purpose of this procedure is to prevent aspiration of food, fluids, secretions, blood, or vomitus.

Caring for a Resident with an Obstructed Airway

Sometimes food or a foreign object is aspirated into the windpipe, or trachea. This causes an

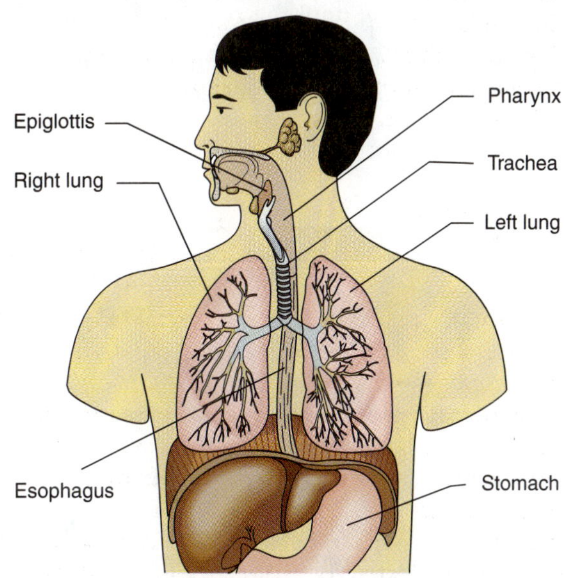

FIGURE 4-18 The trachea and esophagus share a common passage in the throat through which food and air pass.

PROCEDURE

11 Emergency Care for Controlling Bleeding

1. Stay with the resident and call for help.
2. Apply the principles of standard precautions and select personal protective equipment appropriate to the procedure.
3. If the hemorrhage is visible:
   - Apply direct pressure over the site of bleeding with a clean pad or towel and your *gloved* hand.
   - Increase the pressure if the bleeding continues.
   - Do not remove the pad to check the injury. If the pad becomes soaked, add extra padding.
   - Continue direct pressure until you are given further instructions by the nurse.
4. Keep the resident warm and quiet. Have the resident lie flat. Elevate the feet, if possible.
5. Take the blood pressure, pulse, and respirations as directed. You may be instructed to monitor the vital signs frequently until the resident is stable.
6. Do not give the resident anything to eat or drink. The resident may complain of being very thirsty. Thirst is a sign of shock. Notify the nurse of this complaint.
7. Leave the resident in a position of comfort and safety. Leave the call signal and needed personal items within reach.
8. Dispose of items containing blood according to facility policy.
9. Remove gloves and other PPE and dispose of them according to facility policy.
10. Wash your hands.
11. Observe for and report to the nurse:
    - Time the bleeding was discovered
    - Cause of the bleeding, if known
    - Location of the bleeding
    - Emergency measures taken
    - Blood pressure, pulse, and respirations
    - Any additional information required for the incident report
    - Witnesses to the injury
    - Other observations and resident response

PROCEDURE

12 Emergency Care for Vomiting and Aspiration

1. Stay with the resident and call for help.
2. Use standard precautions and select personal protective equipment appropriate to the procedure.
3. Keep the resident's head elevated if possible.
4. Keep the resident's body or head turned to the side to allow fluids to drain from the mouth.

5. Provide an emesis basin if the resident is vomiting.
6. Notify the nurse immediately if the resident:
   - Is choking or is unable to swallow
   - Is unable to spit out the vomitus, blood, or secretions in the mouth
7. The nurse may need to suction the resident or notify the doctor.
8. If the resident begins choking and an airway obstruction occurs, follow the procedure for clearing the obstructed airway (see Procedure 4.8).
9. After the episode, assist the resident with mouth care.
10. Leave the resident in a position of comfort and safety. Leave the call signal and needed personal items within reach.
11. Dispose of items containing blood or other body secretions according to facility policy.
12. Remove gloves and dispose of them according to facility policy.
13. Wash your hands.
14. Observe for and report to the nurse:
    - Difficulty swallowing, bleeding, vomiting, choking, or aspiration.
    - The color and odor of the vomitus, and the presence of undigested food, blood, or coffee-ground appearance (coffee-ground appearance suggests blood in the stomach).
    - Measure or estimate the amount of vomitus or blood, and record on the intake and output record.
    - Do not discard the vomitus or blood until it is seen by the nurse and a specimen obtained, if needed

PROCEDURE 13

Emergency Care for Clearing the Obstructed Airway in a Conscious Adult Who Is Sitting or Standing

1. Ask the resident, "Are you choking?" or "Can you speak?"
2. If the resident can speak or cough, leave him or her alone and see if he or she can cough the obstruction out. Assist the resident if the cough is weak and ineffective and the resident is in obvious distress.
3. Stay with the resident and call for help.
4. Tell the resident that you will help.
5. Stand behind the resident and wrap your arms around his or her waist (Figure 4.20A).

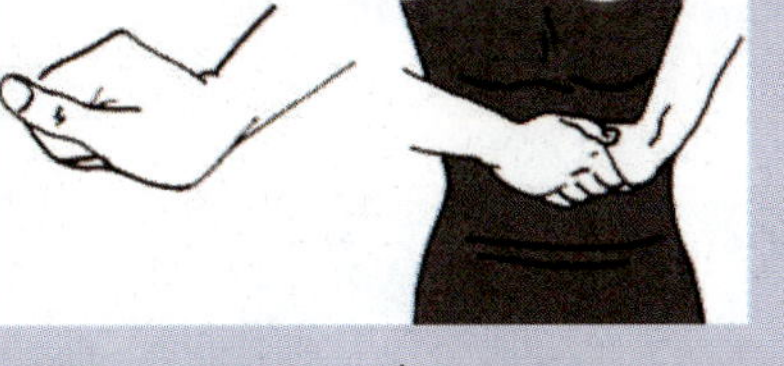

FIGURE 4-20A Place your arms around the abdomen, slightly above the waist. Avoid resting your forearms on the ribs.

6. Make a fist with one hand and place the thumb side of the fist against the abdomen, just above the navel (Figure 4.20B).

(continues)

PROCEDURE 13 Emergency Care for Clearing the Obstructed Airway in a Conscious Adult Who Is Sitting or Standing, *continued*

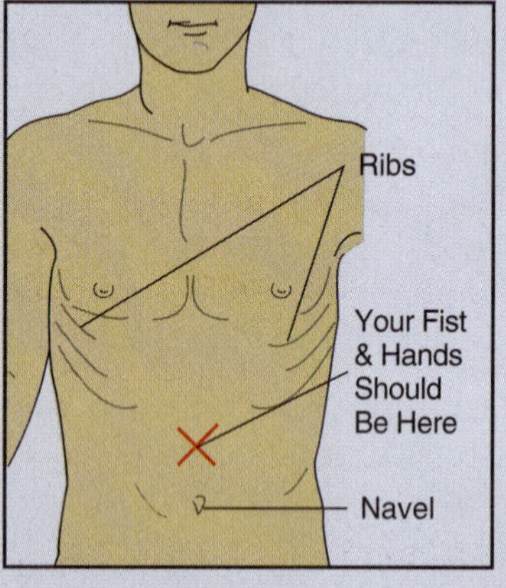

FIGURE 4-20B Turn your thumb inward.

7. Grasp your fist with the other hand. Do not put pressure on the ribs or breastbone with your forearms.
8. Quickly squeeze inward and upward (Figure 4.20C). Each thrust should be a separate and distinct movement done with the intent of removing the obstruction. You are trying to push the diaphragm up to force out the air behind the foreign body. As the air is expelled, it will push the object out.
9. If the resident does not expel the foreign body, continue the inward, upward thrusts. If the resident begins to cough forcefully, wait and see if the object can be expelled.
10. Continue until the foreign body is expelled or the resident loses consciousness.
11. When the foreign body is expelled, stay with the resident, and follow the nurse's directions.
12. Leave the resident in a position of comfort and safety. Leave the call signal and needed personal items within reach. The nurse may instruct you to monitor the resident's vital signs periodically.
13. Wash your hands.

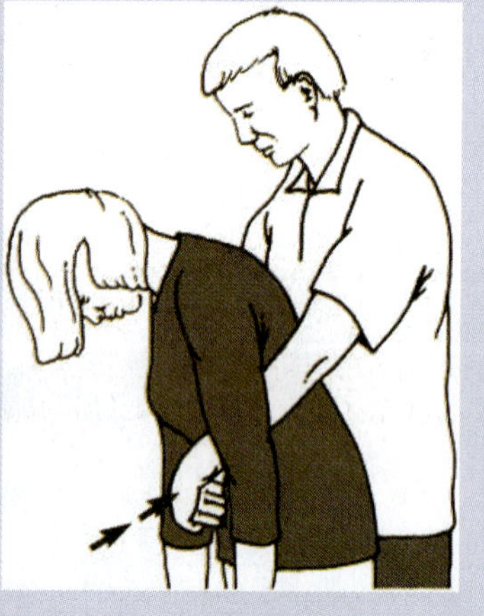

FIGURE 4-20C Squeeze in and up.

PROCEDURE 14 Emergency Care for Clearing the Obstructed Airway in an Unconscious Adult

1. Perform abdominal thrusts (see Procedure 10) until the resident loses consciousness. Activate the emergency response system, if this has not already been done. Send someone else, if possible. Remain with the resident and continue to try to relieve the obstruction.
2. Wear gloves during this procedure and use standard precautions.

3. Position the resident on his or her back on the floor, with his or her head facing up.
4. Kneel beside the resident and open the airway by tilting the head back with one hand while gently lifting the chin and tongue with the other hand. Perform a finger sweep with two fingers of your gloved hand to see if you can feel and remove a foreign body. If you feel an object, take care to avoid pushing it farther into the resident's throat.
5. Open the airway by placing one hand on the forehead. Apply firm, backward pressure to tilt the head back. With your other hand, position your fingers in the bony part of the jaw, under the chin. Avoid pressure on the soft tissue of the neck. Lift the jaw forward so the teeth are in good alignment with the upper jaw.
6. Attempt to give a breath into the resident's mouth through a ventilation barrier device (Figure 4.21). If the air does not go in, reposition the head and attempt to breathe into the resident's mouth again.

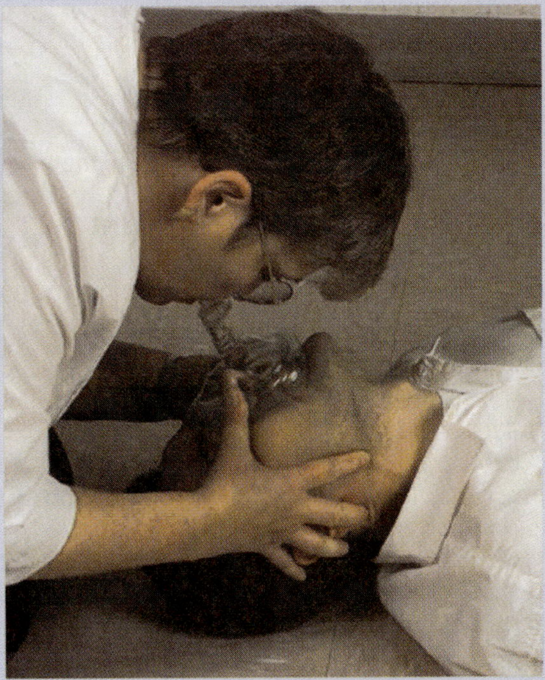

FIGURE 4-21 A pocket mask with a one-way valve is a barrier device for artificial ventilation. You must receive special education in the use of this device.

7. If no air enters the resident after the second attempt at ventilations, straddle the resident's hips.
8. Place the heel of one hand on the resident's abdomen, immediately above the navel. Your fingers should be pointing up toward the head. Do not place your hand on the ribs or breastbone.
9. Place your other hand on top. Position your shoulders directly above the resident's abdomen.
10. Press your hands inward and upward five times.
11. Open the airway by doing a tongue/jaw lift. Check the resident's mouth and perform another finger sweep.
12. Attempt to ventilate.
13. Repeat steps 5 through 12 until the object is expelled.
14. Assist the nurse, code team, or *EMS* (emergency medical services), as appropriate.
15. Dispose of gloves and face shield according to facility policy.
16. Wash your hands.
17. Observe and report to the nurse:
    - Exact time the choking and unconsciousness started and stopped
    - The procedures done and the time that you started and stopped
    - The resident's response
    - Factors related to the cause of choking, if known

    Note: Follow your facility policy for mouth-to-mouth ventilation. To prevent the transmission of disease, standard precautions should be used. This means that a ventilation barrier mask (Figure 4.21) with a valve that prevents the backflow of secretions or resuscitation face shield should be placed between your mouth and the resident's mouth. Familiarize yourself with the devices in your facility. CPR classes are offered to teach you how to use ventilation devices correctly. Attending a CPR class will benefit you personally and professionally.

obstructed airway, which is a serious emergency. The obstruction must be removed immediately, or the resident will die. When a person is choking, putting one or both hands about the throat is instinctive. This is known as the **universal choking sign** (Figure 4.19). If you see a resident with hands on the throat, ask if he or she can speak or cough. If the resident can speak, the airway is not obstructed. Stay with the resident and see if he or she can expel the foreign body on his or her own. If the resident is unable to speak, cough, or breathe, you must take immediate action by performing the obstructed airway procedure. The purpose of this procedure is to remove a foreign object from the airway of an adult. The procedure is different for infants, small children, and pregnant women.

Cardiopulmonary resuscitation. Cardiopulmonary resuscitation (CPR) is an emergency procedure used in health care facilities if the resident's heart and breathing have stopped. CPR is used to keep the resident alive until more advanced life support can be obtained. It is recommended that you attend a CPR course and learn this valuable lifesaving technique. Your facility might require you to become certified in CPR.

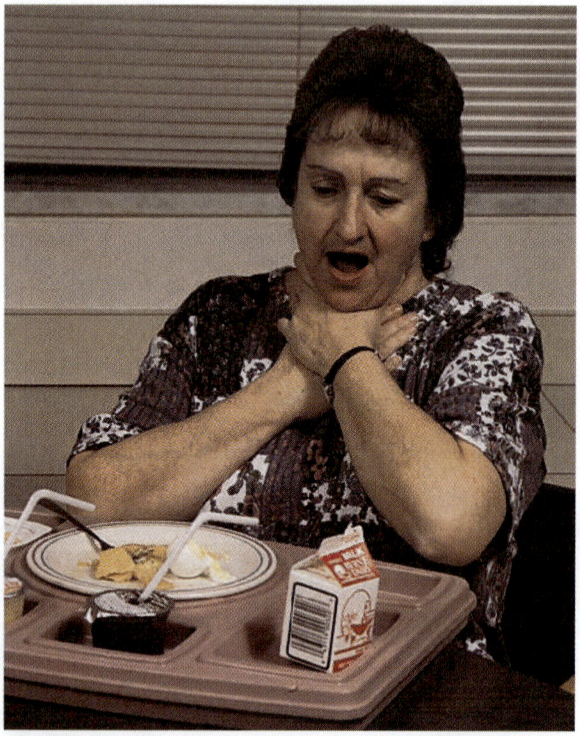

FIGURE 4-19 The universal choking sign.

Early Defibrillation

Public access to **defibrillation** has proven to be highly successful. Defibrillation is a method of treatment that uses an electric shock to reverse disorganized activity in the heart during cardiac arrest. Early defibrillation has proven to be critical to survival in cardiac arrest. Defibrillators are placed in various locations in the community and are used by trained rescuers in the event of cardiac arrest. Some studies have shown that the chance of survival doubles when early access to defibrillation is available. The speed with which defibrillation is performed is the key to success. Early defibrillation (within five minutes) is a high-priority goal in the community. In health care facilities, the goal is to defibrillate within three minutes.

Automatic external defibrillators (AEDs) are computerized devices that are simple to learn to use and operate. The AED is used *only* when a resident is unresponsive, not breathing, and pulseless. When the device is attached to the victim's chest, the unit determines if an electrical shock is necessary to reestablish or regulate the heartbeat. Several different models are available, and the operating instructions are slightly different for each. The four basic steps to using an AED are:

1. Turn the power to the unit on.
2. Apply the electrode pads to the resident's chest.
3. All rescuers stand back to allow the machine to analyze the heart rhythm.
4. All rescuers continue to stand back; the operator of the unit presses the shock button and/or follows the unit's instructions, which are usually audible through a voice-synthesized message.

Hospitals normally use manual, portable defibrillators for caring for resident victims of cardiac arrest. These defibrillators are operated by qualified licensed personnel. The AED is not routinely used in the hospital. However, some long-term care facilities have AEDs available in strategic locations. If your facility purchases an AED, employees will be instructed in its use. Although the AED is simple to operate, only those who are properly trained may use it. CPR and use of the AED are included in basic life support classes for health care professionals.

KEY POINTS IN CHAPTER

- Every employee of the health care facility is responsible for keeping the environment safe.
- Changes in vision, hearing, blood vessels, and reflexes put some residents at high risk for accidents.
- You should correct unsafe conditions, if possible, or report them to the proper person.
- Material safety data sheets give instructions for safe use of chemicals, identify health risks of chemicals, and describe first aid and safety precautions.
- You should answer the call lights of all residents, whether you are assigned to care for the resident or not.
- Identify the resident before giving care.
- Before applying a heat or cold application, know the type of application, area to be treated, length of time the application is to be used, proper temperature, safety precautions, and side effects to watch for.
- The nursing assistant must know and practice oxygen safety.
- Oxygen, fuel, and a spark are necessary to start a fire.
- In a fire emergency, the RACE system is used to remove residents from danger, activate the alarm, and contain and extinguish the fire.
- Know and follow facility policies for tornado, hurricane, earthquake, and bomb threat emergencies.
- The Occupational Safety and Health Administration is an agency that is responsible for overseeing employee safety in the workplace.
- If you discover a resident who is having a medical emergency or is injured, stay with the resident and call for help.
- The universal sign for choking is one or both hands on the throat.
- The speed with which defibrillation is performed is the key to success in cardiac arrest. In the community, defibrillation within five minutes is a goal; in health care facilities, defibrillation within three minutes is the goal.

REVIEW

A. Multiple Choice

Select the one best answer.

1. Safety is the responsibility of the
   a. director of nursing.
   b. housekeeping department.
   c. maintenance department.
   d. entire staff.

2. Physical changes in aging and disease that increase the risk of incidents are
   a. changes in vision, hearing, and reflexes.
   b. chest pain and shortness of breath.
   c. nausea, vomiting, and diarrhea.
   d. hair loss, diabetes, and cancer.

3. When placing the resident's call signal, you should
   a. place the call signal by alert residents only when they are in bed.
   b. never place the call signal near a confused resident.
   c. place the call signal near all residents at all times.
   d. give the resident the call signal only if requested.

4. Chemicals:
   a. are used only in the laundry.
   b. are stored in the clean utility room.
   c. should be kept in their original containers.
   d. are not permitted in the long-term care facility.
5. When using heat and cold applications, you should know
   a. the type of application and area to be treated.
   b. the resident's medical diagnoses.
   c. whether the resident is at risk of heart attack.
   d. the precise temperature preferred by the resident.
6. The three elements necessary to start a fire are
   a. oxygen, fuel, and a spark.
   b. oxygen, chemicals, and fuel.
   c. matches, cigarettes, and chemicals.
   d. matches, candles, and fuel.
7. You answer the facility telephone and the caller advises you that there is a bomb in the nursing home. You should
   a. ask the caller to hold while you get the nurse.
   b. hang up and call the police immediately.
   c. keep the caller on the line and get as much information as you can.
   d. tell the caller not to play silly games with the nursing facility.
8. If you find a resident who is ill or injured, you should
   a. run and get the nurse.
   b. stay with the resident and call for help.
   c. go to the phone and call an ambulance immediately.
   d. leave the room and pretend that you did not see the resident.
9. If you find a resident who has fallen on the floor next to the bed, you should
   a. help the resident back to bed.
   b. go to the desk and fill out an incident report.
   c. tell the resident he or she should have called for help.
   d. reassure the resident while waiting for help to arrive.
10. You find a resident who is having a seizure. You should do all of the following *except*
    a. place an object in the resident's mouth so he or she doesn't swallow the tongue.
    b. stay with the resident and call for help.
    c. loosen tight and restrictive clothing.
    d. move any objects that could harm the resident.
11. A serious complication of hemorrhage is
    a. bleeding.
    b. swelling.
    c. fractures.
    d. shock.
12. The universal choking sign is
    a. waving your hands in the air.
    b. coughing and gagging.
    c. one or both hands on the throat.
    d. clutching the chest.

B. True/False

Answer each statement true (T) or false (F).

13. _______Most accidents cannot be prevented.
14. _______Residents in wheelchairs should be parked across the hall from the linen cart.
15. _______Aging changes in vision make it difficult to see in dim lighting.
16. _______When answering a resident's call signal, you should knock on the door before entering the room.
17. _______Thermal burns are caused by chemicals touching the skin.
18. _______An example of a generalized cold application is an ice bag placed on a swollen ankle.
19. _______ Heat applications dilate the blood vessels.
20. _______Oxygen is necessary for life.
21. _______The first step in the RACE system is to run for help.
22. _______OSHA is responsible for employee safety in the workplace.

C. Fill in the Blanks

Compete each sentence by adding the missing word or words.

23. Syncope is the medical word for _______.

24. The major cause of fire in a health care facility is_______.

25–27. List three safety precautions to take when a resident is using oxygen.

25. _______

26. _______

27. _______

D. Clinical Applications

Answer the following questions:

28. Laura Tyler is walking in her room. She has only nylon stockings on her feet. What should you do?

29. You are assigned to bathe Mrs. Lincoln in the whirlpool tub. The tub has a built-in thermometer that reads 85°. The water is steaming and appears very hot. What should you do?

30. When you go around the corner in Wing A, you notice a large puddle on the floor. The housekeeper is off the unit taking her lunch break. Other personnel are busy passing trays and transporting residents to the dining room. What should you do?

31. Mr. Lake's oxygen concentrator is supposed to be set at two liters per minute. When you check it, you observe that it has been turned up to five liters per minute. Mr. Lake admits that he turned it up so he could "breathe easier." What action should you take?

32. Your facility requires residents to be supervised when smoking. Residents may not keep smoking materials. You enter Mrs. Rose's room and find her smoking a cigarette. She has burn holes in her clothing. How should you handle this situation?

Read the following case study, then answer the questions.

Mrs. Coxon fell three days ago. She has a skin tear on her left forearm, a bruise behind her right ear, and a bump on her head. The resident is normally alert and independent. You enter her room to serve breakfast and find that she is not dressed, which is unusual for this resident. Mrs. Coxon is mentally confused. She asks you to get her mother. She says she feels sick and begins to vomit.

33. How will you respond to the resident's request to get her mother?

34. What action should you take first?

35. What should you do next?

36. What do you think is causing the problem?

UNIT 5

Legal and Ethical Responsibilities

OBJECTIVES

After reading this unit, you will be able to:

- Spell and define key terms.
- Define the purpose of the residents' rights document.
- State the purpose of the advance directive.
- Describe how to assist residents who are physically or mentally unable to exercise their legal rights.
- Define resident abuse and neglect and give one example of each.
- List six other legal considerations of concern to the nursing assistant.
- Explain why understanding the resident's culture is important to the nursing assistant.
- Describe how to promote resident independence and explain why this is important.

Legal Considerations For The Nursing Assistant

Long-term care facilities operate under state, federal, and local laws. Some companies and accrediting organizations have additional requirements. All nursing assistants must operate within the scope of these rules. Each facility has policies and procedures governing employee conduct and resident care within the institution. These policies and procedures are designed to maintain compliance with the various bodies that govern the agency.

Ethical Standards And Legal Standards

Each day, as you carry out your work and relate to patients, coworkers, families, and others from the community, you will be faced with decisions to make about your actions. Some of these decisions involve the moral right or wrong of an action. Other decisions involve the legality of your behavior.

Two sets of rules help govern these moral and legal actions you will take. They are:

1. **Ethical standards**. These are guides to moral behavior. People who give health care voluntarily agree to live up to these standards. When these rules are not followed, the nursing assistant fails to live up to the promise to give safe, correct care and to do no harm.
2. **Legal standards**. These are guides to lawful behavior. When laws are not obeyed, the nursing assistant may be prosecuted and found **liable** (held responsible) for injury or damage. Legal guilt can result in the payment of fines or imprisonment.

The ethical standards and legal standards are established to ensure that only safe, quality care is given. Following these standards also protects the caregiver. Sometimes the rules that govern moral actions and the laws that govern legal actions cover the same area.

Ethics Questions

Probably at no other time in history have the questions of medical ethics been under such scrutiny. Questions health care providers ask include:

- When is life gone from a person on life support systems?
- How much lifesaving or resuscitation effort should be given in situations of terminal illness?
- When does human life actually begin?
- How much assistance should be given to the conception process?
- Should the body organs of a brain-dead person be harvested for transplants for the living?
- Does an unborn baby have rights?
- Is assisting a patient during or after an abortion right or wrong?
- Is euthanasia (assisted death) ever justified?
- Should animals be used in research of potential value to human life?
- Should food and water be withheld to speed death when the patient has expressed the desire to have this action performed?
- Who makes decisions about removing life support systems when there is no direct expression of the patient's wishes or there is conflict within the family?
- How will a choice be made when two or more people could benefit from an organ transplant but only one organ is available?
- How should the limited money available be spent when many serious disease conditions need to be researched?
- Who has the final authority over whether a woman will carry a pregnancy to term?
- Should marijuana be used for medicinal purposes?

Many facilities have ethics committees that advise the staff on ethical matters. The members of the ethics committees often include staff, clergy, interested community members, and advocates for the sick and elderly.

The committee usually does not make recommendations for specific cases. Instead, the committee reviews the ethical problems and principles involved to help guide the staff and family.

Respect for patients and their wishes is the primary concern. Part of this respect for life is shown by having patients actively involved in decisions about their care and future.

As a nursing assistant, you will take directions from the legal and ethical guidelines established by your facility.

Respect For Life

One of the most basic rules of ethics is that life is precious. Everyone involved in the care of patients has the promotion of health and the quality of life as primary goals (Figure 5.1). Death, however, is a natural progression of life. When death is certain, the objective is to keep the dying person comfortable. Today, there is a greater

LEGAL *Alert*

At some point in your life, you probably learned to "Do unto others as you would have them do unto you." Use this principle to guide your nursing assistant practice. You will find many instances in which personal comfort and convenience could potentially interfere with the care you give. By placing the patient's interests ahead of your own, you fulfill the ethical and legal obligations of your practice, protect patient safety, and reduce your risk of legal exposure.

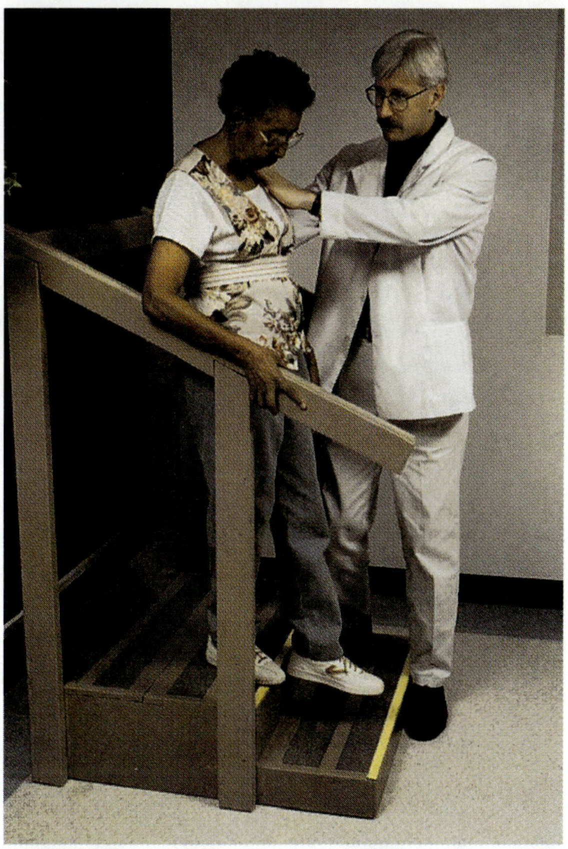

FIGURE 5-1 Promoting good health and quality of life is a primary goal.

appreciation of individual wishes and the quality of life expected. One fact remains clear—the major responsibility of medicine and all members of the health care team is to maintain quality of life and make comfortable those whose lives are limited.

Respect For The Individual

Respect for each patient as a unique individual is another ethical principle. This uniqueness is demonstrated by differences in:

- age
- race
- religion
- gender
- sexual preference
- culture
- attitudes
- background
- response to illness

You may find the differences that make the patient so special also make dealing with the patient challenging or difficult. If you respect each patient as a valuable person, you can learn to accept and work with each one in the best possible way.

Rights of the Resident

The resident has certain legal rights to safe care. Institutional policies vary regarding how residents are informed of these rights. Some facilities present a copy of the rights to residents upon admission and have them sign an acknowledgment that they have received them. Other agencies post copies of the rights in prominent locations throughout the facility. The bill of rights is written in very simple language that all residents can understand. In some communities with large groups of non-English-speaking residents, the bill of rights is translated into the prevalent language in the community. Health care workers must be aware of what the rights of the resident are. All health care providers are obligated to uphold and protect these rights for all residents. The nursing assistant must assist mentally confused residents to exercise their rights.

Residents' Bill of Rights

Residents in long-term care facilities have the same rights as other citizens of the United States. The Omnibus Budget Reconciliation Act (OBRA) of 1987 guarantees residents of nursing facilities certain legal rights. These rights are listed in a document called the **Residents' Bill of Rights**. The nursing assistant must be familiar with,

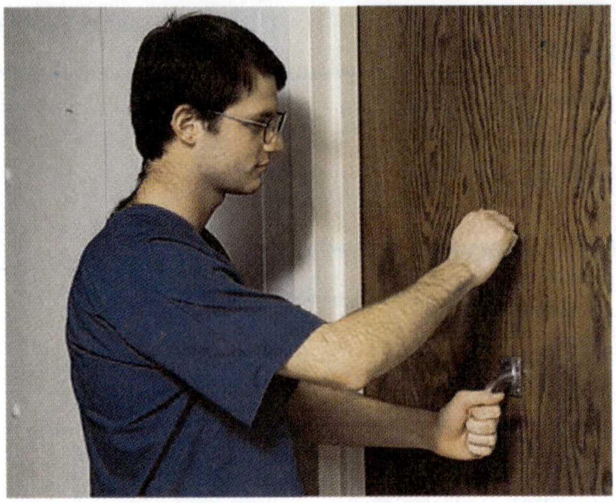

FIGURE 5-2 Knocking on the door and awaiting a response shows respect for the resident's privacy.

respect, and assist residents to exercise their rights. The rights of residents who are mentally confused are no different from the rights of others. The nursing assistant must protect the rights of mentally confused residents. Resident rights are summarized in Table 5.1.

Privacy Residents have the right to privacy. Always knock on the door (Figure 5.2) and allow time for a response before entering the resident's room. When providing care or performing procedures, close the door to the room, the privacy curtain, and the window curtains. The privacy curtain and window curtains must be closed even if the door to the room is closed and no one else is in the room. The nursing assistant must not unnecessarily expose residents when giving care. To protect dignity and prevent embarrassment, drape the resident's body so that only the part you are working on is exposed. A bath blanket is used for draping the body during examinations, treatments, and personal care.

Confidentiality The law guarantees residents **confidentiality** in their medical care and treatment. This means that unauthorized persons may not read the residents' medical records. It also means that health care workers cannot discuss personal information about the residents or their conditions with others. Information about residents should be discussed only in private areas. Do not discuss residents in hallways, on elevators, in the break room, or with others outside the long-term care facility. If a resident tells you something in confidence, you should not tell anyone else unless the information affects the resident's condition or medical care. For example, if a resident tells you something about a private financial matter, you should not tell anyone else. However, if a resident tells you that he or she is secretly spitting out his or her medication, this information should be reported to the nurse. If a visitor asks you for information about a resident, refer the visitor to the nurse for information.

PATIENT INFORMATION

The ethical code asserts that information about patients is privileged and must not be shared with others (Figure 5.3).

1. Discuss patient information only in appropriate places.
    a. It is unwise to discuss a patient's condition while in the patient's room, even if the patient is unresponsive. The patient may be able to hear everything that is said. This could cause the patient unnecessary worry.
    b. Never discuss the patients in your care with your family or in the community.
    c. Never discuss the patients during lunch or coffee breaks, even with your coworkers.
2. Discuss information only with the proper people.
    a. At times you will be approached by others requesting information about a patient. For

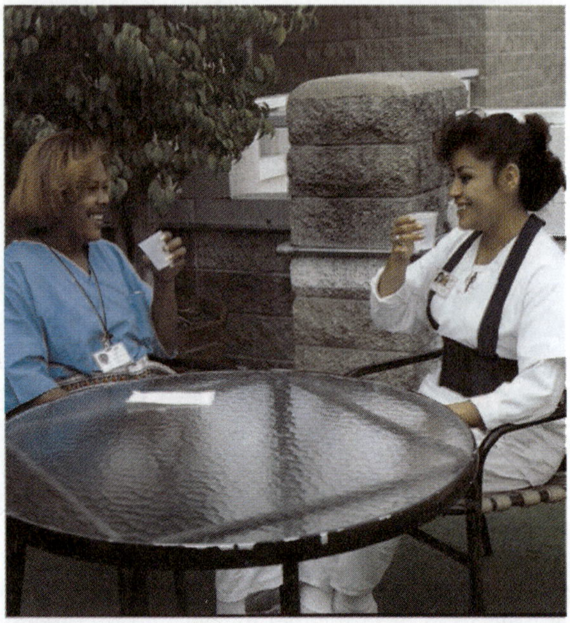

FIGURE 5-3 Information about patients is confidential and must not be discussed casually.

TABLE 5-1 Residents' Rights

- Residents have the right to exercise all their rights as citizens of the state and citizens of the United States, as well as any other rights given them by law.
- The facility must explain the rights to residents both verbally and in writing in a language that the residents understand.
- Residents cannot be discriminated against because of age, sex, race, ethnic origin, religion, or disability.

Privacy, Dignity, and Respect

- Residents have a right to privacy.
- Residents will be treated with consideration, dignity, and respect.
- The resident's likes, dislikes, and special needs and preferences must be considered in the services provided by the facility. This is called **reasonable accommodation**.
- Personal and clinical records must be kept confidential. Residents have the right to refuse to allow others to see these records. Permission to release records is given in writing.
- Residents have the right to communicate both verbally and in writing with anyone of their choosing. This includes family members, other visitors, the ombudsman, attorneys, and representatives of governmental agencies.
- Residents have the right to send and receive personal mail unopened. Residents may request that staff assist them to open and read their mail when it arrives.

Safety and Security

- Residents have the right to a safe environment.
- Residents have the right to care that is free from **misappropriation of property** (theft).

Medical Care and Treatment

- Residents have the right to choose their own physicians. They have the right to be informed of matters affecting their care and to make decisions regarding their care.
- Medical problems must be explained to residents in a language they understand.
- Residents may refuse treatment. If they do refuse treatment, they have the right to be informed of the consequences of their refusal.
- Residents have a right to voice problems and complaints about their care without fear of **reprisal**, or retaliation. The facility is required to respond to these complaints.
- Residents have the right to make choices to withhold life-sustaining treatment in the event of terminal illness.
- Residents may designate someone else to make treatment decisions for them in the event they become unable to make these decisions themselves.

Freedom from Restraint, Abuse, Neglect, and Misappropriation of Property

- Residents have the right to be free from abuse, neglect, and misappropriation of property. The facility is responsible for caring for the resident's health, well-being, and personal possessions.
- Drugs cannot be given for discipline or convenience of the nursing home staff. Any mood-altering drugs given must be required for the treatment of a medical condition.
- Residents cannot be punished, scolded, abused, neglected, or secluded. Their privileges cannot be taken away and they cannot be physically, mentally, or sexually abused.
- Residents cannot be restrained by physical means except for their own safety, the safety of others, during certain medical procedures, or in an emergency.

Financial Matters

- Residents have the right to manage their own financial affairs or may choose another person to manage their money.
- Facilities must account for and properly manage resident money deposited with them.

(continues)

TABLE 5-1 *(continued)*

Freedom of Association

- Residents have the right to have visitors at any reasonable hour.
- Residents do not have to talk to or see anyone they do not want to visit.
- Residents may make and receive private phone calls.
- Married couples have the right to share a room.
- Residents have the right to organize and participate in resident and family councils.
- Residents may meet with others outside the facility.
- Residents may leave the facility for visits or shopping trips.
- Family members may meet with families of other residents in the nursing home.
- Residents have the right to plan and execute their daily activities.
- Residents have the right to vote in elections.

Work

- Residents may choose to work in the facility as part of their activity plan. They have the right to be paid the prevailing rate for the same type of work in the community. Residents may also perform certain duties without pay, if they choose to do so.

Personal Possessions

- Residents may wear their own clothing.
- Residents may bring in furnishings and personal belongings from their own homes.

Grievance

- If residents have problems or complaints, they have the right to speak to those in charge. The complaints may be about care or failure to receive expected services. Residents have the right to a response.
- Residents have the right to contact the **ombudsman** for the facility and the state survey and certification agency. The ombudsman is a resident advocate. He or she can provide information on how to find a facility and how to get quality care. An ombudsman can help solve problems and will assist the resident to file a **grievance**, or complaint, if requested.
- The facility may not retaliate against residents who have complained.

Admission, Transfer, and Discharge

- The facility must advise residents about eligibility for Medicaid. If Medicaid or Medicare pays for any items or services, the resident cannot be charged additional money for these services.
- In the event of the resident's death, the facility must give an accounting of money in the resident's personal account to the person responsible for the estate.
- Residents may not be asked to give up their rights to benefits under Medicaid or Medicare.
- The facility is required to have the same policies and practices regarding services, transfer, or discharge for all individuals, regardless of the source of payment.
- The facility may be required to hold the resident's bed for a specified period if the resident is hospitalized or goes on a therapeutic pass.
- The facility cannot make the resident leave or move to another room unless:
  - The health and safety of the resident or others are affected.
  - The facility cannot meet the resident's needs.
  - The resident's condition has improved so that services are no longer required.
  - The resident has not paid the bill and the facility has given the resident reasonable notice of discharge.
- Residents must be given a 30-day written notice before they can be transferred unless there are medical reasons, or the life, safety, and health of the resident or others is endangered. Residents may waive the right to the 30-day waiting period if they choose.

example, you might be asked for such information by other patients, family members, or members of the public, such as news reporters.

b. Discuss patients and their personal concerns only with your supervisor during conference or report. Make sure you will not be overheard by visitors or other patients.

c. You will learn to evade inquiries tactfully by:

  - Stating that you do not know all the details of the treatment or the patient's condition.
  - Redirecting inquirers to the proper authority.
  - Firmly, but politely, indicating that you do not have the authority to provide the answers they seek.

3. Refer patient requests for information about laboratory results, the patient's condition, or course of the illness to the nurse or doctor.
4. Let the nurse or doctor relay information about a patient's death. Never give information concerning the death of a patient to the patient's family. When done with tact, a refusal of this kind is rarely resented by the family.
5. Follow the ethical code to ensure respect of the patient's personal religious beliefs. People of all faiths or beliefs and those with no proclaimed faith are admitted for care. These differences must be respected. You show your respect when you:

   a. Inform the nurse of requests for clergy visits.
   b. Know correct information about the type of chaplain services available in your facility.
   c. Know if a chapel is open for use by patients and families.
   d. Respectfully treat the patient's religious articles, such as a Bible, crucifix, Koran, or holy pictures.
   e. Avoid imposing your own religious beliefs on patients.
   f. Assist patients to practice their religious beliefs and rituals, if requested.

   When the clergy visits (Figure 5.4), you should:

   a. Be helpful and courteous.
   b. Escort the clergyperson to the patient's bedside.
   c. Draw the curtains or close the door for privacy.
   d. Leave the room.

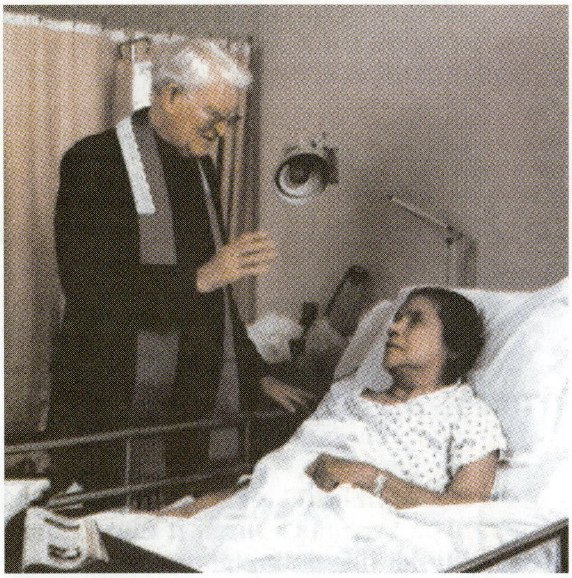

FIGURE 5-4 A private visit from the clergy can be very comforting and reassuring.

Tipping

If you follow the ethical code, the service you give will depend on need. It will *not* depend on the patient's race, creed, color, or ability to pay. There is no place for tipping within the health care system (Figure 5.5).

Patients are charged for the services they receive while in the hospital. The salary you are paid is included in that charge.

Sometimes patients will offer a "little something" to you. A firm but courteous refusal of the money is usually all that is necessary to assure the patient of your meaning.

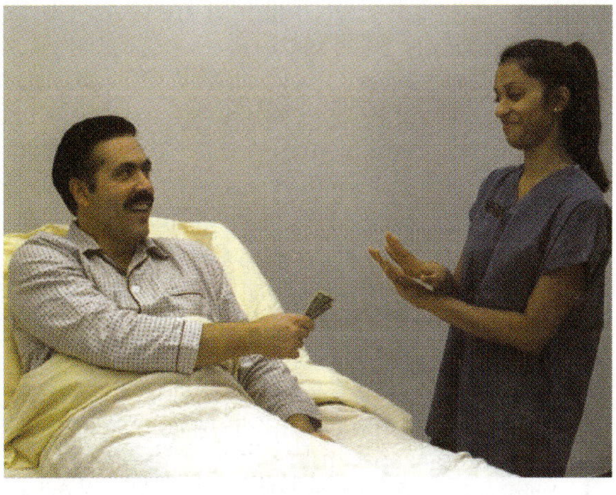

FIGURE 5-5 Tips must be courteously refused.

As you can see, the ethical code ensures that the patient is treated with dignity and respect in ways that always promote safe care.

Legal Issues

Laws are passed by governments (local, state, and federal) and are to be obeyed by citizens. Anyone who fails to obey a law may be liable (responsible) for fines or imprisonment.

You need not fear breaking these laws if you are careful to:

- Stay within your scope of practice and do not overstep your authority.
- Do only those things that you have been taught and that are within the scope of your training.
- Carry out procedures carefully and as you were taught.
- Keep your skills and knowledge up to date.
- Request guidance from the proper person before you take action in a questionable situation.
- Always keep the safety and well-being of the patient foremost in your mind, and act accordingly.
- Make sure you thoroughly understand directions for the care you are to give.
- Perform your job according to facility policy.
- Stay within OBRA guidelines.
- Maintain in-service requirements of OBRA.
- Do no harm to the patient.
- Respect the patient's belongings (property).

Situations you must avoid are negligence, theft, defamation, false imprisonment, assault and battery, abuse, and invasion of privacy.

Assisting Residents Who Cannot Exercise Their Rights

The nursing assistant is responsible for helping residents exercise their rights if they are physically or mentally unable to do so on their own. This involves using a good deal of common sense. For example, a resident with a physical or mental impairment may not be able to cover her body if it is exposed. It is your responsibility to cover the resident. Offer to help residents who cannot do things for themselves. You may notice an unopened card on the resident's table. Offer to open and read the card to the resident. Do not open the card without the resident's permission.

Give residents as much control over care and daily routines as possible. Always explain what you are going to do and how it will be done. Although the resident may be physically incapable of performing certain tasks, he or she may be able to tell you how and when he or she wants them done (Figure 5.6). Giving residents control and offering choices about care and routines is an excellent way to help residents exercise their rights, and promotes healthy self-esteem. It sends a message to residents that you value them as people and respect their opinions. Inform residents of facility practices, policies, and procedures that affect them.

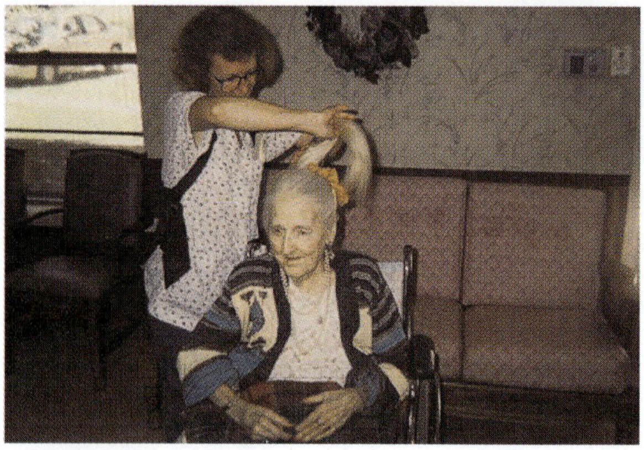

FIGURE 5-6 The resident is mentally alert and able to tell the nursing assistant how she wants her hair styled.

Although residents are guaranteed many legal rights, they are not allowed to infringe upon the rights of others. If the rights of one resident are interfering with the rights of others, try to find a compromise. If you are unable to resolve the situation, consult the nurse.

Abuse and Neglect

Abuse is the willful infliction of injury, unreasonable confinement, intimidation, or punishment that results in physical harm, pain, or mental anguish. Abuse can be physical, verbal, sexual, or mental. **Neglect** is failure to provide needed care or services. It can be deliberate or accidental. An example of neglect is forgetting that you have been assigned to care for a resident and not providing care. All states have laws concerning abuse and neglect of residents in the long-term care facility. You are legally responsible for reporting suspected or actual abuse and neglect of residents. The health care agency must always report abuse to law enforcement authorities and state agencies. This is the nurse manager's responsibility. There are severe penalties for abusing or neglecting residents. Health care workers who witness abuse or neglect and do not report it may be held equally responsible for the situation. If you suspect that a resident has been abused or neglected by a staff member, family, or any other individual, report this information to the nurse immediately.

Abuse and neglect may occur because a nursing assistant or other individual is feeling stressed. Residents may say things that are hurtful or upsetting to you. Remain calm and do not take a resident's behavior or negative remarks personally. Abuse often occurs when a worker is feeling tired, experiencing personal problems, or losing control. If you feel overwhelmed with your duties or with a resident, discuss it with the nurse. Arrange to take a break and compose yourself.

Types of Abuse

Abuse can take many different forms. Sometimes the abuser is not even aware that the behavior or action toward a resident is abusive. The different types of abuse are described in Table 5.2.

Recognizing signs of abuse New bruises, pain, swelling, or other unexplained injuries to a resident may be an indication of abuse and should be reported to the nurse. Other signs of possible abuse include residents responding to the nursing assistant or others with fear and anxiety. Residents who have been abused may show sudden changes in their personality or behavior. You are not required to determine whether the changes in the resident are the result of abuse. Your responsibility is to report the observations to the nurse for further investigation.

ADVANCE DIRECTIVES

A resident of a long-term care facility has the right to execute an **advance directive**. An advance directive is a document that designates the resident's wishes if he or she cannot speak for himself or herself. Advance directives can be in the form of a **living will**, which designates the resident's wishes if he or she is in a terminal condition. The resident also has the right to designate a surrogate decision maker, often called a **health care proxy**. The document that the resident signs is called a **durable power of attorney for health care**. This document allows the health care proxy to make medical decisions on behalf of the resident. State laws vary on how advance directives are implemented, but residents in all states have the right to execute these documents. The long-term care facility informs the resident of this right upon admission. The facility is obligated to follow the written directions of the resident on these documents.

OTHER LEGAL CONSIDERATIONS

Consent means giving permission for treatment when a person is conscious and alert (Figure 5.7). Residents have the right to refuse treatment for any reason. They also have the right to have the

TABLE 5-2 Types of Abuse

Type of abuse	Description
Physical abuse	Willful, nonaccidental injury, such as handling a resident roughly or striking, slapping, or hitting a resident
Verbal abuse	Swearing, using demeaning terms to talk to a resident, or embarrassing a resident
Mental abuse	Threatening to harm a resident or threatening to withhold food, fluid, or care as a form of punishment
Sexual abuse	• Physical force or verbal threats are used to force a resident to perform a sexual act • Touching or fondling a resident inappropriately • Any behavior that is seductive, sexually demeaning, harassing, or reasonably interpreted as sexual by the resident

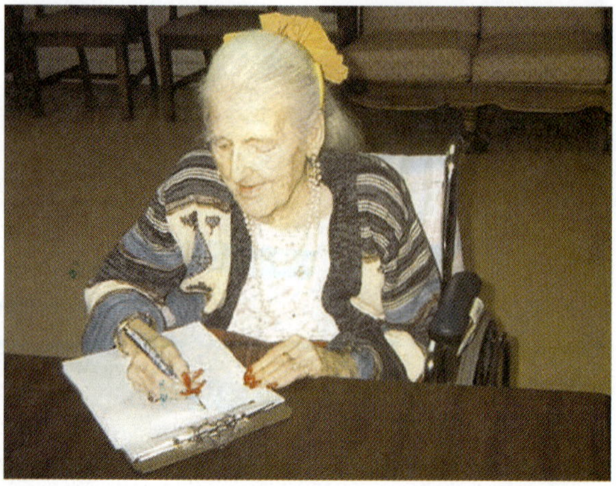

FIGURE 5-7 This alert resident understands her treatment and is able to give permission by signing a consent.

consequences of the refusal explained to them. Spouses or legal guardians have the right to give consent or refuse treatment for residents who are mentally confused. Report to the nurse for further directions if a resident or guardian refuses care.

Consent and the resident's right to refuse treatment can create a dilemma for the nursing assistant if the resident is mentally confused. For example, a confused resident may refuse bathing, grooming, or change of clothing. Residents who are confused have legally appointed guardians or family members who make medical decisions on the residents' behalf. These individuals have consented to nursing facility treatment, including the provision of personal hygienic care. In a refusal situation, gaining the resident's cooperation is always best. Avoid forcing a confused resident. Try different techniques, such as leaving and returning later, or making a fun activity of the procedure by singing, laughing, or joking with the resident. Use good communication skills. If the confused resident persists in the refusal, consult the nurse. Additional methods of working with mentally confused residents are described in Unit 16.

Negligence and malpractice **Negligence** involves breaching the standard of care. This means that a health care worker fails to provide services to residents in the same manner as a reasonably prudent person with the same education would do. An example of negligence is telling a resident it is all right to get up unsupervised even though you know the resident is dizzy and weak. The resident falls and is injured. An attorney can argue that the reasonably prudent nursing assistant should have known that the resident was at risk of injury. The proper course of action would be to instruct the resident to call for help before getting up, and remaining with the resident to assist while he or she was out of bed. To avoid negligence, always perform procedures in the manner in which you were taught, and use good judgment. If you are in doubt about what to do, consult the nurse. Follow your facility policies even if you do not agree with them. Malpractice is negligence that results in harm to the resident. For example, the care plan states that the resident's side rails are to be up at all times when in bed. The nursing assistant forgets to put the rails up and the resident falls from the bed, breaking a hip.

Making False Statements

Defamation of character is making false or slanderous statements about another person. An example is to tell others that your neighbor was admitted to the long-term care facility for treatment for AIDS. The neighbor was actually admitted for recovery after hospital treatment for pneumonia and does not have AIDS. Discussing a resident with someone outside the facility is also a serious breach of the resident's right to confidentiality. Discussions about residents should be limited to only those persons who have a legal right to know the information. **Slander** is a negatively spoken statement. **Libel** is a derogatory written statement.

Abandonment

Abandonment means leaving or walking off the premises. If the nursing assistant must leave the facility for any reason, the nurse should be notified. Before you leave, an equally qualified person must be available to care for your assigned residents. An example of abandonment is leaving the facility before a qualified person has been secured to replace you. You can be accused of abandonment, even if other staff is on duty, if no one else has been assigned to care for your residents.

False Imprisonment and Involuntary Seclusion

False imprisonment means holding or restraining residents against their will. Use of physical restraints and side rails can be considered methods of false imprisonment. To avoid this situation, follow all facility policies about the use of restraints. Consult the care plan before using any restraining device. **Involuntary seclusion** is a form of abuse if used as punishment for the resident. This involves separating the resident from others against his or her will. For example, Mrs. Long swears at Mrs. King in the dining room. Mrs. King is upset. To punish Mrs. Long, the nursing assistant removes her from the dining room and takes her to her room to finish eating lunch alone. Involuntary seclusion can be used in certain circumstances as part of the therapeutic plan of care, but this determination is not made by the nursing assistant.

Standards of Care

Although health care is delivered in many different settings, the legal requirements for nursing assistants are similar in all settings. **Standards of care** are common health care practices based on laws, facility policies, information learned in your classes, and information published in textbooks and journals for nursing assistants. Standards are defined by community, state, and national practices. They are used to measure the worker's performance and permit you to be judged based on what is expected of a nursing assistant with your education and experience. All long-term care facilities have standards of performance that you must follow in your job. In legal situations, you will be held to the same standard of care and judgment as the average worker in your job.

Good Samaritan Laws

All states have **Good Samaritan laws** to protect health care workers who provide emergency care outside their place of employment. If you assist someone at the scene of an emergency, you are protected under these laws if you deliver care that you are qualified to provide. These laws do not apply to workers providing emergency care in the long-term care facility.

Ethical Behavior With Residents And Families

Professional boundaries are limits on how a health care worker acts with residents. Compare these boundaries to the borders between states on a map. They exist, but you cannot see the boundary lines when you are driving down the highway. Professional boundaries are the same way. They exist, but you do not always know when you cross them. Boundaries are lines that define the best behavior of nursing assistants when caring for residents and meeting their needs. The nursing assistant must act professionally, not personally as a family member or friend. Professional boundaries help the nursing assistant act appropriately. You do not want to have too much or too little contact. You must use good judgment and determine the amount of contact that is right for the resident. Consult the nurse if you are uncertain.

The nursing assistant must treat all residents professionally. Residents expect you to act in their best interests and to treat them with dignity. This means you must not take advantage of a resident's situation, and must avoid becoming inappropriately involved in the resident's personal and family relationships. Some relationships with residents and families are not healthy for the resident or the nursing assistant. Unfortunately, it is not always easy to recognize unhealthy relationships until it is too late. Strive to find a balance in your relationships. If any of the situations in the following list have occurred, you have probably crossed boundary lines and are in a relationship danger zone. Seek help from your nurse, pastor, or another professional person with whom you are comfortable speaking.

- Discussing your personal problems with the resident or the resident's family members
- Discussing your feelings of sexual attraction with a resident
- Keeping secrets with a resident and becoming defensive when someone questions your relationship or involvement with the resident's personal life
- Thinking you are immune from having an unhealthy relationship with a resident
- Believing that you are the only nursing assistant who can meet the resident's needs
- Spending an inappropriate amount of time with the resident, including off-duty visits or trading assignments with others to be with the resident
- Reporting only partial information about the resident to the nurse because you fear disclosing unfavorable information or secrets the resident has told you
- Being flirtatious with a resident, including sexual innuendos, jokes that are sexual in nature, or using offensive language
- Feeling that you must protect the resident from other health care workers and always siding with the resident's position
- Feeling that you may become involved in a sexual relationship with the resident

Discussing Facility Business with Others

Discussing facility business with residents, family members, and others outside the facility is not ethical. You must be tactful and professional in disclosing information. For example, it is inappropriate to tell residents or family members that you are "short of staff," or to discuss working conditions, salary, benefits, or other information about the operation of the facility. It is also inappropriate to discuss this information or complain to others in the community. A common expression is "The long-term care facilities' employees are their worst enemies." When employees make negative comments and disclose private information, it sends a negative message about all parties involved. You have a moral and ethical obligation to your employer. Complaining to others does not solve problems. In fact, it can make problems worse. If you have concerns about staffing, working conditions, or other situations, use the chain of command within the facility to resolve them.

CULTURAL INFLUENCES ON HEALTH CARE DELIVERY

Health care workers care for residents from many different **cultures**. A culture is a pattern or lifestyle of a group of people. Residents may come from other countries or communities (Figure 5.8). Their backgrounds, beliefs, values, religions, hygiene, and health care practices may be very different from your own. Do not judge them for their beliefs. Look at this as an opportunity to learn more about others. If you can learn about the resident's culture, you will be in a better position to meet his or her needs. Cultural background may influence the residents' beliefs about illness and preferences in health care. The best way to find out about these preferences is to ask the resident or the family. Asking is not offensive. It shows that you are sensitive, have a sincere desire to learn, and are trying to find ways to help the resident. There is no one good way to meet the needs of an entire cultural group. Trying to place members of a cultural group in a specific category and thinking that they are all alike is called **stereotyping**. Every person is an individual with different wants and needs. Different cultural groups have different beliefs and different ways of meeting their needs. Treat all residents as worthwhile human beings and recognize their individuality!

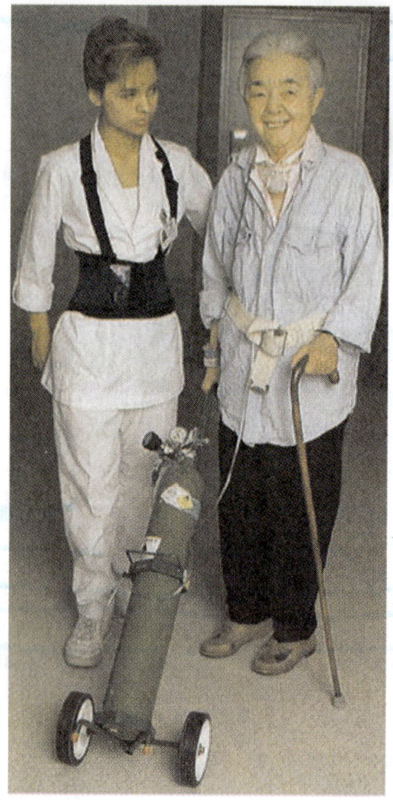

FIGURE 5-8 The resident and nursing assistant are from different cultural backgrounds.

Language Barriers

Always address each resident in English. Speak slowly, gently, and in a respectful manner. If you determine that the resident does not speak English, ask if the resident has a bilingual dictionary. If not, try using gestures or writing. Some residents learn to read English before they learn to speak it. Use simple terms. Drawing pictures may be useful. If you must perform a procedure on a resident, use gestures and a demonstration to make the resident understand. Always ask the resident if he or she understands, or say "Okay?". Do not assume that the resident understands because he or she smiles. A smile may be a polite gesture, indicating a lack of understanding. Be prepared to spend extra time with a resident who does not speak English.

Cultural Influences on Personal Space

Personal space is a comfortable distance for communication. The amount of space necessary varies in different cultures. In the United States, personal space is about 18 to 36 inches. People from other cultures may believe that this distance is too great or too small. In some cultures, personal space is much smaller. Be sensitive to residents' discomfort when you are working closely with them. Their beliefs about personal space may be different from yours. People from some cultures will not permit members of the opposite gender to care for them. Saudi Arabians, for example, will not permit a male caregiver to enter the room if a female resident is alone.

Use of Gestures and Eye Contact

The use of gestures and eye contact are not universal. In some cultures, making eye contact when you speak is offensive. Gestures that are acceptable to residents in the United States may be offensive to those from other countries. In India, the head motions used for "yes" and "no" are the direct opposite of the motions used in the United States. Monitor your body language, use of eye contact, and gestures carefully. If something appears to make the resident uncomfortable, don't do it.

Cultural Influences on Pain

Residents from different cultures react differently to pain. Residents from some cultures are very emotional and react very dramatically to pain. In others, the pain can be severe, but the resident will not show any response. In China and Japan, for example, displaying pain in public is unacceptable. In these cultures, pain is considered a sign of weakness.

Cultural Influences on Hygienic Practices

Some countries have different beliefs about bathing, personal hygiene, and the use of deodorant. They may not bathe regularly or use deodorant to eliminate odor. In the United States, it is normal to bathe and use deodorant daily. Women remove hair from their legs and underarms. This is not true of women in some other cultures. Do not be offended if the resident's hygienic practices differ from yours. This may be a difficult problem for you to deal with. Consult the nurse if you are having difficulty with cultural differences.

Cultural Influences on Clothing

Various pieces of clothing may have cultural or religious significance. Some religions require men to keep their heads covered. Others require women to keep their heads covered. In some cultures, women may not show any skin besides their face and/or hands. All other skin must be covered. A resident from such a culture will be very uncomfortable in a bed wearing only a hospital gown, because of the difference in cultural beliefs. Learning about the resident's culture and trying to make accommodations show that you care and will be greatly appreciated by the resident.

Cultural Influence and Home Remedies

People in some cultures have home remedies that they believe will cure their illness or relieve symptoms. These remedies may consist of wraps, rubs, teas, or inhaling herbs and spices. Friends and family members may practice these remedies on residents in the long-term care facility. In some cases, the remedies may actually interfere with the resident's treatment. Consult the nurse for advice if you observe residents practicing home remedies.

Cultural Influence on Food Preferences

Residents may refuse to eat foods served to them because of their cultural and religious beliefs. Some residents eat certain foods because of beliefs that the food has a healing effect on the body. Other residents will refuse certain foods or food combinations because of their religious beliefs. People of some religions have days during which they fast and do not eat. The dietitian and nurse may be able to arrange to have special foods served to residents to meet their needs.

Promoting Independence

The OBRA legislation requires long-term care facilities to maintain or improve the residents' condition and to promote independence. This is because being independent promotes healthy self-esteem. **Restorative care** is care designed to assist residents to function at their highest level in light of their individual situations. This is a very important part of the OBRA philosophy and is used to help residents attain maximum independence. Restorative care is simply good resident care. It is helpful to all residents and makes them feel good about themselves.

There is a common expression, "If you don't use it, you lose it." This is particularly true of self-help skills. We are not doing residents any favors by performing skills that they are able to complete. If the resident does not use the skill, eventually he or she will lose the ability to perform it. Some residents have low self-esteem because of their inability to care for themselves. Do not underestimate confused residents' abilities to do self-care. Test their ability. Provide support and direction, if needed. You may be surprised to find that they can do a great deal of self-care. Allowing them to do so will help maintain their ability.

The sensitive nursing assistant will give residents every opportunity to perform daily life skills independently. Provide support and encouragement. Set the resident up with the needed materials. Allow as much time as necessary to complete the task. If the resident is unable to complete a task independently, offer to finish it and provide positive feedback for what the resident was able to accomplish. Avoid making residents feel like failures. Always stress the ability and not the disability.

KEY POINTS

- Residents in long-term care facilities have specific legal rights that are guaranteed by the federal government.
- Nursing assistants must respect and protect the residents' rights. If the residents are unable to exercise these rights, the nursing assistant should assist.
- Professional boundaries are limits on how a health care worker acts with residents.
- The residents' culture and religion influence your ability to provide care.
- Restorative care is given to assist the resident to attain and maintain the highest level of independence possible.

REVIEW

A. Multiple Choice

Select the one best answer.

1. An advance directive is a document that
   a. gives consent for treatment and procedures while the resident is hospitalized.
   b. states the resident's wishes for care if the resident cannot speak for himself or herself.
   c. gives the health care worker the right to act in the resident's best interest.
   d. designates another person to make medical, legal, and financial decisions.

2. A health care proxy is
   a. a person who makes health care decisions on behalf of the resident.
   b. the health care worker responsible for diagnostic testing.
   c. the individual who prescribes the resident's medical treatment.
   d. another term for the licensed nurse.

3. The Residents' Bill of Rights guarantee residents treatment that is
   a. negligent.
   b. confidential.
   c. libelous.
   d. above the standard of care.

4. When providing care to a resident,
   a. leave the door open so others will know you are in the room.
   b. closing the door is the only step necessary if the resident is alone in the room.
   c. close the door, privacy curtain, and window curtains.
   d. you may leave the door open if the privacy curtain is pulled.

5. It is acceptable to discuss a resident's condition
   a. at the nurses' station or another private area.
   b. in the elevator.
   c. in the cafeteria.
   d. with your family at home.

6. A visitor asks you what is wrong with Mr. Stone, the resident in room 402. You know that Mr. Stone was recently diagnosed with pneumonia related to AIDS. Your best response is:
   a. "He has AIDS. For further information, consult administration."
   b. "He has pneumonia."
   c. "I'm sorry, but I cannot give you that information."
   d. "Ask the doctor."
7. Mr. Stephens is an alert 24-year-old male resident who is unable to move his arms and legs. He was admitted to the long-term care facility for rehabilitation after a serious automobile accident. He is able to communicate with you. The nurse has instructed you to bathe and shave the resident. You should
   a. ask the resident what time he would like the bath.
   b. encourage the resident to be independent.
   c. set up the supplies and ask the resident to try hard.
   d. bathe the resident when it is most convenient for you.
8. You cared for Mrs. King, a 92-year-old confused resident, on Monday. Mrs. King speaks, but does not make sense. You were off on Tuesday. When you return to work on Wednesday, you are assigned to care for Mrs. King again. When you remove her gown to bathe her, you notice bruises on her upper arms. You should
   a. say nothing, as the bruises must have occurred on your day off.
   b. report your findings to the nurse.
   c. ask Mrs. King why she has bruises.
   d. tell the nurse that Mrs. King was neglected on your day off.
9. Mr. Murray is a 72-year-old confused resident. You are assigned to care for him on the 3 p.m. to 11 p.m. shift. When you make your first round to check your residents, you discover that Mr. Murray is in bed. His sheets are wrinkled and soaking wet. There are brown rings of urine on the bottom sheet, indicating that Mr. Murray's linen has not been changed in quite a while. There is food in the bed, and the resident's face and hands are dirty. It appears that someone forgot to care for this resident. This may be an example of
   a. neglect.
   b. abuse.
   c. false imprisonment.
   d. involuntary seclusion.
10. Signs of abuse may include
    a. nausea and vomiting.
    b. unexplained injuries.
    c. fever.
    d. mental confusion.
11. Negligence that results in harm to the resident is
    A. involuntary seclusion.
    B. slander.
    C. malpractice.
    D. defamation.
12. Walking off duty before a suitable replacement can be obtained is
    a. libel.
    b. abandonment.
    c. neglect.
    d. abuse.
13. Good Samaritan laws are designed to protect
    a. health care workers from liability for care provided at the scene of an emergency outside the place of employment.
    b. licensed personnel who provide emergency care as part of their job responsibility.
    c. health care workers on duty in the nursing facility.
    d. physicians only.
14. Standards of care are based on
    a. information in books, journals, and laws.
    b. what the nurse says.
    c. what the doctor would do.
    d. information provided by other assistants.
15. People who come from other cultures
    a. have incorrect beliefs and values.
    b. may have different beliefs than your own.
    c. are all the same.
    d. have different needs.

16. Mrs. Hernandez is a 64-year-old Hispanic female with ovarian cancer. She is in the last stage of her illness, and her family members are at her bedside. When you are making the bed, you notice a raw egg in a cup under the bed. You should
    a. throw the egg away immediately, because it is unsanitary.
    b. tell the family to remove the egg.
    c. ask the resident or family the purpose of the egg.
    d. tell the resident she cannot have raw eggs.
17. Personal space is
    a. a comfortable distance in which to communicate.
    b. a private area used for dressing.
    c. the bathroom.
    d. the resident's room.
18. When caring for residents, you should
    a. provide all care needed even if the residents can do the care themselves.
    b. practice restorative care.
    c. force the residents to do as much as possible.
    d. always consult the doctor for advice.

B. Fill in the Blanks

19. One way of showing that you respect the resident as a person is to offer ________.
20. Residents in the long-term care facility have the right to ________ during personal care procedures.
21. Something that is personal and not known to other people is ________.
22. ________ is a spoken statement that maligns the resident.
23. ________ is treating residents with honor and esteem.
24. ________ are used to measure nursing assistant performance.
25. Failure to provide services that results in harm to residents is ________

C. Clinical Applications

Answer the following questions.

26. Your friend John is a CNA at another long-term care facility. John tells you that there are much faster ways to do your work than the way you were taught in class. John says that he always gets through with his work early because he has learned all the shortcuts, and offers to teach you what they are. How will you handle this situation?
27. Mary Gray is a mentally confused resident. She goes on an overnight pass with her son and returns after supper the next day. When you are undressing her for bed, you notice bruises on her upper arms and chest. Mary says, "I don't know how I got them." How will you handle this situation?
28. Mr. King is very ill. He has chronic respiratory disease. Mr. King has an advance directive that states that CPR and lifesaving measures will be performed in the event of cardiac arrest or emergency. The resident tells you that he is tired of fighting his illness and has changed his mind. He states he would like to revoke his advance directive. What should you do?
29. You are working the 10 p.m. to 6 a.m. shift. There are two nursing assistants on duty. The other CNA, Mary, has been a close personal friend for a long time. Your friend is upset with the nurse, who corrected her earlier in the shift. She tells you that you should both walk off duty to get back at the nurse. How will you handle this situation?
30. Mrs. Hall is a newly admitted resident. She walks with a strong, steady gait. The nurse instructs you to walk Mrs. Hall to the dining room for supper. Mrs. Hall says, "All the others have wheelchairs, and I want to use a wheelchair, too. I'm paying for it." What should you tell Mrs. Hall?

UNIT 6

Nutrition and Hydration

OBJECTIVES

After reading this unit, you will be able to:

- Spell and define key terms.
- Describe how proper nutrition influences health.
- Name the six classes of Nutrients.
- List the categories in the food pyramid.
- List five common categories of diets served in health care facilities.
- Describe how the nursing assistant assists residents to meet their nutritional needs.
- Describe general care and list the risks for the resident with dysphagia and swallowing problems.
- Identify residents who are at risk of malnutrition and list measures to promote adequate food intake.
- State the purpose of calorie counts and food intake studies.
- List three alternative methods of feeding.
- Explain why elderly individuals are at risk of dehydration and list nursing assistant actions to prevent dehydration.
- Identify the normal daily fluid requirement for adults.
- Demonstrate accurate measurement of oral fluid intake.
- List the general rules for passing fresh drinking water.
- Demonstrate the procedure related to nutrition and hydration.

OBSERVATIONS TO MAKE AND REPORT RELATED TO NUTRITION AND HYDRATION

Sores or ulcers inside the mouth
Difficulty chewing or swallowing food
Unusual or abnormal appearance of feces
Blood, mucus, parasites, or other unusual substances in stool
Unusual color of feces
Hard stool, difficulty passing stool
Extremely small or extremely large stool
Loose, watery stool
Complaints of pain, constipation, diarrhea, bleeding
Frequent belching
Changes in appetite
Excessive thirst
Fruity smell to breath
Complaints of indigestion
Excessive gas (flatus)
Nausea, vomiting
Choking
Abdominal pain
Abdominal distention (swelling)

Oral or rectal bleeding
Vomitus, stool, or drainage from a nasogastric tube that looks like coffee grounds
Increase or decrease in food (caloric) intake
Increase or decrease of body weight
Diabetic residents who do not eat all their food, or who eat more than allowed on diet
Residents on restricted diets who do not adhere to their diet
Refusal to accept meal, supplement, snack
Refusal to accept food substitute for meat or vegetable
Meal intake of less than 50% (or 75%, according to facility policy)
Drinking less than six cups of liquid a day
Dry mouth
Cracked lips
Sunken eyes
Dark urine
Urine output less than usual for resident
Urine dark and concentrated in appearance
New onset of difficulty swallowing food or liquids
Diarrhea, vomiting, or fever
New onset of mental confusion or worsening mental confusion
Weak or tired
Lethargy, difficulty staying awake

Important Observations of Diabetic Residents

Inadequate food intake
Eating food not allowed on diet
Refusal of meals, supplements, or snacks
Nausea, vomiting, or diarrhea
Inadequate fluid intake
Excessive activity
Complaints of dizziness, shakiness, racing heart

Signs and Symptoms of Abnormally High Blood Sugar (Hyperglycemia, Diabetic Coma)

Nausea, vomiting
Weakness
Headache
Full, bounding pulse
Fruity smell to breath
Hot, dry, flushed skin
Labored respirations
Drowsiness
Mental confusion
Unconsciousness
Sugar in the urine

Signs and Symptoms of Abnormally Low Blood Sugar (Hypoglycemia, Insulin Shock)

Complaints of hunger, weakness, dizziness, shakiness
Feeling faint or lightheaded
Skin cold, moist, clammy, pale
Rapid, shallow respirations
Nervousness and excitement
Rapid pulse
Unconsciousness
No sugar in the urine

Introduction

Nutrition is the entire process by which the body takes in food for growth and repair and uses it to maintain health. The signs of good nutrition include:

- Shiny hair
- Clear skin and eyes
- A well-developed body
- An alert expression
- A pleasant disposition
- Healthy sleep patterns
- Appropriate appetite
- Regular bowel habits
- Body weight appropriate to height

Normal Nutrition

Food is normally taken into the body through the mouth. The mouth is the beginning of the digestive tract. **Digestion** is the process of breaking down foods into simple substances that can be used by the body cells for nourishment. These substances are called **essential nutrients**.

Essential Nutrients

To be well nourished, we must eat foods that:

- Supply heat and energy
- Build and repair body tissue
- Regulate body functions

These foods are called **nutrients**. The six nutrients essential to maintain health are:

- Proteins
- Carbohydrates
- Fats
- Minerals
- Vitamins
- Water

Protein

Protein is an essential nutrient. It is the basic material of every body cell. It is the only nutrient that can make new cells and rebuild tissue. The foods that contain the greatest amount of protein come from animals. They include:

- Meat
- Poultry
- Eggs
- Milk
- Cheese

Proteins are made of small building blocks called **amino acids**. The body can manufacture some of the amino acids, but not all of them.

- *Complete proteins* are proteins that contain all the amino acids the body cannot manufacture. Examples of complete proteins are meat, fish, eggs, and poultry.
- *Incomplete proteins*, though still important, do not contain all the essential amino acids. Essential amino acids are those that must be obtained through foods. Examples of incomplete proteins are corn, soybeans, peas, and nuts.

Carbohydrates and Fats

Carbohydrates and **fats** are called energy foods because the body uses them to produce heat and energy. When a person eats more energy foods than the body needs, the remainder is stored as fat. Foods that contain the greatest amount of carbohydrates come from plants (Figure 6.1). They include:

- Fruits
- Vegetables
- Foods that are made from grains, such as breads, cereals, and pasta products

Carbohydrate foods also supply the body with fiber or roughage (**cellulose**). Cellulose is important in maintaining bowel regularity.

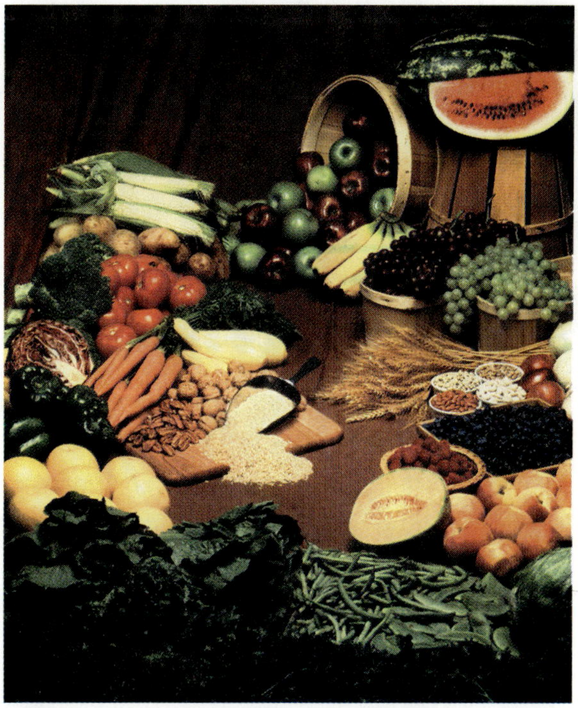

FIGURE 6-1 Fruits, vegetables, grains, and some dairy products are good sources of carbohydrates. (Courtesy of Agricultural Research Service, USDA)

Fats come from both plants and animals. Examples of foods that are rich in fat include:

- Pork
- Nuts
- Cheese
- Butter
- Egg yolk

Vitamins and Minerals

Vitamins and minerals are present in a wide variety of foods. The best way to be sure that you are getting enough vitamins and minerals is to include a variety of foods in your daily diet.

Vitamins are substances that regulate body processes. They help to:

- Build strong teeth and bones
- Promote growth
- Aid normal body functioning
- Strengthen resistance to disease

You probably know the vitamins by their letter names:

- Vitamin A
- B-complex vitamins
- Vitamin C
- Vitamin D
- Vitamin E
- Vitamin K

Fat-soluble vitamins do not dissolve easily in water. They can be stored in the body. Vitamins A, D, E, and K are fat-soluble vitamins.

Vitamins B and C are water soluble. Water-soluble vitamins dissolve in water, so they can be lost in the cooking process. In general, these vitamins are not stored in large amounts in the body. Deficiencies in water-soluble vitamins are more common.

Minerals help to build body tissues, especially the bones and teeth. They also regulate the chemistry of body fluids such as the blood and digestive juices. Minerals needed in the daily diet include:

- Calcium
- Iodine
- Copper
- Phosphorus
- Iron
- Potassium

The Five Food Groups

The U.S. Department of Agriculture revised the guidelines for a balanced food intake. The recommendations include:

- Eat a variety of foods.
- Maintain a healthy body weight.
- Select foods low in fat, saturated fat, and cholesterol.
- Select plenty of vegetables, fruits, and grain products.
- Use sugar in moderation.
- Use salt and sodium in moderation.
- Drink alcoholic beverages in moderation, if at all.

The 2005 Dietary Guidelines for Americans

The *2005 Dietary Guidelines for Americans* were developed by the Dietary Guidelines Advisory Committee, a group of scientists appointed by the Secretaries of the Department of Health and Human Services (HHS) and the United States Department of Agriculture (**USDA**). Primary use of these *guidelines* is to provide information for health care providers, nutritionists, and nutrition educators to develop nutrition-related educational programs. Based on the latest scientific evidence, these *guidelines* provide information that can be shared with the general public for choosing a nutritious diet, maintaining a healthy weight, getting adequate exercise, and avoiding foodborne illness by keeping foods safe. The guidelines emphasize the importance of eating a diet rich in fruits and vegetables, eating whole grain foods and foods containing potassium, drinking adequate fluids, decreasing the intake of added salt, sugars, and alcohol, and limiting the intake of saturated and *trans* fats, and cholesterol. As the basis for a federal nutrition policy, *MyPyramid* was developed to help individuals implement the recommendations contained in the *guidelines*.

The new "food pyramid" that replaces the old version is called *MyPyramid*; it is actually 12 pyramids in one. The central pyramid is divided into six vertical colored bands: (Figure 6.2)

- Orange—grains
- Green—vegetables
- Red—fruits
- Yellow—oils
- Blue—milk products
- Purple—lean meats and beans

Each band represents a different food group; this stresses the importance of variety in the diet. The bands also are different widths to represent the proportion of food to be chosen in each group. The actual quantity of food a person should consume on a daily basis to maintain weight or to lose

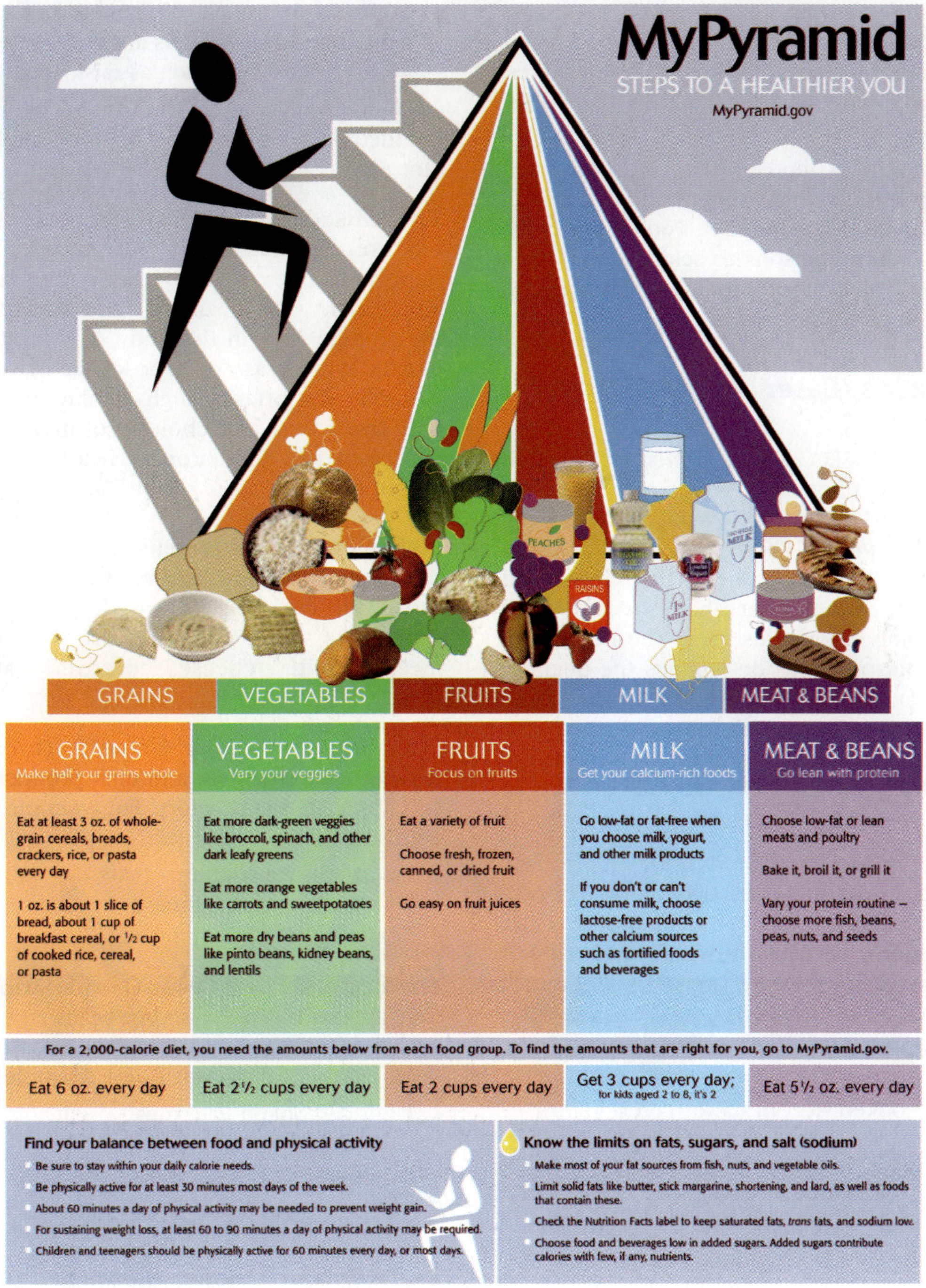

FIGURE 6-2 MyPyramid: Steps to a Healthier You

weight is based on age, gender, and amount of daily exercise. The person climbing stairs on one side of the pyramid shows that exercise and activity are important elements of health. *MyPyramid* becomes personalized when a person goes to the USDA website (*www.mypyramid.gov*) and enters the requested information that is based on the person's age, sex, and level of daily physical activity. Dietary recommendations are generated that are tailored to the individual person's needs.

In general, the USDA Food Guide recommends five food groups, oils, and discretionary calories as follows:

- Grains (3 ounces whole grains + 3 ounces other grains)
- Vegetables (dark green, orange, legumes, starchy or other—5 servings)
- Fruits (4 servings)
- Lean meats and beans (5.5 ounces throughout the day)

- Milk (3 cups, low-fat)
- Oils (6 teaspoons)
- Discretionary calorie allowance (267 calories, i.e., 8 teaspoons added sugar and 18 grams solid fats)

The amount of food used to illustrate each food group is the amount suggested for a person consuming a 2,000-calorie diet. Food choices are flexible and allow persons to select foods based on their individual or cultural food preferences. Figure 6.2 depicts *MyPyramid*.

Food Groups (Based on 2,000-Calorie Diet)

In general, the USDA *dietary guidelines* stress an increase in the amounts of whole grains, vegetables, fruits, and fat-free or low-fat milk and milk products that we eat. These food groups provide an abundant source of nutrients that are needed by the body and that help reduce risk for developing chronic diseases. The number of calories a person needs determines the quantity of the various foods that are consumed. Some persons need to eat fewer calories in order to lose weight or to maintain a healthy weight; the caloric intake, however, should still be rich in nutrients.

The Grain Group (Orange Stripe). It is recommended that a person on a 2,000-calorie diet consume 6 ounce-equivalents of grain products per day (3 ounce-equivalent of whole grain and 3 ounce-equivalent of other grains). A 1-ounce equivalent is:

- 1 cup dry cereal
- 1 slice of bread
- 1½ cup cooked rice, pasta, or cereal

The Vegetable Group (Green Stripe). Eating five (½ cup) servings of vegetables is suggested each day. For example:

- ½ cup cut-up raw or cooked vegetables
- 1 cup raw leafy vegetable
- ½ cup vegetable juice

Because vegetables are so varied in color and type, it is important to eat a variety throughout the week. The USDA suggests:

- Dark green vegetables (3 cups/week)
- Orange vegetables (2 cups/week)
- Legumes (dry beans) (3 cups/week)
- Starchy vegetables (3 cups/week)
- Other vegetables (6 1/2 cups/week)

The Fruit Group (Red Stripe). The recommended intake of fruit is four (½ cup) servings:

- ½ cup fresh, frozen, or canned fruit
- 1 medium fruit such as an apple or banana
- ¼ cup dried fruits such as raisins

Whole fruits rather than fruit juices are recommended because the juices do not contain important fiber.

The Oils Group (Yellow Stripe). Fats and oils are essential to the healthy diet and are important because they carry the fat-soluble vitamins (A, D, E, and K) and carotenoids to the storage sites in the body. The total amount of fats as well as the type of fat or oil that is eaten is important. High intake of saturated fats, *trans* fats, and cholesterol may lead to an increased risk for coronary heart disease. The recommended intake of fats/oils is 6 teaspoons per day.

Remember that the fats we eat are not only the spreads we put on bread or toast but also those we use to cook with and to season vegetables with. Fats/oils are contained in meats, poultry, cheese, ice cream, cakes, and pies.

The Milk Group (Blue Stripe). Three cups of low-fat or fat-free milk and milk products should be chosen in this category. For example, a 1 cup-equivalent is:

- 1 cup milk or yogurt
- 1½ ounces natural cheese
- 1 ounces processed cheese

The Meat and Beans Group (Purple Stripe). The daily allotment of meat and/or beans is 5 ½ ounce equivalents.

A 1 ounce-equivalent is, for example:

- 1 ounce cooked lean meat, poultry, or fish
- 1 egg
- ¼ cup cooked dry beans or tofu
- 1 tablespoon peanut butter
- ½ ounce nuts or seeds

Discretionary Calorie Allowance. For a person who eats a 2,000-calorie diet, 267 discretionary (extra) calories are allowed. A person may prefer whole milk to low-fat milk and could use the extra calories in this way. Another person may prefer more salad dressing or butter with a meal, or extra sugar on cereal, or a small glass of soda.

Alcoholic Beverages. Key recommendations of the USDA dietary guidelines regarding use of alcoholic beverages indicate that persons who choose to drink alcohol should do so in moderation. Moderate alcohol intake for women is one drink per day and two drinks per day for men. One alcoholic beverage is considered to be:

- 12 ounces regular beer
- 5 ounces wine
- 1 ½ ounces distilled spirits (80-proof)

Alcoholic beverages are harmful when consumed in excess. Precautions for older persons include making sure that the use of alcohol does not interact with medications the person may be taking or with specific medical conditions. The physician will decide if the use of alcohol is appropriate for the resident.

Special Populations. There are a number of suggestions for special populations, older persons, and children that have been incorporated into the *guidelines*. Older adults are encouraged to eat fortified foods or take supplements to achieve adequate intake of crystalline vitamin B_{12} (2.4 micrograms/day) and vitamin D (1,000 international units per day). Because of changes in the acid secretion in the stomach, older persons may not be able to adequately absorb the vitamin B_{12} in foods. Older dark-skinned adults, especially the population that is homebound or in nursing homes, may not be exposed to enough sunlight. These persons should eat foods fortified with vitamin D, like milk and milk products, or take supplements. Adequate intake of vitamin D is important to enhance the absorption of calcium and to prevent osteoporosis and risk of fractures. Older adults, African-Americans, and persons with high blood pressure are encouraged to consume no more than 1,500 mg of sodium per day. Salt is sodium chloride; some foods contain a large quantity of salt and should be used in moderation. The dietitian will plan the resident's diet and determine whether salt substitutes or other flavoring agents may be used by the resident. Potassium, on the other hand, can help lower blood pressure by blunting the effects of salt. Potassium-rich foods include leafy green vegetables, as well as a variety of fruits including bananas, oranges, melons, and strawberries. Many vegetables are a good source of potassium as well, especially potatoes, both white and sweet varieties, the squash family, corn, and tomatoes, among others. The potassium found in milk, meats, and cereal products is not as easily absorbed in the body; that is the reason for including adequate amounts of fruits and vegetables to the diet.

The *2005 Dietary Guidelines for Americans* are designed to encourage people to eat a diet with fewer calories, to be more active, and to make wiser food choices. The recommendations begin for Amer-icans who are older than 2 years of age, and they stress the importance of providing for the food preferences of different racial and ethnic groups, as well as vegetarians.

NUTRITIONAL STATUS

Eating to meet nutritional needs is one of the major activities of daily living. Eating also meets important social and emotional needs when dining is carried out in the proper environment and with the proper support. Older people who live independently may prepare foods that satisfy their appetites, yet do not meet basic nutritional needs.

Easy-to-chew, high-calorie foods may provide energy in excess of body needs; the extra energy is stored as fat. Although the person's appetite is satisfied by these foods, they do not necessarily provide the nutrients needed. Essential vitamins, minerals, and proteins may be lacking.

Older people are at risk for becoming malnourished. An important part of the job of a nursing assistant is to monitor and report the food and fluid intake of the residents. Malnutrition can result in unintended weight loss and pressure ulcers. A guide called "Nutrition Care Alerts" has been developed by experts in nutrition and long-term care. The guide is to be used not only by nursing assistants but also by other members of the interdisciplinary health care team. Nutrition Care Alerts list the warning signs for unintended weight loss and dehydration and provides a list of actions that caregivers should take to avoid resident malnutrition.

Warning signs for unintended weight loss:

- Needs help to eat or drink
- Eats less than half of the meals/snacks that are served
- Has mouth pain or dentures that do not fit
- Has a hard time using eating utensils Has a hard time chewing or swallowing
- Has sadness or crying spells, or withdraws from others
- Is confused, wanders, or paces
- Has diabetes, chronic obstructive lung disease, cancer, HIV, or other chronic disease

If any of these signs are present. the nursing assistant should follow these steps:

- Report observations and warning signs to nurse and dietitian
- Encourage resident to eat
- Honor food preferences
- Offer many kinds of foods and beverages
- Help residents who have trouble feeding themselves
- Allow adequate time to finish eating
- Notify nurse if resident has trouble using utensils
- Record meal/snack intake
- Provide oral hygiene before meals Position resident correctly for feeding

Facilities should have a protocol for standards of care for residents who experience weight loss of 5% or more in 30 days or 10% or more in the last 6 months. All residents should be weighed at least monthly and those at risk more often. It is important always to use the same scale, at about the same time of the day, and to take into account the weight of wheelchairs, leg rests, and lapboards.

Health Care Facility Diets

Physicians write diet orders for residents based on the residents' individual medical and nutritional needs. Food served in the health care facility is prepared by the dietary department. A licensed dietitian writes the menus to be sure that diets are well-balanced. The dietitian writes special menus for people with certain diseases to ensure that the nutrients provided meet their needs.

Many types of diets are served in long-term care facilities. Each facility has a listing of the types of diets served. Facilities post the menu each day. Some facilities have a selective menu. This menu allows each resident to select what he or she wants to eat. The common categories for diets served in long-term care facilities are:

- Regular, or general diets
- Liquid diets
- Soft or bland diets
- Mechanically altered diets
- Therapeutic diets

Regular Diets

The **regular diet** is a normal, unrestricted diet. This diet is served to residents with no dietary restrictions. The diet is well balanced and has a variety of foods from the food pyramid.

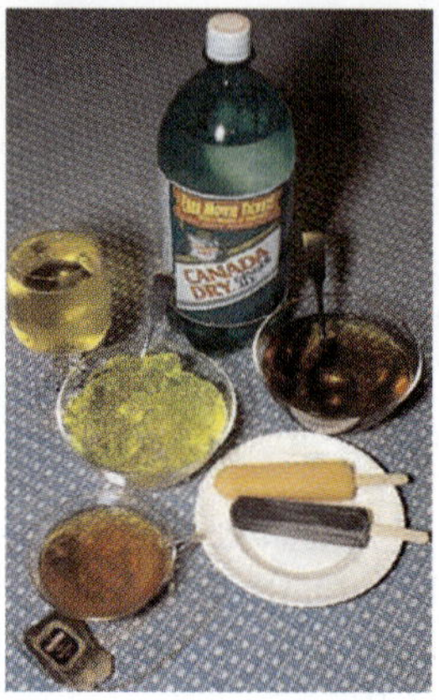

FIGURE 6-3 Items on a clear liquid diet include only liquids that you can see through.

Liquid Diets

Liquid diets are served to residents after surgery, and before some tests. They are also used for residents who have nausea, vomiting, or diarrhea. They are not nutritionally complete and should only be used for a short time. The two main types of liquid diets are:

- **Clear-liquid diet**. This diet is high in water and carbohydrates and consists of liquids that you can see through (Figure 6.3). It includes broth, tea, soup, gelatin, popsicles, and strained fruit juices. Clear soda pop and ginger ale are also served with this diet.
- **Full-liquid diet**. This diet consists of all clear liquids plus milk-based liquids. It includes cream soups, milk, ice cream, eggnog, and yogurt.

Soft Diets

Soft or **bland diets** are served to residents who have conditions of the digestive system or those who cannot eat spiced or seasoned food. A soft diet limits seasoning and is low in residue. Food served on this diet includes soups, white meat and fish, cream cheese and cottage cheese, breads, crackers, and milk products.

Mechanically Altered Diets

Mechanically altered diets are served to residents who have chewing, swallowing, or digestive disorders. Any kind of diet can be blenderized to alter the mechanical consistency of the food. The two main types of mechanically altered diets are:

- **Pureed diet**. This diet is blended with liquid so the food is smooth without large particles (Figure 6.4). It is the consistency of baby food,

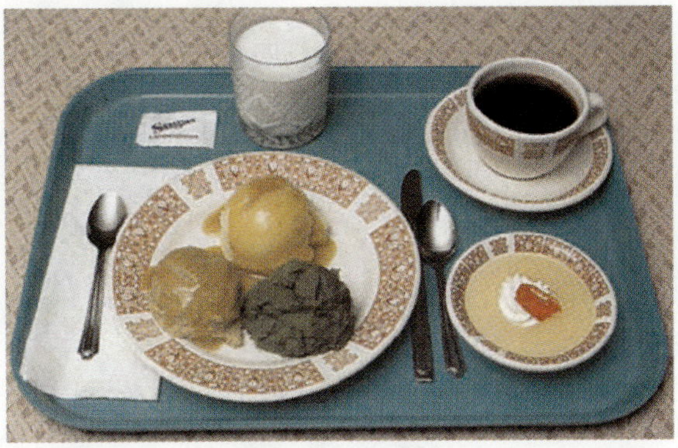

FIGURE 6-4 The pureed diet should have a firm consistency. Liquid should not run from the food.

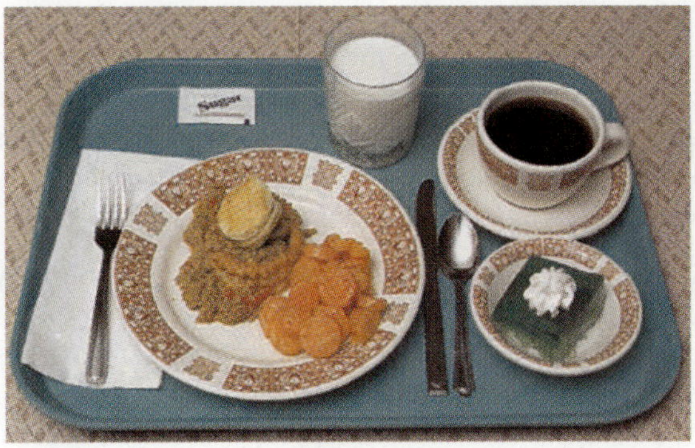

FIGURE 6-5 The mechanical soft diet includes ground meat. Foods that can be easily chewed are not blended.

but should not appear runny or watery. If the diet is blended properly, a plastic spoon will stand upright in the food without falling over.

- **Mechanical soft diet**. This diet is usually served to residents with chewing problems (Figure 6.5). It includes some foods, such as bread, that are not blended. Hard-to-chew items, such as meats, are ground until they are finely chopped. The food is not reduced to liquid in this diet.

Therapeutic Diets

Therapeutic diets are served to treat certain medical diseases or conditions. The licensed dietitian plans these diets very carefully to meet the resident's treatment needs. Regular food is used, but preparation of the food may be different from that of a regular diet. For example, certain foods on a regular diet are prepared with salt. A resident on a salt-restricted diet would have the same food item prepared without salt. Each therapeutic diet has special requirements, and some foods may be restricted on certain diets. There are four common types of therapeutic diets.

Diabetic Diet The **diabetic diet** serves normal foods, but the diet is prepared without sources of free sugar. This type of diet is served to residents with diabetes mellitus. Some diabetic diets count calories. Other diabetics are served a **no concentrated sweets diet**, which restricts forms of concentrated sweets, such as sugar packets, fruits canned in sugar, cakes, pies, and sweetened desserts. The recommended distribution of calories in a diabetic diet is 60 percent carbohydrate, 20 to 30 percent protein, and 20 to 30 percent fat.

Meal intake is very important for the diabetic resident. Meals and snacks must be served in a timely manner to maintain the resident's blood sugar. Diabetics receive medication to control their diabetes based on their food intake. If intake is inadequate, or meals are missed or delayed, serious complications may result. If a diabetic resident does not eat, report this information to the nurse. You will usually be instructed to offer the resident another food of similar nutritive value, to replace the uneaten items.

Calorie-Controlled Diets **Calorie-controlled diets** usually are served to residents who are overweight. These diets are nutritionally complete, but the portions are usually smaller than those of a regular diet. Like the diabetic diet, sugar and forms of concentrated sweets are avoided on this type of diet.

Sodium-Restricted Diets The **sodium-restricted diet** is served to residents with heart or kidney disease. Sodium-restricted diets are some of the most difficult diets to follow. The average American consumes 2 to 6 grams of sodium in food each day. Table salt is a major source of sodium in the diet. The doctor may order a diet prepared completely without sodium (salt), or the resident may be allowed sodium in a limited amount. In this diet, salt packets are not served on trays. Some facilities use salt substitutes if the doctor agrees. Foods that are usually low in sodium are fresh fruits, vegetables, and some cereals. Some foods have a high sodium content and should be avoided. Some examples are:

- Potato chips and similar snacks
- Lunch meats and processed meats, ham, and bacon
- Certain soft drinks
- Pickles and olives
- Many canned foods

Lowfat/Low-Cholesterol Diets **Lowfat** and **low-cholesterol diets** are served to residents with heart, blood vessel, liver, and gallbladder disease. Sources of fat are limited or avoided in food preparation, and fats such as butter, margarine, and oil are limited or restricted. This diet includes lean meats that are baked or broiled, fruits and vegetables, and lowfat dairy products.

Other Types of Diets Residents have many unique needs, and sometimes other types of diets are necessary. Some diets restrict sources of fiber. Others may serve a high or low amount of protein. Some are high in calories. High-calorie diets are commonly served to residents with burns, or those who need extra nutrition for healing. Some residents are on special diets because of religious prohibitions of certain foods. Special dietary requirements of cultural and religious groups in the United States are listed in Table 6.1.

Supplemental Feedings

Supplemental feedings are served to many residents. Supplements are served to meet special nutritional needs. Many residents have poor appetites and are underweight. Supplements are served to assist residents to maintain their weight, and gain if possible. Serving supplements and assisting residents to consume them is a very important nursing assistant responsibility. Sometimes common foods or beverages, such as milkshakes, ice cream, or juices, are served as supplements. Some facilities offer canned beverages, such as Ensure (Figure 6.6). Ensure and other canned supplements require a physician's order for administration. The percentage of supplement the resident consumes is documented on a flow sheet. In some facilities, the nursing assistant is responsible for documenting this. In others, licensed nurses document this information. Know and follow your facility policy. Supplemental feedings are always served between meals. If they are served too close to mealtime, the resident may not be hungry and will not eat. Diabetic residents are often given medication to control their diabetes. If supplements are served to a diabetic, the total calorie value of the supplement is included in the diet. The diabetic medication given is calculated based on the calorie count. Supplements must be given as ordered to maintain a proper balance between the food and medication.

Bedtime Snacks Most facilities offer residents a light bedtime snack, such as milk, juice, graham crackers, cookies, or fruit. This is an important part of the residents' diet, and should be offered to all residents before they go to sleep. Most facilities document that the resident accepted or refused the bedtime snack. Some facilities document snack consumption according to the percentage of the snack consumed. Know and follow your facility policy.

Assisting Residents with Nutrition

Illness and certain medications can affect the resident's appetite. When preparing residents for meals, it is important to make the environment and the food as pleasant and appealing as possible. Washing residents' hands before meals is also important.

Preparing Residents for Meals

Before mealtime, prepare residents for meals so that when meals arrive they can be served quickly. This maintains proper temperature. Food can be a source of infection if the temperature is not maintained. Hot foods should be served hot, and cold foods served cold.

Follow your facility policy for preparing the nursing unit for meals. Some facilities require removal of laundry hampers and housekeeping carts from hallways before tray carts arrive. Bring a clothing protector (Figure 6.7) to the room if needed by the resident. Do not call a clothing protector a bib. "Bib" is a demeaning term to most adults.

When assisting residents to be seated at dining tables, or using an overbed table, proper positioning is very important. The resident should sit upright with feet supported on footrests or the floor. Monitor the resident's distance from the table. The resident should not have to stretch and reach to eat. Monitor the height of the table. Some short residents may be sitting too low. They should not have to eat with their elbows in the air to reach the food. The elbows should be below the level of the hands when eating. Some adjustments in the type of table used, table height, or type of chair may be necessary to make eating easier. If the resident has to work to eat, he or she may not eat as well. It is usually easier to seat the resident in a straight-backed chair than it is to use a wheelchair. A straight-backed chair usually has lower armrests (or no armrests), making it easier to get close to the table. Wheelchair arms may not fit under the table and increase the distance that the resident has to stretch. Chairs that are used in health care facility dining rooms are usually the correct

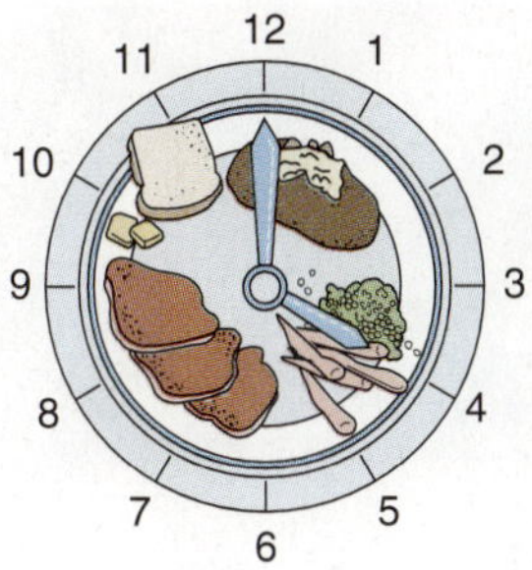

FIGURE 6-8 When serving a tray to a resident with visual impairment, describe the arrangement of the food compared with the face of a clock.

requirement to substitute desserts, breads, and beverages. If these foods are requested by the resident, follow your facility policy for serving them. Use common sense, and do your best to make mealtime satisfying. Know and follow your facility policy for substitutes. Many facilities provide a glass of ice water on food trays. Many confused residents will drink whatever liquids are placed in front of them. Offer residents a second cup of coffee when they are finished with the meal. When dining in a restaurant, a glass of water and additional coffee are always provided. Long-term care residents will appreciate this gesture and benefit from the fluid intake. Making mealtime special will pay off in resident satisfaction.

Serving Meals In most health care facilities, food is served on trays. The trays will be delivered to the dining room and nursing units in carts. Each tray is labeled with the resident's name, room number, and type of diet. After all trays are passed, check on residents while they are eating. If food is not being eaten, offer a substitute. Offer to replace or reheat food that has become cold.

Adaptive Devices for Eating The most common adaptive devices are used to enable residents to feed themselves. Many individual devices are available to meet residents' needs. The most common devices are adaptive silverware (Figure 6.9A and 6.9B), plates (Figure 6.9C), plate guards, and cups (Figure 6.9D). Other items, such as straw holders (Figure 6.9E), may also be necessary.

Mealtime Mealtime is a busy time in the long-term care facility. The nursing assistant has a major responsibility to see that it goes smoothly and pleasantly. You will:

- Make sure the area is pleasant and odor-free.
- Assist residents to reach the dining room.
- Serve trays.
- Help residents who need assistance in eating. Always be sure the resident receives the proper diet (standard or therapeutic) by checking the tray card.

GUIDELINES FOR

Serving Meals

- Plan and organize your time so you are available to pass trays as soon as the cart is delivered. Food must be served promptly to maintain temperature.
- Wash your hands.
- Check the tray card for the resident's name and room number.
- Check the food on the tray to see if it should be served on the resident's diet. If you think a food item is not appropriate, consult the nurse.
- Keep food covered during transportation to maintain temperature and prevent contamination.
- Leave trays on the food cart until you are ready to feed residents. Do not put a tray in front of a resident who must be spoon-fed until you are available to assist with the meal.
- Take the tray to the room, identify the resident, and place the tray on the overbed table.
- Prepare the tray, if necessary, by opening milk cartons, cutting meat, buttering bread, and putting condiments on food.
- Provide adaptive eating devices, if used.
- Feed the resident, if necessary.
- Serve all uneaten trays before returning used trays to the food cart. Do not return used trays if uneaten food remains on the cart.

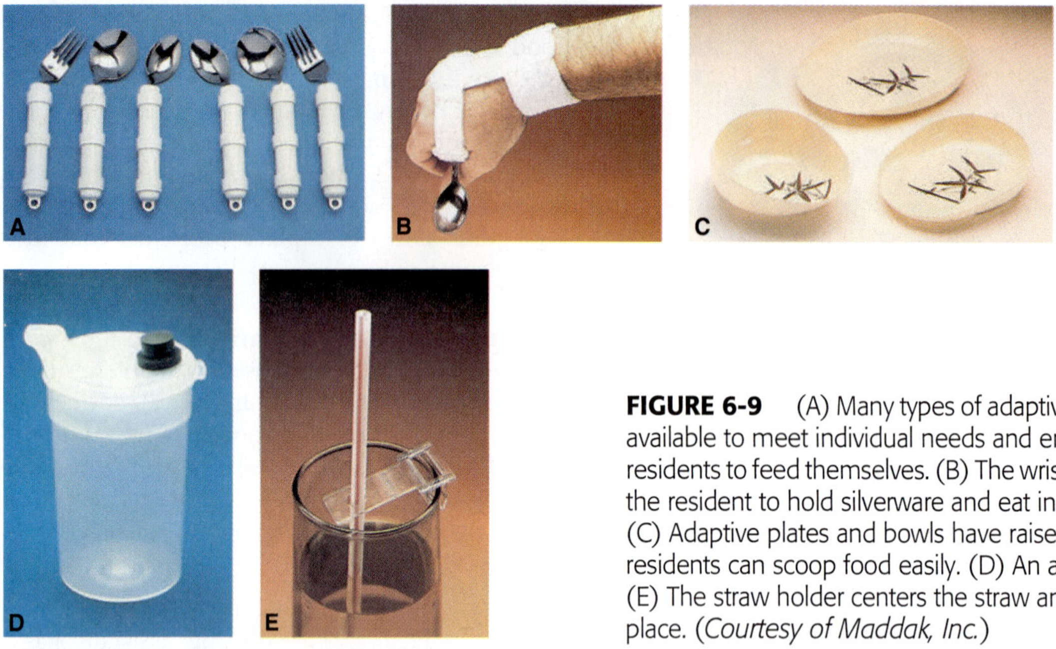

FIGURE 6-9 (A) Many types of adaptive utensils are available to meet individual needs and enable residents to feed themselves. (B) The wrist cuff enables the resident to hold silverware and eat independently. (C) Adaptive plates and bowls have raised edges so residents can scoop food easily. (D) An adaptive cup. (E) The straw holder centers the straw and holds it in place. (*Courtesy of Maddak, Inc.*)

- Offer substitutes if the resident dislikes the food that is served.
- Be sure foods are served at the proper temperature; don't hesitate to warm foods if necessary.
- Make sure that used trays are not returned to the serving cart until all clean trays have been served.

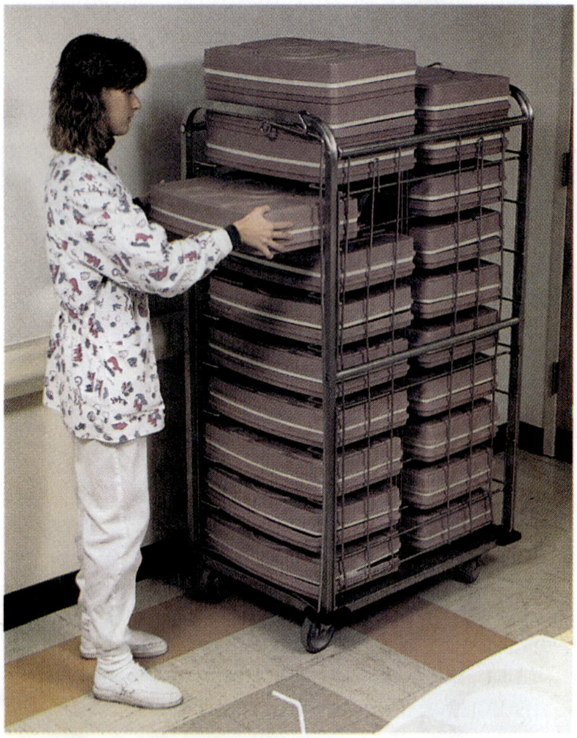

Residents' diets are prepared in the dietary department. The dietary aide takes the marked tray from the cart to serve to the resident. If a dietary aide is not available, the nursing assistant delivers the tray to the resident.

- Keep food trays covered until served.
- Keep housekeeping carts and laundry hampers out of the corridor when food is served or keep them at least two room widths away from the food cart when they are placed in the corridor.
- Place the food cart against the wall when it is brought into the dining room.
- Keep doors to the food cart closed until the trays are served.

Eating may be one of the few generally enjoyable activities left to older persons. In addition to meeting nutritional needs, meals should also be sensually and socially satisfying. Large dining areas permit residents to eat together and promote a social atmosphere. The meals are prepared by the dietary staff in large kitchens and brought to the dining area on tray carts.

In many facilities, special evening meals are organized so that residents who are able will dress up and eat in a restaurant-like atmosphere. Dining tables are set up homestyle and dinner is not served on trays.

This activity meets both social and nutritional needs and is greatly appreciated by residents.

Food Thickeners Residents with certain diseases and disorders may have trouble swallowing beverages, soup, and thin liquids. Residents who have had a stroke, or have Parkinson's disease or multiple sclerosis, are at high risk of choking on liquids.

Food thickeners (Figure 6.10) are nonprescription, powdered products that are mixed into beverages and some foods to make swallowing easier and prevent aspiration. The consistency of

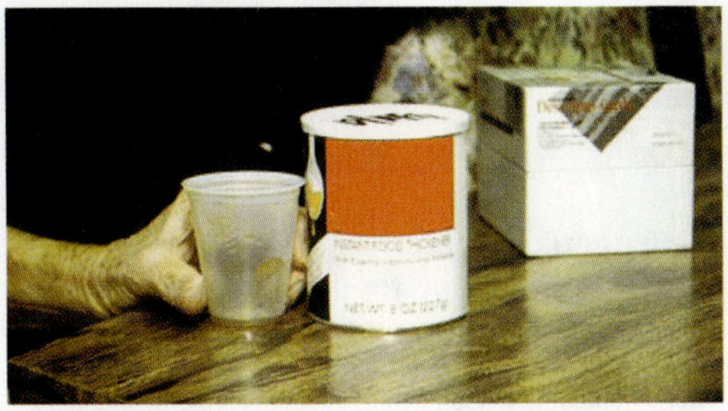

FIGURE 6-10 The speech-language pathologist will order the type of thickener and consistency to use.

the liquid depends on the amount of powder added. It is important to add exactly the amount that has been ordered. Thickeners do not change the flavor of food or liquids, but they may change the intensity, making it taste stronger. Prethickened liquids are also available.

The care plan will specify the type and amount of thickener to use to achieve the necessary texture. For example, the therapist may recommend that liquids be mixed to the consistency of peach juice, nectar, honey, or pudding. Milk products may take longer to thicken than other liquids, and coffee and hot beverages must be stirred very well, because the thickener has a tendency to lump. Add the thickener immediately before serving the product. Follow the therapist's directions exactly. When adding thickeners:

- Use the correct product
- Use the correct amount of thickener in the correct amount of liquid
- Follow manufacturers' directions
- Stir the thickener well (make sure the container is large enough to permit stirring)
- Stir again if product settling occurs
- Allow the beverage to stand for the recommended time to thicken
- Follow the speech therapist's instructions and plan of care for positioning and feeding

Feeding the Resident Some residents are not able to eat by themselves and must be fed. The resident may feel embarrassed and childish. Be sensitive to the resident's feelings.

After Meals After meals, pick up trays and return them to the tray cart. Wipe spilled food off the overbed table, if necessary. Facilities record how much residents have eaten in different ways. Some write "good," "fair," or "poor." Other facilities use fractions or record the percentage of the diet consumed (Figure 6.11). Know and follow your facility policy. Notify the nurse if the resident eats less than 75% of the meal. Follow the nurses'

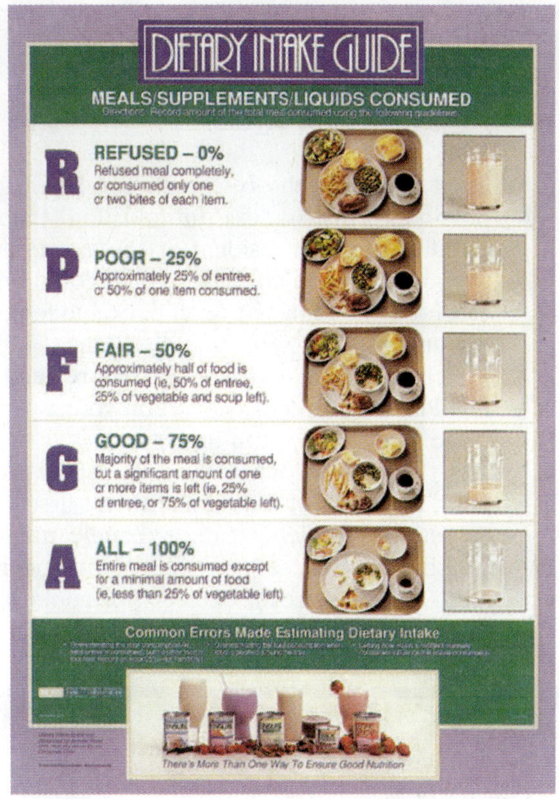

FIGURE 6-11 Accurate documentation of meal intake is an important nursing assistant responsibility. (Used with permission of Ross Products Division, Abbott Laboratories, Columbus, Ohio)

instructions. Record the amount of liquid taken if the resident is on intake and output. Before leaving the room, return the bed to a position of comfort and assist the resident to use the toilet, wash face and hands, and meet other hygienic needs. Make sure that there is no food on the face, hands, or clothing. Change the resident's clothing if soiled. Wait until all uneaten trays have been passed before returning used food trays to the cart.

DYSPHAGIA

Some residents have **dysphagia**, or difficulty swallowing food and liquids. This condition may occur in residents who have:

- Had a stroke
- Neurological diseases
- Cancer of the head, neck, or esophagus
- Undergone radiation therapy to the head or neck
- Dementia

People who take medications that cause sedation or reduce saliva production are also at risk of dysphagia. Signs and symptoms of dysphagia are:

GUIDELINES FOR

Feeding Residents

- Sit at or below the resident's eye level, if possible. This is less intimidating than standing over the resident. It also prevents the resident from choking, which could be caused by bending the head back and looking up at you.
- Check the food temperature before feeding. Place a drop of hot food on your wrist to be sure it is not too hot.
- Tell the resident what is on the tray. Ask what the resident would like to eat first.
- Sometimes residents cannot handle utensils, but are able to eat their own finger foods, such as bread, crackers, or cookies. Encourage them to do this, if able.
- Offer liquids at intervals. Using a straw will make it easier for residents to drink. For some residents, sipping from a small, flexible cup works best. The care plan will list the approach to use.
- Make pleasant conversation while feeding. Avoid making conversation if the resident has difficulty swallowing. Responding to conversation may cause accidental choking.
- Avoid rushing the resident.
- Be emotionally sensitive to the residents' needs. Focus on residents when feeding. Avoid having conversations with others in the room.

- Taking a long time before beginning to swallow
- Swallowing three or four times with each bite of food
- Frequent throat clearing or coughing
- Lack of a gag reflex or weak cough
- Difficulty controlling liquids and secretions in the mouth
- Wet, gurgling voice
- Refusing to eat, spitting food out, or pocketing food in cheeks
- Unintentional weight loss
- Tightness in the throat or chest
- Feeling as if food is sticking in the esophagus or sternal area

If you observe any of these signs or symptoms, inform the nurse. Residents with dysphagia are at high risk of developing malnutrition and dehydration. Consultation with a speech-language pathologist and diagnostic tests for dysphagia may be necessary.

Dysphagia is treated with swallowing exercises, practicing proper swallowing techniques, and altering the consistency of food and beverages. The dietitian will work closely with the speech-language pathologist to ensure that the food is the proper consistency to meet the resident's needs and reduce the risk of aspiration. The goal is to keep the look, taste, and food consistency as close to normal as possible, while considering the resident's safety needs. Extra gravies or sauces may be added to some foods. Adults may be resistant to eating pureed food because it resembles baby food. Molds and special methods of preparation are used to enhance the appearance of pureed foods, making them more acceptable to the resident. You may be instructed to monitor the resident's food and fluid intake accurately. Inform the nurse if the resident has special dietary requests. The physician may order frequent weight monitoring.

Residents with dysphagia will have special approaches for eating and drinking to prevent aspiration and ensure proper intake. The speech therapist works closely with these residents. Liquids are usually the most difficult to swallow. The speech professional may recommend using food thickeners to slow the movement of fluid through the esophagus.

Assisting with Meals for Residents Who Have Swallowing Problems

Residents who have difficulty swallowing may require one-to-one assistance, prompting, or supervision at meals. The speech therapist recommends special techniques and positions for improving swallowing and preventing aspiration. These will be listed on the care plan. The therapist may work closely with each staff member who feeds the resident. In general:

- Before serving food or beverages, make sure the resident is fully awake and alert

- Position the resident in an upright position, as upright as possible
- The head should face forward, with the neck flexed forward slightly
- During the meal, reduce distractions
- Limit conversation. The resident with dysphagia should not try to carry on a conversation while eating. Focus the resident on eating
- Direct the food to the unaffected side of the mouth
- Prompt or feed the resident slowly, offering small bites. Remind him or her to chew and swallow the food well. Check the mouth to make sure the resident has swallowed the food

The speech-language pathologist may order other special positions and exercises, depending on the resident's medical condition and needs. The care plan will provide additional directions, such as reminding the resident to tuck the chin in when swallowing. In some types of dysphagia, this changes the position of the airway, further reducing the risk of aspiration. In other types, this technique increases the risk. Because dysphagia care is highly individualized, many staff members must work as a team to ensure that the resident's nutritional needs are safely met.

MALNUTRITION

Malnutrition is inadequate nutrition due to poor diet or inability to absorb nutrients. This is a serious condition that causes serious complications. It can and does occur in long-term care facility residents, despite their being served a balanced diet and having nutritional supplements available.

Nursing Assistant Actions

Mealtime is very busy in the long-term care facility, especially on the day shift, when two meals are served. Do not get so busy that you overlook residents who are having difficulty or who are not eating. Residents who are at greatest risk of malnutrition and unintentional weight loss are those who:

- Forget what they ate, or if they ate, or forget to eat altogether
- Lose interest or become distracted before the meal is consumed, or during the meal
- No longer know the purpose of food
- Do not know what utensils are used for
- Cannot recognize or identify feelings of hunger or thirst
- Need help eating and drinking
- Eat less than half their meals and/or planned snacks
- Have mouth pain
- Have no dentures, or have dentures that do not fit correctly
- Have difficulty chewing or swallowing or need to be prompted to chew and swallow
- Have difficulty getting utensils or glasses to their mouth
- Cough or choke while eating
- Are sad, have crying spells, or withdraw from others
- Are confused, wander, pace, or have increased calorie needs because of activity
- Have diabetes, lung disease, cancer, HIV, or other chronic diseases

To increase food intake and prevent weight loss and malnutrition, create a pleasant, positive dining atmosphere for the residents. Be aware of each resident's self-feeding ability and changes in eating patterns. Report your observations and changes in residents' conditions and appetite to the nurse. You should also:

- Provide oral care before meals
- Position residents correctly for feeding
- Honor food preferences, likes, and dislikes
- Prompt and cue the resident, if necessary
- Before feeding the resident, use hand-over-hand technique
- Offer substitutes according to facility policy
- Serve meals promptly so that foods are at the proper temperature; check foods by dropping a small amount on your wrist
- Assist residents in using condiments, as allowed on diet
- Offer a variety of foods and beverages
- Help residents who are having trouble feeding themselves
- Provide adaptive utensils and dishes, as ordered
- Notify nursing staff if a resident has difficulty feeding himself or herself, eating, or using utensils
- Encourage residents to eat
- Allow enough time for residents to finish eating; avoid rushing
- Reheat cold food items if necessary
- Ask what's wrong if a resident's appetite decreases, or he or she seems sad
- Accurately record the resident's intake at each meal
- Assist and prompt residents to consume planned, ordered snacks and supplements

Calorie Counts and Food Intake Studies

The physician or dietitian may order special food intake studies for residents who are at

Diet ____________________

CALORIE/PROTEIN SUMMARY

RESIDENT ____ ROOM # ________________

DAY 1					DAY 2					DAY 3				
DATE ___/___/___					DATE ___/___/___					DATE ___/___/___				
	% 0–25	% 25–50	% 50–75	% 75–100		% 0–25	% 25–50	% 50–75	% 75–100		% 0–25	% 25–50	% 50–75	% 75–100
Breakfast					**Breakfast**					**Breakfast**				
Meat					Meat					Meat				
Milk					Milk					Milk				
Fruit					Fruit					Fruit				
Starch					Starch					Starch				
Fat					Fat					Fat				
Other					Other					Other				
AM Supp.					AM Supp.					AM Supp.				
Noon Meal					**Noon Meal**					**Noon Meal**				
Meat					Meat					Meat				
Milk					Milk					Milk				
Juice					Juice					Juice				
Starch					Starch					Starch				
Vegetable					Vegetable					Vegetable				
Bread					Bread					Bread				
Fat					Fat					Fat				
Dessert					Dessert					Dessert				
Other					Other					Other				
PM Supp.					PM Supp.					PM Supp.				
Evening Meal					**Evening Meal**					**Evening Meal**				
Meat					Meat					Meat				
Milk					Milk					Milk				
Juice					Juice					Juice				
Starch					Starch					Starch				
Vegetable					Vegetable					Vegetable				
Bread					Bread					Bread				
Fat					Fat					Fat				
Dessert					Dessert					Dessert				
Other					Other					Other				
PM Supp.					PM Supp.					PM Supp.				
Total Kcal					**Total Kcal**					**Total Kcal**				
Total Pro					**Total Pro**					**Total Pro**				
Avg. for 3 days Kcal:							**Avg. Protein for 3 days:**							

PLEASE RETURN COMPLETED FORM TO NUTRITION CARE MANAGER

FIGURE 6-12 The calorie count provides an accurate picture of the resident's calorie and nutrient intake over a three-day period. The information is used to adjust the resident's diet and nutritional plan of care.

risk of malnutrition, and those with special nutritional needs. The resident's food intake is carefully recorded for a period of time, usually three days. The food intake is analyzed for nutritional adequacy and number of calories consumed. The dietitian uses this information to plan a diet to meet the resident's special medical needs.

If the physician orders a food intake study, a special food documentation form (Figure 6.12) is prepared and placed on the medical record or other designated location. The food intake study

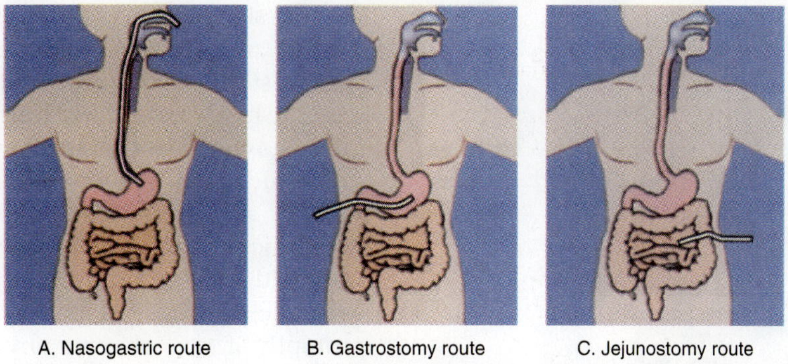

FIGURE 6-13 Enteral feeding methods: (A) Nasogastric feeding (B) Gastrostomy feeding (C) Jejunostomy feeding

usually begins with the breakfast meal on the day after the physician writes the order. In some facilities, each food item is weighed or measured. At the end of each meal, you will accurately record the resident's food intake on the form. Facility policies vary on how food intake is documented, but this is usually done by recording an accurate percentage of each individual meal item. You will also accurately document intake of all snacks, liquid nutritional beverages, and food items brought from home by visitors.

At the end of the study period, the form is returned to the dietitian. He or she will use the information to calculate the amount of protein, carbohydrates, fat, and calories the resident consumed each day. In some facilities, nutrient, vitamin, and mineral intake are also calculated. The dietitian will use this information to adjust the resident's diet and nutritional plan of care. The results of the study and the dietitian's recommendations are communicated to the physician, who may order extra vitamin or mineral supplements necessary for the resident's medical condition. Completing a food intake or calorie count study requires a team effort, good communication, and very accurate documentation.

Alternative Methods of Feeding

Sometimes residents cannot eat solid food and are fed by other methods. The nursing assistant does not administer these feedings, but must have a basic understanding of how to care for residents who are being fed by alternative methods.

Tube Feeding

Feeding tubes (Figure 6.13) are used for residents who have certain medical problems or are unable to swallow. A **nasogastric tube** is inserted through the nose and threaded through the esophagus to the stomach. This tube is for short-term use, usually six weeks or less. A **gastrostomy tube** (Figure 6.14) is surgically inserted through the abdominal wall into the stomach. This tube is inserted when long-term feeding-tube use is necessary. It is often, but not always, permanent. The tube can be removed if the resident regains his or her ability to eat. The resident is fed liquid formula through the tube. Feedings are commonly administered through a pump (Figure 6.15), which delivers the solution at a slow rate over a long period of time. Several other methods of tube feeding may also be used. Keeping the head of the bed elevated at least 30 to 45 degrees while the tube feeding is running is important. The head should remain elevated for 30 to 60 minutes, or

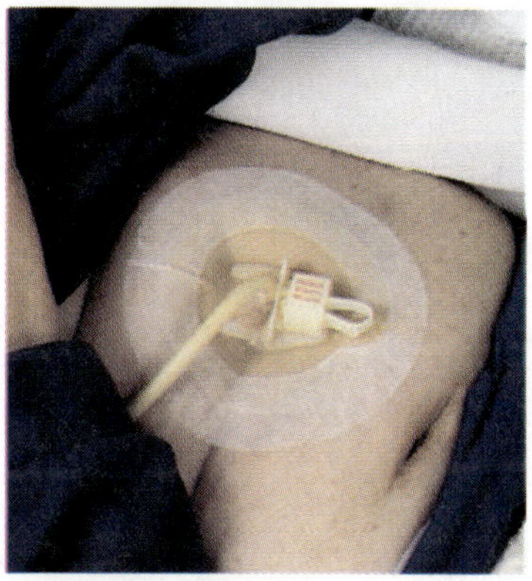

FIGURE 6-14 A gastrostomy tube is surgically inserted into the stomach through the abdominal wall.

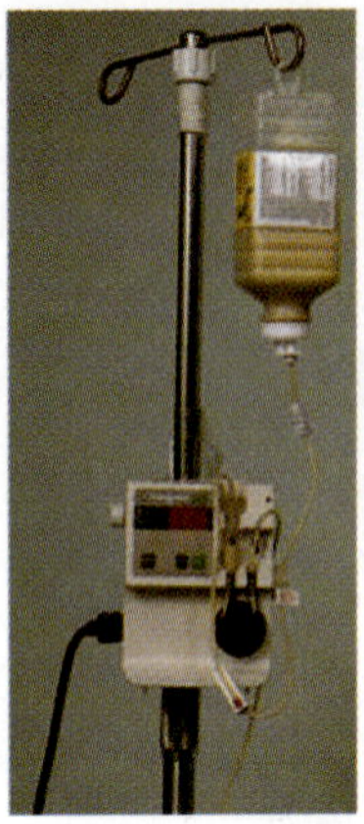

FIGURE 6-15 Most tube feedings are delivered through a pump. The total amount of tube feeding formula is not equivalent to free liquid. Approximately 15 to 20 percent of the formula is considered solid. To prevent dehydration, the dietitian will calculate the free fluid needs based on the resident's weight. Additional water will be given by the nurse.

according to facility policy, after the feeding is completed. For residents who receive continuous feedings on a pump, the head of the bed must be elevated at all times. This increases the risk of skin breakdown on the hips, buttocks, and coccyx area. Anticipate this and plan your care to position the resident correctly and use pressure-relieving devices to avoid breakdown.

The skin around the feeding tube must be kept clean and dry. Sometimes the skin around a gastrostomy tube is covered with gauze. If the resident has a nasogastric tube, it may be clipped to the gown or clothing to prevent pulling.

Residents who are receiving tube feedings are also at nutritional risk. Their medical needs sometimes change, and tube-feeding formula and fluid orders must be adjusted to keep up with their bodies' demands. Inform the nurse promptly if you observe any of these potential problems:

- Nausea
- Vomiting
- Diarrhea
- Swollen stomach
- Constipation
- Excessive flatus, cramping
- Pain, redness, heat, swelling, crusting, or fluid oozing from the site where the feeding tube enters the body
- Coughing, choking
- Wet breathing
- Feeling that something is caught in the throat
- Complaints of dryness or discomfort in the mouth or throat
- Pulling at or removing the feeding tube
- The feeding solution is low or empty
- The pump alarm sounds.

PROCEDURE 15 Feeding the Dependent Resident

1. Perform your beginning procedure actions.
2. Place the tray on the overbed table and sit at or below the resident's eye level.
3. Inform the resident what is on the tray and ask what he or she would like to eat first.
4. Fill the fork or spoon half-full. If the resident has had a stroke, place food in the unaffected side of the mouth.
5. Alternate liquids and solids.
6. Wipe the resident's mouth as often as necessary.
7. Remove the tray when the resident is finished.
8. Wash the resident's hands and face, if necessary.
9. Assist the resident with oral hygiene and toileting after meals.
10. Record the resident's appetite and fluid intake according to facility policy.
11. Perform your procedure completion actions.

Nursing assistant actions to take when residents are at risk of tube-feeding complications are:

- Keep the head of the bed elevated 30° to 45° (Figure 6.16) any time the tube feeding is running, and for one hour after feeding is completed
- Provide frequent oral care
- Follow the nurse's instructions and care plan for care of the skin around the feeding tube
- Move the resident carefully and position to avoid tension or traction on the tube
- Make sure that the tube is not kinked or obstructed
- Give the resident something to hold if he or she is pulling on the feeding tube; notify the nurse promptly
- Turn the resident on the side if coughing or choking
- Report observations and warning signs to the nurse promptly; if the resident is in distress, remain in the room and use the call signal, phone, or other method of getting help

Intravenous Feedings

Intravenous feedings, or **IVs** (Figure 6.17), are sterile liquid and nutrient solutions used for many purposes. Sometimes they are used to give the resident extra fluids or medications. The intravenous solution is attached to a needle or plastic cannula in the vein. The intravenous line may be placed in the veins of the arms, legs, neck, or chest. The solution may flow into the vein by gravity or be measured through an electric pump. For some residents, the intravenous feeding is the only source of nutrition. Intravenous solutions are not nutritionally complete, so this will be used for only a short period of time.

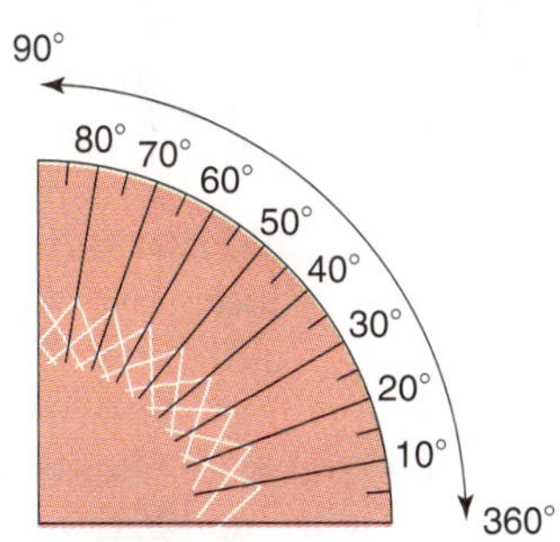

FIGURE 6-16 The head of the bed must be elevated 30 to 45 degrees or as specified on the plan of care whenever the tube feeding is running, and for at least an hour after the feeding is completed. To prevent aspiration, never position the head of the bed lower than 30 degrees.

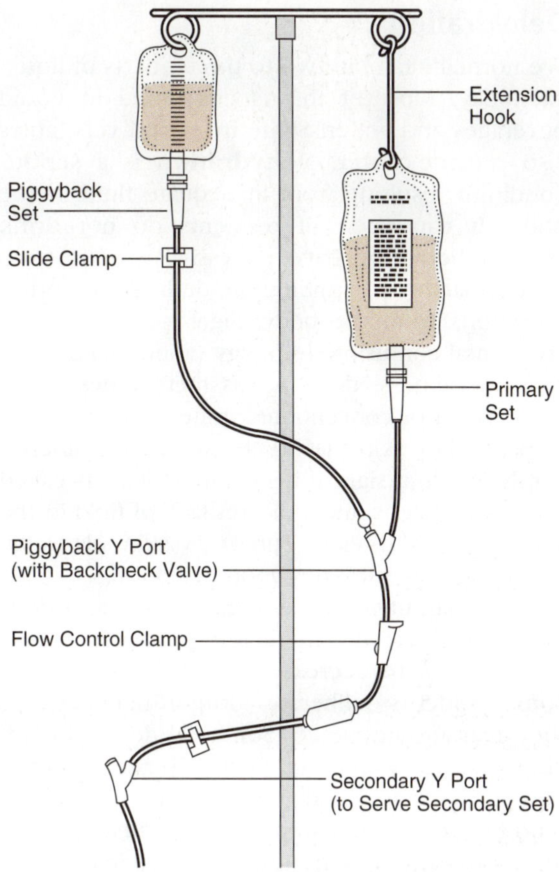

FIGURE 6-17 Residents who receive an intravenous infusion may also be served a meal tray. Oral intake and fluid output will also be monitored.

Residents who are receiving intravenous feedings may also receive a meal tray. Consult the care plan for instructions regarding a meal tray.

Hyperalimentation

Hyperalimentation, also called **total parenteral nutrition (TPN)**, is another type of intravenous feeding that is sometimes used to provide total nutrition.

FLUID INTAKE

An adequate intake of water and other fluids is essential to life. Two-thirds of the body is water. The body uses complex mechanisms to balance the fluid we take in with the fluid eliminated. In sickness and disease, ensuring that the resident drinks enough fluid is important. Fluid eliminated from the body may also be monitored.

Dehydration

We normally take in two to three quarts of liquid each day. Most of this is consumed in liquid beverages and water. Some fruits and vegetables also provide water. **Dehydration** is a serious condition resulting from inadequate fluid in the body. It can occur if residents do not drink enough liquid or have excessive output from urine, diarrhea, vomiting, or drainage of other secretions from the body. Signs of dehydration are mental confusion, **lethargy** (abnormal drowsiness), weakness, dry mucous membranes, rapid pulse, scant or concentrated urine, and low blood pressure. Dry skin that "tents" when you pinch it gently is also a sign of dehydration. This is called poor skin **turgor** and indicates lack of fluid in the subcutaneous tissues. Turgor is skin elasticity. Good elasticity indicates good hydration.

Like malnutrition, dehydration can and does occur in long-term care facility residents. This is partially due to decreased thirst in the elderly. Some residents deliberately forgo fluids because they fear incontinence. Some residents do not like to drink water, but willingly accept other liquids when provided. The majority of residents who become dehydrated do so because of medical illness and the physical or mental inability to ask for liquids. For example, they cannot reach for or hold the cup, pour from the pitcher, or drink from a straw without assistance. Extra fluid is needed by all residents in very hot weather.

Dehydration can be a very serious condition in the elderly. Residents who are at high risk for dehydration are those who:

- Have signs and symptoms of dehydration (see preceding paragraph)
- Drink less than six cups of liquid a day
- Do not like to drink water
- Cannot pour water from a pitcher
- Need help drinking from a glass
- Have trouble swallowing liquids
- Have diarrhea, vomiting, infection, or fever
- Have difficulty communicating and cannot make their needs known
- Are weak or tired
- Take medications to remove water from the body
- Do not consume the liquids on meal trays
- Have depression
- Deliberately do not drink liquids for fear of incontinence
- Consume a large amount of caffeine or alcohol
- Have urinary output that exceeds fluid intake
- Have had a recent unplanned weight loss

Nursing Assistant Actions Nursing assistant actions to prevent dehydration are:

- Offering the resident a drink each time you enter the room; set a goal, such as two to four ounces of liquid each time
- Drinking with the resident, if permitted
- Providing fluids the resident likes, at the preferred temperature, as permitted on the diet
- Making sure fresh water is available, that the resident can reach it, and that the pitcher and cup are light enough to hold
- Providing physical assistance to pour and consume fluids, as needed
- Offering ice chips, if permitted
- Following all swallowing precautions listed on the care plan
- Alternating liquids with solids when feeding meals
- Encouraging the resident to attend activities involving food and fluids
- Accurately monitoring and recording intake and output, when ordered
- Promptly notifying the nurse of your observations

Measuring and Recording Fluid Intake

Because most residents are asleep during the night, most of the liquid taken in should be consumed during the day and the evening. There are two meals on the day shift, so this is usually the time of day when most of the fluids are consumed. Measurements are often taken of how much liquid the resident takes in. Output from urine, vomitus, blood, and other drainage the resident excretes is also measured and recorded. This is called **intake and output (I & O)**. Regardless of whether a resident is on intake and output, taking in enough liquid each day is still important. Offer residents liquids each time you are in the room. Pay particular attention to confused and dependent residents who may not be able to drink without your help. Providing extra liquids in hot weather is particularly important, as fluid needs are increased to keep the body cool.

Fluid intake is all liquid that the resident takes into the body. This includes everything the resident drinks and all fluid given in intravenous feedings and tube feedings. The nurse is responsible for keeping track of fluid intake given through tubes and with medications, but the nursing assistant is responsible for monitoring the oral intake. This includes all fluids consumed in the resident's room, with meals in the dining room, and during activity programs.

When monitoring intake and output, certain food items are also considered liquids, and should

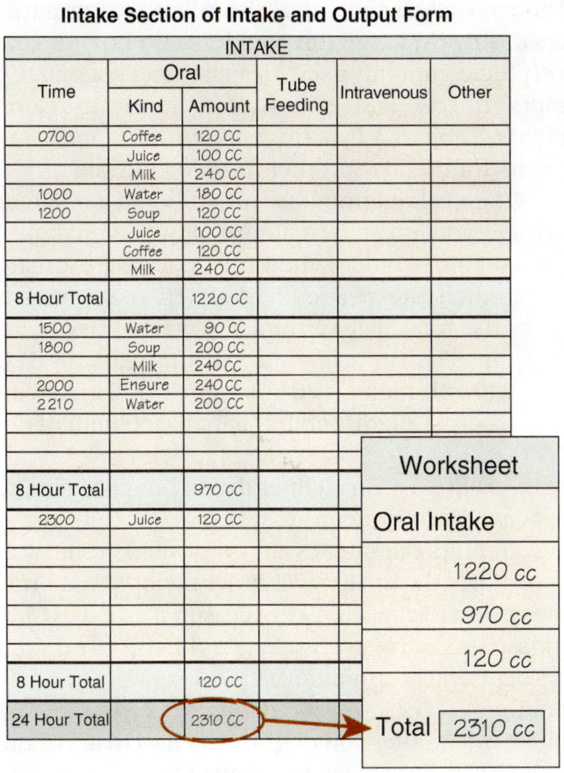

Intake Section of Intake and Output Form

INTAKE					
Time	Oral		Tube Feeding	Intravenous	Other
	Kind	Amount			
0700	Coffee	120 CC			
	Juice	100 CC			
	Milk	240 CC			
1000	Water	180 CC			
1200	Soup	120 CC			
	Juice	100 CC			
	Coffee	120 CC			
	Milk	240 CC			
8 Hour Total		1220 CC			
1500	Water	90 CC			
1800	Soup	200 CC			
	Milk	240 CC			
2000	Ensure	240 CC			
2210	Water	200 CC			
8 Hour Total		970 CC			
2300	Juice	120 CC			
8 Hour Total		120 CC			
24 Hour Total		2310 CC			

Worksheet
Oral Intake
1220 cc
970 cc
120 cc
Total 2310 cc

FIGURE 6-18 The oral intake is on the left side of the form. The type of fluid, time, and amount are recorded. The intake is totaled every 8 hours and cumulated every 24 hours.

be recorded. These are things that would become liquid if allowed to stand at room temperature, such as ice cream, sherbet, gelatin, pudding, custard, and popsicles. Pureed foods and items such as applesauce are not counted as fluid intake.

Force Fluids Residents who require extra fluid often have an order to **force fluids**. This does not mean that you physically force the resident to drink. When this order is written, you will encourage the resident to drink as many fluids as possible. Finding out what beverages the resident likes and providing them may be helpful. Offer the resident a drink every time you are in the room. It may be helpful to offer fluid in small amounts instead of large quantities each time. You will write down the amount the resident drinks. This will be totaled and recorded at the end of your shift. The night shift adds the amounts consumed on all shifts to obtain the 24-hour total (Figure 6.18).

Fluid Restrictions Sometimes residents with heart or kidney disease or other medical problems have **fluid restrictions**. Residents with fluid restrictions can take in a very limited amount of fluid each day. The total liquid allowed in a 24-hour period is calculated carefully. Usually, the total is divided by three shifts, and the care plan lists how much fluid each shift may give the resident. The fluid given

TABLE 6-2 Example container amounts

Container	***Approximate Number of Ounces***	***Approximate Number of mL (cc)***
Water glass	6 oz	180 mL
Styrofoam cup	6 oz	180 mL
Juice glass	4 oz	120 mL
Large glass	8 oz	240 mL
Water pitcher	32 oz (1 qt)	1000 mL (930 mL)
Coffee or tea pot	10 oz	300 mL
Coffee cup	5 oz	150 mL
Milk carton	8 oz	240 mL
Soup bowl (small)	6 oz	180 mL
Soup bowl (large)	10 oz	300 mL
Gelatin	4 oz	120 mL
Ice cream cup	4 oz	120 mL
Creamer	1 oz	30 mL

Note: This is only an example. Your facility will have a listing of specific amounts.

TABLE 6-3 Metric equivalents for common U.S. measurements

Common U.S. Measurement	Metric Equivalent
1 teaspoon	5 mL
1 ounce	30 mL
1/2 pint	250 mL
1 pint	500 mL
1 quart	1000 mL (or 1 liter)
1/2 gallon	2000 mL
1 gallon	4000 mL

includes fluid served on meal trays as well as liquids consumed on the nursing unit. The largest quantity is usually given by the day shift. The night shift may be allowed to give only a very small amount of fluid, because the resident is usually asleep during the night. In some facilities, residents who are on fluid restrictions do not get water pitchers.

Measuring Fluid Intake The metric system is used to measure fluid intake and output. Fluid intake is measured in **milliliters (mL)** or **cubic centimeters (cc)**. The two measurements are equivalent. One ounce is the equivalent of 30 mL or 30 cc. Your facility will have a chart that gives the number of milliliters for containers, such as the cups, dishes, and water pitchers (Table 6.2). You must understand how to convert the commonly used measurements of ounces, pints, quarts, and gallons into metric measurements. Table 6.3 lists the common U.S. measurements for liquids and their metric equivalents.

When calculating how much liquid a resident drinks, you must first know how much liquid the container holds when full. You will estimate how much the resident drank, then subtract it from the total. For example, a water glass holds 240 mL. The resident drinks half a glass, or 120 mL. 240 mL minus 120 mL equals 120 mL. You will record 120 mL under the intake column of the I & O record.

Usually, an estimation of the amount of fluid the resident drinks is adequate. When we measure intake and output, our figures are very close estimates. Sometimes the doctor will order **strict I & O**. This means that the fluid must be measured exactly. Using the same example, the water glass holds 240 mL. The resident drinks approximately half a glass. You will pour this water into a measuring device to see how much is left. After you do this, you find that 118 mL remain in the glass: 240 mL minus 118 mL equals 122 mL. You will record 122 mL on the I & O record. This method of measuring intake and output is more accurate, but as you can see, the figures are very close to the estimated amount in the first example.

You will be assigned to add the total intake at the end of your shift. Remember that most people drink 2000 mL to 3000 mL every 24 hours. Drinking less than this amount may not be enough to meet the body's needs. If the total for your shift

GUIDELINES FOR

Providing Fresh Drinking Water

- Wash your hands before beginning this procedure. If your hands become contaminated, or if you assist a resident, wash your hands again before continuing. Your hands remain clean if you are touching only clean items.
- Follow facility policy and good infection-control practices.
- Avoid contaminating the ice scoop, ice machine, or supply of clean ice with your hands, a cup, pitcher, or ice scoop. Avoid touching the ice scoop against the pitcher when you are filling the pitcher with ice.
- Do not pour water from a cup back into a water pitcher.
- Avoid filling a pitcher or cup directly over the clean ice supply. Ice from the scoop will hit the outside of the container and fall back into the clean ice supply, causing contamination. Fill the pitcher over a plastic bag, sink, or other container.
- Avoid mixing the pitchers and cups if there is more than one resident in the room. Pitchers that are reused should be labeled with the resident's name. Return the correct pitcher to each resident.

seems too low, consult the nurse. Your facility may have guidelines for you to follow. For example, a facility may require you to report to the nurse if the resident takes in less than 1200 mL on the day shift and 1000 mL on the second shift.

PASSING FRESH DRINKING WATER

The nursing assistant is usually assigned to pass fresh drinking water to residents every four to eight hours. Consult the care plan to see if the resident is allowed to have ice. In certain medical conditions, beverages are served without ice. The care plan will also note if the resident needs thickened water. Also check to see if residents are NPO. Most facilities remove the cup and water pitcher from the room while a resident is NPO. The method of passing drinking water and the type of ice dispenser will vary with your facility. However, certain common rules for passing drinking water apply in all facilities.

KEY POINTS

- Water, vitamins, minerals, carbohydrates, fats, and proteins are essential for good health.
- The actual quantity of food a person should consume on a daily basis to maintain weight or to lose weight is based on age, gender, and amount of daily exercise.
- There are five common categories for diets served in health care facilities.
- Therapeutic diets are planned by the licensed dietitian to meet a resident's specific medical needs.
- The nursing assistant is responsible for preparing residents for meals, serving trays, feeding residents, documenting food intake, and removing trays after residents have eaten.
- Dysphagia is a condition in which the resident has difficulty swallowing and is at risk for aspiration. Special techniques are used to prevent inhalation of food and fluids.
- Tube feeding, intravenous feeding, and hyperalimentation are alternative methods of feeding residents who have special needs.
- Residents in long-term care facilities can and do develop malnutrition and dehydration. The nursing assistant must be aware of at-risk residents and take steps to prevent these conditions.
- Adults need 2000 mL to 3000 mL of liquid each day for their bodies to function properly.
- Measuring fluid intake and output is an important responsibility of the nursing assistant.
- The nurse is responsible for recording intake for tube feedings and medications. The nursing assistant is responsible for recording all other fluid intake, including fluids that residents consume in the dining room and at activities.
- The nursing assistant applies principles of medical asepsis when passing fresh drinking water to residents.

REVIEW

A. Multiple Choice

Select the one best answer.

1. How many nutrients are essential for good health?
   a. two
   b. three
   c. five
   d. six

2. Which basic nutrient is essential for tissue building and repair?
   a. minerals.
   b. proteins.
   c. carbohydrates.
   d. fats.

3. Water is a/an

   a. mineral
   b. vitamin
   c. essential nutrient
   d. discretionary calorie

4. Which of the following is part of the meat group?

   a. rice
   b. fish
   c. butter
   d. whole grains

5. You are assigned to serve a full liquid diet to Mr. Johnson. Which of the following would you expect to find on his tray?

   a. vegetable soup
   b. pureed fish
   c. yogurt
   d. peach cobbler

6. Therapeutic diets

   a. are planned by the dietitian for residents with special medical needs.
   b. are rarely used in the health care facility.
   c. have no effect on residents with heart disease or diabetes.
   d. are always limited in sugar.

7. Foods that are high in sodium include

   a. fresh fruit.
   b. fresh vegetables.
   c. bread and grains.
   d. lunch meat and ham.

8. Which of the following is a water soluble vitamin?

   a. vitamin C.
   b. vitamin E.
   c. vitamin A.
   d. vitamin D.

9. If you feel that a food is too hot to feed to a dependent resident, you should

   a. return the food to the tray cart uneaten.
   b. blow on the food to cool it.
   c. leave the food until it cools.
   d. put the food in the refrigerator.

10. When feeding a resident who has a paralyzed side, direct the food

    a. to the unaffected side of the mouth.
    b. to the affected side of the mouth.
    c. in the center of the mouth.
    d. to the back of the throat.

11. Alternative methods of feeding include

    a. therapeutic diets.
    b. tube feeding.
    c. mechanically altered diets.
    d. thickening liquids.

12. When a resident is receiving a tube feeding, the head of the bed should be

    a. flat.
    b. elevated 10 to 20 degrees.
    c. elevated 30 to 45 degrees.
    d. tilted back.

13. When caring for a resident with a gastrostomy feeding, notify the nurse if the

    a. resident is coughing or choking.
    b. head of the bed is elevated more than 45 degrees.
    c. resident needs mouth care.
    d. resident needs to be turned to the side.

14. The normal daily fluid requirement for adults is

    a. 100 to 1000 mL.
    b. 500 to 2000 mL.
    c. 2000 to 3000 mL.
    d. 3500 to 4000 mL.

15. A condition that results from inadequate fluid in the body is

    a. hydration.
    b. dehydration.
    c. mechanical alteration.
    d. dysphagia.

16. Lethargy is

    a. hyperactivity.
    b. abnormal thirst.
    c. abnormal drowsiness.
    d. an indication of overhydration.

17. 1 quart is the same as
    a. 100 mL.
    b. 250 mL.
    c. 500 mL.
    d. 1000 mL.

18. 30 mL is equivalent to
    a. 1 teaspoon.
    b. 1 ounce.
    c. 1 cup.
    d. 1 quart.

19. 8 ounces is equivalent to
    a. 24 mL.
    b. 80 mL.
    c. 240 mL.
    d. 800 mL.

20. 500 mL is equivalent to
    a. 1 pint.
    b. 1 quart.
    c. 1 gallon.
    d. 1 dram.

21. Malnutrition
    a. is a risk in certain residents in long-term care facilities.
    b. is a chronic condition in most elderly individuals.
    c. frequently occurs in residents with diabetes and chronic disease.
    d. never occurs in the long-term care facility.

22. Residents who are at risk of dehydration
    a. drink six cups of fluid each day.
    b. are always confused.
    c. have straw-colored urine.
    d. often have difficulty holding a cup.

23. Food thickeners may be ordered for residents with
    a. malnutrition.
    b. dehydration.
    c. tube feedings.
    d. dysphagia.

24. Residents at risk for dysphagia are those who have had
    a. a stroke.
    b. an amputation.
    c. fluid restriction.
    d. malnutrition.

25. The purpose of a calorie count is to
    a. document the total volume of liquids consumed.
    b. evaluate intake for a 30-day period.
    c. evaluate the intake for one meal.
    d. analyze intake for nutritional adequacy.

26. Sodium-restricted diets
    a. limit concentrated sweets.
    b. contain extra salt.
    c. may be difficult to follow.
    d. are ordered by the nurse.

27. Residents who are on fluid restrictions
    a. must drink 2000 mL to 3000 mL each day.
    b. are on intake and output monitoring.
    c. should not consume more than 500 mL daily.
    d. are usually fed by gastrostomy tube.

28. A nasogastric tube
    a. is threaded through the nose and into the stomach.
    b. is inserted into the mouth and into the lungs.
    c. requires surgical insertion.
    d. enters the stomach through the abdominal wall.

29. When a resident has an order to force fluids, the
    a. nursing assistant should force the resident to drink.
    b. resident must consume at least one pitcher of water each shift.
    c. nurse is responsible for administering fluids.
    d. resident should be encouraged to drink as much as possible.

30. Poor skin turgor may be a sign of
    a. dehydration.
    b. dysphagia.
    c. neurologic disease.
    d. lethargy

B. Clinical Applications

Answer the following questions.

31. Mr. Long has a complete set of dentures. He is on a regular diet. When you serve his meal trays, he picks at his food. He seldom

eats much meat. He always eats his mashed potatoes, pudding, and soft foods. After meals, he commonly removes his dentures and leaves them out. He confides in you that his dentures are loose and make his gums sore when he chews. What should you, the nursing assistant, do?

32. Miss Stewart is an obese diabetic resident who receives insulin injections daily. When you open the drawer of the resident's bedside stand to get her toothbrush, you notice several candy bars. Miss Stewart begs you not to tell anyone about the candy. What should you do?

33. Mrs. Martinez is an elderly resident with a bleeding ulcer. She is on a bland diet. The resident immigrated from Mexico and lived with her daughter in your city for several years before admission. When you pick up her supper tray, you find the food uneaten. Mrs. Martinez tells you that her daughter will be visiting soon and will bring her a special Mexican dinner. She is looking forward to visiting with her daughter and eating her favorite food. What should you do?

34. Will James is a 31-year-old resident. He is on a regular diet, but has been losing weight. He tells you he is tired of institutional food and wants a hamburger, french fries, and a milkshake from the fast-food restaurant. He also says he likes Chinese food. What can a nursing assistant do?

35. Mr. Hall, the nurse, instructs you to encourage fluids for Mrs. Blount. He puts the resident on I & O to evaluate her fluid balance. When you enter the resident's room and offer her water, she tells you that she does not like water. What should you do to make sure Mrs. Blount gets enough liquid on your shift?

36. Mr. Arnold is an underweight resident with pressure ulcers. He is on a regular diet, but his appetite is poor. He receives liquid nutritional supplements several times on your shift. When you serve the supplements, he takes a sip, then puts the container down. He rarely drinks any more after you leave the room. What can you do?

UNIT 7

Common Diseases & Conditions of Body Systems

OBJECTIVES

After reading this unit, you will be able to:

- Spell and define key terms.
- List the aging changes that occur in each body system.
- Describe common disorders of each body system.
- Describe the nursing assistant actions related to the care of patients with disorders for each body system.

Terminology

1. Cell - building blocks of the body
2. Function - specialized activity of cells and tissues
3. Organs - made of specialized tissues
4. Systems - several organs working together
5. Tissues - made of specialized cells

The Skeletal System

1. Arthritis - inflammation of the joints
2. Fracture - break in a bone
3. Joint - where bones meet
4. Ligament - connects bone to bone
5. Osteoporosis - porous bones

The Muscular System

1. Atrophy - wasting away of a muscle
2. Bursitis - inflammation of the bursa
3. Contracture - shortening of a muscle
4. Multiple sclerosis - disease which causes muscle wasting
5. Paralysis - loss of voluntary movement

The Circulatory System (Cardiovascular)

1. Anemia - reduced number of red cells
2. Angina pectoris - chest pain
3. Chambers - four hollow cavities of heart
4. Hypertension - high blood pressure
5. MI- heart attack (Myocardial Infarction)

The Respiratory System

1. Alveoli - thin walled sacs in lung
2. Aspiration - inhalation of foreign object
3. Dyspnea - difficulty breathing
4. Lobe - part of lung
5. URI - Upper Respiratory Infection

The Digestive System

1. Constipation-difficulty in expelling feces (stool)
2. Feces/fecal - referring to waste material from colon
3. Intestines - muscular tube for digestion and expelling waste material
4. Liver - large organ involved with many bodily processes including digestion
5. Peristalsis - rhythmic contractions of intestines

The Urinary System

1. Edema - swelling of tissue due to water retention
2. Dehydration - decreased water in body tissue
3. Frequency - need to urinate often
4. Incontinence - no control of bladder or bowel
5. Renal Calculi - kidney stones

The Endocrine System

1. Glands - secrete hormones
2. Hormones - regulate activities of organs and glands
3. Hyperglycemia - elevated glucose in blood
4. Insulin shock - dangerously low level of glucose in blood
5. Mortality rate - proportion of deaths in population

The Nervous System

1. CVA - stroke (Cerebral Vascular Accident)
2. Dementia - loss of ability to think, remember and reason due to changes in the brain
3. Reflex - automatic response such as sneezing
4. Seizure - generalized muscular spasms as a result of abnormal electrical impulses in brain
5. Tremors - uncontrollable trembling

The Sensory Organs

1. Glaucoma - abnormal pressure within the eye
2. Neuron - basic unit of the nervous system
3. Retina - back of eye that receives light
4. Sensory nerves - specialized nerve endings that allow sight, hearing, touch, smell, and taste
5. Tympanic membrane - ear drum

The Integumentary System

1. Burns - destruction of skin by heat classified as first, second, or third degree
2. Cyanosis - bluish or gray skin color due to lack of oxygen
3. Gangrene - death of tissue resulting from decreased blood supply
4. Diaphoresis - profuse sweating
5. Tactile sense - feeling with sense organs in skin (pain, pressure, heat, cold, pleasure)

The Reproductive System

1. Estrogen - female hormone
2. Herpes Simplex II - sexually transmitted disease similar to cold sores
3. Prostatic hypertrophy - enlarged prostate gland
4. Testosterone - male hormone
5. Vaginitis - inflammation of the vagina due to disease or irritation

AGING CHANGES

Aging begins at birth and continues throughout life. Some aging changes are visible. Others cannot be seen, but affect the functioning of the body and the way people adapt to their environment. Each system of the body has a specific function. These functions are summarized in Table 7.2. Every body system undergoes aging changes. People age at different rates. Some people seem to age quickly. Others can be quite old, but remarkably healthy. The rate at which people age is determined by factors such as heredity, lifestyle, disease, nutrition, and environment.

Effects of Aging Changes on Functional Status

Normal changes of aging affect the way the human body functions. You must look at each resident **holistically**. This means to look at the entire person and realize that something that affects one part or system affects the person as a whole. Aging changes in vision and hearing may cause the resident to feel confused and disoriented. Some aging changes cause the resident to feel a loss of control and loss of self-care ability. Changes in the environment may cause confusion, changes in behavior, feelings of loss of control, stress, and sleep disturbances. An acute illness may cause mental confusion, changes in behavior, and loss of self-esteem. The nursing assistant must understand that these changes are beyond the resident's control and help the resident adapt to them as much as possible.

BASIC HUMAN NEEDS

The nursing assistant has a very important responsibility in helping residents meet their needs. When the resident's needs are not met, you may notice a change in behavior. When needs on a lower level are not met, you will notice physical problems. For example, if the resident needs food and fluids, he or she may be weak and tired. When needs on a higher level are not met, you may notice anger, withdrawal, or other behavior problems. Your care and observations are important to the success of the resident and all team members in meeting the care plan goals. Understanding the nature of human needs will enable you to assist residents in meeting their needs.

The care plan uses a holistic approach and is designed to meet the resident's physical and psychological needs. The interdisciplinary team establishes approaches for all caregivers to use to help residents meet their care plan goals. The team meets periodically to reevaluate whether the resident has met or is making progress toward the goals. You will be required to assist residents to meet needs on many different levels. As the resident's condition improves, he or she will begin to meet more needs on his or her own. This provides a sense of self-satisfaction and accomplishment that aids in meeting psychological needs. Residents who are totally dependent on others for their physical care can still derive mental satisfaction from being in control of their care and making decisions about their routines.

COMMON DISEASES IN LONG-TERM CARE FACILITY RESIDENTS

Because of aging changes, elderly residents are at greater risk of developing chronic diseases. These diseases require a change in lifestyle and a period of time to mentally adjust. Presence of one or more chronic conditions can be frustrating. In some cases, the diseases make self-care difficult or impossible. Many chronic diseases cause pain, fatigue, or immobility, and limit activity. Some interfere with sexual function. A list of common diseases and conditions in elderly long-term care residents is found in Table 7.1.

UNDERSTANDING THE BODY

The reasons for the type of care given to residents are based on an understanding of how the body is made, how it functions normally, and the changes caused by age and disease.

These reasons, or principles, are derived from four sciences:

- Anatomy: the study of structure
- Physiology: the study of function
- Gerontology: the study of aging
- Pathology: the study of disease

ANATOMIC TERMS

Special terms are used to describe the location and relationship of body parts and organs. Know-

TABLE 7-1 Common Diseases/Conditions in Elderly Long-Term Care Residents

Disease or Condition	Description
Alzheimer's Disease	A progressive disease of brain cells in which the resident loses mental and physical ability. The disease is incurable and ends in death.
Amputation	Removal of an extremity. Amputation is usually performed because of diabetes, vascular disease, trauma, or gangrene.
Arteriosclerosis	A narrowing of the inside walls of the arteries that makes them rigid and thick. Adequate blood flow cannot pass through the vessel walls to nourish the body. High blood pressure is common because the heart has to work harder to force blood through the blocked vessels. Residents are at high risk of stroke and heart attack.
Arthritis	A painful inflammation of joints that results in limited movement, swelling, and deformities.
Atherosclerosis	A buildup of plaque, calcium, and fat on the walls of the arteries, which makes them rigid and thick. Adequate blood flow cannot pass through the vessel walls to nourish the body. High blood pressure is common because the heart has to work harder to force blood through the narrow vessels. Residents are at high risk of stroke and heart attack.
Cancer	A malignant tumor or new growth anywhere in the body. Cancer may spread slowly or rapidly.
Cerebrovascular Accident (CVA, Brain Attack, or Stroke)	An incident in the brain caused by a blood clot or bursting of blood vessels, allowing blood to spill out into the brain cavity. Common effects of a stroke are paralysis on one side of the body, loss of bowel and bladder control, and speech impairments. The effects may be temporary or permanent.
Congestive Heart Failure	A condition in which the heart is unable to pump sufficient blood to meet the needs of the body. Characterized by high blood pressure and fluid retention.
Diabetes Mellitus	A disorder of the endocrine system in which the body cannot metabolize carbohydrates, proteins, and fat properly.
Emphysema	A disorder in which the air sacs of the lungs have stretched and lost their elasticity, causing them to be unable to contract to remove excess air.
Head Injury	An injury to the brain that results from falls or trauma. Head injuries may affect mental function, physical function, or both. In the elderly, the effects are often permanent because of brain damage.
Hearing Impairment	Difficulty hearing from a number of causes. Impairment may range from being hard of hearing to complete deafness. Some residents may benefit from use of a hearing aid.
Heart Attack (Myocardial Infarction)	A serious medical emergency in which the blood vessels that nourish the heart muscle are blocked or burst, disrupting the normal flow of blood through the heart.
Heart Block	A condition that may require a pacemaker for treatment. Caused by a disruption in the electrical conduction of the heart in which the heart's own internal pacemaker does not beat regularly.
Hip Fracture	A broken hip that is usually the result of a fall but can result from trauma (such as an auto accident) or osteoporosis. The hip must be

	repaired surgically or by using traction to enable the resident to walk again. This is a serious injury, and there is a known relationship between hip fracture and mortality in the elderly.
Hip Replacement	Removal of the entire hip joint and replacement with a synthetic joint. The resident usually requires skilled therapy and restorative nursing after surgery to enable him or her to return to the former level of function.
Huntington's Disease	A progressive, hereditary disease that results in rapid, involuntary movements and progressive dementia.
Hypertension	High blood pressure. The resident may have no symptoms, or may develop dizziness, headaches, and fatigue. Serious complications can result if hypertension is not treated.
Multiple Sclerosis	A chronic, progressive disease marked by intermittent periods of remission. The resident has loss of muscle control, weakness, incoordination, and speech, visual, and sensory disturbances.
Paraplegia	Paralysis below the waist. The condition is usually caused by trauma, but can be caused by tumors and other conditions.
Parkinson's Disease	A neurological disorder that results in tremors, muscular rigidity, and a shuffling gait.
Peripheral Artery Disease	A condition caused by atherosclerosis that results in insufficient blood flow to the legs. It may result in leg ulcers or necessitate amputation.
Peripheral Vascular Disease	A disorder that is frequently the result of varicose veins. Blood return from the legs is not adequate. The condition commonly results in blood clots and leg ulcers.
Pneumonia and Influenza	Serious infections of the lungs contracted by the droplet method of transmission.
Quadriplegia	Paralysis below the neck. The usual cause is trauma, but can result from tumors, infection, and other conditions.
Transient Ischemic Attack (TIA)	A temporary period of diminished blood flow to the brain. An attack occurs suddenly and usually lasts from 2 to 15 minutes, although it may last longer. Signs and symptoms are similar to those of a stroke but are reversible and temporary. Persons who experience TIA's are at high risk for strokes.
Vision Impairment	Difficulty seeing, caused by any one of a number of causes. Sometimes vision can be improved with glasses or surgery. In some disorders, vision cannot be restored.

ing these terms will help you to study and learn more easily. You will also be able to communicate more accurately as you report and record your observations.

The Anatomic Position

Health care providers must use the same frame of reference when describing the resident's body, the position of the resident, and actions to be taken. For example, everyone who works with the resident must understand and describe precisely where the back of the resident's left wrist is and which is the resident's right hand.

It is helpful to view the resident as if he or she were standing in the anatomic position. This means the resident:

- Is standing
- Is facing the observer

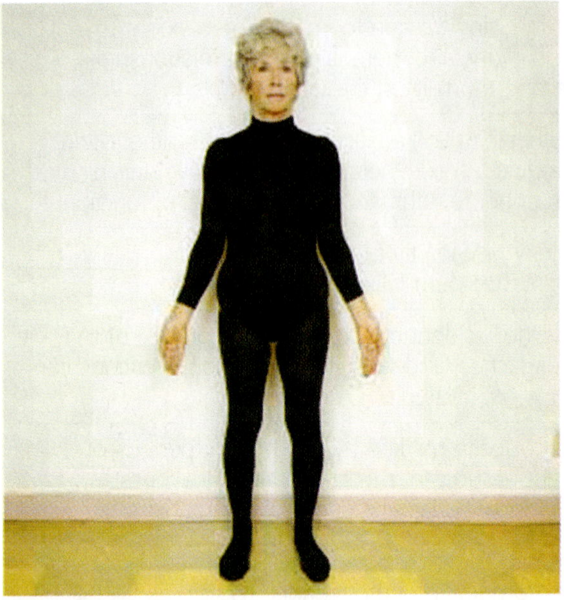

FIGURE 7-1 In the anatomic position, the person is standing, facing forward, with palms forward.

- Has hands at the sides
- Has palms forward (Figure 7.1)

This means that the heels will always be toward the back, even if the resident is resting on the abdomen or lying on the side. The breasts will always be described as facing front even if she is sitting in a wheelchair or walking away from you. Notice also that the resident's left hand will be on the same side as your right hand. It is the same as looking at a mirror image.

Descriptive Terms

Imaginary lines drawn through the body (Figure 7.2) can provide us with other reference terms.

- line drawn down the center of the body from head to foot divides the body into equal right and left sides. This line is called the midline or midsagittal line. Note that the body has the same parts on either side. For example, there is an arm, a leg, an eye, and half of a nose on each side of the line.
- Parts close to this line are medial to the line.
- Parts farther away from the line are lateral to the line.
- For example, in the anatomic position, the thumbs are more lateral to the line and the little fingers are more medial to the line.

Another line drawn parallel to the floor divides the body into upper and lower parts. This line can be drawn at any level on the body as long as it is parallel to the floor. This is the transverse line.

- Parts located above this line are superior to the line.
- Parts located below this line are inferior to the line.
- For example, if the line is drawn between the knees and ankles, the knees are superior to the ankles and the ankles are inferior to the knees.

A third line can be drawn to divide the body into front and back.

- Parts in front of this line are anterior or ventral to the line.
- Parts in back of this line are posterior or dorsal to the line.

Points of Attachment

The arms and legs are called the extremities of the body. The arms are attached to the body at the shoulders. The legs are attached to the body at the hips. Two terms are used to describe the relationship between the parts of the extremities and their points of attachment to the body.

- Proximal—means closest to the point of attachment
- Distal—means farthest away from the point of attachment

Because the upper arm is closest to the shoulder, where it is attached, this part is described as proximal when compared to the fingers, which are farthest away. The fingers are distal or farthest away from the point of attachment of the upper extremity. Figure 7.3 presents a summary of terms.

Abdominal Quadrants

If a resident places his or her hand on the anterior abdominal wall, complaining of pain, you must be able to describe the area in proper terms. For reference, the anterior wall of the abdomen is divided into four parts or quadrants (Figure 7.4). The center of the area is the umbilicus. The abdomen can also be described as having regions (Figure 7.4).

Organization of the Body

All parts of the body are interdependent. The basic unit of the body is the cell. Groups of similar cells are organized into tissues. Different tissues form organs. The organs are organized into systems that perform the body functions.

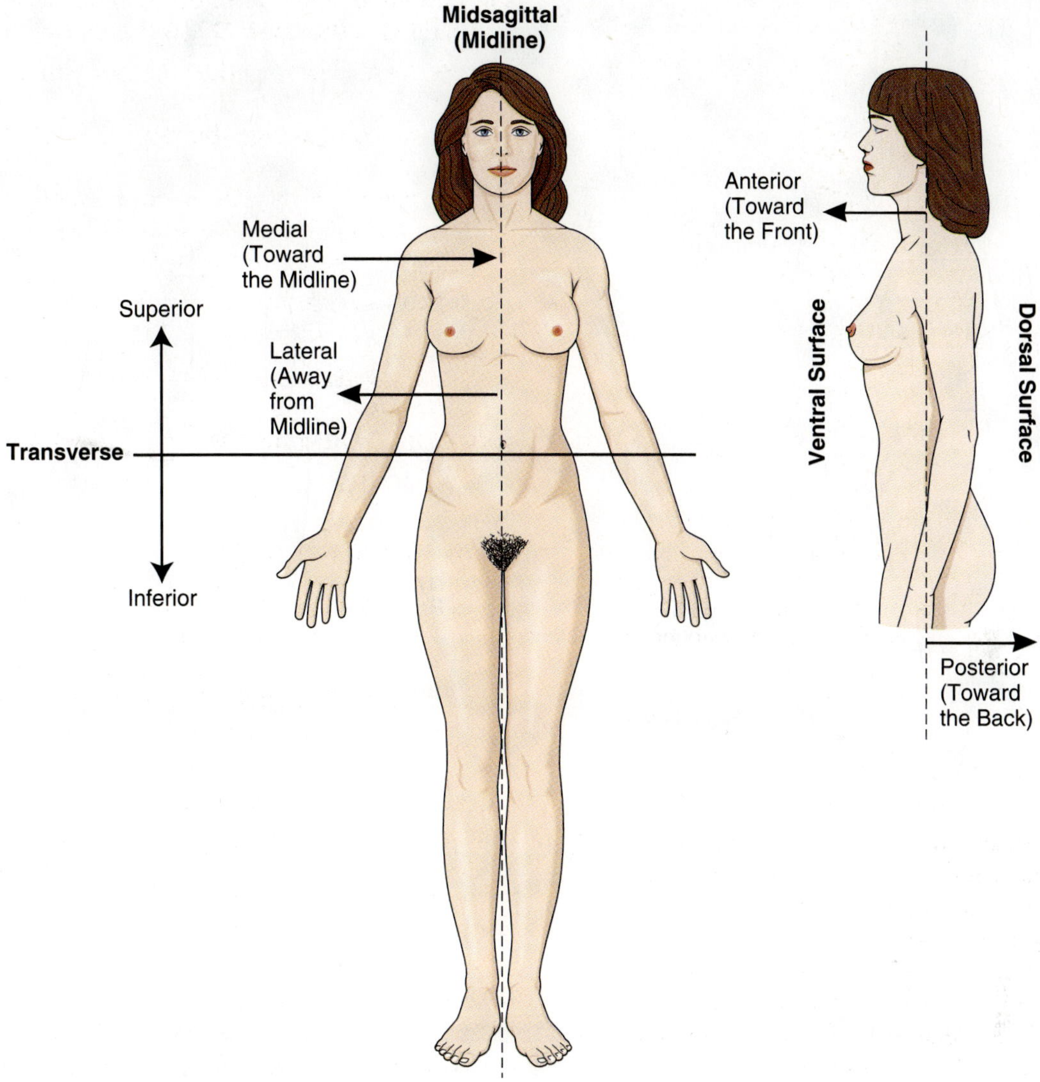

FIGURE 7-2 Imaginary lines can be used to section the body to make it easier to locate parts.

TABLE 7-2 Summary of terms relating to the anatomic position and the location of parts
• Anterior or ventral refers to the front.
• Posterior or dorsal refers to the back.
• Lateral refers to the side (away from the midline).
• Medial refers to the center of the body (midline).
• Proximal means closest to the point of attachment.
• Distal refers to the point farthest away from the point of attachment.
• Midsagittal refers to an imaginary line that divides the body into equal right and left sides.
• Transverse refers to an imaginary line that divides the body into upper and lower areas.

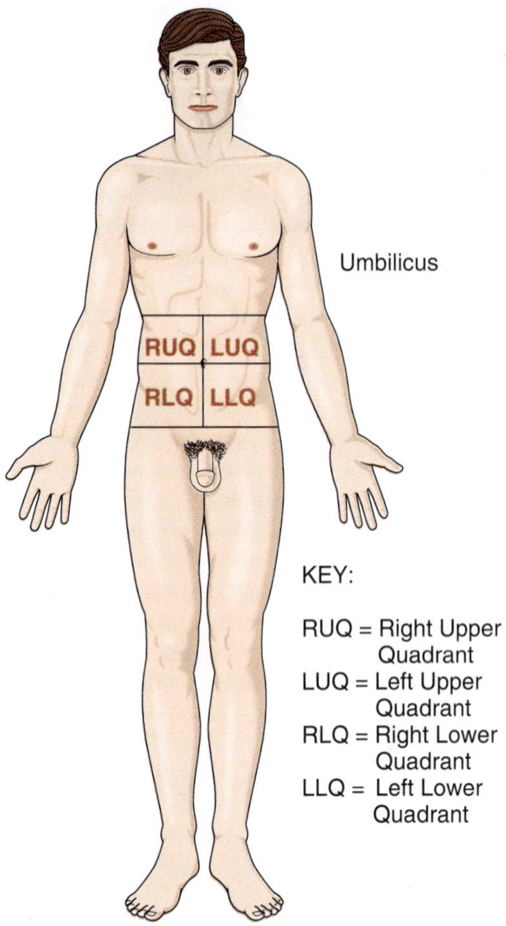

FIGURE 7-3 The abdominal quadrants

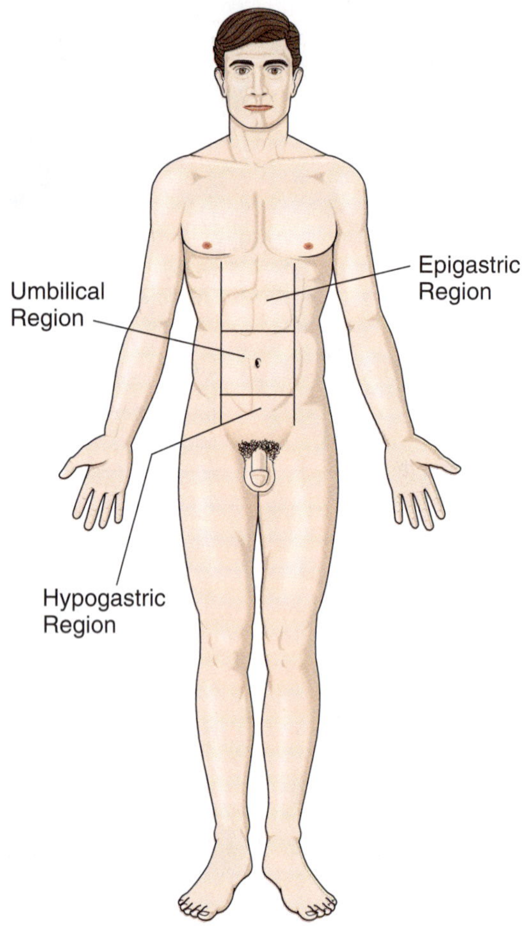

FIGURE 7-4 The abdomen can also be decribed as having three medical regions

Cells

Each cell performs the same basic functions that the total body performs, but on a smaller scale. These functions are breathing (respiration), reproduction, nutrition, and excretion (eliminating wastes). Some cells perform different kinds of work necessary for the body as a whole to function. Some of the various specialized types of cells are:

1. Epithelial cells
2. Nerve cells
3. Muscle cells
4. Connective tissue cells

Epithelial cells, which are very close together, form protective coverings and sometimes produce body fluids.

Nerve cells carry electrical messages to and from the different parts of the body, coordinating activities and making us aware of changes in the environment.

Muscle cells are special in their ability to shorten or lengthen, changing their shape and the position of parts to which they are attached. They also surround body openings, such as the mouth, to control the size of these openings.

Connective tissue cells are present throughout the body in many different types. They support and connect body parts.

Tissues

Groups of similar cells are organized into tissues. The basic tissue types are:

- Epithelial tissue
- Connective tissue
- Nervous tissue
- Muscle tissue

Epithelial tissue is specialized in its ability to absorb, secrete (produce) fluids, excrete (eliminate) waste products, and protect.

Nervous tissue forms the brain and spinal cord and the nerves throughout the body. This tissue is also found in the special sense organs such as the eyes, ears, and tastebuds. The activities of the rest of the body are directed and coordinated through the nervous tissues.

Three kinds of muscle tissue are found in the body:

- Skeletal muscle is attached to bones for movement.
- Cardiac muscle forms the heart wall.
- Smooth muscle (visceral) forms the walls of body organs such as the stomach and intestines.

Connective tissue forms blood, bone, and fibrous and elastic tissues to hold the skin on the body, attach muscles to bones, and support delicate cells throughout the body. Generally, connective tissues support and form connections for other tissue types.

Organs

Each organ is made up of more than one kind of tissue and performs special functions that contribute to the function of the body systems. Some organs, like the kidneys, are found in pairs. Some single organs contribute to more than one system. For example, the pancreas contributes secretions to both the endocrine and digestive systems.

Systems

The body has 10 major body systems. Figure 7.5 lists the organs that contribute to the function of each system. Notice that some organs are included with more than one system. For example, the ovaries contribute to the endocrine system by producing female hormones and to the reproductive system by producing the female egg.

Membranes

Membranes are sheets of epithelial tissues supported by connective tissues. Membranes:

- Cover the body
- Line body cavities
- Produce some body fluids

Important membranes include:

- Mucous membranes
  - Produce a fluid called mucus
  - Line body cavities that open to the outside

TABLE 7-3 Systems of the body

System	Function	Organs
Skeletal	Supports and shapes body, protects internal organs, produces blood cells, acts as levers in movement	Bones, joints, cartilage
Muscular	Protects organs by forming body walls, forms walls of some organs, assists in movement by changing position of bones at joints	*Smooth* muscles—form walls of organs *Skeletal* muscles—attached to bones *Cardiac* muscles—form wall of heart Fascia, tendons
Cardiovascular (Circulatory)	Transports materials around the body; carries oxygen and nutrients to the cells and carries waste products away; part of the immune system that provides protective cells and chemicals to fight current infections and protect against future infections	Heart, arteries, capillaries, veins, spleen, lymph nodes, lymphatic vessels, blood, lymph, tonsils, thymus, specialized blood cells
Respiratory	Brings in oxygen and eliminates carbon dioxide	Sinuses, nose, pharynx, larynx, trachea, bronchi, lungs
Gastrointestinal (Digestive)	Digests, transports food, absorbs nutrients, and eliminates solid wastes	Mouth, esophagus, pharynx, stomach, small intestine, large intestine, salivary glands, teeth, tongue, liver, gallbladder, pancreas

TABLE 7–3 *(continued)*

System	Function	Organs
Urinary	Manages fluids and electrolytes of body, eliminates liquid wastes	Kidneys, ureters, urinary bladder, urethra
Endocrine	Produces hormones that regulate body processes	Pituitary gland, thyroid gland, parathyroid glands, thymus gland, adrenal glands, testes, ovaries, pineal body, islets of Langerhans in pancreas
Nervous	Coordinates body functions, coordinates reception of stimuli, transmits messages throughout body	Brain, spinal cord, spinal nerves, cranial nerves, special sense organs such as eyes and ears
Integumentary	Protects the body from injury and against infection, regulates body temperature, eliminates some wastes	Skin, hair, nails, sweat and oil glands
Reproductive	Reproduces the species, fulfills sexual needs, develops sexual identity	*Male*: Testes, epididymis, urethra, seminal vesicles, ejaculatory duct, prostate gland, bulbourethral glands, penis, spermatic cord *Female*: Breasts, ovaries, oviducts, uterus, vagina, Bartholin glands, vulva

Because the respiratory, digestive, and genitourinary systems all open to the outside they are lined with mucous membranes. The eyelids are also lined with a mucous membrane; a mucous membrane covers the eyeballs.

- Synovial membranes
  - Produce synovial fluid
  - Line joint cavities

The synovial fluid is a clear fluid resembling the white of an egg. It reduces the friction between the bones of active joints and the tendons.

- Serous membranes
  - Produce serous fluid
  - Cover the organs and line the closed cavities of the body

Serous fluid reduces friction as the organs work and move. Important serous membranes are the:

- Pericardium—surrounds the heart
- Pleura—surrounds the lungs and lines the thoracic cavity
- Meninges—cover the brain and spinal cord and line the dorsal cavity
- Peritoneum—covers the digestive organs and lines the abdominal cavity

- Cutaneous membrane (skin)
  - Protects the body
  - Covers the entire body
  - Helps to control body temperature
  - Eliminates wastes through sweat glands
  - Produces vitamin D when exposed to sunlight

Special epithelial cells in this membrane, called glands, secrete perspiration and oils.

Cavities

The body seems like a solid structure, but cavities (spaces) within it contain the organs. Figure 7.5 lists the two main cavities, the dorsal cavity and the ventral cavity. Each of these cavities is lined by and divided into other cavities by serous membranes. These other cavities are also listed in Figure 7.5, as are the organs contained in each.

Figure 7.5 is a simple drawing of the location of these cavities.

TABLE 7-4 Body cavities and the organs contained within each cavity

	Cavity	Organs	
Dorsal Cavity	Cranial	Brain, pineal body, pituitary gland	
	Spinal	Nerves, spinal cord	
Ventral Cavity	Thoracic	Lungs, heart, great blood vessels, thymus gland	
	Abdominal Peritoneal	Stomach, small intestine, most of large intestine, liver, gallbladder, pancreas, spleen	
	Pelvic	*Male* Seminal vesicles, prostate gland, ejaculatory ducts, urinary bladder, urethra, rectum	*Female* Uterus, oviducts, ovaries, urinary bladder, urethra, rectum
	Retroperitoneal Space	Kidneys, adrenal glands, ureters	

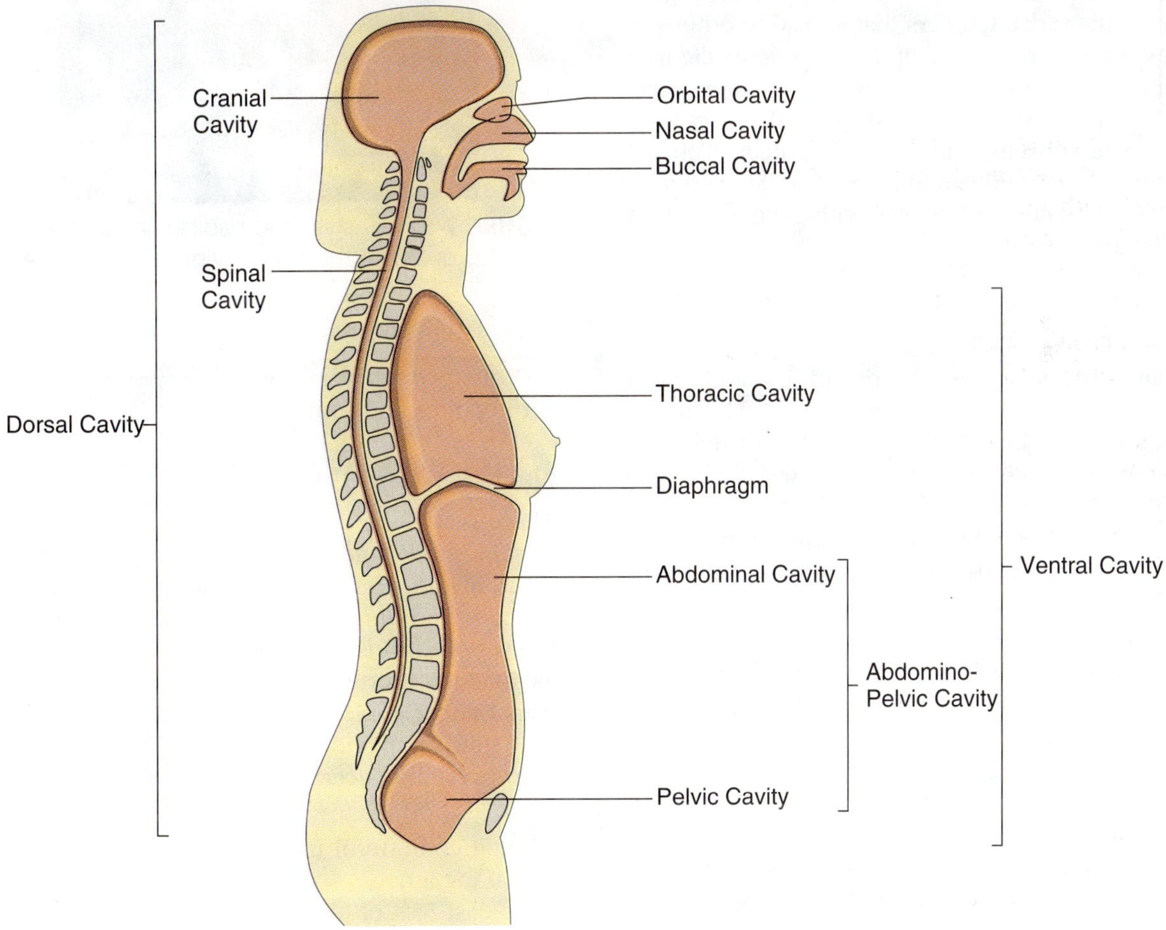

FIGURE 7-5 Lateral view of body cavities

Cancer

Introduction

Cancer is a disease in which the normal mechanisms of cell growth are disturbed. Cells grow abnormally, invade surrounding tissues, and use oxygen and nutrition intended for normal cells. Cancers that stay in one location and do not spread are benign. Benign cancers usually grow slowly. Some types of cancer cells spread to other parts of the body through the blood and lymphatic systems. This is called metastasis. When metastasis occurs, a tumor will eventually grow in another area. Cancers that spread to other part of the body are malignant. Many patients die from metastasis instead of the original tumor. Some malignant cancers spread very rapidly. A carcinogen is a substance that causes cancer. Tobacco is one common carcinogen. The incidence of cancer and death rates vary with geographic location, sex, race, and age.

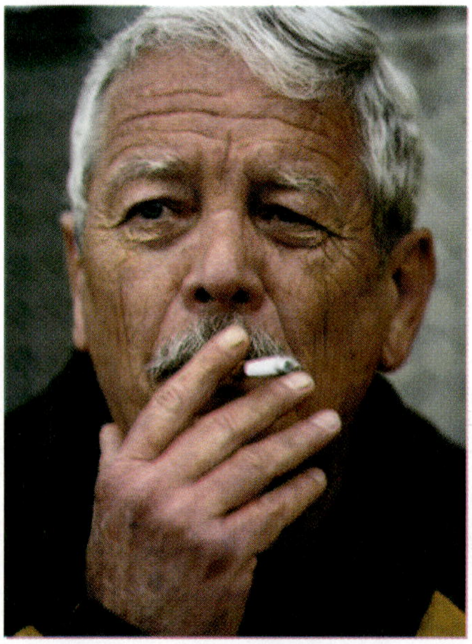

FIGURE 7-6 Lifestyle and habits such as cigarette smoking increase the risk of cancer.

Risk Factors

Many factors increase the risk of developing cancer. Some cancers tend to be genetic. This means they run in families. Breast cancer, ovarian cancer, and pancreatic cancer are examples of cancers that seem to have a hereditary component. Other common risk factors for cancer are:

- Age—this is the most common risk, with most cancers occuring in persons over the age of 55
- Lifestyle and habits:
  - smoking (Figure 7.6) and using smokeless or chewing tobacco
  - alcohol consumption
  - diet
- Family history, genetics
- Environmental pollution
- Harmful substances in the environment
  - asbestos
  - benzene
- Chemicals
- Radiation
- Prolonged sun exposure
- Infections and some viruses

Nutrition and Cancer

There is a direct relationship between intake of certain foods and the development of certain types of cancers. Table 7.4 lists various types of cancers and their relationship to certain food items. Obesity is associated with cancer of the gallbladder, uterus, colon, and breast. The American Cancer Society recommends following the food guide pyramid. These dietary guidelines will help prevent cancer:

- No more than 30% of total calories from fat
- Total cholesterol from diet should not exceed 300 mg a day
- At least 55% of total calories should come from complex carbohydrates, such as fruit, vegetables, cereals, and grains
- Salt from all food sources should not exceed 1 teaspoon a day

TABLE 7-5 Cancer and Food	
Type of Cancer	**Relationship to Food**
Breast	High-fat diet
Prostate	High-fat diet
Colon	High-fat diet, low intake of fruits and vegetables, low fiber, low intake of complex carbohydrates
Esophagus	Low intake of fruits and vegetables, low fiber, low intake of complex carbohydrates, salt-cured foods; also drinking alcoholic beverages
Bladder	Low intake of fruits and vegetables, low fiber, low intake of complex carbohydrates
Stomach	Low intake of fruits and vegetables, low fiber, low intake of complex carbohydrates, high intake of salt-cured food
Larynx	Low intake of fruits and vegetables, low fiber, low intake of complex carbohydrates
Lung	Low intake of fruits and vegetables, low fiber, low intake of complex carbohydrates

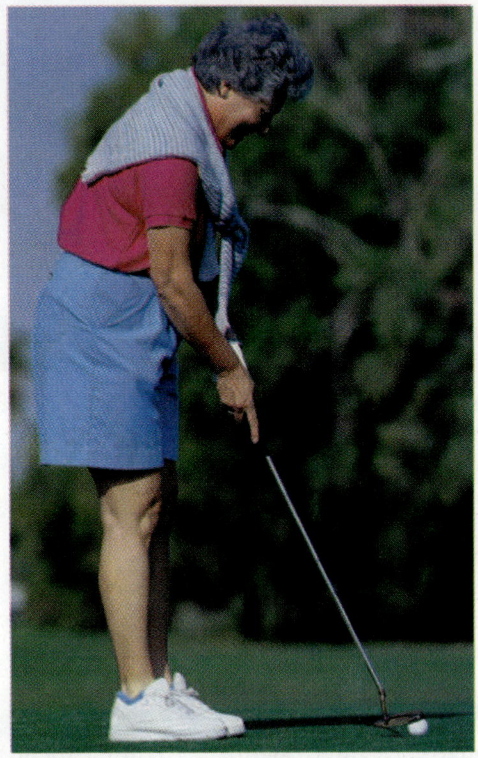

FIGURE 7-7 Regular exercise reduces the risk of cancer and many other diseases.

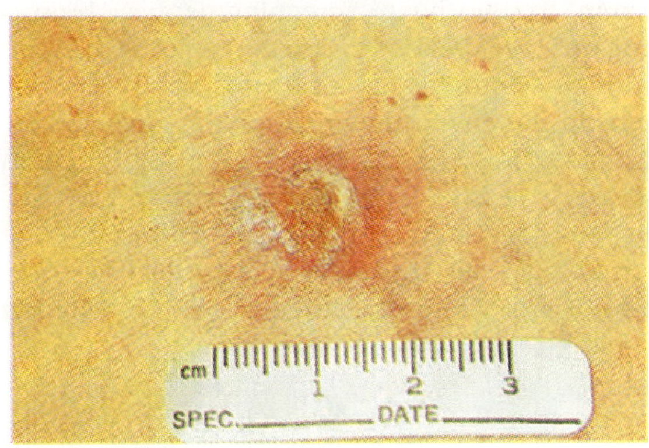

FIGURE 7-8 A sore that does not heal should be examined by the doctor.

Cancer Prevention and Detection

The American Cancer Society recommends certain lifestyle changes and preventive measures. These include:

- not smoking
- limiting the intake of alcoholic beverages
- following the food guide pyramid and eating a healthy diet
- regular exercise (Figure 7.7)
- maintaining a healthy weight
- avoiding sun exposure, particularly between 10:00 am and 3:00 pm.
- getting genetic testing and counseling if at risk for familial cancers

Some patients take various drugs to reduce the risk of cancer. Natural substances, such as vitamin E and selenium, are being researched for their cancer prevention properties.

Signs and Symptoms of Cancer

Each type of cancer has its own signs and symptoms. General signs and symptoms that may indicate cancer spell the word CAUTION:

C = Change in bowel or bladder habits
A = A sore that does not heal (Figure 7.8)
U = Unusual bleeding or discharge
T = Thickening or lump in the breast, testicles, or any part of the body
I = Indigestion or difficulty swallowing

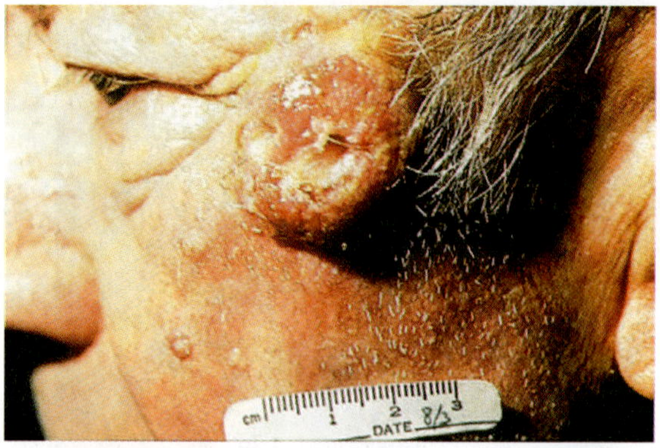

FIGURE 7-9 Change in a wart or mole warrants further investigation.

O = Obvious change in a wart, mole, or skin condition (Figure 7.9)
N = Nagging cough or hoarseness

People with one or more of these warning signs should see a doctor right away.

Screening

Regular screening (Figure 7.10) for cancer is a key to survival, because the outcome is better if the disease is detected early. Many different professional organizations have guide-lines for cancer screening. These vary slightly from one group to the next. Screening is based on a person's age, gender, risk factors, family history, ethnicity, and history of exposure to carcinogens in the environment. Some personal screening tests are recommended monthly, such as breast self-examination for women and testicular self-examination for men. Other routine screening tests are done by physicians. Examples of screening recommendations are listed in Table 7.5

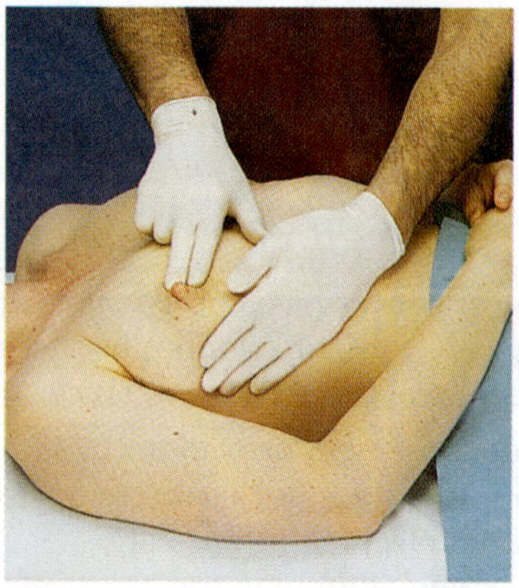

FIGURE 7-10 Regular health screening and early cancer detection are key to survival.

TREATMENT

Many different treatments are used for cancer. In addition, some people use alternative and complementary therapies. The type of treatment is determined by:

- the type of cancer
- location of the cancer
- whether the cancer is malignant
- the stage (how advanced the cancer is)
- general condition of the patient

Surgery

A biopsy is a minor surgery that is sometimes done to diagnose a cancer. A biopsy involves removing a small piece of tissue from a suspicious area. The tissue is sent for laboratory examination. If the biopsy is positive for cancerous cells, a surgical procedure is done with the goal of completely removing the cancer. This may involve removing all or part of an organ, such as a lung, breast, or the uterus. Lymph nodes in the area may also be removed. The surgeon removes as much cancerous tissue as possible.

If removing the entire cancerous area is not possible, a portion is left and is usually treated with other methods.

Reconstructive surgery may be done for cosmetic repair of an area. Sometimes this is done early, or even with the initial surgery. Other times reconstruction is done long after the original surgery. An example of reconstructive surgery is breast reconstruction. Preventive surgery may involve a radical procedure that is done when there is a strong genetic link to cancer. For example, the breasts or ovaries may be removed because of a high risk of developing cancer. Preventive surgery is also done to remove areas, such as rectal polyps, that may develop into cancer later.

Chemotherapy

Chemotherapy uses medications or drugs to destroy the cancer. Unfortunately, healthy cells may also be destroyed. The goals of chemotherapy vary, depending on the type of cancer, stage, and situation. Goals might be to:

- completely eliminate the cancer.
- control and slow the growth of cancer to prolong the patient's life.
- reduce the size of the cancer to eliminate pain and improve quality of life.

Chemotherapy is given by many different routes. Some patients are able to take oral medi-

TABLE 7-6 Screening Recommendations

Location	Screening Test	Age	Frequency of Test
Breast	Mammogram	35–39	Baseline examination
Breast	Mammogram	40 and over	Yearly
Prostate	Rectal exam PSA blood test	50 and over	Yearly
Testicular	Exam by doctor	15 and over	Yearly
Colon/rectal	Digital rectal exam Fecal occult blood test	40 and over	Yearly
Colon/rectal	Sigmoidoscopy	50 and over	Every 3 years
Colon/rectal	Colonoscopy	50 and over	Every 5 years
Cervix	Pap smear	18 and over or at onset of sexual activity	Yearly
Skin	Skin examination	20–39	Every 3 years
Skin	Skin examination	over 40	Yearly
Mouth	Oral examination	20–39	Every 3 years
Mouth	Oral examination	over 40	Yearly

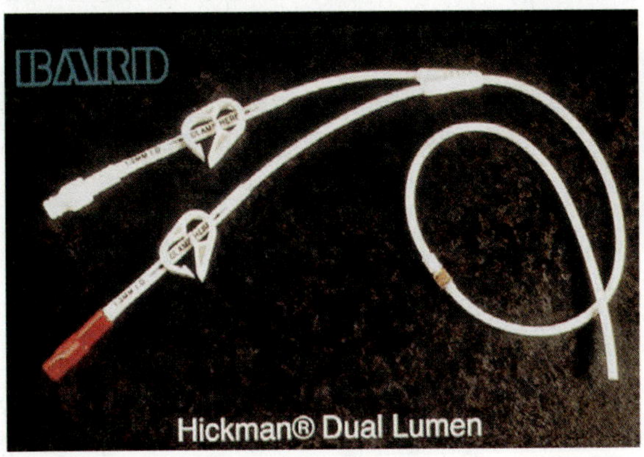

FIGURE 7-11 The central intravenous catheter is commonly inserted to deliver intravenous chemotherapy. (Photo provided by Bard Access Systems. Hickman™ is a registered trademark of Bard Access Systems)

cations. Others must receive the drugs in the muscles, veins, or other organs and body cavities. If the drugs are given intravenously, a central intravenous catheter (Figure 7.11) is often inserted to avoid repeated needlesticks and reduce the risk of vein irritation and collapse.

Chemotherapy drugs are very potent and can irritate the skin, eyes, and mucous membranes of caregivers. Because of this, special measures are used to handle the drugs. Never eat, drink, or chew gum in an area where chemotherapy is being prepared. If you accidentally contact a chemotherapy drug with your hands or mucous membranes, flush well with water and seek medical attention. These drugs and the containers they are dispensed in require special handling and disposal.

Side Effects of Chemotherapy. Chemotherapy targets rapidly regenerating cells, such as cancer cells. The drugs cannot differentiate cancer cells from normal cells, so other cells that regenerate rapidly may also be affected. Other cells in the body that are commonly affected are:

- blood cells, such as red blood cells, white blood cells, and platelets
- hair and nail cells
- gastrointestinal cells

DIFFICULT SITUATIONS

Monitor the chemotherapy patient for bruising and abnormal skin lesions. Inform the nurse promptly if fever is present. Encourage fluids of the patient's choice, as tolerated.

Side effects of cancer drugs can range from mild to lifethreatening. Patients receiving these drugs need special monitoring. Sometimes the dose and scheduling must be changed to reduce side effects. Common side effects are:

- Alopecia (hair loss). This commonly starts within two weeks after chemotherapy begins. It may take up to five or six months to regrow the hair.
- Nausea and vomiting, depending on the drugs used. Sometimes nausea occurs immediately, but it may be delayed until several days after the drug is given.
- Anorexia, or loss of appetite. This sometimes occurs because the drugs cause changes in the tastebuds. In other patients, loss of appetite is due to nausea.
- Anemia, a deficiency of the red blood cells. This is caused by changes in the body due to the chemotherapy drugs. Sometimes special medications are given to reverse the anemia.
- Fatigue. Patients often become very tired. Anemia and reduced number of red blood cells are the most likely cause.
- Low white blood cell count, which increases the risk of infection. This usually starts within a week of the beginning of therapy, and it may last a long time. Precautions are taken to prevent exposure to infection.
- A reduction in the number of platelets in the blood, which increases the risk of bleeding. Precautions must be taken to prevent injury.
- Destruction of the mucous membranes of the mouth. This causes burning, pain, redness, and breakdown inside the mouth.

Many other side effects are caused by chemotherapy drugs. The nurse will advise you what to watch for in each patient.

Disposal of Body Fluids and Wastes. Patients receiving chemotherapy may excrete the drugs in their waste and body fluids. Discard gloves and other protective apparel, if worn, in a leakproof container. Follow facility policies for discarding PPE in a biohazardous waste or other contaminated area. Because the drugs are excreted in body waste, linens that have contacted blood, body fluids, or excretions require special handling. Wear gloves when handling linen, and always apply the principles of standard precautions. Soiled items should be put in specially marked bags before you send them to the laundry.

Special Care of the Chemotherapy Patient. Observe chemotherapy patients for side effects of the drugs and report any possible problems to the nurse promptly. Provide nursing comfort measures, such as good mouth care and daily bathing. Routinely take precautions to prevent injuries and infection. For example, you may be instructed to remind the patient to cough and deep breathe to keep the lungs clear. You may be asked to take vital signs every 4 hours. Rectal temperatures should not be taken in some patients. Check with the nurse before taking a rectal temperature. Report a fever over 101 °F or chilling to the nurse immediately. Other signs of infection to report are:

- swelling, redness, or irritation inside the mouth
- rectal pain or tenderness
- change in bowel or bladder habits
- pain or burning on urination
- redness, swelling, open area, or pain on the skin
- cough or shortness of breath
- decreased level of consciousness
- decreased urine output
- warm, flushed, dry skin
- hypotension (below 100/60, or as instructed)

Because of the risk of bleeding, patients may have to take special precautions, such as blowing the nose gently and using an electric razor. A very soft toothbrush will probably be necessary. Special mouthwash products may be ordered. The care plan and the nurse will provide special directions.

Promoting good nutrition and hydration is very important. You may be asked to serve the patient six small meals a day. High-protein drinks may also be ordered. Encourage fluids, and record intake and output, including emesis. Alternate periods of rest with periods of activity, to reduce fatigue. Plan your care to allow frequent rest periods. Inform the nurse if the patient:

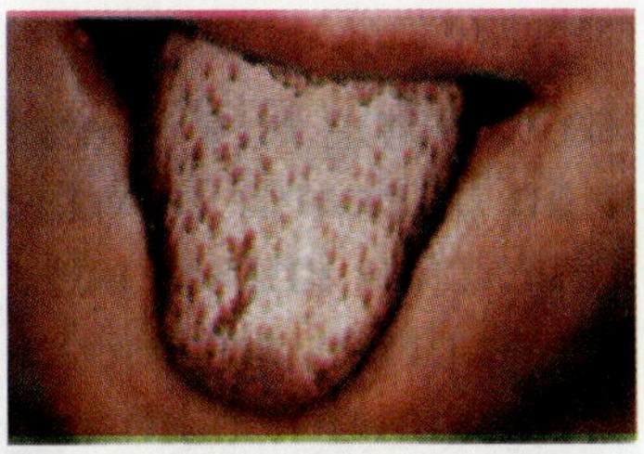

FIGURE 7-12 Monitor for and report white patches in the mouth to the nurse. (Courtesy of Daniel J. Barbaro MD, Fort Worth, Texas)

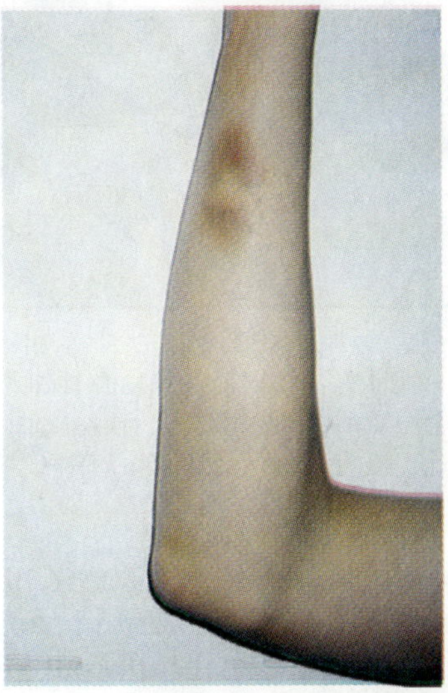

FIGURE 7-13 Report bruises to the nurse promptly.

- has nausea or vomiting
- is not eating or drinking
- complains of changes in the tastebuds, affecting the ability or desire to eat
- constipation or diarrhea
- has white patches or unusual areas inside the mouth (Figure 7.12)
- complains of signs of a vaginal infection
- develops bruising or bleeding (Figure 7.13)

Because the chemotherapy drugs are so toxic, you must observe the patient closely when he or she is receiving them. Inform the nurse promptly if:

- there are signs of intravenous (IV) infiltration, such as redness, swelling, or pain at the needle insertion site
- change in mental status
- change in vital signs

Assisting the Patient with Body Image. Cancer surgery and chemotherapy may change body appearance. This is often very upsetting to the patient. Hair loss may be especially traumatic, particularly in females. Be calm and reassuring. The hair will grow back, although the color or texture may be different. Assist the patient to wear a turban, scarf, or wig, if desired.

Radiation Therapy

Radiation therapy involves the use of high-energy, ionizing beams at the site of the cancer Figure 7.14 The objective is to destroy the cancerous tissue without damaging healthy tissue. Several different types of radiation therapy may be used. Common side effects of radiation that should be reported to the nurse are:

- fatigue
- nausea, vomiting
- diarrhea
- skin redness, irritation, peeling
- change in ability to taste
- irritation of mucous membranes
- cough
- shortness of breath

Special Care of the Radiation Therapy Patient. The patient may have markings on the skin at the site where radiation is delivered. Do not wash these off. The radiation may be very irritating to the patient's skin. Check the skin daily for problems and report them to the nurse, if found. Special skin care may be listed on the care plan. You may be instructed to:

- wash the patient with lukewarm water and mild soap; in some situations no soap is used.
- avoid rubbing or creating friction on the skin.
- avoid shaving areas near the treatment field.
- avoid tape on the patient's skin near the treatment field.
- avoid lotions and cosmetics near the treatment field.
- avoid tight fitting garments; dress the patient in loose, comfortable clothing.

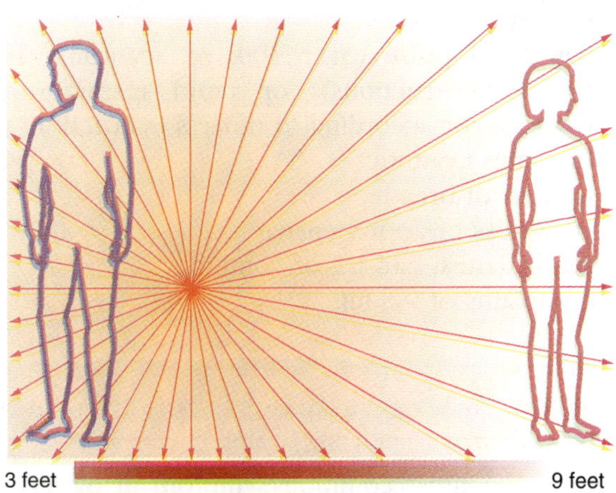

FIGURE 7-14 Radiation therapy is used to treat certain cancers.

Protecting Yourself from Radiation Exposure. Sources of radiation are sometimes implanted inside the patient's body. If this is the case, you will be instructed in special precautions to follow to reduce your risk of radiation exposure. A list of precautions will be placed on the chart or elsewhere. Follow these instructions carefully. In general, you should:

- not remain in the patient's room any longer than necessary.
- stay at least 3 feet away from the patient unless direct care is being delivered.
- inform the nurse if an implant comes out of a body cavity (if so, do not touch it).
- find out if special precautions are necessary for handling soiled linens, tissues, or dressings.
- inform the nurse if you are pregnant, or suspect you may be pregnant.

Immunotherapy

Immunotherapy is another cancer treatment that is done to alter the patient's immune response and eliminate the cancer. Various biologic agents are given to change the normal immune response. The vital signs are regularly and closely monitored when these agents are given. Side effects of therapy usually cease within a week after treatment. Care of the patient receiving immunotherapy involves:

- monitoring vital signs every 4 hours, or more often if instructed.
- monitoring capillary refill as instructed.
- advising the patient to remain in bed if the systolic blood pressure is below 100, or according to the nurse's instructions.
- weighing the patient daily and informing the nurse of weight gain.

Notify the nurse promptly if the patient:

- has fever or chills
- has rapid pulse (over 100, or according to nurse's instructions), or rapid respirations (over 24, or according to nurse's instructions)
- becomes cyanotic
- is short of breath
- is restless or apprehensive
- has diarrhea, nausea, or vomiting
- complains of itching

Pain

Pain is the most common symptom in patients with cancer. The pain may be caused by the cancer, or be a result of the treatment. The pain may cause difficulty sleeping, loss of appetite, depression, and anxiety. Pain over an extended period of time reduces the patient's quality of life. The World Health Organization (WHO) analgesic ladder (Figure 7.15) is used as a model for pain management. Cancer patients should be evaluated for pain regularly. A pain scale is usually used. Narcotic pain-relieving medications may be necessary to control the pain. These are not withheld out of fear of addiction. The incidence of addiction in cancer patients is very low. Pain should be treated before it becomes severe and out of control. Notify the nurse promptly if a patient complains of pain.

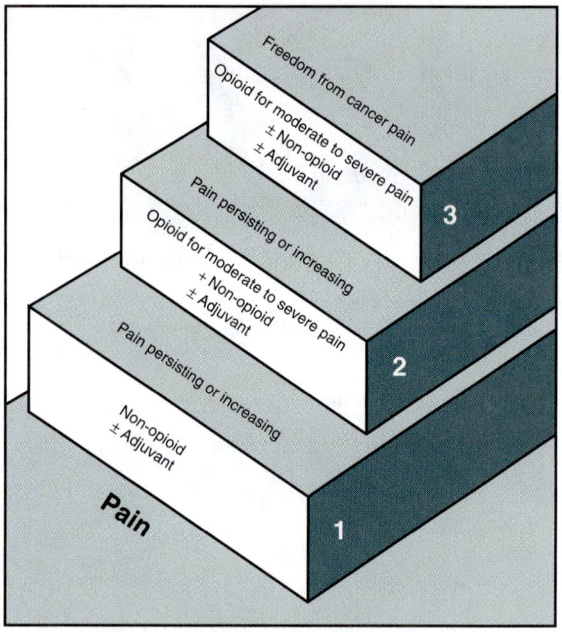

FIGURE 7-15 The WHO three-step analgesic ladder is used for a model in pain management. (Courtesy of World Health Organization, Geneva, Switzerland. Used with permission)

Mental and Emotional Needs

Patients with cancer have a life-altering disease. They often fear dying. They may be anxious or depressed, and they often go through the grieving process. Nursing assistant measures to assist with mental and emotional needs include:

- spending as much time as possible with the patient if he wants to talk.
- allowing the patient to talk about feelings and fears.
- being proficient at providing physical care and assistance with ADLs.
- anticipating patient's needs before they ask.

- respecting the patient's beliefs and wishes.
- providing emotional support.
- respecting the patient's privacy if she wants to be alone.
- making the patient feel respected and valued as a person.

Avoid giving the patient false hope. If you think a patient is losing control, inform the nurse. Just being with the patient and allowing him to talk is very helpful.

PALLIATIVE CARE

Some patients with cancer elect to have palliative care. This care is designed to treat the symptoms of discomfort, but not the disease. The patient will have an advance directive and do not resuscitate (DNR) order. The patient is kept comfortable until death occurs. A hospice may be involved in the patient's care. One goal of this care is to maintain the patient's quality of life for as long as possible.

Nursing Assistant Measures.

Your care is designed to keep the patient clean and comfortable. Use nursing measures, such as positioning and backrubs, to enhance the patient's comfort. Spend time with the patient and allow her to talk, if she wants. Respect the patient's wishes. Provide emotional support. Inform the nurse if the patient is short of breath, anxious, or complains of pain.

COMMUNICATION HIGHLIGHT *Alert*

A cancer diagnosis evokes strong feelings and emotions in patients and their families. These may be difficult to understand and cope with. Patients or families may lash out in anger at you or their loved ones. They are not angry with you. They are angry with their circumstances. Avoid responding with anger. Keep your temper even, and do not take comments personally. Saying, "I see you are upset," or validating their feelings is the best way to respond. Providing compassionate care, listening, and giving sincere, solid, emotional support will help patients and family members cope with this difficult time.

The Cardiovascular System

Structure and Function

The organs of the cardiovascular system include:

1. Heart—a central pumping station
2. Blood vessels
   a. **Arteries**— tubes that carry blood away from the heart. They
      - have muscular, elastic walls with smooth linings.
      - branch to form arterioles with thinner walls. Arterioles then become capillaries.
      - carry blood with a high concentration of nutrients and oxygen to the body cells.

   b. **Veins**— tubes that carry blood toward the heart. They
      - have thinner muscular walls.
      - carry blood back to the heart.
      - carry blood with a lower concentration of oxygen, more carbon dioxide, and more waste products.
      - have cuplike valves that help move the blood.

   c. **Capillaries**—tubes that connect arteries and veins. They
      - have walls only one cell thick.
      - are the site of exchange of nutrients and oxygen from the blood to the cells, and carbon dioxide and waste products from the cells to the blood.
3. **Lymphatic vessels**—tubes that carry lymph or tissue fluid to the bloodstream. Fluid from the bloodstream passes into the tissue spaces, where it is called *tissue fluid*. Some of the tissue fluid returns to the bloodstream by way of the capillaries. Some of it is first drawn off into the lymphatic vessels, where it is called **lymph**. Eventually the lymph is returned to general circulation and once more becomes part of the blood.
4. Lymph nodes—masses of lymphatic tissue along the pathway of the lymph. They filter the lymph.
5. Spleen—a lymphatic organ. The spleen produces some of the blood cells and helps destroy worn-out blood cells. It acts as a blood reservoir or blood bank.
6. Blood—a connective tissue made up of a liquid (plasma) and cellular elements.

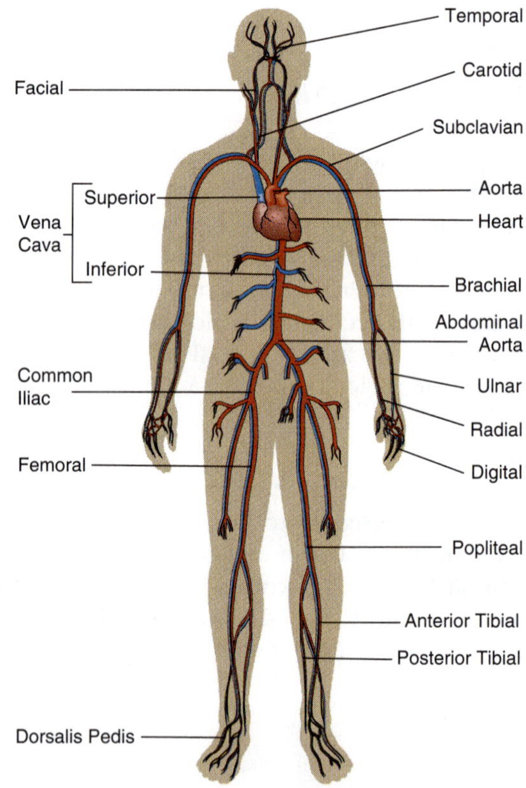

FIGURE 7-16 The cardiovascular system

The Blood

Blood is a red body fluid composed of plasma and cellular elements. The body contains 4 to 6 quarts (liters) of blood. Fifty-five percent of the blood is formed of the liquid plasma. **Plasma** is a watery solution containing:

- Antibodies (gamma globulin)—chemicals to fight infection
- Nutrients—such as glucose, amino acids, fats, salts
- Gases—such as oxygen and carbon dioxide
- Waste products—such as urea and creatinine

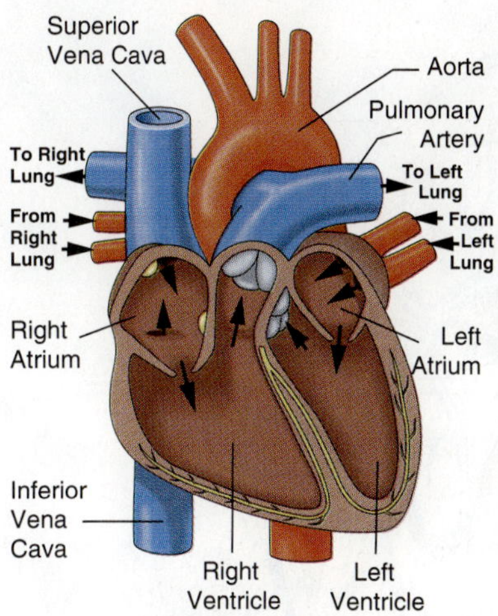

FIGURE 7-17 The heart

The blood cells are produced in the bone marrow and lymphatic tissues of the body. The bone marrow, liver, and spleen destroy worn-out blood cells. The blood cells include red blood cells, white blood cells, and thrombocytes.

- Red blood cells (RBC)—**erythrocytes**—carry most of the oxygen and small amounts of carbon dioxide. There are 4.5 to 5 million RBC per cubic millimeter (mm^3).
- White blood cells (WBC)—**leukocytes**—fight infection. There are 7,000 to 8,000 WBC/mm^3.
- **Thrombocytes** (or platelets)—are not whole cells but only parts of cells. They seal small leaks in the walls of blood vessels and initiate blood clotting. There are 200,000 to 400,000 thrombocytes/mm^3.

The Heart

The heart is a hollow muscular organ about the size of a fist (Figure 7.18). It is divided into a right and left side by a muscular wall called the *septum* and into four chambers. There are three layers in the heart wall. The **endocardium** lines the heart chambers. The **myocardium** is the muscle layer. The **pericardium** is a membranous outer covering.

The four chambers are:

1. The right **atrium** (RA)—(right upper heart chamber) receives blood from all over the body. This blood has a low oxygen content and a relatively high carbon dioxide level. It is called *deoxygenated blood*.
2. The right **ventricle** (RV)—(right lower heart chamber) receives blood from the right atrium and sends it out to the lungs through the pulmonary artery to pick up oxygen and get rid of the carbon dioxide.
3. The left atrium (LA)—(left upper heart chamber) receives oxygenated blood from the lungs and sends it to the left ventricle.

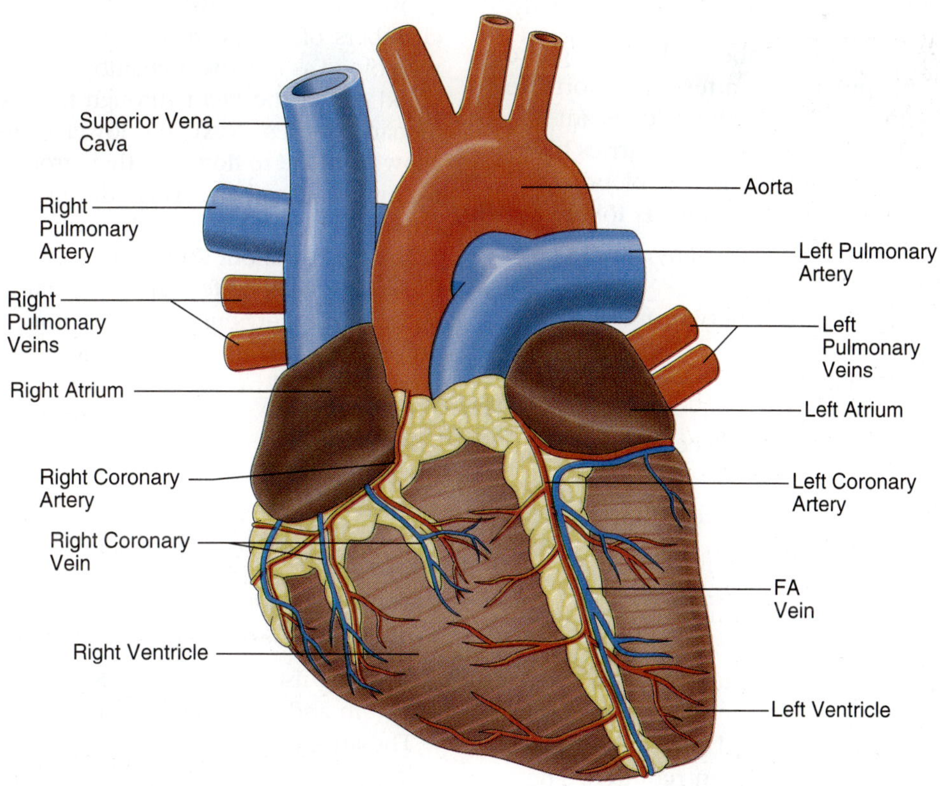

FIGURE 7-18 The heart and blood vessels.

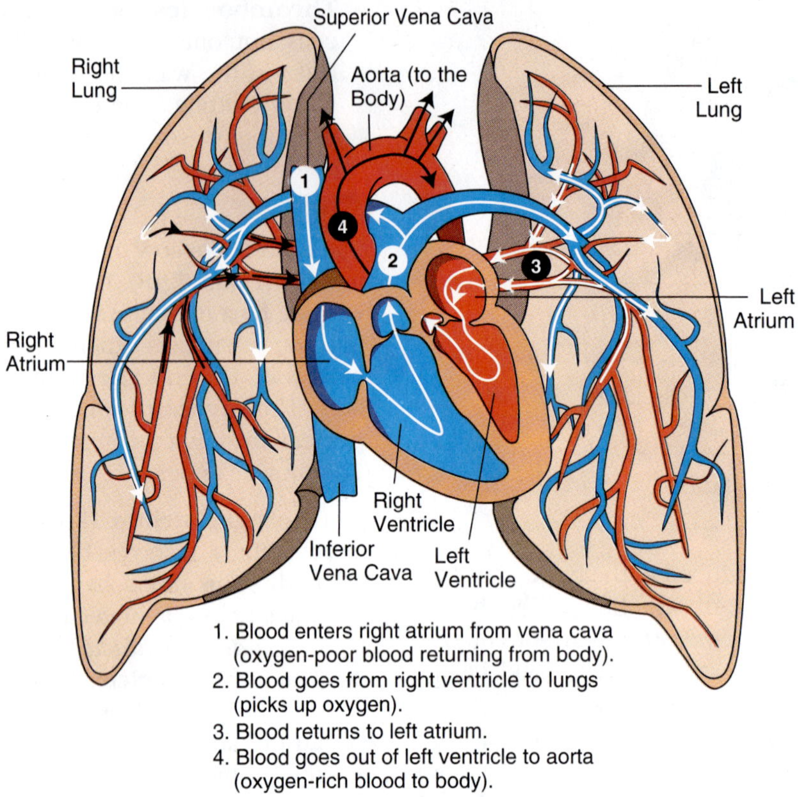

FIGURE 7-19 Flow of blood from the heart to the lungs, to the body, and back to the heart to begin the cycle again.

4. The left ventricle (LV)—(left lower heart chamber) receives blood from the left atrium and sends it out through the aorta to the entire body.

Valves separate the chambers. They also guard the exit of the pulmonary artery and aorta to prevent backflow and maintain a constant forward motion. The pulmonary artery carries blood to the lungs. The aorta is the largest blood vessel in the body. The valves are located as follows:

- Tricuspid valve—between right atrium and right ventricle
- Bicuspid (mitral) valve—between left atrium and left ventricle
- Pulmonary semilunar valves—between right ventricle and pulmonary artery
- Aortic semilunar valve—between left ventricle and aorta

Nerve impulses make the heart contract regularly according to body needs. For example, when you run, your body cells need more oxygen. The cells signal the brain that they need more oxygen. The brain sends a signal to the heart through the nerves, telling it to supply more blood. These nerve impulses cause the heart to beat faster. Thus, more oxygenated blood is pumped to the body cells to supply the oxygen required. These impulses cause the heart to beat faster.

The Cardiac Cycle The heart pumps blood through the body by a series of movements known as the **cardiac cycle**. First, the upper chambers of the heart, called *atria*, relax and fill with blood as the lower chambers contract, forcing blood out of the heart through the aorta and pulmonary arteries. Next, the lower chambers relax, allowing blood to flow into them from the contracting upper chambers. Then the cycle is repeated (Figure 7.19). Each cycle lasts about 0.8 second. This happens about 70 to 80 times per minute.

The pulse you feel at the radial artery corresponds to ventricular contraction. The sounds you hear when listening to the heart and when taking a blood pressure are the sounds made by the closing of the valves during the cardiac cycle.

The rate and rhythm of the cardiac cycle are regulated by the conduction system. The conduction system is made up of special neuromuscular tissue that sends out impulses. The impulses eventually reach the myocardial cells, which respond by contracting.

- The impulses begin at the S-A node in the right atrium and spread across the two atria.
- The atria contract.
- Impulses from the S-A node reach the A-V node in the right atrium.

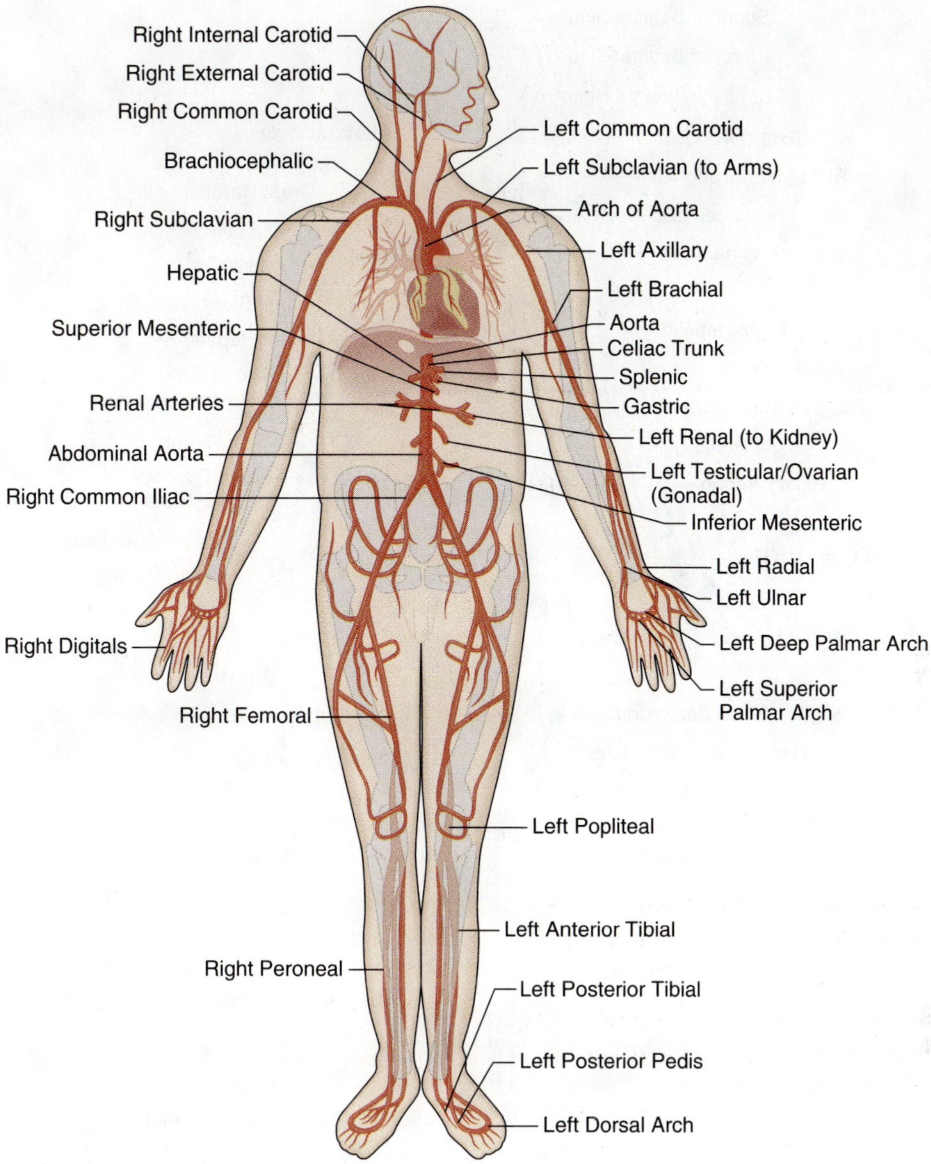

FIGURE 7-20 Arteries of the body.

- Messages from the A-V node then spread through the bundle of His in the septum. From there they go through the Purkinje fibers to the walls of the ventricles.
- The ventricles contract, forcing the blood forward.

An electrocardiogram, called an ECG or an EKG, is a test that traces the electrical impulses of the heart. Heart disease may be detected with this test.

Blood Vessels

Many large arteries and veins take their names from the bones they are near or from the part of the body they serve. For example, the femoral artery and vein run close to the femur (thigh bone). The subclavian arteries and veins are found under the clavicle. The axillary arteries and veins are found in the axillary (armpit) area. Figure 7.20 shows the arterial system that distributes blood from the heart. Figure 7.21 shows the venous system that returns blood to the heart.

Aging Changes in the Cardiovascular System

The cardiovascular system is also called the circulatory system. It is the transportation system for the body. The cardiovascular system transports food and oxygen to every cell in the body

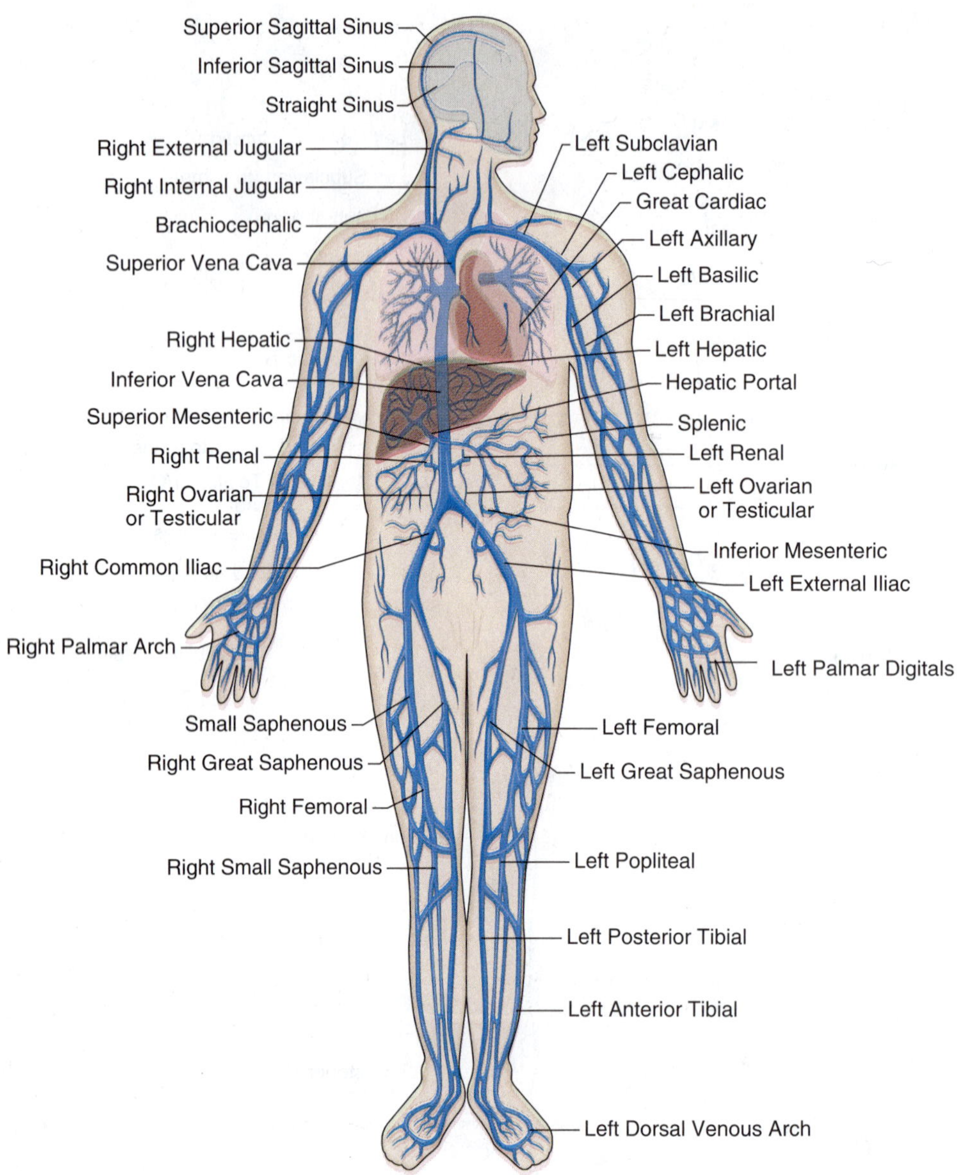

FIGURE 7-21 Veins of the body.

through the bloodstream. This system consists of the heart, which pumps blood throughout the body, and a series of blood vessels. Arteries are blood vessels that carry freshly oxygenated blood to the body parts. Veins are the blood vessels that carry blood from the body parts back to the heart. The immune system is the part of the circulatory system that recognizes foreign germs in the body and helps fight disease.

As the body ages, the following changes occur in the cardiovascular system:

- The heart rate slows, causing a slower pulse and less efficient circulation.
- Blood vessels lose elasticity and develop calcium deposits, resulting in narrowing.
- Blood pressure increases because of changes to the walls of the blood vessels.
- It takes longer for the heart rate to return to normal after exercise.
- Veins become enlarged, causing the blood vessels near the surface of the skin to become more prominent.

Common Circulatory System Disorders

Common disorders of this system include:

- Diseases relating to the blood vessels
- Diseases of the heart
- Blood **dyscrasias** (abnormalities); these diseases can involve the bone, bone marrow, liver, or spleen.

Observations the nursing assistant is to report in patients with disorders of the circulatory system are:

- Color change, pallor or cyanosis, redness
- Cool to touch
- Hot to touch
- Changes in pulse rate or rhythm
- Changes in blood pressure
- Edema
- Disorientation

PERIPHERAL VASCULAR DISEASES

The blood vessels that serve the outer parts of the body, particularly those of the hands and feet, are referred to as **peripheral** (toward the outer part) blood vessels. Diseases of these vessels affect the parts of the body through which they pass. The health of these vessels also influences heart function. Peripheral vascular diseases that affect the arteries diminish the flow of blood to the extremities. Tissues through which the narrowed arteries pass may not get the nourishment they need. Areas affected are the extremities: the arms, legs, and brain. The signs and symptoms associated with decreased peripheral circulation are:

- Burning pain during exercise
- Hair loss over feet and toes
- Thick and rigid toenails
- Dusky red skin or cyanotic, brownish skin
- Dry and scaly or shiny skin
- Chronic edema of the feet and legs
- Cool skin temperature of feet and legs
- Difficulty with ambulation

When the arteries are affected, the blood flow may be seriously interrupted. This condition requires immediate medical treatment. Vascular ulcers may occur. These are sores that start because of the poor circulation of the blood in the legs. These ulcers are difficult to treat and may take months to heal.

Treatment is aimed at:

- Increasing local circulation
  - Positioning and specific prescribed exercises can promote arterial flow and venous return.
  - Sometimes an oscillating (rocking) bed is employed to improve the circulatory flow. The oscillating bed rocks up and down in cycles, raising the patient's feet 6 inches above his head and then lowering them 12 to 15 inches. The steady rhythm provides both passive exercise for the patient and some circulatory stimulation.
  - Nothing that would hamper the patient's circulation is permitted.
- Preventing injuries that may heal poorly.

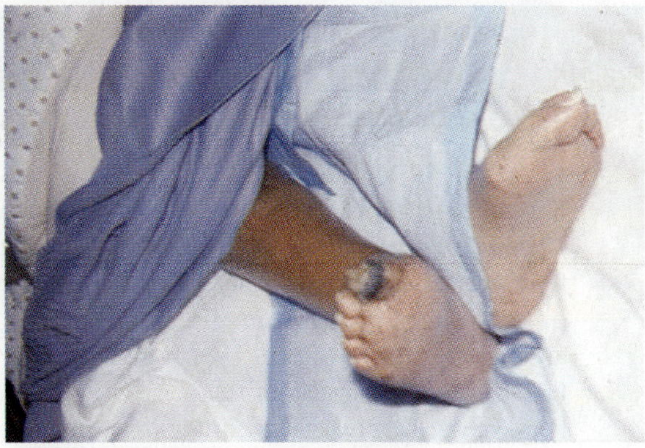

FIGURE 7-22 The big toe is gangrenous. The toe was eventually amputated, but the foot was saved.

Protecting the Feet. Patients with impaired circulation are at great risk of ulceration, gangrene (Figure 7.22), and eventual amputation due to pressure or injuries to the feet and ankles. A small injury or ulcer can lead to major complications. Nursing assistant care for patients with peripheral vascular disease includes:

- Checking the feet and legs daily and reporting abnormalities to the nurse promptly.
- Protecting the feet from injury.
- Making sure the patient is wearing properly fit footwear when out of bed. The patient should always wear socks under shoes. He or she should never ambulate barefoot or wearing only socks on the feet.
- Not cutting toenails; this is a licensed health care provider responsibility. Avoid using sharp objects such as a nail file on the toes.
- Making sure bed linen is not too tight on the feet. Use a bed cradle, if ordered.
- Checking the skin under support hose regularly. Remove the hose periodically, according to the care plan.
- Making sure footwear is not too tight; if footwear fits tightly, notify the nurse.
- Propping bedfast patients' calves on pillows that are positioned lengthwise so that the heels are elevated from the surface of the bed. You may also position the patient so that the heels hang over the end of the mattress, with the soles of the feet against a footboard. Do not position the pillow width-wise under the calves. Heel protectors are excellent for preventing friction and shearing, but they do not prevent pressure on the heels. Other devices are available to keep the heels off the surface of the bed to relieve pressure. Follow the care plan and the nurse's instructions.

GUIDELINES FOR

Caring for Patients with Peripheral Vascular Disease

- Elevate the feet when the patient will be sitting in a chair for a long time. When the feet are not elevated, make sure that the patient's feet are flat on the floor. If they are not, support the feet with a footstool. Discourage the patient from crossing the legs when sitting. Discourage the patient from using circular garters.
- Discourage smoking–it interferes with circulation.
- Avoid using the knee gatch of the bed.
- Avoid using heating pads or hot water bottles. The patient may not feel temperatures that are too hot.
- Maintain body warmth. Make sure the patient has warm clothes, including socks that fit well. Provide blankets for the bed.
- Prevent injury to the feet:
  - Instruct the patient to wear shoes when out of bed.
  - Check to see that the shoes are in good repair and that they fit well.
  - Avoid pressure to the legs and feet from any source.
- Inspect the feet carefully when you bathe the patient or if the patient complains of any discomfort in the feet. Promptly report any signs of inflammation, injury, or circulatory problems:
  - Broken skin
  - Color change (redness, whiteness, or cyanosis)
  - Heat or coldness
  - Cracking between toes
  - Corns or calluses
  - Swelling
  - Pain
  - Loss of function
  - Drainage
- Bathe the feet regularly.
  - Dry thoroughly and gently between the toes.
  - Use a moisturizing lotion on the feet and legs if the skin is dry.
- Do not cut the toenails of patients who have peripheral vascular disease.

- Making sure the feet are supported on footrests when the patient is using a wheelchair; avoid dragging them across the floor.

Atherosclerosis

Atherosclerosis is a common form of vascular disease.

- Roughened areas known as **atheromas**, which are growths developed over deposits of fatty materials, form on the inner walls of the arteries and narrow the vessels.
- The vessels of the heart and brain, and those leading to the legs from the body, are often affected.
- The atheromas gradually grow larger until they eventually block blood flow to the parts and organs served by the affected vessels (Figure 7.23).
- Sometimes clots that have formed over the irregular areas in the vessel walls break off and travel as emboli to block distant vessels.
- The narrowing of vessels can lead to serious complications, such as:
  - Formation of blood clots
  - Angina pectoris
  - Myocardial infarction (MI)
  - Strokes (CVA) (also known as brain attacks)
  - Gangrene

Refer to Figure 7.24.

The exact cause of this vascular disease is unknown, but several factors seem to increase the risk that a person will develop it. These factors include:

- Hypertension
- Diabetes mellitus
- Overweight
- Heredity
- Smoking
- Stress
- Lack of exercise
- Diets high in cholesterol and fats

Treatment includes:

- Exercise
- Proper diet
- Reduction of stress
- Control of smoking and obesity

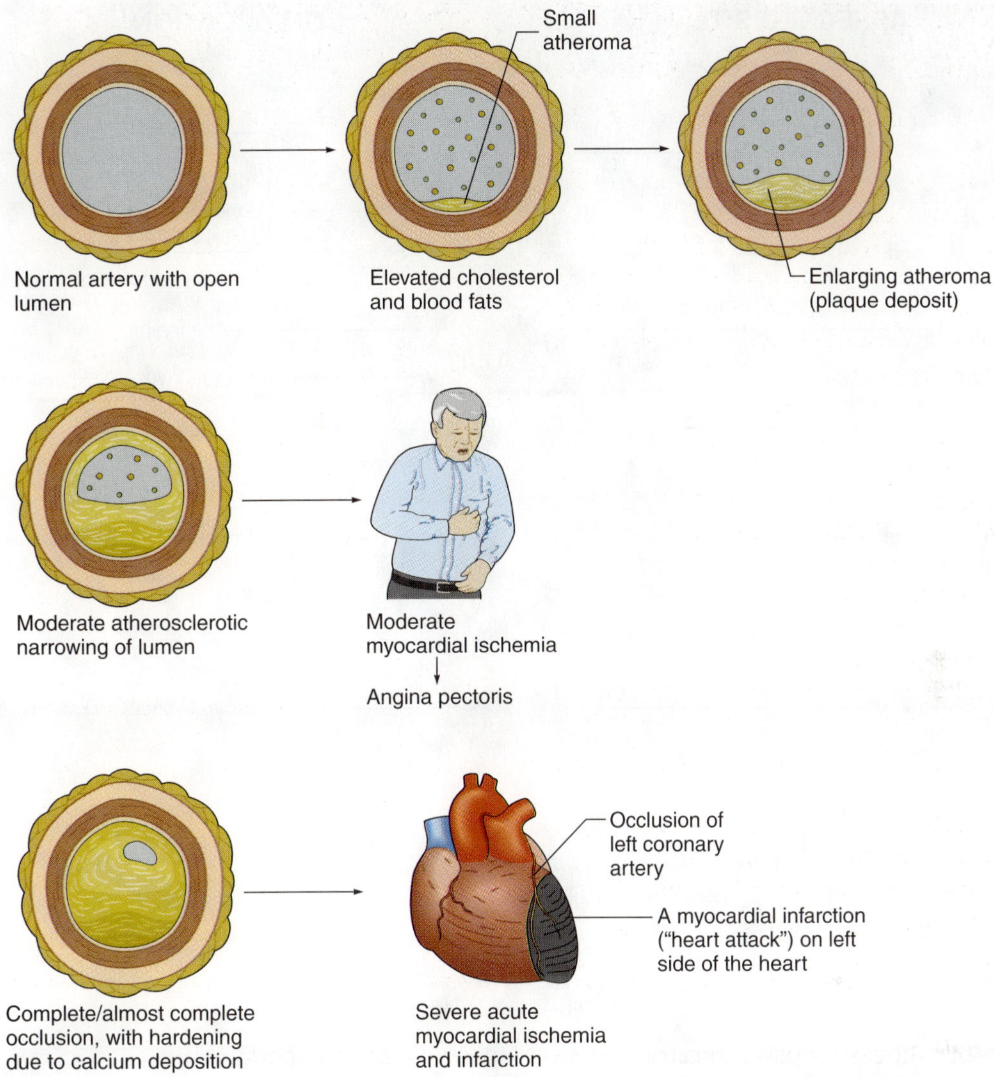

FIGURE 7-23 Cross-sections through a coronary artery that is undergoing atherosclerotic changes.

Varicose Veins

The veins can also cause problems. **Varicose veins** form when the valves in the veins in the legs become weakened (Figure 7.25). This means:

- The blood does not flow through the veins as it should.
- The veins become distended and visible through the skin.
- The veins may become inflamed (**phlebitis**).
- A blood clot may form in the vein.

Report the following signs:

- Pain or aching in the legs
- Signs of inflammation (warmth and redness)

Remember that you *never* rub or massage the area of a varicose vein.

Transient Ischemic Attack

Transient ischemic attack (TIA) is a temporary interruption of the blood flow to part of the brain. The patient may experience:

- Weakness or paralysis of any extremity or the face
- Vision problems
- Difficulty with speech
- Difficulty with swallowing

The attack comes on rapidly and may last from 2 to 15 minutes or for as long as 24 hours. Symptoms are similar to those of a stroke but are temporary and reversible. Transient ischemic attacks may occur once or several times in a lifetime. Persons experiencing TIAs are at risk for eventually suffering a stroke.

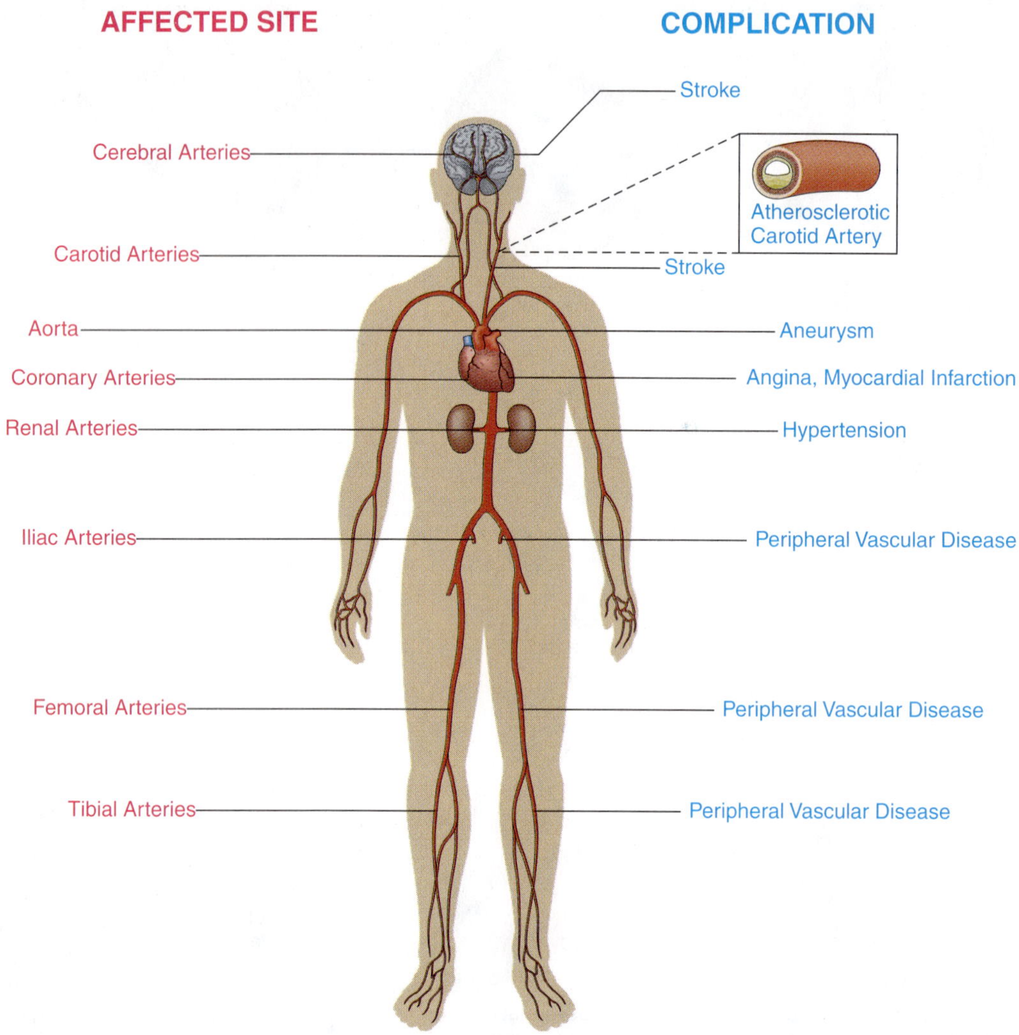

FIGURE 7-24 Atherosclerosis can cause disease in many parts of the body.

Stroke

A stroke is also called a cerebrovascular accident (CVA) or brain attack. It affects the vascular system and the nervous system. The complete or partial loss of blood flow to the brain tissue is frequently a complication of atherosclerosis or brain hemorrhage. Causes of CVA include:

- Vascular occlusion due to a thrombus, atherosclerotic plaques, or emboli that obstruct the flow of blood
- Intracranial bleeding as blood vessels rupture, releasing blood into the brain tissue

Hypertension

Hypertension is another name for high blood pressure. It may have no known origin, or it may follow illnesses that affect such organs as the:

- Blood vessels
- Kidneys
- Liver

High blood pressure:

- Promotes the development of atherosclerosis, which further narrows the vessels. This increases the blood pressure even more.
- Increases the stress on the heart.
- Increases the damage to the blood vessel walls, so they are more apt to rupture.
- Further limits the blood flow to the organs of the body.

Treatment may consist of:

- Drugs that lower the blood pressure
- Diet low in sodium
- Diet that promotes weight loss
- Regular exercise program
- Quitting smoking
- Surgical **sympathectomy** (a procedure in which the nerves that cause blood vessels to constrict are cut. When the nerves are cut, the blood vessels dilate.)

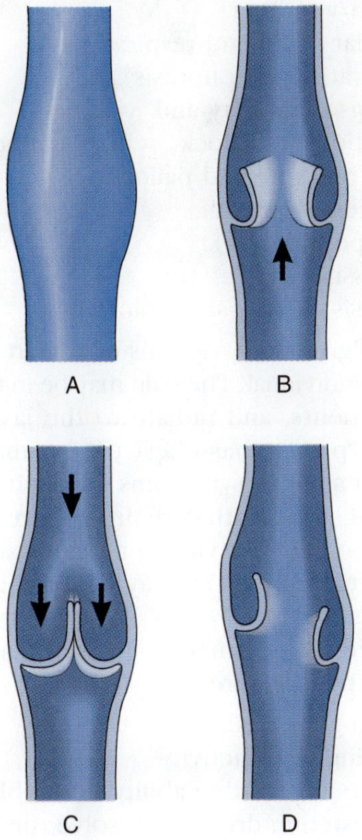

FIGURE 7-25 Veins contain valves to prevent the backward flow of blood. A. External view of the vein shows wider area of valve. B. Internal view with the valve open as blood flows through. C. Internal view with the valve closed. D. Vein with weakened valve that causes a varicose vein.

- Moderation in lifestyle
- Biofeedback techniques to lower the blood pressure

Report immediately any of the signs and symptoms of hypertension:

- Flushed face
- Dizziness
- Nosebleeds
- Headaches
- Changes in speech patterns
- Blurred vision

HEART CONDITIONS

Heart disease may sometimes be due to an infection, but most heart disease develops because of changes in the blood vessels. As the openings of the blood vessels become smaller, the heart must work harder and harder to do its job of pumping blood to the body.

Tips: Always take patient complaints of chest pain seriously. If a patient complains of chest pain, assist him or her to stop all activity and assume a comfortable position. Notify the nurse promptly.

Angina Pectoris

Angina pectoris is known as cardiac "pain of effort." You will recall that the blood vessels nourishing the heart are the coronary arteries. These vessels often are the site of atherosclerotic changes. In an angina attack, the vessels are unable to carry enough blood to meet the heart's demand for oxygen. This may develop:

- gradually over a period of time as atheromas develop.
- suddenly, as the vessels constrict.

Factors that precipitate (bring on) an attack include:

- Exertion
- Heavy eating
- Emotional stress

The signs and symptoms of angina pectoris that you should immediately report include:

- Pain when exercising or under stress. Stress causes a need for an immediate increase in coronary circulation. The pain is described as dull, with increasing intensity. It is usually centered under the breast bone (sternum), spreading to the left arm and up into the neck.
- Pale or flushed face.
- Patient who is freely perspiring.

Signs and symptoms may differ with individuals, but the symptoms are usually the same each time a person experiences an attack.

Treatment of angina pectoris consists of:

- Diagnosing hidden causes. A treadmill stress test is one method of doing this.
- Teaching the patient to avoid stress and sudden exertion.
- Drugs that relax the coronary arteries.
- Coronary artery bypass surgery.
- Angioplasty, a surgical procedure to open the vessels.

You may assist the patient who has angina pectoris by:

- helping the patient to avoid unnecessary emotional or physical stress.
- encouraging the patient not to smoke.
- reporting any signs or symptoms of an attack to the nurse at once.

Myocardial Infarction (Coronary Heart Attack)

The term **myocardial infarction (MI)**, or heart attack, refers to a period in which the heart suddenly cannot function properly. There are different kinds of heart attacks. They differ in their severity and prognosis (expected outcome). Remember that the heart is muscle tissue and may become tired just as any muscle may tire. The cells of the heart require nourishment and oxygen like all other cells.

An acute myocardial infarction occurs when the coronary arteries, which nourish the heart, are blocked. Part of the heart muscle supplied by these vessels becomes **ischemic** (loses its blood supply). Unless circulation is restored quickly, the cells die (**infarction**). If too much tissue dies, the person cannot survive. Coronary heart attack is also called:

- **Coronary occlusion**—blockage of coronary arteries
- **Coronary thrombosis**—when a **thrombus** (stationary blood clot) forms at the site, blocking the blood flow
- **Coronary embolism**—when a moving clot or insoluble particle (**embolus**), which originated elsewhere and has moved, becomes lodged in the artery

Signs and Symptoms. The signs and symptoms of a heart attack include:

- Pain—may resemble severe indigestion. It is often described as "crushing" chest pain that radiates to the jaw and left arm (Figure 7.26).

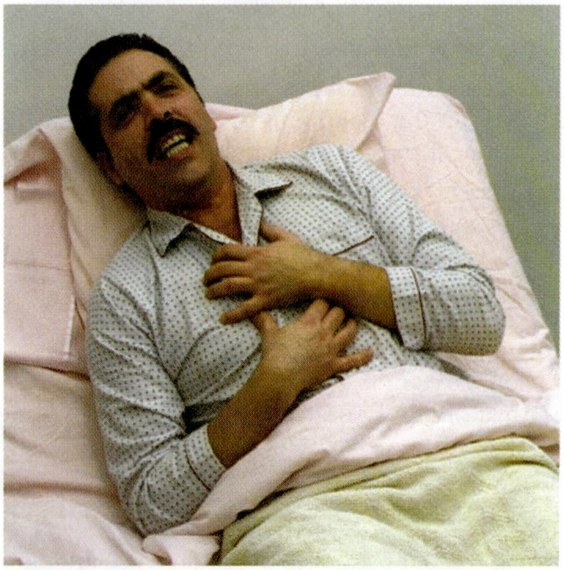

FIGURE 7-26 The patient having a heart attack usually experiences crushing chest pain that is described as, "the worst pain I've had in my life," or "It feels like an elephant is standing on my chest."

- Nausea/vomiting.
- Irregular pulse and respiration.
- Perspiration (diaphoresis).
- Feelings of anxiety and weakness.
- Indications of shock, which include drop in blood pressure and pallor.
- Shortness of breath.
- Syncope (fainting).
- Restlessness.
- Cyanosis or gray skin color.

The signs and symptoms of a heart attack vary with the individual. The pain may be in the chest in some patients, and radiate to the jaw or either arm. If a patient has chest pain combined with any other signs or symptoms, he or she should be evaluated by a health care professional. Have the patient stop any activity immediately and assume a comfortable position. Stay with the patient and call for assistance.

Immediate treatment has saved many people. The treatment is directed toward:

- Relieving the pain
- Reducing heart activity
- Altering the clotting ability of the blood
- Administering drugs to dissolve the clot

Nursing Care. During the acute stage, heart attack patients require professional care. Many hospitals provide intensive cardiac care units for these patients. Nursing care supports the therapy ordered. Special attention must be given to:

- Noting signs of a recurrence and reporting immediately to the nurse
- Watching for bleeding and reporting immediately
- Assisting with activities of daily living
- Monitoring vital signs
- Patient teaching to eliminate risk factors

Congestive Heart Failure (CHF)

The heart, like any other muscle, will enlarge and tire if it has to work against increasing pressure. When blood vessels narrowed by atherosclerosis increase the resistance to blood flow, and when there is severe damage to major organs like the liver and spleen, it is more difficult to maintain the circulation. The heart is not pumping well enough to meet the body's demands for oxygen. The heart muscle may also have been damaged and weakened by myocardial infarction. Other common causes are heredity, longstanding high blood pressure, alcohol abuse, and a virus. The heart must pump harder to maintain the internal flow of blood.

At first, the heart enlarges (**hypertrophy**) and makes up (**compensates**) for the additional workload. Eventually, however, it reaches a point when it can no longer compensate. Heart failure follows.

This form of heart disease is known as **congestive heart failure (CHF)** or **cardiac decompensation**. The condition got its name because of *failure* of the *heart* to pump efficiently, which results in *congestion* of the lungs. The heart tries to compensate for the problem, but this worsens the condition.

Signs and Symptoms. The signs and symptoms are the result of the heart being unable to pump the blood with sufficient force.

- Hemoptysis (spitting up blood)
- Cough
- Dyspnea (difficulty breathing)
- **Orthopnea** (difficulty in breathing unless sitting upright)
- **Ascites** (fluid collecting in the abdomen)
- Neck vein swelling
- Fatiguing easily
- Hypoxia (inadequate oxygen levels)
- Confusion
- Edema (swelling), which develops in dependent tissues and slows blood flow, congesting the vessels and allowing more fluid to enter the body spaces and tissues. It is most common in the abdomen, ankles, and fingers.
- Waking up at night with breathlessness
- Being unable to lie flat at night
- Fluid accumulation in the lungs
- Cyanosis, which occurs because fluid in the lungs makes gas exchange less efficient
- Irregular and rapid pulse.
- High blood pressure
- Palpitations (galloping heartbeat)
- Kidney malfunction in later stages
- Liver malfunction

Treatment. Treatment involves:

- Drugs to help the heart beat more strongly and regularly and to increase the output of fluids (**diuresis**) by the kidneys.
- Minimally invasive procedures may be done to open the arteries. These involve inserting a long tube into an artery in the groin. The tube is threaded through the system to the heart. A balloon on the tube is inflated to open blocked arteries (Figure 7.27A). The balloon-tipped catheter is removed and replaced with a **stent** (Figure 7.27B), a device that keeps the arteries open. This procedure pushes the fatty deposits back against the artery walls, making more room for blood to flow through and preventing heart attack.
- Low-sodium diet.

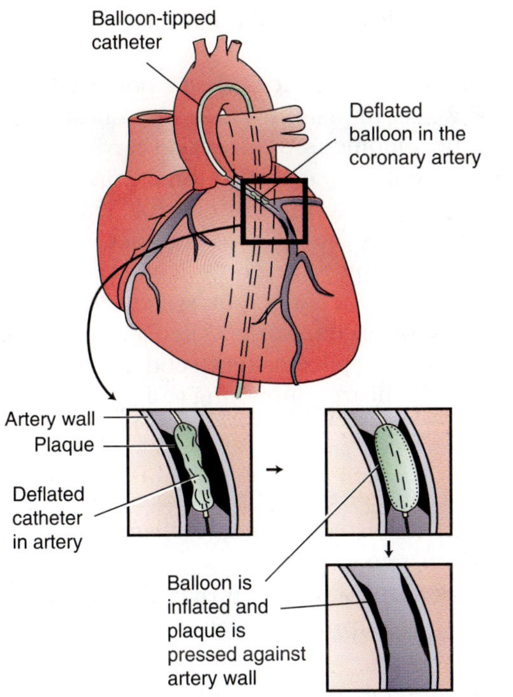

FIGURE 7-27A The balloon presses the plaque against the wall of the artery, making the vessel larger.

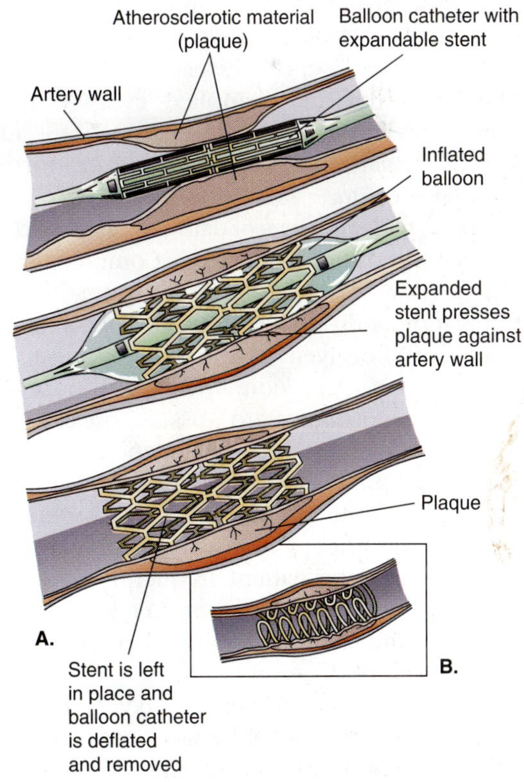

FIGURE 7-27B stent is left in place to keep the artery open and the balloon is removed.

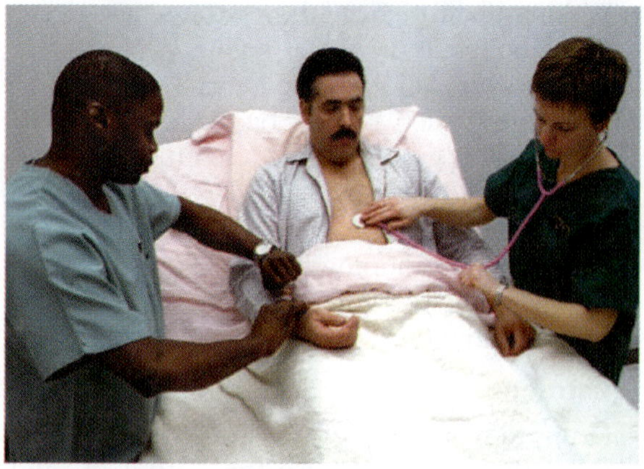

FIGURE 7-28 Ineffective heart contractions may cause a pulse deficit.

- Restriction of fluids, if ordered.
- Weighing the patient daily to monitor level of fluid retention.
- Monitoring the apical pulse and observing for pulse deficit (Figure 7.28).
- Positioning the patient in orthopneic position or high Fowler's supported by pillows, or supported in a chair. The position must be changed frequently, but changes in position should be made slowly. Padded footboards help keep the weight of the bedding off the toes.
- Applying elasticized stockings or **TED hose**. TED hose are elastic anti-embolism stockings. TED hose and Ace bandages help channel blood to the deeper vessels. They must be checked often and reapplied every 6 to 8 hours. Check the extremities carefully for adequate circulation. The skin should be normal color and warm.
- Assisting with activities of daily living as needed.
- Attending to general hygiene. Complete bathing is tiring, but partial baths can stimulate circulation and provide comfort. Special attention must be given to the skin because the combination of position, edema, and poor circulation contributes to tissue breakdown. Allow the patient to be as independent with bathing as possible, unless you are instructed otherwise. Bathing is not normally a strenuous activity, but the patient with CHF may tire easily. Check the patient frequently while he or she is bathing. Be prepared to take over and complete the bath if the patient becomes short of breath or too tired.
- Assisting with oxygen therapy. Oxygen therapy may be provided either by face mask or nasal cannula. Because cardiac patients often breathe through the mouth, the mouth tends to be very dry. Special mouth care may be needed.
- Providing for elimination. A bedside commode is convenient. The use of a commode is less tiring for the patient than using a bedpan for elimination.
- Encouraging adequate nutrition. Small, easily digested meals should be provided. You may need to assist in feeding the patient to prevent fatigue.
- Monitoring and recording fluid intake. Patients with acute heart failure may be given drugs that increase the output of urine and alter the heart rate. Measuring the intake and output and taking daily weights are ways of determining if fluid is being retained. The patient may be on fluid restriction (Unit 26) in the acute phase of the illness.
- Regularly checking vital signs. Sometimes the force of heart contraction, which propels the blood forward into the blood vessels, does not have enough strength to make the vessels expand.
- Keeping the feet elevated when the patient is up in a chair or wheelchair.
- Encouraging regular rest periods throughout the day.
- Assisting with exercise, as specified on the care plan.

Heart Block

Heart block is a condition that develops due to interference in the electrical current through the heart. (The flow of electrical current through the heart muscle makes the normal cardiac cycle possible.)

An electronic device called a **pacemaker** (Figure 7.29) is implanted under the chest muscles or in the abdomen. An electrode carries electrical current from the pacemaker directly into the heart muscle to replace the lost control. The electrical current signals the heart to contract. Some pacemakers send messages only if normal messages carried by the conduction system are delayed. This type of pacemaker is called a *demand pacemaker*. Other pacemakers send regular signals to keep the heart contracting at a preset rate.

When caring for a patient who has a pacemaker:

- count and record the pulse rate.
- report any irregularities or changes below the present rate.
- report any discoloration over the implant site.
- report hiccupping, because this may indicate problems.
- keep the patient away from microwave ovens and cellular phones, because they may disrupt the function of the pacemaker.

Patients usually function very well with pacemakers so long as they are adequately monitored.

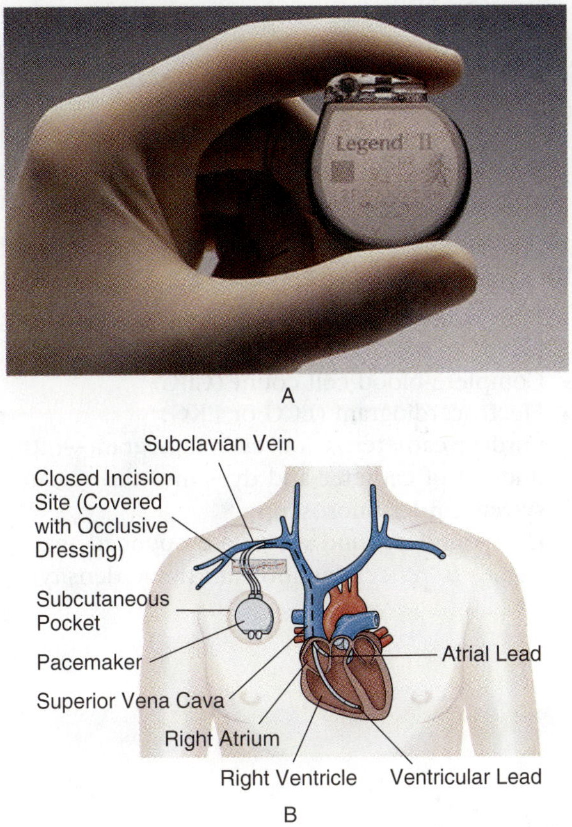

FIGURE 7-29 The electronic pacemaker sends electrical impulses to the heart muscle, causing it to contract. A. A typical pacemaker. B. The pacemaker is inserted under the skin with the electrode placed inside the heart, resting on the heart muscle. *(Courtesy of (Photo courtesy of Medtronic, Inc.)*

Blood Abnormalities

Blood abnormalities are often called *blood dyscrasias.*

Anemia

Anemia is a condition that results from a decrease in the quantity or quality of red blood cells. There are several causes, such as:

- Poor diet
- Low production of new red blood cells
- Blood loss, as in hemorrhage

Types of anemia include:

- Pernicious—inability to absorb vitamin B_{12} (most often seen in the elderly). Vitamin B_{12} is required by the body to produce red blood cells.
- Sickle cell—inability to form normal hemoglobin. Sickle cell anemia is transmitted genetically. It is seen most often in African Americans.
- Deficiency—inadequate intake of iron, inability to absorb iron, or excessive loss of iron.
- Dietary—inadequate intake of iron or vitamins in diet.

Signs and Symptoms. The person with anemia may:

- have little energy.
- be pale or jaundiced.
- have dyspnea.
- experience digestive problems.
- have a rapid pulse.
- complain of light-headedness.
- feel cold.
- experience dizziness.
- have an increased respiratory rate.

Treatment. Treatment is aimed at:

- Improving the quantity and quality of the blood by giving iron supplements
- Eliminating the basic cause of the disease
- Giving blood transfusions as needed
- Providing nutrients and nutritious meals

Leukemia

Leukemia is sometimes called cancer of the blood. The causes of the many forms of leukemia are not known. This disease may strike young or old. The number of white blood cells increases, but the white blood cells may be of poor quality. The number of erythrocytes and platelets decreases. Patients with leukemia are highly susceptible to infection. During the course of the disease, even minor trauma causes bleeding.

Treatment. Treatment is aimed at:

- Easing symptoms and keeping the patient comfortable.
- Maintaining normal blood levels. Transfusions may be needed to combat the anemia that accompanies the condition.
- Combating infection by using antibiotics.
- Slowing the production of abnormal white cells through chemotherapy and/or radiation therapy.

Special Care

Patients who have cancer or anemia require special care. You must:

- Check vital signs
- Encourage rest
- Handle the patient very gently
- Encourage good nutrition
- Give special mouth care, because the mouth and tongue become sensitive
- Be sure to report any signs of bleeding, such as bruises or discolorations, because further blood loss makes the condition worse

INFECTION CONTROL *Alert*

Patients with leukemia are at high risk of infection. Conscientiously apply the principles of standard precautions in all patient care. Notify the nurse promptly if signs or symptoms of infection are present.

- Keep patient warm
- Protect patient from falls that may result from dizziness or weakness
- Change the patient's position often, at least every 2 hours
- Provide emotional support

Diagnostic Tests

Some techniques used to diagnose problems of the cardiovascular system include:

- Blood chemistry tests, such as electrolyte panels
- Complete blood cell count (CBC)
- Electrocardiogram (ECG or EKG)
- Cardiac catheterization and angiogram—introduction of catheter and dyes into the vascular system under fluoroscopy
- Ultrasound—sound waves are bounced against tissues to reflect variations in tissue density

The Respiratory System

Structure and Function

The respiratory system (Figure 7.30) is sometimes called the lifeline of the body. It extends from the nose to the tiny air sacs **(alveoli)** that make up the bulk of the lungs.

The organs of the respiratory system include the:

- Nose
- Pharynx (throat)
- Larynx (voice box)
- **Trachea** (windpipe)
- Bronchi
- Lungs

The sinuses, diaphragm, and intercostal muscles between the ribs are called auxiliary structures.

Air is warmed, moistened, and filtered as it passes through the nasal cavities, which are separated by the nasal septum. The air passes through the **pharynx**, a passageway for both air and food, into the larynx and trachea. It then passes into the **bronchi** to join the upper respiratory tract to the lungs. Within the lungs, the bronchi branch into smaller and smaller divisions called **bronchioles**. The *alveoli* are tiny air sacs that extend from the bronchioles. It is at the level of the alveoli that the exchange of gases takes place

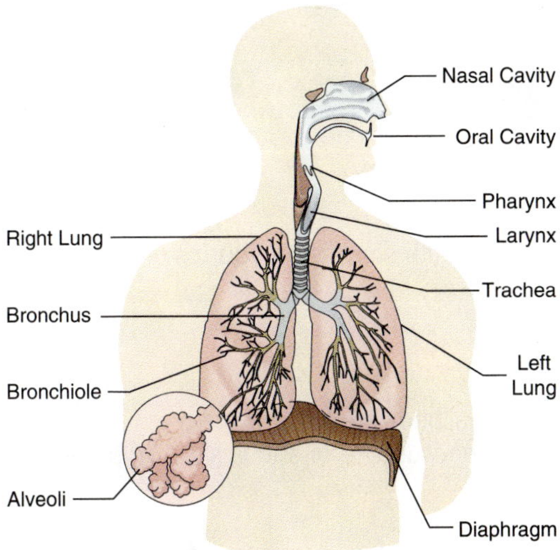

FIGURE 7-30 The respiratory system.

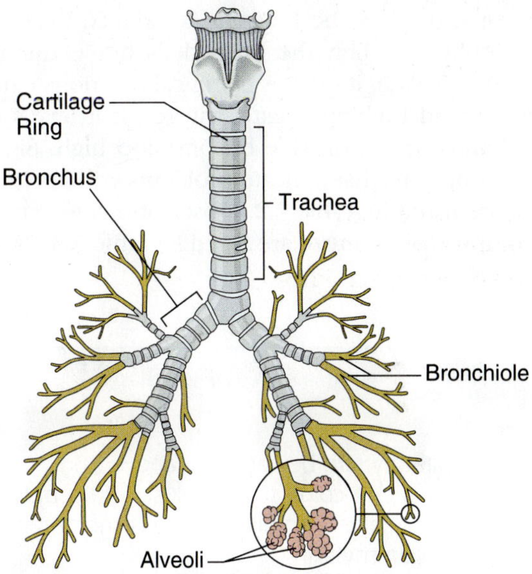

FIGURE 7-31 The lower respiratory tract.

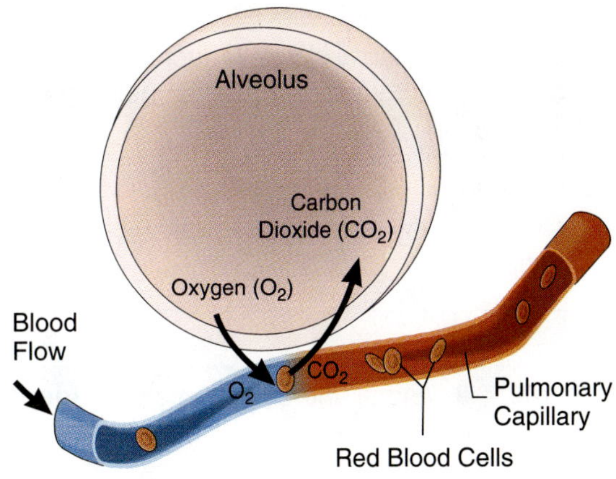

FIGURE 7-32 Oxygen and carbon dioxide are exchanged in the alveoli.

(Figure 7.31). The alveoli, bronchioles, and the important pulmonary blood vessels form the lungs. The way in which oxygen and carbon dioxide are exchanged between the alveoli and the capillaries is shown in Figure 7.32.

The purpose of this system is to bring **oxygen** (O_2) into the body to meet cellular needs and to expel carbon dioxide (CO_2). **Carbon dioxide** is a gaseous, metabolic waste produced by the cells.

Each cell in the body must have a constant supply of oxygen. The oxygen is used to produce the energy for cellular activity.

Nutrients + oxygen yields energy + water + CO_2

There is a close connection between the respiratory and circulatory systems. Oxygen is delivered throughout the body by means of the bloodstream. Every cell in the body produces carbon dioxide. It is transported in venous blood. When it reaches the lungs, it is exhaled into the atmosphere. When the body does not eliminate carbon dioxide, it creates chemical reactions causing an acid buildup. Death will result if levels of acid and carbon dioxide become too high. Signs and symptoms that indicate problems with oxygen use are listed in Table 7.2. Observations to report promptly to the nurse are listed in Table 7.3.

Aging Changes in the Respiratory System

Aging changes in the respiratory system include:

- Lung capacity is decreased because of muscular rigidity in the lungs.
- Cough becomes less effective, allowing pooling of secretions and fluid in the lungs, increasing the risk of infection.
- Shortness of breath may occur on exertion.
- Less effective gas exchange takes place in the lungs.

The Act of Respiration

Two lungs are located in the thorax. Each lung is surrounded by a double-walled membrane called the **pleura**. Between the layers of the pleura is a

TABLE 7-7 Signs and Symptoms of Decreased Oxygenation

- Respiratory rate below 12 or above 20
- Unusual skin color, such as dusky, pale, blue, or gray
- Unusual color of the lips, mucous membranes, nail beds, lining or roof of mouth
- Cool, clammy skin
- Slow, rapid, or irregular breathing
- Shortness of breath or labored breathing
- Noisy breathing
- Gasping for breath
- Changes in mental status, including decreased responsiveness, drowsiness, sleepiness for no apparent reason, restlessness, increased confusion.
- Tachycardia
- Cheyne-Stokes respirations
- Wheezing
- Coughing (dry or moist/productive)
- Retractions

TABLE 7-8 Signs and Symptoms of Inadequate Breathing to Report to the Nurse Immediately

- Movement in the chest is absent, minimal, or irregular.
- Breathing movement appears to be in the abdomen, not the lungs.
- Air movement cannot be detected by listening and feeling for breath sounds on your cheek and ear.
- Respiratory rate is too slow or rapid.
- Respirations are irregular, gasping, very deep, or shallow.
- Respirations appear labored.
- Patient is short of breath.
- Patient's skin, lips, tongue, ear lobes, mucous membranes, or nailbeds are blue or gray.
- Patient is unable to speak at all, or cannot speak in sentences because he or she is short of breath.
- Respirations are noisy.
- Nasal flaring is present during inspiration.
- The muscles below the ribs and/or above the clavicles retract inward during respiration.

small amount of fluid that reduces friction as the lungs alternately expand and contract, filling with and then expelling air.

The size of the thorax depends on the contraction of the diaphragm and intercostal muscles. As the muscles contract, the thorax enlarges, expanding the lungs. Air carrying oxygen enters the lungs. When the muscles relax, the thorax becomes smaller. Air carrying carbon dioxide leaves the lungs and is breathed out.

- *Inspiration* (or inhalation) is the act of drawing air into the lungs.
- *Expiration* (or exhalation) is the act of expelling air.
- **Ventilation** is the combination of these two actions.
- **Oxygenation** is the movement of oxygen from the lungs and into the blood to be carried to the cells.

Voice Production

The **larynx**, or voice box, is part of the respiratory tract. It is important in voice production. Two membranes called the **vocal cords** stretch across the inside of the larynx. As air moves upward through the larynx, it passes through an opening in the vocal cords. Changes in the shape of the vocal cords and the size of the opening permit controlled amounts of air to reach the mouth, nasal cavities, and sinuses, where specific speech sounds are made when formed by the teeth, lips, and tongue.

Patients at Risk of Poor Oxygenation

Hypoxemia is a condition in which there is insufficient oxygen in the blood. Many of the patients who are at high risk for developing hypoxemia are not in the intensive care unit where monitoring is routine. They are on medical and surgical units, in the long-term care facility, or in other patient care areas. Patients who are immobile and those on bedrest have an increased risk of hypoxemia. When hypoxemia develops, immobility makes a positive outcome less likely. Other high-risk conditions are:

- cardiac disease
- pulmonary disease
- being postoperative (for up to a week after surgery)
- sleep apnea
- decreased level of consciousness
- neuromuscular diseases
- morbid obesity
- kyphoscoliosis (curvature of the spine)
- trauma

Checking capillary refill is a quick means of evaluating how well oxygen is getting to body tissues. You may also use the pulse oximeter for monitoring patients with high-risk conditions.

Respiratory Care

Patients with respiratory disorders have many needs that require highly skilled care. The **respiratory care practitioner (RCP)** is a licensed professional who specializes in the care of patients with disorders of the cardiopulmonary system, respirations, and sleep disorders that affect the patient's breathing. The RCP will be highly involved in the care of the patient and the specialized equipment used for treatment.

Upper Respiratory Infections

An **upper respiratory infection (URI)** follows invasion of the upper respiratory organs by microbes. The upper respiratory organs include the nose, sinuses, and throat. A common cold, which is caused by a virus, is an example of an upper respiratory infection. It is one of the most ordinary illnesses found in people. Symptoms include:

- Elevated temperature (fever)
- Runny nose
- Watery eyes

OSHA Alert

We all know that respiratory infections are spread by the airborne and droplet methods of transmission. Handwashing is an often overlooked means of preventing the spread of respiratory infection. Secretions containing pathogens make their way to the environment. You pick up these pathogens on your hands. Good handwashing is the best method for preventing infection, including respiratory infection.

This usually self-limiting disease is best treated by:

- Use of a drug to reduce fever, such as acetaminophen
- Rest
- Increased fluid intake

Patients with respiratory infections should be taught to:

- cover the nose and mouth with a tissue when coughing or sneezing.
- dispose of soiled tissues by placing them in a plastic or paper bag to be burned.
- turn the face away from others when coughing or sneezing.
- wash their hands after handling soiled tissues.

You must take special note of and report the following:

- **Dyspnea** (difficult breathing)
- Changes in rate and rhythm of respiration
- Presence and character, color, and amount of respiratory secretions
- Cough
- Changes in skin color, such as pallor or cyanosis

URIs sometimes move down into the chest and develop into bronchitis or even pneumonia.

Pneumonia

Pneumonia is a serious inflammation of the lungs. It can be caused by a variety of infectious organisms. Three common causes of pneumonia are:

- Viruses
- Bacteria
- Protozoa

Pneumocystis carinii is most often seen in patients who have poorly functioning immune systems. Today, most pneumonias, though serious and potentially life-threatening, respond favorably to antibiotic therapy.

Chronic Obstructive Pulmonary Disease

Chronic obstructive pulmonary disease (COPD) is also called chronic obstructive lung disease (COLD). This term refers to conditions that result in chronic blockage or obstruction of the respiratory system that is not reversible. Several conditions constitute COPD, including:

- Emphysema
- Chronic bronchitis
- Bronchiectasis

It can be very difficult to differentiate asthma from COPD, particularly in older patients.

Asthma

Asthma is a breathing disorder resulting from:

- Constriction of the muscles of the bronchioles
- Swelling of the respiratory membranes
- Production of large amounts of mucus that fill the narrowed passageways

A person having an asthma attack has labored breathing and frequent coughing. An attack may result when the person contacts an allergen. Respiratory infections can also cause an asthma attack. Common allergens are:

- Pollen
- Medications
- Dust
- Feathers
- Foods such as peanuts, eggs, or chocolate

If a patient has known allergies (hypersensitivity to specific items), they should be marked in the patient's health record. Long-term treatment consists of determining the allergen and eliminating it. To relieve the attack, the patient is given medication to decrease the swelling and dilate the bronchioles. Low levels of oxygen may also be given.

Chronic Bronchitis

Chronic **bronchitis** is prolonged inflammation in the bronchi due to infection or irritants. Signs and symptoms include:

- Swollen and red bronchial tissues, resulting in narrowed bronchial passageways
- Persistent cough
- Sputum production
- Respiratory distress

Treatment includes:

- Antibiotics to fight the infection
- Drugs to loosen secretions deep in the respiratory tract
- Techniques to improve ventilation and drainage
- Adequate fluid intake to keep secretions thin so they can be coughed up

Emphysema

Emphysema develops after chronic obstruction of the air flow to the alveoli. The air sacs:

- Become distended
- Lose their elasticity and recoil ability
- Finally become nonfunctional
- Lose the ability to exchange gases

The patient can bring air into the lungs, but it becomes more difficult to expel air from the lungs. As a result, there is less and less room for air to reenter.

Risk factors for emphysema are:

- Genetic
- Airways that are very responsive to irritants
- Exposure to tobacco smoke
- Exposure to dust and chemicals in the workplace
- Exposure to indoor and outdoor air pollution
- Repeated lung infections

Emphysema alone (without chronic bronchitis, which often accompanies it) is a dry disease. There is no sputum production. However, patients with emphysema are at high risk of developing pneumonia. This condition also causes the heart to work harder. The most common sign of respiratory problems in a patient with emphysema is headache. This is caused by increasing carbon dioxide levels in the blood. Other signs and symptoms of emphysema are:

- fatigue
- chronic oxygen deprivation
- difficulty breathing
- loss of appetite and weight loss

General Care. The care of the emphysema patient includes all the care required of any patient with COPD:

- Assisting with the proper breathing techniques, such as pursed-lip breathing
- Encouraging breathing exercises
- Positioning to improve ventilation
- Assisting with postural drainage (this therapy is not commonly used for emphysema)
- Providing care during low-flow oxygen therapy
- Assisting with and encouraging good nutrition
- Treating infections with antibiotics and drugs to loosen and thin respiratory secretions
- Encouraging fluid intake
- Taking annual flu shots and the pneumonia vaccine at the frequency specified by the health care provider
- Encouraging patients to avoid crowds, especially during the flu season
- Encouraging patients not to smoke

Tips: When caring for patients with COPD, pace activities. Help them to conserve energy as much as possible. Minimize activities in which the patient must raise the arms over the head. Avoid exposing patients to aerosol sprays.

Wear gloves if your hands may contact the patient's respiratory secretions. Wear a gown, goggles or face shield, and a surgical mask if the patient is coughing and spraying respiratory secretions into the air.

Special Therapies Related to Respiratory Illness

Nursing assistants aid patient breathing by proper positioning and by helping provide moisture and oxygen. They also are assigned to collect sputum specimens for examinations.

Oxygen Therapy

Oxygen is often ordered by the physician. Remember that when oxygen is in use, special precautions are required to prevent fires and to administer the oxygen safely.

Special safety measures must be emphasized in areas where oxygen is being used:

- Be certain that there are no open flames and that no one smokes or has matches.
- Post "no smoking" or "oxygen-in-use" signs.

Hospitals have a centralized source of oxygen piped to wall units in the patient's room (Figure 7.33). In some facilities, the oxygen is stored in a tank that is brought to the patient's room when therapy is ordered. The amount of oxygen (rate of flow measured in liters) is ordered by the physician. Oxygen is a prescription item, and changing the flow rate is the responsibility of a licensed nurse or RCP.

Caring for a Patient Who is Receiving Oxygen Therapy. The care plan may instruct you to elevate the head of the bed when the patient is receiving oxygen. This will make it easier to breathe. Patients using oxygen masks cannot eat meals while wearing the mask. The physician may order a nasal cannula at meal time. Follow the instructions on the care plan or critical pathway for patient care measures. Being unable to breathe is very frightening.

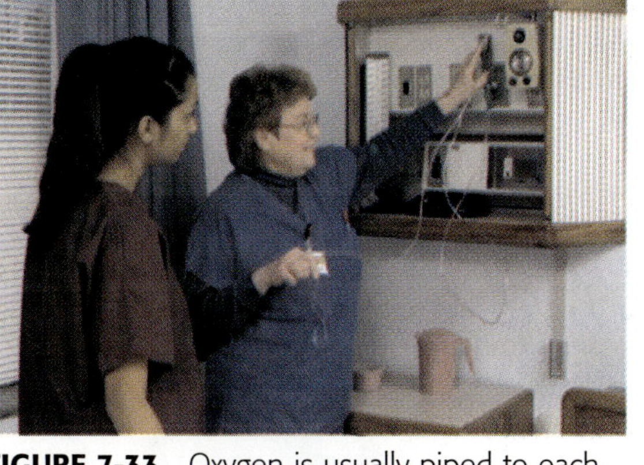

FIGURE 7-33 Oxygen is usually piped to each unit through a central delivery system.

COMMUNICATION HIGHLIGHT *Alert*

Oxygen is a basic need at the lowest level of Maslow's hierarchy of needs. Needs at the lower levels must be fulfilled before needs at the higher levels become important. The patient who is having trouble breathing cannot focus on much else. Keep conversation short and succinct. Give the patient verbal and nonverbal reassurance. Find alternate means of communicating, such as furnishing pen and paper, if necessary.

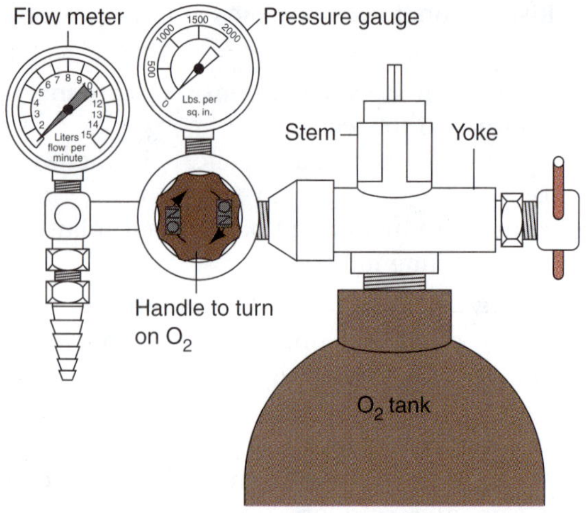

FIGURE 7-34 The flow meter shows the amount of oxygen being delivered. The pressure gauge shows the amount of oxygen remaining in the tank.

Patients who are receiving oxygen may need reassurance and emotional support. Check on the patient frequently and spend as much time in the room as possible. Difficult breathing makes it hard to talk. The patient may be unable to hold a normal conversation. Just being with the patient without talking is very reassuring. If the patient is having trouble breathing, try to ask questions that can be answered "yes" or "no" so it is easier for the patient to communicate with you. You will care for patients using different devices for the administration of oxygen. Carefully check the skin under the device to make sure it is not red or irritated from the elastic that holds the oxygen device in place. Report any skin problems to the nurse. Oxygen is drying, so patients who are receiving oxygen may need extra liquids to drink. They also need frequent care of the mouth and nose. Sometimes patients feel warm and will perspire heavily. Extra bathing and linen changes may be necessary. You may need to adjust the temperature in the room and help the patient change into a hospital gown. Cover him or her with a sheet. The care plan or critical pathway will provide information on patient preferences and needs. When caring for a patient who uses oxygen, you should:

- wear gloves and apply the principles of standard precautions if contact with the patient's oral or nasal secretions is likely.
- know the oxygen flow rate that was ordered and set for your patient.
- be able to read the flow meter for the rate of oxygen delivery if instructed to check the rate by the nurse.
- notify the nurse immediately if there is a change in the flow rate.
- check that the tubing is not obstructed in any way that would prevent oxygen from reaching the patient.
- check for proper position of the catheter, cannula, or mask and that the elastic band around the head is snug but not constricting.
- check whether straps, cannula, or mask are causing skin irritation.
- provide frequent mouth care.
- use a portable tank to transport the patient to other areas of the hospital. Do not remove the oxygen without permission from the RCP or RN.

If a tank is used as the source of oxygen, be sure that:

- there is sufficient oxygen in the tank. Check the gauge each time you visit the patient (Figure 7.34).
- the oxygen is on.
- an additional tank is available to exchange for the tank in use when it is empty.
- empty tanks are marked and stored according to facility policy.
- the tank is upright and secure on the carrier or in the stand.

The Urinary System

Introduction

The urinary system consists of the kidneys, ureters, bladder, and urethra. The functions that this system performs are vital. It:

- excretes liquid wastes.
- manages blood chemistry.
- manages fluid balance.

Because the chemistry of the blood and urine reflect the chemistry of the cells, many tests are performed on urine specimens. It is important that urine samples be obtained and preserved properly.

Structure and Function

The urinary system is shown in Figure 7.35. As the name implies, the organs of this system produce urine—liquid waste—that is excreted from the body. The urinary system also helps to control the vital water and salt balance of the body. Inability to secrete urine by the kidneys is known as **suppression**. Inability to excrete urine that has been produced by the kidneys is called **retention**. The organs of this system include:

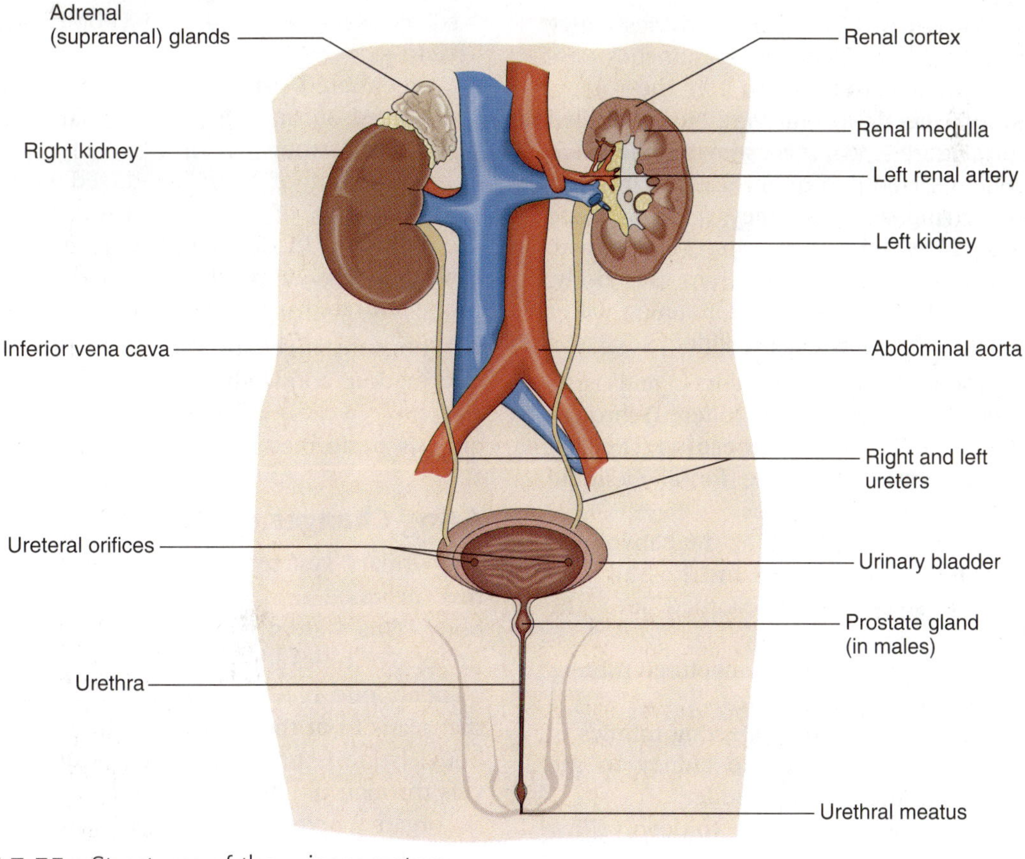

FIGURE 7-35 Structures of the urinary system.

- **Kidneys**: Organs that produce the urine.
- **Ureters**: Tubes that carry the urine from the kidneys to the urinary bladder. These tubes are 10 to 12 inches long and about ¼-inch wide.
- **Urinary bladder**: Holds the urine until expelled. The urge to urinate (micturate or void) occurs when 150 to 300 mL of urine are in the bladder, although the bladder can hold more urine than this.
- **Urethra**: The tube that carries the urine to the outside. The female urethra is about 1½ inches long. The male urethra is about 8 inches long. The opening to the outside is called the external **urinary meatus**. The meatus is guarded by a round sphincter muscle that relaxes to release the urine.

The Kidneys

The two bean-shaped kidneys are located behind the peritoneum. They are held in place by capsules of fat. Each kidney weighs about 5 ounces. The outer portion of the kidney is called the **cortex**. This area produces the urine. The middle area is known as the **medulla**. It is a series of tubes that drain the urine from the cortex. The **pelvis** of the kidney receives the urine and directs it to the ureter.

Urine Production. The renal arteries carry blood to each kidney. Their many branches pass through the medulla to the cortex. In the cortex, urine is produced in filtering units called **nephrons** (Figure 7.36). It is estimated that each kidney contains 1 million nephrons.

Blood arriving at the kidneys carries waste products such as acids and salts. These waste products must be eliminated from the body. Urine is a liquid waste solution containing water and dissolved substances. In the kidneys:

- Waste products, helpful products, and large quantities of water are passed (filtered) through the capillary walls of the **glomerulus** (capillary bed) into **Bowman's capsule**, forming a liquid called *filtrate*.
- The filtrate moves slowly along the convoluted tubules where some water and helpful substances like sugar are reabsorbed into the blood.
- The liquid remaining in the convoluted tubules is urine, which contains wastes.
- The urine passes into the collecting tubules of the medulla, then out of the kidney to the ureter and into the urinary bladder.
- Normal urine is acidic and pale to deep yellow in color.

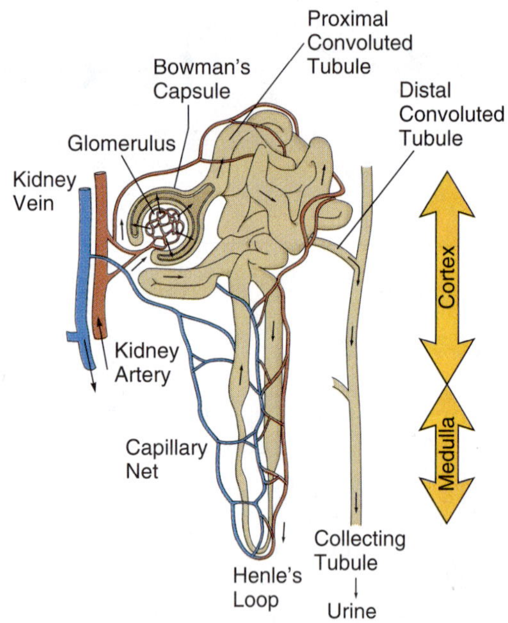

FIGURE 7-36 Nephron and related structures. Small arrows indicate the flow of blood through the nephron. The urine produced by the nephron flows through the collecting tubule.

- Dilute urine has more water and fewer dissolved substances, so it is colorless to pale yellow.
- Concentrated urine has less water and more dissolved substances, so it is darker in color and has a stronger odor.
- The amount of urine produced depends on the amount of intake and various physical conditions. Inadequate water intake leading to dehydration results in a small amount of concentrated urine.

The substances in the urine provide good information about the chemistry of the body and how well it is functioning. Tests are frequently performed on the urine (**urinalysis**).

Aging Changes in the Urinary System

The urinary system is made up of those organs that produce urine and eliminate it from the body. This system consists of two kidneys, two ureters, or tubes leading from the kidneys to the bladder, one bladder, and the urethra, or tube that leads from the bladder to the outside of the body. Urine is produced in the kidneys and travels through the ureters to the bladder, a muscular organ where urine is stored until it is eliminated from the body through the urethra. The urinary system plays a major role in maintaining fluid balance in the body.

Aging changes in the urinary system include:

- Bladder capacity decreases, increasing the frequency of urination.
- Kidney function increases at rest, causing the elderly to get up during the night to urinate.
- Bladder muscles weaken, causing leaking of urine or inadequate emptying of the bladder.
- The prostate gland (a tubular gland that encircles the urethra just below the bladder in the male) frequently enlarges, increasing the frequency of urination and causing dribbling, urinary obstruction, and urinary retention.

Common Conditions

Common conditions affecting the urinary system include inflammations due to ascending or descending infections and obstructions to the normal flow of fluids through the tube structure.

Cystitis

Cystitis, or inflammation of the urinary bladder, is fairly common. It is particularly common in women because of the shortness of the female urethra. Signs and symptoms of cystitis include:

- Frequent urination
- **Hematuria** (blood in the urine)
- **Dysuria** (painful urination and/or burning upon urination)
- Bladder spasm

Treatment. Treatment is aimed at relieving the symptoms and eliminating the cause. Treatment includes:

- Sitz baths
- Rest
- Bacteriostatic agents
- Increased fluid intake
- Antibiotics

Nephritis

Nephritis means inflammation of the kidney. Nephritis:

- May follow an attack of infectious disease or may result from general arteriosclerosis. In either case, kidney cells are destroyed. This results in decreased urine production.
- May follow a disease course that is acute (rapid) or chronic (slow).
- Causes hypertension and edema.

Signs and symptoms of nephritis are:

- Edema
- Hematuria
- Proteinuria (protein in urine)
- Hypertension
- Oliguria (occasionally) (decreased urination)

Treatment. Treatment includes:

- Absolute bed rest
- Low-sodium diet
- Restricted fluid intake, at times
- Frequent checks on vital signs
- Accurate intake and output (I/O) measurement
- Steroid medication in some cases

If both kidneys are involved, the patient will require regular dialysis until the diseased kidneys can be replaced with a healthy kidney (kidney transplant). **Dialysis** is the process of removing the waste products from the blood with a hemodialysis machine, commonly called an artificial kidney.

Many patients on dialysis receive treatment in a hospital dialysis unit or in special outpatient dialysis centers. Portable equipment is brought to the patient's bedside, if necessary. Other patients receive dialysis at home, using portable dialysis machines. The patient's overall physical condition is an important factor in determining if home dialysis is an option.

Renal Calculi

Renal calculi are kidney stones. They can cause obstructions when they become lodged in the urinary passageways.

There may be no sign of the development of renal calculi until some obstruction develops. Then:

- The pain is sudden and intense. It is called **renal colic**.
- Calculi may be passed in the urine.
- As stones pass along the tract, tissue damage may occur, resulting in hematuria (blood in the urine).

Treatment. The goal of treatment is to relieve the blockage and eliminate the stones.

- Encouraging fluids increases urine output. This helps to move the stones along the tract.
- All urine must be strained through gauze or filter paper, which is inspected for stones before it is discarded (Figure 7.37). Stones that are found can be analyzed. With information from the stones, the diet can sometimes be changed to make the formation of stones less likely.

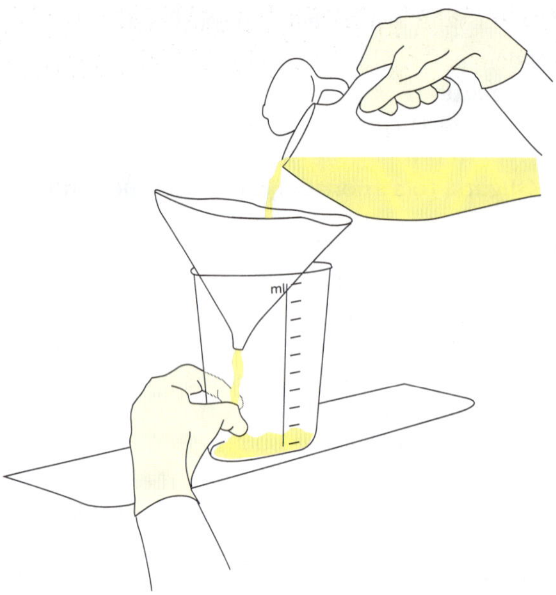

FIGURE 7-37 When the physician writes an order to strain urine, each voiding is poured through filter paper to retrieve kidney stones.

- When it is impossible for the patient to pass the stones, surgery may be necessary. This type of surgery can be done by passing a cystoscope through the urethra or through a surgical incision. With the cystoscope, the physician is able to see inside the bladder and locate the stones. The stones may then be crushed so they can be flushed out in the urine.
- At other times, the stones can be reached and removed only through a surgical incision. When a surgical incision is made, the patient usually returns from surgery with two drainage tubes in place. One tube is inserted in the urinary bladder. The other tube is inserted in the ureter or kidney.
    - The nurse will see that proper drainage is established.
    - In addition to routine postoperative care, you must check frequently to be sure the drainage is not blocked by kinks in the tubes or by the patient's body lying on the tubes.
    - The amount and type of drainage from each area should be carefully noted.
- **Lithotripsy** is a technique that uses carefully directed sound waves to crush the stones without the need for any surgical incision. The patient receiving this form of treatment is usually in the hospital less than 24 hours.

Hydronephrosis

Hydronephrosis results from accumulation of fluid within the kidney. The increasing amount of urine causes pressure on the kidney cells. As a result, kidney cells are destroyed. The fluid accumulates in the kidney because something is blocking its flow. The flow may be blocked by:

- Renal calculi
- Kinking or twisting of the ureters
- Tumors, especially benign prostatic hypertrophy
- Distended bladder

Symptoms may be acute and similar to those of renal calculi, or they may occur so gradually that they go unnoticed until much damage has been done.

Treatment. The condition is treated by draining the urine above the blockage to relieve pressure and then correcting the cause.

Responsibilities of the Nursing Assistant

Be sure you understand the orders for each individual patient before you assist in nursing care. Orders regarding positioning, drainage, and activity for urological (urinary) patients vary.

There are some important measures that will apply to most urinary patients in your care:

- Accurately measure intake and output (Figure 7.38).
- Promptly report signs and symptoms of:
    - Bleeding
    - Chilling
    - Elevated temperature

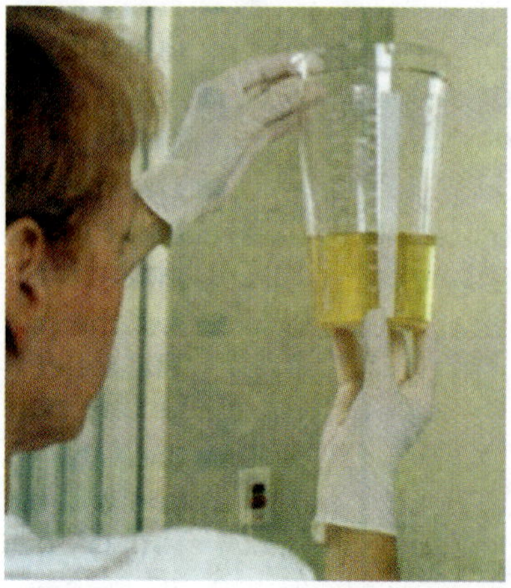

FIGURE 7-38 Accurately measure and record intake and output.

GUIDELINES FOR

Caring for the Patient with Incontinence

Nursing assistant responsibilities include:

- Assisting patients who need help to toilet regularly.
- Answering call lights promptly.
- Always being courteous and patient when assisting patients with toileting.
- Maintaining a positive attitude when changing soiled garments and bed linen and never being critical.
- Performing good perineal care and being sure skin is clean and dry.
- Checking the skin for signs of irritation whenever toileting or bathing a patient or performing perineal care.
- Giving special attention to patients who are confused or forgetful, because they may be unable to clearly state their need for assistance.
- Changing wet linen immediately. This limits discomfort and embarrassment of the patient. Prolonged exposure of the skin to urine is a major cause of skin breakdown. In addition, pathogens grow rapidly on the warmth and moisture and can quickly move upward through the urinary tract, causing life-threatening infection.
- Helping the patient become continent. Little reference should be made to the temporary incontinence. Nursing assistants can do much to give emotional support and reassurance to patients who are incontinent.

  - Reduced output
  - Increased edema
  - Pain
- Properly care for urinary drainage.
- Know the proper steps to take for encouraging fluid intake (forcing fluids) and for limiting fluids.
- When assisting with urination, collecting a urine sample, or recording I/O, note and report the following:
  - Amount of urine
  - Color of urine
  - Odor of urine
  - Presence and type of sediment

Urinary Incontinence

Urinary incontinence (loss of control of urination) may be due to one or a combination of factors. It is not unusual to find more than one factor present at the same time.

- Any interruption of cerebral control can lead to incontinence, including stroke, brain damage that destroys the control centers or pathways, confusion and decreased awareness due to general cerebral degeneration, or aphasia leading to the patient's inability to communicate to others the need for help.
- Incontinence may occur simply because the patient is unable to reach the proper facilities in time. The condition may be related to fecal impaction. Fecal impaction acts as a mechanical obstruction, causing the urine to be retained. The incontinence in this case is actually overflow. Perhaps the most common reason for incontinence is infection. Inflammation irritates sensory nerve endings in the bladder. Mucosal and bladder contractions are increased, causing the incontinence.
- Incontinence may be temporary, lasting only a few days. For example, after a period of illness, continence may improve as the patient becomes more able to respond to the environment. Attention to the underlying causes and the temporary use of incontinence pads may be all that is needed. Every effort should be made to help the patient become continent as soon as possible, with little reference to the temporary incontinence. You can give a great deal of emotional support and reassurance to the patient.
- Incontinence of an established nature continues even though the patient is ambulatory. This is a more difficult, but still not impossible, form of incontinence to treat. Drugs are sometimes used to achieve bladder control. Retraining may also be needed.

The Digestive System

Introduction

The digestive tract extends from the mouth to the anus. It receives the help of the teeth, tongue, salivary glands, liver, gallbladder, and pancreas in breaking food into simpler substances. These substances are used by the body cells to carry on their work of supplying nutrition and eliminating wastes.

Structure and Function

The gastrointestinal system is also called the GI or digestive tract. It extends from the mouth to the anus and is lined with mucous membrane. The organs along the length of this system change food into simple forms that can pass through the walls of the small intestine and into the circulatory system. The circulatory system then carries the nutrients to the body cells. The gastrointestinal system includes the:

- Mouth, teeth, tongue, salivary glands
- Pharynx
- Esophagus (gullet)
- Stomach
- Small intestine
- Liver, gallbladder, pancreas
- Large intestine

In the digestive system:

- proteins are changed to amino acids.
- carbohydrates are changed to simple sugars like glucose.
- fats are changed to fatty acids and glycerol.

These changes are brought about by mechanical action and chemicals called *enzymes*. The nondigestible portions of what we eat are moved along the intestines and are finally excreted from the body as feces. Several organs contribute to the digestive process and many disease conditions affect them.

Mouth

In the mouth (Figure 7.40), food is chewed so it can be swallowed easily. The digestive process begins with the help of the:

- Tongue—a skeletal muscle that is covered by tastebuds. The tongue pushes the food between the teeth to be broken up. It assists in mastication (chewing). It propels the food backward toward the pharynx to assist in swallowing. It also aids in speech formation.
- Salivary glands—secrete saliva containing a digestive enzyme called salivary amylase.
  - Salivary amylase begins carbohydrate digestion
  - 1½ quarts of saliva are secreted daily
  - Saliva moistens food to help in swallowing
- Teeth—mechanically break up the food into smaller particles, forming a **bolus** of food. The bolus is then swallowed. There are two natural sets of teeth. The first set (deciduous or temporary) numbers 20. The second set (permanent) numbers 32 and gradually replaces the deciduous set.
- Pharynx—allows the passage of both food and air. It leads to the esophagus.
- Esophagus—a tube 10 to 12 inches long that carries the food to the stomach. Strong muscular contractions called *peristaltic* waves move the food along the tract. These waves begin in the

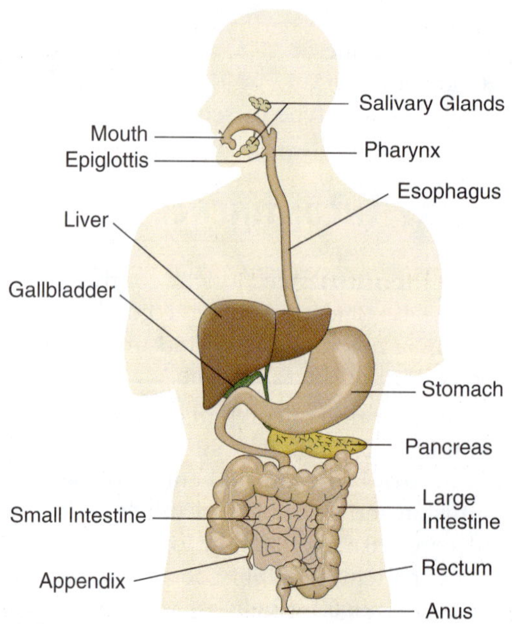

FIGURE 7-39 The digestive system

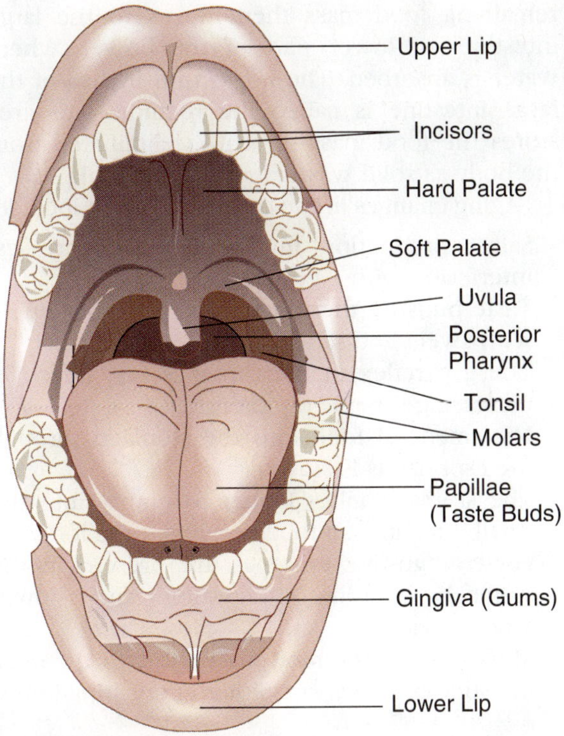

FIGURE 7-40 Mouth.

esophagus and continue throughout the intestinal tract.

The Stomach

The stomach

- Is a hollow, muscular, J-shaped organ
- Is found in the peritoneal cavity
- Is two-thirds to the left of the midline
- Is just below the diaphragm
- Has circular muscles at either end that hold the food while it is thoroughly mixed with digestive enzymes
- Begins the chemical process of digestion
- Holds the food between 3 to 4 hours

The stomach has three parts:

1. Fundus—the area above the entrance of the esophagus
2. Body—holds the food
3. Pylorus—the long, narrowly tapered distal end that connects with the small intestines. The muscle guarding this exit point is called the **pyloric sphincter**. Sometimes in babies this muscle is so tight (pyloric stenosis) that milk cannot get through and the muscle must be cut surgically.

The stomach cells produce gastric juice, which contains:

- Proteolytic enzyme (**pepsin**) to begin protein breakdown
- Hydrochloric acid (HCl)
- Intrinsic factor, needed for the absorption of vitamin B_{12}

The Intestines

When food leaves the stomach, it is in a semiliquid form called **chyme**. Chyme enters the small intestine, where any undigested nutrients are broken down by intestinal and pancreatic enzymes and bile from the liver.

Materials continue to be moved through the intestines by waves of **peristalsis**. Food digestion is completed in the small intestine. Most of the nutrients and food the body needs are absorbed into the bloodstream through the walls of the small intestine.

The small intestine is about 20 feet long. It coils within the peritoneum. There are three main portions:

1. The duodenum—about 12 inches long. Has an opening in the back to receive the bile and pancreatic secretions.
2. The jejunum—about 8 feet long.
3. The ileum—the last 12 to 13 feet. Terminates in the ileocecal valve and is connected to the large intestine. The ileocecal valve prevents food from traveling backward into the small intestine.

The large intestine (colon) is 4½ feet long. It is divided into several sections:

- Cecum
- Ascending colon
- Transverse colon
- Descending colon
- Sigmoid colon
- Rectum
- Anus

No digestive enzymes are secreted in the colon. The colon is the place where:

- Some vitamins are absorbed into the circulatory system.
- More complex carbohydrates are acted upon by bacteria.
- Much of the remaining water is absorbed through the walls of the large intestine, changing wastes to a more solid form. In this way, the large intestine helps to maintain the water balance of the body.

Peristalsis continues to move waste through the large intestine until it reaches the rectum.

When a certain amount has been collected in the rectum, it is eliminated as feces through the anus. This process is called **defecation**.

The Appendix

The appendix is located in the lower right quadrant, attached to the cecum. Its function is not known. When it becomes inflamed, the condition is called *appendicitis*.

Liver and Gallbladder

The liver is a large gland that has four lobes. It is located just beneath the right diaphragm. It carries on numerous metabolic functions. For example, the liver helps control the amount of protein and sugar in the blood by changing and storing excess amounts. It produces blood proteins such as prothrombin and fibrinogen, which are important factors in the blood clotting process. The liver also produces bile, which is carried directly to the small intestine for use in digestion or to the gallbladder for storage. Bile prepares (emulsifies) fats for digestion.

The gallbladder is a small hollow sac that is attached to the underside of the liver. It holds about two ounces of bile that it receives from the liver. It releases bile into the small intestine to help digest a fatty meal. The presence of bile in the digestive tract gives solid wastes their usual brown color.

The Pancreas

The pancreas is a glandular organ that produces both exocrine secretions (digestive enzymes) and endocrine secretions (insulin and glucagon). It extends from behind the stomach into the curve of the duodenum. It manufactures pancreatic juice. The pancreatic juice is sent into the duodenum to aid in the digestion of foods. The pancreas also produces insulin and glucagon. Both insulin and glucagon are sent directly into the bloodstream.

Aging Changes in the Digestive System

The digestive system begins in the mouth and extends all the way through the body to the anus, or external outlet of the intestines. Food is taken into the mouth and moves through the esophagus, or food tube, to the stomach, where it is mixed with fluids that aid in the digestion process. The food continues to move downward through the small intestine, the part of the intestine where digestion is completed. The food is further digested and nutrients are absorbed. The remaining food mass then moves to the large intestine, or lower part of the bowel, where water is absorbed. The last 6 to 8 inches of the large intestine is called the rectum. This area stores the food mass until it is eliminated from the body as solid waste, or fecal material.

Aging changes in the digestive system include:

- Saliva production in the mouth decreases, interfering with digestion of starch.
- Taste buds on the tongue decrease, beginning with sweet and salt.
- The gag reflex in the throat is less effective, increasing the risk of choking.
- Movement of food into the stomach through the esophagus is slower.
- The stomach takes longer to empty into the small intestine, so food remains there longer.
- Fewer digestive enzymes are present in the stomach, causing indigestion and slower absorption of fat.
- Movement of the food mass through the large intestine is slower, resulting in constipation.

Common Conditions

The tubelike mucus membrane structure of the alimentary canal lends itself to the possibility of malignancies, ulcerations, obstructions, and herniations.

Malignancy

Malignancies (cancers) of the gastrointestinal tract are very common. The symptoms they cause depend on their location. Among the symptoms are:

- Obstruction. Blocking of the passageway is sometimes the first major indication of a long-growing tumor.
- Indigestion.
- Vomiting.
- Constipation.
- Changes in the shape of the **stool** (bowel movement).
- **Flatus** (gas).
- Blood in the stool.

Treatment. Malignancies of the intestinal tract are usually treated surgically by removing the affected part. For example:

- Esophagectomy—removal of the esophagus
- Subtotal gastrectomy—removal of part of the stomach
- Colectomy (bowel resection)—removal of a part of the **colon** (large intestine).

- **Colostomy**—creation of an artificial opening in the abdominal wall and bringing a section of the colon to it for the elimination of feces
- **Ileostomy**—creation of an artificial opening in the abdominal wall and bringing a section of ileum through it for the elimination of waste

Ulcerations

An **ulcer** (sore or tissue breakdown) can occur anywhere along the digestive tract. Common places are the:

- Colon—**ulcerative colitis**. In colitis, malnutrition and dehydration are brought about by loss of fluids in frequent, watery, foul-smelling stools with mucus and pus.
- Stomach—**gastric ulcer**.
- Duodenum—**duodenal ulcer**.

Treatment. Treatment of ulcerative colitis includes:

- Medication to slow peristalsis (the wave-like contractions of the intestines) and reduce patient anxiety.
- Modification of diet to include high protein, high calories, and low residue. The low-residue diet is one in which the foods are almost completely digested. There is little waste with this type of diet.
- Medication (steroids) to reduce inflammation.
- Antibiotics to control infection by the microorganism *H. pylori*.

Patients with gastric or duodenal ulcers have periodic burning pain about 2 hours after eating. Most patients improve when they are placed on a diet in which foods that cause distress are not served. Medications are given to neutralize the **hydrochloric acid (HCl)**, to coat the stomach, and to decrease anxiety. It is sometimes necessary to remove part of the stomach (**gastrectomy** or **gastric resection**) or duodenum (**duodenal resection**). Following such surgery, the patient is:

- Placed on NPO. Special mouth care is therefore needed.
- Placed on gastrointestinal drainage. A **nasogastric tube (NG tube)** (Figure 7.41A and 7.41B) is inserted through the patient's nose and into the stomach. The tube is attached to a drainage bottle. Additional tubes are inserted into the intestinal tract. Be careful not to disturb the tubes. Check frequently to ensure that the drainage is not blocked. If drainage becomes blocked, report it to your supervisor at once. The type and amount of drainage are noted and recorded.

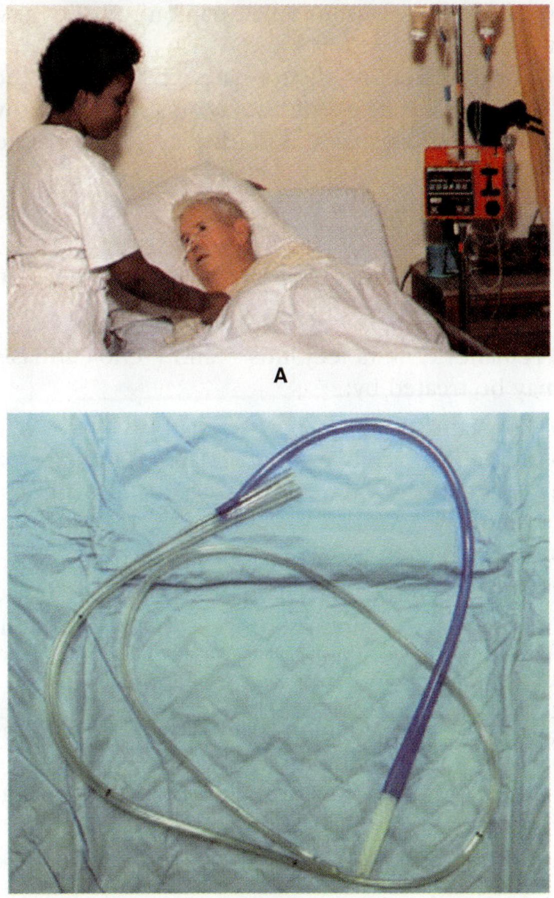

A

B

FIGURE 7-41 A. Materials for feeding tube insertion. B. Double-lumen nasogastric tube.

Hernias

A **hernia** results when a structure such as the intestine pushes through a weakened area in a normally restraining wall. The danger of such abnormal protrusions is that some of the protruding tissue can become trapped in the weakened area. Circulation then becomes limited so that the tissue is in danger of dying. This is called an **incarcerated (strangulated) hernia**.

Frequent sites of herniation are:

- Groin area (inguinal hernia)
- Near the umbilicus (umbilical hernia)
- Through a poorly healed incision (incisional hernia)
- Through the diaphragm (hiatal hernia)

Hernias are usually repaired surgically with a **herniorrhaphy**.

Gallbladder Conditions

Two common conditions affecting the gallbladder are:

- **Cholecystitis**—an inflammation of the gallbladder.
- **Cholelithiasis**—the formation of stones in the gallbladder. The stones may obstruct the flow of **bile** (fluid that aids digestion), giving rise to signs and symptoms such as:
  - Indigestion
  - Pain
  - Jaundice (yellow discoloration of the skin and whites of the eyes)

Treatment. Cholecystitis and cholelithiasis may be treated by:

- Low-fat diet.
- Surgery to remove the gallbladder and stones. This surgical procedure is called a **cholecystectomy**.
- Laser therapy to break up the stones.

Drains are often placed in the operative areas. Initially, large amounts of yellowish-green drainage may be expected.

In addition to routine postoperative care:

- Position the patient in a semi-Fowler's position.
- Do not disturb drains.
- If you notice fresh blood on the dressing, increased jaundice, or dark urine, report it immediately to your team leader.

Common Problems Related to the Lower Bowel

The frequency of bowel elimination varies with the individual. Some people have more than one bowel movement (BM) a day, but others have a BM every two or three days. **Fecal material** (solid body waste, bowel movement, BM) is normally brown, but the color can be affected by certain foods, medications, and diseases. The bowel movement is normally soft and formed. If it passes through the colon too quickly, it is loose and watery. Multiple watery stools is called **diarrhea**. If stool passes through the colon too slowly, the fecal material becomes hard, dry, or sticky and pasty in consistency. This is referred to as **constipation**.

Certain foods, medications, infections, and diseases can cause constipation and diarrhea. As foods move through the gastrointestinal tract by peristalsis, gas is formed. When the gas is expelled from the body, it is called "passing flatus" or flatulence. If the gas is not passed, it accumulates in the intestine. The abdomen will enlarge and appear bloated. This is called **abdominal distention**, and is an important observation to report to the nurse. Abdominal distention may also be caused by constipation and urinary retention.

Changes in Function of the Gastrointestinal System Associated with Aging and Disease

Change in bowel function may be caused by aging, disease, surgery, diet, and medications. Lack of privacy may also affect the patient's ability to have a bowel movement. As a person ages, movement in the colon is decreased. Food absorption is slowed and fewer digestive juices are produced. Constipation is a common problem. Other factors that affect bowel function are:

- Bedrest
- Inactivity
- Inadequate exercise
- Inability to chew foods properly
- Loose or missing teeth
- Inadequate fluid intake
- Stress
- Change in environment
- Change in diet
- A diet that does not contain enough fiber, fruits, or vegetables

Observations to Make when Assisting Patients with Bowel Elimination

You must observe the amount/quantity, color, odor, character, and consistency of the patient's bowel movement before discarding it. Notify the nurse if the fecal material has an unusual color or odor, if there is an unusual amount, or if there is blood, mucus, parasites, or food particles (except corn and raisins) in the stool. If you think a stool is abnormal, save it for the nurse to assess.

Constipation and Fecal Impaction

Report problems with constipation to the nurse. The patient is probably constipated if he has not had a bowel movement in more than three days, strains, or passes hard, marble-like stools. **Fecal impaction** (Figure 7.42) is the most serious form of constipation. It is caused by retention of stool in the rectum, where water is absorbed. Over time, the stool becomes hard and dry. The patient may be unable to pass it. The dried waste irritates the bowel. Mucus dissolves the hard, outer part of the mass. The rectum becomes so full that the fluid escapes around the impaction and is eliminated from the rectum as diarrhea. The patient may complain of:

- abdominal or rectal pain
- nausea
- loss of appetite
- feeling the need to have a bowel movement, but cannot

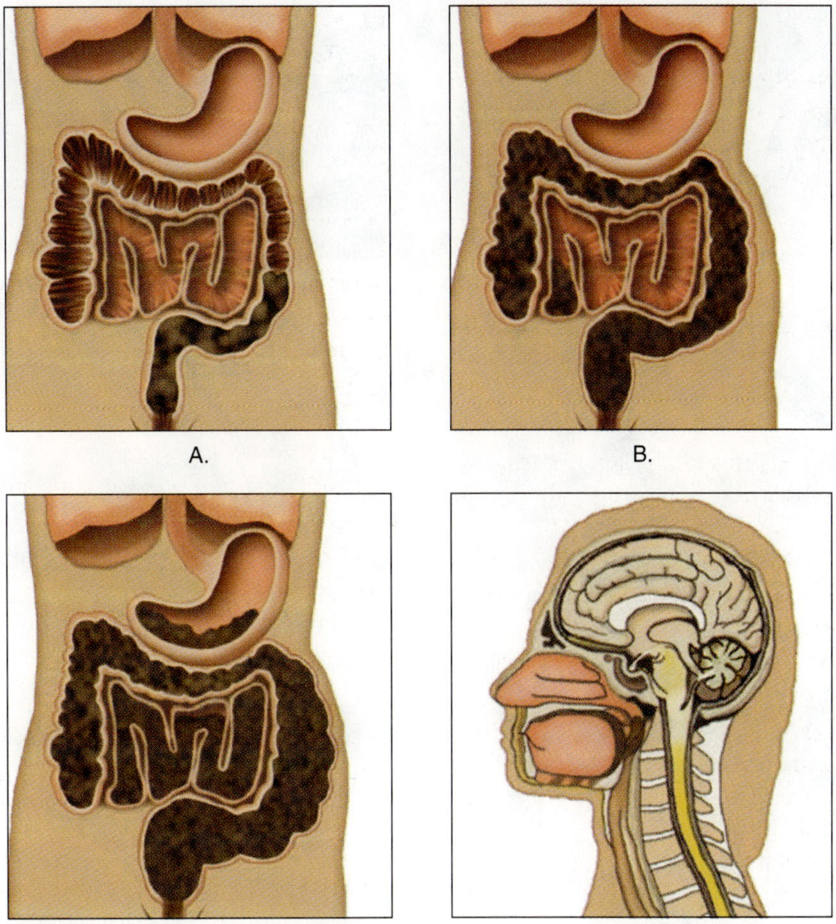

A. B. C. D.

FIGURE 7-42 Progression of a fecal impaction, a life-threatening condition. A. A fecal impaction blocks the rectum. The rectum and sigmoid colon become enlarged. B. The colon continues to enlarge. C. Fecal material fills the colon. Digested and undigested food back up into the small intestines and stomach. The patient has signs and symptoms of acute illness, including lethargy, distention, constipation, and pain that is dull and cramping. D. The entire system is full, and the patient vomits fecal material. The feces are commonly aspirated into the lungs.

Other signs and symptoms of impaction are:

- passing excessive flatus
- bloating and abdominal distention
- frequent urination
- inability to empty the bladder
- leaking around the catheter
- mental confusion
- fever
- liquid stool or mucus seeping from the rectum

Fecal impaction is a very serious condition that is usually treated by manual removal of the mass by the nurse or advanced care provider. Laxatives and enemas are also used to treat fecal impaction. The best thing to do is observe the patient's bowel elimination carefully and prevent fecal impaction from developing.

Diarrhea

Diarrhea occurs when peristalsis in the intestines is very rapid. The need to defecate is usually very urgent if the patient has diarrhea. Some patients may become incontinent because of the force with which the fecal material moves through the intestines. The patient may also complain of abdominal pain and cramping.

Diarrhea can cause dehydration and other serious medical problems if undetected or untreated. Most health care facilities have a definition of diarrhea, such as three or more loose stools within a defined period of time. One loose stool is not diarrhea. Remember to be objective in reporting your observations. When reporting loose stools to the the nurse, report the color,

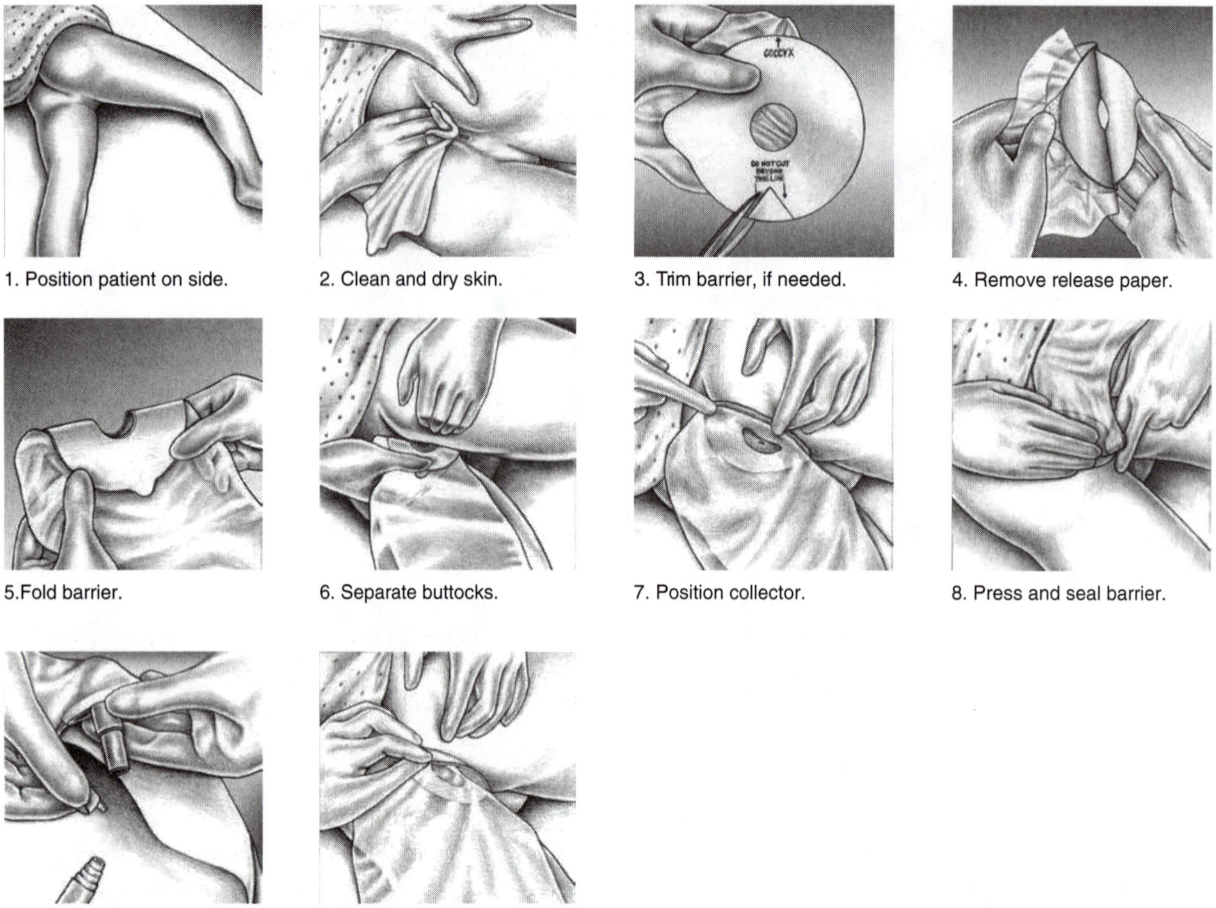

1. Position patient on side. 2. Clean and dry skin. 3. Trim barrier, if needed. 4. Remove release paper. 5.Fold barrier. 6. Separate buttocks. 7. Position collector. 8. Press and seal barrier. 9. Connect to bed side collector. 10. Remove.

FIGURE 7-43 Fecal incontinence collection system. *(Courtesy of (Permission to reproduce this copyrighted material has been given by the owner, Hollister, Inc., Libertyville, Illinois)*

odor, consistency, character, amount, and frequency of stools. Also report any patient complaints of pain or other discomfort.

Bowel Incontinence

Bowel incontinence is involuntary passage of fecal material from the anus. It has many causes, including trauma, neurological diseases, inability to reach the toilet on time, and mental confusion. It is not as common as urinary incontinence. Fecal material is very irritating to the skin, so the patient must be cleansed well after each episode of incontinence. Skin exposed to fecal material will break down quickly. Bowel incontinence may lower the patient's self-esteem. Be professional, compassionate, and understanding when assisting patients with bowel elimination and incontinence.

Patients with bowel incontinence may be placed on a bowel retraining or incontinence management program. If this is ineffective, a fecal incontinence collector (Figure 7.43) may be used.

COMMUNICATION HIGHLIGHT *Alert*

Remember that bowel activity is a normal body function. Do not show disgust in your facial expressions or body language when assisting patients with elimination. Documenting bowel activity is a very important responsibility. Unrelieved constipation is a serious, uncomfortable condition. The nurse depends on the accuracy of your documentation in the elimination record. The nurse will use this record to contact the physician, and administer medications and other treatments related to bowel elimination.

GUIDELINES FOR

Assisting Patients with Bowel Elimination

- Apply the principles of standard precautions when assisting with bowel elimination. Avoid environmental contamination from your gloves.
- Encourage patients to consume an adequate amount of fluid. Maintaining fluid intake is as important for bowel elimination as it is for urinary elimination.
- Encourage patients to eat a well-balanced diet.
- Allow adequate time for patients to eat meals.
- Encourage patients to chew food well. Cut it into small pieces if necessary. Report chewing problems to the nurse for further assessment.
- If you observe that a patient has not eaten fiber foods, fruits, or vegetables, offer a substitute. The dietitian may visit the patient to discuss likes and dislikes and assure that the patient will eat the foods served.
- Encourage exercise and activity, as allowed and as tolerated.
- Assist patients with toileting at regular intervals and provide privacy.
- Position patients in a sitting position, if allowed, for bowel elimination.
- Use a bath blanket to cover a patient who is using the bedpan or commode, for privacy and warmth.
- Leave the call signal and toilet tissue within reach and respond to the call signal immediately.
- Allow adequate time for defecation.
- Provide perineal care as needed, or according to facility policy. Feces are very irritating to the skin and prolonged contact promotes skin breakdown and infection.
- Assist patients with cleaning the anal area (this may be called the rectal area by some health care providers).
- Assist patients with handwashing and other personal hygiene after bowel elimination.
- Monitor bowel elimination and report irregularities.
- Record bowel movements on the flow sheet or other designated location. If a patient is independent with bowel elimination, ask if she has had a bowel movement each day.
- Report to the nurse: frequent stools, absence of stools, pain, cramping, excessive flatulence, abnormal color or consistency of stool, extremely small amounts of stool, hard, dry stool, or enlargement of the abdomen.
- Specific abnormalities in stools to report are presence of blood, pus, mucus, black or other unusual color, undigested food (except corn and raisins), or presence of parasites.

Role of the Nursing Assistant in Assisting Patients with Bowel Elimination

Assisting with bowel elimination is a very important responsibility. Always apply the principles of standard precautions when assisting with elimination. Avoid contaminating environmental surfaces with your gloves. Wear a gown, eye protection, and face mask if splashing is likely.

The Nervous System

Structure and Function

The nervous system controls and coordinates all body activities, including the production of hormones. Special parts of the nervous system are concerned with maintaining normal day-to-day functions. Other parts act during emergency situations. Still others control voluntary activities. Neurological conditions require highly specialized nursing care. You will assist with the less technical aspects of that care.

Neurons

Cells of the nervous system are called **neurons** (Figure 7.44A). They are specialized to conduct electriclike impulses. The neuron has extensions called **axons** and **dendrites**. Impulses enter the neuron only through the dendrites and leave only through the axon.

Although neurons do not actually touch each other, the axon of one neuron lies close to the dendrites of many other neurons. In this way, impulses may follow many different routes. The space between the axon of one cell and the dendrites of others is called a **synapse**. Axons and dendrites in the periphery are covered with *myelin*, which acts as insulation.

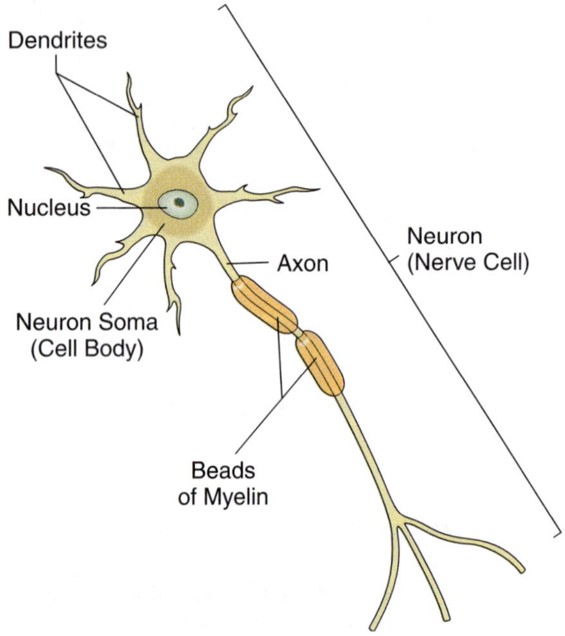

FIGURE 7-44A The neuron.

Neurotransmitters

Neurotransmitters are chemicals that enable messages (nerve impulses) to pass from one cell to another (Figure 7.44B). If the chemicals are not produced in the right amounts, the message pathway becomes confused or blocked.

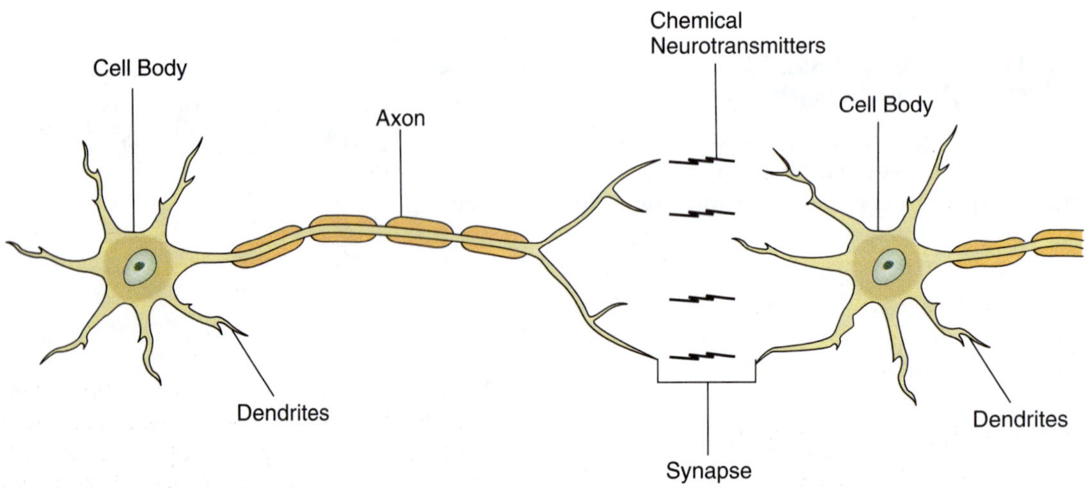

FIGURE 7-44B Chemicals called neurotransmitters help pass the message across the synapse from one neuron to another.

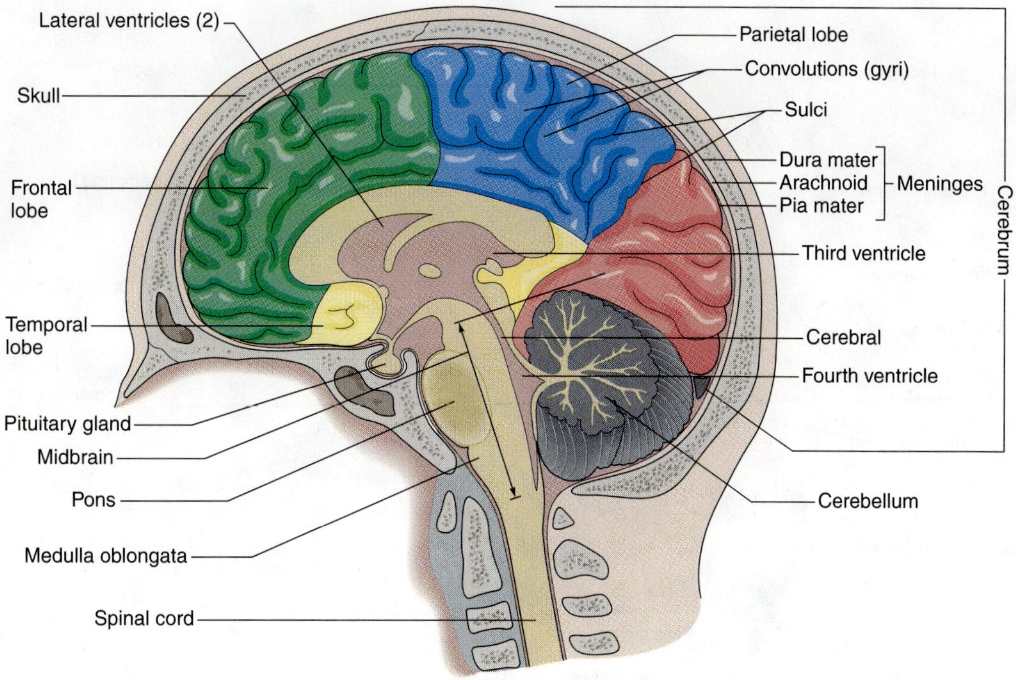

FIGURE 7-45 The central nervous system is composed of the brain and the spinal cord.

Nerves

Some axons and dendrites are long. Others are short. Axons and dendrites of many neurons are found in bundles. The bundles are held together by connective tissue. These bundles resemble telephone cables and are called **nerves**. The cell bodies of the axons and dendrites in these nerves may be found far from the ends of the nerves in clusters called *ganglia*.

Sensory nerves are made up of dendrites. They carry sensations to the brain and spinal cord from the various body parts. Feeling is lost when these nerve impulses are interrupted. Motor nerves carry impulses from the brain and spinal cord to muscles that cause body activity. Paralysis or loss of function occurs when these nerves are damaged.

For easier study, the nervous system can be divided into two parts: the central nervous system (CNS) and the peripheral nervous system (PNS). The CNS is composed of the brain and spinal cord (Figure 7.45). The PNS is composed of the 12 pairs of cranial nerves and 31 pairs of spinal nerves that reach throughout the body (Figure 7.46). Remember, though, that the nervous system is one interwoven system, a complex of millions of neurons.

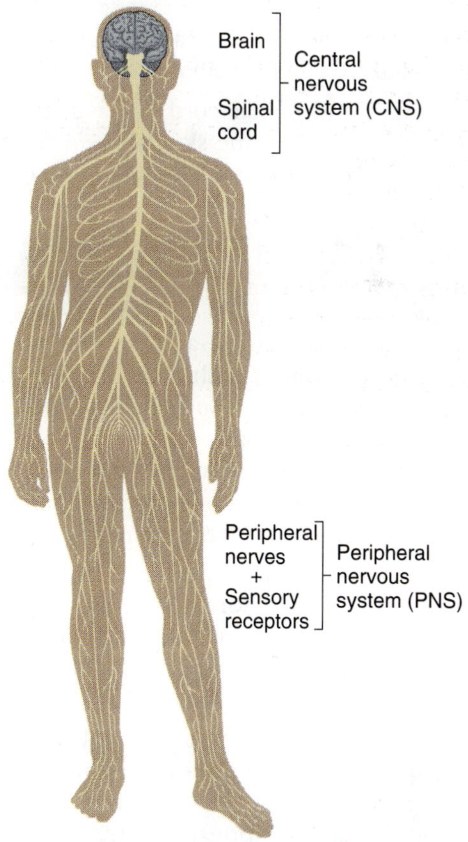

FIGURE 7-46 The peripheral nervous system connects the central nervous system to the various structures of the body. Messages are relayed from these structures back to the brain through the spinal cord.

The Central Nervous System

The brain and spinal cord are:

- Surrounded by bone

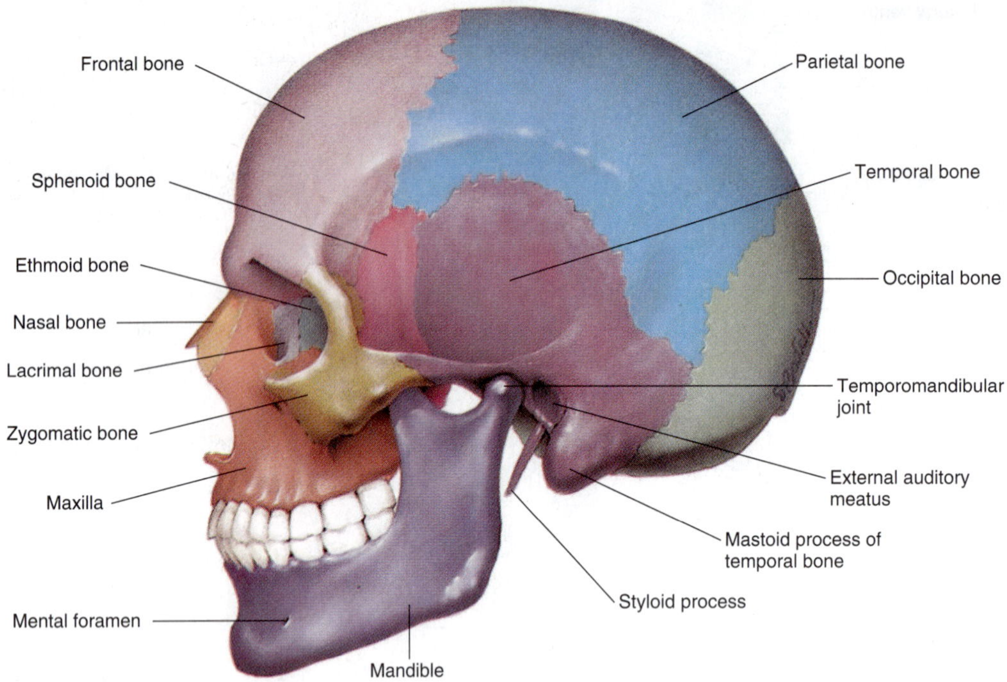

FIGURE 7-47 The lobes of the brain are named according to the skull bones.

- Protected by membranes called *meninges*
- Cushioned by cerebrospinal fluid (CSF)

The brain and spinal cord are a continuous structure found within the skull and spinal canal. The spinal cord is about 17 inches long. It ends just above the small of the back. Nerves extend from the brain and the spinal cord.

The Brain

The brain (encephalon) is a large, soft mass of nerve tissue contained within the cranium. It is composed of gray matter and white matter. Gray matter consists principally of nerve-cell bodies. White matter consists of nerve cells that form connections between various parts of the brain.

The brain can be further subdivided into the:

- **Cerebrum**—The largest portion of the brain. The outer portion is formed in folds known as convolutions and separated into lobes. The lobes take their names from the skull bones that surround them (Figure 7.47).
  - The outer portion, the cerebral cortex, is composed of cell bodies and appears gray.
  - The inner portion is composed of axons and dendrites and so appears white.
  - All mental activities—thought, direction of voluntary movements, interpretation of sensations, and experience of emotions—are carried out by cerebral cells (Figure 7.48). Certain activities are centered in each lobe.

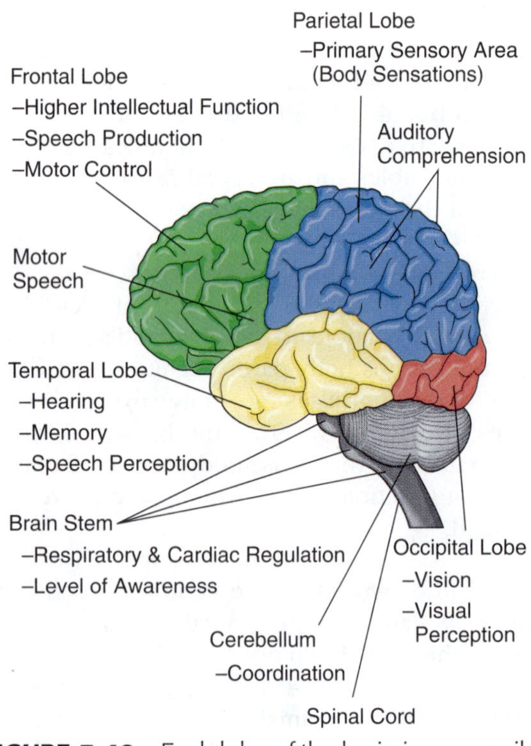

FIGURE 7-48 Each lobe of the brain is responsible for a different function.

  - In general, the right side of the cerebrum interprets for and controls the left side of the body and vice versa.
- **Cerebellum**—Found beneath the occipital lobe of the cerebrum. It too has an outer

layer of gray cell bodies. This portion of the brain coordinates muscular activities and balance.

- **Brain stem**—The midbrain, pons, and medulla are in the brain stem. They are composed mainly of axons and dendrites. These fibers serve as connecting pathways between the control centers in the cerebrum and cerebellum and the spinal cord. Control centers are found within the brain stem for involuntary movements of such vital organs as the:
  - Heart
  - Blood vessels
  - Lungs
  - Stomach
  - Intestines

The Spinal Cord

The spinal cord (Figure 7.49) extends from the medulla to the second lumbar vertebra in the spinal canal, which is above the small of the back, a distance of about 17 inches. Nerves entering and leaving the spinal cord carry impulses to and from the control centers. Certain reflex activities performed without conscious thought are controlled within the cord. Pulling your hand away from something hot is an example of this type of reflex activity (Figure 7.50).

The Meninges

Three membranes, called **meninges**, surround both the brain and the spinal cord. They are the

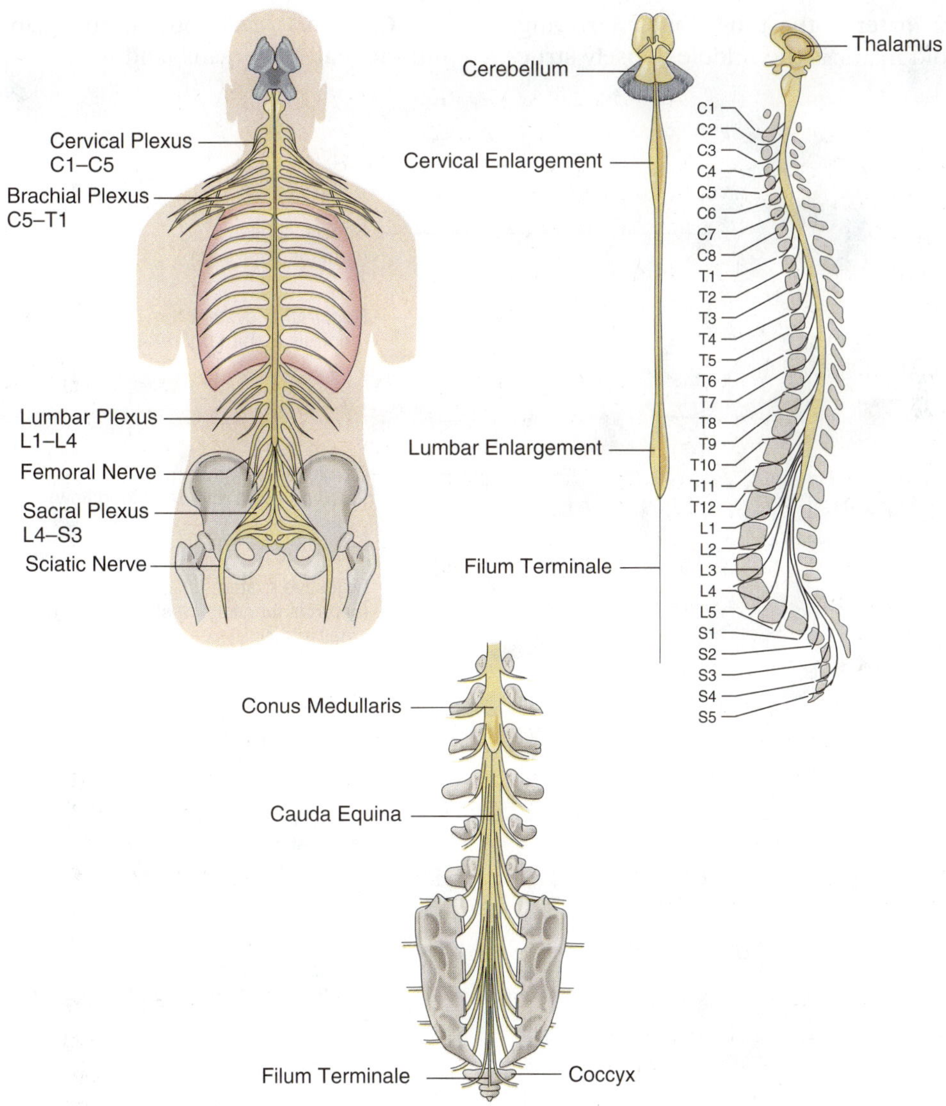

FIGURE 7-49 Spinal cord and nerves.

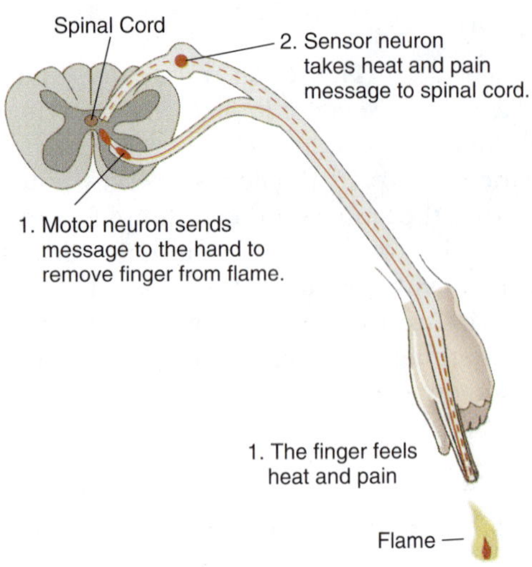

FIGURE 7-50 Reflex arc.

dura mater, the arachnoid mater, and the pia mater.

The dura mater is the tough outer covering. The arachnoid mater is the middle, loosely structured layer. It is filled with cerebrospinal fluid. The pia mater is the innermost, delicate layer. It is very vascular (contains many blood vessels) and clings to the brain, spinal cord, and nerve roots.

Cerebrospinal Fluid

Ventricles are cavities within the cerebrum that are lined with highly vascular tissue. These tissues produce **cerebrospinal fluid (CSF)**, which flows around the brain and the spinal cord. The cerebrospinal fluid bathes the central nervous system as tissue fluid and cushions it against shock and possible injury.

Special Relationships: The Autonomic Nervous System

The phrase *autonomic nervous system (ANS)* refers to special pathways that travel in cranial and spinal nerves (Figure 7.51). The control center is in the brain stem. The pathways begin in the CNS and reach out to the glands, smooth muscle walls of organs, and heart.

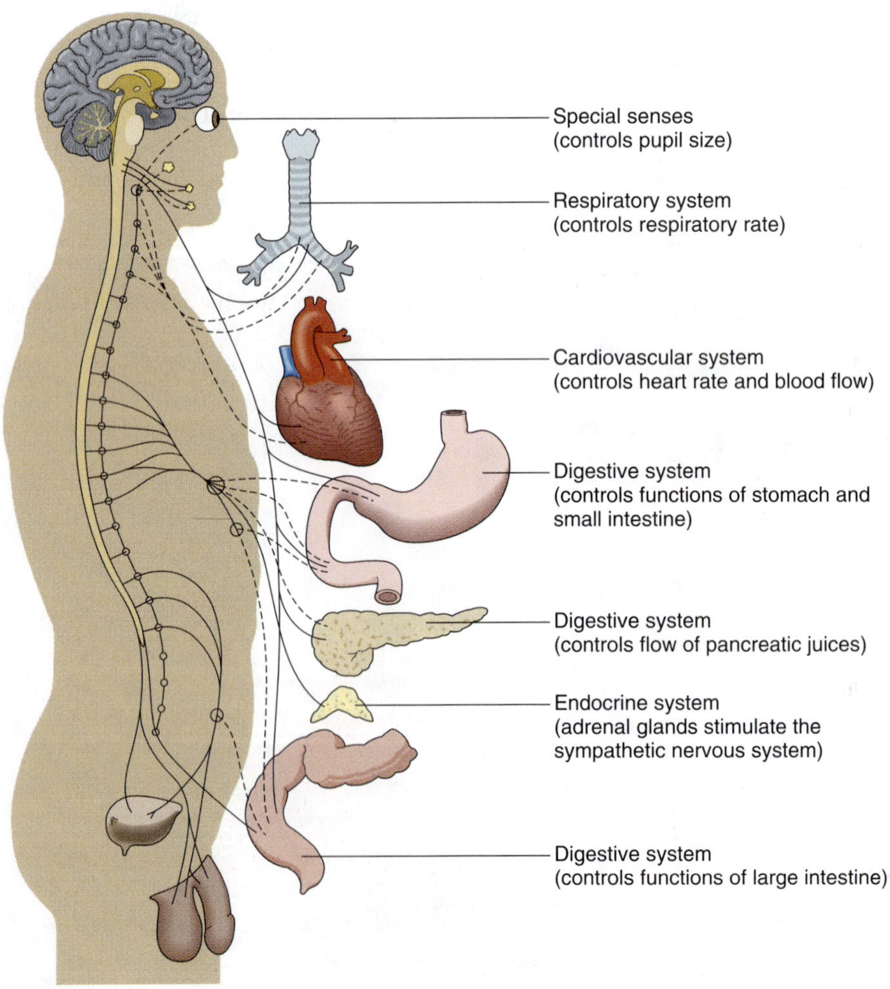

FIGURE 7-51 Autonomic nervous system.

The autonomic nervous system consists of two parts: sympathetic fibers and parasympathetic fibers. Sympathetic fibers stimulate activities that prepare the body to deal with emergency situations. It is called the mechanism of "fight or flight." Parasympathetic fibers control the usual functions of moderate heartbeat, digestion, elimination, respiration, and glandular activity.

Sensory Receptors

The ends of the dendrites carrying sensations to the central nervous system are found throughout the body.

- Some begin in joints and bring information about body positions to the brain.
- Others in the skin carry sensations of pain, heat, pressure, and cold.
- Those in the nose carry the sense of smell.
- The dendrites in the tongue carry the sense of taste.

Sensory dendrites also receive stimulation through two very special end organs, the eye and the ear. All of these structures are called sensory receptors because they carry information about the outside world to the brain. The brain interprets and processes the information.

The Eye

The eye (Figures 7.52A and 7.52B) is a hollow ball filled with two liquids called the *aqueous humor* and the *vitreous humor*. The wall of the eye is made up of three layers:

- The sclera: A tough, white outer coat that is protective. The **cornea** is the transparent portion in the front. Light rays pass through the cornea into the eye.

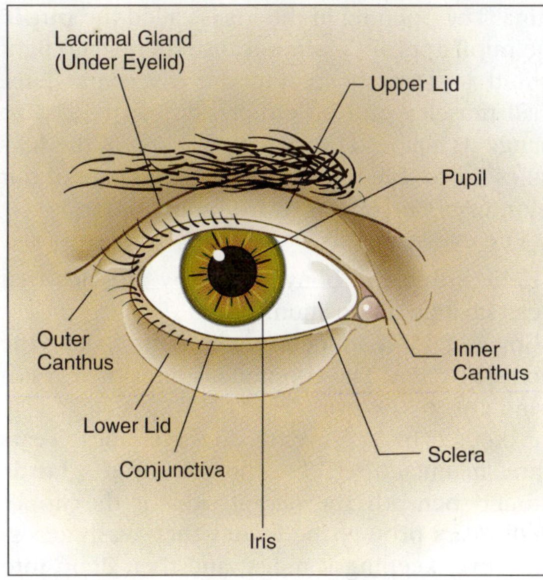

FIGURE 7-52A External view of the eye.

- The choroid: The nutritive layer found beneath the sclera. The choroid nourishes the eye tissues through its large number of blood vessels.
- The retina: The innermost layer is made up of neurons that are sensitive to light. The neurons join together and their axons leave the eye as the optic nerve. The two nerves cross beneath the brain and carry their impulses to the occipital lobe of the cerebrum to let us know what we are seeing.

Seeing. We see as light enters the eye through the cornea. The amount of light entering the eye is controlled by the iris. The **iris** is the colored portion of the eye. It is found behind the cornea. Fluid between the cornea and iris helps to bend the light rays and bring them to focus on the

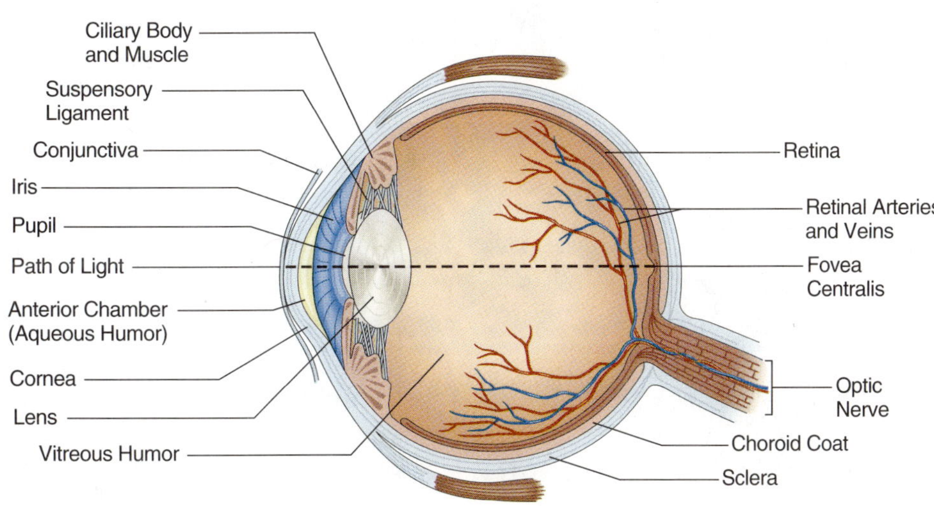

FIGURE 7-52B Internal view of the eye.

retina. The opening in the iris is called the **pupil**. The pupil appears black because there is no light behind it. Directly behind the iris is the lens. Small muscles pull on either side of the lens to change its shape. The changing shape of the lens makes it possible for us to adjust the range of our vision from far to near or from near to far.

The eye is:

- Held within the bony socket by muscles that can change its position.
- Covered by a mucous membrane, called the **conjunctiva**. The conjunctiva lines the eyelids and covers the eye.
- Protected by the eyelids and eyelashes. Tears are manufactured by the **lacrimal glands** found beneath the lateral side of the upper lid. Tears protect the eye as they wash across the eye, keeping it moist, and then drain into the nasal cavity.

The Ear

Just as the eye is sensitive to light, the ear is sensitive to sound (Figure 7.53). The ear functions in hearing and equilibrium (balance). The ear has three parts: the outer ear, the middle ear, and the inner ear. The outer ear consists of the visible external structure known as the *pinna* and a canal, which directs sound waves toward the middle ear. At the end of the canal is the eardrum, or **tympanic membrane**. Sound waves cause the eardrum to vibrate.

The middle ear is made up of three tiny bones called **ossicles**. The ossicles form a chain across the middle ear from the tympanic membrane to an opening in the inner ear. These bones are known as the:

- Incus or anvil
- Malleus or hammer
- Stapes or stirrup

Small tubes, called the **eustachian tubes**, lead from the nasopharynx into the middle ear to equalize pressure on either side of the eardrum. Sound waves pushing against the tympanic membrane cause the ossicles to vibrate and push against the opening of the inner ear. This motion starts fluid moving in the inner ear.

The inner ear is a very complex structure. It has two main parts: the cochlea and three semicircular canals. The **cochlea** looks somewhat like a coiled snail shell. Within the cochlea are the tiny dendrites of the hearing or auditory nerve.

Fluid covers the dendrites. When the fluid is set in motion by the vibration of the middle ear bones, it stimulates the dendrites with sound sensations. The auditory nerves, one from each ear, carry the sensations to the temporal lobe of the cerebrum to let us know what we are hearing.

The three **semicircular canals** also contain liquid and nerve endings. When these nerve endings are stimulated, impulses about the position of the head are sent to the brain. This helps us keep our balance.

Aging Changes in the Nervous System

The nervous system (Figure 7.62) is vital to the body's ability to communicate internally, as well

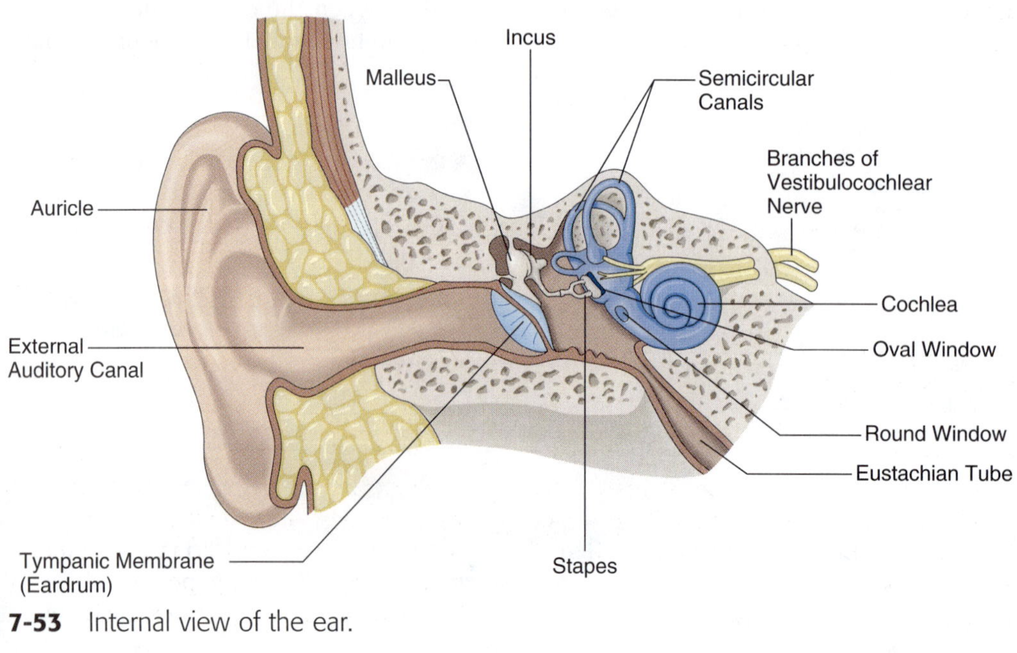

FIGURE 7-53 Internal view of the ear.

as with the environment. The nervous system consists of the brain (Figure 7.63), spinal cord, and all the nerves in the body. Messages travel back and forth from the nerves, spinal cord, and brain. These messages control how the body functions (Figure 7.49). They also tell the body how to react to environmental conditions. For example, if you touch something very hot with your hand, the nerves send a message to the brain (Figure 7.54). The brain sends a message back telling you to pull your hand away.

Aging changes in the nervous system include:

- More time is needed for tasks involving speed, balance, coordination, and fine motor activities, such as those involving the fingers.

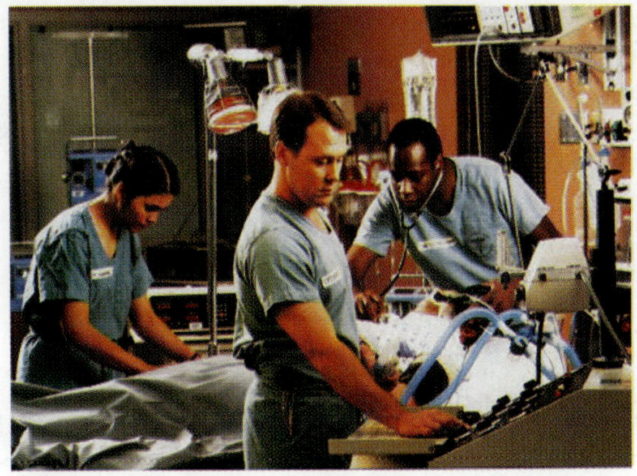

FIGURE 7-54 Critical care nursing. "Be All You Can Be." *((Courtesy of United States Government, as represented by the Secretary of the Army)*

Common Conditions

The nervous system usually remains healthy. However, injury or disease to the brain, spinal cord, or nerves requires appropriate treatment.

Increased Intracranial Pressure

The structures within the skull normally exert a certain amount of pressure, called the **intracranial pressure**. The pressure is due to:

- Nervous tissue
- Cerebrospinal fluid
- Blood flowing through cerebral vessels

Any change in the size or amount of these components changes the pressure. Increased intracranial pressure can result from:

- Head injury. Bleeding from damaged blood vessels and edema puts pressure on the delicate nervous tissue.
- Inflammation or infection plus edema.
- Intracranial bleeding due to ruptured blood vessels. This is called a cerebrovascular accident (CVA).
- Toxins.
- High temperature.
- Blockage of the normal flow of cerebrospinal fluid.
- Tumors.

Signs and Symptoms. Indications of increased intracranial pressure include:

- Alteration in pupil size and response to light. In the normal eye, the pupil becomes smaller when a flash-light is directed at each eye. The equality of the pupils and their ability to react to light is an important observation when a head injury occurs.
- Headache.
- Vomiting.
- Loss of consciousness and sensation.
- **Paralysis**—loss of voluntary motor control.
- **Convulsions** (seizures)—uncontrolled muscular contractions that are often violent.

How long all or part of the symptoms remain depends on the extent and cause of damage to the brain cells. Remember also that paralysis is not always accompanied by sensory loss.

Specific Nursing Care. Patients who are acutely ill with head injuries or increased intracranial pressure require skilled nursing care (Figure 7.54). The nurse is responsible for monitoring the patient's:

- Level of consciousness
- Degree of orientation to time and place
- Reaction to pain and stimuli
- Vital signs

If you note any change in the patient's response or behavior as you are assisting in care, bring it to the nurse's attention immediately. Changes that might be very significant include:

- Incontinence
- Uncontrolled body movements
- Disorientation
- Deepening or lessening in the level of consciousness
- Dizziness
- Vomiting
- Alterations in speech
- Change in ability to follow directions

Once improved, the patient may be moved from a critical unit to an intermediate unit. From there, the patient may go to a long-term care facility for a possibly long period of convalescence. The patient may require extensive rehabilitation to regain functional skills. The nursing measures first established in the critical care unit must be maintained throughout this extended period.

Loss of sensation and decreased mobility make these patients more prone to pressure sores, infection, and contractures. You must continue to:

- Give special skin care.
- Carry out range-of-motion exercises.
- Check skin over pressure points frequently.
- Change the patient's position regularly.
- Report early signs of infection.
- Monitor elimination. Loss of muscle tone and inactivity may lead to constipation and impaction.
- Check drainage tubes such as indwelling catheters. They must receive careful attention.
- Provide reality orientation as needed.
- Be alert to any signs of mood change and plan extra time to provide essential support. Patients recovering from these illnesses often experience anxiety and depression.
- Keep a careful check on vital signs of any patient with a head injury. A special record (neurological monitoring record) may be kept for recording all observations.

Transient Ischemic Attack

A **transient ischemic attack (TIA)** is a temporary period of diminished blood flow to the brain. The attack comes on rapidly and may last from 2 to 15 minutes or for as long as 24 hours. Symptoms are similar to those of a stroke but are temporary and reversible. Transient ischemic attacks may occur once or several times in a lifetime. Persons experiencing TIAs are at risk for eventually suffering a stroke.

Stroke

A **stroke** is also called a **cerebrovascular accident (CVA)** or **brain attack**. It affects the vascular system and the nervous system. The complete or partial loss of blood flow to the brain tissue is frequently a complication of atherosclerosis or brain hemorrhage. Causes of CVA include:

- Vascular occlusion due to a thrombus, atherosclerotic plaques, or emboli that obstruct the flow of blood
- Intracranial bleeding as blood vessels rupture, releasing blood into the brain tissue

Remember, most nerve pathways cross. Therefore, damage on one side of the brain results in signs and symptoms on the opposite side of the body. Symptoms vary depending on the extent of interference with the circulation and on the area and amount of tissue damaged. Patients with damage to the right side of the brain will exhibit:

- Paralysis on the left side of the body (left **hemiplegia**).
- **Spatial-perceptual deficits**. This means it is difficult to distinguish right from left and up from down. The world may appear "tilted" to the person with right-brain damage. The patient will have problems propelling a wheelchair, setting down items, and carrying out the activities of daily living.
- Change in personality. The individual with right brain damage becomes very quick and impulsive.

If the left side of the brain is damaged, you will note:

- Paralysis on the right side of the body (right hemiplegia) (Figure 7.55).
- **Aphasia**—an inability to express or understand speech.
- Change in personality. The individual becomes very cautious, anxious, and slow to complete tasks.

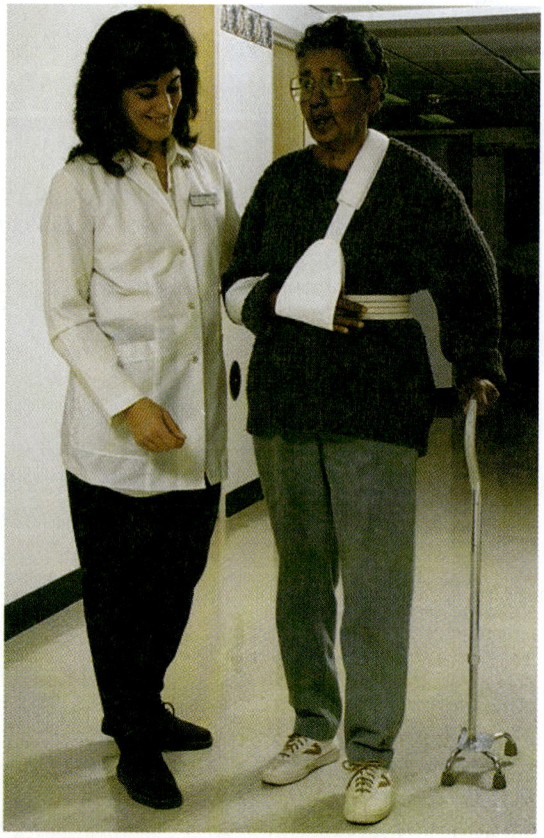

FIGURE 7-55 Right hemiplegia.

Other symptoms may be present with either right- or left-brain damage. These include:

- Sensory-perceptual deficits
  - Loss of **position sense**. The person cannot tell, for example, where an affected foot is or what position it is in without looking at it.
  - The inability to identify common objects such as a comb, a fork, a pencil, or a glass.
  - The inability to use common objects. The patient may know what an item is, such as a fork, but be unable to pick it up and use it. This is not a result of paralysis but is due to brain damage.
- **Unilateral neglect**. The patient ignores the paralyzed side of the body. For example, the affected arm may hang over the side of the wheelchair without the patient realizing where the arm is.
- **Hemianopsia**. This is impaired vision. Both eyes have only half vision. For example, if the patient has left hemiplegia, the left half of both eyes is blind (Figure 7.56). Remember this if a patient who has had a stroke eats the food on one side of the tray and leaves the food on the other side. The patient probably cannot see it. Turn the tray around.
- **Emotional lability**. Patients who have had a stroke may start to cry or laugh for no apparent reason. They have very little control over this and may be embarrassed.
- **Cognitive impairments**. There may be changes in the patient's intellectual function. This may affect memory, judgment, and problem-solving abilities.

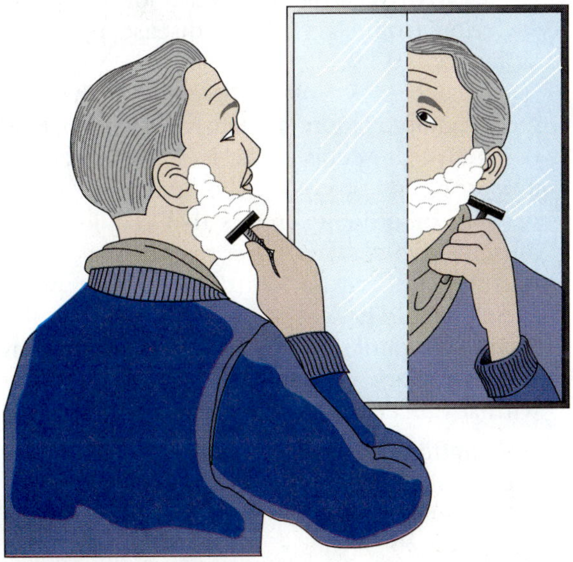

FIGURE 7-56 Hemianopsia is a common problem after a stroke.

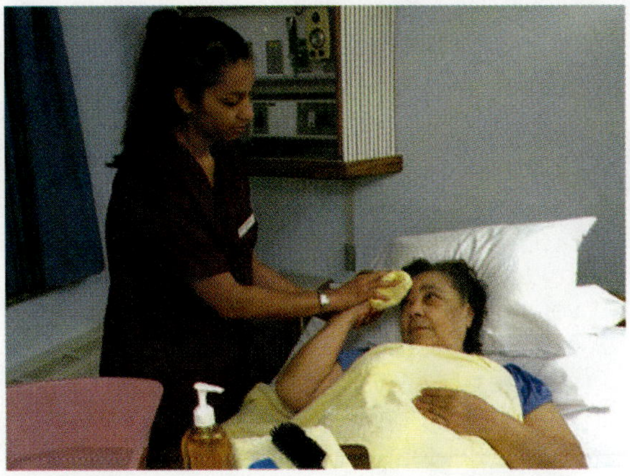

FIGURE 7-57 The patient who has had a stroke may need to relearn activities of daily living.

Nursing Care The goals of poststroke care include:

1. Maintaining the skills and abilities that the patient has left.
2. Preventing complications caused by immobility:
   - Contractures
   - Pressure ulcers
   - Pneumonia
   - Blood clots
3. Helping the patient regain functional abilities:
   - Activities of daily living (Figure 7.57)
   - Bowel and bladder control
   - Mobility
   - Communication skills

During Recovery. Recovery from a stroke is often a very frustrating experience for the patient. Caregivers must be patient. In your approach to the patient, remember two things:

1. The patient has more than enough frustration for both of you, so be careful not to let yours show. The last thing the patient needs is your silent reinforcement of his helplessness.
2. The degree and speed of recovery are directly related, in most cases, to the patience and encouragement of the caregivers with whom the patient has close contact.

Other interventions during recovery include:

- Physical therapy to increase independent mobility: bed movement, getting to the side of the bed, standing by the side of the bed, transferring out of bed and into a chair, and ambulation.
- Occupational therapy to regain the ability to perform the activities of daily living, such as bathing, grooming, dressing, and eating, with little or no assistance.

COMMUNICATION HIGHLIGHT Alert

Try to develop rapport with the patient on your first contact. At times, this is difficult because a stroke often causes mood changes. If the patient is newly dependent, he may also have mood or behavior problems. Be consistent and avoid becoming discouraged. Try to remember that the illness is causing the problem. Find the most effective means of communicating the information you need to convey. Ask yes or no questions whenever possible. Avoid treating the patient like a child and do not correct his speech. If you must repeat yourself, do so quietly and calmly. Use gestures, if necessary.

- Speech therapy to regain or to learn different methods of communication. The speech therapist also works with swallowing problems caused by the stroke.
- Nursing care to:
  - Implement bowel and bladder training programs, or give catheter care if necessary
  - Implement pressure ulcer prevention programs
  - Reinforce the programs provided by the therapists
- Care to prevent contractures by:
  - Positioning the patient appropriately and changing positions at least every 2 hours
  - Performing passive range-of-motion exercises as directed
  - Applying splints or braces as ordered

All staff can help with rehabilitation efforts by:

- Encouraging the patient to communicate
- Maintaining a positive and supportive attitude at all times
- Providing only the assistance that the patient needs
- Following approaches consistently as outlined in the patient's care plan

Convalescence is often long. The nursing care is demanding, requiring much patience and understanding.

Aphasia

Stroke victims often suffer from aphasia or language impairment. They have difficulty forming thoughts or expressing them in coherent ways. This is extremely frustrating and frightening for the patient and family.

- **Receptive aphasia** means that the person cannot comprehend communication.
- **Expressive aphasia** means that the person cannot properly form thoughts or express them coherently.
- **Global aphasia** means that the person has lost all language abilities.

Parkinson's Disease

Parkinson's disease is believed to be caused by not having enough neurotransmitters (dopamine) in the brain stem and cerebellum. The symptoms are progressive over many years. Some people will show minor changes. Others will have much more obvious symptoms (Figure 7.58).

Signs and Symptoms. Signs and symptoms of Parkinson's disease include:

- **Tremors** (uncontrolled trembling). Tremors of the hands commonly affect the fingers and thumb in such a way that an affected person will appear to be rolling a small object (such as a pill) between them. These tremors occur frequently. They usually begin in the fingers, then involve the entire hand and arm, and finally affect an entire side of the body. Starting on one side, the tremors eventually involve both sides of the body. Tremors are more evident when the person is inactive. A typical posture of a patient suffering from Parkinson's disease is shown in Figure 7.44.
- Muscular rigidity (loss of flexibility). The muscular rigidity is more evident when the patient is inactive. It seems to be lessened when the person sleeps or engages in activities such as walking or other exercises that require large-muscle involvement. The rigidity makes the person with Parkinson's disease more prone to falls and injury.
- **Akinesia** (difficulty and slowness in carrying out voluntary muscular activities). Persons with advanced Parkinson's typically have:
  - A shuffling manner of walking
  - Difficulty starting the process of walking
  - Difficulty stopping smoothly once walking has started
  - Affected speech, causing words to be slurred and poorly spoken (enunciated)

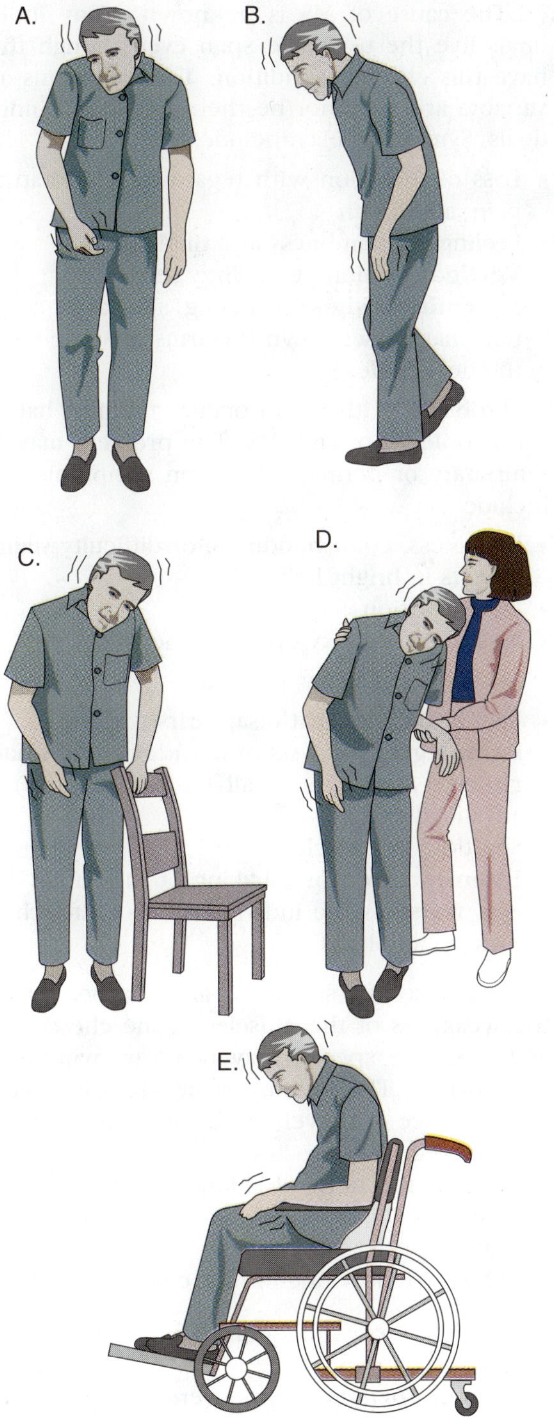

FIGURE 7-58 Progression of Parkinson's disease. A. The patient leans slightly forward and develops flexion of the affected arm. B. The patient stoops forward slightly and walks with a shuffling gait. C. As the disease progresses, the patient needs support to prevent falling. The patient tends to shuffle faster and faster, leaning farther forward until he falls on his face. D. The disease progresses to the point where the patient needs assistance for ambulation. E. The patient has profound weakness and severe tremors. Ambulation becomes impossible.

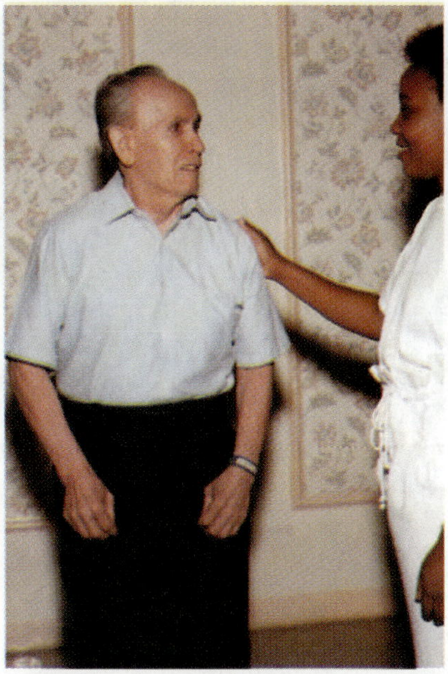

Ventral view

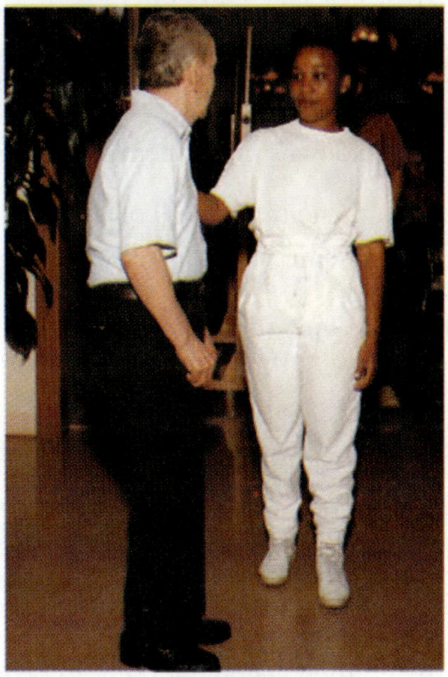

Lateral view

FIGURE 7-59 The typical posture of a patient with Parkinson's disease. In addition to the standing posture, note the patient's hands.

- Facial muscles that lose expressiveness and emotional response
- Loss of autonomic nervous control. Because of loss of autonomic nervous control, persons with Parkinson's may:
  - drool.
  - become incontinent.
  - become constipated.
  - retain urine.

DIFFICULT SITUATIONS

Patients with Parkinson's disease may have inconsistent needs for physical support and assistance. If the patient is tired, he may need more support than when he is rested. When the patient is stressed, the tremors may worsen, increasing the need for hands-on assistance.

- Mood swings and gradual behavioral changes. A patient may appear happy and positive one moment, and then be depressed the next. The depression tends to be progressive. Personality and behavioral changes may occur that cause psychotic breakdowns and dementia in later stages.

Treatment. The treatment consists of:

- Surgery for some younger persons
- Drug therapy
- Therapy to limit the muscular rigidity and to meet the basic physical and emotional needs

Nursing Care. Nursing care of the person with Parkinson's disease includes:

- Maintaining a calm environment. Symptoms are more intense when the patient is under stress.
- Assisting and supervising the activities of daily living. For example, directing food into the mouth and then keeping it there to be chewed and swallowed is very difficult for many persons with Parkinson's disease.
- Providing emotional support and encouragement.
- Carrying out a program of general and specific exercises.
- Providing protection for patients with dementia.

Multiple sclerosis

Multiple sclerosis (MS) generally occurs in young adults. It is the result of the loss of insulation (myelin) around central nervous system nerve fibers. This interferes with the ability of the nerve fibers to function.

The cause of MS is unknown. Many individuals live the usual life span even though they have this chronic condition. The symptoms are variable and may not be the same for all individuals. Symptoms may include:

- Loss of sensation with regard to temperature, pain, and touch
- Feelings of numbness and tingling
- **Vertigo** (a spinning or dizzy sensation)
- **Lhermitte's sign** (a tingling, shock-like sensation that passes down the arms or spine when the neck is flexed)

Problems with vision occur in almost half of the people who have MS. The problem may be temporary or permanent. Vision symptoms may include:

- Blurriness, color blindness, or difficulty seeing objects in bright light
- Double vision
- **Nystagmus** (jerky eye movements)

Mobility is usually affected:

- Pain in the legs that disappears with rest
- **Paraplegia** (paralysis of both legs) and **quadriplegia** (paralysis of all four extremities) in advanced cases
- Spasticity of muscles
- **Intention tremor** (shaking of the hands that gets worse as the individual tries to touch or pick up an object)

In severe MS, speech is affected because of the weakness of the muscles in the chest, face, and lips. The speech may be slow, with poor articulation. The mind usually remains alert. Incontinence of bowel and bladder are common in advanced cases.

One of the most disabling features of MS is fatigue. The fatigue is very real and is not psychological.

MS may follow one of four courses:

- *Benign course:* mild attacks with long periods of no symptoms.
- *Exacerbating-remitting:* Severe attacks (exacerbations) followed by periods of partial or complete recovery (remissions). Often the periods of exacerbation get longer and more severe with shorter periods of remission.
- *Slowly progressive:* slow, steady deterioration.
- *Rapidly progressive:* deterioration is rapid and progressive and may be life-threatening.

Nursing Care. Nursing care of the patient with multiple sclerosis includes:

1. Implement pressure ulcer prevention program.

DIFFICULT SITUATIONS

A warm bath or shower is often very relaxing to a patient with multiple sclerosis. However, you must make sure that the water is not too hot, which temporarily intensifies some symptoms of MS. Keeping bath water at about 100°F to 105°F is best. Take your responsibility for assisting with range-of-motion exercises seriously. ROM is especially important in patients with MS to maintain joint mobility and muscle tone, reduce spasticity, improve coordination, and boost self-esteem.

2. Implement contracture prevention programs through consistent changes of position and passive range-of-motion exercises. Apply splints correctly, if ordered.
3. Pay careful attention to catheter care if the patient has an indwelling catheter, to prevent bladder infections.
4. Encourage independence. Follow instructions from the nurse or the therapists for specific techniques to use.
5. Help the patient maintain a balanced schedule of rest and activity.
6. Provide emotional support and encouragement.

Treatment. There is no known way to stop the progression of the disease. Treatment consists of maintaining functional ability as long as possible through general health practices and physical therapy.

Post Polio Syndrome (PPS)

Polio is a very serious neurological disease that has been with us since at least 1350 B.C. This disease is caused by a virus. The virus attacks the motor neurons in the spinal cord. Muscles affected by these neurons no longer function properly, resulting in weakness and paralysis. Some patients had respiratory paralysis, and needed a special ventilator to breathe. Others had speech and swallowing problems. Most had paralysis and weakness in the arms and legs. Many people died as a result of polio. Most of those who survived learned to overcome their disabilities and lead productive lives.

There were large annual outbreaks of polio in the United States every summer. The largest was in 1952. In 1955, an injectable vaccine was developed to prevent polio. Because of the severity of the condition, most children received the vaccination. In 1962, an oral polio vaccine was developed. Both vaccines continue to be used today. Because of the effectiveness of the vaccines, infectious polio has been eliminated in the United States.

Post polio syndrome (PPS) is a neurologic condition marked by increased weakness and abnormal muscle fatigue in persons who had polio many years earlier. Estimates are that 30 to 70% of all polio survivors will develop this condition. There are several theories about the cause of PPS. The most common involves the motor neurons. Most polio survivors have about half as many motor neurons as others who were not affected by polio. It is believed that motor neurons that were not destroyed by the initial polio infection compensated by sprouting new connections. Some of the new neurons adapted to innervate areas that are five to seven times larger than normal. These neurons may be slowly dying, perhaps because of years of overuse. As the neurons die, they lose their muscle connections, and muscles stop responding.

Signs and Symptoms. Signs and symptoms of PPS range from annoying to debilitating. Onset may be sudden, following trauma, infection, surgery, a fall, or a stressful event. The new injury puts stress on the remaining motor neurons, causing further reduction in function, pain, and fatigue. Signs and symptoms include:

- fatigue that may be debilitating.
- new joint and muscle pain.
- new weakness in muscles affected by polio; unaffected muscles are also affected. The new weakness may be more prominent on one side of the body.
- new dyspnea and other respiratory problems.
- severe cold intolerance, even with mild cold exposure. This causes the muscle weakness to worsen, the arms or legs to become pale or cyanotic, and the extremities to feel cold to the touch. The patient may say, "It's so cold it hurts."
- muscle spasms and cramps that are sometimes severe and painful.

- difficulty swallowing.
- difficulty falling asleep and waking frequently during the night.

Some PPS patients become anxious when they are hospitalized. Emotional expressions of discouragement and displays of anger are fairly common. The patient may be fearful. Health care practices and attitudes were very different during the era of the polio epidemic. Many PPS patients were children during the original infection. They were in the hospital for a long time, and may have been forcibly separated from their parents. This was traumatic and caused them to feel isolated. Sadly, some were physically, emotionally, and sexually abused by hospital personnel. When a person with PPS is in the hospital, old feelings and fears sometimes return. The patient may experience feelings of fear and powerlessness that she cannot or will not talk about. Provide reassurance and emotional support, and report the patient's behavior to the nurse.

Most PPS patients experience pain daily. Muscle spasms often worsen the pain. Use nursing comfort measures, such as positioning and a backrub, to relieve pain. Inform the nurse of the patient's complaints of pain. Reducing strain and adjusting activities to conserve energy also help relieve pain. You may be asked to provide a heat treatment, which also relieves pain.

Many polio survivors have disturbed sleep because of muscle spasms, pain, or anxiety. Some experience sleep apnea, but are not aware of it. Body positioning is important during sleep to support weakened areas and deformities. Certain positions may be painful for the patient and extra pillows may be needed for support. Observe the patient's sleep at night and manage problems as they arise. Report your observations to the nurse.

Fatigue occurs daily, and can be debilitating. It may worsen as the day progresses. Some require more sleep than others who are not affected by PPS. Encourage the patient to rest and nap periodically throughout the day. Help the patient pace her activities and use measures to conserve energy. Therapy may be ordered to teach the patient to conserve energy.

About one-fifth of all PPS patients have swallowing problems. This increases the risk of choking. Position the patient as upright as possible while he is eating, and for 30 to 60 minutes after meals. Monitor the patient while eating and teach her to avoid talking while eating. Encourage her to alternate food and fluid, and to avoid swallowing when her head is tipped back. Assist with oral care after meals to remove retained food particles.

Patients with PPS have serious problems with cold because the nerves that control blood vessel size were destroyed by the virus. The legs and feet are commonly affected. One theory is that people with PPS function as if it were 20 degrees colder than the actual temperature. Their legs and feet turn bright red following a hot bath. When the patient stands up, she may become dizzy or faint as blood pools in the legs, causing the blood pressure to drop. If the patient complains of cold, assist her with socks or extra blankets. You may be instructed to soak the feet in warm water, or assist with a warm bath. Caution the patient to call for help before getting out of the tub.

Surgical Procedures. Post polio patients who are admitted for surgery have many special needs. They are much more sensitive to anesthesia than persons who have not had polio. They require less medication and half the anesthesia, yet take twice as long as other patients to recover from the anesthesia. Because of this, the patient with PPS must be monitored closely for other problems. Patients may:

- Shiver violently after surgery. Provide warm blankets.
- Have side effects from common drugs. Monitor closely for abnormalities, and report to the nurse promptly.
- Have problems from blood loss, even a small amount. Monitor the operative site and vital signs carefully and report to the nurse.
- Have respiratory problems because of muscle weakness and lung problems. Encouraging the patient to cough and deep breathe after surgery is very important.
- Be unable to reposition themselves in bed. Assist the patient as needed.
- Have positioning problems because of deformities or discomfort. Do your best to make the patient comfortable. Use pillows and props for comfort and support.
- Vomit. This may cause fainting if the patient is upright. Monitor for choking. Report nausea or vomiting to the nurse.
- Choke on secretions. Position the patient on his side until he is fully awake. Monitor closely.
- Have problems with transfers and ambulation after surgery. Instruct the patient to call when she is ready to get out of bed. Have the patient dangle before rising. Use a transfer belt for safey.

Nursing Assistant Care. Patients with post polio syndrome are usually in the hospital for treatment of another condition. The problems caused by post polio are seldom severe enough to require hospitalization. However, they complicate the care of other conditions and procedures. Remember that these patients have lived with their polio condition for years and have found ways to adapt to it. Overall, they are experts in their own care. Respect their expertise. Coping with the new problems from PPS is often much more difficult than the recovery from the original illness. Be prepared to help with activities of daily living, bed mobility, transfers, and ambulation. Patients with post polio syndrome may have many special needs. They may not complain because most were taught that part of their recovery includes being "normal." They have spent their lives trying to appear normal. Asking for help may be very difficult for these patients.

Most PPS patients have their homes arranged so they can function independently. Temporarily staying in a different environment, such as a hospital, can be very troublesome for the patient. She may need help with tasks that she could do independently at home. Most PPS patients fear becoming dependent on others. The patient may have great difficulty asking for help. Anticipate her needs and ask if assistance is needed. Do not be surprised if the patient refuses your offer of help. Respect the refusal, but advise the patient that accepting assistance is different from being dependent. In fact, assistance may help the patient to remain independent. Even if the patient refuses your help, stand by to see if she can perform the task or procedure safely. Adapt the environment, whenever possible, for optimal independent function. You may do this by moving furniture, or bringing a bedside commode, for example. Most polio survivors are in tune to what their bodies are telling them. If the patient says she cannot do something, pay attention.

Amyotrophic Lateral Sclerosis (ALS)

Amyotrophic lateral sclerosis (ALS) is a progressive neuromuscular disease that causes muscle weakness and paralysis. It is a disease of the motor nerves that control voluntary movement. The cause is unknown. There seems to be a familial link in about 10% of the cases. ALS occurs in all races and both genders, although it is more common in men. The most common age of onset is 55, but it can occur in persons of any age. It is a progressive condition for which there is no cure. ALS is almost always fatal. In the United States, ALS is also called Lou Gehrig's disease, after a famous baseball player. Other names may be used in other countries. About half of the patients diagnosed with ALS die within 18 months, although some may live for many years. One drug has been successful in slowing progression of the disease, but there is no known cure. Some medications are used to relieve the symptoms.

Signs and Symptoms. ALS takes months to diagnose because the signs and symptoms are similar to those of other neurologic conditions. Common signs and symptoms of ALS are:

- stumbling, tripping, and falling
- loss of strength and muscle control in hands, arms, and legs
- difficulty speaking
- difficulty swallowing
- drooling
- breathing becoming progressively more difficult
- muscle cramping, shaking, and twitching, progressing to spasticity
- muscle weakness and atrophy
- abnormal reflexes

ALS is not a painful disease, but the effects of ALS often cause pain. These are:

- muscle cramps
- contractures
- constipation
- burning eyes
- swelling feet
- muscle aches
- pressure sores

ALS does not affect the entire body. The patient's mental acuity is intact. Depression is common. The heart, bowel and bladder control, and sexual function are not affected. The eyes are the last muscles affected and are sometimes not affected at all.

Progression of ALS. Progression of ALS varies with the patient. Worsening occurs over several months to several years. A common pattern is:

- Difficulty walking, causing the patient to use a cane, then a walker, then a wheelchair.
- As the legs weaken, the hands and arms also become weaker.
- The patient loses the ability to write and feed herself.
- The patient experiences difficulty speaking, chewing, swallowing, and talking.
- Eventually a feeding tube becomes necessary.
- The patient needs an alternate communication system.
- Chest and diaphragm muscles weaken, causing lung problems.
- The patient needs a ventilator to stay alive.

DIFFICULT SITUATIONS

ALS is a particularly cruel disease that causes fairly rapid degeneration of the nervous system, making the patient dependent. The mind remains intact and alert, so the patient is aware of each small change and its implications. Strive to develop a good rapport with the patient and provide generous emotional support and compassion.

Nursing Assistant Care. Most ALS patients are cared for at home, with brief hospitalizations to manage complications. Because of this, ALS often involves the whole family. Patients are taught to manage their own illness. Allow the patient to be in control of daily routines, and respect his intelligence. Adaptive equipment is used to maintain independence for as long as possible.

Many ALS patients are not bedridden, despite being completely paralyzed. Special wheelchairs and portable ventilators are often used so patients can get out of bed. Follow the patient's care plan for mobility. If the patient does not get out of bed, reposition and turn her at least every 2 hours, or more often, as instructed.

Nursing care is designed to prevent complications of immobility. The most common problems are constipation, contractures, and pressure ulcers. You will also take measures to prevent choking and infection. Care of the patient is largely determined by the stage of the patient's disease at hospital admission. Follow the care plan and the nurse's instructions. Care of the typical ALS patient involves:

- Attention to positioning. An upright position (such as high Fowler's) may be ordered to ease respirations.
- Range-of-motion and light exercises to prevent deformities and maintain the strength of muscles that are not yet affected.
- Assisting the patient to use the incentive spirometer.
- Having the patient rest before meals to conserve muscle strength and reduce the risk of choking.
- Providing small, frequent feedings.
- Taking swallowing precautions when feeding the patient. The speech therapist may have taught the patient positions and techniques to use to prevent choking. Commonly, the patient is as upright as possible, with the neck flexed slightly forward.
- Not washing solid foods down with liquids. This increases the risk of choking and aspiration in the ALS patient.
- Checking the mouth after meals to make sure that no food particles remain. They can cause choking later. Provide mouth care promptly after each meal.
- Scheduling rest and activities to preserve the patient's strength and energy.
- Using good infection control measures, handwashing, and standard precautions to reduce the risk of infection.

Seizure Disorder (Epilepsy)

Seizure disorder (convulsions, **epilepsy**) involves recurrent, transient attacks of disturbed brain function. It is characterized by various forms of convulsions called *seizures*. Not all seizures are alike. A seizure occurs when one or more of the following is present:

- An altered state of consciousness, which may be momentary or prolonged
- Convulsive uncontrolled movements
- Disturbances of feeling or behavior Seizures may develop:
- congenitally, associated with a difficult birth.
- following a head injury.
- as a result of increased intracranial pressure.
- as a result of lesions of the brain such as tumors.
- as a result of cerebrovascular accidents.
- as a result of high fever or infection, especially in infants and children.
- from taking certain medications or street drugs.

Some persons experience an aura just before the seizure occurs. An **aura** involves one of the senses. The person may smell an unusual odor or hear a sound. The aura is usually consistent and remains the same each time it is experienced. For some people the aura serves as a warning so the person can get to a safe place. Other people may not remember the aura.

Some people have service dogs that warn them of an impending seizure so they can take safety precautions before the seizure begins. A dog's sense of smell is much more sensitive than a human's. It is believed that the dog smells a chemical reaction that signals the onset of a

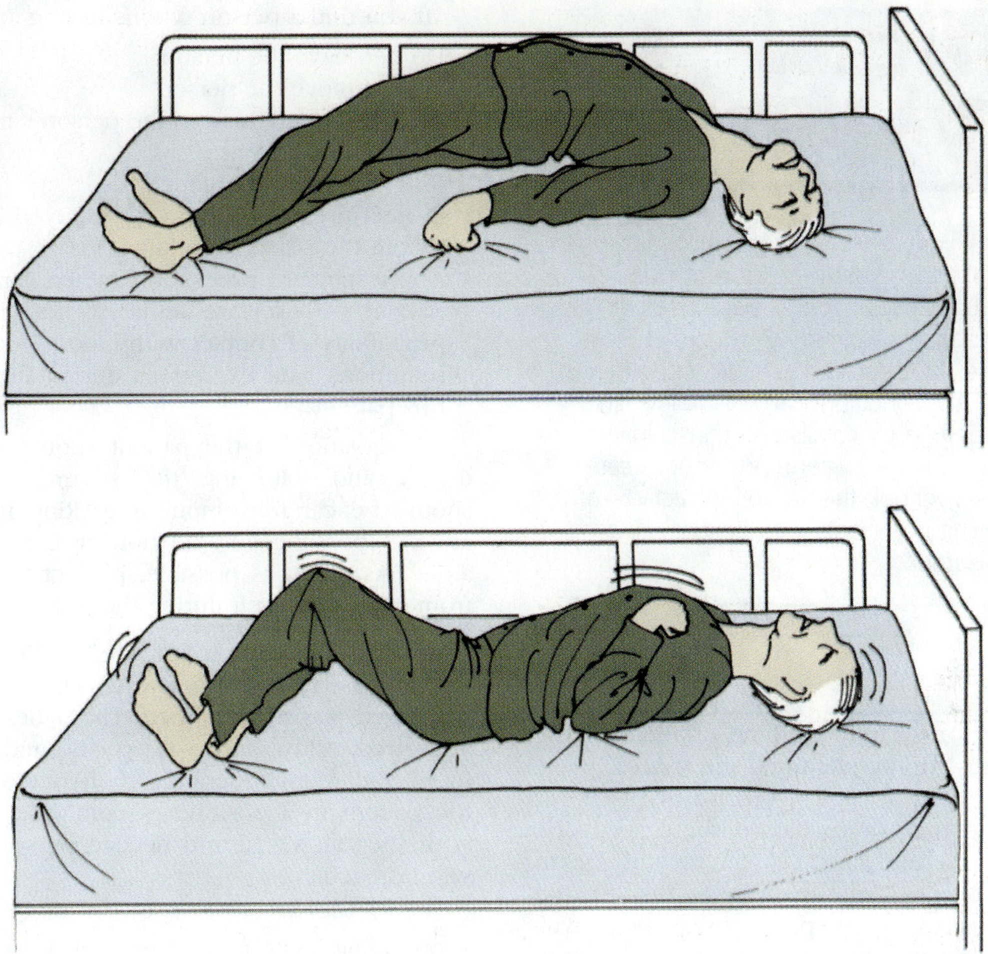

FIGURE 7-60 Generalized tonic-clonic seizures involve the entire body. Side rails should be padded for patients with seizure disorder. The side rails are down in this picture for clarity.

seizure. All states have access laws regarding service animals, but these vary widely. Your facility may have policies regarding the use of service animals while patients are hospitalized.

There are many different types and categories of seizure activity. The most common types of seizure activity are classified as follows:

- Partial seizures
  - There may or may not be loss of consciousness.
  - Seizures generally begin in one part of the body and involve only one side of the body.
- Generalized seizures (Figure 7.60)
  - These include **grand mal seizures**. There are also called **generalized tonic-clonic seizures**. There is bilateral generalized motor movement and muscular rigidity. Consciousness is lost and special awareness may or may not precede convulsive movements. The sensory awareness or aura may be in the form of lights, sounds, or aromas and is part of the seizure. When this seizure begins, the patient cries out, then falls to the floor. The muscles stiffen (tonic phase), then the extremities begin to jerk and twitch (clonic phase). The patient may lose bladder control. Consciousness returns slowly. After this seizure, the patient may feel tired, or be confused and disoriented. This state may last from a few minutes to several hours or days. The patient may fall asleep, or gradually become less confused until full consciousness returns.
- **Petit mal seizures** are characterized by momentary loss of muscle tone. These are also called **absence seizures**. The seizure begins without warning, and consists of a period of unconsciousness, in which the patient blinks rapidly, stares blankly, breathes rapidly, or makes chewing movements. The seizure lasts 2 to 10 seconds, then ends abruptly. The patient usually resumes normal activity immediately. Because these seizures are mild, they may go unnoticed. Children with absence

DIFFICULT SITUATIONS

Patients with epilepsy commonly take a drug called phenytoin to prevent seizures. This drug causes hyperplasia of the gums, a condition in which the normal cells increase, causing excess bulk and thickness. This condition can be relieved to some degree by consistent, conscientious attention to oral hygiene and mouth care. Do not overlook this important activity of daily living in patients with epilepsy or seizure disorder.

seizures may have learning problems if the seizures are not identified and treated.

- *Status epilepticus* is a seizure that lasts for a long time, or repeats without recovery. It is a serious medical emergency. Death may result if the patient is not treated immediately. Status epilepticus can be convulsive (tonic-clonic) or nonconvulsive (absence). A person in nonconvulsive status epilepticus may become confused or appear dazed. The highest incidence of status epilepticus occurs during the first year of life and after age 60. In elderly adults, most cases are related to cerebrovascular accidents.

Nursing Care During Seizures. The main nursing focus during a seizure is to:

- Prevent injury by:
  - Staying with the person
  - Assisting the person to lie down, if there is time
  - Making no attempt to restrain the person's movements or to put anything in her mouth
  - Moving away any object the person might hit, to protect the person from injuring herself
- Maintain an airway by:
  - Loosening clothing, particularly around the neck
  - Turning the person's head or body to one side so that saliva or vomitus drains out
  - Opening an airway, if necessary, by lifting the person's shoulders and allowing the head to tilt back

If you find a person who is having a seizure:

- Do not leave the person.
- Do not move the person.
- Do not put anything in the person's mouth.
- Maintain an airway.
- Ring or call for assistance.
- Protect the person from self-inflicted injury.
- Watch the person carefully.
- Apply standard precautions when caring for a patient with seizure activity. There is a high probability of contact with blood, body fluids, secretions, and excretions during the care of this patient.

Observation of the patient should be made during and following the seizure. Breathing should be carefully monitored. Ring for assistance, if possible, but do not leave the patient alone. As much as possible, protect the patient from injuring herself during the seizure.

Nursing Care after a Seizure. When the seizure stops, tell the patient where she is and what happened. Assist her to bed. The patient will be very tired. Allow her to sleep. She may be confused and require periodic reorientation. Leave the patient in a position of comfort and safety with the call signal and needed personal items within reach.

Other care includes:

- providing incontinent care, if necessary.
- checking the vital signs as instructed; you may take vital signs frequently until the patient is stable.
- monitoring the patient closely for return of seizure activity.
- assisting the nurse to administer oxygen or suctioning, if needed.

Report to the nurse:

- any change in the patient before the seizure, such as an aura, confusion, or change in behavior.
- a description of the way the seizure looked, including the body parts involved.
- loss of bowel or bladder control, eyes rolling upward, rapid blinking, biting tongue.
- the time the seizure started and stopped, if known.
- condition of the patient after the seizure.
- vital signs.

Spinal Cord Injuries

Injuries to the spinal cord result in loss of function and sensation below the level of the injury. These patients are particularly prone to contractures and pressure ulcers. Special terms have been given to the conditions resulting from such injury:

- Quadriplegia—both arms and legs are paralyzed (paralyzed from the neck area down)
- Paraplegia—lower part of the body is paralyzed

Flaccid paralysis involves loss of muscle tone and absence of tendon reflexes. Some patients have **spastic paralysis**. These patients have no voluntary movement. The extremities move in an involuntary pattern, similar to muscle spasms. The patient is aware of the movements, but cannot stop them. The type of paralysis is determined by the level of injury. Patients with upper motor injuries are more likely to exhibit spastic paralysis.

Signs and Symptoms. Signs and symptoms of paralysis vary with the level of the injury. The patient will be paralyzed below the level where the spinal cord was damaged. For example, an injury to the upper vertebrae in the neck will cause respiratory depression. The patient will be unable to move the arms and legs. He or she will lose bowel and bladder control. An injury near the waist will also cause loss of bowel and bladder control. The patient will be unable to move the legs.

Treatment. Treatment depends on the level of injury. Overall, treatment is directed at:

- preventing complications of immobility.
- preventing deformities.
- restoring the patient to the highest degree of independence possible.

Responsibilities of the Nursing Assistant. - Patients with spinal cord injury need long-term nursing care, which includes:

- Listening. Many persons with spinal cord injury are taught to give directions to caregivers who are doing for the person what the individual cannot do for himself.
- A consistently calm and patient approach, because the loss of sensory and motor functions often makes self-care difficult.
- Acceptance of the patient's expressions of anger, fear, and depression, as well as clumsy attempts at self-care. Remember that the patient's ability to think is not necessarily impaired. Frustration is even greater because these patients can no longer will their actions.
- Careful skin care, because:
  - Incontinence not only causes the patient embarrassment and discomfort but also makes the skin prone to breakdown
  - The lack of nervous stimulation decreases circulation to the skin
  - Pain and pressure cannot be felt

OSHA Alert

Patients with spinal cord injury can provide limited to no assistance with positioning, moving, and transfers. To prevent injury to your back, never move a patient who has a spinal cord injury by yourself. Make sure that another assistant is available to help you. The use of lift sheets, mechanical lifts, and other adjunctive devices makes moving the patient easier for both the patient and the nursing assistant.

- Attention to elimination needs. For example, suppositories may be given daily. A catheter may be inserted into the bladder, so catheter and drainage care will be needed. Special pads within plastic incontinence pants may also be used.
- Avoidance of contractures and deformities, which occur rapidly after the onset of paralysis. When moving and positioning patients with paralysis, move the extremities slowly and gently. Rapid, rough movements will cause spasticity. If a patient's extremities move into a position of flexion, position them in extension. If the extremities move into a position of extension, position them in flexion. Positioning devices may be necessary to maintain position. Attention to proper positioning is very important. This is a major key to preventing contractures and deformities in these high-risk patients.
- Provision of ROM exercises. These will be needed for the rest of the patient's life.
- Proper attention and care to prevent:
  - Respiratory infections
  - Urinary tract infections
  - Pressure ulcers

Autonomic Dysreflexia. Autonomic dysreflexia is a potentially life-threatening complication of spinal cord injury. It usually occurs in patients with injuries above the mid-thoracic area. It indicates uncontrolled sympathetic nervous system activity. Problems that seem minor can trigger this condition. As a rule, injuries that would normally cause pain below the level of spinal injury can set this life-threatening chain of events in motion. For example:

- overfull bladder (this is the most common cause)
- urinary retention
- urinary infection
- blocked catheter
- overfilled urinary drainage bag
- constipation or fecal impaction
- hemorrhoids
- infection or irritation in the abdomen, such as appendicitis or acute abdominal conditions
- pressure ulcers
- prolonged pressure by an object in the chair, shoe, wrinkled clothing, and the like
- minor injury, such as a cut, bruise, or abrasion
- ingrown toenails
- burns, including sunburn
- pressure on skin from tight or constrictive clothing
- menstrual cramps
- labor and delivery
- overstimulation during sexual activity
- fractured bones

Signs and symptoms of autonomic dysreflexia are:

- extremely high blood pressure, over 200/100
- severe headache
- red, flushed face
- red blotches on the skin above the level of spinal injury
- sweating above the level of spinal injury
- stuffy nose
- nausea
- bradycardia (pulse below 60)
- goose bumps below the level of injury
- cold, clammy skin below the level of injury

If you observe any of these signs and symptoms, notify the nurse immediately. Treatment for this condition involves identifying the offending stimulus and removing it. If you believe something has triggered the condition, inform the nurse. Remove tight and constricting clothing and shoes. Check the catheter and drainage bag. Follow the nurses' instructions.

Meningitis

Meningitis is an inflammation of the meninges. It is usually caused by microorganisms.

The signs and symptoms of meningitis are:

- Headache
- Nausea
- Stiffness of the neck
- Seizures
- Chills
- Elevated temperature

This condition is treated with antibiotics. If it is communicable, droplet precautions are used.

Cataracts

Cataracts (Figure 7.61) are the leading cause of vision loss in adults over the age of 55. Because of this, cataract surgery is one of the most common surgeries in the United States today.

Cataracts cause the normally clear lens of the eye to become cloudy. The cloudy (opaque) lens will not allow light rays to pass through. Therefore, the person is no longer able to see.

Treatment. Removal or replacement of the lens permits light rays to enter the eye. Sight is then restored. The lens is needed to adjust vision to different distances. The latest innovations in cataract surgery increase comfort and convenience for the patient. Until recently, most surgery for cataracts involved removing the center (nucleus) of the lens through a larger incision. Currently, most surgeons remove cataracts with a small incision and ultrasound.

The surgery is performed either as an outpatient procedure or in a day surgery center. The patient is admitted to the center in the morning and remains for one to two hours after the surgery, or until vital signs are stable. Eye drops are used to numb the eye. In this surgery, the cataract is removed. A plastic, silicone, or hydrogel lens is usually implanted (Figure 7.62A and 7.62B), and the incision is naturally sealed. Stitches are not used. Some surgeons apply a patch to the eye, but most do not.

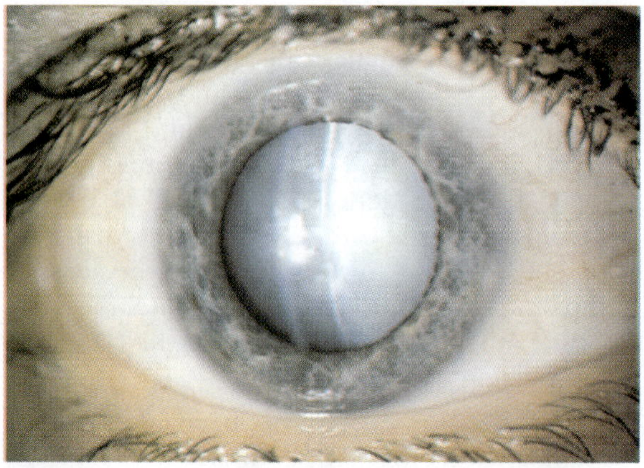

FIGURE 7-61 When the patient develops a cataract, the lens is cloudy instead of transparent. *(Courtesy of (Photo courtesy of Linda Jaakobovitch, Cincinnati Eye Institute)*

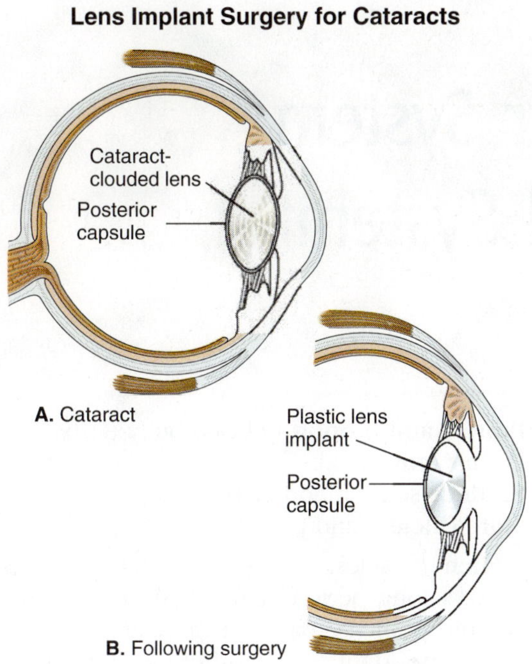

FIGURE 7-62A The lens is removed and the plastic intraocular lens is permanently placed in the eye.

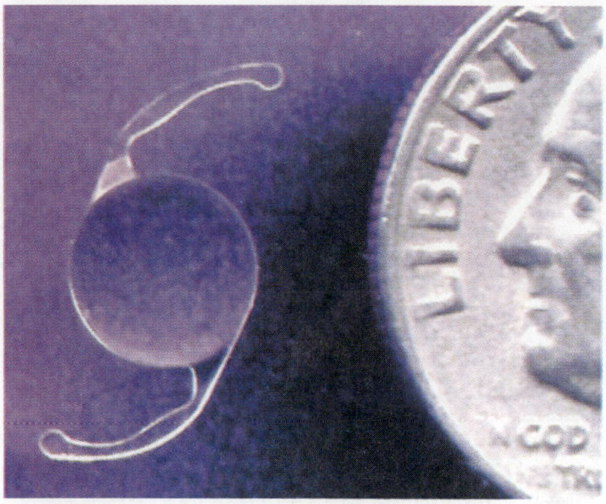

FIGURE 7-62B The lens implant is left in place. The patient cannot feel it after the eye heals. The lens implant is similar to a contact lens and is smaller than a dime. *(Courtesy of (Photo courtesy of Linda Jaakobovitch, Cincinnati Eye Institute)*

Nursing Care. Nursing care of the cataract patient includes:

- Routine postoperative care.
- Relief of pain. Discomfort is usually mild. If pain worsens, the patient complains of sharp pain, or vision decreases, promptly notify the nurse.
- Being sure all needed items, such as signal cords, are within easy reach.
- Taking extra precautions if the patient is confused or restless.
- Checking vital signs until stable.
- Keeping the surgical site undisturbed. After surgery, the patient may feel as if something (such as an eyelash) is in the eye. The patient may complain of itching. Slight fluid discharge may be present, and the eye may be sensitive to light and touch. Instruct the patient not to rub or squeeze the eye.
- Helping the patient to adapt to temporarily blurred vision. This is normal due to the bright lights used in surgery and drops used to dilate the eyes. The problem should resolve on its own promptly.
- Assisting the patient with initial ambulation, if needed. Many patients are able to walk without help immediately after surgery.

After the patient is stable, he or she is usually discharged home.

Orders regarding postoperative activity usually include:

- Protecting the eye from injury for the first four weeks.
- Avoid straining activities such as bending over, lifting objects that weigh more than 20 pounds, or strenuous coughing. Bending increases pressure in the eye. The patient can usually walk, climb stairs, and do light housework. The surgeon or nurse will instruct the patient on the level of activity.
- Using medicated eye drops for several weeks to promote healing and control pressure. These may sting a little, but the medication is necessary to promote a successful outcome.
- Wearing an eye shield at night, if instructed by the doctor.
- Informing the physician if there is an increase in pain or loss of vision.

The Muscular System
The Skeletal System

THE MUSCULOSKELETAL SYSTEM

The bony frame of the body is called the *skeleton*. Tissue that is made up of contractile fibers (fibers that contract and relax) or cells that produce movement are called *muscles*. Together, the skeleton and muscles are termed the musculoskeletal system.

The musculoskeletal system includes:

- Skeletal muscles
- Bones
- Joints
- Tendons
- Ligaments

The system functions to:

- Give shape and form to the body
- Protect and support delicate body parts
- Permit movement
- Produce some blood cells
- Store calcium and phosphorus

When muscles, bones, or joints have been injured, a long period of rest and inactivity may be required for the part to heal. During this period, it is important that all other moving parts get sufficient exercise. Bones that are not stressed lose calcium and become less functional.

Structure and Function

Bones. It will be helpful for you to learn the names and general location of the bones of the body. To learn the names, study the skeleton in Figure 7.63A and the skull in Figure 7.63B. Note

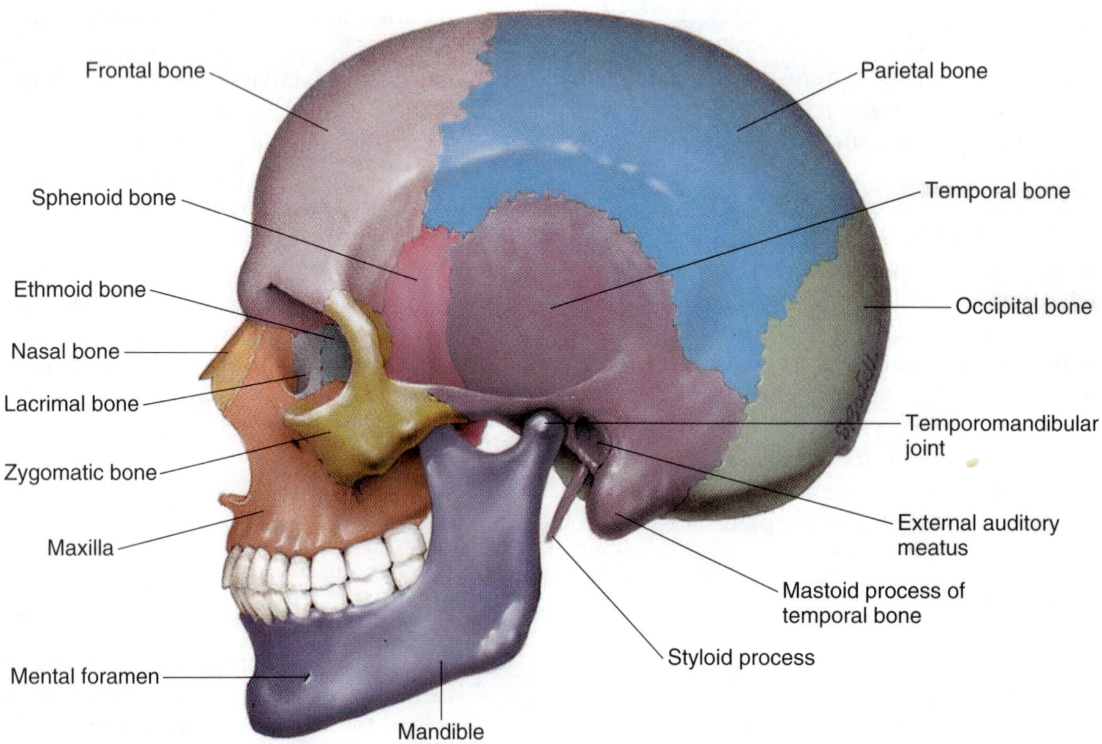

FIGURE 7-63B Bones of the skull.

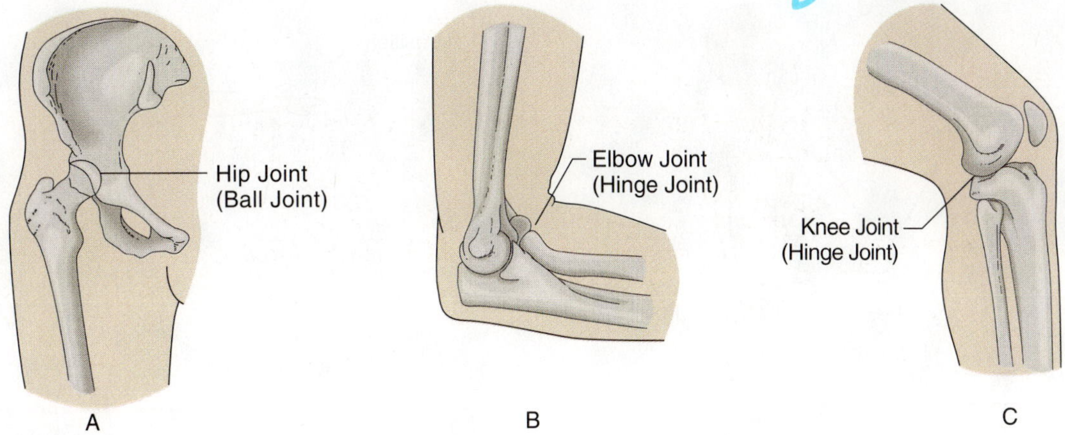

FIGURE 7-64 Types of joints: A Ball joint. B. and C. Hinge joints.

that the same number and kinds of bones are found on one side of the midline as on the other.

The bones:

- Number 206
- May share the same name. For example, there are:
  - 24 ribs helping to form the chest
  - 56 phalanges, the finger bones
  - 2 femurs, the thigh bones
  - 31 bones (**vertebrae**) in the spinal column. Small discs or pads of **cartilage** with soft, gel-like centers between the vertebrae help to cushion these bones. The anterior (front) of the vertebrae support the head and body. The posterior (rear) portions form a tunnel that surrounds the delicate spinal cord and nerves.
- Are of different shapes and sizes, such as
  - long, like the femur, humerus, ulna, and radius
  - short, like the phalanges, carpals, and tarsals
  - flat, like the scapula and cranial bones
  - irregular, like the vertebrae and mandible
- Meet one another to form joints

Joints. Joints are points where bones come together and there is the possibility of movement. Without movable joints, walking, bending, lifting, and sitting would not be possible. Joints are capable of different movements depending upon the type of joint (Figure 7.64). **Ligaments** are strong bands of fibrous tissues that hold the bones together and support the joints. **Bursae** are small sacs of synovial fluid that are located around joints and help reduce friction.

Special terms are used to describe the different movements in a diarthrotic joint.

- **Flexion**: Decreasing the angle between two bones (Figure 7.65A). For example, bending the elbow.

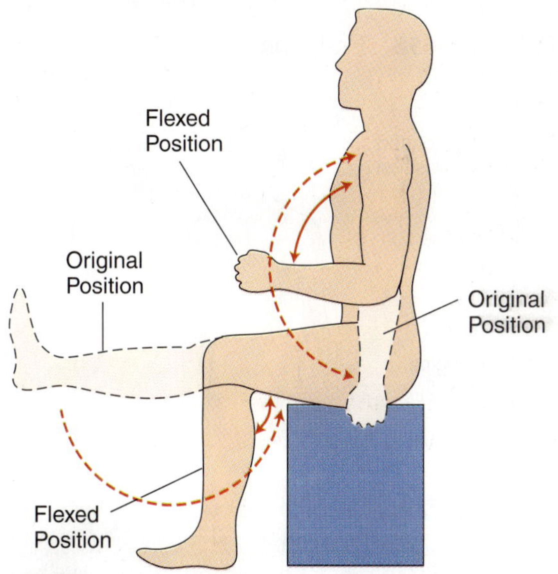

FIGURE 7-65A Flexion—bending a joint.

- **Extension**: Increasing the angle between two bones (Figure 7.65B). For example, straightening the elbow.
- **Rotation**: Circular motion in a ball-and-socket joint (Figure 7.65C). For example, the shoulder and hip joints, which can move in all directions.
- **Abduction**: Moving away from the midline (Figure 7.65D).
- **Adduction**: Moving toward the midline (Figure 7.65E).

Muscles. There are more than 500 muscles in the body (Figure 7.66A and 7.66B). The muscles work in groups. There are three kinds of muscles:

1. **Cardiac muscle** forms the wall of the heart.
2. **Voluntary muscles** are skeletal muscles that are attached to bones. When we wish to pick up something, for instance, we can make our

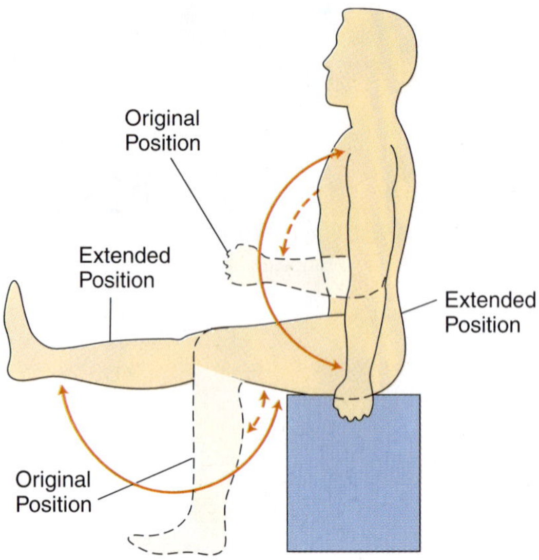

FIGURE 7-65B Extension—straightening a joint.

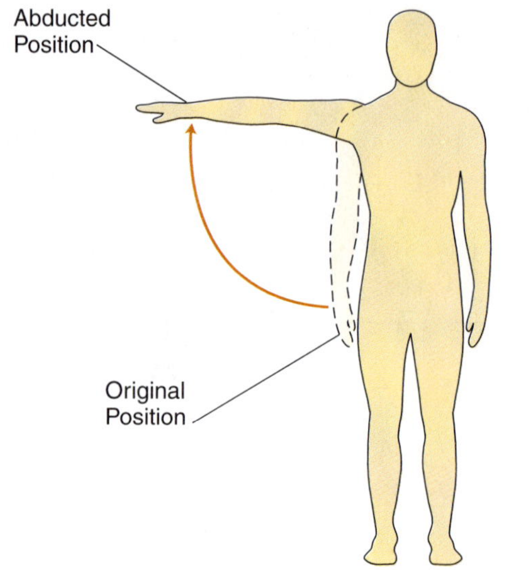

FIGURE 7-65D Abduction—moving an extremity away from the body.

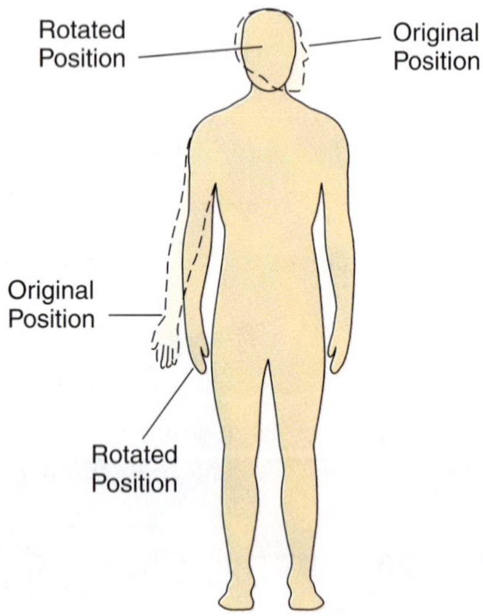

FIGURE 7-65C Rotation—moving a joint in a circular motion.

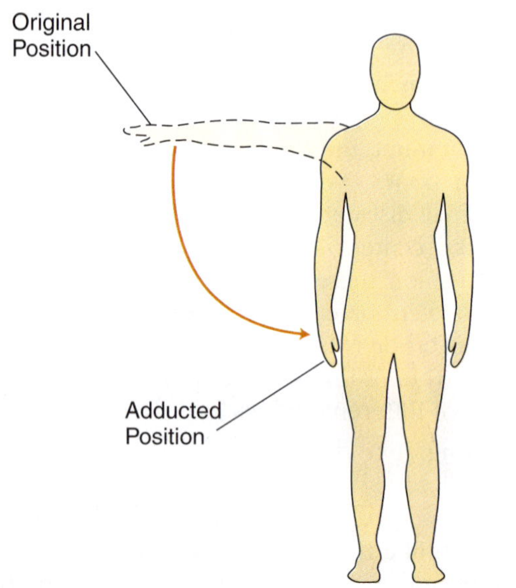

FIGURE 7-65E Adduction—moving an extremity back toward the body.

muscles contract and perform the necessary movements.

3. **Involuntary** or **visceral muscles** form the walls of organs. These muscles operate without our conscious control.

Muscles receive their names in three ways:

1. Their location. For example, rectus femoris near the femur
2. Their shape. For example, trapezius—trapezoidal shape
3. Their action. For example, flexors—bring about flexion

You can easily locate the major muscle groups responsible for an activity if you remember that:

- Muscles can only shorten (contract) and lengthen (relax). Contraction occurs when nerves bring the message **(stimulus)** to the muscle cells. Muscles relax when there is no stimulus.
- Muscles have two points of attachment to the bone. As they stretch from one point **(origin)** to the other **(insertion)**, they cross over one or more joints.
- Muscles are not inserted directly into bones. Rather, they are connected to the bone by strong, fibrous bands of connective tissues called **tendons**. Ligaments support bones at joints.

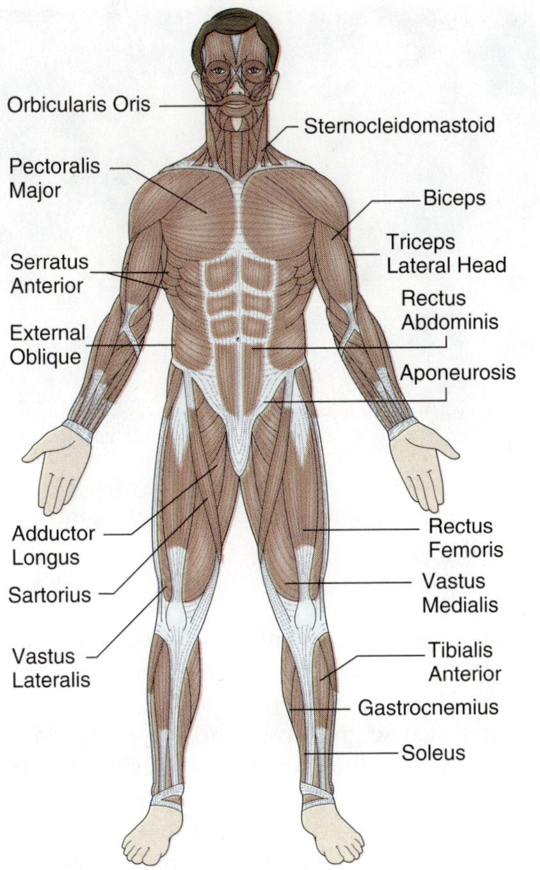

FIGURE 7-66A Major muscles of the body, anterior view.

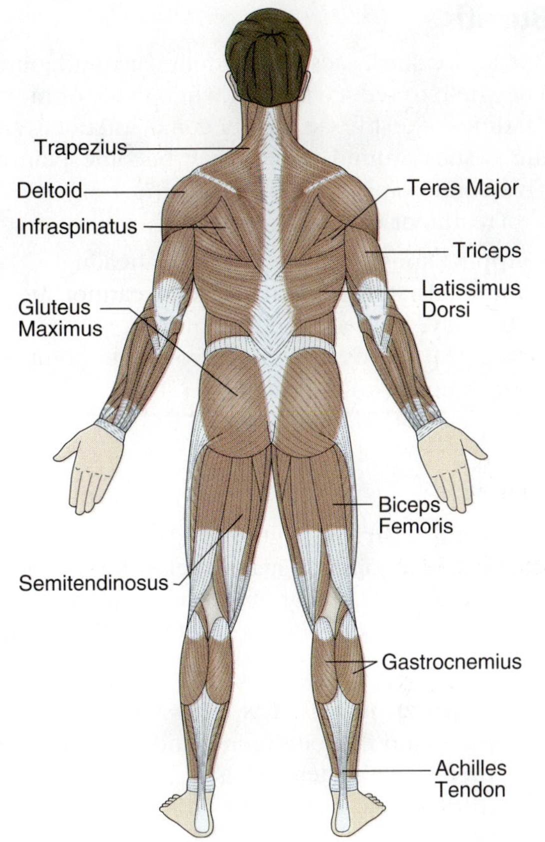

FIGURE 7-66B Major muscles of the body, posterior view.

- As muscles contract, they shorten, pulling their points of origin and insertion closer together. For example, bending the forearm at the elbow takes place when the biceps muscle contracts. The biceps muscle is on the anterior arm and extends from the shoulder to below the elbow. At the same time, the triceps muscle relaxes. This muscle is attached to the posterior shoulder and to the arm below the elbow. To straighten the arm at the elbow, the triceps contracts and the biceps relaxes.
- The more muscles are used, the more powerful they become. The less muscles are used, the weaker they become.

Aging Changes in the Musculoskeletal System

The musculoskeletal system actually consists of two systems, the muscular system (Figure 7.55A) and the skeletal system (Figure 7.55B). They function together to move and protect the body and are commonly referred to together. The skeletal system consists of 206 bones; its function is support, movement, protection, blood cell formation, and calcium storage. The muscular system produces body heat, maintains posture, and permits movement.

Aging changes in the musculoskeletal system include:

- A decrease in strength, endurance, muscle tone, and reaction time is caused by loss of elasticity of muscles and decrease in muscle mass.
- Bones lose minerals, become brittle, and break more easily.
- The spine is less stable, less flexible, and more easily injured.
- Posture may become poor because of weakness in back muscles.
- Degenerative changes, or deterioration, occur in the joints, resulting in limited movement, stiffness, and pain.

Common Conditions

Many conditions can affect the bones, muscles, tendons, ligaments, and joints. Often, when one of these structures is diseased or injured, the surrounding tissues are also involved.

Bursitis

Bursae are small sacs of fluid found around joints. They help to reduce friction when muscles move. At times, the bursae can become inflamed and the tissues around a joint may become painful. This condition is known as **bursitis**.

Treatment of bursitis includes:

- Applications of heat to promote healing
- Immobilization so that the joint cannot move, to relieve pain around the joint
- Removal of excess fluid from the joint by aspiration with a needle
- Administration of steroids

Arthritis

The term **arthritis** (Figure 7.67) means inflammation of the joints. It may develop following an acute injury, or it may be chronic and progressive. The most common forms of chronic arthritis are:

1. **Rheumatoid arthritis (RA)** affects the joint tissues and the joint lining, and can affect any other body system. It is a serious form of arthritis that can occur in persons of any age. The cause is not specifically known. It is believed to be an autoimmune response. It usually follows an intermittent course. RA has **exacerbations**, or times in which the condition seems to worsen, and **remissions**, or times in which the disease appears stable. The involved joints may feel hot to touch. The condition causes reduced joint function and deformities. These can be severe and disabling.
2. **Osteoarthritic joint disease (OJD)** or **degenerative joint disease (DJD)** affects the cartilage covering the ends of the bones that form a joint. Cartilage breaks down and the ends of the bones rub together, causing pain and deformity. The joints most often affected are the weight-bearing joints. Several factors seem to contribute to the disease process, including:
   - Aging
   - Trauma
   - Obesity

   The most common symptom of osteoarthritis is pain. This is usually described as a deep, aching pain that occurs after exercise, weight bearing, or exertion. It is often relieved by rest. Changes in the weather may also cause pain. Other symptoms include limited ability to move and stiffness, particularly upon arising in the morning. This also may occur after strenuous exercise or physical overactivity. In some individuals, an audible grating sound can be heard in the joints during movement. Osteoarthritis may cause redness and swelling in the joints. Conditions such as obesity and stress aggravate the symptoms.

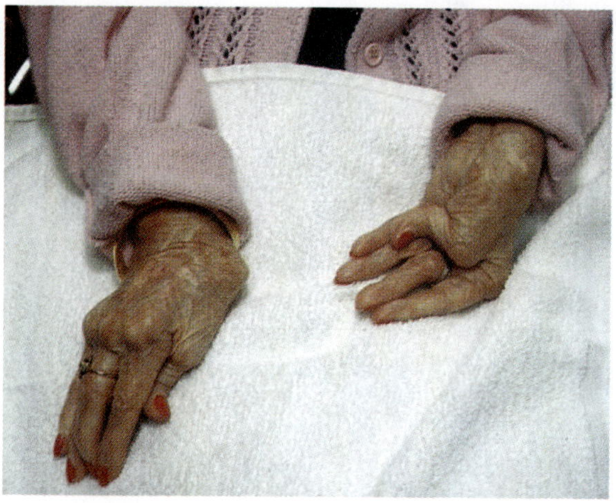

FIGURE 7-67 These deformities, caused by rheumatoid arthritis, make hand movement difficult.

3. **Gout** (gouty arthritis) is a metabolic disease that can be severely disabling. It is caused by increased uric acid in the bloodstream, which deposits in the joints and forms crystals that cause pain. It can occur in any joint, but is most common in the feet and legs. The great toe is often the first joint affected. Gout also follows a course of remission and exacerbation. It can lead to complete disability, hypertension, and chronic renal disease. The cause is unknown, but it is thought to be caused by a genetic defect in the ability to metabolize uric acid. The affected joints may be red or cyanotic in appearance. The patient may have a low-grade fever during this time. After the initial, painful period, symptoms subside. The condition goes into remission and the patient will be pain-free for a period of time. The next attack is usually more painful and severe than the first. Eventually, chronic disease sets in. It is marked by constant pain, tenderness, and swelling in the joints. Other body systems may be affected in this stage. Dietary restrictions are used to reduce the uric acid level in the blood. The dietitian will plan a diet that restricts the amount of red meat and foods rich in purines.

Arthritis can cause mild discomfort to severe deformities and disability. Patients with arthritis

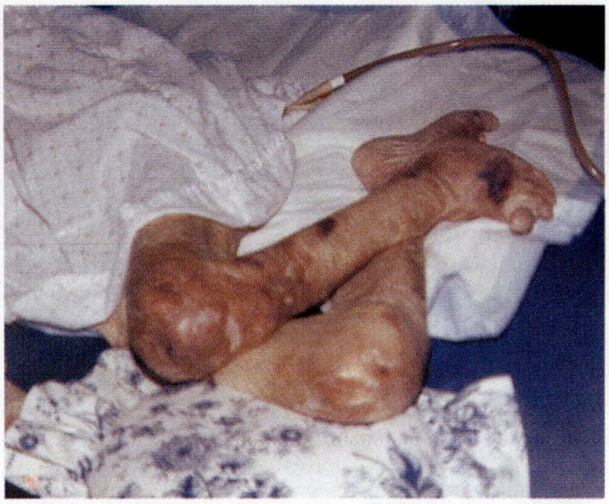

FIGURE 7-68 This patient has many problems with her legs, including arthritic deformities and contractures.

are at high risk of contractures (Figure 7.68). If permitted by your facility, place patients with this condition in the prone position periodically. This reduces the risk of contractures of the hips and knees. Avoid placing pillows under the knees or elevating the knee area of the bed. Using a small, flat pillow under the head and neck is best. A large pillow pushes the neck into a position of flexion. You may be assigned to perform range-of-motion exercises on patients with arthritis. Be very gentle. Avoid moving joints past the point of resistance.

Treatment of arthritis includes:

- Relief of pain
- Balance of rest and exercise
- Joint immobilization where there is pain
- Weight control to relieve pressure on the joints
- Medication to relieve pain and reduce the inflammation
- Physical therapy when inflammation subsides, to maintain joint mobility
- Replacement of badly damaged joints by surgery
- Use of splints, braces, and adaptive equipment to enable the patient to get the most range of motion from injured joints
- Exercise of arthritic joints in warm water (with or without whirlpool action) to maintain function and relieve pain
- Prevention of deformities and contractures

Osteoporosis

Osteoporosis is a metabolic disorder of the bones. It is most common in elderly females, but can occur in males. Bone mass is lost, causing bones to become porous and spongy. Because of this, affected bones are at very high risk for fracture. Fractures can occur spontaneously, such as when the patient is walking. They can also occur by moving or turning the patient in bed or during transfers.

The cause of osteoporosis is unknown. It is thought to result from years of inadequate calcium intake. Other potential causes are declining adrenal function, faulty protein metabolism, estrogen deficiency, and lack of exercise or activity.

Signs and Symptoms. The first sign of osteoporosis is usually a fracture. Commonly, the patient moves or lifts something and hears a "pop" or snapping sound in a bone. This frequently occurs in the lower back or hip. The patient who is walking may suddenly fall. In this case, the fall is the *result* of the fracture; in most falls, the opposite is true. After the initial incident, the area is very painful, particularly upon movement. Sometimes the onset of osteoporosis begins with a curvature of the spine and loss of height. The back progressively weakens, straining the neck, hips, and low back. Spontaneous fractures may occur during movement or as a result of a minor injury.

Treatment. The goals of treatment are to prevent further fractures and control pain. Gentle range-of-motion and other exercises may be ordered. Splints, braces, and other devices may be ordered to support weakened bones. Patients are given estrogen replacement and other drugs to replace calcium and bone mass. You must handle the patient very gently. If you are assigned to perform range-of-motion exercises, do so slowly and carefully. Avoid stretching the joint past the point of resistance. Use a mechanical lift for transfers whenever possible. This is less traumatic than pulling on the patient. Make sure you have extra help for all procedures in which you will be moving or positioning the patient. Follow the care plan exactly in the care of the patient.

Fibromyalgia

Fibromyalgia is a common chronic pain syndrome for which there is no known cause or cure. It affects more women than men. The area between the shoulder blades and the bottom of the neck is often painful. The pain is described as either a general soreness or a gnawing ache, and stiffness is usually worst in the morning. Although this is a common problem, it is very controversial. Some physicians believe that there is no physical cause, and that psychiatric

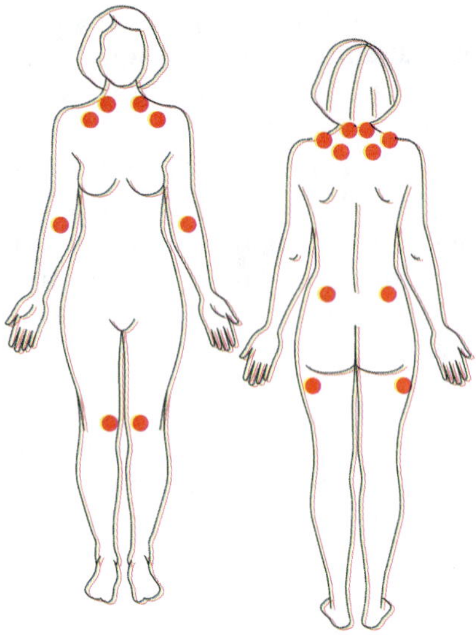

FIGURE 7-69 The patient must have pain at 11 of 18 specific areas of the body for a diagnosis of fibromyalgia.

problems or sleep disorders are responsible for the patient's symptoms. The condition can be very painful and interfere with the patient's quality of life and daily activities. To be diagnosed with this condition, the patient must meet certain criteria, such as:

- having pain on both sides of the body
- having pain both above and below the waist
- having pain upon palpation in at least 11 of 18 specified body sites (Figure 7.69)

Signs and Symptoms Signs and symptoms of fibromyalgia are:

- pain and stiffness
- feeling abnormally tired
- waking up tired
- pain upon touch in certain areas of the body

Treatment Treatment involves pain medications and exercise. Muscle-relaxant medications and antidepressants are sometimes used. Some patients use alternative and complementary therapies to relieve pain and stiffness. The most common complementary therapies used to treat this condition are:

- massage
- biofeedback
- acupuncture
- hypnosis
- relaxation, meditation, and other forms of stress management

Because the cause of fibromyalgia is not known, there is no prevention or cure for this condition. Fibromyalgia complicates treatment for many other medical problems because of the underlying pain and difficulty in assuming some positions necessary for examination and treatment.

Tips: Most patients with fibromyalgia are middleaged women. They are often very deconditioned because pain and fatigue have caused them to limit movement and stop exercising. The pain and fatigue of fibromyalgia often improve with mild exercise, and the physician will usually order some type of exercise program. Encourage the patient to adhere to the program, but not to push to the point of exhaustion. Patients should start exercising slowly, and should not try to keep the same exercise pace as they did before the fibromyalgia developed. A restful night's sleep will improve comfort and mood. Be attentive to the patient's needs for uninterrupted sleep. Plan your care to allow the patient to sleep for prolonged periods without interruption.

Fractures

A **fracture** is any break in the continuity of a bone. Falls are the most common cause of fractures. If the bone breaks through the skin, the injury is called an *open compound fracture*. If the bones do not break through the skin, the fracture is known as *closed*.

Fractures (Figure 7.70) are classified by the type of break in the bone and whether or not the skin is broken:

- A **complete fracture** involves a break across the entire cross-section of the bone. It is often displaced, or improperly aligned, and must be reduced and straightened.
- An **incomplete fracture** involves only part of the cross-section of bone.
- A **closed** or **simple fracture** (Figure 7.70A) occurs when the skin is intact and not broken.
- An **open** or **compound fracture** (Figure 7.70B) occurs when the skin over the fracture is broken. The bone may or may not protrude.
- A **pathologic fracture** is a fracture in a diseased bone.

It occurs as a result of osteoporosis, a tumor, or cancer. The pattern of a fracture describes the manner in which the bone is broken:

- A **greenstick fracture** (Figure 7.70C) occurs when only one side of the bone is broken and the other side is bent. This fracture is common in children, whose bone growth is incomplete. The bones tend to bend like young trees; hence the name "greenstick" fracture.

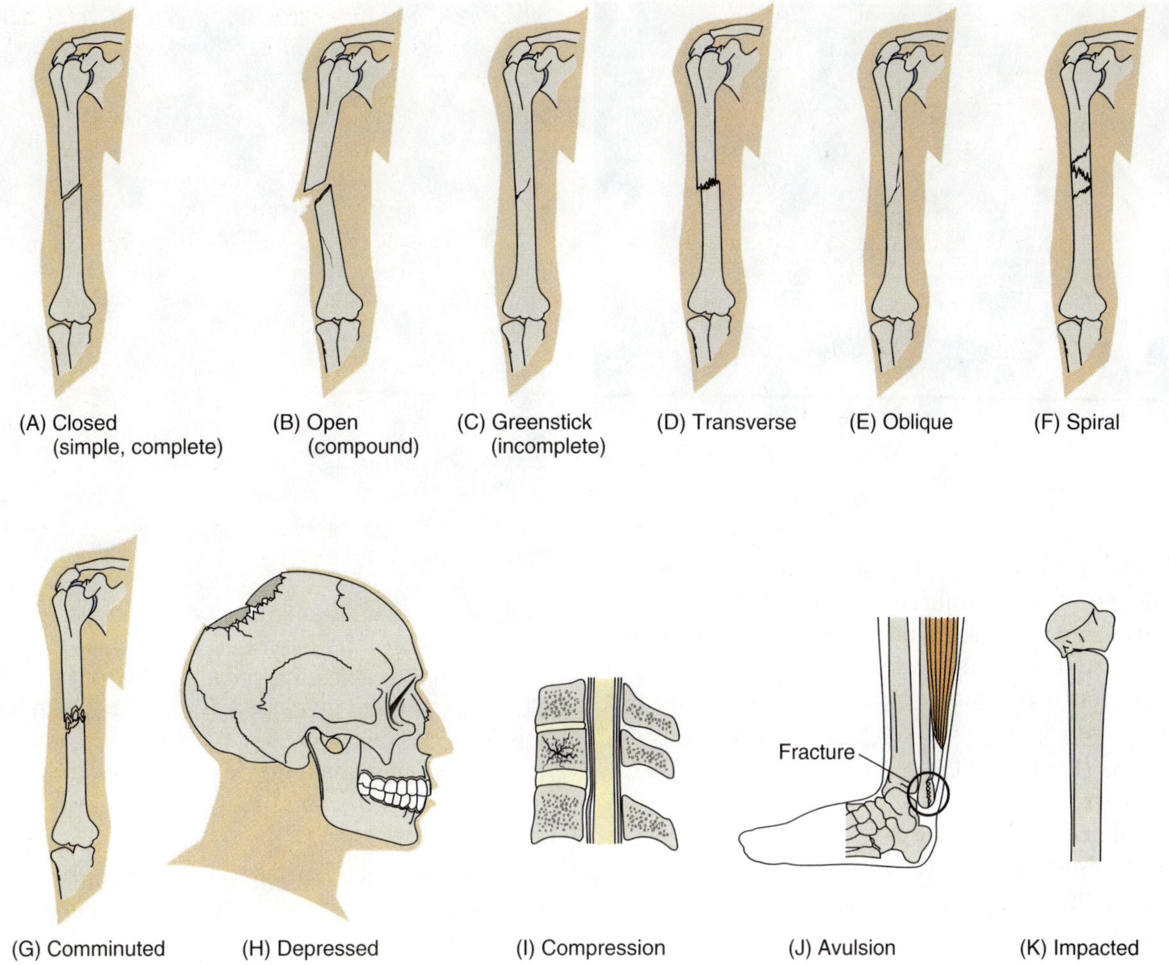

FIGURE 7-70 Types and patterns of fractures.

- A **transverse fracture** (Figure 7.70 D), breaks completely across the bone.
- An **oblique fracture** (Figure 7.70E) runs at an angle across the bone.
- A **spiral fracture** (Figure 7.70F) twists around the bone.
- A **comminuted fracture** (Figure 7.70G) involves shattering and splintering of the bone into more than three fragments.
- A **depressed fracture** (Figure 7.70H) is seen only in fractures of the skull and face. This type of fracture depresses the bone and drives fragments inward.
- A **compression fracture** (Figure 7.70I) is seen only in the vertebrae of the spine. This type of fracture collapses the bone inward.
- An **avulsion fracture** (Figure 7.70J) occurs when a bone fragment is pulled off at the point of ligament or tendon attachment.
- An **impacted fracture** (Figure 7.70K) occurs when the fragment from one bone is wedged into another bone.

Signs and Symptoms. Signs and symptoms of fractures will vary with the type of fracture and location. Fractures are painful conditions. Movement is limited, or the patient may be unable to move the injured area. The skin surrounding the fracture may appear deformed. Edema is common. **Ecchymosis**, or bruising, may occur. Some parts of the body, such as the area over the femur, are very **vascular**. Areas that are vascular contain many blood vessels. They bleed readily under the skin. An ecchymosis the size of an adult's fist over the femur indicates loss of approximately one pint of blood.

Treatment. A new fracture is usually treated in the hospital emergency department. Admission for surgical correction of the fracture may be necessary. The immediate goals of care are to:

- control pain
- prevent complications of immobility
- prevent or reduce edema
- keep the fracture in good alignment
- keep the fractured extremity immobile

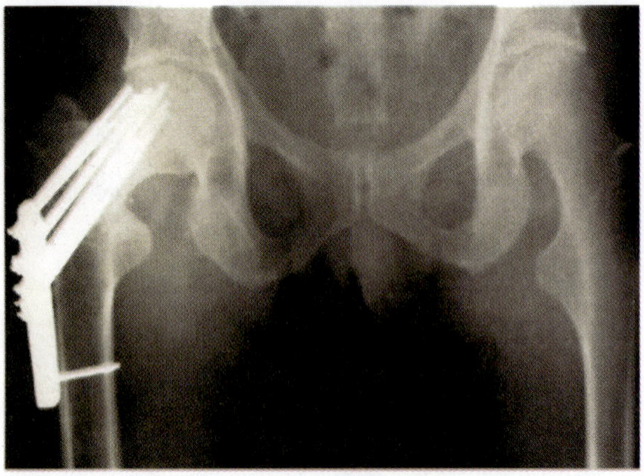

FIGURE 7-71 Certain fractures are repaired using plates, pins, or screws.

Fractures of any kind are treated by keeping the part that is injured immobilized in proper position until healing takes place. Injured bones take from several weeks to several months to heal. Immobilization is achieved through the use of:

- Pins (Figure 7.71)
- Screws
- Splints
- Bone plates
- Casting
- Traction

Special beds and attachments are used to make nursing care easier. The patient may be placed on a Stryker frame or the CircOlectric® bed.

Be sure you know how to operate each bed and attachment before attempting care. In many facilities, an RN must be present when the bed is turned. Know and follow the policy of your facility.

You will assist patients who have fractures with range-of-motion exercises several times each day. Check with the nurse or care plan for specific instructions. In most cases, you will not exercise the fractured extremity. You may be assigned to exercise the patient's joints above and below the cast to keep them mobile. For fractured arms and legs, you may be permitted to exercise fingers and toes. Exercising the rest of the patient's body is important. The exercise prevents complications related to immobility and inactivity.

You may also assist the patient with coughing and deep breathing exercises to prevent pneumonia. When working with patients with fractures, encourage adequate fluid intake. The increased fluid liquefies secretions that accumulate in the lungs. Coughing and deep breathing exercises are the same as those used in postoperative care. A **trapeze** (Figure 7.72) may be attached to the bed to assist the patient with movement. Your supervisor will teach you how to move and reposition the patient without interfering with the traction. The casted extremity is elevated on pillows if traction is not used.

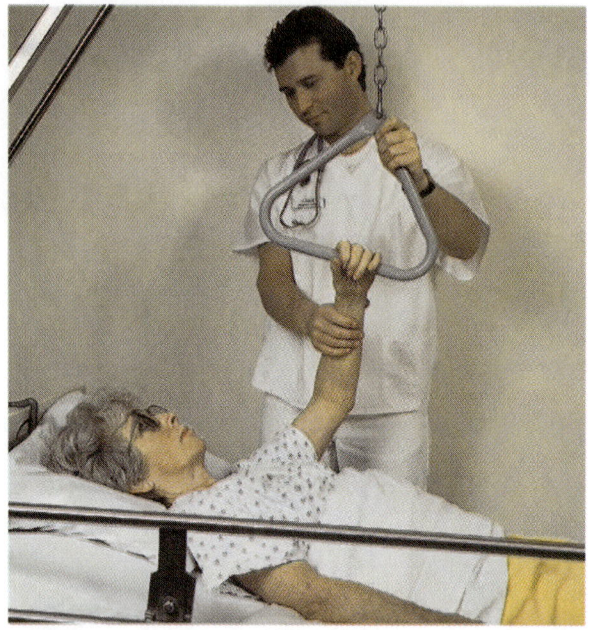

FIGURE 7-72 The overhead trapeze is a helpful adjunct that enables the patient to move in bed. The trapeze is not used for some patients with back injuries and back surgeries, because independent positioning can worsen the condition or cause further injuries.

Treatment for patients with fractures begins soon after admission. The type of treatment is determined by the location and type of fracture, and method of fracture reduction. Patients with fractures will be evaluated by the physical and occupational therapists. Therapists will design rehabilitation programs to meet the patients' needs and help them to regain as much mobility as possible.

Care of Patients with Casts. Two types of cast materials are commonly used:

1. Plaster of Paris, which can take up to 48 hours to dry completely
2. Fiberglass, which dries very rapidly

Cast material is wet when it is applied. During the drying period, the cast gives off heat. Special care for the newly casted patient includes:

- Supporting the cast and body in good alignment with pillows covered by cloth pillowcases, and keeping the cast uncovered.
- Elevating the casted extremity on a pillow as instructed. When positioning a patient with a

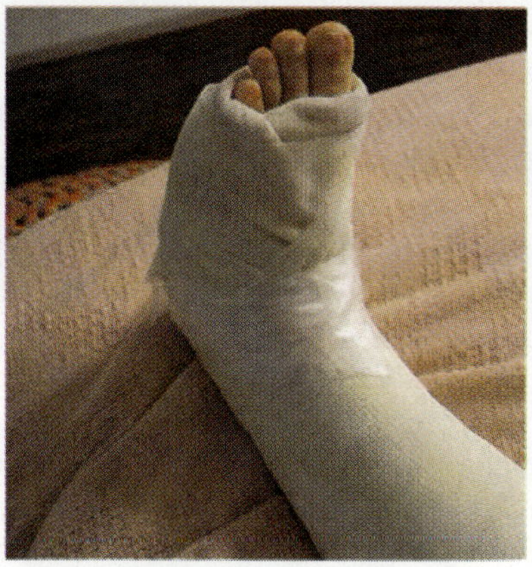

FIGURE 7-73 Check the skin around the edges of the cast regularly for signs of irritation. Check the circulation in the toes.

leg cast, elevate the foot higher than the hip. The fingers should be higher than the elbow. Avoid placing the cast on a flat surface. Avoid placing anything plastic under a wet cast. Check the skin distal to the cast frequently for signs of poor circulation.

- Turning the patient frequently to permit air circulation to all parts of the cast. Maintain support. Use the palm of your hand, not your fingers, to support the wet cast.
- Not positioning the cast against the footboard or side rail. Leaving the cast open to air until it dries is best. If the patient is cold, cover the cast loosely with a sheet. Avoid tucking the sheet under the mattress. A bed cradle may be used, if necessary. The greatest area of heat loss is the head. Covering the upper body and back and top of the head with a blanket may help keep the patient warm.
- Closely observing the uncasted areas of the extremities, such as the fingers and toes, for signs of decreased circulation. Report coldness, cyanosis, swelling, increased pain, numbness, or tingling immediately.
- Closely observing skin areas around the cast edges for signs of irritation (Figure 7.73). Rough edges should be covered with adhesive strips to prevent skin irritation.

Recall the following key of reportables when checking the patient:

- C = color
- M = motion
- E = edema
- T = temperature

Special Care After Cast Is Dry. After the cast has completely dried:

SAFETY *Alert*

A fiberglass cast dries immediately. A plaster arm or leg cast will take 24 to 48 hours to dry completely. A plaster body or spica cast will take 48 to 72 hours to dry. Proper positioning of the cast is essential during the drying period to prevent depressions that can cause pressure and edema. Never use a table or hard object to support the cast during the drying period. Avoid rubber or plastic pillows, which increase heat under the cast. When the cast is dry, it will look white and shiny. It will not appear soft or damp.

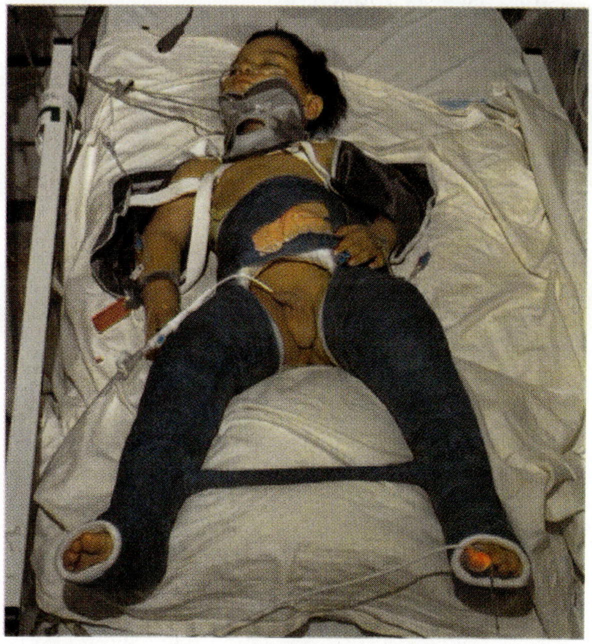

FIGURE 7-74 The spica cast is a full-body cast that is commonly used to treat hip fracture and after hip surgery in children.

- Turn the patient to the noncasted side. This is particularly important in moving a patient with a body cast (**spica cast**) (Figure 7.74) because turning to the casted side may crack the cast.
- Always support the cast when turning or moving a patient.

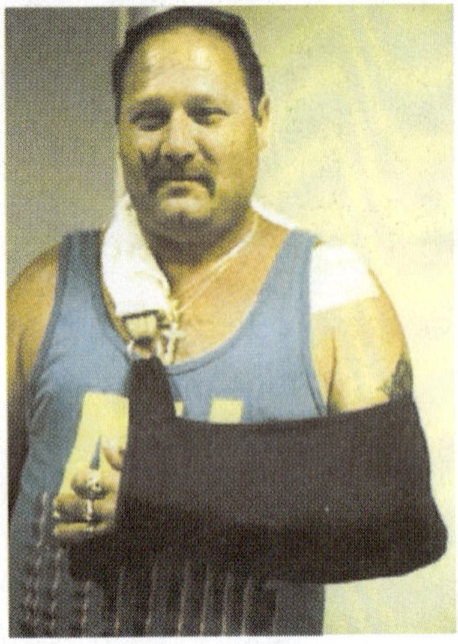

FIGURE 7-75 A sling may be ordered to elevate the hand and wrist.

- Encourage use of a trapeze to assist the patient in helping herself.
- Tape edges of casts to prevent pressure and abrasive areas, if edges were not covered when the cast was applied.
- Use plastic to protect cast edges that are near the genitals and buttocks, to help prevent soiling during toileting.

After the cast dries, you may observe changes that indicate infection or ulceration under the cast:

- odor from the cast
- drainage through the cast

The care plan may instruct you to keep the casted extremity elevated to prevent edema. A sling (Figure 7.75) may be used to elevate an arm cast when the patient is out of bed. A wheelchair with an elevated leg rest is used for patients with leg casts. Cover the cast with plastic during bathing. Keep small objects from getting inside the cast. The patient may complain of an itching sensation under the cast. Discourage him or her from placing objects down the cast to scratch. This could cause a skin injury and infection. Report complaints of itching to your supervisor.

Care of Patients in Traction. Traction is designed to pull two body areas slightly apart to:

- relieve pressure.
- help tightly contracted (spasmodic) muscles relax.
- keep them in proper position as healing takes place.

Traction is of two types:

- Skin traction, where traction is applied to the skin or outside of the body (Figure 7.77)
- Skeletal traction, where traction is applied through the skin to the bone

Traction is applied by attaching weights to a part of the body above or below the area to be treated. The patient's body weight serves as **countertraction** by pulling in the direction opposite to the traction. Belts, head halters, or tapes may be applied to the patient's skin to hold the traction. Traction may be applied continuously or intermittently.

Skeletal traction (Figure 7.78) uses tongs or pins placed into bones with weights applied to the tongs or pins. Skeletal traction is always continuous once applied. The weights for skeletal traction must not be lifted or removed until the traction is to be discontinued.

When patients are in traction:

- Review the correct placement of straps and weights with the therapist or nurse. Get instructions for moving the patient up in bed and turning to the sides, as ordered.
- Do not disturb the weights or permit them to swing, drop, or rest on any surface. Avoid moving, dropping, or releasing the weights. They should not touch the bed, swing back and forth freely, or rest upon any object or surface. The water bag or weight hangs motionless at the end of the bed.
- Keep the patient in good alignment in the center of the bed. Make sure that the body is acting properly as countertraction by keeping the head of the bed low. The feet should not rest against the end of the bed.
- Check under straps and belts for areas of pressure or irritation.
- Make sure straps and belts are smooth, straight, and properly secured.
- Keep bed covers off ropes and pulleys.

Not all patients remain in traction continually. If **pelvic belt traction** (Figure 7.79), or **cervical traction** with a head halter (Figure 7.80), is to be discontinued, take the following steps:

- Slowly raise the weights to the bed. Avoid abrupt or jerking movements, as this may cause the patient pain. If two sets of weights are being used, raise them at the same time and rate.
- Remove the weight holder and weights from the connection with the halter or belt and place them on the floor. Remove the head halter or pelvic belt.
- To reapply traction, reverse the procedure.
- Remember never to jerk or drop the weights quickly or lower them unevenly. Always apply weights smoothly to avoid causing the patient pain.

PROCEDURE

16 Applying an Arm Sling

1. Carry out beginning procedure actions.
2. Gather equipment:
   - arm sling or triangular bandage
   - padding for neck, if needed
3. Position the affected arm at a 90° angle.
4. Apply the sling:
   - If a triangular bandage is used, place one end of the triangle over the unaffected shoulder. Position the point of the triangle under the affected elbow. Bring the other end of the triangle over the shoulder on the affected side, covering the arm. Adjust the bandage so the fingers are elevated, and tie the ends of the bandage in back. Position the knot slightly to the side so it is not directly over the spine. Pad the skin under the knot to prevent pressure and irritation. Fold the extra fabric over at the elbow. Secure it on the inside with pins or tape.
   - If a commercial sling is used, support the affected arm. Guide the sling up over the hand until the elbow is covered and the fingers are exposed. Wrap the strap around the patient's neck, then fasten it to the buckle on the sling. Adjust the strap so the fingers are elevated. Pad the strap under the neck (Figure 7.76) to prevent pressure and irritation.
5. Carry out procedure completion actions.

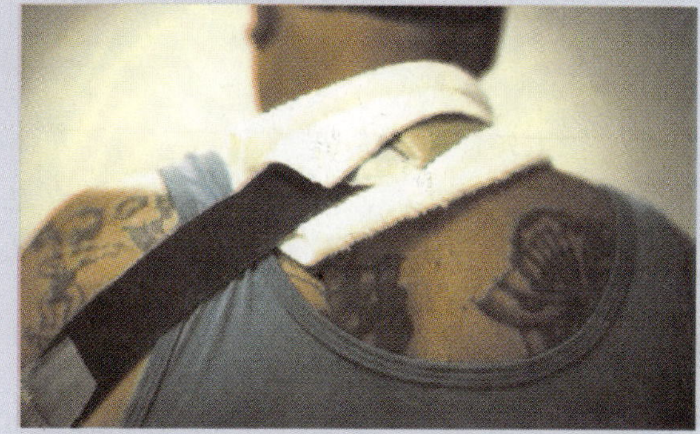

FIGURE 7-76 Pad the neck strap of the sling to prevent pressure and irritation from the weight of the cast.

SAFETY *Alert*

If the patient has an arm sling, monitor the skin at the back of the neck for irritation and breakdown from the strap. Monitor the skin under the arm daily for redness and breakdown. Make every effort to keep the underarm area clean and dry.

Bedmaking. Bedmaking for orthopedic patients varies according to the type of traction.

- Two half sheets are often used in place of a large sheet for the bottom.
- Bottom linens may be changed from top to bottom rather than side to side.
- The top linen is arranged according to the patient's special needs. Half sheets and folded bath blankets can be worked around the traction to keep the patient covered and comfortable.

Fractured Hip

Hip fractures are the most common type of fracture in the elderly. It is not unusual for a patient to be admitted to the hospital for treatment of another problem, then fall and break a hip. The

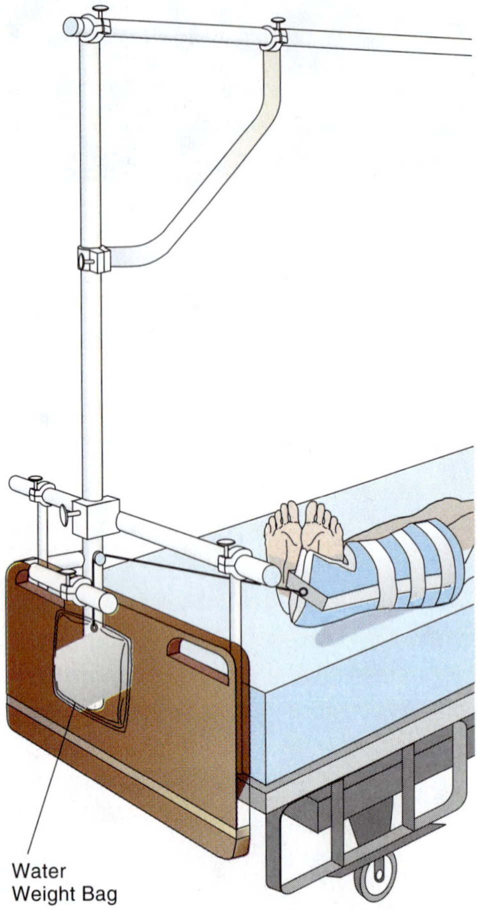

FIGURE 7-77 Buck's traction is a type of skin traction that may be used for a hip fracture.

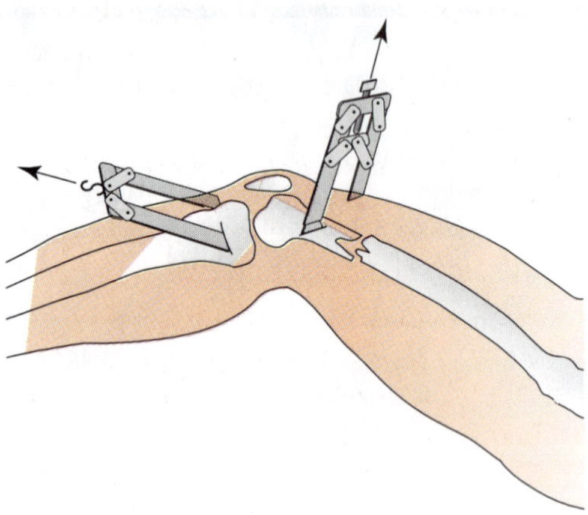

FIGURE 7-78 Skeletal traction immobilizes a body part by attaching weights directly to the patient's bones with pins, screws, wires, or tongs.

most common cause of hip fractures is falls, but fractures may also occur because of osteoporosis. In this case, the patient may hear a popping sound in the bone, then fall. An x-ray will reveal

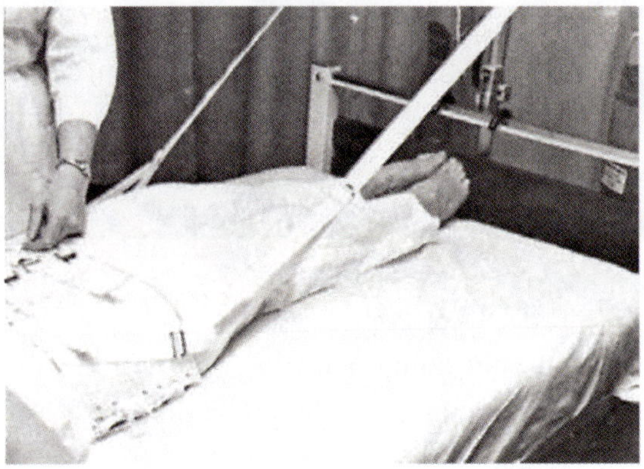

FIGURE 7-79 Pelvic belt traction. A bag filled with water is used as a weight.

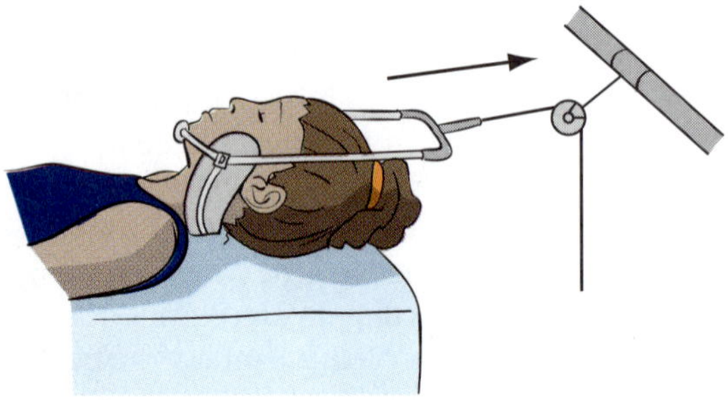

FIGURE 7-80 Cervical traction.

a fracture. The term "hip fracture" really is not accurate. This term refers to a fracture anywhere in the upper third or head of the femur.

Signs and Symptoms of Hip Fracture. A patient with a fractured hip is usually found on the floor. He or she will be unable to get up or move the injured leg. The leg on the affected side may be shortened and in a position of external rotation. In this position, the toes point outward. The shortening and rotation occur because the strong muscles in the upper leg contract. This causes the bone ends to override each other.

The patient will complain of severe pain in the hip. The pain of a hip fracture is usually localized in the hip. Some patients complain of pain in the knee. This may be confusing or misleading. Edema and ecchymosis may be present in the hip, thigh, groin, or lower pelvic area.

Emergency Care. Avoid moving the patient until you are instructed to do so by a nurse. You will use a sheet, backboard, or other device to move the patient. Avoid excessive movement, which can worsen the injury. Moving a patient with a hip fracture requires four or five individuals. The patient is logrolled onto the lifting device. The device is lifted to the bed or

DIFFICULT SITUATIONS

A patient who has had hip surgery will probably have physician orders for antiembolism hosiery and an incentive spirometer. A pressure-relieving mattress may be ordered. Following hip surgery, the patient will be at high risk for pressure ulcer development, particularly on the heels. Take active measures to prevent pressure. Follow the care plan. Check the skin regularly for redness, irritation, and breakdown.

stretcher. You may be assigned to monitor the patient's vital signs and check for signs of shock. Some patients are treated with Buck's traction.

Open Reduction/Internal Fixation. The most common treatment for a fractured hip is a surgical procedure called **open reduction/internal fixation**. This means the surgeon makes an incision, manipulates the fractured bone into alignment, and then inserts a device such as a nail, pin, or rod to hold the ends of the fractured bone in place. If you are assigned to a patient who has had this surgery, you must:

- Know how to position the patient in bed. It is important to avoid adduction and internal and external rotation of the affected hip.
- Know the correct procedure if the patient is allowed to ambulate. The patient is usually not allowed to bear weight on the affected side for a few weeks after surgery.

Total Hip Arthroplasty

Total hip arthroplasty (THA), or insertion of a hip prosthesis (artificial body part), is a common procedure. This surgery is done because the patient:

- has fractured a hip and the bone cannot be set by traditional methods
- has degenerative arthritis that has caused the hip joint to deteriorate

The patient's hip joint is surgically removed and a metal or synthetic ball and socket are inserted (Figure 7.81). There are specific body positions that the patient must avoid to prevent damage to the new joint.

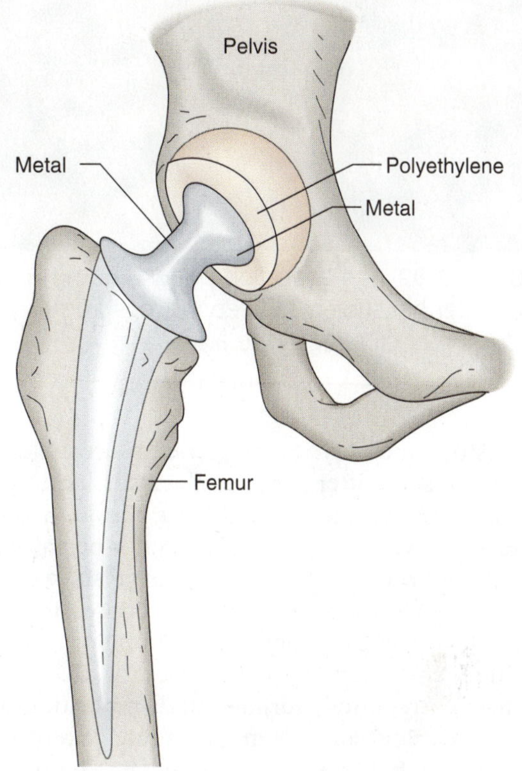

FIGURE 7-81 A hip prosthesis replaces the ball of the femur and the socket when the patient has a total hip arthroplasty.

Caring for the Patient with Hip Surgery. After hip surgery, the following general procedures are commonly ordered:

- A trapeze is attached to the bed to assist with movement. The patient is instructed not to press down on the foot of the affected leg when using the trapeze.
- Antiembolism stockings are applied.
- A fracture bedpan is used initially for elimination. When the patient is able to use the toilet, an elevated toilet seat is used.
- The head of the bed is not elevated more than 45 degrees without a specific order.
- Avoid acute flexion of the hip and legs. The physician will give directions for positioning and the degree of flexion permitted.
- Patients who have had hip replacement surgery will usually have a special pillow, called an **abduction pillow**, to keep the legs apart (Figure 7.82). This is particularly important when the patient is turned on the side. The patient will be instructed to avoid crossing the legs, which can cause a dislocation.

The physician will specify how long the patient must avoid weight bearing after surgery. The physical therapist will work with the patient

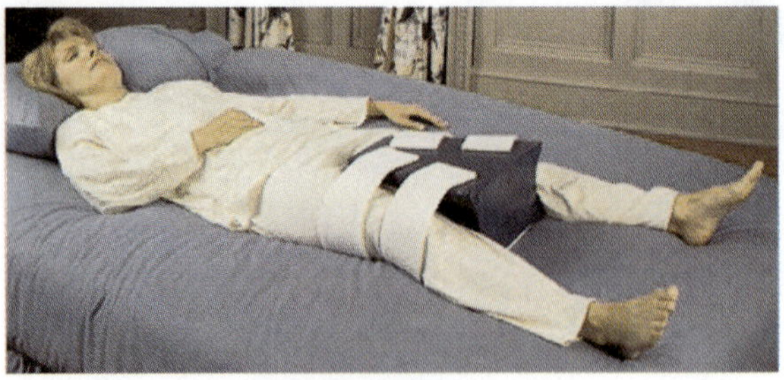

FIGURE 7-82 An abduction pillow is commonly used after hip surgery to keep the legs from adducting or crossing at the ankles.

to restore mobility. Some patients are able to ambulate soon after surgery. A walker, crutches, or cane are commonly used for a period of time after surgery. Some physicians do not permit full weight bearing for as long as four to six weeks. Initially, you will assist with procedures to prevent the complications of immobility. These include range-of-motion exercises of the unaffected extremities, turning and repositioning, and coughing and deep breathing exercises. Patients with hip surgery are at very high risk of developing heel pressure ulcers. Follow the care plan and get specific instructions from the nurse for positions and techniques to use for turning and repositioning the patient. Relieve pressure from the heels and check the patient's skin carefully each day for signs of red or open areas.

Total Joint Replacement

Sometimes joints are completely replaced because of arthritis or severe damage to the joint. The goal of joint replacement surgery is to relieve pain, which is often so severe that the patient avoids using the joint as much as possible. This weakens the muscles and worsens the problem. Hip and knee replacements are the most common, but joint replacement surgery can be done on the ankle, foot, shoulder, elbow, and fingers. Postoperative care will vary with the surgical procedure. General care for joint replacement surgery includes:

- preventing infection
- preventing blood clots
- administering anticoagulant medication to thin the blood
- applying antiembolism hosiery
- doing exercises to increase blood flow in the leg muscles, if not contraindicated
- using sequential compression therapy

DIFFICULT SITUATIONS

A patient who has had hip replacement surgery may usually have the head of the bed elevated up to 45 degrees for comfort. Never elevate the head more than this without specific permission from the nurse. Some physicians will permit greater elevation. Try to limit elevation of the head to 30 minutes at a time, if possible. In any event, do not let the patient remain in a position of hip flexion for more than 90 minutes, because longer periods increase the risk of prosthesis dislocation. Positioning the patient in the supine position, with the affected leg in extension, for 1 hour three times a day will help prevent contractures of the hip joint.

Continuous Passive Motion **Continuous passive motion (CPM)** therapy (Figure 7.84) may be ordered following joint replacement and other orthopedic procedures. Moving a joint is painful for most patients postoperatively. If the patient fails to move the joint, stiffness and limited range of motion will occur. Months of physical therapy will be necessary for the patient to fully recover. CPM therapy prevents stiffness by delivering a form of passive range-of-motion exercise so the joint is moved without the patient's muscles being used. CPM therapy is effortless for the patient. A machine moves the affected joint through a prescribed range of motion for an extended period of time. CPM therapy:

- enhances circulation, which lowers the risk of blood clots
- reduces edema
- promotes collagen formation within the joint, which enhances healing
- reduces scarring
- decreases stiffness
- improves range of motion (which decreases postoperatively without movement)
- reduces the risk of complications in the joint, such as contractures and adhesions
- helps reduce pain

GUIDELINES FOR

Caring for Patients with THA

The patient should **not**:

- Flex the hip more than 90 degrees (Figure 7.83A).
- Cross the affected leg over the midline of the body, whether in bed or sitting in a chair (Figure 7.83B).
- Internally rotate the hip on the affected side (Figure 7.83C).

Never do passive range-of-motion exercises on a joint that has had surgery, unless you are specifically instructed to do so–and then only if you have been given instructions as to which actions can safely be performed. The patient will have limited weight bearing on the affected leg for several days or weeks after surgery.

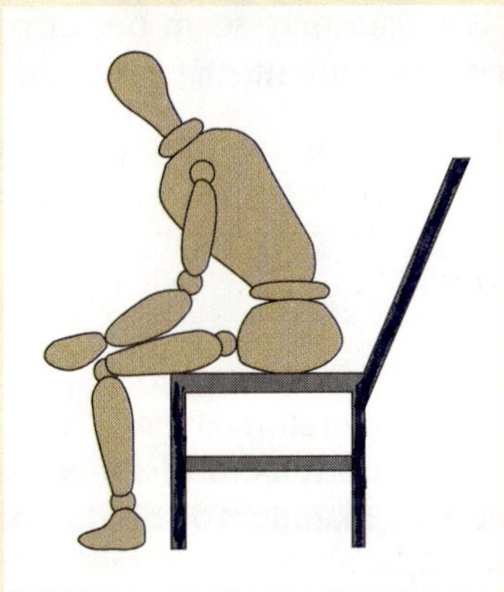

FIGURE 7-83A The patient with a new hip prosthesis should never flex the affected hip more than 90 degrees.

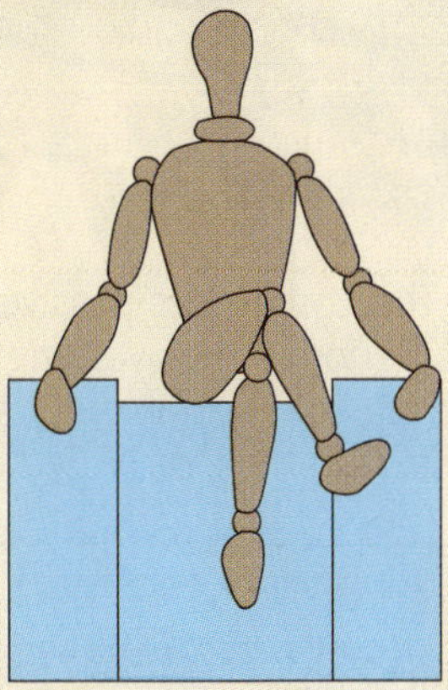

FIGURE 7-83B The patient with a new hip prosthesis should never cross the affected leg over the midline of the body.

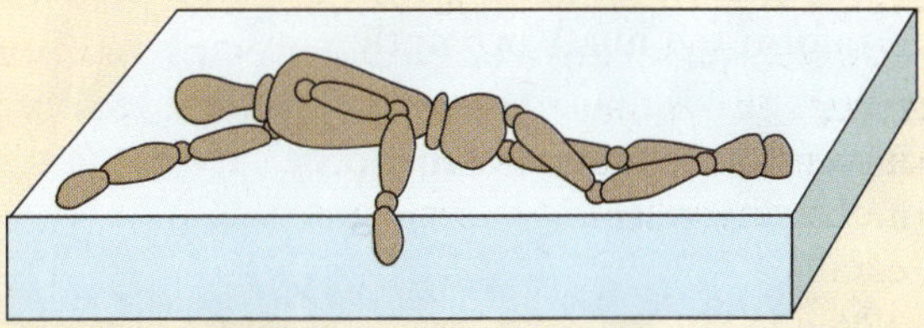

FIGURE 7-83C The patient with a new hip prosthesis should never internally rotate the hip on the affected side.

Many orthopedic surgeons prescribe CPM therapy following knee replacement and other surgical procedures. CPM devices are available for the knee, ankle, toes, jaw, shoulder, elbow, wrist, and hand. Indications for using CPM therapy are:

- Crush injuries of the hand without fractures or dislocations
- Burn injuries
- Stable fractures
- Joint and tendon repair
- Surgical release of contractures
- Knee or hip replacement
- Reconstructive surgery on bone, cartilage, tendons, and ligaments
- Prolonged joint immobilization

The physician prescribes how the CPM unit should be used. He or she orders the settings on the CPM unit that control the speed, duration of use, range of motion, pause settings, hours of use per day, and rate of increase of motion. The directions for use will vary slightly depending on the body area being treated, the type of CPM machine used, and physicians' orders. In some facilities, this procedure is done only by licensed nurses. In others, the nursing assistant can set up the unit, but the nurse must check the settings for accuracy. This is a key step. Improper settings can damage reconstructive work in the joint. Follow your facility policies and procedures. Contraindications for CPM therapy include:

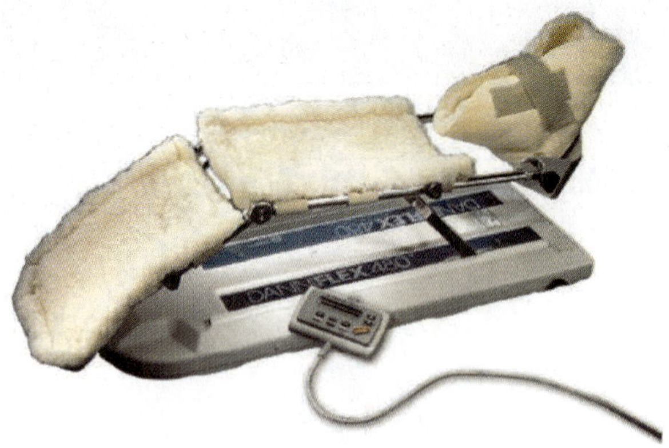

FIGURE 7-84 The continuous passive motion (CPM) machine performs passive range-of-motion exercises on the affected joint without straining the patient's muscles. *(Courtesy of of OrthoRehab, Inc.)*

- untreated infections
- unstable fractures
- known or suspected blood clots (deep vein thrombosis)
- hemorrhage

If the patient develops any of the following signs or symptoms upon using the device, stop the unit and inform the nurse promptly:

- fever
- increasing redness or irritation
- increasing warmth
- edema
- bleeding
- increased or persistent pain

Do not proceed with treatment until the nurse informs you that the physician has approved continued use of the device. Check the patient periodically when using the CPM machine. Each time the settings are changed, stay with the patient for several cycles to be sure she tolerates the change. Check the skin every 2 hours for signs of redness, irritation, or breakdown. Report problems and abnormalities to the nurse.

Compartment Syndrome

Compartment syndrome is a very painful condition that occurs when pressure within the muscles builds up, preventing blood and oxygen from reaching muscles and nerves. This is a very serious complication that may develop following an injury or surgical procedure. It may also occur following athletic injuries, burns, snake bites, IV infiltration, frostbite, and musculoskeletal conditions in which there is no fracture. Patients of all ages can be affected.

Compartment syndrome is usually seen after a traumatic injury, such as a long bone fracture. It may develop if an injury or surgical site swells after a cast has been applied. A tough membrane, called **fascia**, surrounds the muscles in the arms and legs. Fascia does not expand readily. Compartment syndrome develops gradually over several hours. Bleeding or swelling occurs in the muscle tissue, under the fascia. In some cases, pressure from a cast or compression device also increases the pressure from the outside. If the swelling is not relieved, pressure on the muscles and nerves builds. Eventually, the pressure inside the fascia compartment will exceed the blood pressure, causing the capillaries to collapse. Blood flow to the muscles and nerves stops. If it is not restored promptly, tissue death begins.

Signs and Symptoms. The most common symptom of acute compartment syndrome is severe pain, especially when the muscle is moved. The pain may seem out of proportion to the injury. The patient may also complain of

- severe pain when the muscle is gently stretched
- tenderness when the area is touched gently
- pain during deep breathing
- tingling
- burning
- numbness
- feeling tight or full in the affected muscle
- abnormal sensations in the affected area
- weakness or inability to use the muscle

You may observe:

- The color of the extremity may appear pale, cyanotic, or red
- The skin of an extremity with no cast may feel warm to touch
- The fingers or toes of a casted extremity may feel cool to touch
- Edema (swelling)

Loss of the pulse in the extremity is a late sign. Rapid identification and treatment of this condition is necessary.

Nursing Assistant Responsibilities. Follow the care plan and monitor patients with musculoskeletal injuries and casts frequently. Monitor for changes in the extremity. Check the color and temperature of the extremity distal to a cast. Notify the nurse if the color is abnormal. Ask the patient if he or she is able to move the fingers or toes. Notify the nurse promptly of any unusual findings. If the patient complains of severe pain, or if the pain is not relieved after the patient

PROCEDURE

17 Procedure for Continuous Passive Motion

Note: Be sure this is a nursing assistant procedure at your facility.

Note: These instructions are generic and are not device-specific. The person setting up the device should be trained on use of the specific device, and have an operating manual for that device.)

1. Carry out beginning procedure actions. Apply the principles of standard precautions during this procedure if contact with wound drainage or nonintact skin is likely.
2. Gather equipment:
   - CPM unit
   - soft goods kit, if available OR
   - sheepskin foot pad
   - tibia/femur sling
   - hip pad
   - Velcro fasteners
3. Check the unit for safety and stability. Make sure that the attachments are tight, the frame is stable, and the electric controls work. Have the nurse adjust the settings according to the doctor's orders, or follow facility policy for setting the speed and degree of flexion. (In some facilities, assistants are permitted to adjust the settings. If this is the case, have the nurse check the settings before proceeding.) Stop the machine in full extension.
4. Raise the side rail on the side of the bed where you will be placing the unit.
5. Position the CPM unit on the bed and secure the attachment, depending on the type of device being used.
6. Fasten the foot pad to the foot plate with a Velcro fastener.
7. Attach the tibia/femur sling (wide section toward the footrest). Fasten the Velcro closures under the sling.
8. Apply the hip pad to the hinge area of the adjustment bar. Position the femur sling straps over the hinges, then fasten underneath with Velcro.
9. Fit the CPM machine to the patient's leg length by lengthening or shortening the frame.
10. Align the knee joint with the knee hinge, then position the knee approximately 1 inch below the knee joint line (Figure 7.85A).
11. Center the leg on the unit. Avoid pressure on the side and middle of the knee joint.
12. Adjust the foot pad so the patient's foot is comfortable and well supported. The leg should be lifted at the thigh with no pressure on the foot. Secure the Velcro straps across the thigh and top of foot (Figure 7.85B).
13. When the leg is in the proper position, give the patient the control (Figure 7.85C). Instruct the patient to start the unit. Instruct the patient to turn the unit off and use the call signal if the exercise causes extreme pain, or the unit malfunctions.

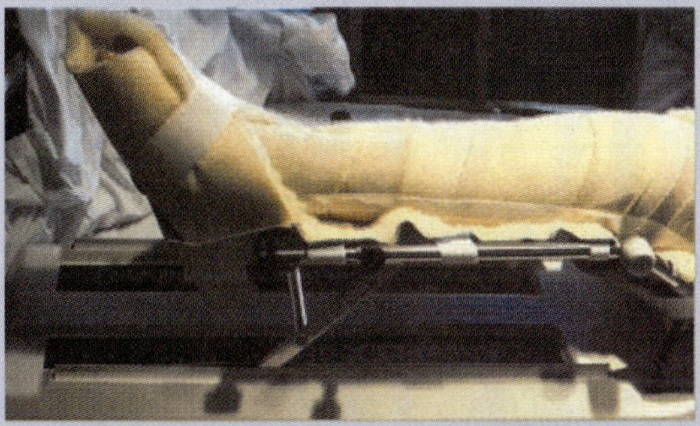

FIGURE 7-85A Position the leg straight, with the toes upright. Line the knee up with the marking at the hinge.

(continues)

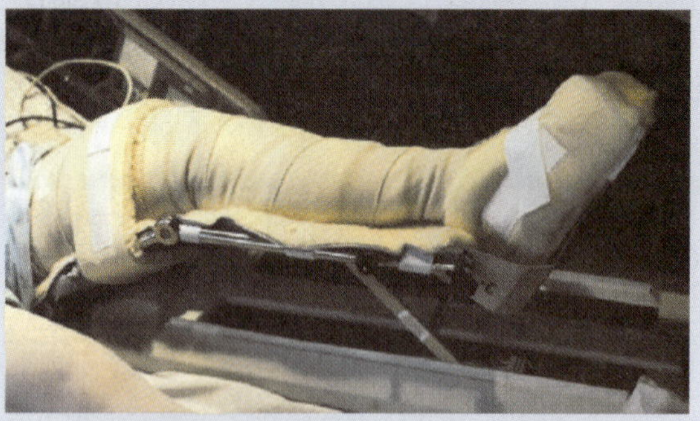

FIGURE 7-85B Secure the straps across the leg and foot. Make sure the strap is not too tight.

14. Stay with the patient for at least two full cycles to make sure she tolerates the procedure.
15. Return to check on the patient frequently when the unit is in use. Some devices have compliance monitors that allow you to check usage of the device. After the patient is experienced in the use of the CPM machine, he or she may be instructed to keep a record of the times the unit is used, or you may be required to document this information.
16. Carry out procedure completion actions.

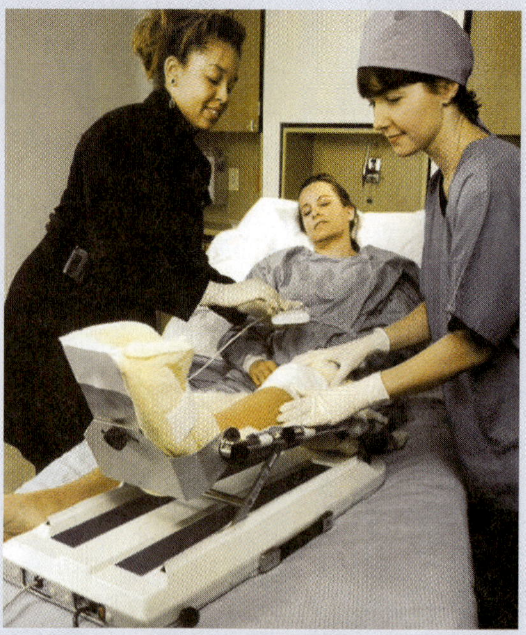

FIGURE 7-85C Show the patient how to turn the unit on, then give her the switch. Stay in the room until the machine goes through at least two cycles if the unit is being used for the first time. *((Courtesy of of OrthoRehab, Inc.)*

DIFFICULT SITUATIONS

The most common location of compartment syndrome in adults is in a fractured tibia. The most common location of compartment syndrome in children is the humerus.

receives pain medication, notify the nurse promptly. This condition is frightening for the patient. Provide emotional support.

Compartment syndrome is a surgical emergency. The nurse will assess the patient and notify the physician of the findings. If compartment syndrome is suspected, the patient will be taken to surgery quickly to relieve the pressure. Follow facility policies and the nurse's instructions for preparing the patient for surgery.

Ruptured or Slipped Disc

It is possible for a disc to bulge (slip) out of place or for the soft center to rupture. In either case, pressure is placed on the spinal nerves (Figure 7.86). Depending on which disc is injured, the patient may experience, in different parts of the body:

- Pain
- Numbness
- Tingling
- Weakness of one or more muscles

Treatment. Treatment attempts to relieve pressure on the nerve roots. Early treatment is very conservative and includes rest, medication, ice,

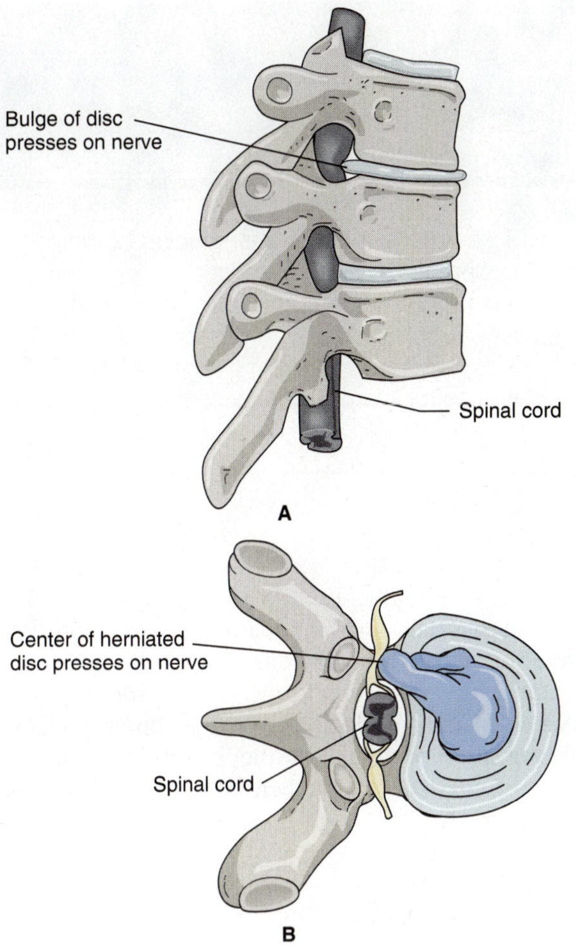

FIGURE 7-86 A. Uneven pressure causes the disc to bulge, putting pressure on the nerve root (slipped disc). B. A herniated (ruptured) disc applies pressure on the nerve root as the gel-like center oozes backward.

compresses, physical therapy, and exercise. Some people use complementary and alternative therapies, most commonly:

- acupuncture
- chiropractic
- massage
- yoga
- biofeedback

If conservative attempts to relieve pressure fail, other methods will be used to relieve pressure on the spinal cord. These are:

1. Traction. This is an older treatment that is seldom used nowadays.
2. Surgery to remove the protruding portion of the disc (**laminectomy**). The surgery sometimes includes a fixation (**fusion**) of the vertebral bones.
3. A surgical procedure called **nucleoplasty**. This is a minimally invasive procedure with rapid recovery. In this procedure, a tiny wand is inserted through the back into the disc. Tissue is removed through the wand, and the channel is thermally sealed. The wand is then removed. This may be done as an outpatient surgery in some facilities.

Lower Extremity Amputation

You may care for patients who have had one or both legs surgically removed (amputated). A leg may have to undergo **amputation** because of circulatory problems, a malignancy, or an accident in which the leg was severely damaged.

It is common for people to experience **phantom pain** after the removal of a limb. Patients with phantom pain may feel pain or tingling where the limb used to be. These feelings may persist for months. The pain is real, although it is difficult to explain.

When you are positioning a patient who has had an amputation of the lower extremities, remember:

- Avoid abduction and flexion of the patient's hip—because the weight of the lower leg is not there, the hip on the affected side will quickly become contracted if flexion is allowed.
- If the patient has a below-the-knee amputation (BKA), avoid flexion of the knee, so that a contracture does not form.
- Avoid placing pillows under the amputated extremity. Position the leg flat on the bed.
- Avoid elevating the head of the bed for prolonged periods.
- Keep the legs in a position of adduction. A trochanter roll is helpful. Avoid positioning the patient with pillows between the legs.
- Assist the patient to lie in the prone position twice a day, if permitted.
- Encourage and assist the patient to move in bed frequently.

After the surgery, the patient will either have the stump wrapped with elastic bandage or will wear a stump shrinker. It is important that these be on at all times except during the bath. It is the nurse's responsibility to apply either of these items. If you notice that the bandage or shrinker is loose or needs to be reapplied, notify the nurse. The purpose of these items is to make sure that the stump heals in the appropriate shape.

If you bathe a patient with an amputation:

- Gently wash the stump with soap and warm water, rinse well, and pat dry.

- Observe the stump for:
  - redness
  - swelling
  - drainage from the incision
  - open areas in the incision or anywhere else on the stump
- Do not apply lotion to the stump. Lotion softens the skin, making safe prosthesis use difficult.
- Make sure the skin is protected before applying the prosthesis. Never apply a prosthesis over unprotected skin.

After an amputation, some patients are fitted with an artificial leg (prosthesis). They have to learn how to walk and sit when the prosthesis is worn. A prosthesis is custom-made for the person who will be wearing it. A special health care professional measures the patient and makes the prosthesis. The physical therapist teaches the patient how to apply the prosthesis and how to use it. If you are responsible for helping a patient put on a prosthesis, be sure you know how to attach and secure it, because each device is different. Various types of materials are used to make prostheses. They need to be cleaned regularly, and the method of cleaning depends on what materials were used to make the prosthesis. Wipe the inside of the prosthesis daily with a damp, soapy cloth to remove sweat and body oils. Rinse with a second damp cloth. Dry the inside of the socket well. Avoid placing a damp prosthesis on a patient. Never attempt to adjust the prosthesis. Consult your supervisor if you believe an adjustment is necessary.

SAFETY *Alert*

Make sure that the stump shrinker or wrap is smooth, with no wrinkles or exposed skin. Inform the nurse promptly if the patient complains of throbbing under the stump shrinker. Throbbing is an indication of impaired circulation, a potentially serious complication.

The Integumentary System

Structure and Function

The integumentary system includes:

- Skin
- Hair
- Nails
- Sweat glands
- Nerves
- Oil glands

The outermost layers of the skin make up the epidermis. The dermis lies under the epidermis. The **subcutaneous tissue** that attaches the skin to the muscles lies under the dermis. The nails are horny cell structures found on the dorsal, distal surfaces of the fingers and toes. They protect the sensitive fingers and toes. The teeth are formed from the tissues of the **integument** (body shell).

Epidermis

The **epidermis** consists of dead outer cells that are constantly shed as new cells move upward from the dermis. There are no blood vessels in the epidermis, so injury to this layer does not cause bleeding. Nerve endings reach into this outer layer. The nerves are sense organs that keep us in contact with changes in the environment. Nerve endings called **receptors** receive information about:

- Heat
- Cold
- Pain
- Pressure

Dermis

The **dermis** contains blood vessels, nerve fibers, and two kinds of glands:

- Sweat glands (**sudoriferous glands**)
- Oil glands (**sebaceous glands**)

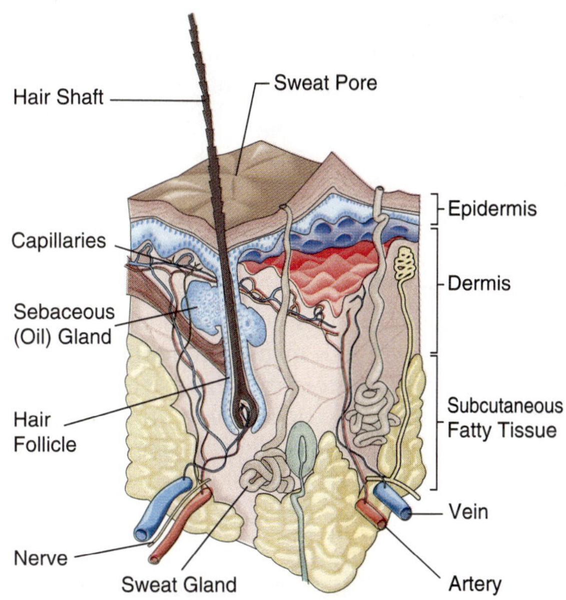

FIGURE 7-87 The skin is the largest organ in the body. It protects the underlying structures, and provides temperature regulation and elimination.

DIFFICULT SITUATIONS

When the stump is healed and the patient prepares to use the prosthesis, the physician may order special care. This involves not shaving the stump, as shaving increases the risk of rash and irritation. Bathing of the stump may be ordered at bedtime, because warm water may increase swelling, and make application of the prosthesis difficult. The physician may also order alcohol rubs to the stump several times a day to toughen the skin. Avoid powders and lotions, which soften the skin. Monitor the stump for irritation and report to the nurse, if present. The stump sock may require frequent changing to avoid wetness. The socks must be handwashed. Muscle-strengthening exercises will be ordered to prepare the patient to lift the weight of the prosthesis.

Sweat Glands

The sweat glands produce perspiration that reaches the skin surface through tubes or ducts that end in openings called pores. Heat from deep in the body is brought to the skin by blood vessels. This heat is transferred to the perspiration. At the skin surface, the perspiration and the heat are lost through the pores to the air. The heat of the body is controlled by changes in the size of the blood vessels in the skin.

- When the central opening of a blood vessel becomes enlarged (dilated), more heat is brought to the body surface.
- When the central opening of a blood vessel becomes smaller (constricted), less heat is brought to the body surface.

Oil Glands and Hair

Oil glands lubricate and keep flexible the hairs found in the skin. Hair covers almost all body surfaces except for the palms of the hands and the soles of the feet.

Skin Functions

The skin has many functions that are critical to the well-being of the body:

- Protection—forms a continuous membranous covering for the body and regulates body temperature
- Storage—stores fat and vitamins
- Elimination—loses water, salts, and heat through perspiration
- Sensory perception—contains nerve endings that keep us aware of environmental changes

The skin tells us much about the general health of the body.

- A fever may be indicated by hot, dry skin.
- Unusual redness—**rubra**, or flushing of the skin—often follows strenuous activity.
- **Pallor**, which is less color than normal, is a sign associated with many conditions.
- The oxygen content of the blood can be noted quickly by the color of the skin. When the oxygen content is very low, the blood is darker and the skin appears bluish or **cyanotic**.

Aging Changes in the Integumentary System

Aging changes in the integumentary system include:

- The skin thins and becomes less elastic; wrinkles appear, and the skin becomes irritated and breaks more easily.
- Blood vessels that nourish the skin become more fragile and break more easily, resulting in bruising, senile purpura, and skin tears. Skin tears are irregular-shaped injuries in which the top layer of the skin peels back. Senile purpura are dark purple bruises that appear on the backs of hands and forearms in the elderly.
- Blood flow in vessels that nourish the skin is reduced, resulting in slower healing.
- Oil glands that supply the skin secrete less, causing drying of the skin and itching.
- Perspiration decreases, and the body's ability to regulate temperature is impaired.
- Subcutaneous fat diminishes.
- Blood supply to the feet and legs is reduced.
- Fingernail and toenail growth slows and nails become brittle.
- Hair thins and turns gray.

Common Conditions

Skin Lesions

Injury or disease can cause changes in skin structures. These changes are called **lesions**. The lesions may be caused by disease, trauma, wear, or the aging process. When caring for patients with skin lesions, standard precautions are followed. Some of the most common skin lesions or eruptions are:

- **Macules**—flat, discolored spots, as in measles (Figure 7.88)
- **Nodules**—small, knotlike protrusions; small masses of tissue
- **Papules**—small, solid, raised spots, as in chickenpox
- **Pustules**—raised spots filled with pus, as in acne
- **Vesicles**—raised spots filled with watery fluid, such as a blister (Figure 7.89)
- **Wheals**—large, raised, irregular areas frequently associated with itching, as in hives
- **Excoriations**—portions of the skin appear scraped or scratched away
- **Crusts**—areas of dried body secretions, such as scabs

Skin lesions may be a result of systemic responses:

- Communicable disease—diseases that are easily transmitted, directly or indirectly, from person to person. Measles and chickenpox are

AGE-APPROPRIATE CARE *Alert*

Aging changes cause the skin to become very dry and fragile. The skin of elderly persons often tears, breaks, and bruises readily. Handle elderly patients very gently to avoid accidental injury to the skin. Many elderly individuals avoid soap for routine bathing. Some use clear water, and many others use lotion-based cleansing products. Ask the patient what he or she prefers. Keep the skin well lubricated with lotion to prevent dryness. This may involve applying lotion to dry areas several times during your shift. Rub and pat lotion into the skin gently. Avoid vigorous massage of the legs. Apply lotion to the feet as well. Avoid the area between the toes.

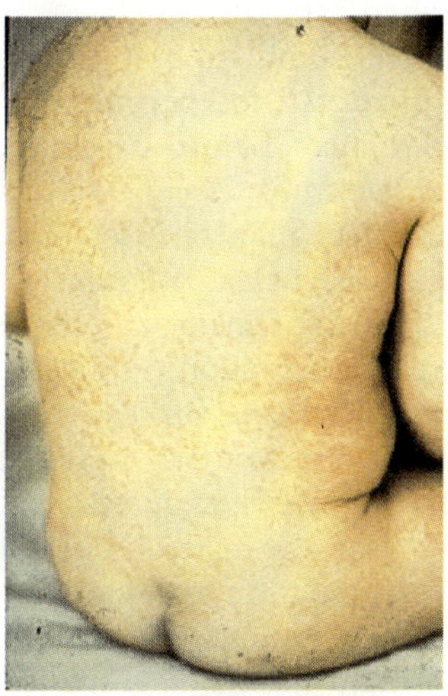

FIGURE 7-88 The macules of German measles. *((Courtesy of of the Centers for Disease Control and Prevention [CDC], Atlanta, Georgia)*

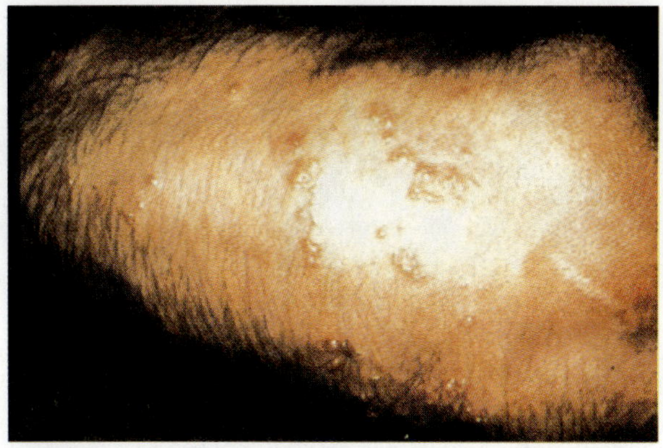

FIGURE 7-89 The fluid-filled vesicles of poison ivy. *((Courtesy of of the Centers for Disease Control and Prevention [CDC], Atlanta, Georgia)*

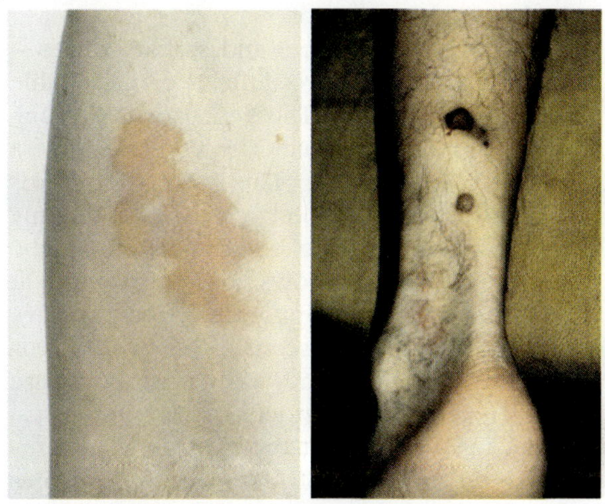

FIGURE 7-90 A. Typical lesions of Kaposi's sarcoma. B. Raised lesions of Kaposi's sarcoma. *(Courtesy of (Both courtesy of Daniel J. Barbaro, MD, Fort Worth, Texas)*

two such diseases. Each has characteristic skin lesions called **skin eruptions** or **rashes**.

- Immune system problems—Persons whose immune systems are depressed, such as those suffering from HIV infection, may develop a specific type of cancer called **Kaposi's sarcoma** (Figure 7.90). It appears as lesions in the skin and eventually in other organs. The skin lesions begin as macules, papules, or nodules that gradually become bigger and darker. The lesions are reddish-purple to dark blue in color. In addition to persons with HIV disease, Kaposi's sarcoma (Figure 7.90A and Figure 7.90B) is most common in men over 60 years of age. Recent research suggests that it is caused by a herpes virus, and may be spread by kissing an infected person. Kaposi's lesions can also appear in the mouth and internal organs. Progression of the disease may be slow or rapid.
- **Allergies**—also called *sensitivity reactions*, may have associated skin lesions. The vesicles of poison ivy are well known. The material causing the sensitivity is called an **allergen**. Individuals respond to allergens in different ways.

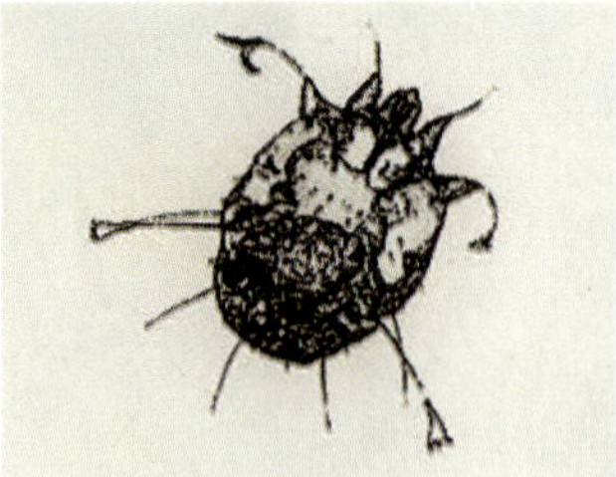

FIGURE 7-91 The scabies mite cannot be seen with the eye. *((Courtesy of of L.E. Morris and Donna J. Lewis, "Management of Chronic, Resistive Scabies: A Case Study,"* Geriatric Nursing *16 (Sept./Oct. 1995): 230–37)*

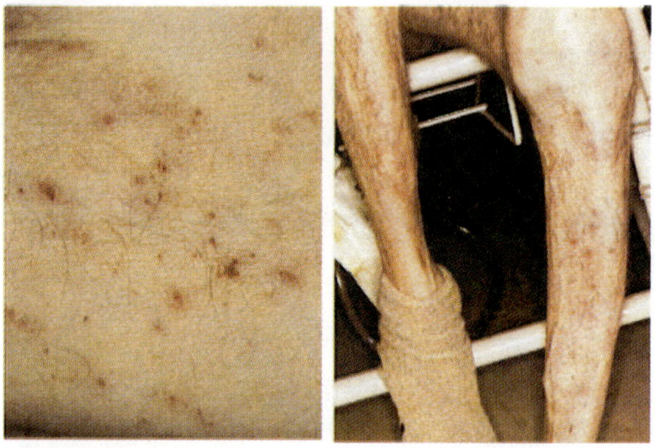

FIGURE 7-92 A. Scabies rash on the back. B. Scabies rash on the knees and lower legs. *(Courtesy of (Both courtesy of L.E. Morris and Donna J. Lewis, "Management of Chronic, Resistive Scabies: A Case Study,"* Geriatric Nursing *16 (Sept./Oct. 1995): 230–37)*

- **Anaphylactic shock**—a severe, sometimes fatal, sensitivity reaction.
- **Pediculosis** (body lice) and scabies **mites**—these tiny parasites are difficult or impossible to see (Figure 7.91). The patient usually complains of intense itching. The skin may have a rash-like appearance. The rash of scabies usually follows the blood vessels. It commonly appears in the webs of the fingers, inside the wrists, outside the elbows, in the underarm, at the waist, and in the nipple area (Figure 7.92A). It is also sometimes seen in the genital area in men, and around the knees (Figure 7.92B) and lower buttocks. One type of scabies causes scaling of the skin on the palms of hands and soles of feet. Lice and scabies are highly infectious and are spread by direct and indirect contact with an infected person or object.

Some lesions commonly occur when the skin is injured:

- **Abrasions** are injuries that result from scraping the skin.
- **Contusions** are mechanical injuries (usually caused by a blow) resulting in hemorrhage beneath the unbroken skin.
- An ecchymosis is a bruise.
- A **hematoma** is a localized mass of blood that is confined to one area.
- Lacerations are accidental breaks in the skin.
- **Senile purpura** are dark purple bruises on the forearms and backs of hands. These are common in elderly individuals.
- **Skin tears** are shallow injuries in which the epidermis is torn. The shape is often irregular. These injuries are also common in elderly individuals.

Observation of the skin and accurate descriptions of what you see must be carefully charted.

Care of Skin Lesions

When skin lesions are present, certain general nursing care is indicated. Take the following precautions when caring for these patients.

- Closely observe the patient's skin on admission, but do not remove any dressings. Any changes noted should be reported immediately and described accurately.
- Soap and water and rubbing lotions are often **contraindicated** (not permitted). Check the nursing care plan before bathing the patient or giving a backrub.
- Special products may be used for bathing or soaking the skin, such as *colloidal oatmeal*. This product is used for many different skin conditions to relieve irritation, reduce itching, and moisturize, soften, and protect the skin. When bathing the patient, you may be instructed to use **tepid** (lukewarm) water instead of hot water. Make sure that the patient does not get the treated bath water in the eyes. The product may make the tub slippery. Instruct the patient to use the hand rail when rising from the tub, and provide assistance as needed.
- Wear gloves when contact with blood, body fluids (including drainage from blisters or skin lesions), or nonintact skin is likely.
- Do not attempt to remove any crusts from skin lesions without special instruction from your supervisor.
- Handle the patient gently. Avoid rubbing the skin.
- Special bed linen may be used, such as sterile linen, linen that has been washed in special detergent, or disposable linen. Special bedding will be listed on the care plan.

OSHA Alert

Become familiar with the appearance of scabies and body lice on the skin. These microscopic parasites often appear as numerous, tiny scabs on the skin surface. These areas commonly itch, and the patient may scratch them. If the patient has multiple, tiny scab-like areas, wear gloves when care requires skin contact. Report the presence of these lesions to the nurse for further assessment.

- A bed cradle may be placed on the bed to prevent the sheet from contacting the open skin areas.
- Notify the nurse if the:
  - skin lesions are draining
  - nature of the drainage changes
  - amount of drainage increases
  - drainage becomes **malodorous** (having a bad or foul odor)
  - drainage changes in color

Pressure Ulcers (Dermal Ulcers)

Pressure ulcers, commonly called bedsores or **dermal ulcers**, may occur in patients of any age. You may also hear them called **decubitus ulcers**. This is an older term that continues to be used. It is not as accurate as *pressure ulcers*. Pressure ulcers are open areas that develop on the skin over a bony prominence as the result of pressure. If there is pressure on the skin for a prolonged period, ulceration can occur, regardless of the patient's position. *Decubitus* is Latin for lying down. Because ulcers can occur when a patient is not in bed, the descriptive terminology was changed to "pressure ulcer" for accuracy. They are particularly common in patients who are:

- Elderly
- Very thin
- Overweight (**obese**)
- Unable to move
- Incontinent
- Debilitated
- Poorly nourished (eats less than half of meals and snacks)
- Confined to bed or wheelchairs
- Disoriented
- Dehydrated
- In prolonged contact with moisture
- Circulation-impaired
- Has discolored, torn, or swollen skin
- Subjected to shearing

Shearing (Figure 7.93) occurs when the skin moves in one direction while the structures under the skin, such as the bones, remain fixed or move in the opposite direction. This can happen when patients are dragged rather than lifted up in bed, when positions are changed, or when patients slide down in bed or in a wheelchair (Figure 7.94). Blood vessels become twisted and stretched, causing the tissues being served to lose essential oxygen and nutrients, leading to breakdown. In addition, shearing may cause actual tears in fragile skin. These skin tears are painful, a portal of entry for infectious pathogens, and commonly lead to further breakdown. **Friction** (rubbing the skin against another surface, such as bed linen) also contributes to pressure ulcer formation. It usually occurs when the patient is being moved.

Pressure ulcers are caused by prolonged pressure on an area of the body that interferes with circulation. The tissue first becomes reddened. As the cells die (undergo **necrosis**) from lack of nourishment, the skin breaks down and an ulcer forms. The resulting pressure ulcers may become large and deep.

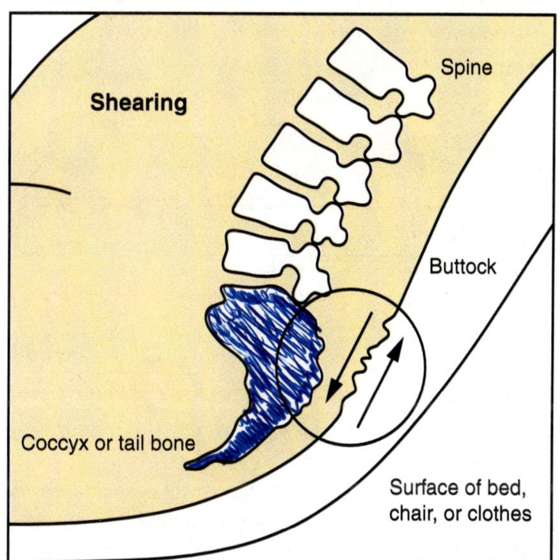

FIGURE 7-93 Shearing occurs when the skin is stretched in one direction and the underlying structures move in the opposite direction.

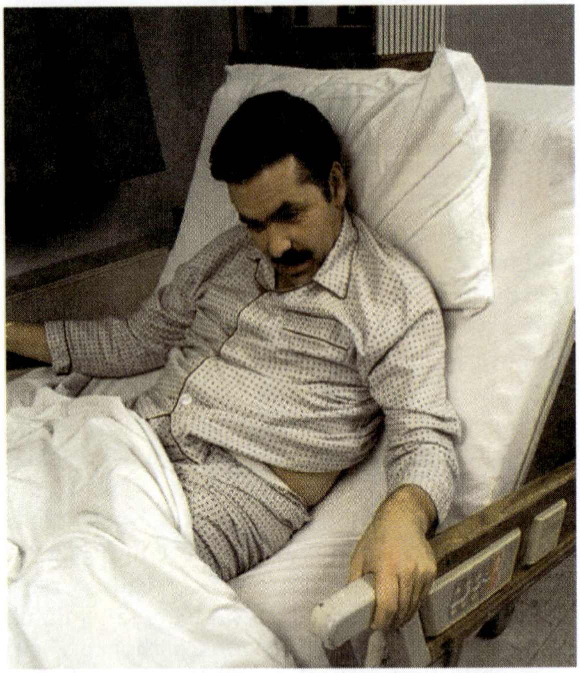

FIGURE 7-94 Shearing occurs when a patient slides down or is improperly pulled up in bed.

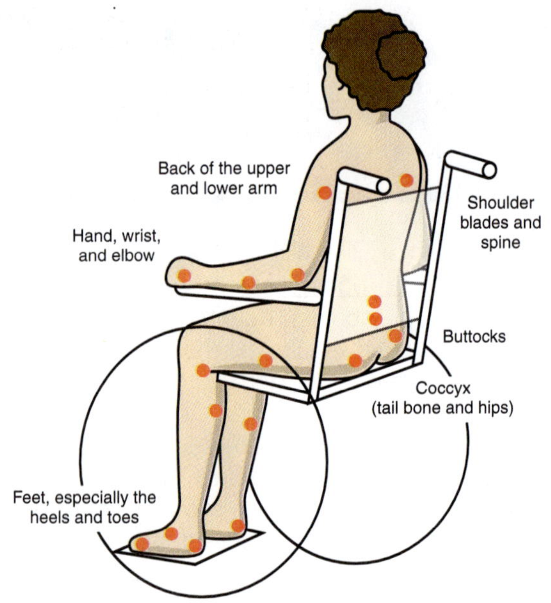

FIGURE 7-95B Potential areas of pressure when a patient is in a chair or wheelchair.

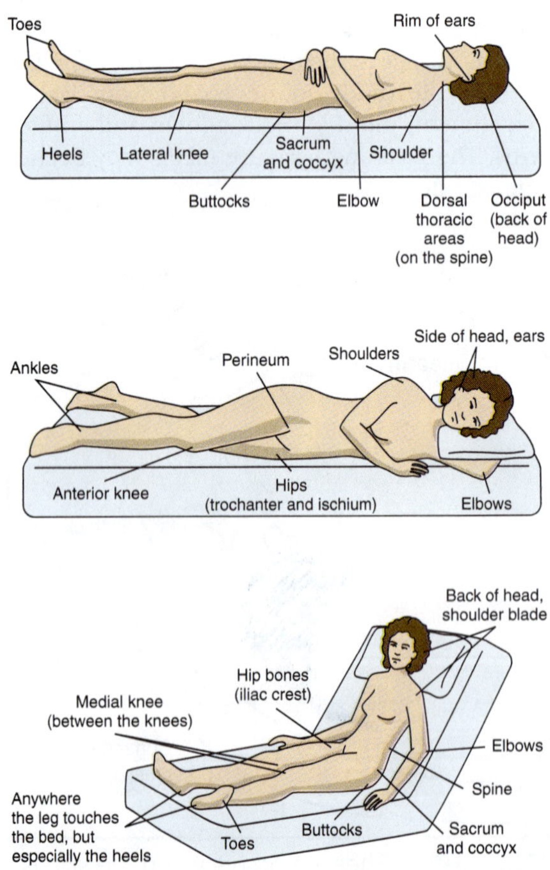

FIGURE 7-95A Potential areas of pressure when a patient is in bed.

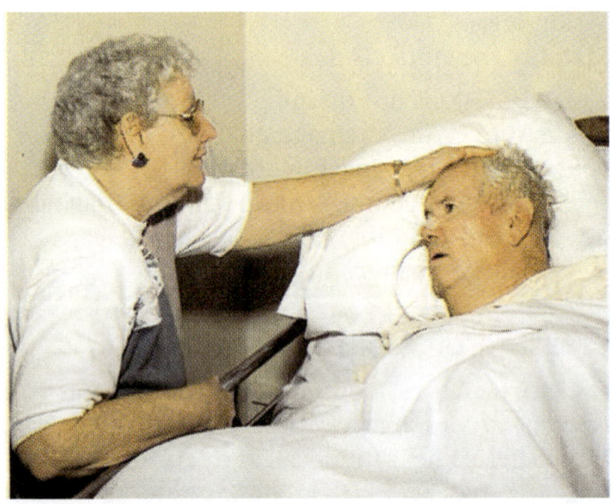

FIGURE 7-96 Rubbing and presure from tubes can cause irritation and skin breakdown.

Pressure ulcers occur most frequently over areas where bones come close to the surface. The most common sites (Figure 7.95A and 7.95B) are the:

- Elbows
- Heels
- Shoulders
- Sacrum, coccyx
- Hips
- Buttocks
- Ankles
- Ears
- Knees (inner and outer parts)
- Toes

Patients tend to develop pressure ulcers where body parts rub and cause friction. Common sites are:

- Between the folds of the buttocks
- Legs
- Under the breasts
- Abdominal folds
- Ankles
- Knees

The rubbing of tubing and other equipment used in the care of patients over a long period can also cause pressure sores. (Figure 7.96).

Preventing Pressure Ulcers. Because pressure ulcers are far easier to prevent than to cure, everyone participating in the patient's care has a responsibility to prevent skin breakdown.

When a patient is admitted, the nurse will assess the patient's current status and potential for skin breakdown. This assessment gives a baseline against which all future assessments may be measured. The assessment may be described on the patient's chart in words, pictures, diagrams, or as a score. Pressure ulcers will be discussed in more detail in Unit 14.

The Endocrine System

Structure and Function

The **endocrine glands** (Figure 7.97):

- secrete hormones.
- control body activities and growth.
- are found as distinct glands or clusters of cells.
- are subject to disease that can result in **hyposecretion** (underproduction) or **hypersecretion** (overproduction) of hormones.

Hormones are chemicals that regulate the body's activities.

Pituitary Gland

Because it controls most of the other glands, the **pituitary gland** is called the master gland.

The pituitary gland has two portions called *lobes*. Each of the lobes secretes more than one hormone.

1. The anterior lobe secretes:
   - STH (somatotropic hormone)—a growth hormone that stimulates the growth of long bones
   - TSH (thyroid-stimulating hormone)—stimulates the thyroid gland

FSH(follicle-stimulating hormone)—promotes

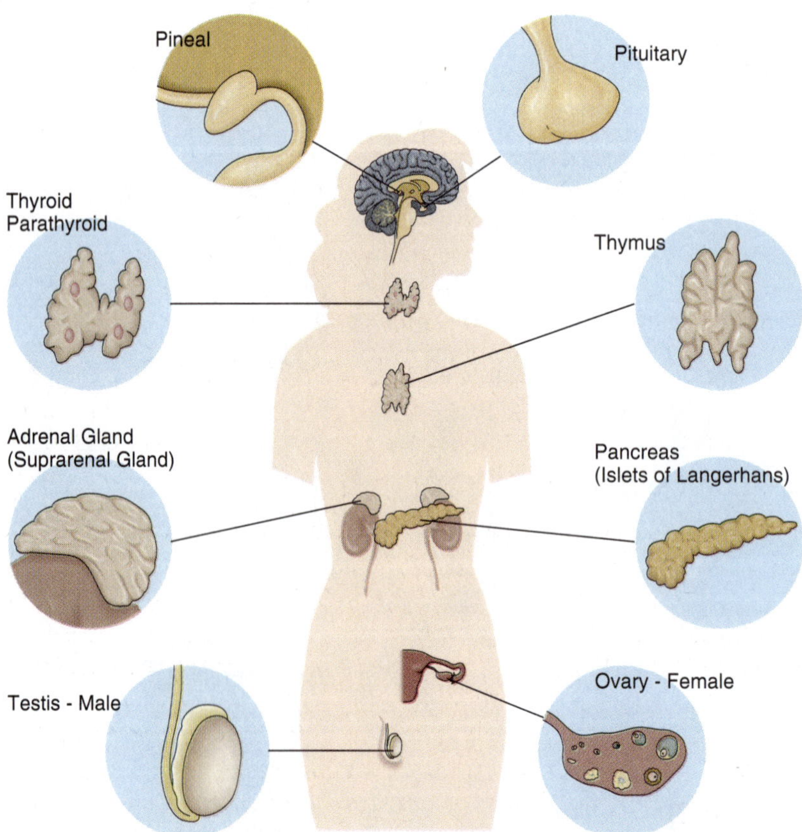

FIGURE 7-97 Endocrine system.

- FSH (follicle-stimulating hormone)—promotes growth of the ovarian follicle inwhich the egg develops during the menstrual cycle
- ACTH (adrenocorticotropic hormone)—stimulates production by the adrenal gland
- LH (luteinizing hormone)—in females, helps stimulate ovulation during the menstrual cycle
- ICSH (interstitial cell-stimulating hormone)—stimulates the male testes
- Lactogenic hormone (LTH)—stimulates milk production in pregnant women

2. The posterior lobe secretes:
   - ADH (antidiuretic hormone)—acts on kidneys to prevent excess water loss
   - Pitocin (oxytocin)—stimulates uterine contractions during childbirth

Pineal Body

The **pineal body** is a small gland that is also located in the skull beneath the brain. Very little is known about this gland. It is thought to be related somehow to sexual growth, because it tends to get smaller at maturity. It produces:

- Glomerulotropin, which influences the adrenal gland
- Serotonin, which acts in the brain
- Melatonin, which keeps sexual maturity from occurring too early and may affect the sleep/wake cycle.

Adrenal Glands

There are two **adrenal glands**. One gland is located on top of each kidney. Each gland has two distinct portions that secrete separate hormones.

1. The adrenal medulla (inside) produces norepinephrine (noradrenalin) and epinephrine (adrenalin), which stimulate the body to produce energy quickly during an emergency.
2. The adrenal cortex (outside) produces:
   - Glucocorticoids—elevate blood sugar levels and control the response of the body to stress and inflammation. They also depress inflammation.
   - Mineral corticoids—manage sodium and potassium levels.
   - Gonadocorticoids—influence both male and female sex hormones.

Gonads

The term **gonads** refers to the male and female sex glands. The female gonads (two **ovaries**):

- Are located within the pelvic cavity on either side of the uterus.
- Produce two hormones, **estrogen** and **progesterone**.These hormones are responsible for the development of female characteristics such as:
  - Breast development
  - Pubic and axillary hair
  - Onset and regulation of menstruation
  - Pregnancy

The male gonads (two **testes**):

- Are located on the outside of the body in a pouch called the **scrotum**.
- Produce the hormone **testosterone**. This hormone is responsible for secondary male characteristics such as:
  - Muscular development
  - Deepening voice
  - Hair growth

The male and female gonads also produce special cells—in the female, the **ovum** and in the male, the **sperm**. These cells unite during fertilization to form the embryo that becomes a new human being.

Thyroid Gland

The **thyroid gland** has two lobes and is found in the neck, anterior to the larynx. Hormones secreted by this gland are thyroxine and thyrocalcitonin. **Thyroxine** regulates metabolism. **Iodine** is an important component of this hormone. **Thyrocalcitonin** regulates calcium and phosphorus levels.

Parathyroid Glands

The tiny **parathyroid glands** are embedded in the posterior thyroid gland. The hormone they manufacture is called parathormone. **Parathormone** helps control the body's use of two minerals, calcium and phosphorus. Insufficient amounts of calcium result in severe muscle spasms or tetany. Untreated tetany can lead to death.

Islets of Langerhans

The **islets of Langerhans** are small groups of cells found within the pancreas. These cells produce two hormones: insulin and glucagon. **Insulin** lowers blood sugar. **Glucagon** elevates blood sugar.

Aging Changes in the Endocrine System

The endocrine system Figure 7.98 produces hormones. The hormones are released into the bloodstream to all parts of the body. Hormones are chemical messengers responsible for growth and development, reproduction, and stress responses. They play an important role in regulating fluid and energy balance in the body.

Aging changes in the endocrine system include:

- Blood sugar level increases because of delayed release of insulin, a hormone that regulates sugar use in the body.
- The amount of calories needed for the body to function normally decreases because of a lower metabolism rate, or slower body function.

Diabetes

Diabetes is a chronic disease of the endocrine system, affecting as many as 50 percent of all elderly adults. Diabetes affects the utilization of sugar in the body. Sugar (glucose) production in the body is regulated by insulin, a hormone secreted by the pancreas. Diabetes results from a deficiency of insulin or a resistance to the effects of insulin, causing the body to be unable to properly process food into energy. As the blood sugar level rises, more insulin is secreted to regulate the sugar level in the blood. In a person with diabetes, the output or use of insulin is not adequate. The glucose from the food breakdown remains in the blood, resulting in elevated blood sugar (too much glucose in the blood). Proteins and fats are not broken down correctly. Dehydration and fluid imbalances can result. Indications that the resident has diabetes are extreme thirst, hunger, frequent urination, fatigue, itching, slow healing, infections of the skin, and changes in vision. Overweight and obesity are common. Diabetes is treated with an injection of insulin, or oral drugs that lower the blood sugar level. The resident is placed on a special diet and is not given free sugar or extra snacks. The resident's blood sugar is monitored by a finger stick test in the long-term care facility.

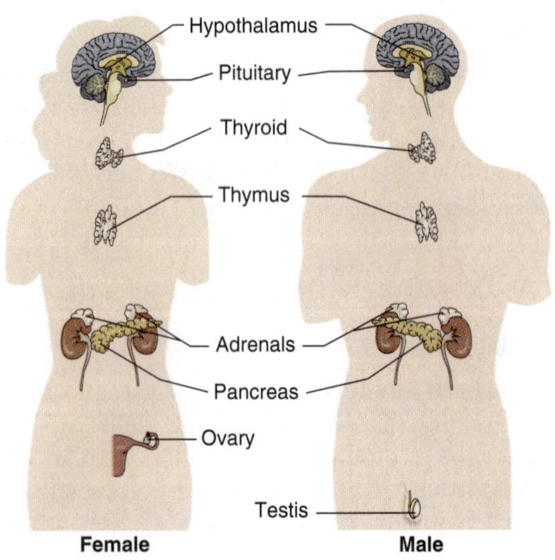

FIGURE 7-98 The endocrine system

TABLE 7-9 Signs and Symptoms

Hyperglycemia	Hypoglycemia
Nausea, vomiting	Complaints of hunger, weakness, dizziness, shakiness
Weakness	
Headache	Cold, moist, clammy, or pale skin
Full, bounding pulse	
Fruity smell to breath	Rapid, shallow respirations
Hot, dry, flushed skin	
Labored respirations	Nervousness and excitement
Drowsiness	Rapid pulse
Mental confusion	Unconsciousness
Unconsciousness	No sugar in the urine
Sugar in the urine	Low blood sugar by finger stick
High blood sugar by finger stick	

Complications of diabetes. Diabetes has two very serious complications. Hyperglycemia, or too much sugar in the blood, occurs when there is not enough insulin to meet the body's needs. Hypoglycemia, or too little sugar in the blood, occurs when the blood sugar level is too low. Both of these conditions can be life threatening. Persistent elevated glucose levels affect the blood vessels and nerves, making the person with diabetes more likely to develop heart attack, stroke, blindness, renal disease, and other serious complications and conditions. If you notice signs of diabetes-related problems developing, report them to the nurse immediately. Signs and symptoms of hyperglycemia and hypoglycemia are listed in Table 7.4.

Common Conditions of the Thyroid Gland

The thyroid gland may secrete too much or not enough hormones. Either situation is treatable. If not treated, severe illness or death will occur.

Hyperthyroidism

Hyperthyroidism, or overactivity of the thyroid gland, results in production of too much thyroxine (hypersecretion). The person shows:

- Irritability and restlessness
- Nervousness
- Rapid pulse
- Increased appetite
- Weight loss
- Sensitivity

Nursing Assistant Actions. When caring for these patients, the nursing assistant must be understanding and have patience. The room should be kept quiet and cool. The patient's increased nutritional needs should be met with foods that are liked.

Treatment. Treatment of hyperthyroidism is designed to reduce the level of thyroxine through:

- Surgical thyroidectomy
- Radiation to reduce the number of functional cells

Thyroidectomy. It may be necessary to treat hyperthyroidism with surgery. You may be assigned to assist in the postoperative care. Following surgery:

- The patient is placed in a semi-Fowler's position, with neck and shoulders well supported. Remember at all times to support the back of the neck. Hyperextension of the neck may damage the operative site.
- Assist with oxygen, if ordered, using all oxygen precautions.
- Give routine postoperative care.
- Check for and report the following:
  - Any signs of bleeding (this may drain toward the back of the neck). The pillows behind the patient should be checked, as well as the dressings.
  - Signs of respiratory distress.
  - Inability of the patient to speak. Initial hoarseness is common, but any increase should be reported.
  - Greatly elevated temperature and pulse, pronounced apprehension, or irritability.
  - Numbness, tingling, or muscular spasm (**tetany**) of the extremities.

Hypothyroidism

Hypothyroidism results in an undersecretion of thyroxine. Recall that iodine is an essential component of thyroxine. A lack of iodine in the diet can result in low thyroxine production.

- The condition is called **simple goiter**.
- The thyroid gland enlarges (**hypertrophies**).
- Secretions produced have low thyroxine content.

Hypothyroidism can usually be successfully managed with thyroxine replacement.

Common Conditions of the Parathyroid Glands

Parathormone, secreted by the parathyroids, regulates the levels of electrolytes, calcium, and phosphates. Hypersecretion of this hormone results in:

- Excessively high levels of blood calcium (**hypercalcemia**)
- Developmental of renal calculi (kidney stones)
- Loss of bone calcium

Hypersecretion is usually caused by tumors. Tumors can be treated by surgical removal.

Hyposecretion can lead to:

- Abnormal muscle-nerve interaction
- Severe muscle spasm (tetany)

This can be an emergency situation, requiring management of the muscle spasms and administration of calcium. In the chronic state, calcium replacements and increased dietary calcium are prescribed.

Common Conditions of the Adrenal Glands

The adrenal gland secretions regulate:

- Development and maintenance of sexual characteristics
- Carbohydrate, fat, and protein metabolism
- Fluid balance
- Electrolyte levels of sodium and potassium

Hypersecretion results in **Cushing's syndrome**, which is characterized by:

- Weakness due to loss of body protein
- Increased blood sugar levels (hyperglycemia)
- Edema
- Hypertension
- Loss of potassium and retention of sodium
- Masculinization of a female

Therapy is primarily surgical and supportive.

Hyposecretion results in **Addison's disease**, which is characterized by:

- Loss of sodium and retention of potassium
- Abnormally low blood sugar (hypoglycemia)
- Dehydration
- Low stress tolerance

Addison's disease is treated by hormone replacement therapy and techniques to combat dehydration.

DIABETES MELLITUS

In the United States, 17 million people have diabetes mellitus. Approximately 5.9 million of these have not been diagnosed yet. Diabetes occurs in people of all ages and races, but is most common in African Americans, Native Americans, Latinos, Asian Americans, and Pacific Islanders. The incidence of diabetes increases with age.

Diabetes mellitus is a chronic disease that results from a deficiency of insulin or a resistance to the effects of insulin. The problems with insulin cause the body to be unable to properly process food into energy. The glucose from the food breakdown remains in the blood, resulting in elevated blood sugar. Persistent, elevated glucose levels affect the blood vessels and nerves, making the person with diabetes more likely to develop heart attack, stroke, blindness, renal disease, and other serious complications and conditions.

The reason why diabetes develops is not fully understood. Factors that seem to play a role in the incidence of diabetes are:

- Heredity
- Obesity
- Age
- Diet
- Lack of exercise

All diabetics should wear or carry a Medic Alert® identification so that proper and immediate care can be provided in an emergency. It is also recommended that the diabetic carry food that provides a quick source of carbohydrates.

Disease Mechanism

In diabetes, the normal metabolism of fats, carbohydrates, and proteins is unbalanced. Normally, when carbohydrates are absorbed into the bloodstream, the blood sugar (glucose) level rises. The pancreas responds to an increase of **glucose** by secreting more insulin. Insulin is the hormone primarily responsible for:

- Lowering the blood sugar level by allowing glucose to cross the cell membrane.
- Increasing the oxidation of glucose by the tissues.
- Stimulating the conversion of glucose to glycogen by the liver. **Glycogen** is a storage form of energy.
- Decreasing glucose production from amino acids.
- Stimulating glucose formation into fat for storage.

In diabetes, there is insufficient insulin for these metabolic functions.

- Glucose cannot be properly utilized for energy.
- Fats and proteins are incompletely broken down. This leads to an accumulation of ketone bodies, and nitrogenous waste products.
- The excess glucose is eliminated, along with water and salts, through the kidneys. This causes dehydration and electrolyte imbalance.
- The characteristic symptoms of excessive thirst, hunger, and increased urination are directly related to the loss of fluids, electrolytes, and sugar.

Types of Diabetes Mellitus

Diabetes mellitus is typed and named according to the need for insulin. Examples are insulin-dependent diabetes mellitus (IDDM) and non-insulin-dependent diabetes (NIDDM). IDDM appears more commonly in the young and NIDDM is more common in older people.

Insulin-dependent diabetes mellitus (IDDM) (Type I) accounts for approximately 5% to 10% of diabetes. This type tends to run in families. It is most common in children and young adults. Symptoms may mimic the flu in young children. People with Type I diabetes must take daily insulin injections to stay alive. Typical signs and symptoms are:

- **Polyuria** (excessive urination)
- **Polydipsia** (thirst)
- **Polyphagia** (hunger)
- **Glycosuria** (sugar in the urine)

Non–insulin-dependent diabetes mellitus (NIDDM) (Type II) is a metabolic disorder that occurs when the body does not make enough insulin, or does not properly use insulin. This is the most common form of diabetes. It accounts for 90% to 95% of all diabetes. It is said to be nearing epidemic proportions due to the high incidence of obesity and sedentary lifestyles. People usually develop Type II diabetes after age 45, but may not be aware they have the condition until symptoms become severe or complications develop. The risk for Type II diabetes increases with age. More than 20 percent of the United States population aged 65 and older has diabetes. Common signs and symptoms of Type II diabetes are:

- Easy fatigue
- Skin infections
- Slow healing
- Itching
- Pruritus vulvae (itching of the vulva)
- Burning on urination
- Vision changes
- Obesity

Often only one or two symptoms are apparent in the elderly person. The older person may:

- complain of constant fatigue.
- have a skin lesion that takes an unusually long time to heal.
- experience vision changes that may be mistakenly attributed to aging.

Care of the diabetic is directed toward maintaining a normal blood glucose level so that complications may be prevented. To regulate blood glucose, the diabetic person must:

- eat a healthful, well-balanced diet as prescribed by the physician.
- exercise regularly in a manner appropriate for the person's age and ability.
- check the blood sugar regularly
- use insulin or oral antidiabetic agents correctly if ordered by the physician.

For some persons this may require lifestyle changes. Nurses and dietitians are responsible for teaching patients who are newly diagnosed with diabetes how to care for themselves. People with diabetes who are knowledgeable about the disease and who are willing to manage their lives accordingly can live happily and productively (Figure 7.99).

Diet

Diet is an important part of diabetic treatment. Physicians do not fully agree as to how strictly a diet must be followed by all patients.

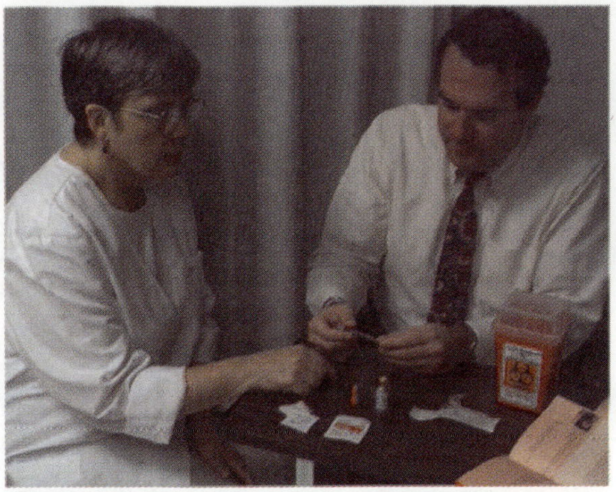

FIGURE 7-99 Patients are taught to manage their diabetes by the nurse.

- Weight reduction is favored.
- Weight reduction alone may be sufficient to bring the condition under control in NIDDM.

Meal Planning. The dietitian is a key member of the health care team for patients with diabetes. The dietitian helps the patient plan meals in keeping with the patient's goals, lifestyle, laboratory values, caloric and nutritional needs, and food preferences. Many diabetics use the diabetic food guide pyramid (Figure 7.100). This is similar to the USDA Food Guide Pyramid, but portion sizes and the total number of portions per day have been adjusted. The dietitian will work with the patient to develop a healthy meal plan.

The goals of the diet include maintaining near-normal blood sugar, optimal fat levels, and adequate calories based on individual needs. Meal plans are flexible. The diet should be well balanced, with sufficient fiber.

The diabetic exchange system of foods was formulated by a committee with representatives from the American Diabetic Association and the diabetic branch of the U.S. Public Health Service. The exchanges are available through the registered dietitian or diabetes educator. Although the exchange list system has been used for years, it is regularly updated to reflect new trends. The lists provide maximum flexibility in planning a healthy diet. The dietitian teaches the patient the importance of reading food labels, and how to interpret them. Common household measures are used to determine portion size.

Exercise

Exercise is an important part of the overall treatment. The amount and type of exercise the

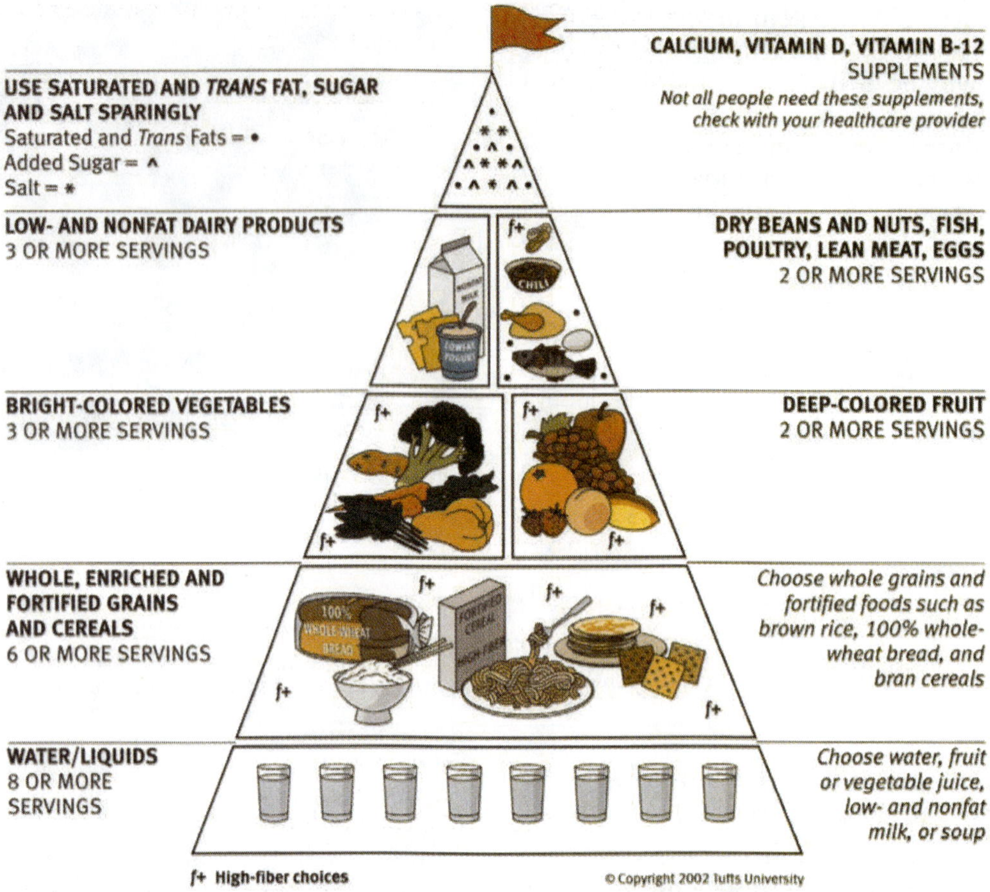

FIGURE 7-100 The diabetic food guide pyramid. *(Copyright 2002 Tufts University)*

patient routinely engages in are balanced by the food intake and insulin or hypoglycemic drug requirements.

Hypoglycemic Drugs

Diabetes mellitus is treated by one of two main drug groups. One is administered subcutaneously or intravenously. The other is given orally.

At present, there are several types of insulin. They vary in their:

- Speed of action
- Duration
- Potency or strength

Insulin is:

- Administered by the nurse. The nurse rotates the administration sites.
- Given by injection.
- Increasingly given through use of an insulin pump. The insulin pump delivers a prescribed amount of insulin on a regular basis into the patient's body.
- Used to treat IDDM and some patients with NIDDM.

Persons living at home are taught to administer their own insulin.

Note: When insulin is self-administered, it is important to report any missed injections or signs of infection around the administration site.

Oral hypoglycemic drugs are:

- Administered by the nurse.
- Given by mouth.
- Used to treat NIDDM.

Complications

Because persistent, increased glucose levels cause damage to the nerves and blood vessels, the following complications can occur:

- Renal disease
- Circulatory impairments that often result in gangrene (Figure 7.101) and amputation
- Poor healing
- Hypertension
- Cardiovascular problems
- Diabetic coma
- Insulin shock (hypoglycemia)
- Vision problems and blindness

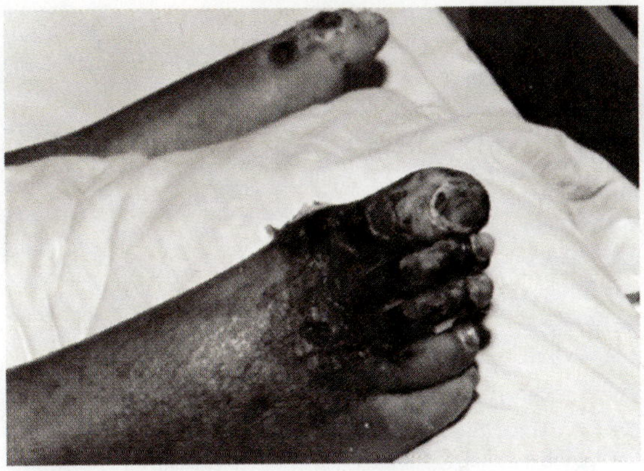

FIGURE 7-101 Gangrene of the feet and toes will require amputation. In most cases, the leg is amputated below the knee.

Hypoglycemia (Low Blood Sugar)

Hypoglycemia occurs when the blood glucose level is below normal. It:

- May occur rapidly.
- Is referred to as *insulin reaction* or *insulin shock* when due to an overdose of insulin.

Hypoglycemia can be brought on by:

- Skipping meals
- Unusual activity
- Stress
- Vomiting
- Diarrhea
- Omission of planned snack or meals
- Interaction of drugs
- Too much insulin or antidiabetic medication

Signs and Symptoms. The signs and symptoms of hypoglycemia include:

- Complaints of hunger, weakness, dizziness, shakiness
- Skin cold, moist, clammy, pale
- Rapid, shallow respirations
- Nervousness and excitement
- Rapid pulse
- Unconsciousness
- No sugar in the urine
- Low blood sugar results from fingerstick test

If the patient is awake and alert, treatment includes intake of orange juice, milk, or another easily absorbed carbohydrate such as hard candy. If the patient is unconscious, the physician or nurse may give glucagon, which causes a rapid elevation of blood sugar.

Hyperglycemia (High Blood Sugar)

Hyperglycemia (diabetic coma):

- Occurs when there is insufficient insulin for metabolic needs.
- Usually develops slowly, sometimes over a 24-hour period.
- May be seen as confusion, drowsiness, or a slow slippage into coma in a patient who is confined to bed.

Hyperglycemia may be brought on by:

- Stress
- Illness such as infection
- Dehydration
- Injury
- Forgotten medication
- Intake of too much food

Signs and Symptoms The signs and symptoms of diabetic coma include:

- Early headache, drowsiness, or confusion
- Sweet, fruity odor to the breath
- Deep breathing, labored respirations
- Full, bounding pulse
- Low blood pressure
- Nausea or vomiting
- Flushed, dry, hot skin
- Weakness
- Unconsciousness
- Sugar in the urine
- High blood sugar results from fingerstick test

Treatment includes administration of insulin, fluids, and electrolytes.

Other Complications

Persons with diabetes should have regular health monitoring so that complications may be detected early and treated promptly. Health monitoring should include:

- Eye examinations by an ophthalmologist for early detection of diabetic retinopathy, which can lead to impaired vision and eventually blindness.
- Urinalysis and other urological examinations to evaluate the condition of the kidneys.
- Cardiac evaluation; monitoring of heart action and blood pressure.
- Circulatory evaluation.
- Care and treatment of any wounds.
- Blood sugar monitoring.

Nursing Assistant Responsibilities

- Know the signs of insulin shock and diabetic coma.
- Be alert for the signs of diabetic coma or insulin shock and report them immediately to the nurse.

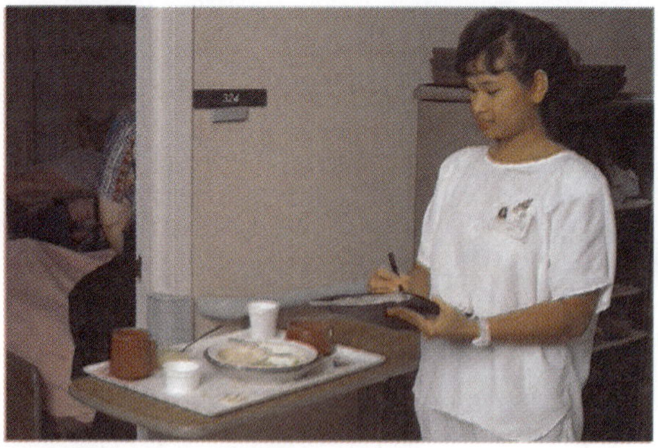

FIGURE 7-102 The amount and type of food consumed by patients with diabetes is closely observed and recorded.

- Know the storage location of orange juice or other easily **assimilated** (absorbed) sources of carbohydrates.
- Keep easily assimilated carbohydrates, such as orange juice, crackers, hard candy, or Karo syrup, available if caring for a diabetic patient at home.
- Make sure you serve the patient proper trays of food.
- Do not give extra nourishments without special permission.
- Document food consumption, on the patient's chart.
- Report uneaten meals to the nurse (Figure 7.102).
- Give special attention to care of the diabetic patient's feet.
  - Wash daily, carefully drying between toes
  - Inspect feet closely for any breaks or signs of irritation.
  - Report any abnormalities to the nurse.
  - Do not allow moisture to collect between toes.
  - The toenails of a diabetic should be cut only by a nurse or a podiatrist, a specialist who is trained in foot care.
  - Shoes and stockings should be clean, be free of holes, and fit well. Anything that might injure the feet or interfere with the circulation must be avoided.
  - Do not allow the patient to go barefoot.

Difficult Situations

Attention to personal hygiene, oral care, and cleanliness is particularly important in individuals with diabetes. Diabetics must bathe regularly to prevent localized skin infections. However, they should avoid prolonged soaking in a tub, which can soften the tissues and lead to breakdown. If you observe unusual areas, such as yellowish pimples or boils, on a diabetic patient's skin, or angry-looking red areas in skin folds (such as under the breasts, underarms, or groin), inform the nurse. Assist the patient with toothbrushing and flossing. The teeth have five surfaces, and toothbrushing only reaches three. Flossing effectively cleans the areas that are not accessible with the brush. Good foot care and drying well between the toes are essential. Report signs and symptoms of infection, even if they seem minor.

Blood Glucose Monitoring

Bedside glucose testing has become very common in the management of patients with diabetes. Many individuals perform this testing at home several times each day. The antidiabetic medication may be adjusted according to the patient's blood sugar. A blood sample is taken from a capillary. The test meter will display the blood sugar value in one minute or less. This is a convenient, accurate method of monitoring the blood sugar. Nursing assistants perform this procedure in some facilities. Know and follow your facility policy.

The physician will order specific times for blood sugar testing. The specimen may be collected at a fixed time, such as before meals. The nurse may administer insulin to the patient based on the blood sugar value. Collect the capillary sample exactly as ordered. Specimens that are not collected at the proper time can cause misinterpretation of the results. Always report the value to the nurse, and document according to facility policy.

If the nurse suspects that a patient is having complications related to diabetes, he or she may ask you to obtain a star blood sugar. This test must be performed immediately. Report the results immediately.

The Reproductive System

STRUCTURE AND FUNCTION

Both the male and female reproductive organs have dual functions. They:

1. Produce reproductive cells. The male produces **sperm**. The female produces the **ovum**.
2. Produce hormones that are responsible for sex characteristics.
   a. Males produce testosterone.
   b. Females produce estrogen and progesterone.

In the reproductive process, the:

- male and female engage in sexual intercourse.
- male ejaculates (propels) the sperm and the seminal fluid in which they swim into the female vagina.
- sperm and egg meet in the female fallopian tube. One sperm penetrates the egg and conception takes place.
- baby (fetus) develops in the uterus until birth.
- female breasts (mammary glands) produce milk to nourish the newborn.

The Male Reproductive Organs: Structure and Function

The male organs (Figure 7.103) include the:

- **Testes**: Two glandular organs located in the scrotum. The testes produce sperm and the hormone testosterone.
- **Epididymis**: A 20-foot-long coiled tube located on the top and back of each testis. The epididymis stores the sperm and allows them to mature.
- **Vas deferens**: A tube that leads from the epididymis. It carries the sperm upward into the pelvic cavity to the seminal vesicles during ejaculation. The vas deferens is accompanied by nerves and blood vessels. Together, they form the spermatic cord.
- **Seminal vesides**: Located behind the bladder. They receive and store the sperm from the vas deferens. They contribute nutrients to the seminal fluid. The small ejaculatory duct leads from the seminal vesicles to the urethra just below the prostate gland.
- **Ejaculatory duct**: Carries the fluid produced in the seminal vesicles. Fluids are added as the sperm are propelled forward. The sperm and fluid form the seminal fluid or ejaculate. The fluid contains nutrients and other substances needed by the sperm.
- **Prostate gland**: Found just below the urinary bladder surrounding the urethra. It secretes a fluid that increases the ability of the sperm to move in the seminal fluid. Enlargement of the prostate gland may prevent urine from passing through the urethra. This is a fairly common occurrence in older men.
- **Cowper's glands**: Two small glands located beside the urethra. They produce mucus for lubrication.
- **Penis**: Composed of special tissue that can become filled with blood, making the organ enlarge and become stiffened so that it may enter the vagina to deposit seminal fluid. Loose-fitting skin (the prepuce or foreskin) covers the penis.

The male urethra passes through the penis and serves two purposes. It carries:

- Reproductive fluid during intercourse
- Urine during voiding

The two activities cannot occur at the same time because they are under the control of different parts of the nervous system.

The Female Reproductive Organs: Structure and Function

The external female structures (**genitalia**) (Figure 7.104) include the:

- **Vulva**: Made up of two liplike structures, the **labia majora** and **labia minora**. When the labia are separated, other external structures may be seen.
- **Clitoris**: A very sensitive structure found just behind the juncture of the labia minora. It functions during sexual stimulation to begin the rhythmic series of contractions associated with female climax (orgasm).

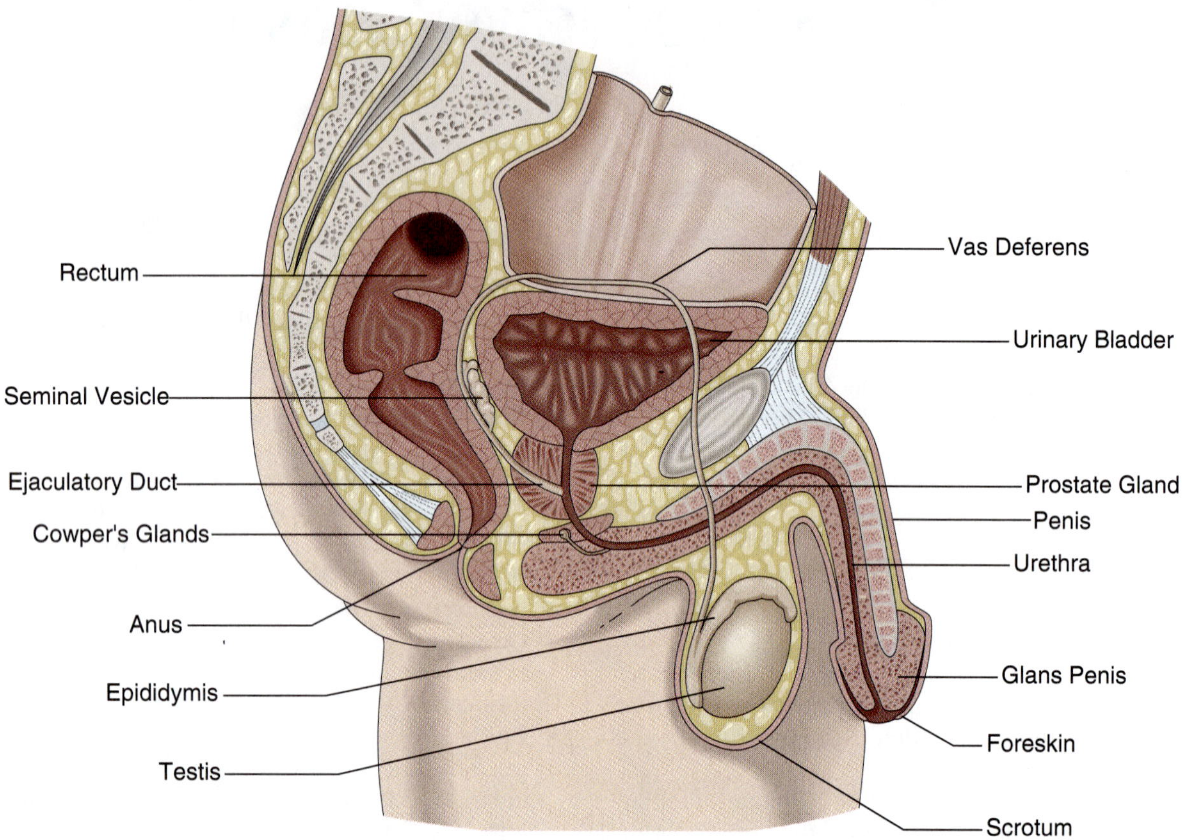

FIGURE 7-103 Cross-section of the male reproductive system.

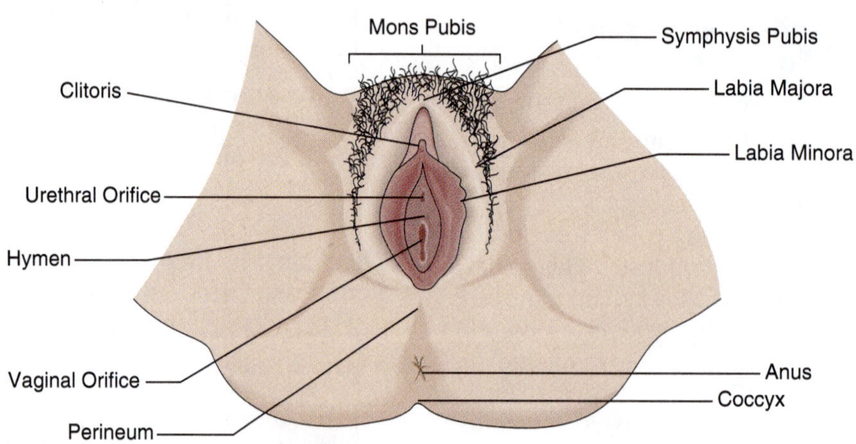

FIGURE 7-104 External female reproductive organs

- Urinary meatus: The opening of the urethra to the outside.
- Vaginal meatus: The opening to the vagina or birth canal.

The Internal Female Structures

The internal female reproductive organs (Figures 7.105 and 7.106) include the following structures.

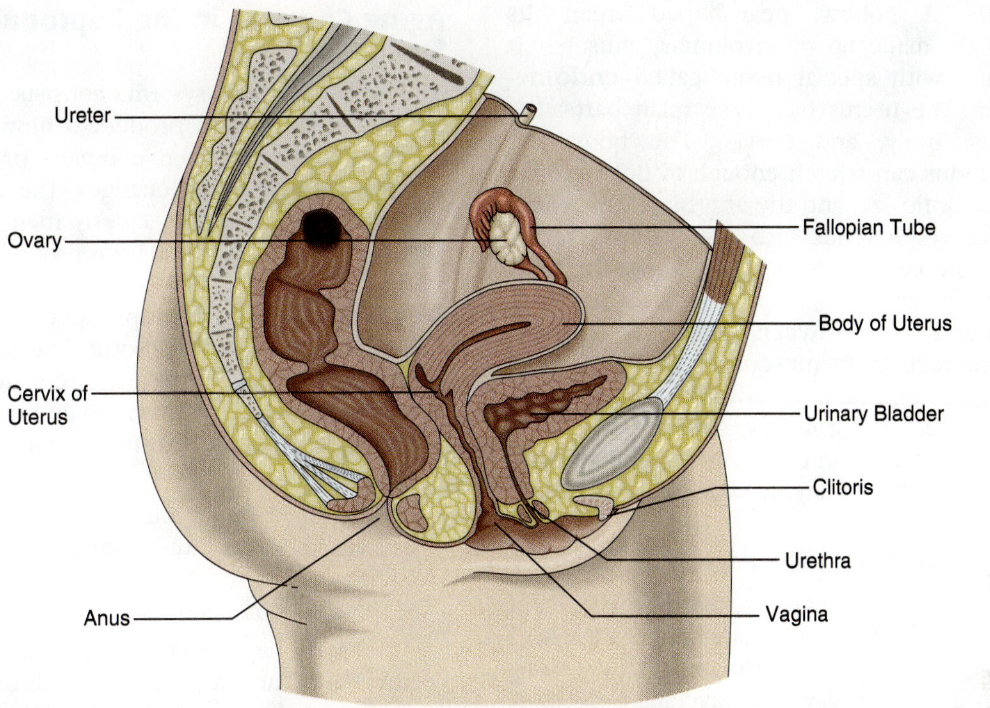

FIGURE 7-105 Cross-section of internal female reproductive system.

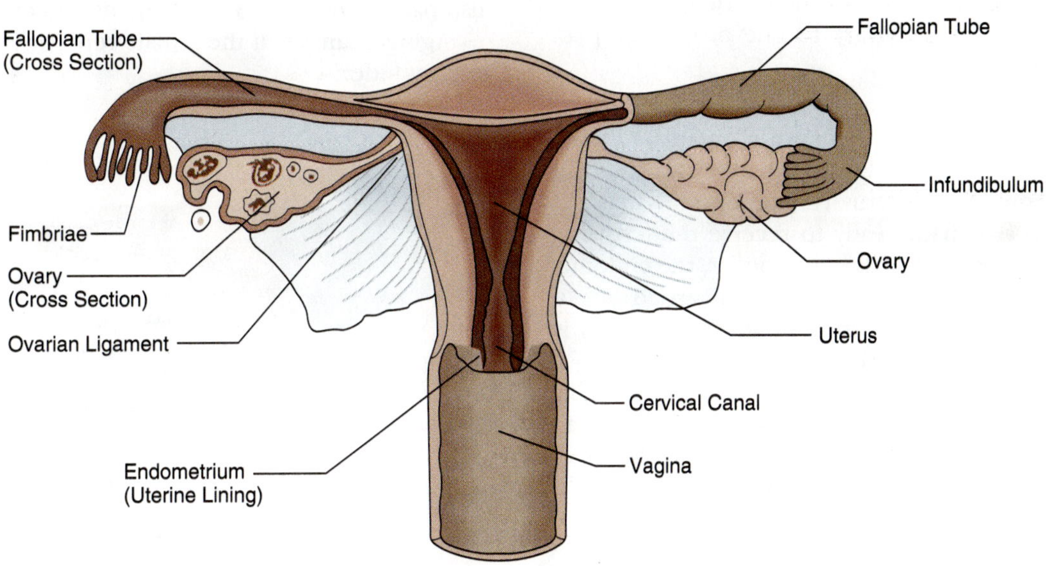

FIGURE 7-106 Anterior view of interior female reproductive organs.

- **Ovaries**: Two small glands, found on either side of the uterus, at the ends of the oviducts (fallopian tubes) in the pelvis. They produce two hormones, estrogen and progesterone, and the egg (ovum). The eggs are contained in many little sacs called follicles. About once each month, a follicle matures and releases an ovum. The ovum makes its way into one of the four-inch-long oviducts. This process is called **ovulation**. The cells of the follicles that are left produce progesterone. The progesterone causes changes within the uterus, readying it for the possibility of receiving a fertilized ovum.
- **Fallopian tubes (oviducts)**: Two tubes, approximately four inches long, that serve as a pathway between the ovary and uterus. The sperm and egg meet in the tubes. Fertilization takes place here.

- **Uterus**: A hollow, pear-shaped organ. Its walls are made up of involuntary muscles. It is lined with special tissue called **endometrium**. The uterus has three main parts: the fundus, body, and cervix. The body and the fundus can stretch enough to hold a fetus, the amniotic sac, and the afterbirth (placenta). The cervix extends into the vagina. During labor, the cervix opens up to allow the baby to be delivered.
- **Vagina**: Found between the urinary bladder and the rectum. Its muscular walls are capable of much stretching. It is lined with mucous membrane. Two glands known as Bartholin's glands are found on either side of the external vaginal opening. They provide lubrication.

Menstruation and Ovulation

The menstrual cycle (female sexual cycle) begins at **puberty**. Puberty occurs in girls between the ages of 9 and 17. The cycle varies in length, usually between 25 and 30 days. The average is 28 days, which is why it is considered a monthly cycle.

During the menstrual cycle, a mature egg, or ovum (plural, ova):

- is released from one of the ovaries.
- travels from the ovary to one of the fallopian tubes.
- may be fertilized by a male sperm.

At the same time that the ovum is being matured and expelled from the ovary (ovulation), the lining of the uterus (endometrium) is being built up and made ready to receive the fertilized ovum. If fertilization does not occur, the endometrium is no longer needed, so it is carried out of the body as the menstrual flow. This process is known as **menstruation**.

Unlike the sperm cells, all the special cells that will become the ova exist when a woman is born. When the last ova are released, the menstrual cycle ceases and **menopause** begins.

Menopause

As women age, the menstrual cycle becomes irregular and gradually ceases altogether. This is called the menopause, or **climacteric**, or change of life.

Menopause usually occurs around the age of 55 and involves a natural series of changes that stops the menstrual cycle. These changes are not abrupt, but usually take place over a period of years. Because eggs are no longer being matured and released, pregnancy cannot occur.

Some women may undergo menopause earlier in life after surgical removal of the ovaries.

Aging Changes in the Reproductive System

The reproductive system consists of organs whose function is to produce a new individual. Some of the reproductive organs produce hormones. Despite aging changes, the elderly can enjoy an active sex life. Elderly men are able to father children. The primary reproductive organs in the male (Figure 7.107) are the penis, which is the male organ used for reproduction and urinary elimination, and the scrotum, a small ovoid pouch containing the testes. The testes produce sperm for reproduction, and male hormones.

Aging changes in the male reproductive system include:

- Hormone production decreases, causing decreased size of testes and a lower sperm count.
- More time is needed for an erection to occur.

The main reproductive organs in the female (Figure 7.107) are two ovaries, glands that produce hormones and eggs for reproduction; the uterus, the organ where a baby grows and receives nourishment; the vagina, or birth canal; and the vulva, or external genitalia (Figure 7.108) The breasts are also part of the female reproductive system.

Aging changes in the female reproductive system include:

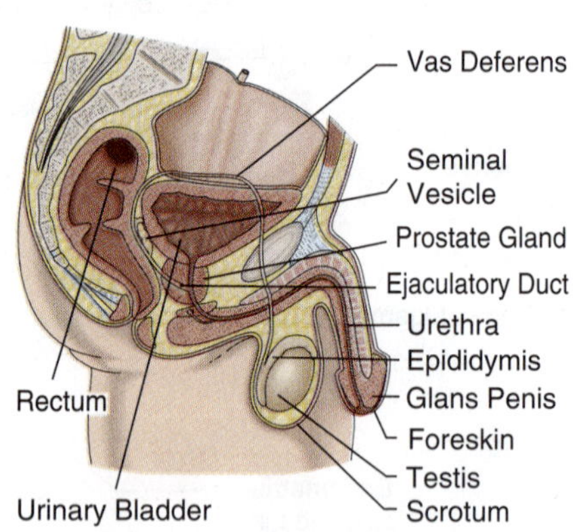

The male genitourinary system

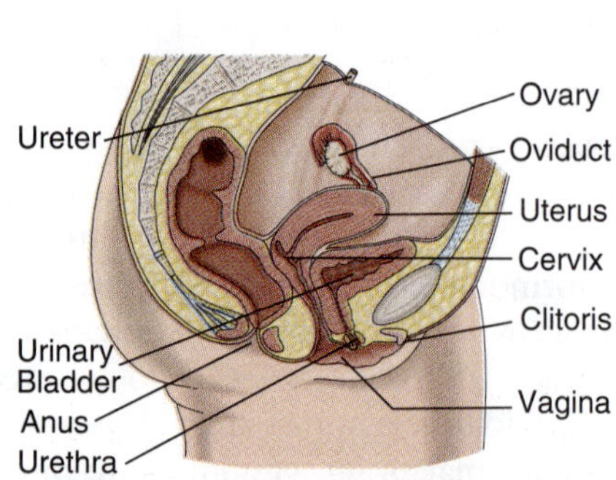

FIGURE 7-107 The female genitourinary system

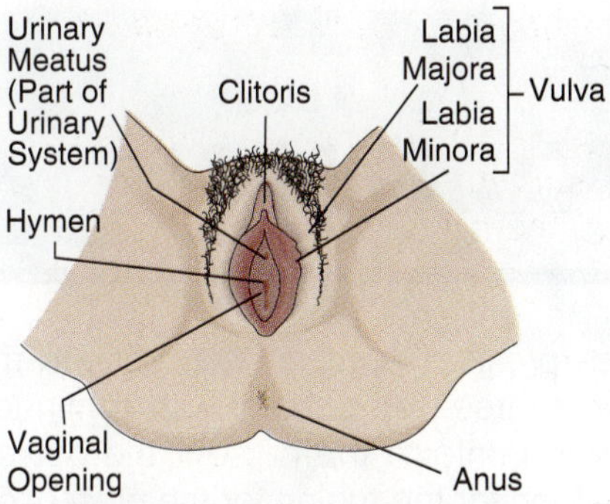

FIGURE 7-108 The female genitourinary system

- Fewer female hormones are produced.
- Menstruation stops.
- The vagina becomes shorter and narrower.
- Vaginal secretions decrease.
- Breast tissue decreases and the muscles supporting the breasts weaken.

Conditions of the Male Reproductive Organs

The male organs are subject to the same kinds of disease processes that affect other body parts. Examples of these conditions are tumors and infections. A very common problem experienced by many men involves the prostate gland.

Prostate Conditions

Benign prostatic (of the prostate gland) **hypertrophy** (Figure 7.109):

- is an enlargement of the prostate gland without tumor development.
- causes narrowing of the urethra, which passes through the center of the prostate gland.
- can cause sufficient enlargement to cause urinary retention.
- is noncancerous.

Signs and symptoms of prostate conditions include difficulty in starting the stream of urine or in emptying the bladder completely.

Prostate cancer is the second leading cause of cancer deaths in males. A blood test, the prostate specific antigen (PSA), is used to screen for abnormalities. Because of the widespread use of the blood test, many prostate cancers are caught early, and the outcome is usually favorable. Prostate cancer usually grows very slowly. In the early stages, there may be no symptoms. As the condition progresses, signs and symptoms develop. The most common are:

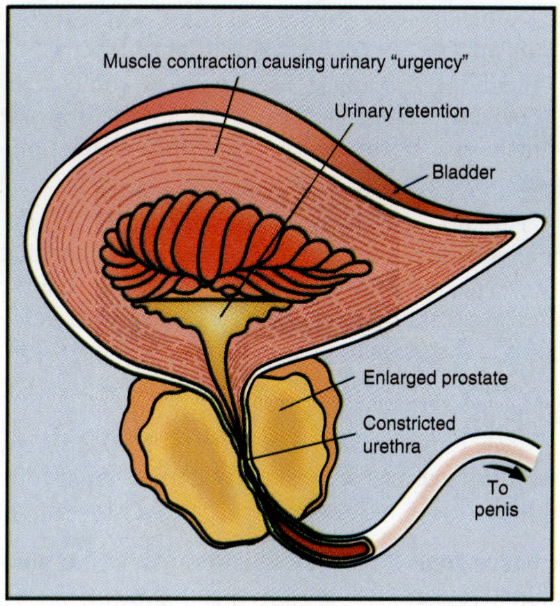

FIGURE 7-109 Cell growth causes the prostate to enlarge, constricting the urethra. The bladder may not empty completely, causing discomfort and increasing the risk of infection.

- difficulty with urination
- decreased force of the urine stream
- frequency of urination
- urgency (an intense need to urinate)
- urinary retention
- repeated urinary tract infections
- blood in the urine or semen

Treatment. Various surgical approaches are used to remove all or part of the prostate gland (**prostatectomy**) to relieve urinary retention.

- Transurethral prostatectomy (TURP)—only enough of the gland is removed, working from inside the urethra, to permit urine to pass.
- Perineal prostatectomy—the entire gland is removed through surgical incisions in the perineum.
- Suprapublic prostatectomy—an incision is made just above the pubis and part of the gland is removed.
- Radiation therapy consists of five to seven weeks of treatments in which radiation is directed to the prostate gland.
- **Brachytherapy** is another form of radiation therapy in which tiny radioactive seeds or pellets are implanted directly inside the prostate gland. This treatment is very successful and

preferred over traditional radiation therapy because it has fewer side effects.

- Hormone therapy is used to treat some prostate cancers. This treatment suppresses the male sex hormone (testosterone) that stimulates the cancer to grow.

Patients are likely to be disturbed by the necessity of prostate surgery. Men often fear that they will not be able to have sexual intercourse after a prostatectomy. They feel that their manhood is threatened.

Urinary incontinence is also a common problem and a great concern. In most cases, the rate of leakage decreases over time. Nevertheless, incontinence has a substantial impact on quality of life.

Postsurgical Care. In addition to routine postoperative care, the prostatectomy patient:

- will have a Foley catheter in place following the surgery.
- may have a suprapubic drain through the suprapubic incision.
- may have a perineal drain in the perineal incision.

The nursing assistant should:

- Wear personal protective equipment and apply the principles of standard precautions if contact with blood, body fluids, mucous membranes, or nonintact skin is likely.
- Be careful that the tubes do not become twisted, stressed, or dislodged when positioning the patient.
- Carefully note the amount and color of drainage from all areas.
- Report at once any sudden increase in bright redness or the appearance of clots that seem to block the tube.
- Report to the nurse if dressings become wet with urinary drainage.
- Be patient and understanding of the patient's emotional stress.
- Refer questions about possible sexual limitation and urinary incontinence to the nurse so that the patient can get information and support.

At times, it will be necessary to irrigate (wash out) the drainage tubes. This is a sterile procedure that will be carried out by the nurse or physician.

Cancer of the Testes

Cancer of the testes is fairly common. Treatment may require removal of the testicles (**orchiectomy**). This procedure is performed when there is testicular malignancy. When an early diagnosis is made, treatment can be started early. Orchiectomy can then be avoided.

Testicular self-examination (Figure 7.110) is an important way to locate lumps or changes in the testes. This procedure should be performed by all adult males:

- At least once each month
- During a warm shower so the scrotum will be relaxed
- With soapy fingers
- By palpating each testis between the fingers and thumb

DIFFICULT SITUATIONS

After prostate surgery, the patient may have a three-way catheter with continuous irrigation. Inform the nurse if the bottle is low. Monitor the tubing for the presence of blood clots. Monitor the patient for signs of excess bleeding, cold or clammy skin, pallor, restlessness, falling blood pressure, orrapid pulse. If noted, report promptly.

Conditions of the Female Reproductive Organs

Like the male organs, female reproductive organs are subject to disease processes, including tumors and infections.

Rectocele and Cystocele

Rectoceles and cystoceles are hernias. They usually occur at the same time.

- **Rectoceles** (Figure 7.111) are a weakening of the wall shared between the vagina and the rectum. These hernias frequently cause constipation and **hemorrhoids** (varicose veins of the rectum).
- **Cystoceles** (Figure 7.112) are a weakening of the muscles between the bladder and the vagina. Cystoceles cause urinary incontinence.

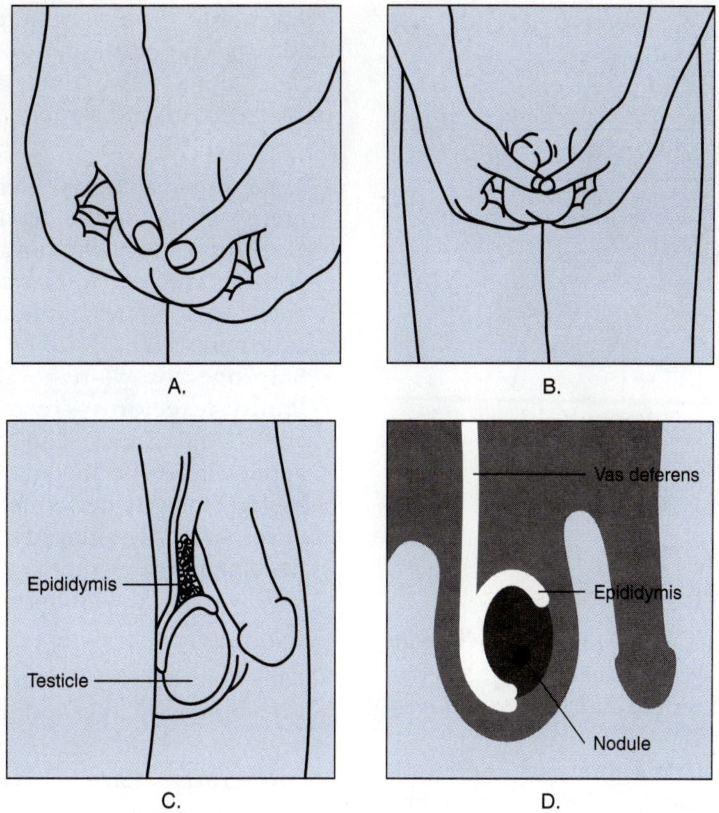

FIGURE 7-110 TSE should be performed once a month after a warm bath or shower. The heat will relax the scrotum, making it easier to find abnormalities. A. Stand in front of the mirror. Look for swelling on the skin of the scrotum. B. Examine each testicle with both hands. Position your index and middle fingers under the testicle with the thumbs on top. Gently roll the testicle between your thumbs and fingers. (Having one testicle larger than the other is normal.) C. Find the epididymis (the soft, tubelike structure at the back of the testicle). Do not mistake the epididymis for an abnormal lump. D. If you find a lump, notify your doctor right away. Most lumps are found on the sides of the testicle, but some are located on the front. Testicular cancer is highly curable when detected early and treated promptly.

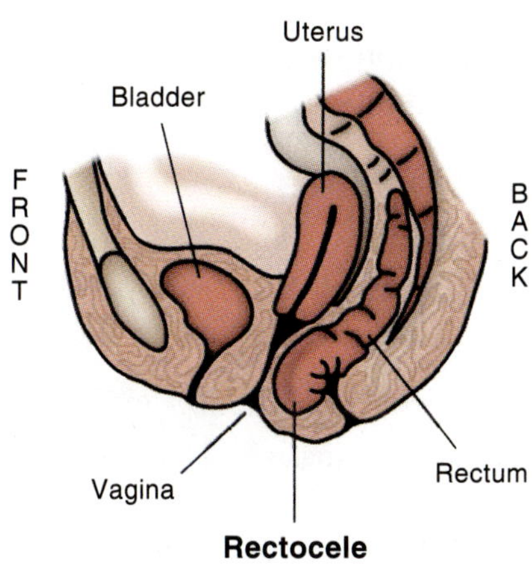

FIGURE 7-111 A rectocele causes the rectum to bulge into the vagina.

Treatment and Nursing Care. A surgical procedure called **colporrhaphy** tightens the vaginal walls.

In addition to routine postsurgical care, you may assist in:

- Applying ice packs
- Giving sitz baths
- Giving vaginal douches (irrigations)
- Checking carefully for signs of excessive bleeding or foul discharge

Vulvovaginitis

Vulvovaginitis is most often caused by a fungal infection of *Candida albicans*.

- There is a thick, white, cheesy vaginal discharge.
- Inflammation and itching are intense.
- Douches are not given for this condition.
- Special drugs and creams are prescribed to fight the infection.

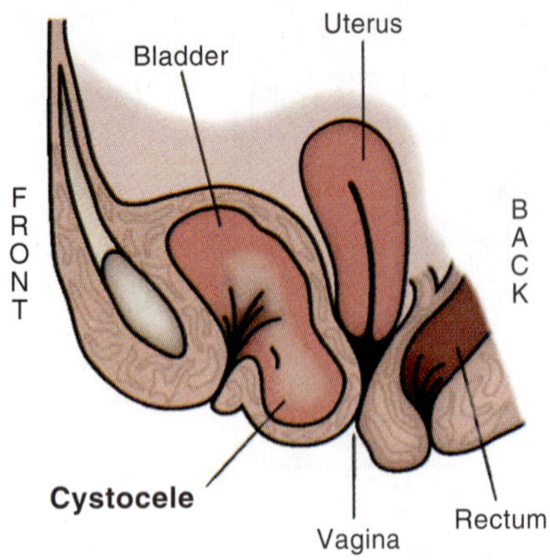

FIGURE 7-112 A cystocele causes the bladder to bulge into the vagina.

Tumors of Uterus and Ovaries

Benign and malignant tumors of the uterus and ovaries are frequent. Malignancies of the cervix are very common. The cure rate is very high if treated in time.

The most common indications of tumors of the uterus and ovaries are changes in the menstrual flow, such as:

- **Menorrhagia** (excessive flow)
- **Amenorrhea** (lack of menstrual flow)
- **Dysmenorrhea** (difficult or painful menstrual flow)
- **Metrorrhagia** (bleeding at completely irregular intervals)

Ovarian cancer is very dangerous because there are no symptoms until it is well advanced and has spread beyond the ovaries. Even then, the symptoms are often mild, such as bloating, and may be attributed to other problems. It usually cannot be detected by a pelvic examination. This cancer accounts for more deaths than any other cancer of the female reproductive system. The disease has a strong familial link, and is most common in women over age 50. Women who have never had children and those who have taken fertility drugs are also at high risk. Women who take birth control pills have a lower risk.

Signs and Symptoms of Ovarian Cancer. Signs and symptoms of ovarian cancer may include:

- abdominal discomfort and pain
- bloating
- nausea
- diarrhea
- frequent urination
- sudden weight gain or loss
- abnormal vaginal bleeding

Treatment. Several different types of procedures may be performed to treat tumors of the female reproductive tract, including chemotherapy, radiation, and surgery. Some surgical procedures are:

- Total **hysterectomy**—removal of the entire uterus, including the cervix.
- **Oophorectomy**—removal of an ovary. In younger women, at least a portion of the ovary is left to continue hormone production whenever possible.
- **Salpingectomy**—removal of a fallopian tube.
- **Panhysterectomy**—removal of the uterus and both ovaries and tubes. The surgical approach may be abdominal or vaginal. If a panhysterectomy is performed, the patient experiences surgically induced menopause. The more uncomfortable symptoms of menopause are usually relieved with hormone supplements.

Nonsurgical forms of treatment include:

- Radiation therapy, if cancer is present
- Chemotherapy, if cancer is present

Postoperative Care. In addition to the usual postoperative care, the care following a hysterectomy will include:

- caring for catheter drainage.
- possibly caring for a nasogastric tube, which may be in place to relieve abdominal distention and nausea.
- giving special attention to maintaining good circulation, because slowing of the blood supply to the pelvis may result in clot formation.
- introducing fluids and foods gradually after the initial nausea subsides.
- carefully observing the patient for low back pain.
- monitoring urine output and bleeding.
- checking both the abdominal incisional area and the vagina for presence and type of drainage.
- providing emotional support

Tumors of the Breast

Tumors, both benign and malignant, are commonly found in the breasts. Breast cancer is the second most common cancer in women. However, men can also develop breast cancer. Signs and symptoms of breast tumors include:

- Painless lump or mass
- Nipple discharge
- Retraction of nipple
- Scaly skin around nipple
- Dimpling of the skin
- Enlarged lymph nodes

Treatment. **Mastectomy** means removal of the breast. All or part of the breast tissue may be removed in a mastectomy.

- A **simple mastectomy** removes the breast tissue only.
- A **radical mastectomy** includes the breast tissue, underlying muscles, and the glands in the axillary area.

This procedure is not performed as often as it was previously.

- A **lumpectomy** removes the abnormal tissue and only a small amount of the breast tissue.

Nonsurgical forms of treatment include:

- radiation therapy
- chemotherapy
- hormonal chemotherapy, which blocks estrogen from entering the breast cancer cells

Any form of mastectomy requires a great deal of psychological adjustment for the patient. There is the fear of disfigurement and the fear of loss of femininity. Many excellent breast forms are now available to restore the outward physical appearance of the mastectomy patient. Breast implants are another way of restoring the physical form of the breast. There are also support groups to aid in the psychological adjustment.

Postoperative Care. In addition to routine postoperative care, you will:

- Wear personal protective equipment and apply the principles of standard precautions if contact with blood, body fluids, mucous membranes, or nonintact skin is likely.
- Avoid taking the blood pressure on the side where the surgery was done.
- Realize that because a large amount of blood can be lost during a mastectomy, transfusions are likely to be ordered. Monitor a blood transfusion as you would monitor an intravenous infusion.
- Check pressure dressings frequently for signs of excess bleeding.
- Check the bed linen, because blood may drain to the back of the dressing.
- Report immediately numbness or swelling in the arm of the operative side.
- Be ready to offer support; walking may be difficult for the patient, who may feel unbalanced.
- Offer your fullest emotional support.
- Assist the patient in rehabilitative exercises.
- Refer questions about disfigurement and loss of femininity to the nurse, who will see that the patient is provided with accurate information and support.

Sexually Transmitted Disease (STD)

Sexually transmitted diseases (STDs) affect both men and women. Although most sexually transmitted diseases can be treated and cured, patients do not develop immunity to repeated infections. It is possible to transmit the organisms causing STDs from:

- Mucous membrane to mucous membrane, such as from genitals to mouth or genitals
- Mucous membrane to skin, such as genitals to hands
- Skin to mucous membrane, such as hands to genitals

Using standard precautions correctly will protect the nursing assistant from contracting these diseases when caring for patients.

Any disease that is transmitted mainly in this way is an STD. There are many sexually transmitted diseases. Some are seen more commonly than others. It is important to realize that patients may:

- not always be aware that they have been infected.
- be too embarrassed to tell you about the problem.
- not realize the serious damage these infectious diseases can do to the body.

The most common sexually transmitted diseases are gonorrhea, herpes simplex II, and syphilis. Other sexually transmitted diseases are caused by chlamydia, human papilloma virus, HIV, and the trichomonas parasite.

Trichomonas Vaginitis

Trichomonas vaginitis is caused by a parasite, *Trichomonas vaginalis*. This condition:

- is sexually transmitted.
- may affect the male reproductive tract with no signs and symptoms.
- in females, causes a large amount of white, foul-smelling vaginal discharge called **leukorrhea**.
- can be controlled with medication.
- requires that both sex partners receive treatment.

Gonorrhea

Gonorrhea is a serious STD caused by the bacterium *Neisseria gonorrheae*. The disease causes an acute inflammation. In the male:

- Greenish-yellow discharge appears from the penis within two to five days after contact.
- There is burning on urination.
- The disease can spread throughout the reproductive tract, causing **sterility** (inability to reproduce).

In the female:

- 80% may have no signs or symptoms for quite a while. Thus, it is possible to spread the disease before the woman is aware of being infected.
- **Pelvic inflammatory disease (PID)** can lead to formation of abscesses and sterility.

It is important for all sex partners to be treated with antibiotics. When a pregnant woman has gonorrhea, her baby's eyes may be permanently damaged if they are contaminated by the disease during birth. As a preventive measure, all babies' eyes are routinely treated with silver nitrate drops or antibiotics shortly after birth.

Syphilis

Syphilis is caused by the microorganism *Treponema pallidum*. Both sexes show the same effects of the disease. If untreated, this disease passes through three stages.

1. First stage—a sore **(chancre)** develops within 90 days of exposure. The chancre heals without treatment. Because it is not painful, it may go entirely unnoticed.
2. Second stage—may be accompanied by a rash, sore throat, or other mild symptoms suggestive of a viral infection. Again, the signs and symptoms disappear without treatment. The disease is infectious during the first and second stages and may be transmitted to a sexual partner. By this time, the microorganisms have gained entrance into vital organs such as the heart, liver, brain, and spinal cord.
3. Third stage—permanent damage is done to vital organs, though the damage may not appear for many years.

An additional danger of syphilis during pregnancy is that the microorganism can attack the fetus, causing it to die or be seriously deformed.

Herpes

Herpes simplex II (genital herpes) is an infectious disease caused by the herpes simplex virus (Figure 7.113). It is transmitted primarily through direct sexual contact. The person who has herpes:

- may develop painful, red, blister-like sores on the reproductive organs.

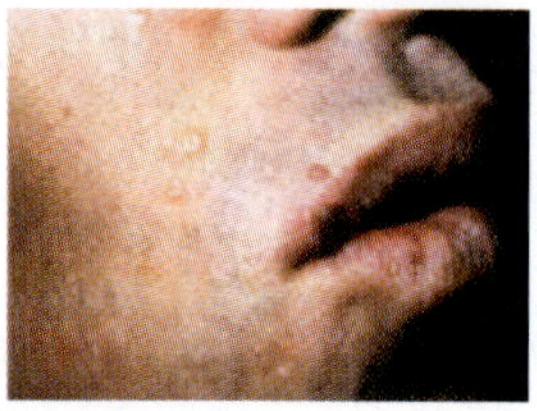

FIGURE 7-113 Oral herpes can be spread to the genital area, just as genital herpes can be spread to the mouth. *(Courtesy of Daniel J. Barbaro MD, Fort Worth, Texas)*

- has sores that are associated with a burning sensation.
- usually has sores that heal in about two weeks.
- must remember that the fluid in the blisters is infectious.
- may transmit (shed) organisms even when an outbreak is not present.

People with the herpes infection may have only one episode or may have repeated attacks. In many cases, repeated attacks are milder. Individuals who have weakened immune systems often develop chronic cases of herpes In addition to the local discomfort:

- There seems to be a greater incidence of cancer of the cervix and miscarriages among female sufferers than among women who do not have this condition.
- Newborn children can be infected when the mother gives birth.
- The baby of a mother with an active case of herpes simplex II is usually delivered by cesarean section.

Because herpes is caused by a virus, there is no cure. Medications are available to stop the replication of the virus, which makes an outbreak subside more quickly. Topical creams are available to relieve discomfort and reduce the danger of spreading the infection.

Venereal Warts

Venereal warts are caused by a virus.

- Lesions develop on the genitals, on both skin and mucous membranes.
- The warts are cauliflower-shaped, raised, and darkened.
- They may be removed by ointments or surgery but often recur.
- They may cause discomfort during intercourse and may cause bleeding when dislodged.
- Warts predispose the patient to development of cancerous changes.

- Venereal warts are one of the most rapidly growing forms of STD.

Chlamydia Infection

Chlamydia are small infectious organisms that can invade mucous membranes of the body. These organisms can be:

- Introduced into the eyes, infecting the conjunctiva. This causes inflammation (conjunctivitis) and a more serious condition called trachoma. Trachoma can lead to blindness.
- Sexually transmitted; this commonly causes infections of the reproductive tract.
- The cause of serious pelvic inflammatory disease (PID), with scarring and even systemic infections. The scarring can result in sterility.
- Responsible for signs and symptoms similar to those of gonorrhea, except that the discharge is usually yellow to whitish in color.
- Treated with antibiotics.

Patients with pelvic infections are usually checked for gonorrhea. If they are found negative for gonorrhea, they are frequently diagnosed as having nongonorrheal urethritis (NGU) or nonspecified urethritis (NSU), because many different organisms may cause the infection. However, chlamydia organisms are the most common cause.

Human Immunodeficiency Virus (HIV) Disease

HIV is a viral disease. It is transmitted primarily through direct contact with the bodily secretions of an infected person. Therefore, it can be transmitted through direct sexual contact. HIV disease destroys the immune system. There is no cure for this condition, although drugs can slow the damage to the body. If the disease progresses, the immune system is severely weakened. This stage of HIV disease is called AIDS (acquired immune deficiency syndrome).

Diagnostic Tests

Techniques used to diagnose problems of the reproductive system include:

- Cultures for microorganisms.
- Urinalysis for hormone levels.
- **Pap smear**—test using cells from the cervix to detect possible cancer of the cervix. The test:
  - is painless.
  - can be performed in the physician's office during the routine pelvic examination.
  - should be done regularly.
- **Dilatation and curettage (D & C)**—a surgical procedure used to help diagnose conditions of the uterus, including tumors. In a D & C, the opening of the cervix is stretched open (dilated) and the uterus is scraped with a surgical instrument known as a curette.
- **Biopsy** (examining a sample of living tissue) is used to make a diagnosis. The biopsy sample is obtained through a needle. The procedure may be performed in the physician's office or in the hospital.
- Blood tests for cancer of the prostate.
- MRI and CT scans to help define the presence and extent of tumors.
- Ultrasound, a painless diagnostic tool that uses sound waves to diagnose ovarian cancer and other tumors.
- Cystoscopy—used to evaluate prostate conditions.
- Self-examination.

  Breast self-examination should be performed:
  - by all adult females .
  - each month on the last day of the menstrual flow.
  - on one selected day of the month, after menopause.
  - Faithfully in a routine manner.

  Testicular self-examination should be performed:
  - by all adult males.
  - at least once each month.
  - during a warm shower so the scrotum will be relaxed.
  - with soapy fingers.
  - by palpating each testis between the fingers and thumb.
- Mammography—x-rays of the breasts. A **mammogram**:
  - can identify the presence of tumors up to two years before the tumor can be felt during self-examination.
  - Should be performed when the woman is between the ages of 35 and 40 years, to provide a baseline evaluation.
  - Thereafter, should be performed every one to two years until age 50.
  - Should be performed yearly after age 50.

Vaginal Douche

A vaginal **douche** is an irrigation of the vagina with fluid or medication. It is done by physician's order.

PROCEDURE

18 Breast Self-Examination

1. Disrobe above the waist and stand or sit in front of a mirror. Observe breasts for changes in shape or size (Figure 7.114A).
   Note: *Some women prefer to perform breast self-examination standing in the shower.*
2. Raise arms above your head and clasp your hands (Figure 7.114B). Press inward with your hands while observing your breasts. Note any "dimpling" of the breast tissue.
3. Fold a small towel.
4. Lie on the bed with the towel under your right shoulder.
5. Flex your right arm and bring it over your head.
6. With the fingers of the left hand, examine the right breast (Figure 7.114C).
   - Use your fingertips.
   - Use a rolling motion.
   - Start at the nipple and work around the entire breast so that all tissue is examined (Figure 7.114D).
7. Examine the right axilla in the same way.
8. Repeat the procedure with the opposite breast and axilla.

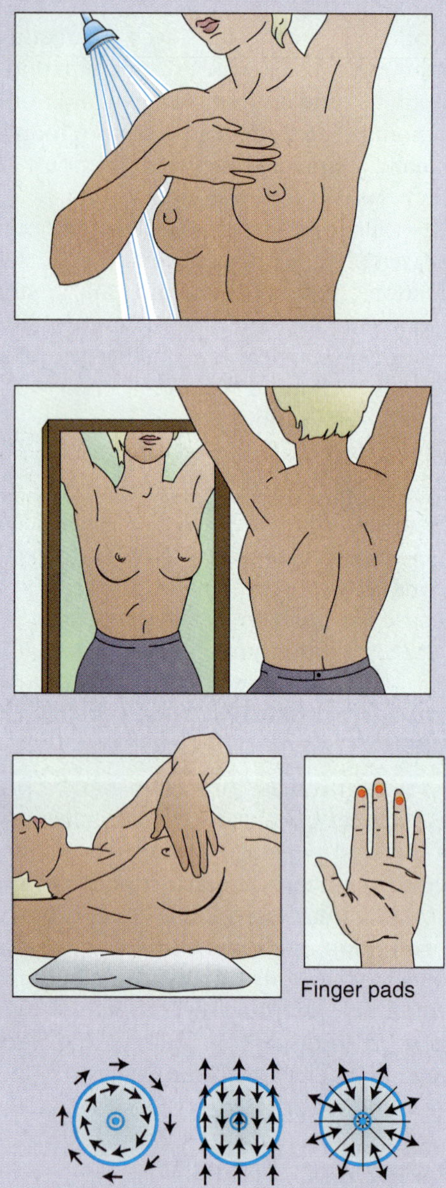

FIGURE 7-99 Breast self-examination. Each breast is examined systematically. A. With the fingers flat, check for a knot, lump, or thickening. B. Raise your arms and compare breast shape. C. Lie down with a small pillow under the shoulder and one arm behind the head. Check again for any knot, lump, or thickening. Move your fingers in a circular motion, inward toward the nipple. Use the pads of the fingers. D. Direction of motion of fingers over breast during examination. *(Courtesy of the American Cancer Society)*

PROCEDURE

19

Giving A Nonsterile Vaginal Douche

1. Carry out beginning procedure actions.
2. Assemble equipment:
    - disposable gloves
    - disposable douche
    - bed protector
    - toilet tissue
    - bath blanket
    - cotton balls
    - disinfectant
    - cup
    - irrigating standard
    - bedpan and cover
    - plastic bag
3. Pour a small amount of the specified disinfecting solution over the cotton balls in the cup.
4. Measure water into the douche container. The temperature should be about 105 °F. Add powder or solution as ordered.
5. Hang the douche bag on the standard. Close the clamp on the tubing. Leave the protector on the sterile tip.
6. Place a bed protector on the chair and assemble equipment where you can reach it. Screen the unit.
7. Elevate the bed to a comfortable working height and put up the side rails for safety.
8. Wash your hands and put on gloves. Lower the side rail on the working side.
9. Assist the patient into the dorsal recumbent position.
10. Place a bed protector beneath the patient's buttocks.
11. Remove the perineal pad (if used) from front to back and discard it in a plastic bag.
12. Drape the patient with a bath blanket (Figure 7.115). Fanfold top bedding to the foot of the bed.
13. Place a bedpan under the patient and ask her to void. Follow facility policies for emptying bedpan, if necessary.

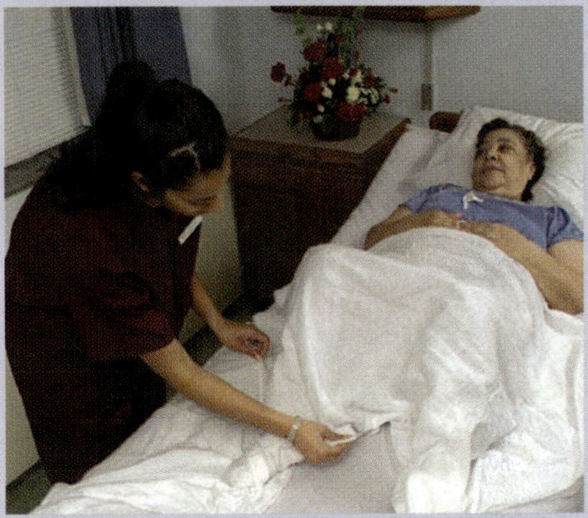

FIGURE 7-115 Drape the patient.

14. Cleanse the patient's perineum.
    - Use one cotton ball with disinfectant for each stroke.
    - Cleanse from the vulva toward the anus.
    - Cleanse the labia majora first.
    - Expose the labia minora with your thumb and forefinger and cleanse.
    - Give special attention to folds.
    - Discard used cotton balls in a plastic bag.
15. Replace the bedpan, if necessary. Position the patient in the dorsal recumbent position and readjust the bath blanket, if necessary. Elevate the head slightly for comfort, if desired.

16. Open the clamp to expel air. Remove the protector from the sterile tip of the disposable douche.
17. Allow a small amount of solution to flow over the inner thigh and then over the vulva. Do not touch the vulva with the nozzle.
18. Allow solution to continue to flow and insert the nozzle slowly and gently into the vagina, with an upward and backward movement, for about 3 inches.
19. Rotate the nozzle from side to side as solution flows.
20. When all solution has been given, remove the nozzle slowly and clamp the tubing.
21. Have the patient sit up on the bedpan to allow all the solution to return.
22. Remove the douche bag from the standard and place it on the bed protector.
23. Dry the perineum with tissue. Discard used tissue in the bedpan.
24. Cover the bedpan and place it on the bed protector on the chair.
25. Have the patient turn on her side. Dry her buttocks with tissue.
26. Place a clean pad over the vulva from front to back. Do not touch the inside of the pad.
27. Remove the bed protector and bath blanket. Replace with top bedding.
28. Observe the contents of the bedpan. Note the character and amount of discharge, if any. Discard the contents of the bedpan according to facility policy. Care for equipment according to facility policy. Remove gloves and dispose of them according to facility policy. Wash your hands.
29. Carry out procedure completion actions.

A vaginal douche requires standard precautions. When a douche is given to administer medications, it is given by the nurse. Other douches may be given by the nursing assistant if it is the policy of the facility. Be sure to check. Vaginal douches are given to:

- Remove odor or foul discharge
- Stop bleeding
- Relieve inflammation and pain
- Neutralize vaginal secretions
- Disinfect the vagina
- Cleanse the vagina before surgery or examination
- Administer antiseptic drugs

REVIEW

Multiple-Choice

Select the one best answer.

A. 1. The term *geriatrics* means

a. care of residents in the hospital
b. care of the elderly.
c. care of the client in the home.
d. care of middle-aged adults.

2. An example of an aging change in the cardiovascular system is

a. lung capacity increases due to muscular rigidity.
b. blood pressure increases.
c. the heart rate increases.
d. reaction time slows down.

3. An example of an aging change in the urinary system is

a. bladder capacity decreases.
b. kidney function increases during the day.
c. fewer hormones are secreted.
d. kidney stones are common.

4. An example of an aging change in the digestive system is

a. movement of food through the stomach increases.
b. the stomach stretches, enabling it to hold more food.
c. the gag reflex is less effective.
d. waste travels through the colon more rapidly.

5. An example of an aging change in the musculoskeletal system is

a. the ability to feel pressure and temperature increases.
b. bones become more porous and break easily.c. endurance increases.
d. muscles become more elastic.

6. The outer layer of the skin is called the

a. dermis.
b. epidermis.
c. subcutaneous layer.
d. external membrane.

7. Aging changes in the integumentary system include

a. the skin thins and becomes less elastic.
b. oil glands secrete more.
c. blood vessels no longer nourish the skin.
d. the skin no longer provides protection.

8. The prostate gland

a. is not affected by aging.
b. controls urination.
c. may enlarge and obstruct the urethra.
d. shrinks and becomes less effective.

9. The brain and spinal cord make up the

a. central nervous system.
b. peripheral nervous system.
c. sensory organs.
d. cerebrospinal fluid space.

10. When the lens of the eye becomes cloudy and impairs vision, it is called

a. glaucoma.
b. macular degeneration.
c. diabetic retinopathy.
d. cataract.

11. Persons with Parkinson's disease generally have

a. pain.
b. rigidity.
c. spasticity.
d. hearing impairment.

12. A person who has had a stroke on the left side of the brain will

a. have left hemiplegia.
b. become quick and impulsive.
c. have aphasia.
d. have no personality changes.

13. The person who has had a stroke on the right side of the brain will

a. have left hemiplegia.
b. have aphasia.
c. become slow, anxious, and cautious.
d. have hearing loss in the right ear.

14. Patients with stroke

a. need proper positioning to prevent contractures.
b. must be repositioned every 4 hours.
c. will be unable to speak during the acute phase.
d. will always be NPO.

15. You come into a room and find a patient having a seizure. You should

a. leave and find help.
b. restrain the patient's movements.
c. raise the foot of the bed.
d. remove any object the patient might hit.

16. To help ensure adequate circulation to prevent skin breakdown, you could

a. change the patient's position frequently.
b. position the patient on bony prominences.
c. rub red areas well.
d. apply rubbing alcohol to the skin after bathing.

17. Scabies and body lice are commonly spread by

a. air and droplets.
b. direct and indirect contact.
c. fomites and common vehicles.
d. viruses and bacteria.

18. In a dark-skinned patient, a Stage I pressure ulcer may appear

a. red or pink.
b. gray or green.
c. blue or black.
d. shiny and oily.

19. Patients with respiratory disease should

a. cover the nose and mouth when coughing.
b. turn the face toward others when sneezing.

c. wash their hands only after toileting.
d. dispose of soiled tissues by dropping them in the nearest trash can.

20. When assigned to perform ROM, you should

a. exercise every joint.
b. exercise joints to the point of pain.
c. check with the nurse for any limitations before starting.
d. perform each exercise four times.

21. A greenstick fracture

a. occurs mainly in children.
b. fragments the bone.
c. occurs mainly in the elderly.
d. twists around the bone.

22. While a leg cast is drying,

a. cover it tightly so moisture will not be lost.
b. maintaining general alignment is not important.
c. carefully observe the extremities for circulation.
d. use only fingertips to handle the cast.

23. Your patient has a ruptured disc. You should note and report

a. crossing of the legs.
b. ambulation in the room.
c. numbness and tingling.
d. complaints of feeling tired.

24. The most common symptom of osteoarthritis is

a. swollen joints.
b. pain.
c. redness.
d. limited mobility.

25. Gout is caused by

a. renal disease.
b. hypertension.
c. arthritic changes in aging.
d. elevated uric acid levels in the blood.

26. Position the patient with an amputation

a. with the legs in abduction.
b. with pillows between the legs.
c. with the head elevated at least 90 degrees.
d. with the legs in adduction.

27. You suspect the patient needs immediate attention for a possible heart attack because the person

a. has chest pain.
b. complains of not feeling well.
c. has ankle edema.
d. has pink nailbeds.

27. Nursing care of the patient with anemia might include

a. blood letting.
b. good nutrition.
c. pacemaker.
d. chemotherapy.

29. The patient with anemia has a

a. high energy level.
b. pink, rosy skin.
c. low energy level.
d. slower than normal respiratory rate.

30. An attack of angina pectoris could be brought about by

a. bathing in the evening.
b. resting in bed.
c. emotional stress.
d. walking in the hallway.

31. Your patient has renal calculi. One of your care tasks will be

a. saving all urine.
b. straining urine.
c. limiting fluids.
d. inserting a catheter

32. Indwelling catheter care is

a. a licensed nurse responsibility.
b. performed during AM care.
c. safely omitted as long as the patient is in bed.
d. performed twice a week.

33. Enemas are given

a. after the patient showers.
b. at bedtime.
c. before diagnostic testing.
d. after surgery.

34. Urgency is a term that means

a. need to urinate.
b. need to empty the bowel.
c. pain from flatus.
d. need to vomit.

36. You are to give a nonsterile douche. You will remember to
    a. place the patient in a high Fowler's position.
    b. use a solution with a temperature of about 115 °F.
    c. insert the nozzle about 3 inches into the vagina.
    d. allow the nozzle to touch the vulva.
5. Breast self-examination should be performed
    a. daily.
    b. weekly.c. monthly.
    d. yearly.
37. Your patient has just returned from a suprapubic prostatectomy. You know that
    a. there will be no incision.
    b. there will be a Foley catheter drain.
    c. the patient must be assisted to void every 2 hours.
    d. the patient will be NPO for 2 to 3 days.
38. Testicular self-examination should be
    a. done daily.
    b. performed while lifting the commode.
    c. performed with soapy fingers.
    d. performed only by males over age 50.
39. Lack of iodine in the diet can result in
    a. hypothyroidism.
    b. hyperthyroidism.
    c. diabetes mellitus.
    d. ketosis.
40. The pituitary gland is responsible for secreting hormones that
    a. stimulate ovulation during the menstrual cycle.
    b. manage sodium and potassium levels.
    c. control calcium and phosphorus.
    d. regulate blood sugar.
41. Your patient is an insulin-dependent diabetic. You know this
    a. is a stable form of the disease.
    b. affects only older persons.
    c. requires hypoglycemic drugs.
    d. is a less stable form of the disease.
42. Insulin is an important hormone because it
    a. lowers blood sugar.
    b. raises blood sugar.
    c. stimulates the conversion of glycogen to glucose.
    d. breaks fat down to form glucose.

B. Fill in the Blank

43. _______care focuses on the whole person, with many strengths and needs.
44. _______ are conditions with the potential to cause a person's health to worsen.
44. The hormone secreted by the pancreas that regulates glucose metabolism is _______.
45. Dark purple bruises on the back of the hands and forearms are_______.

C. Clinical Applications

Please read the following case study, then answer the questions.

47. Mr. Hoover is a 78-year-old resident with a diagnosis of arteriosclerosis. He is mentally confused, but pleasant. He spends most of the day sitting in his armchair, watching television. Mr. Hoover walks with a walker from his chair to the bathroom. He uses a wheelchair for longer distances. You are assigned to walk him 50 feet in the hallway each day using a gait belt and his walker. He accomplishes this well. Mr. Hoover's skin is very dry. If he accidentally bumps his arms or legs, they bruise easily. Mr. Hoover's appetite is good. He uses three packages of sugar in his coffee. His son tells you that he used to use only one package of sugar in his coffee when he was younger. The care plan states to monitor and make sure Mr. Hoover has a bowel movement daily. If he does not, report to the nurse. Mr. Hoover urinates frequently. The care plan states that he has an enlarged prostate gland. Mr. Hoover takes pride in his appearance and likes to receive compliments about how nice he looks.
48. Which of the conditions listed in this case study are related to the normal aging process?
49. Mr. Hoover is able to walk in his room with a walker. Why is it important to walk him a longer distance in the hallway each day?
50. Why does Mr. Hoover use three packages of sugar in his coffee when he formerly used only one?

52. What is a potential explanation for Mr. Hoover's frequent urination?
53. At the end of your shift, you realize that you forgot to see if Mr. Hoover had a bowel movement today. The care plan states that the nursing assistant should monitor for a BM each day and report to the nurse if the patient does not have one. The resident's memory is poor, so he cannot tell you. What action should you take?

D. Matching

Choose the correct term from Column II to match the phrases in Column I.

Column I	Column II
53. _______inflammation of the lungs	a. emphysema
54. _______an example of COPD	b. sputum
55. _______difficult breathing	c. pneumonia
56. _______cough up	d. dyspnea
57. _______material brought up from lungs	e. spirometer
	f. expectorate

Column I	Column II
58. _______correct position	a. arthritis
59. _______small fluid-filled sacs found around joints	b. spica
60. _______name given to a cast covering hips and one or both legs	c. closed
61. _______fracture where bone breaks through skin	d. bursae
62. _______inflammation of joints	e. simple
	f. alignment
	g. open

Column I	Column II
63. _______inflammation of a vein	a. hypertension
64. _______death of the heart muscle	b. edema
65. _______another term for stroke	c. myocardial infarction
66. _______high blood pressure	d. plasma
67. _______blocking of the blood supply to the heart	e. phlebitis
	f. CVA
	g. hypotension
	h. coronary occlusion

Column I	Column II
68. _______indwelling catheter	a. void
69. _______inability to expel formed urine	b. hematuria
70. _______urinate	c. cystitis
71. _______inflammation of the bladder	d. retention
72. _______blood in the urine	e. dysuria
	f. Foley catheter
	g. suppression

Column I	Column II
73. _______gas	a. stool
74. _______yellow discoloration of skin	b. flatus
75. _______large bowel	c. cholelithiasis
76. _______feces	d. cyanosis
77. _______gallstones	e. cholecystectomy
	f. colon
	g. jaundice

Column I	Column II
78. _______inability to reproduce	a. dysmenorrhea
79. _______inflammation of the vagina	b. mastectomy
80. _______painful menstruation	c. circumcision
81. _______removal of a breast	d. leukorrhea
82. _______whitish discharge	e. sterility
	f. vaginitis

Column I	Column II
83. _______internal secretion produced by glands	a. polydipsia
84. _______diabetic coma	b. polyphagia
85. _______excess thirst	c. polyuria
86. _______sugar in the urine	d. glycosuria
87. _______produces hormones	e. endocrine gland
88. _______excess hunger	f. hormone
89. _______blood sugar	g. obesity
90. _______overweight	h. glycogen
91. _______master gland	i. NIDDM
92. _______located above the kidneys	j. insulin shock
	k. glucose
	l. adrenal glands
	m. pituitary gland

UNIT 8

The Residence Environment

OBJECTIVES

After reading this unit, you will be able to:

- Spell and define key terms.
- Describe the furniture found in a typical resident unit.
- Describe how to maintain separation of clean and soiled items in the resident's unit.
- List the nursing assistant's responsibilities in keeping the unit safe and clean.
- Demonstrate procedures related to care of the environment.

OBSERVATIONS TO MAKE AND REPORT RELATED TO CARE OF THE ENVIRONMENT

Residents have a call signal within reach at all times

Call signals are answered promptly

Doors to rooms are closed when care is being provided

Privacy curtain and window curtains are closed when care is being provided

Residents are covered completely in bed, chair, or hallways so they are not exposed

Staff knock on the door before entering a room and wait for a response

If the resident's door is open, staff knock on the door frame or other surface, and wait for permission to enter

Residents have fresh water at least once a shift and as requested

Water pitchers are always covered with lids

Water pitchers are washed regularly

Water pitchers are identified by resident name, bed number, or other method

Staff pours water for residents; offers to assist, assists dependent residents

Staff offers fluids each time they enter the room, or according to facility policy

Bedpans and urinals are marked with residents' names and properly stored

Bedpans and urinals are covered during transport

Gloves are not worn in public areas

One-glove technique or other method is used to prevent contamination of environment

Personal care items, such as combs, toothbrushes, and hygienic supplies, are properly stored and labeled with residents' names

Clean and soiled items are separated in bedside stands

Clean and soiled equipment are separated by at least one room's width in the hallway

Housekeeping carts and soiled linen hampers are removed from the hallway when meals are being served, or stored according to facility policy

Items in the refrigerator are covered, labeled, and dated

Refrigerator thermometer is present, temperature is below 45°F

Food and beverages are not stored in the same refrigerator with medications or laboratory specimens

Food and beverages are covered when carried in a hallway

PPE is readily available in areas of use

Gloves and PPE are available in a variety of sizes; nonlatex and powder-free products are available upon request

Standard precautions are consistently used in the care of the environment and cleaning procedures

Staff avoid environmental contamination with soiled gloves

Gloves and other PPE are discarded in covered containers, or according to facility policy

Sharps containers are available in areas of use

Fire exists are marked; evacuation plan is posted

Only clean items are stored in clean utility room

Chemicals are properly labeled and stored in locked areas

Soiled utility room is used for soiled items only

Staff carry clean and soiled items away from uniforms

Clean linen is at least 18 inches from ceiling in clean linen storage room

Clean linen carts are covered when not in use

Only needed linen is taken into resident rooms

Linen hampers and barrels are not overflowing; lids fit tightly

Soiled linen is never placed on the floor

Facility policies describe routine cleaning tasks, dating and labeling of clean items

Tubs, shower chairs, and permanent equipment items are disinfected before and after each use

Medication room is not accessible to unauthorized persons

Charts and medical records are not accessible to unauthorized persons

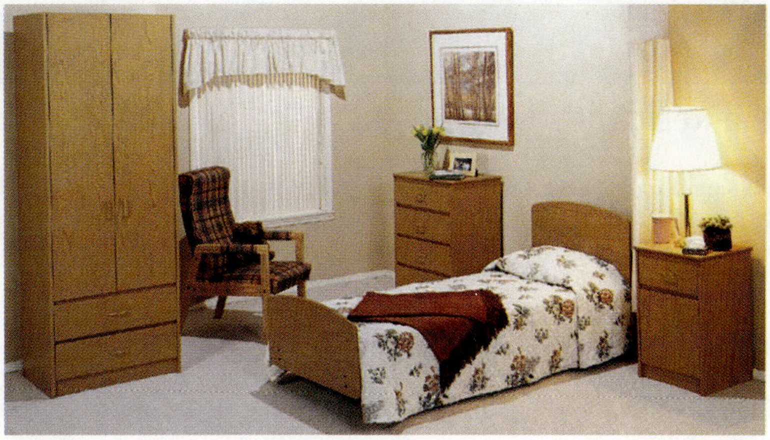

FIGURE 8-1 The resident's unit should be neat and tidy when the resident is admitted. Encourage residents to bring in personal items to create a comfortable, homelike environment. *(Courtesy of Medline Industries, Inc. 1-800-MEDLINE)*

Resident's Unit

The resident's **unit** is the area for the resident's personal use (Figure 8.1). The unit is the resident's personal space, consisting of a bed, chair, overbed table, bedside stand, wastebasket, dresser, and closet. Most of the personal care you deliver is done here. Caring for the resident includes caring for the unit. Some health care facilities also provide a telephone, television set, or radio as part of the unit. In others, residents who use these items provide their own.

The resident has a right to be treated with respect and dignity. You protect this right by knocking on closed doors and providing privacy when visitors are present. When providing personal care in the room, you must close the door, pull the privacy curtain, and close the drapes on the window, even if no one else is present.

Safety and Infection Control

Think *safety* when you enter and leave the room. The nursing assistant is responsible for keeping the unit safe.

Bedside Stand

The **bedside stand** is an important piece of furniture that is used to store personal items and articles used to deliver care. Bedside stands vary in design. Most have at least one drawer. The lower part of the stand may have a cupboard-type door or several drawers. Clean and soiled items must be kept separate in the cupboard and drawers. For example, the drawer in the top of the bedside stand is often used to store personal hygiene items, such as a toothbrush, brush, and comb. These items should not come into contact with each other. The lower part of the bedside stand usually stores the washbasin, bedpan and urinal. The washbasin is considered a "clean" item. It should not be stored next to the bedpan or urinal, which are considered "soiled." The inside of the cupboard-type bedside stand is divided by two shelves. Most facilities store the washbasin on the top shelf and the bedpan and urinal on the bottom shelf. In bedside stands with drawers, store these items in separate drawers (Figure 8.2).

Overbed Table

The **overbed table** is a narrow table on wheels that is used to hold only clean items. The height of the table can be adjusted to a high or low position. It is also used for meal trays, if the resident eats meals in bed. The resident's drinking water may also be placed here. Wipe the top of the overbed table as often as necessary to keep it clean at all times.

The Hospital Bed

The hospital bed is the most important piece of furniture in the resident's unit. As a nursing assistant, you must learn to meet all basic personal care needs for bedfast residents. This may mean adapting some normal procedures, such as bathing. For the bedfast resident, the hospital bed becomes the focal point for care. The bed will have some type of a privacy barrier, such as a curtain or screen. This curtain must be closed when personal care is being provided, even if you are alone in the room with the resident.

GUIDELINES FOR

Caring for the Resident's Unit

- Check the call signal daily. The call signal should be within the resident's reach at all times, even if the resident is mentally confused.
- When the resident is in bed or in a chair, place the call signal, water, tissues, and other needed personal items within reach. This reduces the risk that the resident will reach for an item and fall.
- Cleaning the unit is usually the job of other departments. The nursing assistant is responsible for caring for the resident's personal items. You are expected to wipe tabletops after care, if food is spilled, or if soiling occurs.
- Controlling odors is very important. The best way to do this is to eliminate the source of the odor.
- Follow all infection control guidelines for separation of clean and soiled items in the resident's unit. Know which surfaces can be used to hold clean and soiled items.
- Follow your facility policy for disposing of gloves. Many facilities require that gloves be discarded in a closed container, and not in the open wastebasket in the unit.
- Always respect the resident's choices about arrangement of personal items. Avoid moving the resident's personal belongings without permission. This shows you care about the resident as a person.
- Know and follow your facility policy for storage of food, hygienic products, chemicals, and over-the-counter medications in the unit.
- Some long-term care facilities allow residents to self-administer medication. The medication may be kept in the unit. If this is the case, it must be stored in a secure location.
- Respect the resident's right to privacy when you are performing a procedure that involves exposing the body. Even if all the curtains and doors are closed, use of a **bath blanket** is necessary to preserve the resident's dignity. A bath blanket is a soft cotton or flannel blanket used to protect resident privacy and provide warmth during procedures in which the body is exposed.
- Check the floor for items and equipment that could cause the resident to fall.
- Clean spills on the floor immediately, and place a "wet floor" sign until the floor dries. Follow your facility policies for cleaning and disinfecting blood and body fluid spills.
- If you feel that an electrical or mechanical safety hazard exists, follow your facility policy for having the equipment locked and tagged out until it can be removed and repaired.
- If the resident uses the bathroom at night, leave a night light on.

The hospital bed may be electric or manual. Specialty (therapeutic) beds may be used for medical treatments, such as pressure ulcer management and care of the resident with pneumonia. You must learn the purposes of any specialty beds used in your facility and how to operate them when you are caring for the residents.

The head and knee areas can be raised or lowered in all regular hospital beds. Changing the angle of the head or knee of the bed is done for resident comfort, and to meet medical needs. Most beds also have a high-low function that raises and lowers the height of the bed. This feature has no therapeutic benefit for the residents. Always keep the height of the bed in the lowest horizontal position for resident use. Using the high-low feature makes your job easier and reduces the risk of injury to your back when you are working at the bedside. The bed is raised only when you are providing care, or performing a procedure such as making the bed. It is lowered when you are finished, before you leave the room. You must become familiar with the operation of the hospital beds used in your facility:

- The **gatch handles** are used to change the height of manually operated beds. The gatch handles are at the foot of the bed (Figure 8.3A). They are turned clockwise to raise the bed and counterclockwise to lower the bed. The handle on the left raises and lowers the head of the bed. The handle on the right raises and lowers the foot of the bed. The center handle is used

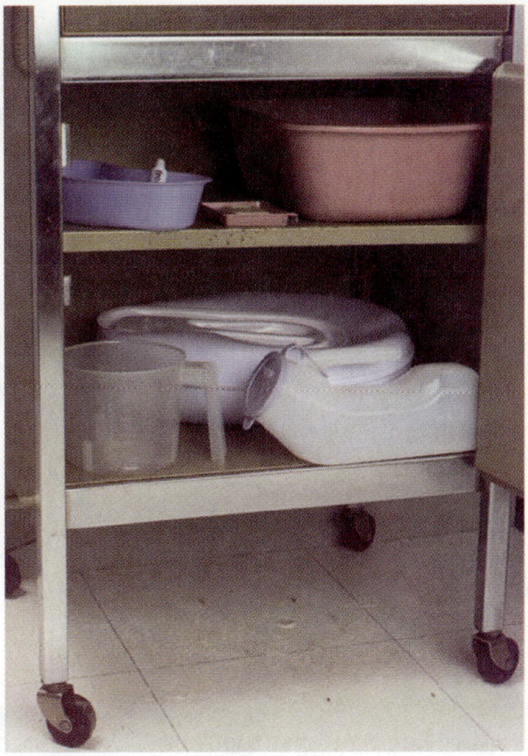

FIGURE 8-2 Clean and soiled items must be separated in the bedside stand.

to control the horizontal height of the bed. Use this handle to adjust bed height so the bed is in a comfortable working position for you. To prevent injuries to residents and staff, always fold the gatch handles under the bed when not in use (Figure 8.3B).

- Wheels on the hospital bed enable you to move the bed, if necessary. All four wheels should be locked in place, except when the bed is being moved.
- Hospital beds are designed to be used with side rails. Some beds have a full-length rail on either side of the bed. Others have two small half rails on each side, one at the head and one at the foot. You must elevate the rails when you are caring for the resident with the bed in the highest horizontal position. Lower the rail only when you are at the bedside providing care. Raise it if you must step away, even for a moment. Keep the rail up on the opposite side of the bed. Some residents use the bed rails to pull on when positioning and turning in bed. Aside from these two situations, side rails may not be used for some residents. Check the care plan for instructions for each of your assigned residents.
- Many facilities use electric beds. Switches are used to change the position of the head, knee, and horizontal bed height. In some beds, these controls are permanently mounted on the bed rail.
- Always check the bed carefully for lost items before removing the linen. Items such as dentures, glasses, and hearing aids are commonly left on the bed. These items are very expensive and will not survive a trip through the washer and dryer.

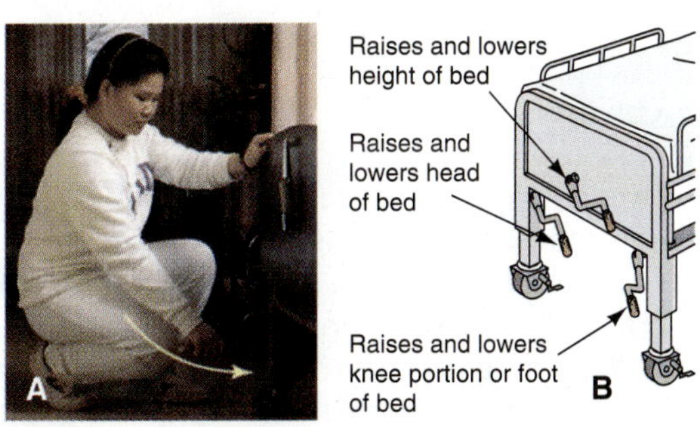

FIGURE 8-3 (A) For safety, fold the gatch handles under the bed when not in use. (B) Gatch handles

Low Beds

Low beds (Figure 8.4) are commonly used in health care facilities for residents at risk of falls, for whom use of side rails is not desirable. The bed frame is four to six inches from the floor to the top of the frame deck. These beds reduce the risk of injury if the resident falls from the bed. Some facilities place pads on the floor next to the bed to further reduce the risk of injury.

Low beds are wonderful tools for reducing resident injuries, but the nursing assistant must

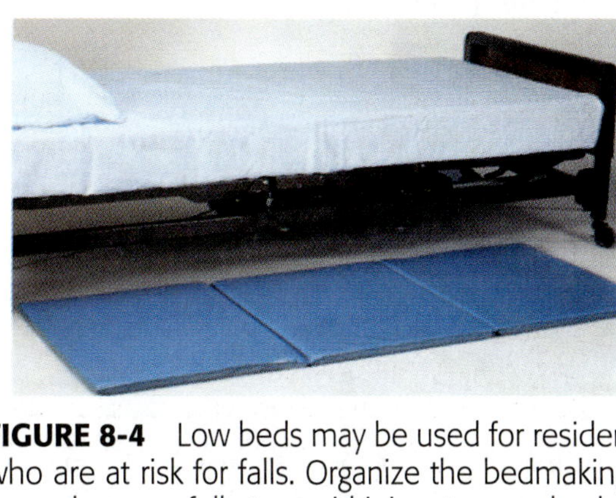

FIGURE 8-4 Low beds may be used for residents who are at risk for falls. Organize the bedmaking procedure carefully to avoid injury to your back. *(Courtesy of Skil-Care Corporation, Yonkers, NY, (800) 431-2972)*

use good body mechanics and common sense to prevent back injuries when lifting, moving, and caring for residents, and when making beds. Some low beds have high-low features, but many are stationary, which increases the risk of back injury. If the bed you are using has a high-low feature, use it whenever caring for the bedfast resident, transferring the resident, and making the bed. A mat on the floor reduces the risk of injury when a resident falls, but it can also be a trip hazard. Move slowly and carefully when working near a floor mat. Avoid entering the room in the dark. Leave a nightlight on, or turn the light on when entering. Squat or kneel on the floor mat when caring for the resident, to reduce back strain caused by bending at the waist. Use good body mechanics, a transfer belt, or a mechanical lift when assisting residents into and out of low beds, to prevent back injuries. The care plan will provide resident-specific instructions. Avoid bending at the waist when moving the resident.

The bedmaking procedure is the same as it is for hospital beds. To make this task easier:

- Mentally plan and prepare yourself for the procedure.
- Organize your work well to reduce the total number of motions required to complete the task.
- Make sure you have everything you need before entering the room.
- Elevate the bed, if possible.
- Place linen and needed items on the resident's chair or within close reach.
- Maintain a neutral posture and bend from the legs, not the waist. Avoid twisting.
- Slowly remove the bed linen several pieces at a time. Avoid trying to remove all the linen in one bundle. The weight of the linen and your posture increase the risk of back injury.
- Make one side of the bed at a time. This is faster, more efficient, and conserves energy.
- Use a fitted bottom sheet to reduce the number of movements necessary for making the bed, thereby lowering the risk of back strain.

Making the Bed

The nursing assistant is responsible for making the bed each day. A clean, wrinkle-free bed promotes resident comfort and prevents skin breakdown. If the resident is out of bed, the unoccupied bedmaking procedure is used. A wide variety of linen is available for bedmaking. Flat sheets may be used on both the top and bottom. Many facilities use fitted sheets on the bottom. Most facilities place draw sheets (lift sheets) under residents who must be turned by the staff. Disposable or reusable underpads are placed under the buttocks if the resident is incontinent or uses the bedpan or urinal in bed. A plastic or rubber draw sheet covered with a cotton sheet may also be used, but many facilities have eliminated these in favor of large underpads. Thermal blankets are usually used for warmth. Many different types of bedspreads are available.

You may be instructed to make the bed in several different ways. Table 8.1 describes different bedmaking methods.

Planning Your Work

Plan your work before making the bed. Bring all necessary linen into the room and stack it in the order of use. Before making the bed, adjust the height so that it is comfortable for you. Lower the head and knee so the bed is flat. Avoid walking around the bed many times. Make one side of the bed at a time, then go to the other side to complete the bedmaking procedure. It may take a little practice to learn to make the bed this way, but it saves your strength and energy and reduces fatigue and injury to your back.

Making the Occupied Bed

Sometimes residents have conditions that require them to stay in bed all the time. When residents are confined to bed, you must make the bed using the **occupied bedmaking** procedure. Sometimes only part of the linen is changed while the resident is in bed. If the resident is bedfast, you will have to check the bed linen and straighten it as often as necessary during your shift. Keeping the linen clean, dry, and wrinkle-free enhances resident comfort and reduces the risk of skin breakdown.

Always apply the principles of standard precautions when changing the bed. Wear gloves if contact with blood, body fluids (except sweat), secretions, or excretions is likely. Wear a gown if your uniform will have substantial contact with linen contaminated by these substances.

TABLE 8-1 Bedmaking Methods

Method of Bedmaking	Procedure Variations	Rationale
Unoccupied bed	Most common type of bedmaking procedure; used for making all types of beds.	Making the unoccupied bed is easier and faster for the nursing assistant. It is more comfortable for the resident.
Occupied bed	Used when the resident is confined to bed.	Changes wet or soiled linen for resident comfort and prevention of skin breakdown; provides fresh, clean linen for feeling of comfort and security.
Closed bed	The bed is made with the top sheet, blanket, and spread pulled all the way to the top. The pillow may be covered or placed on top of the spread, depending on facility policy. The open end of the pillow case faces away from the door.	Used when the resident is expected to be out of bed all day or when making a bed after the resident has been discharged; presents a neat, tidy appearance.
Open bed	The bed is made in the normal manner. The top sheet and spread are fan-folded to the foot of the bed.	This procedure is used when the resident is temporarily out of bed. The resident can be covered easily and quickly upon return to bed.

GUIDELINES FOR

Handling Clean and Soiled Linen

- Wash your hands before handling clean linen.
- Carry all linen (clean or soiled) away from your uniform.
- Bring only the necessary amount of linen to the room. Extra linen cannot be removed and used for other residents until it has been washed.
- Do not shake linen. Unfold clean linen.
- Check the bed linen for lost articles before removing it from the bed.
- Roll soiled linen with the soiled side in.
- Wash your hands immediately after handling used linen, even if it is not visibly soiled.
- Follow your facility policy for placement of clean and soiled linen in the resident's room.
- Soiled linen is never placed on the floor. Some facilities allow the soiled linen hamper in the room and some do not. If you cannot bring the hamper into the room, you may be able to place soiled linen in a plastic bag or pillowcase draped over the back of the chair. Follow your facility policy.
- If you are handling linen contaminated with blood, body fluids, secretions, or excretions, you must wear gloves (Figure 8.5). Wear a gown if your uniform will have substantial contact with soiled linen.
- Linen contaminated with blood or body fluids may be placed in plastic bags that are tied or secured at the top. If the outside of the bag accidentally becomes contaminated during the bagging process, the first bag should be placed in a clean outer bag. If the outside is not contaminated or torn, double bagging is not necessary.
- Some facilities use water-soluble bags for wet linen contaminated with blood or body fluids. These bags dissolve in the washer. Water-soluble bags must always be double-bagged inside a regular plastic bag. The wet linen may cause the water-soluble bag to dissolve before it reaches the laundry.

(continues)

GUIDELINES FOR

Handling Clean and Soiled Linen, *Continued*

- After you have discarded the soiled linen, remove your PPE and wash your hands. Doing this will prevent contamination of clean linen and other environmental surfaces. Gloves are not necessary for handling clean linen.
- Keep the lids on soiled linen hampers. Soiled linen should not overflow under the lid. Most facilities require that hampers be taken to the laundry when they are three-quarters full, to avoid overflowing.
- Clean and soiled linen should never touch each other.
- Follow your facility policy for separation of clean linen carts and soiled linen hampers in the hallways. Most facilities require a one room-width separation of clean and soiled equipment.
- Follow your facility policy for removal of linen hampers from the hallways when food carts are on the unit.

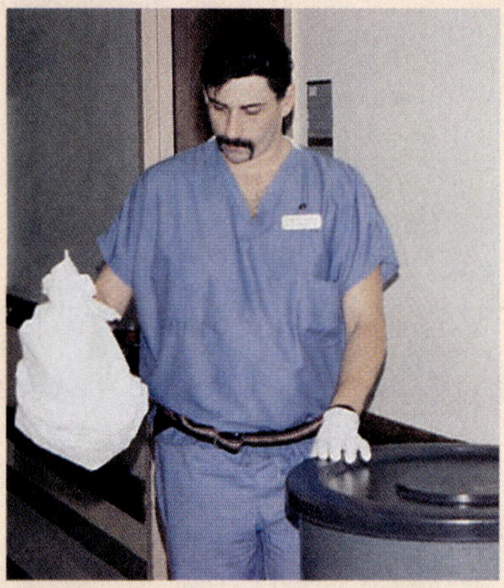

FIGURE 8-5 Wear gloves when handling linen soiled with blood, body fluids, secretions, or excretions. Hold soiled linen away from your uniform.

PROCEDURE

20 Making the Unoccupied Bed

1. Perform your beginning procedure actions.
2. Gather needed supplies: disposable gloves, mattress pad (if used), two large sheets (or one flat and one fitted sheet), a linen draw sheet (if used), underpad (if used), pillowcase, laundry bag or hamper, and blanket or bedspread (if needed). Stack the linen in the order of use.
3. Carry clean linen away from your uniform (Figure 8.6).
4. Stack the linens on a clean area near the bed in the order of use, with bottom linen on top.
5. Lower the head so the bed is flat.
6. Remove and fold the bedspread if you are reusing it.
7. Apply gloves if linen is wet or soiled.
8. Check the linen for lost items. Remove the soiled linen from the bed by rolling it in a ball, soiled side facing in. Follow your facility policy for wiping the mattress. If the mattress is soiled with excretions or secretions, it should be wiped with disinfectant.
9. Place soiled linens in the hamper or laundry bag. Avoid contaminating environmental surfaces with your gloves during this procedure.
10. Remove gloves and discard them according to facility policy.

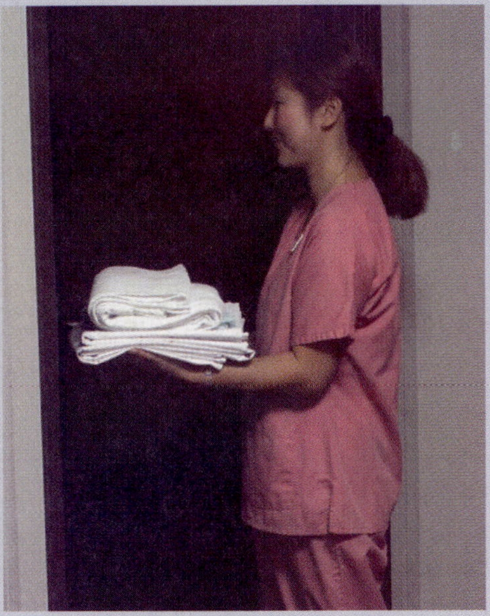

FIGURE 8-6 Carry clean linen away from your uniform.

11. Wash your hands.
12. Straighten the mattress pad (if used). Center the lengthwise middle fold of the bottom sheet in the middle of the bed.
13. Open the sheet.
14. Place the end with the small hem even with the foot of the mattress (Figure 8.7).
15. Tuck the top of the sheet under the mattress.
16. **Milter** the corner (Figure 8.8) by folding it at a 45° angle perpendicular to the mattress, or tuck the corners of the fitted sheet over the edge of the mattress.

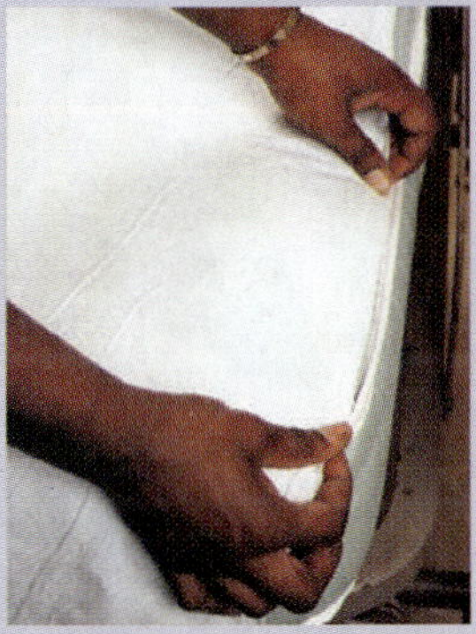

FIGURE 8-7 Place the rough edge down, even with the end of the mattress.

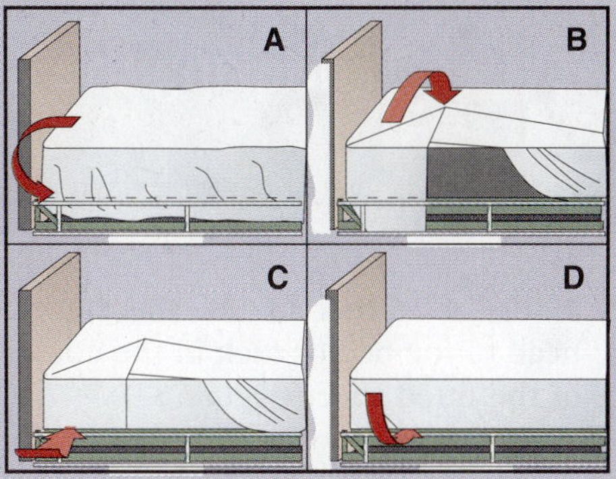

FIGURE 8-8 Making a mitered corner. (A) The sheet is hanging loose at the side of the bed. (B) Pick up the sheet about 12 inches from the head of the bed to form a triangle. (C) Tuck in the sheet at the head of the bed. Pick up triangle and place your other hand at the edge of the bed, near the head, to hold the edge of the sheet in place. Bring triangle over the edge of the mattress and tuck smoothly under the mattress. (D) Tuck in the rest of the sheet along the side of the mattress. Make sure the sheet is wrinkle-free.

17. Beginning at the head of the bed, tuck in the sheet, working from head to foot.
18. Place the draw sheet across the center of the bed.
19. Tuck the edge of the sheet under the mattress.
20. Center the lengthwise middle fold of the top sheet in the center of the bed.
21. Open the sheet and position it so the top edge is even with the top of the mattress.
22. Place the blanket or bedspread on the bed.
23. Miter linens at the foot of the bed by tucking the sheet in at a 45° angle perpendicular to the mattress.
24. Move to the other side of the bed.
25. Pull and straighten the bottom sheet.
26. Pull the sheet tightly, and tuck the bottom sheet under the mattress at the head of the bed.

(continues)

PROCEDURE

21 Making the Occupied Bed, *continued*

34. Pull the bottom sheet tightly and tuck it under the mattress.
35. Pull the draw sheet tight, and tuck it in. If an underpad is used, smooth and straighten it.
36. Help the resident roll on his or her back. Keep the resident covered with the bath blanket.
37. Place the top sheet over the bath blanket, centering the center fold.
38. Pull the bath blanket out from under the clean sheet without exposing the resident.
39. Place the blanket and bedspread over the sheet.
40. Fold the top sheet over the edge of the blanket.
41. Tuck the top linens under the foot of the mattress, allowing room for the resident's toes. Make a **toe pleat** by folding the top linen over two to three inches at the end of the bed (Figure 8.11). The toe pleat provides extra space and keeps the linen from pulling the feet downward. This is more comfortable for the resident and reduces the risk of contractures, such as foot drop.
42. Miter the corner of top linens at the foot of the bed.

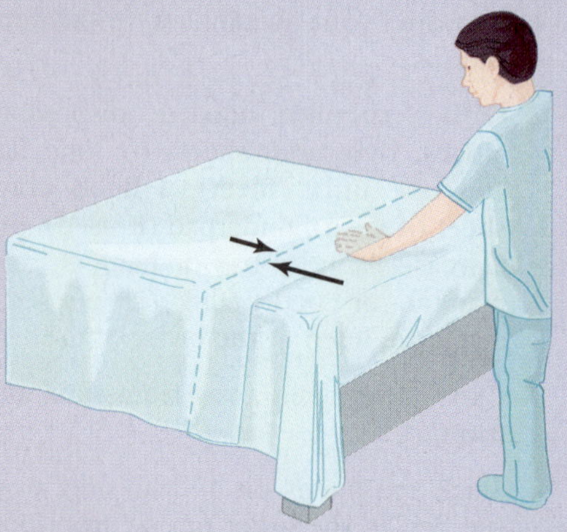

FIGURE 8-11 The toe pleat provides space for movement of the feet. The resident will be more comfortable, and the risk of contractures is reduced.

43. Raise the side rail.
44. Go to the other side of the bed.
45. Lower the side rail.
46. Miter the corner of the top linens at the foot of the bed.
47. Remove the pillow and soiled pillowcase.
48. Place a clean pillowcase on the pillow.
49. Fold and store the bath blanket or place in the soiled linen hamper, according to facility policy.
50. Perform your procedure completion actions.

Other Important Areas

The residents' rooms are part of a larger nursing unit. The area may be called a nursing station, section, hall, floor, or unit. Other important resident care and service areas on the larger nursing unit are:

- Nurses' station—This is a work area for nursing personnel. Reports and assignments are usually given at the nurses' station. Medical records are stored here, and documentation is completed in this area (Figure 8.12). Remember that resident records and documents are confidential. These things should be protected from access by unauthorized persons. Lists of resident names, such as the nourishment list, restraint list, bowel and bladder records, and assignment sheets, should not be placed where they can be viewed by the public.

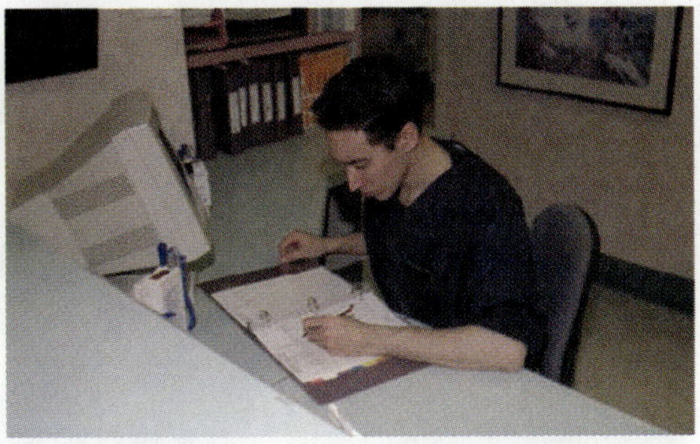

FIGURE 8-12 The nurse's station is a work area for personnel. Medical records are stored behind the station where they are not accessible to the public.

- Medication room—This is a smaller, locked area in the nurses' station. Access is limited to nurses, certified medication aides (if permitted by state law), and other licensed personnel. Other employees (such as the housekeeper) can enter this room only under the direct supervision of a licensed nurse. This room is used for storage and preparation of medications. The door is kept locked when not in use.
- Clean utility room—This area is used only for storage of clean and sterile supplies. New personal care items, such as lotions, toothpaste, and denture cups, may be stored here. Soiled items should never enter this room.
- Soiled utility room—The soiled utility room is used for cleaning soiled supplies. Clean items are removed as soon as they are washed, disinfected, and dried. Clean supplies must never be brought into this room. Personal protective equipment (PPE) should be available for use during cleaning procedures. Apply the principles of standard precautions and select the PPE appropriate to the procedure. A hopper or utensil washer may be available for washing bedpans and urinals. Disinfectants and other chemicals will be stored here. These should be kept in locked cupboards when not in use. (Some facilities keep the door to the soiled utility room locked as well.) Make sure chemicals are stored in the original, labeled containers. Use them only according to manufacturers' directions. Some facilities use this area as a holding room for soiled linen until it is transported to the laundry.
- Linen room—This room is used for clean linen storage. Linen should not be stored on the top shelf closer than 18 inches to the ceiling. If linen is closer than this, the sprinkler system will not be effective in a fire. Most facilities have a central linen storage area. Smaller amounts of linen are removed and placed on wheeled carts that are pushed into the hallways (Figure 8.13). The door to the linen room should be kept closed. The smaller linen carts should be covered except when linen is being added or removed.

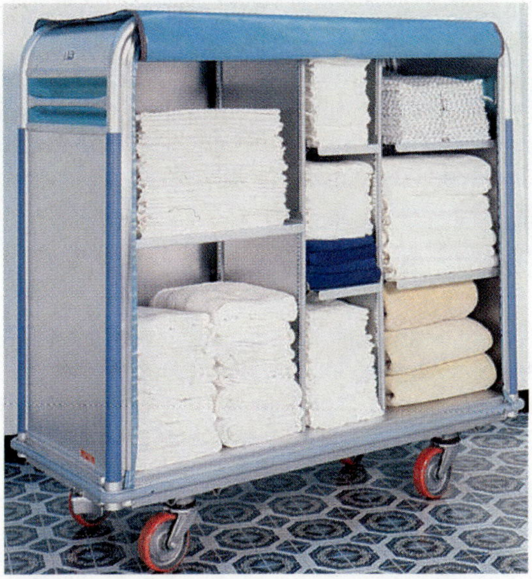

FIGURE 8-13 The clean linen room holds the primary linen supply. Linen is loaded onto smaller carts for use in the hallways. Keep the door closed when not in use. Always keep the carts covered in the hallway, except when removing clean items. *(Courtesy of Medline, Inc. 1-800-MEDLINE)*

- Dining room—Most residents eat their meals in a community dining area. Some facilities have a dining room on each nursing unit, whereas other facilities have a larger dining room that is used by residents from all nursing units. The unit dining room may also be used as a day room, television lounge, and activity room. Eating is a social occasion. Most people do not like to eat alone. Residents' appetites are usually better if they eat their meals with others in a pleasant community area.
- Tub/Shower room—Residents are bathed in community tub and shower areas in some facilities. Shower curtains, privacy curtains, or doors are used to separate residents who are using the room at the same time. Take care to avoid exposing residents in this community area. These are clean areas, and soiled linen should not be placed on the floor.
- Pantry—Some facilities also have a pantry area on each unit in which resident snacks are stored. In many facilities, the ice machine or clean ice chest is stored in the pantry. The refrigerator in the pantry will have a thermometer. Refrigerator temperatures must be checked daily. Temperature should not exceed 45°F. This is a clean area and soiled items

should not be stored here. The refrigerator is for food items only. Laboratory specimens and medications are not stored in this refrigerator. Food items should be covered, wrapped, and sealed. Open items should be dated and discarded according to facility policy.

Cleaning Assignments

Nursing assistants are usually given a cleaning assignment that is completed during or at the end of the shift. You may be responsible for tidying the service areas listed here (Figure 8.14). In some facilities, items such as bedpans, urinals, and wheelchairs are cleaned on a regular schedule. Your assignment may include these responsibilities during your shift. All nursing personnel are responsible for maintaining a clean, homelike, sanitary environment on the nursing unit.

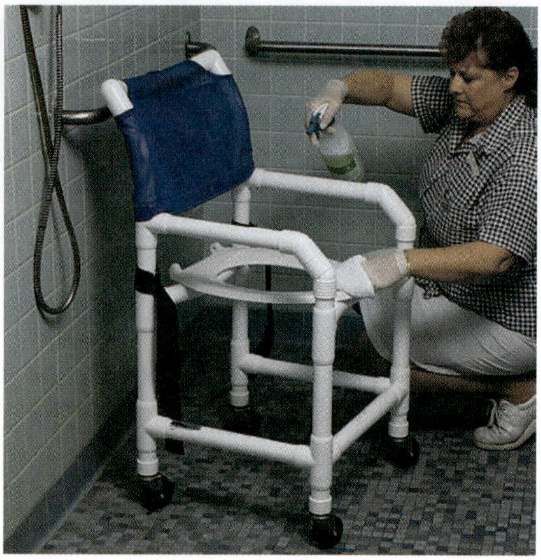

FIGURE 8-14 All staff must complete a cleaning assignment during their shift.

KEY POINTS

- The resident's unit is an area for personal use.
- Respect the resident's rights when giving care and handling personal belongings.
- Think safety when you enter and leave each resident's room.
- Follow your facility infection-control policies for separation of clean and soiled items.
- Follow your facility policies for handling soiled linen.
- Practice the principles of standard precautions when making the bed if contact with blood, moist body fluids (except sweat), secretions, or excretions is likely.
- Personal protective equipment is removed after soiled linen is discarded. The hands are washed before handling clean linen and touching other environmental surfaces.
- The nursing assistant is responsible for keeping resident rooms tidy. You may also be responsible for routine cleaning assignments that must be completed during or at the end of the shift.

REVIEW

A. Multiple Choice

Select the one best answer.

1. When giving personal care to the resident,
   a. close the door only; there is no need to close the privacy curtain unless someone else is in the room.
   b. always drape the resident with a bath blanket even if no one else is present in the room.
   c. you may leave the door open after visiting hours, but close the privacy and window curtains.
   d. close the door and privacy curtain; closing the window curtain is not necessary during daylight hours.
2. The following is true about the use of side rails:
   a. Side rails should be kept up for all residents.

b. Side rails should be kept down for all residents.
c. Consult the care plan to see if side rails are indicated.
d. The resident always determines if side rails are used.

3. The overbed table is used for

a. clean items, food, and water.
b. holding soiled linen and toilet articles.
c. storing the bedpan and urinal.
d. medical procedures only.

4. When caring for a resident in a bed with gatch handles, which handle always elevates the head of the bed?

a. Right.
b. Left.
c. Center.
d. It varies with the bed.

5. Which of the following is true about storing items in the bedside stand?

a. The hairbrush and urinal are stored on the top shelf.
b. The washbasin and bedpan are stored on the bottom shelf.
c. The washbasin and urinal are stored on the top shelf.
d. The bedpan and urinal are stored on the bottom shelf.

6. Which of the following is true about handling linen?

a. Clean and soiled linen are always carried away from your uniform.
b. Extra linen in a room can be removed and used for another resident.
c. Soiled linen may be placed on the floor.
d. Gloves are used for handling both clean and soiled linen.

7. You are assigned to make an unoccupied bed in room 931. The linen is saturated with fresh blood. Select the correct personal protective equipment to wear:

a. Mask, gown, gloves.
b. Gown, gloves.
c. Gloves, mask, face shield.
d. Mask, face shield.

8. When making the unoccupied bed,

a. raise the bed to a comfortable working height.
b. raise the side rail on the side opposite from where you are working.
c. elevate the head of the bed at least 30 degrees when you are done.
d. roll the resident from side to side so you can tighten the bottom sheet.

9. Clean linen should be

a. stored at least 8 to 12 inches from the ceiling.
b. covered when being transported on carts in the hallway.
c. placed next to the soiled linen hamper in the hallway for convenience.
d. carried from one resident's room to the next in a stack.

10. A toe pleat

a. makes the finished bed look neater.
b. is used only in the unoccupied bedmaking procedure.
c. reduces resident discomfort and complications.
d. is an older method that is no longer used.

11. The temperature of the pantry refrigerator should be

a. 45° F or below.
b. at least 50° F.
c. appropriate for laboratory specimens.
d. 36° F or below.

12. Soiled linen

a. should be placed on the floor when making an occupied bed.
b. is put on the overbed table until it can be removed.
c. is not the nursing assistant's responsibility.
d. should be placed in a plastic bag or covered hamper.

B. True/False

Answer each statement true (T) or false (F).

13. ____ Shake soiled linen before placing it in the hamper to check for lost items.

14. ____ The call signal is placed close to alert residents only, because residents who are mentally confused don't know how to use it.

15. ____ A bath blanket is used to drape the resident when providing personal care.

16. ____ Only authorized personnel can access the medication room unless directly supervised.

17. ____ Instruments used in resident care are brought to the clean utility room for cleaning.

18. ____ Chemicals in the soiled utility room must be stored in locked cabinets.

19. ____ Licensed nurses are responsible for the personal care of residents using specialized (therapeutic) beds.

20. ____ The nursing assistant should check the bed for lost items before removing soiled linen.

C. Clinical Applications

Answer the following questions.

21. Beverly Fry's room is very cluttered. She has food, newspaper, trash, and numerous personal items in disarray all over the room. The nurse states that the room is a health hazard and assigns you to clean it. When you enter the room, Beverly starts yelling at you and tells you to get out. She says she will sue you if you throw anything away. What should you do?

22. You are making an occupied bed. The bed linen is soiled and must be changed. The resident is lying on his side. You remove the soiled linen behind his back. No one else is in the room to assist you. There is no soiled linen hamper in the room. What do you do with the soiled linen until you can take it to the hallway and discard it in the hamper?

UNIT 9

Personal Care and Grooming

OBJECTIVES

After reading this unit, you will be able to:

- Spell and define key terms.
- Describe how personal care affects self-esteem.
- List four daily care routines and describe the type of care given in each.
- Demonstrate routine oral hygiene, special oral hygiene, and care of dentures.
- List the general guidelines for assisting residents with bathing and perineal care.
- Demonstrate the back rub procedure.
- List the guidelines for assisting residents with personal grooming.
- Demonstrate hand, foot, and nail care.
- Demonstrate correct application of antiembolism stockings.
- Describe measures to protect the resident's arms and legs from injury.
- Demonstrate dressing and undressing a dependent resident.
- Demonstrate procedures related to personal care skills.

OBSERVATIONS TO MAKE AND REPORT RELATED TO PERSONAL CARE SKILLS

Rash
Redness
Redness of the skin that does not go away within 30 minutes after pressure is relieved from a bony prominence or pressure area
In dark- or yellow-skinned residents, spots or areas that are darker than normal skin tone
Pressure ulcers, blisters
Abrasions, skin tears, lacerations
Irritation
Bruises
Skin discoloration
Swelling
Lumps
Abnormal skin growths
Change in color of a wart or mole
Abnormal sweating
Excessive heat or coolness to touch
Open areas/skin breakdown
Drainage
Foul odor
Complaints such as numbness, burning, tingling, itching
Signs of infection
Unusual skin color, such as blue or gray color of the skin, lips, nail beds, roof of mouth, or mucous membranes
Skin growths
Poor skin turgor, tenting of skin on forehead or over sternum
Sunken, dark eyes

Personal Care of the Resident

Good personal **hygiene** (cleanliness) is essential to maintaining or restoring health. Good hygiene prevents infection, eliminates odors, promotes relaxation, stimulates circulation, and enhances self-esteem. Hygienic habits and practices are developed over a person's lifetime. They may be influenced by culture or religion. Some adaptations of routines and customary practices may be necessary in the long-term care facility. Even minor changes can be upsetting to the resident. Personal care and hygiene is a very private matter for most people.

Providing personal care is a major responsibility of the nursing assistant. It is also an area in which you must be sensitive to the needs, feelings, emotions, and cultural practices of others. Most personal care involves exposing and touching the resident's body. Often, you are bathing and caring for private areas. Think of how you would feel if someone else had to do these things for you. Remember, the resident feels this way, too. The resident may feel embarrassed or ashamed because he or she is unable to care for himself or herself. Be kind, compassionate, and sensitive to the resident's feelings and do not show disgust if you must care for a resident who has lost control of bowel or bladder. If you react in a negative way, this will further lower the resident's self-esteem. Always provide privacy. Use proper terms when referring to elimination. Avoid slang, which may be degrading to the resident.

Activities of Daily Living

Activities of daily living, or **ADLs**, are personal care activities that people do every day to meet their human needs. Examples of ADLs are bathing; shaving; caring for the hair, mouth, and nails; and applying makeup. Dressing, eating, and toileting are also activities of daily living. These activities fall at the lower levels of Maslow's hierarchy of needs, so they are the most basic. If the resident cannot meet these needs independently, the nursing assistant must assist or provide care that meets them. Personal care of the resident includes care of the mouth, teeth, skin, hair, nails, and feet. It may involve cleaning body excretions if a resident is **incontinent**. Incontinence is the inability to control the bowel, bladder, or both, and is often the result of a medical problem over which the resident has no control. It may be temporary. A resident who becomes incontinent may feel guilty and embarrassed. You must be sensitive to the resident's feelings. Personal care also involves bathing, dressing, and grooming the resident. Good personal hygiene prevents skin breakdown; gives the resident a secure, comfortable feeling; and enhances self-esteem.

The resident has carried out ADLs throughout his or her life. Sometimes the resident is able to continue to do all or part of these skills. If so, he or she should be encouraged to continue. You must provide the supplies needed and arrange them conveniently so the resident can use them. It may take longer, but you will reinforce the resident's feelings of self-worth by allowing him or her to do these things. Organize your work so that you can do something else while the resident is performing self-care skills. This makes good use of your time. If the resident is unable to complete a task, you will finish it for him or her. This is part of providing restorative nursing care.

Daily Care Routines

Personal care is given as often as necessary to maintain comfort and keep residents clean. Residents who can be out of bed may be able to continue with their regular routines, but you must assist residents who are weak, mentally confused, or bedfast.

Routine care is given at certain times. The names for the procedures may differ slightly in your facility, but the care given at certain times of day is an important part of the daily routine for all residents. You may be assigned to give AM care, morning care, afternoon care, or HS care. Staff on duty in the early morning are responsible for providing **AM care**. Residents are prepared for breakfast early in the morning. Routine bathing and skin care measures are usually done during **morning care**. Many residents like to have **afternoon care** before visitors arrive. **HS care** may also be called evening care or bedtime care. This care makes the resident comfortable and improves the ability to rest and relax. A summary of the routine hygienic measures performed is found in Table 9.1.

Changing the Resident's Gown. Most residents are up and dressed during the day. Some bedfast residents wear hospital gowns. The gown may have to be changed frequently if it becomes wet or soiled. Avoid exposing the resident during this procedure.

Oral Hygiene

Oral hygiene involves cleaning the mouth, teeth, gums, and tongue. One of your responsibilities is to provide good mouth care for the resident. Residents need mouth care even if they have no teeth and no dentures. When a person is ill, there may be a bad taste in the mouth caused by the

TABLE 9-1 Routine care tasks	
Type of Care	**Responsibilities**
AM care (may also be called early AM care)	1. Assisting with using the bathroom, bedpan, or urinal. 2. Cleaning incontinent residents and changing wet or soiled linen. 3. Assisting the resident to wash face and hands for breakfast. 4. Providing oral care, or assisting the resident to brush teeth. 5. Straightening the bed. 6. Assisting the resident to dress, or put on robe and slippers if getting out of bed for breakfast. 7. Transferring the resident to the chair, or assisting the resident to a comfortable position for eating in bed, if necessary. 8. Tidying the unit and removing unnecessary articles before breakfast. 9. Passing fresh drinking water and assisting the resident to drink, if necessary. 10. Clearing and wiping the overbed table in preparation to receive the breakfast tray, or assisting the resident to go to the dining area.
Morning care (may also be called AM care)	1. Assisting with using the bathroom, bedpan, or urinal. 2. Cleansing incontinent residents and changing wet or soiled linen. 3. Assisting the resident to wash face and hands immediately after breakfast. 4. Providing oral care, or assisting the resident to brush teeth after breakfast. 5. Providing bed baths, partial baths, perineal care, whirlpool baths, tub baths, and showers. 6. Shaving male residents. 7. Assisting female residents to put on makeup. 8. Performing range-of-motion exercises if indicated on the care plan. 9. Assisting residents to change pajamas or dress in street clothes, according to preference and facility policy. 10. Brushing and caring for the hair and nails. 11. Assisting residents with walking and other activity. 12. Transporting residents to other areas for treatments and activities. 13. Changing the bed linen, or making the bed, according to facility policy. 14. Tidying the unit.
Afternoon care (may also be called PM care)	1. Assisting with using the bathroom, bedpan, or urinal. 2. Cleansing incontinent residents and changing wet or soiled linen. 3. Assisting the resident to wash face and hands after lunch. 4. Providing oral care, or assisting the resident to brush teeth after lunch. 5. Changing the resident's clothing, if necessary. 6. Assisting residents to return to bed for a nap. 7. Assisting residents out of bed after they have rested. 8. Assisting residents to brush hair or freshen makeup, if desired. 9. Assisting residents with ambulation. 10. Performing range-of-motion exercises if indicated on the care plan. 11. Straightening the bed linen. 12. Passing fresh drinking water and assisting the resident to drink, if necessary.
HS care (may also be called evening care)	1. Assisting with using the bathroom, bedpan, or urinal. 2. Cleansing incontinent residents and changing wet or soiled linen. 3. Assisting with a bedtime snack, supplement, or nourishment. 4. Assisting the resident to wash face and hands before bedtime. 5. Providing oral care, or assisting the resident to brush teeth at bedtime. 6. Assisting residents with a partial bath before bedtime. 7. Assisting residents into gowns or pajamas for bed (or change, if necessary or desired). 8. Giving back rubs. 9. Straightening the bed linen. 10. Tidying the unit. 11. Passing fresh drinking water and assisting the resident to drink, if necessary.

PROCEDURE 22 Changing the Resident's Gown

1. Perform your beginning procedure actions.
2. Reach behind the resident and untie the gown strings.
3. Remove and loosen the gown under the resident's body.
4. Unfold the clean gown and drape it across the resident's chest, on top of the bath blanket or top sheet.
5. Remove the resident's arms from the sleeves of the gown, but keep the chest covered. If the resident cannot pull the arms from the sleeves, insert your hand into the sleeve to support the resident's hand, and pull the sleeve down and off.
6. Assist the resident to insert the arms into the sleeves of the clean gown. If the resident has a paralyzed arm, place that arm in the sleeve first. If the resident cannot place the arms in the sleeves, put your hand in the sleeve on the outside of the gown. Grab the resident's hand. Slide the gown off your hand, then up over the resident's hand and arm.
7. After both arms are in the sleeves, remove the soiled gown by pulling it under the clean gown, without exposing the resident.
8. Tie the strings and straighten the clean gown under the bedding.
9. Perform your procedure completion actions.

GUIDELINES FOR

Giving Oral Hygiene

- Encourage the resident to do as much self-care as possible.
- Allow the resident to brush his or her own teeth. Take the resident to the bathroom sink, if possible.
- Always wear gloves when performing oral hygiene. Avoid contaminating environmental surfaces and clean supplies with your gloves.
- Observe and report any signs of irritation, sores, loose teeth, pain, swelling, or other abnormalities to the nurse.

illness or medication. The tongue may be coated with a substance that spoils the appetite. One purpose of oral hygiene is to remove food particles and make the mouth feel fresh and clean. Having a clean mouth helps the resident's appetite, prevents bad breath and mouth odor, and reduces the incidence of pneumonia and some other medical conditions to which elderly persons are susceptible.

Good oral hygiene also reduces the buildup of **plaque**, an acidic, decay-causing substance. Everyone has bacteria in the mouth. Many foods cause the bacteria to produce acids. Sugars and starches are the worst culprits, but other foods in combination with bacteria produce plaque as well. Plaque also irritates the gums, making them red, tender, or bleed easily. The gums may pull away from the teeth. Pockets form and fill with pus and more bacteria. Untreated, the condition worsens until the bone around the teeth is destroyed. The teeth may become loose or have to be removed. Gum disease is a leading cause of tooth loss in adults.

Many elderly persons have reduced saliva, which causes the mouth to be dry and uncomfortable. Residents who breathe mainly through the

PROCEDURE

23 Brushing and Flossing the Resident's Teeth

1. Perform your beginning procedure actions.
2. Gather supplies needed: disposable gloves, fresh water, disposable drinking cup, straw, soft-bristle toothbrush, toothpaste, mouthwash, **emesis basin**, and towel. (An emesis basin is a kidney-shaped basin used for oral care procedures.)
3. Sit the resident upright, or elevate the head of the bed as much as possible. Drape the towel across the resident's chest.
4. Mix equal parts of water and mouthwash in the cup.
5. Let the resident rinse his or her mouth with mouthwash.
6. Hold the emesis basin under the chin so the resident can spit out the mouthwash.
7. Wet the toothbrush and apply toothpaste.
8. Gently insert the toothbrush in the mouth with the bristles pointing down. Then rotate the toothbrush so the bristles face the teeth. Brush all surfaces of the teeth. The bristles must reach into the space between the teeth and the gums. Hold the brush at a 45° angle against the teeth, then scrub *gently*, using a short back-and-forth motion, or small circular motion. Scrubbing too hard will damage the gums—be gentle!
9. Brush all surfaces of the teeth (Figure 9.1). Do the outside, insides, bottom, and top. Clean all areas where food can get stuck. To reach the upper front teeth, use the "toe" end of the brush. Rotate the brush vertically, then use the bristles near the end. Move the brush gently up and down.
10. Brush the tongue gently, avoiding the back of the tongue. Contact with the back of the tongue or throat may cause the resident to gag.
11. Hold the emesis basin under the chin and allow the resident to spit out the toothpaste.
12. Break off about 18 inches of dental floss. Wind most of it around the middle finger of one gloved hand. Wind the remaining floss around the middle finger of the other hand. Use this finger to take up the used floss as it becomes dirty. Hold the floss tightly between your thumbs and forefingers.
13. Keep your fingers close to the resident's teeth for good control. Gently guide the floss between the resident's teeth, using a gentle rubbing motion. Avoid snapping the floss into the gums. When you reach the gum line, curve the floss into a C-shape against one tooth. Slide it gently into the space between the tooth and the gum.
14. Hold the floss tightly against the tooth. Gently rub the side of the tooth, using an up-and-down motion as you move the floss away from the gum. Continue until you have flossed all teeth.
15. Let the resident rinse his or her mouth with the mouthwash solution.
16. Hold the emesis basin under the chin and allow the resident to spit out the mouthwash.
17. Wipe the mouth with a towel.
18. Perform your procedure completion actions.

(continues)

PROCEDURE 23 Brushing and Flossing the Resident's Teeth, *Continued*

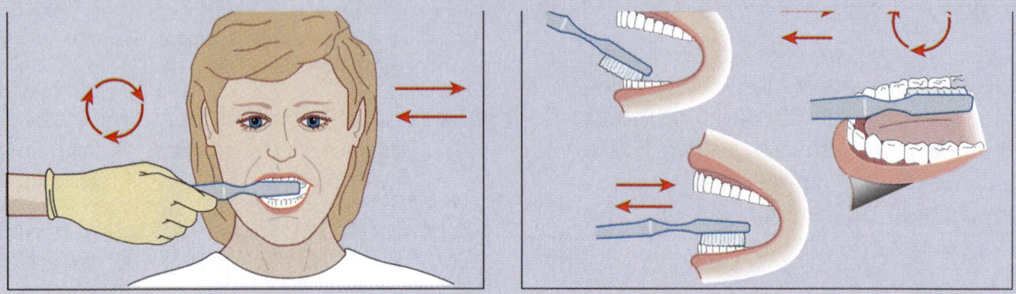

FIGURE 9-1 Gently brush all surfaces of the teeth and gums.

mouth also have dry mucous membranes. Providing mouth care is partly a comfort measure that creates a feeling of well-being. It is also an opportunity for observation. While assisting with oral care, you have an opportunity to observe the resident's mouth and inspect it for abnormalities and pocketed food.

Special Oral Hygiene

You will recall that NPO is the abbreviation for "nothing by mouth." Residents who are NPO, unconscious, receiving tube feeding, or using oxygen require more frequent mouth care. The mucous membranes of the mouth dry out quickly and become coated with mucus. Sometimes they crack and bleed. The purpose of providing special oral hygiene is to keep the mucous membranes and lips moist. This procedure may also be used for residents who have no teeth.

Care of Dentures

Dentures are artificial teeth made of a hard plastic material. Most are removable. Some are permanently attached inside the mouth. They are neces-

PROCEDURE 24 Special Oral Hygiene

1. Perform your beginning procedure actions.
2. Gather supplies needed: disposable gloves, emesis basin, two towels, commercially prepared swabs, lubricant for lips, plastic bag. If commercial swabs are not available, obtain tongue depressors, gauze sponges, a disposable cup, mouthwash, and water.
3. Cover the pillow with a towel. Use the second towel to cover the resident's chest.
4. Turn the resident's head to the side. Tip the head forward slightly so that fluid and secretions will not run down the throat.
5. Place the emesis basin against the resident's chin.

6. Gently open the mouth.
7. Dip the prepared sponge applicators into water, mouthwash, or solution used by the facility. Press against the side of the cup to remove extra fluid. Limit the amount of fluid used if the resident is unable to spit or swallow.
8. If prepared applicators are not available, wrap a gauze sponge around the tongue depressor. Dip the depressor into a cup containing a solution of half water and half mouthwash. Press the applicator against the side of the cup to remove extra solution.
9. Wipe the gums, teeth, tongue, and inside of the mouth with applicators.
10. Discard the used applicators in the plastic bag.
11. Apply lubricant or lip balm to the lips.
12. Perform your procedure completion actions.

GUIDELINES FOR

Giving Special Oral Hygiene

- This procedure is done for bedfast residents who are unresponsive or poorly responsive.
- Always wear gloves when performing this procedure.
- Explain the procedure to the resident even if he or she is confused or unresponsive.
- Turn the resident's head to the side when cleaning the mouth, to avoid getting liquids into the lungs.
- Moisten the lips with lip balm or other lubricant according to facility policy. If oxygen is in use, use a water-soluble lubricant.

GUIDELINES FOR

Denture Care

- Always wear gloves when performing this procedure. Avoid contaminating environmental surfaces and clean supplies with your gloves.
- Handle dentures carefully.
- Let the resident remove the dentures from the mouth, if able.
- Dentures must be brushed daily. Soaking dentures in solution does not eliminate the need for daily brushing.
- Rinse dentures well before brushing under running water. Do not rinse them in standing water in the sink.
- If you must place items such as the toothbrush, toothpaste, or dentures on the counter, put them on a clean paper towel. Never place them in the sink or on an unprotected countertop.
- Check the dentures for cracks, chips, or loose teeth.
- Store dentures in a marked denture cup. Some dentures are stored dry, but most are stored in water. Follow the directions for the type of dentures you are caring for. If in doubt, store the dentures in clean, cool water. Avoid hot water, which will cause them to warp. Consult the nurse if necessary.
- Change the soaking solution and wash the denture cup with soap and water daily. Rinse well.
- The tissues and gums in the mouth must be brushed daily, even if the resident has no teeth. Use a soft-bristle brush to clean the mouth. This improves circulation and removes oral debris.

PROCEDURE

25 Denture Care

1. Perform your beginning procedure actions.
2. Gather supplies needed: disposable gloves, emesis basin, denture cup, denture brush or soft-bristle toothbrush, denture paste or powder, towel, tissues, a disposable cup, paper towels, mouthwash, and water. If you will be removing the dentures, obtain a gauze sponge to place under your gloved hand. The gauze gives you a firm grip on the dentures to avoid slipping. Obtain a small plastic bag to dispose of the gauze sponge and gloves.
3. Drape the towel across the resident's chest.
4. Line the emesis basin with paper towels. A washcloth or hand towel may also be used.
5. Ask the resident to remove the dentures, if able, and place them in the emesis basin.
6. Offer the resident a tissue to wipe the mouth after removing the dentures.
7. If the resident is unable to remove the dentures, apply gloves. Cover your fingers with a gauze sponge and grasp the center of the upper denture with the thumb and index finger of your hand. An alternative is to place your index fingers on both sides at the back of the denture plate. Gently move the denture up and down to break the seal. Pull the denture out of the mouth and place it in the emesis basin.
8. To remove the lower denture, cover your gloved fingers with a gauze sponge and gently grasp it with your thumb and index finger. Turn it to the side slightly and lift it from the mouth. Place it in the emesis basin. Discard the gauze sponge in the plastic bag.
9. Raise the side rail.
10. Line the bottom of the sink with paper towels, a washcloth, or a hand towel. Fill the sink half-full of cool water so the dentures do not break if they drop (Figure 9.2). You may also place the dentures in an emasis basin under running water.
11. Rinse the dentures well under cool running water to remove food particles and other debris.
12. Wet the toothbrush and apply the denture paste or powder. If you have not yet applied gloves, do so at this time.
13. Hold the dentures securely and brush all surfaces.
14. Rinse the dentures well under cool running water. Place them in the denture cup.
15. Return to the bedside and lower the side rail.

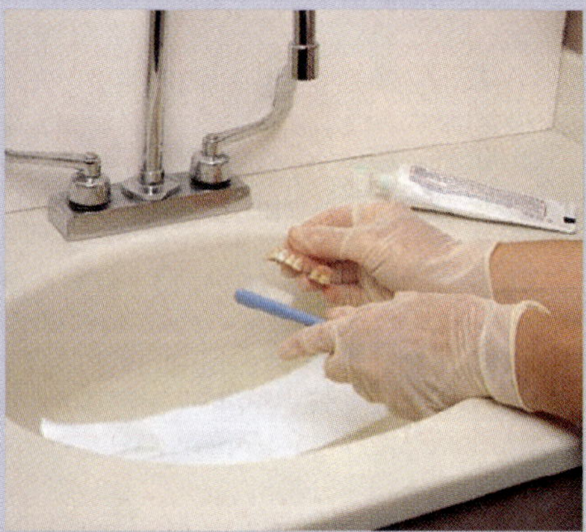

FIGURE 9-2 Line the sink with a paper towel and fill it half-full with water to avoid breakage if the dentures accidentally drop.

16. Let the resident brush his or her gums and tongue, then clean and rinse the resident's mouth with a solution of equal parts water and mouth-wash before replacing the dentures.
17. Hold the emesis basin under the chin and allow the resident to spit out the solution.
18. Hand the resident the denture cup and ask him or her to insert the dentures, if able. Some residents may ask for denture paste or powder to hold the dentures in place. Apply it according to the directions on the package. For a paste, a dot on each back corner and a dot in the front center are usually enough.
19. If the resident is unable to insert the dentures, grasp the middle front of the upper denture firmly with your thumb and index finger. Raise the upper lip with your other hand and slide the denture into the mouth. Place both index fingers in the mouth on each side of the upper denture and press firmly to ensure that the denture is in place.
20. Grasp the middle front of the lower denture securely with your thumb and index finger. With your other hand, pull the lower lip down and slide the denture into the mouth. Place both index fingers in the mouth on each side of the denture and press firmly to ensure it is in place.
21. Raise the side rail.
22. Remove the towel and discard according to facility policy.
23. Rinse and dry the denture cup and return it, with your other supplies, to the top drawer of the bedside stand. If the resident does not want the dentures in his or her mouth, store them in the cup in the bedside stand. Some dentures are stored dry, but most should be kept moist. Ask the resident how the dentures should be stored. If in doubt, fill the cup with clean, cool water, and place the dentures in it. Cover the cup and place it in the bedside stand.
24. Perform your procedure completion actions.

sary for eating, retaining the shape of the face and jaw, and giving the resident a sense of well-being. Many people are sensitive about wearing dentures and will not allow others to see them without their teeth. Always provide privacy when caring for dentures. Dentures are very expensive and break easily if dropped, so handle them carefully.

Bathing the Resident

Bathing is done to eliminate odor, stimulate circulation, provide mild exercise, and refresh and relax the resident. Bath time is an excellent time to inspect the resident's skin for redness, irritation, or other problems. If skin problems are observed, notify the nurse. Washing removes secretions, excretions, dirt, and oil that are harmful to the skin. Bath time is a good time for you to communicate with the resident.

Types of Baths

Many types of baths are given in health care facilities. A **complete bath** is given when washing the entire body is necessary. Some facilities give all residents a **partial bath** at bedtime. A partial bath consists of washing the face, hands, under-arms, back, and genital area, and may be given as often as necessary to meet the resident's needs. Follow your facility policy for washing the hair. Some facilities do not consider a shampoo part of the bathing procedure, and may require a doctor's order to wash the hair. Some female residents have their hair done at the beauty parlor each week. If this is the case, get permission from the nurse before washing their hair. Doing so will remove the curl and style the beautician has created.

Most residents can take a tub, shower, or whirlpool bath. Some facilities require a doctor's order for certain types of baths, so follow your facility policy. Special shower chairs are available for residents to sit in while taking a shower. Tub baths and showers are given two or more times a week, according to your facility policy and individual resident needs. Some facilities have special tubs that may be used to immerse bedfast residents in water for bathing (Figure 9.3). These are very comforting and appreciated by the residents. Refer to the care plan for information about the type of bath and other special hygiene and grooming needs.

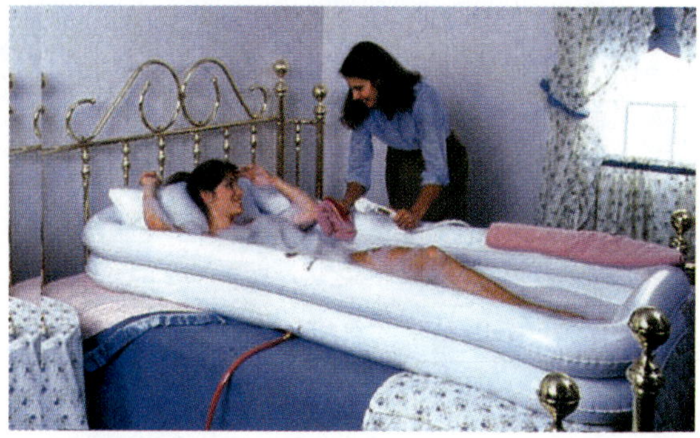

FIGURE 9-3 Special tubs may be used to bathe bedfast residents. (*Courtesy of* Medline Industries, Inc. 1-800-MEDLINE)

GUIDELINES FOR

Bathing Residents with the Waterless Bathing System

- Commercially prepared waterless bathing products are designed to be used for one bath. A full-size kit contains eight cloths. Smaller kits containing four cloths are also available for partial baths and perineal care. The package may be resealed if you do not use all the cloths.
- The washcloths may be used at room temperature, but many facilities microwave them for comfort. Monitor the temperature carefully to prevent over-heating and intermittent hot spots that could injure the resident.
- Peel the label back or open the package before heating to avoid bursting in the microwave.
- Follow manufacturers' directions for heating the package. One minute is usually sufficient to warm the contents to a comfortable temperature.
- The cloths in the package are for a single use only.
- The procedure is similar to a bed bath, with cleansing done in the same order:
  1. Face and neck
  2. Far arm and hand
  3. Chest and abdomen
  4. Near arm and hand
  5. Far leg and foot
  6. Near leg and foot
  7. Back and buttocks
  8. Perineum
- Discard used cloths properly, according to facility policy. Avoid flushing them down the toilet. A plastic bag at the bedside works well for cloth disposal.
- If you have extra cloths at the end of the procedure, reseal and date the package. Discard unused cloths within 72 hours of opening, or immediately if they are dry.

GUIDELINES FOR

Assisting with Bathing and Personal Care

- Consult the care plan for information about the type of bath to be given, special information, resident's self-care ability, routines, use of adaptive devices or other equipment, resident needs, goals related to bathing and grooming, and general care. Your care should be consistent with the care plan goals.

- Gloves are worn for part of the bathing procedure. You will have to change your gloves and wash your hands several times during a complete bath to apply the principles of standard precautions.
- If you have open cuts or sores on your hands, you will have to wear gloves for the entire bathing procedure. To apply the principles of standard precautions, you must remove your gloves, wash your hands, and reapply clean gloves immediately before contacting mucous membranes or nonintact skin.
- Moving the resident to the side of the bed near you may be helpful, if you are bathing the resident in bed.
- Provide privacy by closing the door, window curtains, and privacy curtain.
- Many personal care procedures involve exposing the resident, so be sure the room is warm and comfortable.
- Before beginning a procedure, organize your work. Anticipate what you will need and gather it in advance.
- Keep the resident's body covered with a bath blanket for modesty and warmth and expose only the part of the body on which you are working.
- Bathe only one part of the body at a time, keeping the rest of the resident covered.
- Offer the resident choices. Personal care should be given according to the resident's preference, considering medical needs. Also consider culture, religion, social, and familial practices, as well as individual preference.
- If you find a technique that improves resident self-esteem or independence, share this information with other members of the interdisciplinary team.
- Change the water if it cools off or becomes soapy or dirty.
- Soap can be irritating and drying to the skin. Be sure it is rinsed off.
- When not using the soap, keep it in the soap dish and not in the wash basin.
- If you will be using liquid soap from a dispenser mounted on the wall, avoid putting the soap directly into the bath water. Dispense some soap into a small cup and carry it to the bedside. Pour the liquid soap onto the washcloth as needed.
- In some facilities, bar soap is not permitted. If refillable liquid soap bottles are used, each resident should have a bottle labeled with his or her name. The soap from that bottle is used for that resident only.
- The shower bath is commonly given in the long-term care facility. Keep the spray of warm water on the resident's body during the entire procedure to prevent chilling.
- If you wash the resident's hair in the shower, placing cotton in the ears will prevent problems if the spray is misdirected. Bring an extra towel and wrap the resident's head after rinsing out the shampoo.
- A bottle of lotion can be placed in the bath water at the beginning of the bath to warm it. After the bath it can be used on the resident's hands, arms, and back.
- When applying lotion to resident's arms and legs, rub or pat it on lightly. Avoid vigorous up-and-down massage, as this may cause circulatory complications.
- After the bath, dry the skin well. Pay special attention to skin folds, creases, and the area between the toes. Drying helps prevent infection and skin breakdown.
- Follow your facility policy for use of powders. If permitted, use sparingly. Too much powder is not good for the skin. Powder can cause respiratory problems if inhaled.
- Apply deodorant after the bath, unless the resident objects.
- Upon completion of the bathing procedure, dress the resident in appropriate clothing. If the resident must wear a hospital gown or other nightwear, cover the body as much as possible.
- Clothing should be appropriate for the resident's age and gender. Consider the season and color-co-ordinate clothing as much as possible. Let the resident select the clothing, if possible.
- Assist the resident to put on proper undergarments. Avoid using a hospital gown under clothing in place of undergarments.
- If the resident will be getting out of bed, put socks and footwear appropriate to the floor surface on the feet.

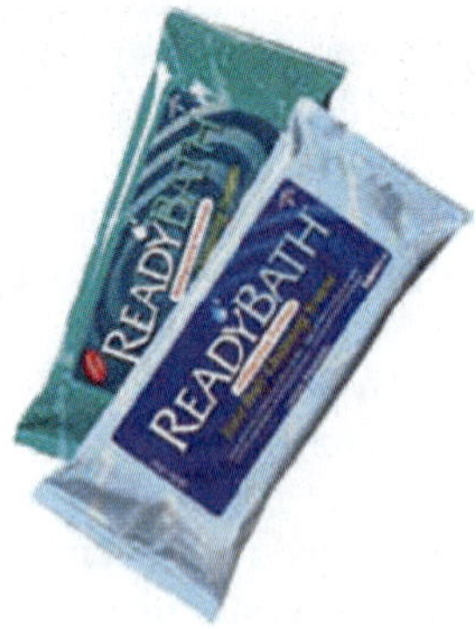

FIGURE 9-4A A waterless bath or "bag bath" is a popular, comfortable, time-saving alternative to the traditional bed bath. (*Courtesy of Medline Industries, Inc. 1-800-MEDLINE*)

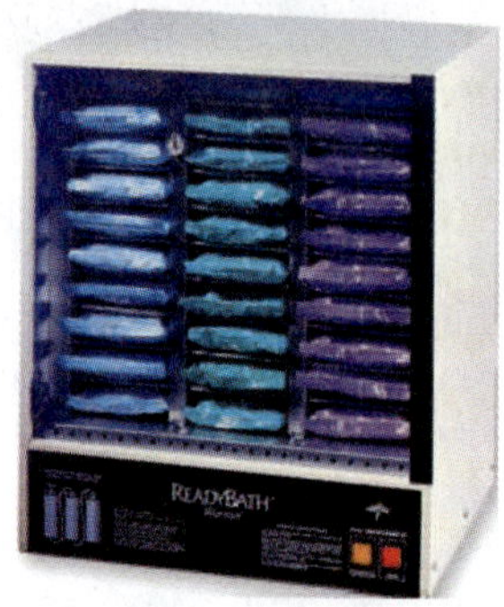

FIGURE 9-4B Warmed bag bath is very comfortable and soothing for the resident. The commercial warmer reduces the risk of hot spots and overheating in the microwave. (*Courtesy of Medline Industries, Inc. 1-800-MEDLINE*)

Residents who must stay in bed or are either too weak or ill to receive a tub bath or shower are given a **bed bath**. The nursing assistant cleans the resident's entire body, one part at a time, while the resident remains in bed. The resident who receives a complete bed bath probably will be unable to assist you.

Waterless Bathing

When residents are bathed in bed, a basin of water and soap are traditionally used. Over the past few years, a newer system of bathing, developed by a nurse, has become popular. This system is called **waterless bathing**. It may also be called basinless bathing or bag bath. The waterless bathing system is prepackaged (Figure 9.4A). A package of moistened washcloths is used in place of the water basin and soap. The package may be used at room temperature, or heated in a microwave or commercial warmer (Figure 9.4B), according to facility policy and resident preference. Advantages to the waterless bathing system include:

- Faster and more economical for the facility; each bath takes approximately 8 to 10 minutes
- Less fatiguing for the resident
- Conserves moisture, reduces drying, and is gentler to skin than soaps
- Less friction, because the cloths are softer than regular washcloths and towels, and drying is eliminated

Perineal Care

The **perineum** is the area between the anus and vagina in the female; the area between the anus and scrotum in the male. **Perineal care** is also

SAFETY GUIDELINES FOR

Personal Care Procedures

- Test the temperature of the bath water with a thermometer. As a rule, water that is 105 °F is comfortable for bathing. Use common sense with water temperature. Ask the resident if the temperature is comfortable for him or her. Check the temperature with your elbow or wrist to make sure it is not too hot.
- If you will be transporting the resident in the hallway to a tub or shower room, be sure that the resident's body is covered.
- Use the transfer belt over the clothing to move the resident.
- Use safety belts on tub lifts and shower chairs.
- Make certain that bath mats are secure.
- Help residents in and out of the tub and shower.
- *Never leave the resident unattended in the bathtub, whirlpool, or shower.*
- If the resident becomes weak or dizzy in the tub or shower, stay in the room and pull the emergency call signal. Begin to drain the water from the tub. Cover the resident with a bath blanket for warmth.

INFECTION CONTROL GUIDELINES FOR

Personal Care Procedures

- Apply the principles of standard precautions and wear gloves and other personal protective equipment when indicated.
- Use of gloves is not necessary or desirable for the entire bathing procedure. Use them only when contact with blood, body fluids (except sweat), secretions, excretions, mucous membranes, or nonintact skin is likely. Change gloves as often as necessary to comply with standard precautions.
- If you are wearing gloves, remove them, wash your hands, and reapply new gloves *immediately before* contact with mucous membranes or nonintact skin. Mucous membranes are found in the eyes, nose, mouth, and **genital area**. The genital area is the part of the body where the external reproductive organs are located.
- Avoid contaminating equipment or items in the room and environment with gloves used for resident care.
- Dispose of gloves according to facility policy.
- Wash from the cleanest area to the least clean.
- Change water, washcloth, and gloves after washing a contaminated or "dirty" area.
- Once a towel has been used below the waist, avoid using it above the waist.
- The handheld shower spray should be placed on the hook when not in use. Do not let it hang down or touch the floor, which is always considered dirty.
- Disinfect the tub, shower chair, or whirlpool according to facility policy before and after each use.
- Follow your facility infection-control policies for handling clean and soiled linen. Soiled linen or towels should not be left on the tub or shower room floor.

PROCEDURE 26 Giving a Bed Bath

1. Perform your beginning procedure actions.
2. Gather supplies needed: basin, bath thermometer, soap, washcloth, two towels, clean gown or clothing, bath blanket, lotion, comb or brush, disposable gloves, and plastic laundry bag or hamper.
3. Place clean equipment on the resident's overbed table. Follow your facility policy for covering the overbed table with a barrier.
4. Check the temperature of the room. Make sure it is not too cold.
5. Offer the resident the bedpan or urinal before beginning the procedure. If you will be assisting, apply the principles of standard precautions.
6. Remove the bedspread and blanket. Fold and place them on the chair.
7. Place the bath blanket over the top sheet. Ask the resident to hold the blanket in place. Remove the sheet by pulling it down from underneath the blanket. Avoid exposing the resident. Place the soiled sheet in the hamper or dispose of it according to facility policy.
8. Remove the gown and dispose of it according to facility policy. Keep the resident covered with the bath blanket. Expose only the part on which you are working.
9. Raise the side rail.

(continues)

PROCEDURE 26

Giving a Bed Bath, *continued*

10. Fill the basin with warm (105 °F) water. Check the temperature with a thermometer.
11. Return to the bedside and lower the side rail.
12. Place a towel across the resident's chest.
13. Allow the resident to wash his or her own face, if possible. If the resident is unable, you will wash the face. Check for the resident's preference regarding soap. Some people do not use soap on the face.
14. Apply disposable gloves to wash the eyes.
15. Make a mitten by folding the washcloth around your hand (Figure 9.5).
16. Wash the eyelids from the inner corner to the outer corner, using plain water without soap. Use a separate part of the washcloth for each eye.
17. Dry the washed area.
18. Rinse the washcloth.
19. Remove the gloves and discard according to facility policy.
20. Wash and dry the remainder of the face, neck, and ears.
21. Place a towel lengthwise under the resident's arm farthest from you.
22. Hold the arm up. Wash the arm from the shoulder to the wrist and fingertips, using long, firm, circular strokes.
23. Rinse and dry the arm.
24. Wash, rinse, and dry the armpit, or **axilla**.
25. Repeat for the other arm.
26. If possible, place the resident's hands in water. Wash, rinse, and dry hands, fingers, and nails. Clean under the nails with an orange stick, if soiled.
27. Place the towel across the chest (Figure 9.6). Pull the bath blanket down to the abdomen.
28. Fold the towel to expose half the chest.
29. Wash, rinse, and dry the chest. In the female resident, dry under the breast well. Repeat for the other side of the chest.
30. Cover the chest with the towel.
31. Pull the bath blanket down to expose the abdomen.
32. Wash, rinse, and dry the abdomen.

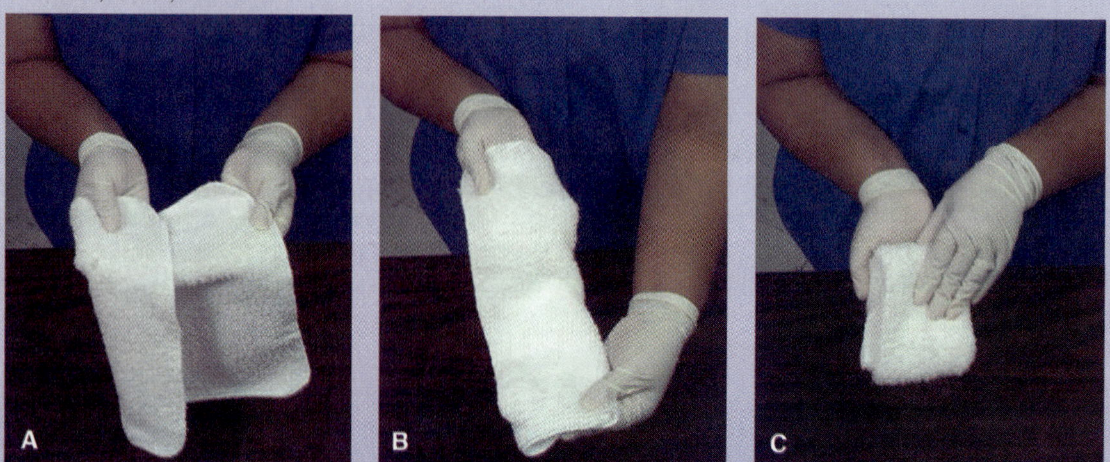

FIGURE 9-5 Make a washcloth mitt. Wear gloves if there is potential for contact with blood, body fluids, secretions, excretions, mucous membranes, or nonintact skin.

(continues)

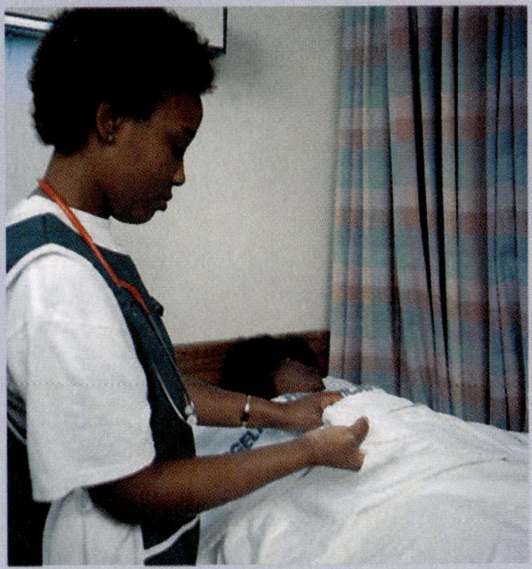

FIGURE 9-6 Respect the resident's modesty by covering her body with a towel and draping with the bath blanket.

33. Cover the resident with the bath blanket.
34. Remove the towel from under the blanket.
35. Uncover the leg farthest from you. Place the towel lengthwise under the leg. Bend the knee and place the foot on the bed, if the resident is able.
36. Wash, rinse, and dry the leg from the groin area to the toes.
37. Repeat for the other leg.
38. If the resident is able, place the basin on the towel and place the feet in the basin one at a time (Figure 9.7).
39. Wash, rinse, and dry the feet. Wash, rinse, and dry well between the toes. Check the appearance of the toes and skin between the toes for redness, cracking, or irritation.
40. Cover the legs with the bath blanket.
41. Raise the side rail.
42. Empty the basin, rinse, and refill with clean (105 °F) water.
43. Return to the bedside and lower the side rail.
44. Assist the resident to turn so that his or her back is toward you.
45. Place the towel lengthwise on the sheet against the resident's back.

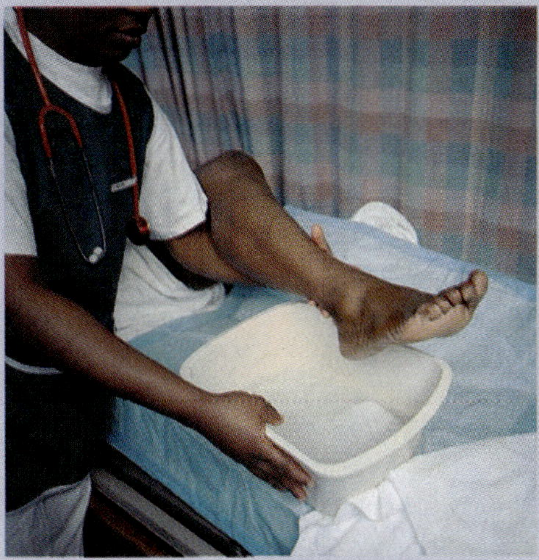

FIGURE 9-7 If the resident is able, soak the feet in a basin, one at a time.

46. Wash, rinse, and dry the back and outer buttocks. Observe for signs of redness, irritation, or skin breakdown.
47. Put lotion on the resident's back.
48. Remove the towel and assist the resident to turn on his or her back.
49. Ask the resident if he or she would like to wash the genital area. If the resident is unable, apply disposable gloves.
50. Wash, rinse, and dry the genital area from the front to the rectal area.
51. Place the soiled linen in the hamper or plastic bag, according to facility policy.
52. Remove gloves and dispose of them according to facility policy.
53. Apply deodorant and put a clean gown on or dress the resident.
54. Raise the side rail.
55. Wash your hands.
56. Return to the bedside and put the side rail down.
57. Comb the hair and assist with other grooming requests.
58. Replace bed linens, if indicated, or straighten the bed.
59. Perform your procedure completion actions.

PROCEDURE 27 Giving a Partial Bath

1. Perform your beginning procedure actions.
2. Gather supplies needed: basin, soap, washcloth, two towels, clean gown or clothing, bath blanket, lotion, comb or brush, hamper or plastic laundry bag for soiled linen, and disposable gloves.
3. Place the equipment on the overbed table. Follow your facility policy for covering the overbed table with a barrier.
4. Offer the resident the bedpan or urinal. Apply the principles of standard precautions if you will be assisting with this procedure.
5. Remove the bedspread and blanket. Fold and place them on the chair.
6. Place the bath blanket over the top sheet. Ask the resident to hold the blanket in place. Remove the sheet by pulling it down from underneath the blanket. Avoid exposing the resident. Place the soiled sheet in the hamper or dispose of it according to facility policy.
7. Fill the basin with warm (105°F) water. Check the temperature with a thermometer.
8. Remove the gown and dispose of it according to facility policy
9. Place a towel across the resident's chest.
10. Allow the resident to wash his or her own face, if possible. If the resident is unable, you will wash the face. Check for the resident's preference regarding soap.
11. Apply disposable gloves to wash the eyes, because of the potential for mucous membrane contact.
12. Make a mitten by folding the washcloth around your hand.
13. Wash the eyelids from the inner corner to the outer corner, using plain water without soap. Use a clean area of the washcloth for each eye.
14. Dry the washed area.
15. Rinse the washcloth.
16. Remove the gloves and discard according to facility policy.
17. Wash the remainder of the face, neck, and ears.
18. Place the towel under the hand farthest from you.
19. Wash, rinse, and dry the hand.
20. Repeat for the other hand.
21. Place the towel under the axilla.
22. Wash, rinse, and dry the axilla.
23. Repeat on the opposite side.
24. Assist the resident to turn so that his or her back is toward you.
25. Place the towel lengthwise on the sheet against the resident's back.
26. Wash, rinse, and dry the back and outer buttocks. Observe for signs of redness, irritation, or skin breakdown.
27. Put lotion on the resident's back, following the guidelines in Procedure 11.
28. Remove the towel and assist the resident to turn on his or her back.
29. Use gloves to wash the genital area. Wash from the front of the genital area to the rectal area.
30. Place the soiled linen in the hamper or plastic bag, according to facility policy.

31. Remove gloves and dispose of them according to facility policy.
32. Apply deodorant, if desired, and put a clean gown on the resident.
33. Raise the side rail.
34. Wash your hands.
35. Return to the bedside and put the side rail down.
36. Comb the hair and assist with other grooming requests.
37. Replace bed linens, if indicated, or straighten the bed.
38. Perform your procedure completion actions.

PROCEDURE 28

Waterless Bed Bath

1. Perform your beginning procedure actions.
2. Gather supplies needed: disposable gloves, bed linen; bath blanket; hospital gown/resident's night-clothes; bath towel; lotion for back rub; waterless bathing product (heated according to facility policy or resident wishes); basin of warm water for soaking hands (optional); comb; brush; supplies for oral hygiene, as needed; supplies for nail care, as needed; deodorant; small plastic bag to discard used bathing cloths; large plastic bag or hamper for soiled linen.
3. Place clean supplies on overbed table.
4. Offer the bedpan or urinal. Put on gloves if you will be assisting with this procedure.
5. Lower the head of the bed and the side rail on the side where you will be working.
6. Loosen the top bedclothes. Remove and fold the blanket and spread and place them over the back of the chair.
7. Place the bath blanket over the top sheet and remove the sheet by sliding it out from under the bath blanket. Place the sheet in the laundry hamper.
8. Leave one pillow under the resident's head. Place any extra pillows on the chair.
9. Remove the resident's gown and place it in the laundry hamper.
10. Assist the resident to move to the side of the bed near you.
11. Open the package of bathing cloths. (If a microwave was used to heat the package, check cloths for hot spots.) Remove one cloth and cleanse the resident's face and neck. (Solution can safely be used around the eyes.)
12. Place a towel over the resident's chest. Fold the blanket down to the waist and cleanse the chest. Be sure that the area under the breasts is carefully cleaned.
13. Fold the bath blanket down to the pubic area and wash the abdomen. Replace the bath blanket over the abdomen and chest. Remove the towel by sliding it out from under the bath blanket. Discard the used cloth in a plastic bag.

(continues)

PROCEDURE

28 Waterless Bed Bath, *Continued*

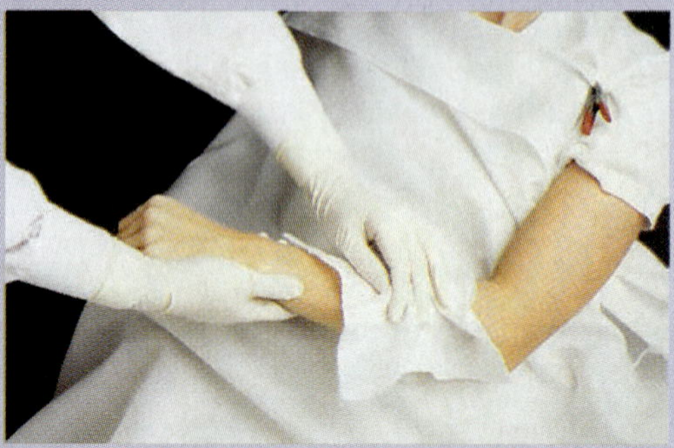

FIGURE 9-8 Wash the far arm and hand. The waterless bath product is kind to the skin and dries quickly. (*Courtesy of Sage Products, Inc.*)

14. Uncover the far arm. Remove another cloth from the package and wash the arm and hand (Figure 9.8). Soaking the opposite hand in a basin of warm water, while you wash one arm, is a nice touch. This is refreshing to the resident if he or she cannot be out of bed to bathe. Wash the axilla. Apply deodorant. Discard the used cloth in a plastic bag. Cover the arm with the bath blanket.
15. Uncover the near arm. Remove a new cloth from the package. Wash the arm, hand, and axilla. Apply deodorant. Discard the used cloth in a plastic bag. Cover the resident with the bath blanket.
16. Provide nail care as needed.
17. Ask the resident to flex the far leg, if possible. Fold the bath blanket up to expose the thigh, leg, and foot. Remove a new cloth from the package. Cleanse the thigh, leg, and foot. Be sure the area between the toes is left dry. Discard the used cloth in a plastic bag. Cover the leg and foot with the bath blanket.
18. Repeat step 17 with the near thigh, leg, and foot.
19. Make sure the side rail on the opposite side of the bed is up. Help the resident turn on the side away from you. Place a bath towel lengthwise next to the resident's back.
20. Remove a new washcloth from the package. Draw the bath blanket back to expose the back. Wash the back and outer buttocks. Discard the used cloth in a plastic bag. A back rub may be given at this time. Cover the resident with the bath blanket.
21. Assist the resident to turn on the back. Position a towel under the buttocks by asking the resident to lift the hips, if possible. Remove a new cloth from the package. Hand the resident the cloth and instruct him or her to wash the perineum. Assist if necessary. (Wear gloves if you will be assisting). Discard your used gloves and the cloth in a plastic bag. Remove the towel.
22. Wash your hands.
23. Assist the resident to put on a clean gown.
24. Cover the pillow with a towel. Comb or brush the hair. Assist with oral hygiene if needed.
25. Change the bed linen, following the occupied bedmaking procedure. Put soiled linen in a plastic bag or the linen hamper.
26. Perform your procedure completion actions.

PROCEDURE 29 Assisting The Resident with a Tub or Shower Bath

1. Perform your beginning procedure actions.
2. Check to see if the tub or shower room is available. Disinfect the tub or shower chair according to facility policy. Adjust the temperature in the room, if necessary. Place a bath mat on the floor of the tub or shower, and a disposable or cloth bath mat in front of the tub.
3. Gather supplies needed: disposable gloves, plastic laundry bag or hamper, washcloth, two or three towels, bath blanket, bath thermometer, soap, lotion, and personal grooming supplies.
4. Go to the resident's room and assist with toileting, if necessary. Apply the principles of standard precautions if you will be assisting with this procedure.
5. Assist the resident to the tub or shower room.
6. Regulate the water temperature. Always turn the cold water on first and off last. Check the water temperature with a thermometer. It should be comfortably warm, or 105 °F. Double-check the temperature by allowing the water to run over your inner forearm or wrist.
7. If the resident is taking a tub bath, fill the tub half-full of water.
8. Assist the resident to undress, if necessary. Give the resident a towel to place in front of the waist and lower abdomen.
9. Assist the resident to transfer to the tub or shower chair. If the resident is being transferred to a chair with a footrest, push the footrest back during the transfer, then pull it out to support the resident's feet.
10. Push the shower chair into the shower and position it so you can support the resident from the front if he or she starts to fall. In the tub, position the resident so that he or she faces the controls.
11. Lock the wheels to the shower chair in position so the chair will not move.
12. Wash the back.
13. Allow the resident to complete the bath. If unable, you will wash and rinse the resident. Apply the principles of standard precautions if contact with blood, body fluids, secretions, excretions, mucous membranes, or nonintact skin is likely. You may have to change your gloves several times during this procedure to avoid cross-contamination.
14. Assist the resident in washing the lower legs and feet, if necessary. Make sure to wash and rinse well between the toes. Discard the washcloth in the hamper.
15. Assist with washing the hair, if needed. If you will be doing this procedure, bring an extra washcloth, towel, and two cotton balls into the shower room. Place the cotton balls in the resident's ears before beginning, and remove them when finished. Give the resident a clean, dry washcloth to cover the face. Wrap the resident's head with the towel after rinsing to prevent chilling.
16. Assist with perineal care, if necessary. Apply gloves. Wash the genitalia from the front of the chair. Then squat down and wash the remainder of the perineum by reaching underneath the chair. Wash the rectal area from the back of the chair. Always wash from front to back (most clean to least clean). Turn the cloth frequently. Rinse well.

(continues)

PROCEDURE 29 Assisting The Resident with a Tub or Shower Bath, *continued*

17. Upon completion of the bathing procedure, assist the resident out of the tub or shower. Wrap with a bath blanket for modesty and warmth.
18. Pat the resident dry, or allow the resident to dry independently. Make sure to dry the perineal area and the areas between the resident's toes well.
19. Apply lotion to the back, and to other areas if the resident desires. Avoid the area between the toes. Applying lotion to this area promotes fungal growth.
20. Return to the resident's room and assist with dressing and other personal care needs. Keep the resident's body completely covered in the hallways. You may dress the resident in the shower room as facility environment and procedures permit.
21. Perform your procedure completion actions.
22. After the resident is safe and comfortable, return to the tub or shower room. Discard the linen according to facility policy. Wear gloves when removing wet linen. Clean and disinfect the tub, shower chair, and handrails.

GUIDELINES FOR

Giving a Whirlpool Bath

- Check with the nurse before giving a whirlpool bath to a resident with an infection, surgical incision, or pressure ulcer.
- If the resident is combative or disoriented, check with the nurse before giving the resident a whirlpool bath. The noise from the whirlpool may worsen agitation in some residents.
- Disinfect the whirlpool tub immediately before and after each use.
- The water temperature in the whirlpool tub is usually set at 97 °F to 100 °F because the temperature in the tub remains constant. (Use common sense; if the tub is steaming, the water is probably too hot. Use a thermometer to check the water temperature.) The constant movement of warm water stimulates the resident's circulation.
- Never leave the resident alone in the whirlpool tub, even for a minute (Figure 9.9).
- Always fasten the safety belt when moving a resident into or out of a whirlpool tub with a hydraulic lift seat. The safety belt should remain fastened throughout the procedure.
- The resident may be frightened when using the hydraulic lift for the first time. Explain the procedure and reassure the resident.
- Drape the resident's genital area with a bath towel for modesty during the whirlpool bath.
- Use low-suds or no-suds products that are designed specifically for whirlpool use.
- Never pour liquid soap or shampoo into the whirlpool tub. Even a tiny bit of liquid soap will result in an abundance of suds. If the resident accidentally creates a suds problem, rub a bar of soap against the walls of the tub to reduce the bubbles.

- The whirlpool activity provides a cleansing action. However, if you will be assisting the resident with bathing, apply the principles of standard precautions.
- Wrap the resident with a bath blanket for warmth and modesty immediately after removing him or her from the whirlpool tub.
- The jets in some whirlpool tubs have the potential to harbor dangerous pathogens. Follow facility policies for carefully cleaning the tub with the proper disinfectant solution. Make sure that you follow directions correctly and run the disinfectant through the tub for the correct length of time.
- When the bath is completed, raise the lift seat out of the soapy water and rinse with the hose, using comfortably warm water.

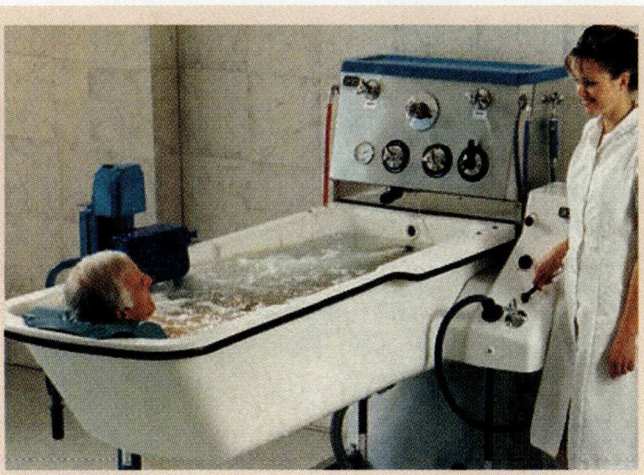

FIGURE 9-9 Never leave the resident alone in the whirlpool. Keep the safety belt fastened on the lift chair. If the resident becomes ill, use the call signal to get help. Drain the tub.

GUIDELINES FOR

Giving Peri-Care

- Always wear gloves during this procedure. Be careful not to contaminate clean supplies and environmental surfaces with your gloves.
- Be kind and sensitive. Most people are very uncomfortable about having someone else clean their genital area.
- Protect the resident's modesty and privacy by exposing only the part of the body on which you are working.
- If the perineum is soiled with excretions, remove them with tissues or disposable wipes. Place them in the bedpan for removal. Change the underpad if it is wet or soiled. If the resident is wet, place on a dry underpad before beginning. After the heavy soiling is removed, discard your gloves. Wash your hands and reapply clean gloves before continuing the procedure.
- Use warm, soapy water. Wash the cleanest area first. In the female, this means you will wash from front to back. In the male, begin at the end of the penis and move down toward the body, under the scrotum, then back to the rectum. Turn the washcloth so you are using a clean section each time you move to a new area. Use a second washcloth if necessary. Avoid rubbing back and forth. Rinse the soap off well and dry thoroughly. Some facilities use special products for peri-care. Follow your facility policy.
- If the resident has a catheter, wash it gently to remove urine, stool, mucus, or dried secretions. Catheter care is described in Unit 11.
- When washing the catheter, begin at the urinary meatus and wash downward three to four inches on the catheter. Do not rub back and forth.
- In the female resident, keep the labia separated as much as possible during the procedure. Avoid placing your fingers on an area after washing it. You may need several washcloths to perform the procedure without contamination. (Some states require a second, clean washcloth for rinsing; the used cloth is not put back into the water basin.)

(continues)

- If using a mitt is difficult for you, an alternate method is to fold the washcloth in fourths. One edge will have corners that can be folded down separately. Wet the washcloth and squeeze out excess water. Place a drop of liquid soap on each corner of the edge. Fold these corners back, one at a time, to expose a clean area of the cloth with each stroke. Turn the cloth around and use the other area of the washcloth to cleanse the perineum.
- Usually, the nursing assistant is expected to give perineal care to residents of both sexes.
- Many facilities apply barrier products to protect the skin after performing perineal care. Know and follow your facility policy. Some barrier products contain alcohol. Avoid applying these products to red or broken skin. If you are applying barrier cream after perineal care, remove your gloves, wash your hands, and apply new gloves. Your gloves become contaminated during the peri-care procedure, and you must use new (clean) gloves to apply barrier cream.

PROCEDURE

30 Female Perineal Care

Note: The guidelines and sequence for this procedure vary slightly from state to state. Your instructor will inform you if the sequence in your state differs from the procedure listed here. Know and follow the required sequence for your state.

1. Perform your beginning procedure actions.
2. Gather supplies needed: basin, soap, washcloth, towels, clean gown or clothing, bath blanket, bed protector, hamper or plastic laundry bag, and disposable gloves.
3. Place the equipment on the overbed table. Follow your facility policy for covering the overbed table with a barrier.
4. Offer the resident the bedpan or urinal. Apply the principles of standard precautions if you will be assisting with this procedure.
5. Remove the bedspread and blanket. Fold and place them on the chair.
6. Place the bath blanket over the top sheet. Ask the resident to hold the blanket in place. Remove the sheet by pulling it down from underneath the blanket. Avoid exposing the resident. Place the soiled sheet in the hamper or dispose of it according to facility policy.
7. Remove the gown and dispose of it according to facility policy.
8. If the linen is wet or soiled, remove and dispose of it according to facility policy. Be sure the resident is lying on a clean, dry surface.
9. Assist the resident to raise her hips. Place a bed protector under the buttocks. Remove the soiled bed protector, if present. Wear gloves if you will be handling a wet or soiled bed protector.

10. Raise the side rail.
11. Fill the basin with warm (105°F) water. Check the temperature with a thermometer.
12. Return to the bedside and lower the side rail.
13. Position the bath blanket so the area between the legs is exposed.
14. Assist the resident to separate and bend the knees, placing the feet on the bed, if able.
15. Put on disposable gloves.
16. Make a mitten by folding the washcloth around your hand.
17. Wet the washcloth and apply soap. Avoid using too much soap, which can be irritating to the skin.
18. Separate the labia with one hand. If a urinary catheter is present, hold the tubing securely to one side and support against the leg to avoid unnecessary movement or traction on the catheter. Keep the tubing and drainage bag below the level of the bladder.
19. With the other hand, wash the center of the labia, using a single downward stroke from top to bottom (Figure 9.10). Stop at the base of the labia.
20. Turn the washcloth to a clean area.

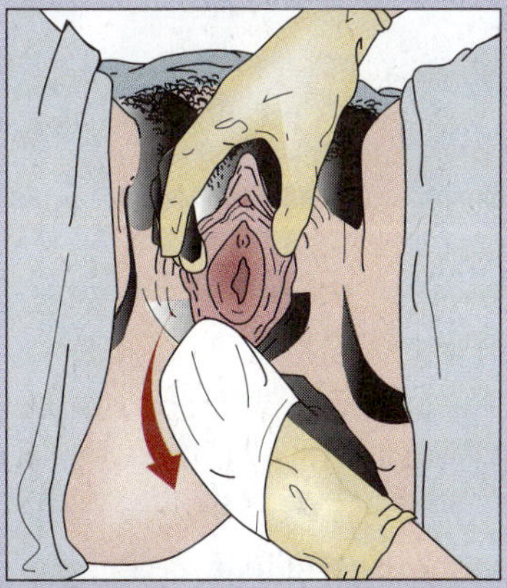

FIGURE 9-10 Wash from top to bottom with a single stroke. Avoid rubbing back and forth. Use a clean section of the washcloth for each downward stroke.

21. Wash the far side of the labia, using a single downward stroke from top to bottom.
22. Turn the washcloth to a clean area.
23. Wash the near side of the labia, using a single downward stroke from top to bottom.
24. Continue to alternate from side to side, working outward to the thighs, using the same technique. Turn the washcloth or use a new washcloth, if necessary, so a fresh section is used to cleanse each area.
25. If a urinary catheter is present, wash, rinse, and dry the perineal area surrounding the urinary meatus and catheter. Change the washcloth. Wash the catheter beginning at the urinary meatus, down the catheter approximately three to four inches. Use a single downward stroke. Do not rub back and forth. Rinse and dry in the same direction. Hold the catheter firmly to avoid pulling and traction. After washing the catheter, continue with perineal care.
26. Rinse the area from top to bottom with the washcloth. Rinse in the same sequence, beginning in the center and moving outward from side to side. Turn the washcloth so a clean surface is used for each downward stroke. Avoid rubbing back and forth.
27. Gently pat the area dry with a towel. Dry in the same sequence, beginning in the center and moving outward from side to side. Position the towel so a clean surface is used for each downward stroke. Avoid rubbing back and forth.
28. Assist the resident to turn on the side away from you. Flex the upper leg forward, if possible.
29. Wet the washcloth and make a mitt. Apply soap.
30. Expose the anal area.
31. Wash the area gently, wiping from the perineum to the tailbone, or **coccyx** (Figure 9.11).

(continues)

PROCEDURE

30 Female Perineal Care, *continued*

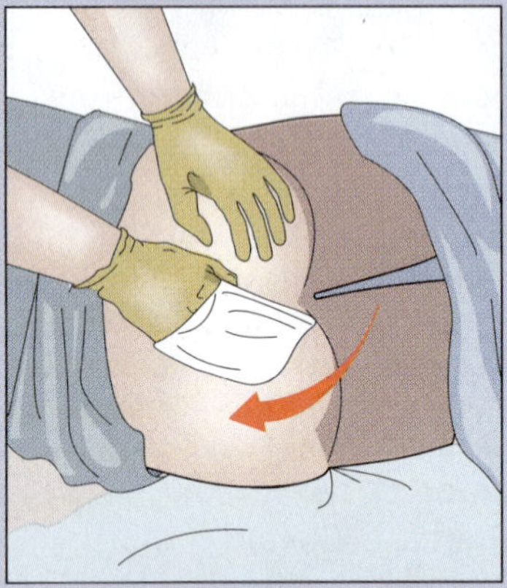

FIGURE 9-11 Turn the resident on the side and wipe from the rectal area to the coccyx.

32. Rinse the washcloth, then rinse the area well.
33. Gently pat dry with a towel. Avoid rubbing back and forth.
34. Assist the resident to return to her back.
35. Remove and dispose of the bed protector according to facility policy.
36. Place the soiled linen in the hamper or plastic bag, according to facility policy.
37. Remove one glove and raise the side rail with the ungloved hand. Dispose of both gloves according to facility policy.
38. Wash your hands.
39. Return to the bedside and lower the side rail.
40. Replace the top covers and remove the bath blanket.
41. Help the resident into a clean gown or other clothing of choice.
42. Perform your procedure completion actions.

PROCEDURE

31 Male Perineal Care

Note: The guidelines and sequence for this procedure vary slightly from state to state. Your instructor will inform you if the sequence in your state differs from the procedure listed here. Know and follow the required sequence for your state.

1. Perform your beginning procedure actions.
2. Gather supplies needed: basin, soap, washcloth, towels, clean gown or clothing, bath blanket, bed protector, hamper or plastic laundry bag, and disposable gloves.
3. Place the equipment on the overbed table. Follow your facility policy for covering the overbed table with a barrier.
4. Offer the resident the bedpan or urinal. Apply the principles of standard precautions if you will be assisting with this procedure.
5. Remove the bedspread and blanket. Fold and place them on the chair.

6. Place the bath blanket over the top sheet. Ask the resident to hold the blanket in place. Remove the sheet by pulling it down from underneath the blanket. Avoid exposing the resident. Place the soiled sheet in the hamper or dispose of it according to facility policy.
7. Remove the gown and dispose of it according to facility policy.
8. If the linen is wet or soiled, remove and dispose of it according to facility policy. Be sure the resident is lying on a clean, dry surface.
9. Assist the resident to raise his hips. Place a bed protector under the buttocks. Remove the soiled bed protector, if present. Wear gloves if you will be handling a wet or soiled bed protector.
10. Raise the side rail.
11. Fill the basin with warm (105°F) water. Check the temperature with a thermometer.
12. Return to the bedside and lower the side rail.
13. Position the bath blanket so the area between the legs is exposed.
14. Assist the resident to separate and bend the knees, placing the feet on the bed, if able.
15. Put on disposable gloves.
16. Make a mitten by folding the washcloth around your hand.
17. Wet the washcloth and apply soap. Avoid using too much soap, which can be irritating to the skin.
18. With one hand, grasp the penis gently and wash. Wash the urinary meatus in a circular motion.
19. Continue to wash down the penis and the rest of the perineal area, including the scrotum, using downward strokes and working out-ward to the thighs (Figure 9.12). Lift the scrotum and wash the perineum.
20. If the resident is not circumcised, gently pull the foreskin back and wash it (Figure 9.13). Rinse the penis, dry gently, and replace the retracted foreskin.
21. If a urinary catheter is present, wash, rinse, and dry the area surrounding the urinary meatus and catheter. Wash the catheter beginning at the urinary meatus, down the catheter approximately three to four inches. Use a single downward stroke. Do not rub back and forth. Rinse and dry in the same direction. Avoid pulling on the catheter.
22. Wash the scrotum, then gently lift it and wash the perineum.

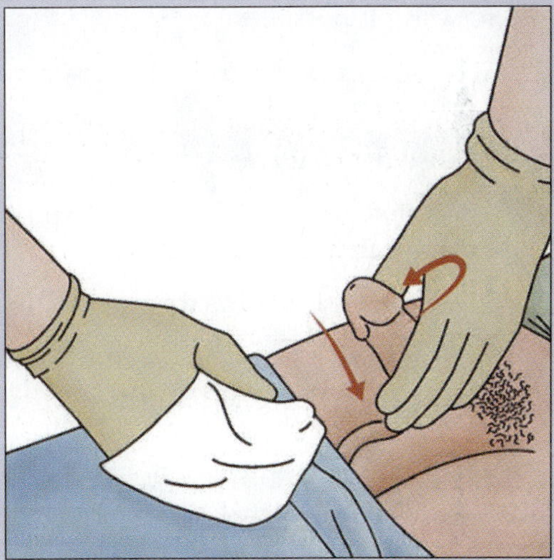

FIGURE 9-12 Wash the meatus area in a circular motion. Wash the shaft using downward strokes.

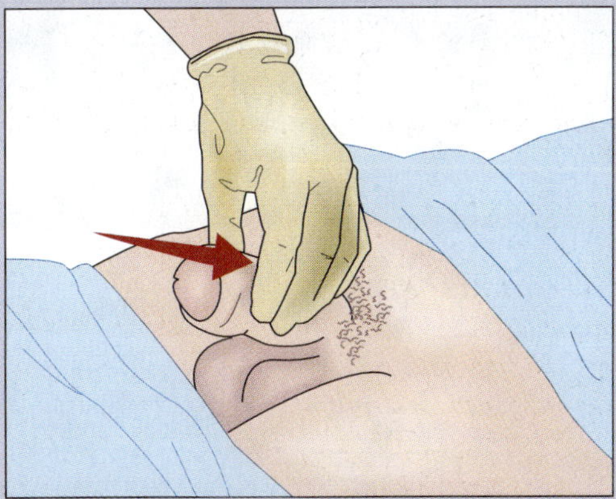

FIGURE 9-13 Gently push the foreskin back to wash the head of the penis.

(continues)

PROCEDURE 31 Male Perineal Care, *continued*

23. Rinse the washcloth.
24. Make a mitten. Gently rinse the urethra, shaft of penis, scrotum, and perineal area well, working in the same direction until the entire area is clean and soap-free.
25. Gently dry the area with a towel.
26. Assist the resident to turn on the side away from you. Flex the upper leg forward, if possible.
27. Wet the washcloth and make a mitt. Apply soap.
28. Expose the anal area.
29. Wash the area, stroking from the perineum to the coccyx.
30. Rinse the washcloth, then rinse the area well.
31. Gently pat the area dry with a towel.
32. Assist the resident to return to his back.
33. Remove and dispose of the bed protector according to facility policy.
34. Place the soiled linen in the hamper or plastic bag, according to facility policy.
35. Remove one glove and raise the side rail with the ungloved hand. Dispose of both gloves according to facility policy.
36. Wash your hands.
37. Return to the bedside and lower the side rail.
38. Replace the top covers and remove the bath blanket.
39. Help the resident into a clean gown or other clothing of choice.
40. Perform your procedure completion actions.

PROCEDURE 32 Giving a Back Rub

1. Perform your beginning procedure actions.
2. Gather supplies needed: basin of water (105 °F), soap, washcloth, towel, hamper or plastic laundry bag for soiled linen, and disposable gloves if contact with nonintact skin or any moist body fluid is likely.
3. Place the equipment on the overbed table. Follow your facility policy for covering the overbed table with a barrier.
4. Assist the resident to turn on the side away from you. Expose the back and upper buttocks.
5. Place the bottle of lotion in the basin of water to warm it (Figure 9.14).

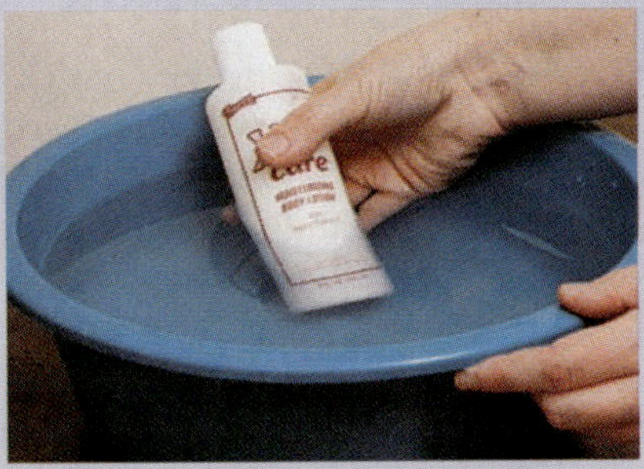

FIGURE 9-14 Warming the lotion in the bath water for a few minutes makes it much more comfortable for the resident.

6. Wash, rinse, and dry the back.
7. Apply a small amount of lotion to one hand.
8. Warm the lotion by rubbing it between your hands, if necessary.
9. Apply lotion to the back.
10. Rub the back with both hands, using gentle, firm strokes in a circular motion. Massage from buttocks to shoulders:
    a. Begin at the base of the spine and rub up the center of the back with long, soothing strokes.
    b. Move your hands in a circular motion as you massage down from the shoulders to the buttocks.

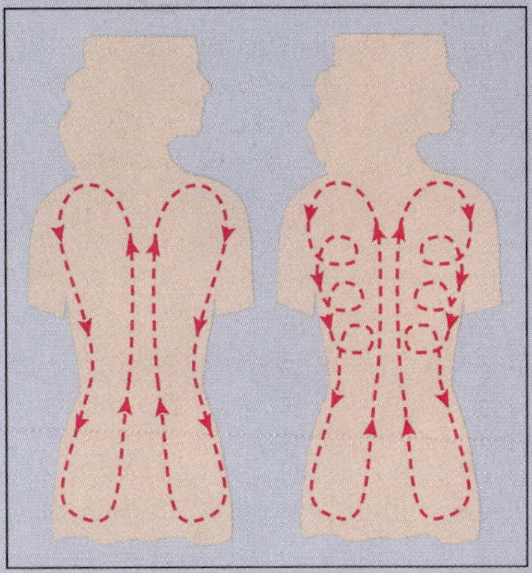

FIGURE 9-15 The back rub is very soothing to the resident. It stimulates circulation and prevents skin breakdown. Avoid rubbing red or open areas.

    c. Repeat this procedure for three to five minutes (Figure 9.15).
11. Wipe off excess lotion.
12. Close and retie the gown, or change the gown if necessary.
13. Straighten and tighten the bottom sheet and draw sheet.
14. Assist the resident to a comfortable position.
15. Perform your procedure completion actions.

called **peri-care**. This procedure involves washing the genital area. Peri-care must be given frequently when residents are incontinent. Urine and stool are very irritating and will promote skin breakdown.

Shampooing the Resident's Hair

Follow your facility policy for washing the resident's hair. Some facilities require a doctor's order for this procedure. If permitted, the hair can be washed in the tub or shower. Offer the resident a washcloth or towel to hold over the face when washing and rinsing hair. For residents on complete bed rest, this procedure must be done in bed. Some facilities use dry chemical shampoos that are brushed out. No-rinse shampoos are also available for bedfast residents.

Shampoo caps (Figure 9.16) are a popular alternative for bathing bedfast residents. These are most comfortable for residents if they are warmed in a microwave for 30 seconds or less, or in the product warmer. The cap is placed on the resident's head, then rubbed gently for one to two minutes for short hair and four to five minutes for long hair. After this time, the cap is removed and the hair towel-dried and combed. Shampoo caps reduce tangling and do not leave residue like some dry chemical products.

Care of African American Residents' Hair

African American residents have special hair care needs. Hair texture of these residents can vary from soft and silky to coarse and thick. Residents

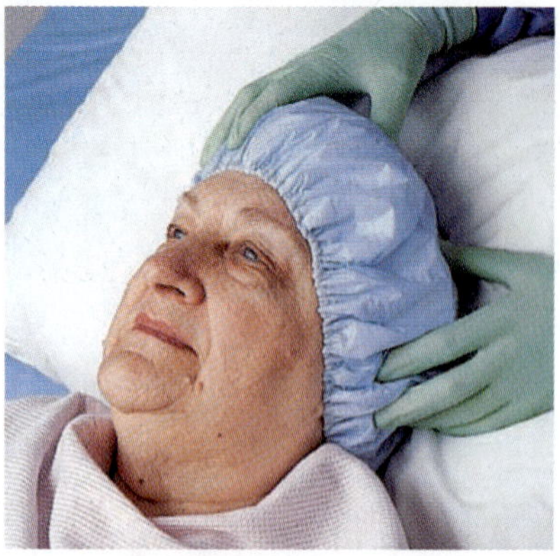

FIGURE 9-16 Shampoo caps simplify the hairwashing procedure for bedfast residents. The products leave the hair feeling clean and tangles are reduced. (*Courtesy of Medline Industries, Inc. 1-800-MEDLINE)*

with coarse hair need special care to prevent damage, tangling, and breaking. Asking the resident or family how to care for the hair is not offensive. In fact, it shows that you care about meeting the resident's needs. They have been caring for the hair for years, and are experts at it. They also know what products work and which do not.

In general, avoid using hair products designed for Caucasian persons. Most of these are designed to eliminate oil. Eliminating the oil from the hair is one of the worst things to do when caring for a person of color. Use a shampoo marketed specifically for "black hair." In most cases, the resident or family will provide a product that works. Wash the hair once every week or two, as specified on the care plan. Washing more often than this dries the hair and causes breakage. If a special shampoo is not available, baby shampoo works best. Use a detangling conditioner according to product directions. After washing the hair, gently towel-dry. Cover the shoulders with a dry towel. Use a wide-toothed comb or pick to comb through the damp hair. Be gentle and patient. It may take time to work through the tangles.

Persons of color need additional oil on the hair at all times. Some residents use products they refer to as hair "grease." If the resident does not have a product preference, apply baby oil *to the scalp, not the hair*. Then, using a soft brush, brush from the scalp to the ends of the hair until all the hairs are covered with oil. You may need to apply this heavily. If it is too oily, wipe the excess with a towel. If you use enough, the hair will appear shiny.

The resident's hair can be braided while damp. Run the wide-toothed comb through the hair to remove tangles. Gently twist the hair and apply a hair tie. Avoid using rubber bands, if possible. These cause breakage and damage hair. If a rubber band must be used, apply hair grease or baby oil liberally to your fingers. Roll the rubber band around in the hair grease until it is well coated, then apply it to the hair. Style the hair in a pony tail, then section and braid it. When you get to the end, apply more grease. Wrap the ends around a barrette and snap it shut, or use a hair tie or grease-coated rubber band.

Applying Lotion To The Resident's Skin

Massaging the resident's skin is comforting and refreshing. Massage can stimulate circulation and helps prevent skin breakdown. Refer to the care plan to see if massage is indicated. Each facility has a house lotion used for massaging residents' skin. Applying moisturizing lotion immediately after the bath helps to seal moisture in the skin, preventing dryness. Always massage the skin in smooth, light strokes. Do not massage red areas that may be Stage I pressure ulcers. Massaging these areas causes tissue destruction. Avoid massaging the legs. Massaging the legs can cause complications related to blood clots. If the resident uses lotion on the legs, pat it on.

Grooming the Resident

Proper grooming is important for the resident's self-esteem. Grooming includes combing hair, shaving, nail care, and applying makeup.

Shaving Residents

Most men shave daily as part of the morning routine. If the resident can shave himself, provide the equipment and supplies and allow him to do it. If the resident is weak or unable, you will shave him. Check the care plan before shaving residents. Some residents may not be shaved

PROCEDURE

33 Shampooing the Hair

1. Perform your beginning procedure actions.
2. Gather supplies needed: shampoo, conditioner, cotton balls, washcloth, two towels, pitcher if needed for rinsing, comb or pick, hair dryer (optional). Additional supplies for bed shampoo include shampoo tray, waterproof bed protector, pitcher of warm (105 °F) water.
3. Place cotton balls in the resident's ears. Remove the resident's hearing aid(s) and glasses, if worn.
4. Have the resident cover the face with the washcloth.
5. Tip the resident's head back, if possible.
6. Use the shower head or pitcher of water to wet the resident's scalp and hair well (Figure 9.17A).
7. Apply shampoo to the palm of your hand. Rub your hands together. Apply the shampoo to the resident's scalp, rubbing with your fingertips (not fingernails) to work up a lather (Figure 9.17B). Wash all areas of the scalp well, using gentle, massaging motions.
8. Have the resident tip the head back. Rinse with warm water from the shower head or water pitcher.
9. Continue rinsing until all soap is removed.
10. Apply conditioner, if the resident desires, or as needed to remove tangles. Follow directions for the product used. Rinse or leave in according to product instructions. (An alternate to reduce tangling is to use a solution of one part white vinegar to five parts warm water. Apply to hair and rub in well. Rinse with warm water. Avoid vinegar if the resident has a fresh permanent; it may remove the curl.)
11. Towel-dry the hair.
12. Wrap the hair with a dry towel.
13. Remove the towel and comb or pick hair following the guidelines in Procedure 45. Avoid brushing wet hair.
14. Dry with a hair dryer if permitted. Hold the dryer 8 to 10 inches from the head. Follow all safety precautions and facility policies for use of the hair dryer. Direct the heat to the hair, not the scalp. Keep the dryer moving. Use the dryer only on the low heat setting. Never use a handheld hair dryer in a wet area. Avoid placing the hair dryer on the resident's lap.
15. Finish styling the resident's hair when it is dry.
16. Perform your procedure completion actions.

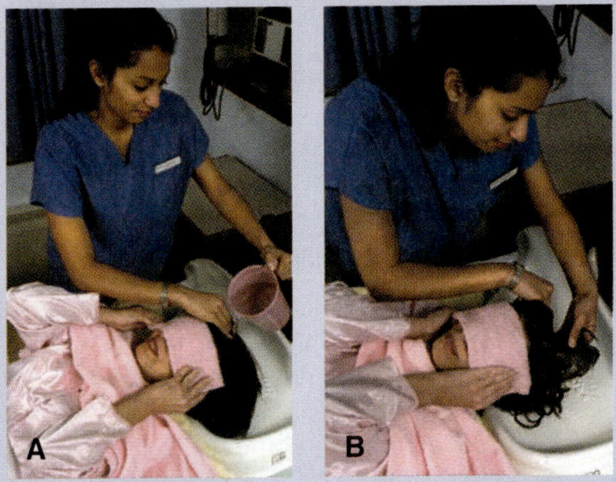

FIGURE 9-17 (A) Cover the eyes with a washcloth and pour water over the hair to wet it thoroughly. (B) Use your fingertips to work up a lather. Wash all areas of the scalp.

GUIDELINES FOR

Assisting Residents with Grooming

- Allow the resident to determine the routine. Respect the resident's preferences and choices.
- Encourage self-care. Assist by setting up supplies and providing equipment.
- Provide privacy.
- Dress and groom the resident appropriately for age, gender, and season, within the limitations of the resident's condition.
- Keep clean grooming items separate from soiled supplies.
- Clean all grooming items after using them.
- Discard disposable razors in the puncture-resistant sharps container.

PROCEDURE 34

Combing the Hair

1. Perform your beginning procedure actions.
2. Gather supplies needed: towel, comb, and brush.
3. Cover the pillow with a towel, or place the towel over the shoulders if the resident is sitting in a chair.
4. Section the hair with one hand. Begin at the scalp and work toward the end of the hair (Figure 9.18).

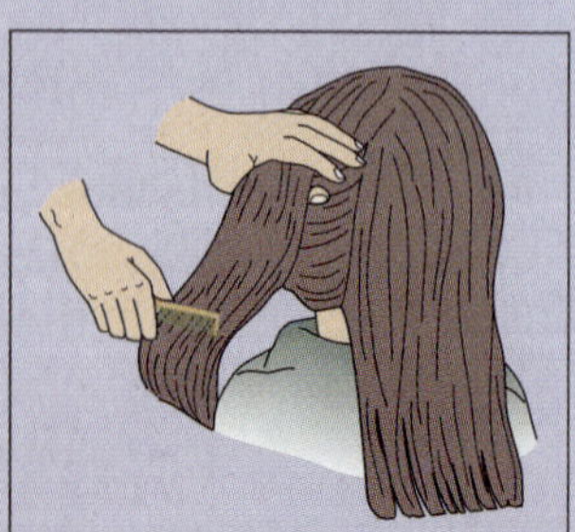

FIGURE 9-18 Beginning at the scalp, comb each section downward.

5. Brush the hair well.
6. If the resident is in bed, assist him or her to turn away from you so that you can brush the back of the hair.
7. If the hair is tangled, separate it with the comb. Start with a small section of hair. Beginning at the end, comb downward. Hold the hair above where you are combing with your other hand so you do not pull on the resident's scalp. Continue working upward until you reach the scalp.
8. Style the hair attractively. If the resident has long hair, consider braiding it or putting it up. Coarse, tightly curled hair may require special treatment.
9. Remove the towel and discard according to facility policy.
10. Perform your procedure completion actions.

PROCEDURE

35 Shaving the Male Resident

1. Perform your beginning procedure actions.
2. Gather supplies needed: disposable gloves, washcloth, towel, electric or safety razor, shaving cream or preshave lotion, basin of water (105 °F), mirror, and aftershave lotion.
3. Place the equipment on the overbed table. Follow your facility policy for covering the overbed table with a barrier.
4. Provide privacy.
5. Drape a towel across the resident's chest.
6. Fill the washbasin with warm (105 °F) water and place it on the table.
7. Soften the beard by placing a warm, moist washcloth over it for two to three minutes. Apply preshave lotion if using an electric razor.
8. Moisten the face with water and apply shaving cream.
9. Put on disposable gloves.
10. Hold the skin taut in front of the ear (Figure 9.19).
11. Starting at the sideburns, move the razor down over the cheeks to the chin, using short, even strokes. Continue until the entire cheek is shaved. Rinse the razor between strokes.
12. Repeat with the other cheek.
13. Ask the resident to tighten the upper lip. Shave from the nose to the upper lip in short, downward strokes.
14. Ask the resident to tighten the chin. Shave the chin in downward strokes.
15. Assist the resident to tip his head back.
16. Apply shaving cream to the neck.
17. Hold the skin taut under the chin, and shave the neck area in short, smooth, upward strokes.
18. Wash and dry the face and neck.
19. Apply aftershave lotion if the resident desires.
20. Remove the basin, empty and dry it, and return it to its storage place.
21. If you accidentally nick the resident, apply a small piece of tissue over the cut to stop the bleeding. Report the cut to the nurse.
22. Perform your procedure completion actions.

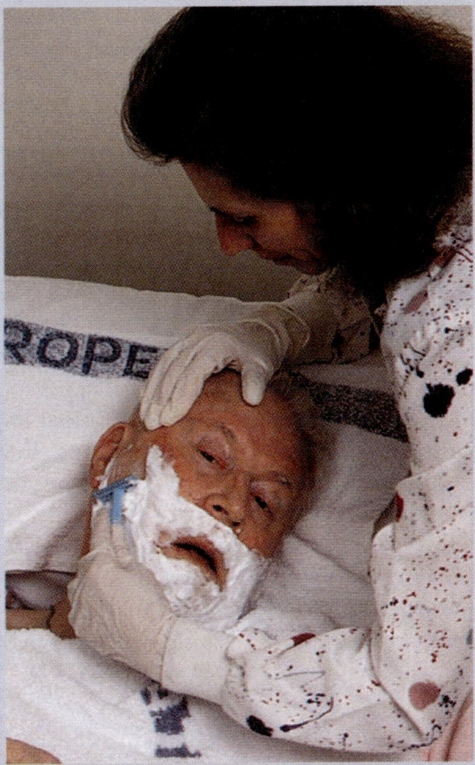

FIGURE 9-19 Hold the skin taut with one hand while shaving in a downward motion with the other.

GUIDELINES FOR

Providing Hand, Foot, and Nail Care

- Know and follow your facility policy for who is allowed to clip and clean nails.
- Cleaning and trimming nails is easier immediately after they are soaked or bathed.
- Avoid the use of nail files and other sharp objects for cleaning nails. An orange stick is a disposable, pointed, wooden stick that can be used safely.
- If your facility allows you to clip fingernails, use clippers, not scissors.
- When trimming nails, be very careful not to accidentally clip or damage the skin surrounding the nail.
- If you observe any abnormalities, such as redness, cracking, or signs of infection by the finger or toenails, report this finding to the nurse.
- Fingernails are clipped straight across, then rounded at the edges with an emery board (Figure 9.20A).
- Push the cuticles back with a washcloth or the dull end of the orange stick (Figure 9.20B).
- After washing the feet, dry well between each toe and inspect for red or cracked areas. Moisture promotes fungal growth and skin breakdown, which can lead to more serious complications.
- Lotion may be applied to the hands or feet if the skin is dry. Do not apply lotion between the toes, as this promotes fungal growth.

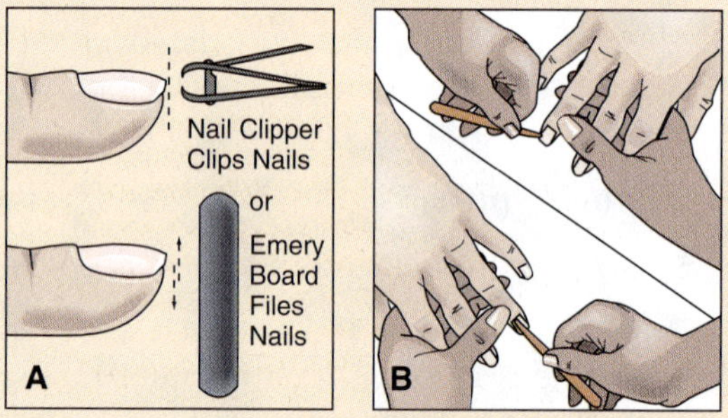

FIGURE 9-20 (A) Clip the nails straight across, then use an emery board to round the edges. (B) Gently push the cuticles back.

because of their medical condition or medications they are taking.

Elderly women may grow facial hair as a result of hormonal changes in aging. Coarse hair is common on the chin. Most women prefer to have facial hair removed. Many women also prefer to have hair removed from their legs and underarms. Honor the resident's preferences. Know your facility policy for removing facial hair from female residents. Some facilities use depilatories. Some facilities shave women in the same manner in which men are shaved.

Shaving may be done with an electric razor or a disposable razor. Electric razors are usually the residents' personal property. They are used for one resident only and cleaned according to manufacturer's directions after each use. This usually involves brushing the heads with a small brush designed for this purpose. All hair should be removed from the head of the razor. Some electric razors must be recharged periodically. Electric razors are expensive. Handle the razor carefully and avoid dropping it. If the electrical cord is frayed or worn, report to the nurse and remove the razor from use. If an electric razor is not available, a disposable safety razor is used. If you are using a disposable razor, always wear gloves because of the high probability of contact with blood during this procedure. Do not recap the razor. Discard the used razor in the sharps container.

Caring for the Resident's Hands, Feet, and Nails

Nails and feet require special attention to prevent injury and infection. In many agencies, only licensed personnel are allowed to cut fingernails, although the nursing assistant is expected to clean them. As a rule, the nursing assistant is not allowed to cut toenails, but is responsible for keeping the feet clean and dry.

PROCEDURE 36 Hand and Fingernail Care

1. Perform your beginning procedure actions.
2. Gather supplies needed: disposable gloves if contact with moist body fluid or nonintact skin is likely, soap, towel, disposable bed protector, basin of warm water (105 °F), lotion, nail clippers, orange stick, and emery board.
3. Cover the overbed table with a bed protector. Place the equipment on the overbed table.
4. Position the overbed table in front of the resident and adjust the height.
5. Fill the washbasin with warm (105 °F) water and place it on the table.
6. Instruct the resident to place his or her hands in the water. A soft brush can be used to clean under the nails when the hands are soaking.
7. Soak the hands for 10 minutes. Placing a towel over the resident's hands and the basin will keep the water warm. Add more warm water if necessary. (Remove the resident's hands when adding water.)
8. Ask the resident to wash his or her hands. Gently push the cuticles back.
9. Lift the hands out of the water and dry them with the towel.
10. Clip the nails if permitted by facility policy. The nail clippings will fall on the bed protector to the discarded later.
11. Round the edges of the nails with the emery board. Apply fingernail polish if requested by a female resident.
12. Rub the hands with lotion.
13. Remove the basin, empty and dry it, and return it to its storage place.
14. Remove the bed protector containing the nail clippings and discard according to facility policy.
15. Perform your procedure completion actions.

The resident's feet require special care. Poor blood circulation to the feet is common, particularly in the elderly and people with diabetes. Ingrown toenails cause pain and breaks in the skin, which can lead to infection. The skin on the feet heals slowly if injured. Protecting the feet from injury is important. Know and follow your facility policy for foot and toenail care. Report to the nurse if the nails need to be cut or if other abnormalities are noted.

Support Hosiery

Support hosiery is used for residents who have circulation problems. It is also used during and after surgery to prevent blood clots and other complications. Support hose may also be used to prevent edema. The hose apply pressure to the legs, increasing the blood flow. The stockings are made of stretchable elastic and fit tightly. Support stockings may be knee length or cover the entire leg. They are called **antiembolism stockings**, or often referred to by the brand name, such as TED Hose.

Protecting the Arms and Legs

Some residents have very fragile, paper-thin skin. The skin bruises easily and commonly tears if it is bumped even slightly, such as on the side rail. Skin tears are unsightly and painful for the resident. They can occur when the resident is transferred into and out of the wheelchair.

PROCEDURE 37 Foot and Toenail Care

1. Perform your beginning procedure actions.
2. Gather supplies needed: disposable gloves if contact with moist body fluid or nonintact skin is likely, soap, towel, bed protector, basin of warm water (105 °F), lotion, orange stick or soft brush.
3. Place the equipment on the overbed table. Follow your facility policy for covering the overbed table with a barrier.
4. Transfer the resident to a chair at the bedside. Remove the resident's shoes and socks.
5. Place a bed protector on the floor under the resident's feet.
6. Fill the washbasin with warm (105 °F) water and place it on the bed protector.
7. Assist the resident to place his or her feet in the water.
8. Soak the feet for 10 minutes. Placing a towel over the resident's feet and the basin will keep the water warm. Add more warm water if necessary. Check the temperature of the water you add. It should be no more than 105 °F. Remove the resident's feet from the water temporarily while you add more water, to avoid accidental burns.
9. Wash the resident's feet. Gently clean under the toenails with the orange stick or a soft brush.
10. Wash the feet with soap, and rinse well.
11. Lift the feet out of the water and dry them with the towel. Dry well between the toes.
12. Inspect the feet for red, dry, cracked, or open areas. Check for bruises, corns, or other abnormalities.
13. Rub the feet gently with lotion. Avoid vigorous massage. Avoid applying lotion between the toes.
14. Apply nail polish if requested by a female resident.
15. Remove the basin, empty and dry it, and return it to its storage place.
16. Assist the resident to put on socks and shoes.
17. Remove the bed protector and discard according to facility policy.
18. Perform your procedure completion actions.

GUIDELINES FOR Applying Antiembolism Stockings

- The care plan will specify the wearing schedule for the stockings, according to physician orders and facility policies. For most residents, the hosiery is applied during the day and removed at bedtime. The care plan will specify when the stockings should be put on and removed.
- It is best to apply the stockings before the resident gets out of bed in the morning. Elevating the legs for 20 to 30 minutes

before applying the hosiery will reduce swelling and make stockings easier to apply.

- Antiembolism stockings come in several sizes. The resident is measured with a tape measure to find the correct size. The hose must fit well to be effective.
- To preserve the life of the stockings, avoid contact with lotions, ointments, or oils containing lanolin or petroleum products. These products deteriorate the elastic.
- Do not apply the hosiery over open areas, fractures, or deformities. If the resident has an open or abnormal skin area, fracture, or deformity on the legs or feet, inform the nurse.
- The stockings must be applied smoothly with no wrinkles.
- A light application of powder or cornstarch on the feet and legs will make the hosiery easier to apply.
- Placing a plastic sandwich bag over the foot allows the hosiery to slide on easily. After the hose are applied, remove the bag through the opening in the toe area.
- Check the stockings periodically to be sure the tops have not rolled or turned down. Keep the fabric straight.
- Most elastic stockings have a hole in the toe end to allow access for circulation checks. In some stockings, the hole is on the top of the foot, and in others it is on the bottom. As long as the heel is centered, the hole will be in the correct place.
- Monitor circulation in the resident's toes every four hours, or as specified on the care plan. Note color, sensation, swelling, temperature, and ability to move. Report abnormalities to the nurse.
- Follow your facility policy for washing antiembolism stockings. These must be hand-washed and drip-dried. The hose are damaged by the commercial washers and dryers used in the health care facility.

PROCEDURE 38 Applying Antiembolism Stockings

1. Perform your beginning procedure actions.
2. Obtain hosiery in the correct size.
3. Expose one leg.
4. Insert one hand into the stocking as far as the heel pocket. Holding the heel pocket, turn the stocking inside out.
5. Carefully position the stocking over the foot and heel.
6. Place the index and middle fingers of both hands into the stocking foot.
7. Face the resident and ease the stocking up over the foot, stretching sideways as you go. Center the heel pocket. An acceptable alternative is to face the foot, then pull the stocking up, similar to the manner in which you apply your own socks.
8. Continue pulling the stocking up over the ankle and calf, smoothing and stretching the elastic. The top of a knee-high stocking should be one to two inches below the knee. The top of a thigh-high stocking

(continues)

PROCEDURE

38 Applying Antiembolism Stockings, *continued*

should be one to three inches below the groin.

9. Check the fit to be sure the stocking is even and that there are no wrinkles. Pull up slightly on the toes to ensure that the stocking is not too tight (Figure 9.21).
10. Expose the other leg.
11. Repeat the procedure.
12. Perform your procedure completion actions.

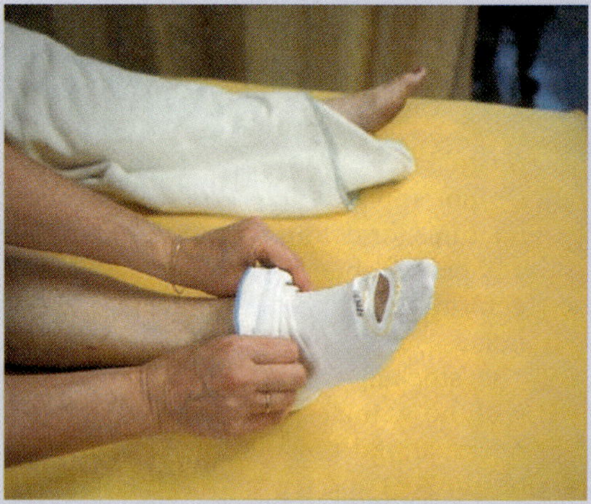

FIGURE 9-21 Roll the stocking up the leg and smooth any wrinkles.

Keeping the skin moisturized and well lubricated will reduce the risk of injury slightly, but some residents need additional protection. The care plan will specify measures to use, such as wearing long sleeves or keeping the arms and legs covered. Many residents use skin sleeves (Figure 9.22). The skin sleeve protects fragile skin. Some skin sleeves have additional padding. They are available in light and dark flesh tones to match the resident's skin color as closely as possible. The sleeve covers the hand and arm, leaving the fingers free. It may also be used as a restraint alternative, to prevent the resident from pulling out an IV or other medical device. To apply a skin sleeve:

- Grasp the sleeve near the upper arm opening.
- Roll and gather the sleeve until you reach the thumb opening.
- Slip the resident's hand into the sleeve, fitting the fingers into the large opening, and the thumb into the smaller opening for the hand.
- Unroll the sleeve up over the arm. Smooth the fabric so it is wrinkle-free.

The care plan will specify when the sleeve is to be worn. Monitor the resident's skin under the sleeve when it is removed. Report skin tears, bruises, or other injuries to the nurse. The skin sleeves should be hand-washed or machine-washed on a gentle cycle. Hang them to dry.

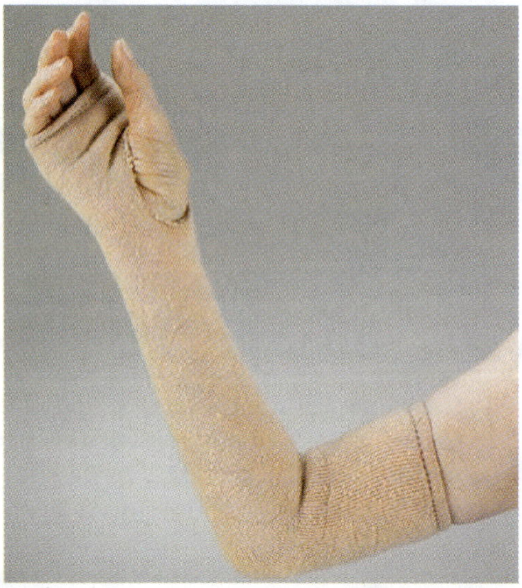

FIGURE 9-22 Skin sleeves offer excellent skin protection against skin tears and bruises. Leg protectors are also available. *(Courtesy of Skil-Care Corporation, Yonkers, NY (800) 431-2972)*

GUIDELINES FOR

Caring for a Resident Who Has a Prosthesis

- Always check the care plan for special instructions regarding applying, removing, and caring for the prosthesis.
- The prosthesis and the skin under the prosthesis must be kept clean and dry.
- Check the skin under the prosthesis. Notify the nurse of any redness, irritation, dark spots, open areas, or blisters.
- Follow the directions on the care plan for covering the extremity under the prosthesis. A **stump sock** is a garment used to protect the extremity from irritation caused by rubbing against the prosthesis and is usually worn under artificial limbs.
- For residents with lower extremity amputation, position the remaining joints in extension (as straight as possible). Residents with leg amputation are at risk for contracture development. Follow the positioning instructions on the care plan. Avoid elevating the stump on pillows.
- Report to the nurse if you feel that the prosthesis needs repair. Do not attempt to fix it yourself.
- An artificial eye is usually cared for by the nurse or resident. If you will be caring for residents with artificial eyes, make sure you are properly trained. Follow facility policy. Handle the eye carefully. The eye socket and the artificial eye must be cleaned as indicated on the care plan. Apply the principles of standard precautions when inserting, removing, and cleaning the eye.

GUIDELINES FOR

Dressing and undressing Residents

- Provide privacy and avoid exposing the resident.
- Wear gloves and apply the principles of standard precautions if you anticipate contact with blood, body fluids (except sweat), secretions, excretions, mucous membranes, or nonintact skin.
- Check the care plan for special instructions and use of adaptive equipment.
- Encourage the resident to do as much self-care as possible.
- Allow the resident a choice of clothing. The clothing should be appropriate for age and season, and color-coordinated. Follow your facility policy for having torn items replaced or repaired. Do not put torn clothing on a resident.
- If the resident has one paralyzed or weak side, remove the clothing from the strong side first. Put clothing on the weak side first. Always support the weak or paralyzed extremity.
- It is easier to dress residents who can assist if they are standing or sitting.
- It is easier to dress a dependent resident in bed.
- Residents who are dressed in street clothes should wear proper undergarments. Apply underwear and socks first.
- When dressing residents who use catheters or tubes, treat the tubes as part of the person's body. Avoid pulling on them or obstructing them. Do not disconnect them. Avoid elevating a urinary catheter above the level of the bladder during the dressing procedure. Consult the nurse for assistance.
- Gather the pant legs and sleeves before putting them on the resident.

Prosthesis Care

Some residents use a prosthesis to replace a body part. Many types of prostheses are used. A resident may have an artificial eye or breast. Others have artificial arms, hands, legs, or feet. The prosthesis helps the resident function as normally as possible. Remember, the prosthesis is part of the resident's body and should be treated with care. You will be responsible for keeping the prosthesis clean. This usually involves washing with mild soap, rinsing, and drying. Follow the instructions on the care plan or check with the nurse.

Dressing and Undressing the Resident

Most residents in the long-term care facility can be up and dressed each day. Self-esteem is improved when the resident is dressed and well-groomed. It also affects other people's perception about the resident's health. All people dress and undress several times a day. In the morning, we remove night clothing and dress in day wear. At bedtime, we remove clothing and put on night wear. Sometimes in health care, more frequent changes of clothing are necessary due to tests, procedures, medical treatments, and accidental soiling of clothes. Some residents cannot dress and undress themselves. Others may need limited assistance. Residents with paralysis have special dressing needs.

Procedure 39 Assisting the Resident with Dressing

1. Perform your beginning procedure actions.
2. Gather needed supplies: bath blanket, clothing, deodorant, and disposable gloves.
3. If the resident has a weak or paralyzed arm, work from the strong side.
4. Cover the resident with the bath blanket and remove the upper linens without exposing the resident.
5. For pants:
   a. Put one foot at a time into underwear. Slide them up over the feet and ankles.
   b. Gather the leg of the pants on the weak side. Slide the pant leg over the foot and ankle. Repeat with the strong leg.
   c. Slide the pants and underwear up the resident's legs.
   d. Ask the resident to raise the hips and buttocks while you pull underwear and pants into position.
   e. If the resident is unable to assist, roll him or her onto the strong side. Pull the underwear and pants up on the weak side (Figure 9.23). Turn the resident to the weak side and finish pulling the clothing up. Fasten at the waist, if necessary.

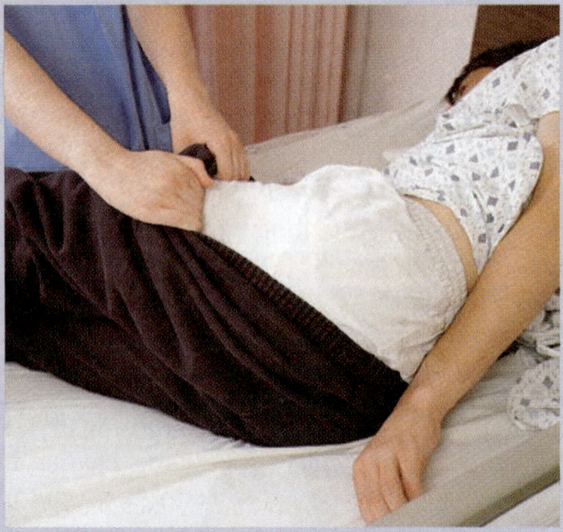

FIGURE 9-23 Pull the pants up on the weak side first.

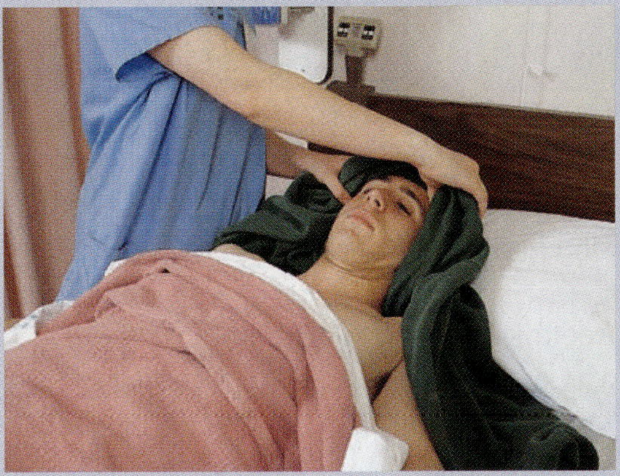

FIGURE 9-24 Stretch the neck and pull the garment over the resident's head.

6. Apply deodorant before putting on a shirt or sweater.
7. To put on garments that go over the arms or head:
   a. Stretch the garment neck as wide as possible and pull it over the resident's head (Figure 9.24).
   b. Put your hand into the sleeve of the garment on the resident's weaker side. Grasp the resident's weak hand. Slide the sleeve off your wrist and pull the resident's hand and wrist through the sleeve.
   c. Pull the sleeve up and adjust it at the shoulder.
   d. Lift the resident's arms and shoulders. Adjust the garment in the back.
   e. Ask the resident to put the strong arm into the other sleeve. If unable, repeat step 7b.
   f. Lift the resident's arms and shoulders, or roll the resident to the side. Pull down the garment and adjust it in back.
8. To put on a shirt or blouse that opens in front:
   a. Put your hand into the sleeve of the garment on the resident's weaker side. Roll the sleeve over your wrist. Grasp the resident's weak hand. Slide the sleeve off your wrist and over the resident's hand and wrist.
   b. Pull the garment up the arm and adjust it at the shoulder.
   c. Lift the resident's head and shoulders and pull the garment around the back. If you cannot lift the resident, roll him or her toward you and tuck the garment under him or her. Turn the resident away from you and pull the garment out. Then return the resident to the supine position.
   d. Ask the resident to put his or her strong arm into the other sleeve. If unable, repeat step 8a.
   e. Pull the garment up the arm and adjust it at the shoulder.
   f. Fasten the garment in the front.
9. Gather the sock back from the opening to just below the heel. Support the foot and slip the sock over the toes. Pull it up and over the heel. Straighten and smooth the top over the calf. Repeat with other sock. (You may find it easier to apply the socks first, when you apply the undergarments. This is an acceptable alternative.)
10. Loosen shoe laces and pull the tongue up in shoes. Slip the resident's foot into the shoe and adjust for comfort. Repeat with the other shoe. If possible, have the resident stand before adjusting laces and tying shoes. If the resident is unable to stand, tie the shoe immediately after putting it on.
11. Perform your procedure completion actions.
12. Reverse the procedure for undressing the resident. Remember to remove clothes from the strong side first.

KEY POINTS

- Good personal hygiene is essential to proper health.
- Activities of daily living are things people do every day to meet their health and hygiene needs.
- The nursing assistant assists residents to meet health and hygiene needs when they are unable to take care of these needs independently.
- Oral hygiene is the cleaning of the resident's mouth, teeth, gums, and tongue.
- Special oral hygiene is given frequently to residents who are unconscious, NPO, receiving tube feedings, or receiving oxygen.
- Dentures are artificial teeth that require special care and handling.
- Bathing is done to cleanse the skin, stimulate circulation, provide exercise, and refresh and relax the resident.
- Bath time is an excellent time to make observations of the resident's skin and body.
- Bath water temperature is checked with a thermometer. A comfortable temperature for bathing is 105 °F.
- When bathing residents, wash from clean to dirty areas.
- The bed bath is given to residents who are on complete bed rest. The resident's entire body is cleaned.
- The partial bath involves washing the resident's face, hands, underarms, back, and genital area.
- When giving perineal care to a female, wash from front to back. Avoid rubbing back and forth.
- When giving perineal care to a male, wash from the tip of the penis to the rectum.
- Massaging the resident's back is comforting, refreshing, and stimulating to circulation. Giving a back rub helps prevent skin breakdown.
- In most agencies, the nursing assistant does not cut fingernails and toenails.
- Antiembolism hose increase blood flow to the legs and prevent blood clots, edema, and other complications.
- A prosthesis is used to replace a missing body part.
- The resident's self-esteem is enhanced when he or she is dressed and well-groomed.

REVIEW

A. Multiple Choice

Select the one best answer.

1. Hygienic habits
   a. are easily changed.
   b. are not influenced by culture and religion.
   c. are a private matter for most people.
   d. are determined by the nursing assistant.

2. ADLs are
   a. all daily learning.
   b. activities of daily living.
   c. all done lovingly.
   d. activities during life.

3. Incontinence is
   a. loss of bowel or bladder control.
   b. difficulty breathing.
   c. inability to move or feel a body part.
   d. not a medical condition.

4. Always brush the resident's teeth with
   a. a stiff-bristle toothbrush.
   b. an abrasive cleanser.
   c. a soft-bristle toothbrush.
   d. the brush vertical to the teeth.

5. You are assigned to give Mr. Lee a partial bath. You know this means to wash the
   a. face, abdomen, legs, underarms, and feet.
   b. face, hands, underarms, back, and perineum.

c. face, arms, hands, perineum, and legs.
d. face, underarms, perineum, and feet.

6. When bathing residents, always wash

a. vigorously in a circular motion.
b. from the dirtiest area to the cleanest.
c. from clean to dirty.
d. the weakest side first.

7. The temperature of bath water should be

a. 85 °F.
b. 95 °F.
c. 105 °F.
d. 115 °F.

8. Which of the following is *not* true about wearing gloves during the bathing procedure?

a. Gloves are worn for the entire procedure.
b. Gloves are changed immediately before contact with nonintact skin.
c. Gloves are changed immediately before performing perineal care.
d. Gloves should be changed if they become heavily soiled.

9. When assisting the female resident with perineal care, wash

a. from back to front.
b. in a back-and-forth motion.
c. in a circular motion.
d. from front to back.

10. You are assigned to bathe Mrs. Lloyd. You notice that her toenails are long and dirty. You should

a. clean and cut the nails.
b. clean the nails and consult the nurse.
c. do nothing, as you are not allowed to care for nails.
d. clean the nails and file them with an emery board.

B. True/False

Answer each statement true (T) or false (F).

11. ________Massage stage I pressure sores well with lotion.

12. ________Shave a man's face using downward strokes.

13. ________Assist the resident to sit up in a chair before applying antiembolism stockings.

14. ________Always dress and undress the paralyzed arm first.

15. ________A prosthesis is an artificial body part.

16. ________HS care is given to prepare the resident for bed at night.

17. ________Always wear gloves when giving oral care.

18. ________It is not necessary to wear gloves when shaving residents with a disposable razor.

19. ________Always brush dentures while they are in the resident's mouth.

20. ________Wear gloves when washing the resident's eyes.

C. Clinical Applications

Answer the following questions.

21. You are assigned to give Mrs. Green a tub bath. After you transfer Mrs. Green into the bathtub, she tells you that she wants privacy and asks that you leave her alone in the tub. Your facility policy is that residents are not to be unattended in the bathtub. What should you do?

22. Mr. Hill is a mentally confused resident with very poor personal hygiene. He does not like to bathe. If his soiled clothes are not removed from the room when he goes to bed at night, he will put them on again the next morning. Today is Mr. Hill's shower day. He tells you he does not want to take a shower. What should you do?

23. Helen Spencer is at high risk of skin breakdown. She is frequently incontinent of bowel and bladder. Helen will not tell anyone when she is wet or soiled. Her skin becomes red and breaks down quickly. What can a CNA do?

24. Carmen Hernandez has arteriosclerotic heart disease. She has a history of blood clots. Carmen has very dry skin. She asks you to massage lotion on her legs to relieve the dryness. What actions should you take?

25. When you arrive on duty at 7 a.m., Mrs. Street is sitting up in the chair in her room. After breakfast, you give her a shower. After the shower, you are dressing the resident and discover that her feet and lower legs are very edematous. The care plan states that Mrs. Street must wear antiembolism stockings when she is out of bed. What should you do?

UNIT 10

Basic Nursing Skills

OBJECTIVES

After reading this unit, you will be able to:

- Spell and define key terms.
- Define vital signs and explain why accurate measurements are important.
- Identify abnormal vital signs.
- Demonstrate procedures related to measuring vital signs, height, and weight.
- Demonstrate procedure for measuring and recording intake and output.

OBSERVATIONS TO MAKE AND REPORT RELATED TO MEASURING VITAL SIGNS, HEIGHT, AND WEIGHT, INTAKE AND OUTPUT

Elevated or subnormal temperature
Pulse rate below 60 or above 100
Pulse irregular, weak, or bounding
Blood pressure below 100/60 or above 140/90
Unable to hear blood pressure or palpate pulse
Pain over center, left, or right chest
Chest pain that radiates to shoulder, neck, jaw, or arm
Shortness of breath, dyspnea, or any abnormal respirations
Headache, dizziness, weakness, paralysis, vomiting
Cold, blue, or gray appearance
Cold, blue, numb, painful feet or hands
Feeling faint or lightheaded, losing consciousness
Respiratory rate below 12 or above 20
Irregular respirations
Noisy, labored, respirations
Dyspnea
Shortness of breath
Gasping for breath
Cheyne-Stokes respirations
Wheezing
Coughing (dry or moist/productive)
Retractions
Blue color of lips or nail beds, mucous membranes
Change in weight of 5 or more pounds (increase or decrease) compared with previous month
Decreased urine output
Swelling of feet, ankles, hands, finger, face
Bleeding, vomiting, excessive perspiration

VITAL SIGNS

Vital signs are an indication of body function. Vital signs are measurements of **temperature**, **pulse**, **respiration**, and **blood pressure**. They are called vital signs because they are measurements of the most vital functions of the body. Temperature is a measurement of heat within the body. The pulse measures how fast the heart is beating. The pulse is checked by feeling the expansion and contraction of an artery with your fingertips. The blood pressure is a measurement of how hard the heart is working. This pressure is measured using the walls of the artery in the upper arm. Measuring respirations is an indication of how fast the person is breathing. Vital signs fall within certain normal ranges. Readings above or below these values may be symptoms of illness and disease. Measurement of vital signs provides an indication of whether a resident's condition is improving, worsening, or staying the same. The physician depends on these readings to order diagnostic tests and make changes in the treatment regimen. Accurate measurement of vital signs is an important responsibility.

Vital Signs in Pediatric Residents

Many long-term care facilities have infant and child residents. Policies and procedures for taking vital signs in these residents may be different than they are for the adult population. Temperature values are less stable in children. Normal values for vital signs are different as well. The values vary with the age of the child.

TEMPERATURE

Temperature indicates how much heat is in the body and is measured with an instrument called a **thermometer**. In some conditions, such as infection, the temperature will be elevated. In other conditions, the temperature will be low. These are important findings. The body attempts to regulate temperature on its own. If you feel hot, your body will sweat and you will feel thirsty. If you feel cold, you will shiver to stimulate circulation and increase your temperature. Diseases and medications affect temperature within the body. Many other factors can also affect the body temperature. Some changes in temperature require immediate attention from the nurse or physician.

Long-term care facilities use many different types of thermometers. Temperature is measured by different methods, depending on the needs of the resident. Your facility will teach you how to use its equipment, which recording scale to use, and how to document your findings.

The nursing assistant must use good judgment in deciding which method to use for taking the temperature. You must evaluate the resident's condition and other safety factors, and select the method that is safe for the resident and will give you the most accurate reading. Four methods are used to measure body temperature:

1. **Oral temperature** is taken by inserting a thermometer in the mouth under the tongue. This is the most common method.
2. **Rectal temperature** is taken by inserting the thermometer into the anus. This method is used for adults only when the temperature cannot be taken orally. In some facilities, this procedure is done only by licensed nurses. Know and follow your facility policies.
3. The **axillary temperature** is taken by placing the thermometer under the arm. An alternate site to use is the groin. This is the least accurate method and is used only when taking the temperature by other methods is not possible.
4. The **aural** or **tympanic temperature** is taken in the ear. This method is controversial. It is an accurate, safe method of taking temperature and is faster than other methods. However, variations in equipment and technique can affect the reading. Some facilities previously used this method, but have now eliminated it because the technique used may affect the accuracy of the reading.

Temperature Values

Health care facilities use different methods of recording temperatures. The **Fahrenheit scale** is the method used most commonly. In the Fahrenheit scale, the boiling point of water is 212 degrees. Writing an F after the temperature value indicates a Fahrenheit reading. Writing a C after the value indicates the **Celsius**, or **centigrade**, **scale**. In the Celsius scale, the boiling point is 100 degrees. In the United States, we commonly use figures in the Fahrenheit scale. The formulas used to convert temperature readings between the two scales are found in Table 10.1. Both scales are recorded in degrees. The symbol for degree is "°," so a properly recorded temperature would be written *98.6°F* or *37°C*.

The normal temperature range for adults is listed in Table 10.2. Memorize these values. If a resident's temperature falls outside the values, report to the nurse immediately.

TABLE 10-1 Formulas for converting Fahrenheit and Celsius temperature readings		
	Celsius (C)	**Fahrenheit (F)**
Conversion Formulas	F to C $C = \frac{5}{9}(F - 32)$	C to F $F = \frac{9}{5}C + 32$
For example: *To convert a Celsius temperature of 100 to Fahrenheit, follow the procedure:* $\frac{9}{5} \times 100 + 32 = \frac{900}{5} + 32 = 180 + 32 = 212°F$		
For example: *To convert a Fahrenheit temperature of 212 to Celsius, follow the procedure:* $\frac{5}{9} \times (212 - 32) = \frac{5}{9} \times 180 = 100°C$		

TABLE 10-2 Normal vital sign ranges for adults

Temperature	Normal	Range	Report Changes Above	Report Changes Below
Axillary temperature	97.6°F	96.6–98.6°F	99°F	96°F
Oral temperature	98.6°F	97.6–99.6°F	100°F	97°F
Rectal temperature	99.6°F	98.6–100.6°F	101°F	98°F
Pulse	76	60–100	100	60
Respiration	16	14–20	20	12
Blood pressure	120/80	100/60–140/90	140/90	100/60

Note: These values are guidelines only. Your instructor will inform you if facility reporting values are different in your area. Know and follow your facility reporting guidelines.

Reporting. It is important to report abnormally high or low temperatures to the nurse promptly. Elevated temperature usually occurs as a result of infection. Elderly individuals do not mount a strong immune response because of normal aging changes. Because of this, even a small elevation in temperature can indicate serious illness. Other common causes of temperature elevation are dehydration and hot environmental temperature.

Abnormally low body temperature (below 95°F) can also be very significant in the elderly. This condition is called **hypothermia**. Some elderly persons do not adjust well to environmental temperature changes and do not tolerate cold environments well. Many feel cold in room temperatures that are comfortable for younger persons. Hypothermia develops as a result of exposure to cold, ingestion of alcohol and some medications, sepsis, and shock. This can be extremely serious. In fact, abnormally low body temperature can cause death in elderly individuals. Signs and symptoms of hypothermia are not specific to this condition, so having an accurate temperature reading is very important. Symptoms worsen as temperature decreases. Once hypothermia is identified, special treatment is necessary to prevent further complications. Keeping residents warm and reporting abnormally low temperature values promptly is the best means of prevention.

Documentation. Facilities have different methods of recording temperatures. Some facilities list the method by which the temperature was taken in parentheses next to the reading. Writing the letter O indicates an oral reading. If recording in this manner is your facility policy, you would record the oral temperature value listed above as *98.6°F (O)*. The common abbreviations for vital signs, height, and weight are listed in Table 10.3.

Gloves. Facility policies vary greatly regarding whether gloves should be worn for measuring

TABLE 10-3 Abbreviations used in documentation of vital signs	
Abbreviation	**Vital Sign**
VS	Vital signs, vitals
TPR	Temperature, pulse, and respiration
BP or B/P	Blood pressure
(O) or (PO)	Oral temperature
(R)	Rectal temperature
(Ax) or (A)	Axillary temperature
No abbreviation, (AU), (A), or (T), depending on agency policy	Aural (tympanic) temperature
F	Fahrenheit
C	Celsius or Centigrade
°	Degrees
T	Temperature
P	Pulse
R	Respiration
Ht	Height
Wt	Weight
mm Hg	Millimeters of mercury

temperature. The principles of standard precautions should be followed at all times. Gloves are always worn when taking a rectal temperature with either glass or electronic thermometers. Many agencies require gloves for the oral temperature procedure with a glass thermometer because of the possibility of contacting saliva, which is a body fluid, and the mucous membranes in the mouth. Use of gloves with an oral electronic thermometer is usually not necessary. Standard precautions do not call for the use of gloves for contact with perspiration (sweat), so your agency may not require glove use for taking an axillary temperature. However, if you are using this method to take the temperature in the groin, gloves are worn. Wearing gloves when using a tympanic thermometer is not necessary. Know and follow your facility policy, but remember that there may be exceptions to the rule. Your facility may not require gloves for oral temperatures. However, if the resident has open lesions in or around the mouth or is drooling excessively, use good judgment and apply gloves. You are taught the principles of standard precautions so that you can apply them as needed in procedures to protect yourself. In health care, there are so many variables that the rules must be flexible. Using the one-glove technique is convenient for taking temperatures. If your ungloved hands accidentally contact a body fluid or mucous membrane during this, or any, procedure, wash them immediately.

Types of Thermometers

Three basic types of thermometers are used in long-term care facilities. The nursing assistant must be able to operate and read all three types. Although variations exist among thermometers and manufacturers, they all operate in basically the same way.

Glass Thermometers. Glass thermometers are thin, hollow tubes with a column of liquid inside that provides the temperature reading. Three types of glass thermometers are used: oral, security, and rectal. Figure 10.1 compares glass thermometers. As you can see, the sizes and shapes of the bulbs are different. Oral thermometers are marked with a blue or clear dot on the end. Rectal thermometers are marked with a red dot. Security thermometers are commonly used in health care facilities.

Facilities that use glass thermometers usually cover them with plastic, disposable **sheaths**

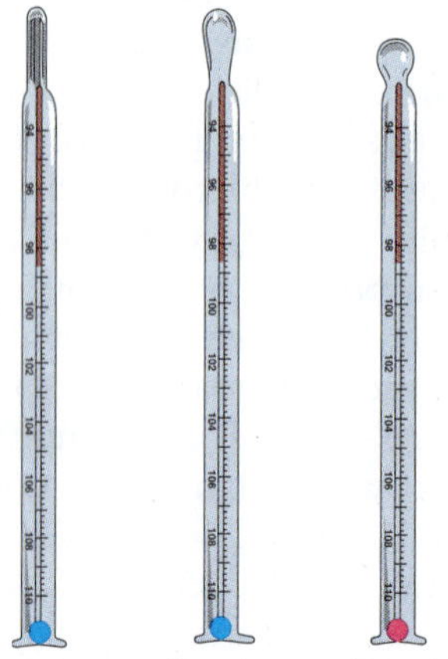

FIGURE 10-1 Clinical thermometers from left to right: oral, security, rectal.

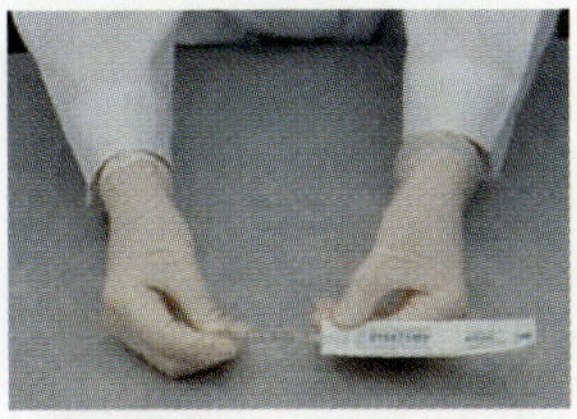

FIGURE 10-2 The disposable sheath is used for safety and infection control.

(Figure 10.2). Although glass thermometers are normally disinfected between each use, the sheath provides further protection against pathogens. It also protects the resident by containing the glass if the thermometer is accidentally cracked or broken.

Reading the Glass Thermometer. The glass thermometer is read by measuring the level of liquid on the inner column. The liquid rises and falls to indicate the temperature value. Most thermometers begin with 94°F. Each long line on the thermometer is one degree. Every other long line (or degree) is marked with a number. There are four short lines between each long line. Each short line indicates $\frac{2}{10}$ of a degree, or 0.2 degrees.

To read the thermometer, hold it at eye level. Rotate it gently between your thumb and index finger until you can clearly see the liquid column. Find the sharp edge where the liquid ends. Take the temperature reading at this point (Figure 10.3). When taking temperatures with a glass thermometer, the value is recorded as an even number. If the reading falls between the lines, use the higher number.

Mercury. Mercury thermometers have been used for many years. However, the recent trend in health care has been to avoid the use of products containing mercury, because they can be very toxic to humans and wildlife if broken. This is true even if mercury exposure occurs in very small amounts.

A mercury thermometer is a small glass tube containing liquid mercury, a silvery-white substance that registers body heat. Alternative products are being used in many glass thermometers because of mercury's potential for toxicity. Some thermometers contain a red or blue liquid. These are alcohol thermometers and contain no mercury. Another, less common thermometer contains galinstan, a substance that is similar to mercury in appearance. These thermometers are mercury-free, however, and are generally marked as such.

Mercury can be toxic in small amounts, particularly if it vaporizes and is inhaled. Even small mercury spills must be cleaned up properly to prevent contamination and illness. If you accidentally break a mercury thermometer or other device containing mercury, inform the nurse promptly. Follow facility policies and procedures for picking up mercury. If no procedures are available, apply gloves, face mask, and eye protection. Pick up broken glass and other debris and place in a puncture-resistant container. Use an index card to consolidate the mercury droplets, then seal them in a plastic bag or covered container. Small droplets can be picked up with adhesive tape or wet paper towels. Seal the container and affix a label identifying the material as "mercury spill debris." Consult the nurse for information regarding where to discard this material.

Electronic Thermometers. Many facilities use electronic thermometers (Figure 10.4). These thermometers are battery operated and stored in a charger when not in use. They are quick, easy to use, and accurate. Electronic thermometers usually have a plastic neck strap on the end. This is worn around your neck when taking temperatures or walking in the hallway. The unit is very sensitive and can be damaged if it is dropped or bumped. Wearing it around your neck frees your hands and helps avoid accidents. The electronic thermometer displays the temperature digitally

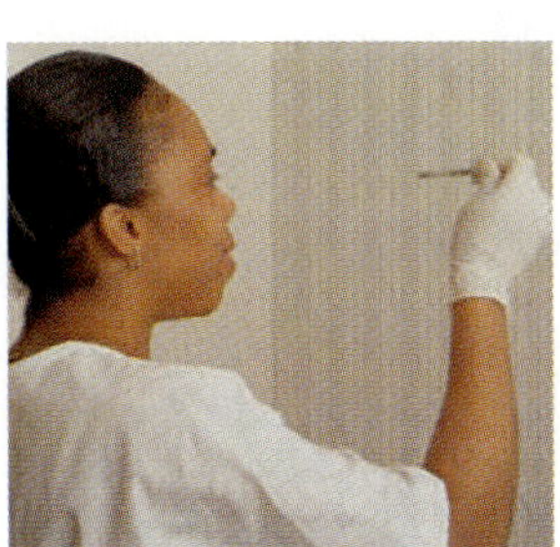

FIGURE 10-3 Hold the thermometer at eye level, then rotate it until you can read the column of liquid.

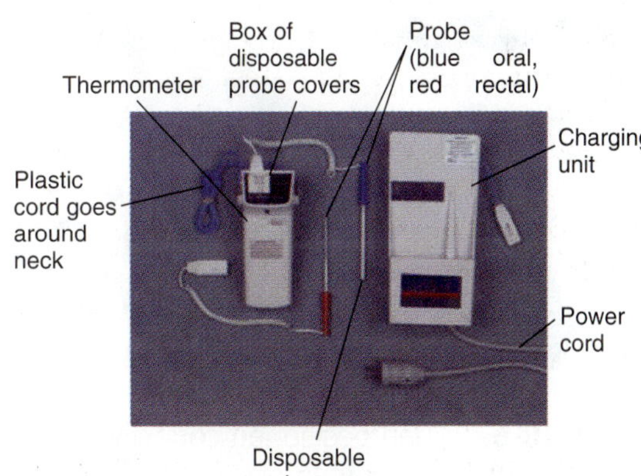

FIGURE 10-4 The electronic thermometer is fast and accurate.

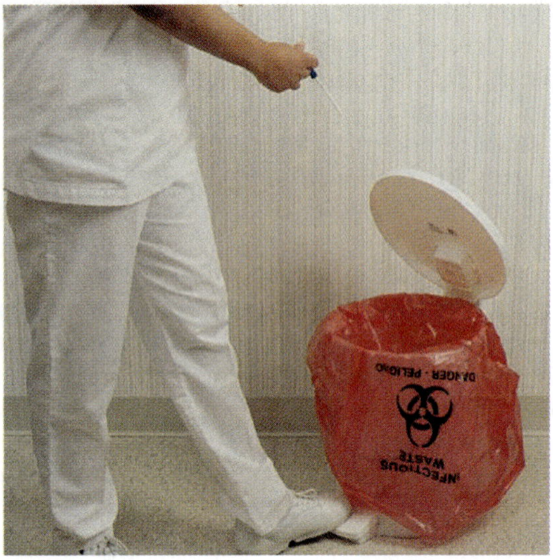

FIGURE 10-5 Dispose of the probe cover properly.

on a screen. The unit will beep or blink when the temperature reading is completed.

The electronic thermometer consists of a main thermometer unit. You will attach an oral or rectal **probe** to record the temperature. The oral probe is colored blue and the rectal probe is red. The probe is covered by a heavy plastic disposable **probe cover** that is used for one resident and then discarded (Figure 10.5). The unit can be used for many different residents by changing the probe cover.

Tympanic Membrane Thermometers. The **tympanic thermometer** (Figure 10.6) is a battery-operated unit. It is held in your hand and inserted into the resident's ear. The ear piece of the thermometer is covered with a protective sheath to prevent infection. The sheath is discarded after each use. The temperature reading is displayed digitally on the handset. Tympanic thermometers can be set to provide the equivalent of either an oral or a rectal reading. They can also be set for a Fahrenheit or Celsius value.

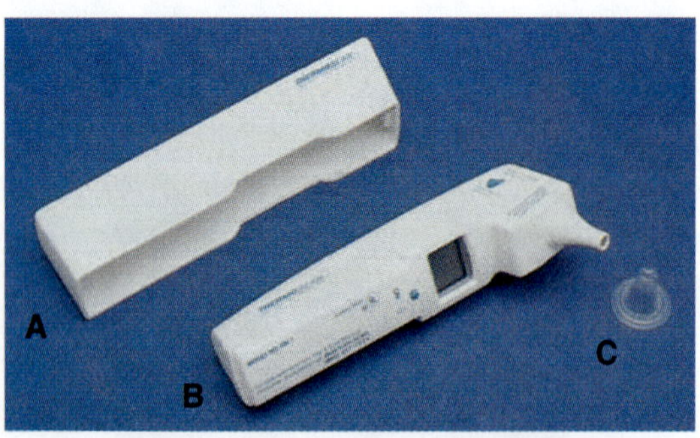

FIGURE 10-6 When positioned correctly, the tympanic thermometer is the fastest and most accurate method of taking the temperature. (A) Holder (B) Tympanic thermometer (C) Disposable speculum or cover

Other Types of Thermometers. Other types of thermometers are available, but they are not as widely used or as accurate as the instruments and methods listed earlier. Another type of thermometer is a paper or plastic, chemically treated, disposable unit (Figure 10.7). Dots on the thermometer are read to obtain the temperature value. This thermometer is used following the guidelines for taking an oral temperature with a glass thermometer. A disposable sheath is not necessary, because the thermometer is discarded after use. This thermometer is commonly used for residents who are in isolation. The disposable thermometer is made of rigid plastic. Remove the thermometer from the resident's mouth *slowly*. Pulling the thermometer out rapidly from between closed lips can cause painful tears of the lips and mucous membranes in the mouth. Small, handheld, battery-operated thermometers are also available (Figure 10.8). These are covered with plastic sheaths. The guidelines for taking the temperature with this thermometer are the same as those for using an electronic thermometer. Follow facility policies for disinfecting the thermometer between residents.

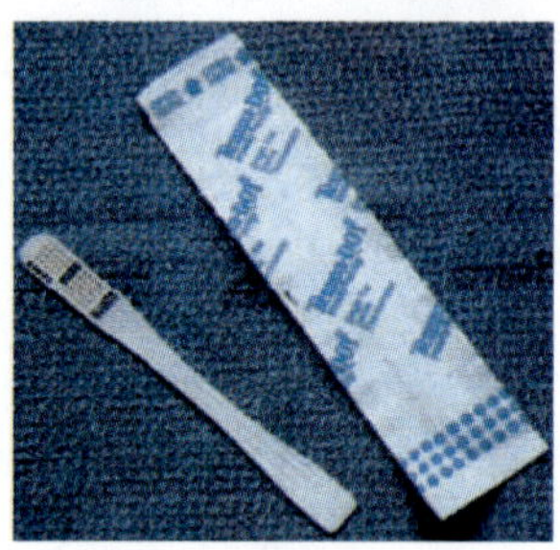

FIGURE 10-7 The chemical-dot thermometer is used only for oral temperatures. It is used once, then discarded.

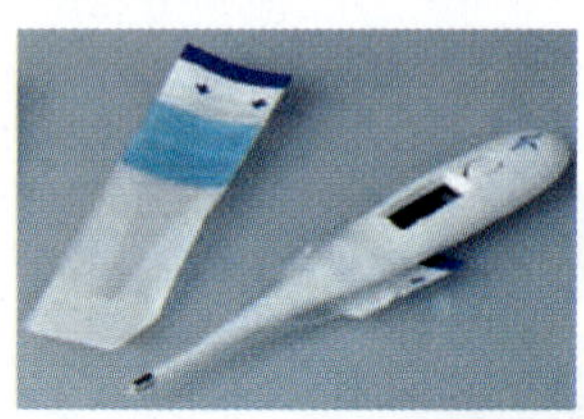

FIGURE 10-8 The battery-operated digital thermometer is commonly used in long-term care facilities. Always cover the thermometer with a disposable probe cover before use. (*Courtesy of Medline Industries, Inc. 1-800-MEDLINE*)

GUIDELINES FOR

Measuring Temperature

- Apply the principles of standard precautions.
- Check glass thermometers for chips and cracks.
- Make sure electronic thermometers are fully charged and that you have the correct probe for the type of temperature you are taking.
- If a glass thermometer is accidentally broken, follow your facility policy for cleaning and disposing of it. Mercury is poisonous and glass must be discarded in a puncture-resistant container. Wear gloves.
- When using a glass thermometer, shake the liquid down below 96°F before inserting the thermometer. Stand away from the resident or surfaces you might hit when shaking the thermometer.
- Use a probe cover or disposable sheath, depending on the type of thermometer you are using.
- Use a clean probe cover for each resident.
- Lubricate the rectal thermometer before inserting it.
- Hold the oral electronic thermometer probe in place, as the probe is heavy and the resident may not be able to hold it between the lips.
- When using the tympanic thermometer, make sure it is securely inside the ear canal. If it is not placed correctly, the reading will not be accurate.
- Hold a rectal thermometer in place with your gloved hand. Hold an axillary thermometer in place (use your judgment and apply the principles of standard precautions as to use of gloves).
- Leave the glass thermometer in place for the length of time specified by your facility for the type of temperature you are taking.
- Follow your facility policy for cleaning, disinfecting, and storing glass thermometers.
- A glass thermometer is used for one resident only, then is disinfected. This is true even if a plastic thermometer sheath was used. Electronic thermometers with probe covers may be used for more than one resident if the cover is changed.
- Use cold water to clean glass thermometers. Hot water may cause breakage.
- The containers used for clean and soiled glass thermometers must be disinfected regularly. Your facility will have policies and procedures for cleaning them.

Oral Temperature

Oral temperature is taken by placing the thermometer in the resident's mouth. If the resident has recently had something to eat or drink, this may affect the temperature reading. Temperature is also affected by smoking. If the resident has had something to eat, drink, or smoke, instruct the resident not to have anything further, and return in 15 minutes to check the temperature.

Oral temperatures are usually taken in alert, cooperative adults. Oral temperatures should not be taken in residents who are:

- Mentally confused
- Uncooperative
- Combative
- Chilled or shivering
- Coughing or sneezing
- Unconscious
- Restless
- Receiving heat or cold treatments about the neck or face
- Mouth-breathing or cannot keep the mouth closed around the thermometer
- Short of breath or having difficulty breathing
- Unable to breathe through the nose
- Receiving oxygen by mask
- On seizure precautions
- Recovering from surgery on or an injury to the nose or mouth
- Using a nasogastric tube
- Under the age of six

If you are in doubt, check with the nurse. The oral thermometer is left in place for a minimum of three minutes.

Oxygen. Each facility has policies and procedures for taking an oral temperature when the resident is using oxygen. In general, if the resident is using oxygen by mask, you should avoid

PROCEDURE 40 Measuring an Oral Temperature with a Glass Thermometer

Note: The guidelines and sequence for this procedure vary slightly from state to state, and from one facility to another. Your instructor will inform you if the sequence in your state or facility differs from the procedure listed here. Know and follow the required sequence for your state and facility.

1. Perform your beginning procedure actions.
2. Gather supplies needed: glass thermometer, disposable plastic sheath, notepad and pen, gloves, container for used thermometers.
3. Rinse the disinfectant off the thermometer and dry it.
4. Shake the thermometer down to 96°F.
5. Cover the thermometer with a plastic sheath.
6. Apply gloves.
7. Place the bulb under the resident's tongue and instruct the resident to close his or her lips.
8. Leave the thermometer in place for three minutes, or according to facility policy.
9. Remove the thermometer.
10. Discard the sheath according to facility policy.
11. Hold the thermometer at eye level and read the liquid column. Note the reading.
12. Shake the thermometer down to 96°F.
13. Place the thermometer in the container for used thermometers or disinfect it according to facility policy.
14. Remove gloves and discard them according to facility policy. Wash your hands.
15. Record the reading.
16. Perform your procedure completion actions.

PROCEDURE 41 Measuring an Oral Temperature with an Electronic Thermometer

1. Perform your beginning procedure actions.
2. Gather supplies needed: electronic thermometer, oral probe, plastic probe cover, notepad and pen.
3. Insert the probe into the probe cover.
4. Place the tip of the probe under the resident's tongue and instruct the resident to close his or her lips.
5. Hold the end of the probe in place.
6. When the alarm sounds, note the reading and remove the probe.
7. Dispose of the probe cover according to facility policy.
8. Insert the probe into the side of the thermometer.
9. Record the reading.
10. Perform your procedure completion actions.

taking an oral temperature. If the resident uses oxygen through a nasal cannula, the temperature reading may be slightly (approximately 0.3 degrees) lower because of the oxygen. Consult the nurse if you are unsure of how to take the temperature of a resident who is using oxygen.

Rectal Temperature

Rectal temperature is commonly taken when oral methods cannot be used. It is also routinely used for taking the temperature of children below the age of six. The rectal temperature registers one degree higher than the oral value. If the oral temperature is 98.6°F, the rectal temperature in the same resident would be 99.6°F.

Times when a rectal temperature *should not* be taken are:

- If the resident is having diarrhea
- If the resident has constipation or fecal impaction
- If the resident has had a colostomy
- If the resident is combative
- If the resident has rectal bleeding, hemorrhoids, or some other rectal condition, or has had rectal surgery
- If the resident has recently had prostate surgery
- If the resident has severe heart disease or has recently had a heart attack

PROCEDURE 42 Measuring a Rectal Temperature with a Glass Thermometer

Note: The guidelines and sequence for this procedure vary slightly from state to state, and from one facility to another. Your instructor will inform you if the sequence in your state or facility differs from the procedure listed here. Know and follow the required sequence for your state or facility.

Note: In some states, nursing assistants are not permitted to perform this procedure. Additionally, the policies of some facilities state that only licensed nurses may perform rectal treatments, including taking temperatures. Perform this procedure only if you are permitted to do so by state law and facility policies.

1. Perform your beginning procedure actions.
2. Gather supplies needed: glass (rectal) thermometer, disposable plastic sheath, lubricant, notepad and pen, gloves, container for used thermometers.
3. Rinse the disinfectant off the thermometer, and dry it.
4. Shake the thermometer down to 96°F.
5. Cover the thermometer with a plastic sheath.
6. Position the resident in the Sims' position.
7. Apply gloves.
8. Place a small amount of lubricant on a tissue or paper towel. Use the tissue to lubricate the bulb of the thermometer (Figure 10.9). Some plastic sheaths are prelubricated.

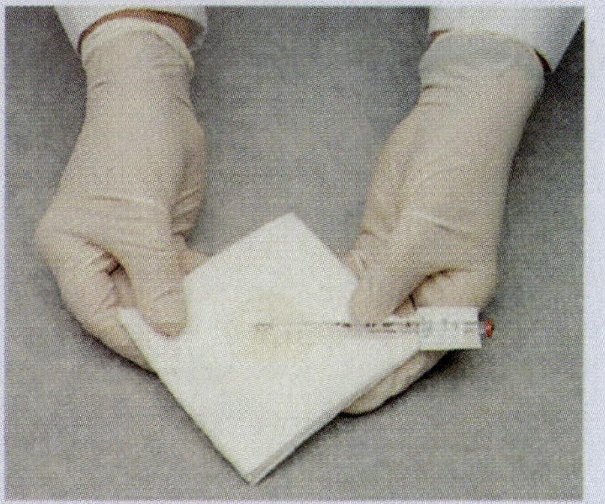

FIGURE 10-9 Lubricate the rectal thermometer well.

(continues)

PROCEDURE 42

Measuring a Rectal Temperature with a Glass Thermometer, *Continued*

9. Separate the buttocks with one hand.
10. Insert the bulb into the rectum one inch (Figure 10.10).

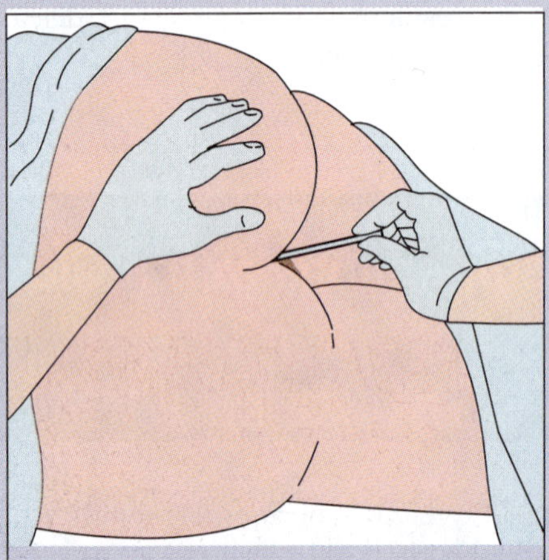

FIGURE 10-10 Spread the buttocks, then gently insert the lubricated thermometer one inch into the rectum.

11. Hold the thermometer in place for three minutes, or according to facility policy.
12. Remove the thermometer.
13. Discard the sheath according to facility policy.
14. Hold the thermometer at eye level and read the liquid column. Note the reading.
15. Place the thermometer in a container for used thermometers or disinfect it according to facility policy.
16. Remove gloves and discard them according to facility policy. Wash your hands.
17. Record the temperature reading.
18. Perform your procedure completion actions.

PROCEDURE 43

Measuring a Rectal Temperature with an Electronic Thermometer

Note: The guidelines and sequence for this procedure vary slightly from state to state, and from one facility to another. Your instructor will inform you if the sequence in your state or facility differs from the procedure listed here. Know and follow the required sequence for your state or facility.

Note: In some states, nursing assistants are not permitted to perform this procedure. Additionally, the policies of some facilities state that only licensed nurses may perform rectal treatments, including taking temperatures. Perform this procedure only if you are permitted to do so by state law and facility policies.

1. Perform your beginning procedure actions.
2. Gather supplies needed: electronic thermometer, rectal probe, plastic probe cover, lubricant, notepad and pen, gloves.
3. Position the resident in the Sims' position.

4. Apply gloves.
5. Place a small amount of lubricant on a tissue or paper towel. Use the tissue to lubricate the bulb of the thermometer.
6. Separate the buttocks with one hand.
7. Insert the probe into the probe cover. Lubricate the end.
8. Insert the tip of the probe cover into the rectum one inch, or according to manufacturers' directions. (Some manufacturers recommend inserting it 1/4 to 1/2 inch.)
9. Hold the probe in place until the alarm sounds.
10. Note the reading and remove the probe.
11. Discard the probe cover according to facility policy.
12. Insert the probe into the side of the thermometer.
13. Wipe excess lubricant from the anal area.
14. Remove gloves and discard according to facility policy. Wash your hands.
15. Record the reading.
16. Perform your procedure completion actions.

PROCEDURE 44 Measuring an Axillary Temperature with a Glass Thermometer

Note: The guidelines and sequence for this procedure vary slightly from state to state, and from one facility to another. Your instructor will inform you if the sequence in your state or facility differs from the procedure listed here. Know and follow the required sequence for your state and facility.

1. Perform your beginning procedure actions.
2. Gather supplies needed: glass thermometer, disposable plastic sheath, towel, notepad and pen, gloves, container for used thermometers.
3. Rinse the disinfectant off the thermometer, and dry it.
4. Shake the thermometer down to 96°F.
5. Cover the thermometer with a plastic sheath.
6. Apply gloves, if this is your facility policy.
7. Dry the axilla with the towel.
8. Insert the thermometer into the center of the axilla, then lower the resident's arm and bend it across the abdomen. Hold the thermometer in place, if this is your facility policy.
9. Leave the thermometer in place for 10 full minutes.
10. Remove the thermometer.
11. Discard the sheath according to facility policy.
12. Hold the thermometer at eye level and read the liquid column. Note the reading.
13. Remove gloves, if worn, and discard them according to facility policy. Wash your hands.
14. Record the reading.
15. Place the thermometer in a container for used thermometers or disinfect it according to facility policy.
16. Perform your procedure completion actions.

Gloves are always worn when taking a rectal temperature. The thermometer is lubricated before insertion. The glass thermometer must be held in place for three full minutes, or according to facility policy.

Axillary Temperature

Axillary temperatures are not taken as commonly as oral and rectal temperatures because they are not as accurate. They are used only when the temperature cannot be obtained by other methods. The axilla must be dry. An oral thermometer is used. The thermometer is placed in the center of the armpit and must remain in place for 10 full minutes. The axillary value is normally one degree less than the oral reading. If the oral temperature in a resident is 98.6°F, the axillary temperature in the same resident would be 97.6°F.

Tympanic Membrane Temperature

The temperature inside the ear is the most accurate temperature in the body. It is often preferred by health care workers because it is quick and convenient. The temperature reading is taken by holding the thermometer next to the tympanic membrane, which is close to the core of the body. It takes one to three seconds to obtain a tympanic temperature. The end of the thermometer is covered with a plastic sheath or cover before it is inserted into the ear.

The tympanic, or aural, thermometer is inserted into the ear by gently lifting the top of the outer ear up and back. This straightens the ear canal. Insert the end of the thermometer as far as it will go. For the temperature to be accurate, the detector at the end of the thermometer must be flat against the tympanic membrane. The reading will not be accurate if it is tipped to the side. The thermometer is held in place until the display flashes. The thermometer is removed and the protective cover discarded.

The tympanic temperature is the fastest and most convenient method, but it can also provide inaccurate readings if the user's technique is not precise. To ensure an accurate reading, insert the probe tip into the ear as far as it will go. Next, rotate the probe handle until it is aligned with the jaw, as though it were a telephone handset. Quickly press the "scan" button. Using this method will help ensure accurate temperature readings.

PROCEDURE 45 Measuring an Axillary Temperature with an Electronic Thermometer

Note: The guidelines and sequence for this procedure vary slightly from state to state, and from one facility to another. Your instructor will inform you if the sequence in your state or facility differs from the procedure listed here. Know and follow the required sequence for your state and facility.

1. Perform your beginning procedure actions.
2. Gather supplies needed: electronic thermometer, oral probe, plastic probe cover, notepad and pen, gloves.
3. Insert the oral probe into the probe cover.
4. Apply gloves, if this is your facility policy.
5. Dry the axilla with the towel.
6. Insert the probe into the center of the axilla, then lower the resident's arm and bend it across the abdomen. Hold the probe in place, if this is your facility policy.
7. When the alarm sounds, remove the probe. Note the reading.
8. Dispose of the probe cover according to facility policy.
9. Insert the probe into the side of the thermometer.
10. Remove gloves, if worn, and discard them according to facility policy. Wash your hands.
11. Record the reading.
12. Perform your procedure completion actions.

GUIDELINES FOR

Using a Tympanic (Ear) Thermometer

- Make sure the thermometer lens is clean and there is no dirt or debris on the lens at the end of the probe tip.
- Use each probe cover only once. Make sure the cover is on snugly, without ripples.
- Store the thermometer out of the path of cold air flow. If the thermometer is in a cold area, allow it to warm up before use, or it may read low.
- Make sure the resident is not directly in the path of cold air or being fanned. This action cools the ears, which can cause a low temperature reading.
- The tympanic thermometer can be set to oral, core, or rectal mode. In most cases, oral is appropriate. The mode will be shown in the readout screen. If the screen says "CAL," the thermometer is in the unadjusted mode, which is used only for calibration and other bench work.
- If the resident is lying on one side, use the opposite ear to take the temperature. If this is not possible, turn the resident's head so the ear is uncovered. Wait several minutes before taking the temperature.
- Remove hearing aids from the resident's ears. Wait several minutes before taking the temperature. (Lying on the ear or having a hearing aid retains heat in the ear canal. Repositioning the resident or removing the hearing aid is similar to taking the lid off a pan on the stove to allow heat to escape).
- Insert the probe tip into the ear as far as possible, then rotate the handle to the correct position, in alignment with the jaw. This step is very important for ensuring an accurate temperature reading.

Ear thermometers are similar to cameras. They provide the temperature of what you point them at. If the thermometer is not used correctly, you will get an inaccurate reading. Common causes of inaccurate tympanic temperatures are:

- Pressing the scan button before the probe is fully inserted
- Using a probe cover more than once
- Using a thermometer without a probe cover
- Improper cleaning of the thermometer lens
- Not following manufacturer's instructions for placing the probe tip into the ear; following instructions for the thermometer you are using is important
- Using a thermometer with a broken or missing lens (the shiny disk at the end of the probe tip through which the infrared energy must pass to be processed)

PROCEDURE 46

Measuring a Tympanic Temperature

1. Perform your beginning procedure actions.
2. Gather supplies needed: tympanic thermometer, probe cover, gloves if needed.
3. Check the lens of the thermometer to make sure it is clean.
4. Cover the thermometer lens with a clean probe cover.
5. Select the appropriate mode on the thermometer.
6. Gently pull the outer ear up and back to straighten the ear canal (Figure 10.11).

(continues)

PROCEDURE 46

Measuring a Tympanic Temperature, *Continued*

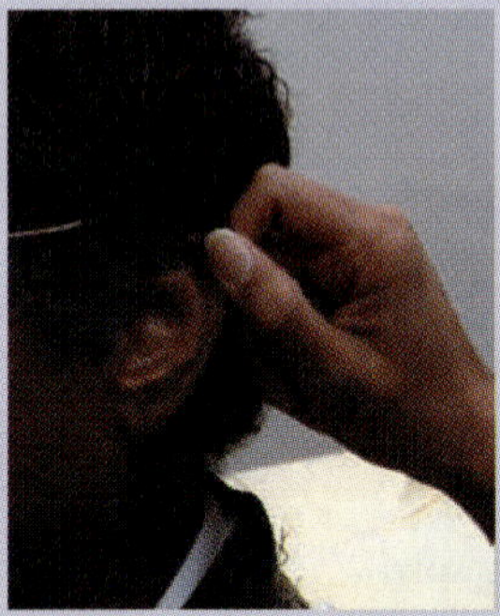

FIGURE 10-11 Gently pull the pinna up to straighten the ear canal.

7. Insert the thermometer, aiming it toward the tympanic membrane (ear drum). Insert until the tip seals in the ear canal. Rotate the probe handle slightly until it is aligned with the jaw, as though speaking on the telephone (Figure 10.12).
8. Press the activation (scan) button. Hold the thermometer in place until the display flashes or the thermometer indicates that you have a reading.
9. Remove the thermometer and discard the probe cover according to facility policy.
10. Document the reading.
11. Perform your procedure completion actions.

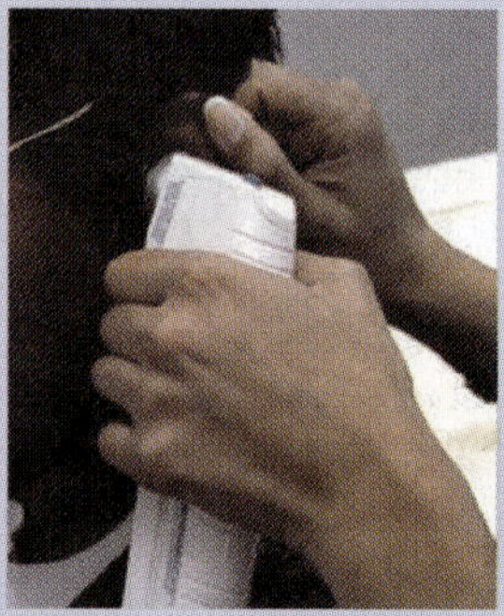

FIGURE 10-12 Insert the thermometer until it seals in the ear canal, then rotate it until it is positioned like a telephone receiver.

Pulse

The pulse is a measurement of how fast the heart is beating. Each time the heart beats, the arteries in the body expand and contract, forcing blood through the system. The pulse is taken in locations where arteries can be easily compressed against the bones underneath, called **pulse points.** Figure 10.13 shows common pulse points. The **radial pulse** at the wrist is used by most health care workers for counting the pulse. The pulse can also be heard by placing a **stethoscope** directly over the heart. The stethoscope is an instrument used to listen to sounds in the body. The **apical pulse** in the heart is usually taken by the licensed nurse or advanced care provider.

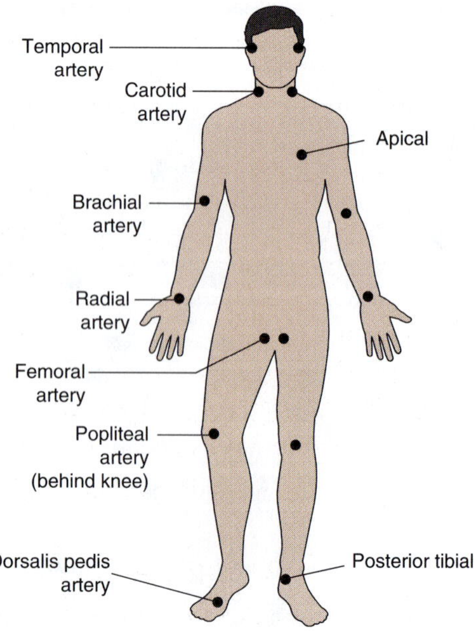

FIGURE 10-13 Pulse locations

Observations of the Pulse

Counting the pulse reveals things about the condition of the heart and circulatory system. When we "take the pulse," we are doing more than counting the number of beats per minute. We are also gathering other information that is important in treating the resident's condition. Some electronic blood pressure devices count the pulse and display the rate. Feeling the pulse is still necessary, however, to make other important observations.

Pulse Rate. We count the number of beats in the pulse to determine how fast the heart is beating. The number of beats per minute is called the **pulse rate**. The normal pulse rate in an adult is between approximately 60 and 100 beats per minute. Pulse rates outside this range may indicate a problem and should be reported to the nurse immediately. Pulse rates lower than 60 beats per minute are called **bradycardia**. Pulse rates above 100 beats per minute are called **tachycardia**.

Pulse Rhythm and Force. The **rhythm** of the pulse is an indication of how regularly the heart is beating. The rhythm should always be regular. Pulse beats should repeat at approximately the same time interval. Beats should not be missed, skipped, or come early in the cycle. If you observe that the pulse is irregular, count it for one full minute and report your findings to the nurse immediately for assessment.

The **force** of the pulse is the strength of the beat. The pulse beat is normally strong and full. If the pulse is weak and hard to feel, this may indicate a problem that should be reported to the nurse. Pulses that feel thready or bounding (full) should also be reported promptly.

Counting the Pulse

The radial pulse is located on the thumb side of the wrist (Figure 10.14). It is easily accessible and commonly used to take vital signs. To count the

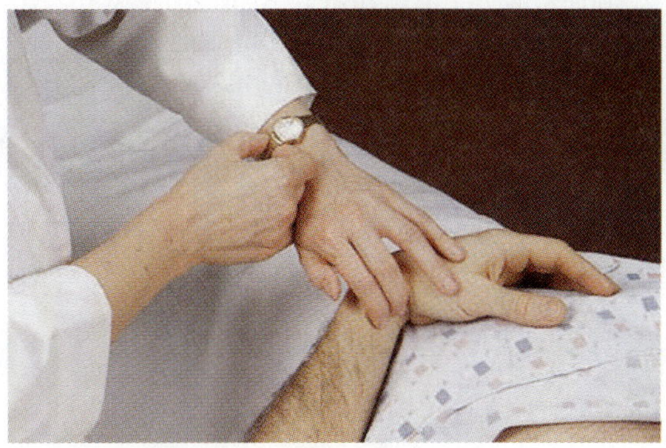

FIGURE 10-14 The radial pulse is on the thumb side of the wrist.

PROCEDURE 47 Taking the Radial Pulse

Note: The guidelines and reportable values for this procedure vary slightly from state to state, and from one facility to another. Your instructor will inform you if the guidelines or reportable values in your state or facility differ from those listed here. Know and follow the required guidelines for your state and facility.

1. Perform your beginning procedure actions.
2. Gather needed supplies: watch with second hand, notepad and pen.
3. Support the resident's arm on a secure surface.
4. Locate the radial pulse and place the first three fingers of your hand on it. Position your thumb on the other side of the wrist to keep it from moving.
5. Look at your watch and begin counting.
6. Count the number of pulse beats for 30 seconds.
7. Multiply the number of beats in 30 seconds by two. Record this figure.
8. If you are taking respirations, you will leave your fingers on the pulse. If you are also counting the respirations, do not stop to record the pulse rate. Remember the number and document it when you are finished.
9. If you are not counting the respirations, perform your procedure completion actions.

PROCEDURE 48 Counting Respirations

Note: The guidelines and reportable values for this procedure vary slightly from state to state, and from one facility to another. Your instructor will inform you if the guidelines or reportable values in your state or facility differ from those listed here. Know and follow the required guidelines for your state and facility.

1. Perform your beginning procedure actions.
2. Count the resident's pulse and remember the number.
3. After you have counted the pulse, glance at the chest, while continuing to look at your watch.
4. Count one inhalation and one exhalation as one respiration.
5. Count the number of respirations in 30 seconds and multiply this number by two.
6. Record the resident's pulse and respirations on your note pad.
7. Perform your procedure completion actions.

radial pulse, gently put the first three fingers of your hand on top of the pulse. Avoid pressing too hard or you will obliterate the pulse. Never count the pulse beat with your thumb, which has a pulse of its own. With the second hand of your watch, count the beat for 30 seconds. If the pulse is strong and regular, stop after 30 seconds. Multiply the number of beats counted in 30 seconds by two to obtain the pulse rate for one minute. The pulse rate documented on the medical record is always recorded in number of beats per minute. If the pulse is weak, irregular, very slow, or very rapid, or if counting for a full minute is your facility policy, count for one full minute and do not multiply the number. Report the abnormality to the nurse.

RESPIRATIONS

Respiration is the act of breathing. **Inhalation**, or **inspiration**, is the act of taking air in. **Exhalation**, or **expiration**, is the act of breathing air out. One respiration is counted as one inhalation and one exhalation. Normal adult respirations are smooth, regular, and unlabored. The normal respiratory rate in adults is about 14 to 20 per minute. If you observe a resident with a respiratory rate under 12 or over 20, report this information to the nurse.

Respiratory Distress

Difficulty breathing, or **dyspnea**, means labored respirations. **Cheyne-Stokes respirations** are seen in critically ill and dying residents. They are irregular and are followed by periods of **apnea**, or no respirations, before the resident starts breathing again. If you observe abnormal or difficult respirations, notify the nurse immediately.

Because respiration involves bringing fresh oxygen into the body, the skin of a Caucasian resident who is breathing normally is pink. A dark bluish or purplish discoloration of the skin and mucous membranes is called **cyanosis**. This condition is caused by inadequate oxygen in the blood. If the skin or nail beds appear cyanotic (blue, gray, or dusky in appearance), the resident is having a serious problem with the intake and use of oxygen. In dark-skinned residents, problems with oxygenation are noted by looking at the nail beds, lips, and mucous membranes inside the mouth. If the color is abnormal, notify the nurse immediately.

Counting Respirations

Respiration is under voluntary control. The resident should not be aware that you are counting the respirations. Placing the resident's arm across the chest or abdomen when counting the pulse is helpful. After you have counted the pulse for

GUIDELINES FOR

Using a Stethoscope

- Clean the ear pieces and diaphragm of the stethoscope before using it.
- Clean the stethoscope tubing if it contacts the resident or bed linen.
- Check the ear pieces of the stethoscope for wax, and remove it if present.
- Check the stethoscope tubing. Do not use if it has cracks or holes in it.
- The ear pieces of the stethoscope should face forward.
- The diaphragm of the stethoscope should not come in contact with the resident's clothing, blood pressure cuff, or other device.
- Place the diaphragm of the stethoscope flat against the resident's skin and hold it in place. If the diaphragm is at an angle, you will not be able to hear the sounds.
- Apply firm but gentle pressure when holding the diaphragm in place. If you press too hard, you may be unable to hear the sound.

30 seconds, glance at the resident's chest to count respirations. Continue looking at your watch while you count. Remember, one respiration consists of one inhalation and one exhalation. If you are unable to see the resident breathing, count how many times the abdomen rises and falls.

When counting respirations, you may count for 30 seconds and multiply this number by two. Like the pulse, the respiratory rate recorded is for one full minute. If the respirations are slow, labored, irregular, or unusual, count them for one full minute and report this information.

Using a Stethoscope

A stethoscope is a medical instrument used to listen to sounds inside the body. It intensifies sounds so they can be heard clearly. The parts of the stethoscope are seen in Figure 10.15. Many health care workers use stethoscopes on many residents. This creates the potential for infection to be passed to both workers and residents. Before and after using the stethoscope, wipe the ear pieces and diaphragm with an alcohol sponge or other disinfectant. If the tubing of the stethoscope contacts the resident or bed linen, wipe the tubing as well.

You will use the stethoscope to take blood pressures. Your health care facility may teach you other procedures with the stethoscope, including taking an apical pulse.

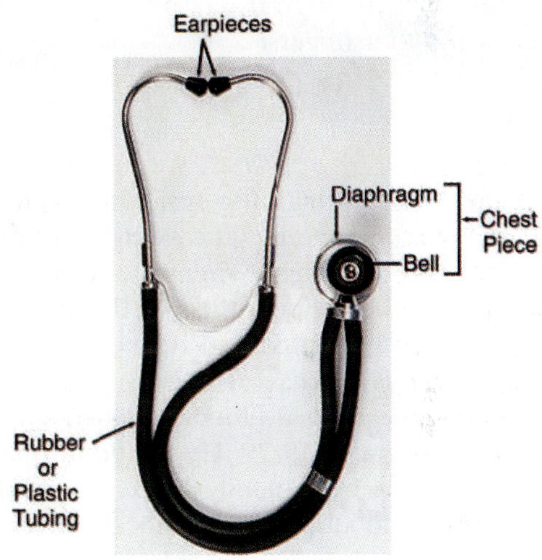

FIGURE 10-15 The stethoscope is used to listen to sounds inside the body.

Blood Pressure

The blood pressure is a measurement of how the heart is working. It measures the force of the blood on the inside of the arteries. The **systolic blood pressure** is a sound you hear during the working phase of the heart cycle. The systolic sound is the first sound heard when the heart contracts and forces blood through the body. The **diastolic blood pressure** is the sound you hear when the heart is resting. This sound is heard when the heart relaxes and refills with blood. Blood pressure is often called the fourth vital sign. If the nurse instructs you to obtain the

PROCEDURE 49

Using the Stethoscope

1. Perform your beginning procedure actions.
2. Gather needed equipment: stethoscope, alcohol sponges, notepad and pen, watch with second hand.
3. Wipe the ear pieces and diaphragm of the stethoscope with the alcohol sponge.
4. If the diaphragm is cold to touch, rub it against your clothing to warm it.
5. Feel the pulse you will be listening to with your fingers.
6. Place the ear pieces of the stethoscope in your ears.
7. Place the diaphragm of the stethoscope over the pulse.
8. Listen to the sound and count if necessary.
9. Remove the stethoscope from your ears and record your findings.
10. Wipe the ear pieces and diaphragm of the stethoscope with the alcohol sponge.
11. Perform your procedure completion actions.

vital signs, you will take the resident's TPR and blood pressure. Sometimes the doctor will order blood pressure readings when the resident is both sitting and standing. Most of the time, the resident should be seated and relaxed when the blood pressure is taken.

In adults, the normal blood pressure range is between 100/60 and 119/79. **Hypertension** is the medical term for high blood pressure, or values over 140/90. Blood pressure values above this value should be reported to the nurse. **Prehypertension** is a blood pressure reading between 120/80 mmHg and 139/89 mmHg. Having this condition means you are likely to develop high blood pressure in the future. People with prehypertension should take steps to decrease their risk. **Hypotension** is the medical term for low blood pressure, or values below 100/60.

Blood pressure classifications are listed in Table 10.4. When systolic and diastolic blood

TABLE 10-4 National Heart, Lung, and Blood Institute blood pressure definitions 2003

	Blood Pressure Level (mmHg)		
Category	**Systolic**	*	**Diastolic**
Normal	< 120	and	< 80
Prehypertension	120–139	or	< 80
High Blood Pressure			
Stage I Hypertension	140–159	or	90–99
Stage II Hypertension	≥ 160	or	≥ 100

Legend:
< means less than
≥ means greater than or equal to
Source: National Heart, Lung, and Blood Institute, National Institutes of Health 2003.
For additional information, see http://www.nhlbi.nih.gov/hbp/index.html.

pressures fall into different categories, the higher category is used to classify blood pressure level. For example, 172/78 mmHg would be stage 2 hypertension (high blood pressure).

Measuring Blood Pressure

Blood pressure is measured with an instrument called a **sphygmomanometer**. Several different types of sphygmomanometers are used in long-term care facilities (Figure 10.16). The technique for measuring blood pressure is the same with most of the units. Many blood pressure units use an **aneroid gauge**. This is a spring-loaded dial marked with numbers to display the reading. The mercury blood pressure cuff also has numbers marked on it. With this unit, the blood pressure is measured by reading the level of a column of mercury. A mercury unit must be placed on a flat surface and read at eye level for readings to be accurate. Some facilities use electronic units. However, no truly satisfactory alternative has been found for mercury in blood pressure devices, so these are still in use in health care facilities. Use mercury devices carefully to avoid breakage.

The fabric blood pressure cuff is wrapped around the resident's upper arm about one inch above the brachial artery. After the cuff is wrapped around the arm, a stethoscope is placed over the **brachial artery** in front of the elbow to obtain the reading.

Reading the Blood Pressure Gauge. The gauge on the sphygmomanometer is marked with

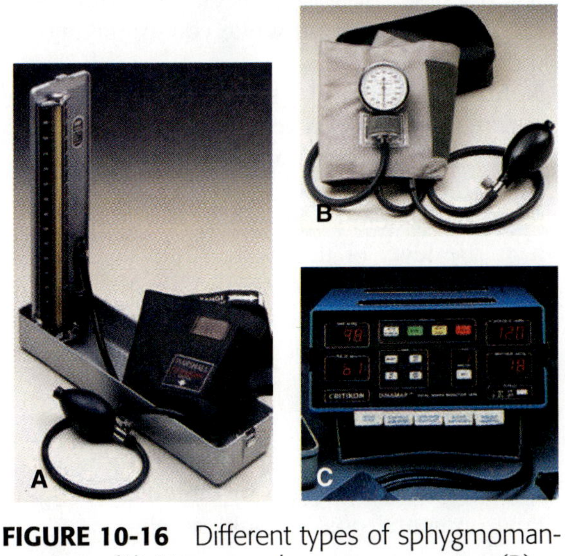

FIGURE 10-16 Different types of sphygmomanometers. (A) Mercury sphygmomanometer (B) Dial (aneroid) sphygmomanometer (C) Electronic sphygmomanometer

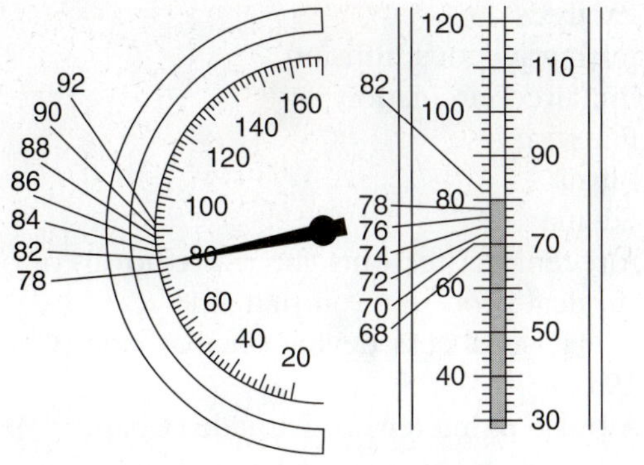

FIGURE 10-17 Read the pressure at the closest line. The pressure on both these gauges is 80.

a series of lines. A number is marked on the gauge in increments of 10 or 20, depending on the unit you are using. If the gauge is marked in increments of 20, a long line appears in the center of each 20 units. The long line represents a value of 10. Each short line on the gauge represents a value of 2. Figure 10.17 demonstrates how to read the gauge on both an aneroid and a mercury blood pressure unit. The number on the gauge is 80 for both units. If the dial or mercury was one small line above 80, the reading would be 82. If the dial or mercury was one small line below 80, the value would be 78. Blood pressure is always recorded in even numbers.

When measuring blood pressure, you use your vision and hearing. You inflate the cuff, then release it slowly, so the gauge falls in increments of 2 mmHg. The stethoscope is placed over the brachial artery and you listen for a sound while simultaneously looking at the gauge. The first sound you hear is the systolic value. The last sound you hear is the diastolic value. The difference between the two numbers is called the **pulse pressure**. In healthy adults, the difference is about 40 mmHg. The normal range is between 30 and 50 mmHg. For example, if the systolic pressure is 118 and the systolic pressure is 78, 118 minus 78 equals 40. The pulse pressure in this case is 40.

Accuracy of Blood Pressure. The blood pressure value is a very important measurement that the physician uses to measure the resident's progress and determine treatment. It is important that blood pressure values be accurate. Blood pressure should not be measured in an arm with a **shunt**. A shunt is a surgically implanted passage between two blood vessels. It is used for **dialysis**, which is a process of removing waste products from the blood for residents with kidney disease.

Do not take a blood pressure on an arm with:

- Paralysis
- An intravenous infusion
- Impaired circulation
- Fracture
- Burns
- Edema
- A recent mastectomy (breast removal) or other surgical procedure on that side
- A dialysis access device on that side (Chapter 19)
- A pulse oximeter on that side (Chapter 19)

Causes of inaccurate blood pressure readings include:

- Use of the wrong size cuff
- An improperly wrapped cuff
- Incorrect arm position
- Not using the same arm for all readings
- Not viewing the gauge at eye level
- Deflating the cuff too rapidly or too slowly
- Being distracted by noise in the room, such as the resident talking, a radio, or a television
- Rapidly inflating and deflating the cuff several times in a row

Ask the resident not to talk, which makes it difficult for you to hear, and may change the reading. The temperature in the room should be comfortable. Changes in temperature may alter the reading.

GUIDELINES FOR

Taking Blood Pressure

Blood Pressure Cuff

- Be sure the cuff is the correct size to fit the resident.
- Check the screw valve to be sure it opens and closes easily.
- Close the valve and pump the cuff. Make sure the gauge rises.
- Place the center of the bladder in the cuff over the brachial artery, or use the arrows on the cuff to guide you.

Aneroid Sphygmomanometer

- Check the placement of the needle on the gauge. It should be exactly at zero. The needle is very delicate and will change position if the gauge is bumped or dropped. If the needle is not on zero, the reading will not be accurate.
- Place the gauge flat against the cuff where you can see it.

Mercury Sphygmomanometer

- Check to be sure you can see the mercury in the glass tube.
- Make sure the glass tube is not cloudy.
- Check the mercury level. It should be at zero.
- Place the unit on a flat surface where you can read it at eye level.
- When you inflate the cuff, the mercury should rise readily. If it is slow to respond, this indicates a problem with the unit, and the reading may not be accurate.

Resident

- Have the resident sit and relax.
- Some facilities prefer to measure the blood pressure in the left arm, if possible, because it is closest to the heart.
- Remove the resident's blouse or shirt, or pull up the sleeve. Do not roll up the sleeve so tightly that it constricts the arm, which will alter the reading. *The cuff must be wrapped around the bare skin.*
- Ask the resident not to talk and to turn the radio or television off while you are taking the blood pressure.
- Notify the nurse if the resident was in pain or uncomfortable when the reading was taken. Pain, anxiety, and discomfort may affect the reading.
- Flex the resident's arm slightly and support it at the level of the heart while you are taking the blood pressure. If the arm is not supported, or is above or below heart level, the accuracy of the reading will be affected.

The Environment

- The temperature should be comfortable.
- Environmental noise should be eliminated when ever possible.

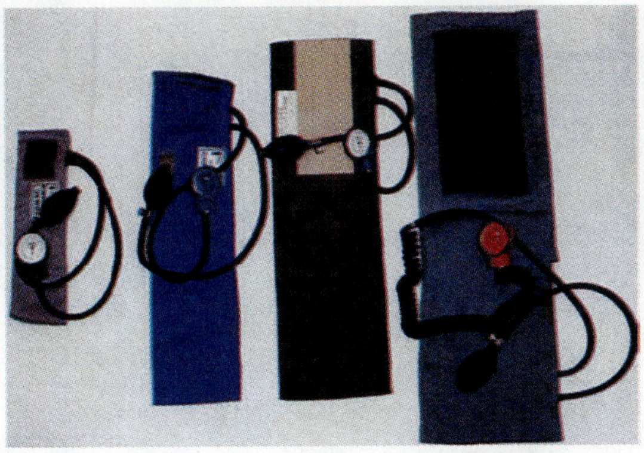

FIGURE 10-18 Select a cuff that fits the resident's arm.

The technique you use for measuring the blood pressure affects the accuracy of the reading. The cuff must fit the resident correctly. Cuffs come in many different sizes (Figure 10.18). Although there is a standard size adult cuff, some residents require an extra-large cuff. Very small residents require a pediatric cuff. If the cuff is too large or small, the reading will be incorrect. To check the size of the cuff, compare the length of the rubber bladder (Figure 10.19) with the resident's arm circumference. The bladder should be at least 80% of the circumference of the arm. If it is larger or smaller, obtain a different size cuff.

Wrap the cuff snugly around the resident's arm. If it is too loose or too tight, the reading will be affected. Most cuffs have arrows marked on the fabric near the tubing. The arrows and markings show you where to place the cuff in relation to the brachial artery. When reading the value on the blood pressure gauge, be sure the gauge is flat and not tipped. Always read the gauge at eye level.

Documenting Blood Pressure. Blood pressure is recorded in millimeters of mercury. The abbreviation for this is *mmHg*. Blood pressure is recorded in fraction form. Because the systolic sound is the first sound you hear, it is the first number recorded. The diastolic reading is the second number recorded. An example of how to record the blood pressure is 118/78. The systolic value is 118. The diastolic value is 78.

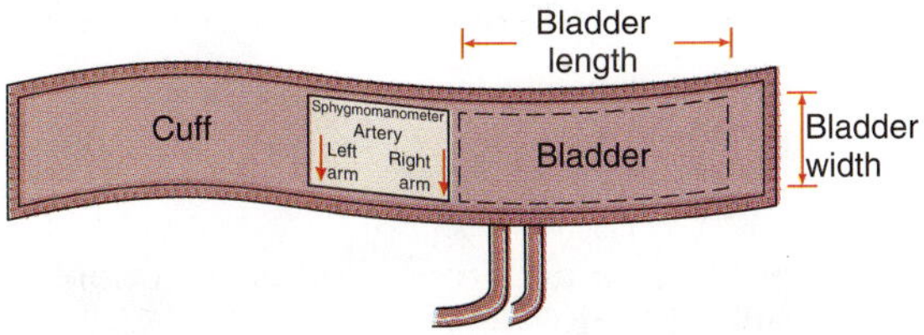

FIGURE 10-19 For an accurate reading, the bladder inside the cuff should be 80% the circumference of the resident's arm.

Facility policies vary as to the order in which to record vital signs. For example, some facilities require you to record the blood pressure first. In these facilities, the vital signs would be recorded in this order:

- blood pressure
- temperature
- pulse
- respirations

In this facility, the vital signs would be recorded as *120/80-98.6°F(O)-88-16*. Some facilities document the blood pressure last. Know and follow your facility policy.

MEASURING AND RECORDING HEIGHT AND WEIGHT

Measuring the resident's height and weight is often the responsibility of the nursing assistant. Many members of the interdisciplinary team need to know the resident's height and weight to perform their assessments and plan care. The dietitian uses the information to plan the diet. The physician uses the information to calculate doses of medications. Most facilities measure the height and weight of residents upon admission, then weigh residents monthly thereafter. This gives the team members baseline information to compare with. Residents who have heart and kidney disease may be weighed daily to monitor for rapid weight gain, which indicates a fluid balance problem. Residents who are under-weight are usually weighed weekly.

Weight loss can be a serious problem in the elderly. Weight loss is a risk factor for skin breakdown and other conditions. Progressive, unplanned weight loss may be a symptom of a more serious problem. Aggressive measures are taken when unplanned weight loss is detected. Accurate measurement and recording of weight is an important responsibility that you must take very seriously. The physician is notified of unplanned weight loss, and steps are taken to prevent additional loss. Know and follow your facility policies for reporting weight loss or gains.

Methods of Weighing Residents

Many different scales are available. Some are mechanical balance scales. Others are electronically operated. Most of the balance scales must be leveled or balanced before they are used, to assure an accurate reading. Check your facility

PROCEDURE

50 Measuring the Blood Pressure

Note: This is the "two-step" procedure recommended by the American Heart Association (AHA) as of 1993. The AHA considers the two-step procedure the most reliable for normal blood pressure measurement. (The most accurate values are obtained by internal monitoring, in which a catheter is placed in an artery. The internal method is not practical for most clinical situations.) In some states, nursing assistants use a one-step procedure for measuring blood pressure. In some facilities, electronic blood pressure monitoring equipment is used.

Note: The guidelines and reportable values for this procedure vary slightly from state to state, and from one facility to another. Your instructor will inform you if the guidelines or reportable values in your state or facility differ from those listed here. Know and follow the required guidelines for your state and facility.

1. Perform your beginning procedure actions.
2. Gather supplies needed: sphygmomanometer, stethoscope, alcohol sponges, notepad and pen.
3. Wipe the ear pieces and diaphragm of the stethoscope with the alcohol sponge.
4. Locate the brachial artery on the thumb side of the inner upper arm.
5. Wrap the cuff around the arm, centering the arrow over the brachial artery. The cuff should be one inch above the artery in the **antecubital space**, in front of the elbow.
6. Locate the radial pulse on the thumb side of the wrist. Keep your fingers on it.
7. Close the screw on the hand set and inflate the bulb until you can no longer feel the radial pulse. Mentally add 30 to the number on the gauge.
8. Open the screw and deflate the cuff.
9. Wait 30 seconds.
10. Place the stethoscope in your ears. Place the diaphragm of the stethoscope over the brachial artery. (You will not hear a sound until you inflate the cuff and open the valve.)
11. Close the screw and rapidly and steadily inflate the cuff to 30 points higher than where the radial pulse was last palpated.
12. Slowly release the screw so the pressure in the cuff falls at 2 mmHg increments.
13. Listen for a sound. When you hear it, note the closest number on the gauge. This is the systolic pressure.
14. Continue to listen until the sound stops. Note the closest number on the gauge. This is the diastolic pressure. Continue to listen for 10 mmHg below this sound.
15. Open the screw completely and deflate the cuff.
16. Remove the stethoscope from your ears.
17. Remove the cuff from the resident's arm.
18. Record your findings.
19. If you are unsure of the blood pressure, wait one to two minutes, then check it again.
20. Wipe the ear pieces and diaphragm of the stethoscope with the alcohol sponge.
21. Perform your procedure completion actions.

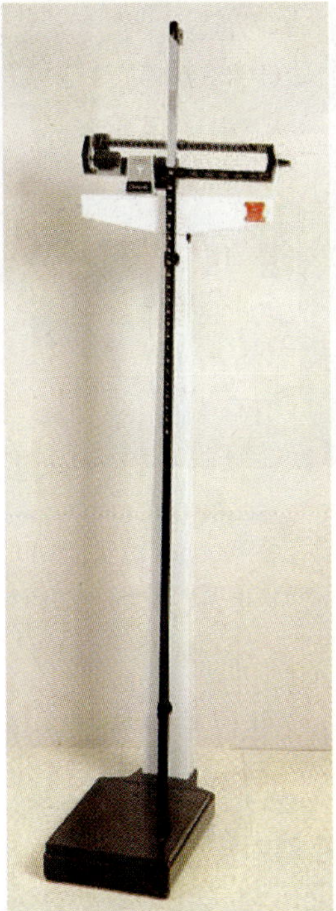

FIGURE 10-20 The balance scale is used for ambulatory residents who can stand unassisted.

policy and learn how to balance the type of scale you are using.

Standing Balance Scale. The standing balance scale (Figure 10.20) is commonly used if residents are able to stand and balance unassisted. Shoes are usually removed and the resident stands on a paper towel.

To weigh a resident on the balance scale, you must understand how to calculate the weight by adding the reading on the two bars. The lower bar is marked with lines every 50 pounds. The upper bar has single pound readings. Even numbers are marked on the bar every 2 pounds. Each long line indicates an odd-numbered pound. Each short line on the upper bar is 1/4 of a pound. You will adjust the weights on each balance bar until the rod hangs free on the end. To obtain the total weight, add the number of pounds on each bar (Figure 10.21).

Chair Scale. The chair scale has a chair permanently attached to it. The resident is transferred to the chair to be weighed. Some chair scales use a balancing mechanism, similar to the standing balance scale. Others read the weight electronically and display a digital readout on a screen.

Wheelchair Scale. When using the wheelchair scale (Figure 10.22) three steps are required to obtain an accurate weight. First, the wheelchair is weighed empty. The weight of the chair is recorded. The resident is transferred to the chair and weighed. The weight is recorded. The empty weight of the chair is subtracted from the total weight. This figure gives you the resident's weight. Most wheelchair scales are balance scales. Some facilities have removable ramps that are placed over the standing balance scale so it can be used for wheelchairs. Some wheelchair scales are electronically operated.

If the resident uses a lap tray on the wheelchair, remove the tray before weighing the resident. If the tray cannot be removed, weigh the tray and the wheelchair together during the first step of the procedure, then subtract the combined weight from the total. Lap trays can add as much as five pounds to the total weight.

Bed Scale. There are several types of bed scales. The electronic bed scale has a sling attached. The resident is placed in the sling, which is suspended from the bed. Both the resident and the sling must be lifted completely off the surface of the bed for the weight to be

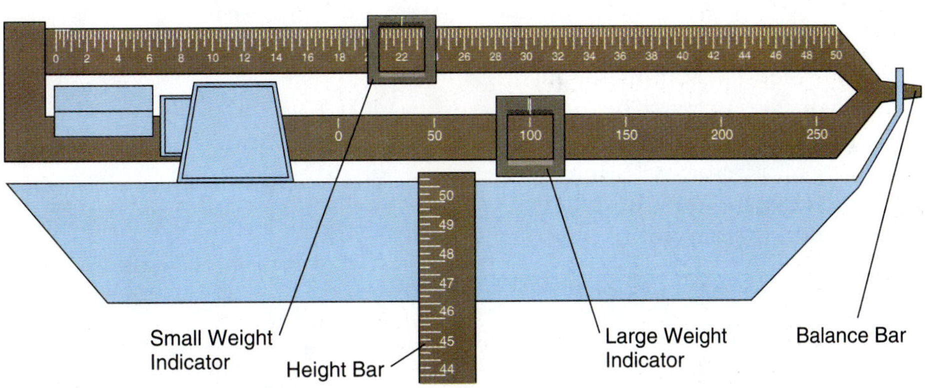

FIGURE 10-21 Add the number of pounds on the upper bar to the weight on the lower bar to obtain the resident's total weight.

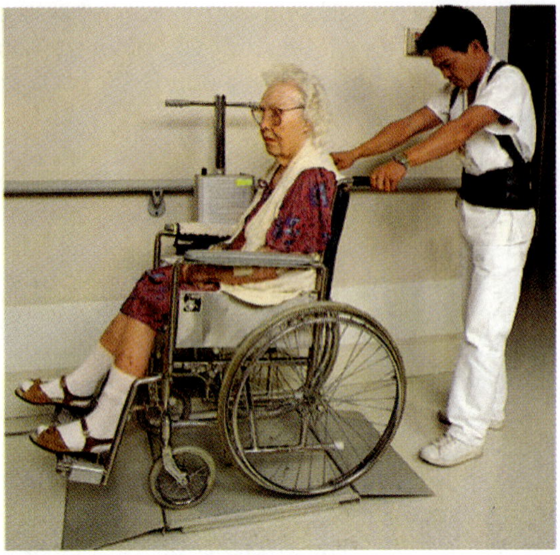

FIGURE 10-22 This wheelchair scale uses a ramp over the balance scale. The wheelchair weight is subtracted from the total weight.

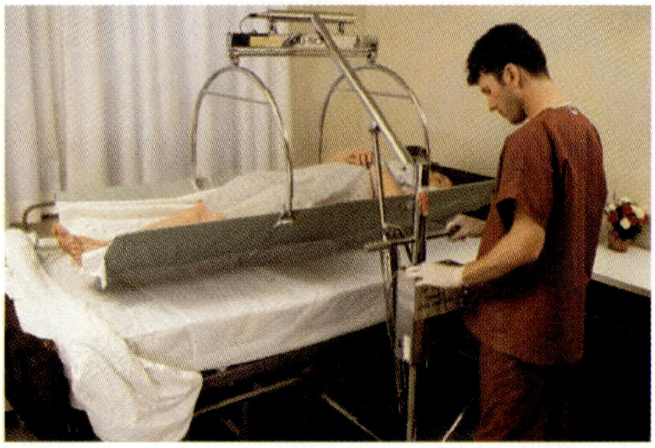

FIGURE 10-23 The bed scale is used for nonambulatory residents who cannot sit in a chair. Make sure the sling is not touching the bed when you take the weight reading.

accurate. After the resident is suspended above the bed, the scale electronically records the weight.

Another type of bed scale is attached to the mechanical lifting device. The resident is transferred to the mechanical lift and the lift is elevated until the resident is above the surface of the bed. This type of scale usually has a detachable dial, balance mechanism, or electronic gauge to record the weight. A similar electronic bed scale (Figure 10.23) uses a canvas sling for residents who must remain supine.

Methods of Measuring Height

Knowing the resident's height is important for determining if the resident is within the ideal weight range. The height is usually taken on admission. It is not checked again because it does not change. You must learn several methods of measuring the resident's height.

Height may be measured in either centimeters or inches, depending on your facility policy. One inch equals 2.5 centimeters. If your facility uses a centimeter measurement, multiply the number of inches by 2.5.

PROCEDURE 51

Measuring Weight and Height

Note: These procedures are generic and apply principles used for common types of scales. Follow the instructions for the specific scale you are using. The operating instructions are slightly different for each. Your instructor will inform you if the directions for the equipment you are using differ from those listed here.

1. Perform your beginning procedure actions.
2. Gather supplies needed: scale, paper towels, notepad and pen.
3. Standing scale
   a. Balance the scale.
   b. Place a paper towel on the scale platform.
   c. Assist the resident to remove shoes and stand on the platform.
   d. Adjust the weights on the scale until the bar hangs freely on the end.
   e. Add the weight on the two bars to determine the weight. Write this down on your notepad or remember it.

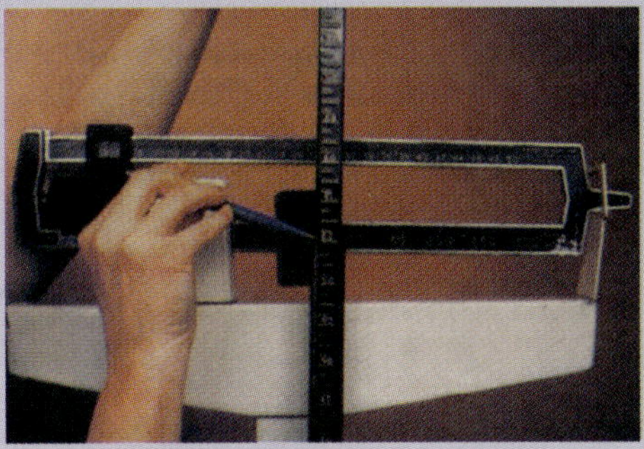

FIGURE 10-24 Read the height at the movable part of the ruler bar.

f. Assist the resident to turn around, facing away from the scale.

g. Raise the height bar until it is level with the top of the head.

h. Record the measurement in the center of the height bar (Figure 10.24).

i. Help the resident down from the scale and assist him or her to put on shoes, if necessary.

j. Remove and discard the paper towel.

4. Chair scale

a. Balance the scale.

b. Assist the resident to transfer from the wheelchair to the chair scale.

c. Place the resident's feet on the footrest of the chair.

d. Move the weights until the balance bar hangs freely, or read the electronic display screen. Remember this number or write it down on your notepad.

e. Transfer the resident back to the wheelchair.

5. Wheelchair scale

a. Balance the scale.

b. Obtain a wheelchair and take it to the scale and weigh it. Write down the weight.

c. Take the wheelchair to the resident's room and assist the resident to transfer into it.

d. Take the resident to the scale. Roll the wheelchair up the ramp and lock the brakes.

e. Adjust the weights until the balance bar hangs freely on the end. Write down this number on your notepad.

f. Unlock the brakes and slowly guide the wheelchair down the ramp.

g. Return to the resident's room and assist the resident to transfer out of the wheelchair.

h. Subtract the weight of the empty wheelchair from the total weight of the resident and chair and record this number.

6. Bed scale

a. Balance the scale. The scale should be balanced with the canvas seat, chains, or straps attached.

b. Remove the sling from the scale and position the resident on the sling.

c. Connect the straps and elevate the lift above the level of the bed. Raise the sling so the resident's body and the sling hang freely over the bed.

d. Adjust the weights until the balance bar hangs freely on the end, or read the electronic display screen. Remember this number or write it on your notepad.

e. Lower the resident back into the bed and remove the sling.

7. Perform your procedure completion actions.

GUIDELINES FOR

Weight and Height Measurements

- Weigh residents at the same time of day.
- Use the same scale each time.
- Balance the scale before weighing the resident.
- Have the resident wear similar clothing each time he or she is weighed.
- Have the resident empty the bladder before being weighed.
- If the resident is wearing an incontinent brief, make sure it is dry before weighing.
- If the resident has an indwelling catheter, make sure the bag is empty before weighing.
- If the resident has a cast, has recently had a cast removed, or has new-onset edema, consult the nurse about possible weight discrepancies.
- If you are taking a standing weight and height on a balance scale, have the resident remove his or her shoes and stand on a paper towel.
- If you are responsible for documenting the weight on the resident's chart, compare it to the previous weight. If there is a difference of five pounds or more (or according to facility policy), recheck the resident's weight. If, after rechecking the weight, there continues to be a difference, inform the nurse.

Standing Height. The standing balance scale has a height bar that can be used for residents who can stand. An adjustable height bar is lifted up from the scale and the height is measured.

Measuring Height in Nonambulatory Residents. There are several methods of measuring a resident who cannot stand. The simplest is to use a tape measure while the resident is lying supine in bed. Before beginning, smooth and straighten the bottom sheet so it is tucked in tightly and is wrinkle-free. Straighten the resident's back, arms, and legs so he or she is lying as straight as possible. Make a small mark on the sheet with your pen at the top of the resident's head. Measuring the distance between the two marks with the tape measure will give you the height.

Measuring and Recording Intake and Output: Fluid Balance

Fluid balance is the balance between liquid intake and liquid output. Because two-thirds of the body's weight is water, there must be a balance between the amount of fluid taken into the body and the amount lost under normal conditions. Generally, we do not need to concern ourselves about this balance. It usually takes care of itself.

The metric system is used for fluid measurements: milliliters (mL) or cubic centimeters (cc). A mL and a cc are the same amount. Table 10.5 provides a comparison of U.S. customary and metric measurements.

TABLE 10-5 Comparison of U.S. Customary and Metric Measurements

U.S. Customary Units	Metric Units
1 minim	0.06 milliliter (mL)
16 minims	1 mL
1 ounce	30 mL
1 pint	500 mL
1 quart	1,000 mL (1 liter)
2.2 pounds	1 kilogram (kg)
1 inch	2.5 centimeters (cm)
1 foot	30 cm

Intake

We take in approximately 2½ quarts (2,500 mL) of fluid daily:

a. In liquids such as water, tea, and soft drinks.
b. In foods such as fruits and vegetables.
c. Artificially, such as by intravenous infusions or gavage.

Most adult patients need to consume an average 600 to 800 mL of fluid during each eight-hour shift. Because patients may sleep during most of the night shift, additional fluids must be provided during waking hours to keep the body in balance. Excessive fluid retention is called **edema**. Inadequate fluid intake results in **dehydration**, or the lack of sufficient fluid in body tissues. Some disease conditions may change the amounts of fluid the patient is allowed to have.

Output

Typical output equals about 2½ quarts daily in the form of:

- Urine, 1½ quarts (1,500 mL)
- Perspiration
- Moisture from the lungs
- Moisture from the bowel

Excessive fluid loss results in dehydration. This can occur through:

- Diarrhea
- Vomiting
- Excessive urine output (**diuresis**)
- Excessive perspiration (**diaphoresis**)
- Wound drainage or blood loss

Recording Intake and Output

An accurate recording of **intake and output (I&O)**, or fluid taken in and given off by the body, is basic to the care of many patients. Intake and output records are kept when specifically ordered by the physician and when patients:

- are dehydrated.
- receive intravenous infusion.
- have recently had surgery.
- have a urinary catheter.
- are perspiring profusely or vomiting.
- have specific diagnoses such as congestive heart failure or renal disease that require accurate monitoring of I&O.

Fluid intake may have to be encouraged in some patients. This is called **push fluids** or **force fluids**. In some situations (as in kidney disease), fluid intake may have to be restricted. Fluid intake and output is calculated by measuring and recording the fluids the patient takes in and the fluids the patient **excretes** (eliminates from the body) (Table 10.6). Because the fluids taken in by the patient cannot actually be measured, an estimate is made and recorded. This is done by:

- Knowing what the liquid container holds when full.

Note: Sizes of containers vary. Learn the fluid content of the containers used at your facility. Remember that there are 30 mL per ounce (240 mL ÷ 30 mL = 8 oz).

TABLE 10-6 Computing Intake and Output

Intake	
IV	1,500 mL
By mouth	2,000 mL
Total	3,500 mL
Output	
Urine	1,500 mL
Vomitus	500 mL
Drainage	600 mL
Total	2,600 mL

- — Coffee/tea cup, 8 oz = 240 mL
- — Water carafe, 16 oz = 480 mL
- — Foam cup, 8 oz = 240 mL
- — Water glass, 8 oz = 240 mL
- — Soup bowl, 6 oz = 180 mL
- — Jello, 1 serving = 130 mL
- — Ice chips, full 4 oz glass = 120 mL

- Estimating how much is gone from the container (what the patient drank), such as one-third of a glass of juice or half of a cup of coffee
- Converting this to mL. *Example*: A water glass holds 240 mL when filled. The patient drinks $^3/_4$ of the glass of water $^3/_4 \times 240 = 180$ mL. Intake for the glass of water is recorded as 180 mL. Fluids that are calculated and recorded include all liquids, such as water, juices, soda, coffee, tea, milk, and soup. Also included are foods that melt at room temperature: ice cream, sherbet, and gelatin.

Note: Containers may vary from one facility to the next. Each facility should have a chart available that tells you what each size of glass, cup, and bowl holds when full.

Fluids taken by mouth, through intravenous infusion, or through gastric feeding are all recorded separately (Figure 10.25). At the end of each 8-hour shift and the end of 24 hours, the figures are totaled.

Fluid output amount is obtained by measuring all fluids excreted from the body. This includes urine, **emesis** (vomitus), and drainage from body cavities, such as gastric drainage. A container called a **graduate** is marked in mL or cc. The

Date	Time	Method of Adm.	Solution	Intake Amounts Rec'd	Time	Output Urine Amount	Others: Kind	Others: Amount
7/16	0700	PO	water	120 mL		500 mL		
	0830	PO	coffee	240 mL				
			or. ju.	120 mL				
	1030	PO	cran.ju.	120 mL				
	1100					300 mL		
	1230	PO	tea	240 mL				
	1400	PO	water	150 mL				
Shift Totals	1500			990 mL		800 mL		
	1530	PO	gelatin	120 mL				
	1700	PO	tea	120 mL				
			soup	180 mL				
	2000					512 mL		
	2045						vomitus	500 mL
	2205						vomitus	90 mL
Shift Totals	2300			420 mL		512 mL		590 mL
	2345						vomitus	80 mL
	0130	IV	D/W	500 mL				
	0315					400 mL		
Shift Totals	0700			500 mL		400 mL		80 mL
24 Hour Totals				1910 mL		1712 mL		670 mL vomitus

FIGURE 10-25 Sample intake and output record.

substance is poured into the graduate to determine the amount of output. Urine and any other excretions are recorded separately.

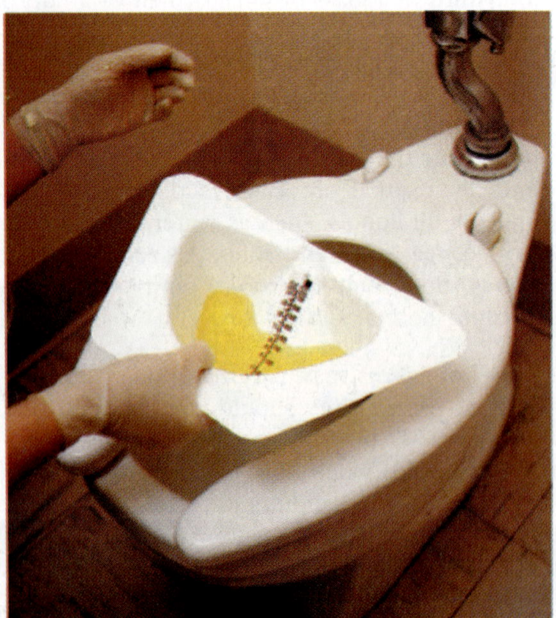

FIGURE 10-26 The specimen collection container is placed under the toilet seat when the patient eliminates. Wear gloves when measuring output, then clean and replace the collection device.

Note: Standard precautions must be followed when measuring any body excretion. Gloves are required for measuring all forms of output (Figure 10.26).

Changing Water

It is important to provide fresh water for patients, because water is essential to life. In all cases, you should know whether a patient is allowed ice or tap water and if water is to be especially encouraged. Even without an order to force fluids, you must encourage patients to take 6 to 8 glasses of fluids daily, unless the patient is NPO (nothing by mouth) or on restricted fluids. Give special attention to confused patients, patients who may not be able to reach a source of water, and the elderly. The need for adequate water intake cannot be overstressed. Because patients often do not drink enough water, sometimes the physician will leave orders that fluids are to be forced to a specific number of mL per day. **Forcing fluids** is an old term that is not quite accurate. Patients should never actually be forced to consume water or other beverages. When "force fluids" is ordered, encourage the patient to drink each time you are in the room. Offer to assist, if necessary. Some patients will not drink water. Find out

INFECTION CONTROL Alert

Avoid contaminating the ice chest or ice scoop when filling pitchers and passing drinking water. Keep the ice scoop covered when not in use. Note that the handle is contaminated and should not touch the clean ice supply. Avoid filling the pitcher over the source of clean ice. (If ice hits the rim of the pitcher and drops back into the clean ice supply, it is contaminated.) Do not allow the scoop to touch the pitcher. Always keep water pitchers covered at the bedside. If more than one patient shares the room, make sure each pitcher and cup are labeled with a single patient's name.

what beverages the patient likes, and provide these, if possible.

Providing fresh water is one way to encourage the patient to increase intake of fluids. The procedure for providing fresh water varies greatly.

- In some hospitals, the water pitcher and glass are replaced with a new disposable set each time water is provided.
- In others, the pitcher and glass are washed, refilled, and returned to the patient's bedside table.

In all cases, be sure you know whether a patient is allowed ice or tap water.

DEHYDRATION

Water in adequate amounts is essential to normal body functioning. Most older adults need to consume about 2,000 to 3,000 mL or 2 to 3 quarts of liquid each day. If the body is functioning properly, the amount of fluids taken in will be balanced by the amount lost.

Dehydration (inadequate fluid level in the body) develops when fluid intake is not adequate. In addition, some drugs cause excessive amounts of fluids to be lost from the body. It is important to recognize the signs of dehydration. All signs of dehydration must be reported immediately so corrective actions can be taken.

Warning Signs of Dehydration. The Nutrition Care Alerts have identified the warning signs of dehydration:

- Drinks less than 6 cups of liquids daily
- Has one or more of the following:
  - dry mouth
  - cracked lips
  - sunken eyes
  - dark urine
- Needs help drinking from a cup or glass
- Has trouble swallowing liquids
- Frequent vomiting, diarrhea, or fever
- Is easily confused or tired

Many residents do not take in enough fluids. This is especially true when they feel ill, have a fever, or have a decreased appetite. An essential task of nursing assistants is to remind and encourage residents to drink water or other fluids frequently.

- Always follow the care plan for each resident for fluid intake. Some residents may be on limited intake because of their medical conditions and should not be offered fluids.
- For other residents, be sure fresh water is within reach. Keep pitchers full. Some residents may request that ice be added to the water.
- Remind the resident to drink whenever you have contact with the resident.
- A resident who has a fever requires careful monitoring of fluid intake.
- Increase attention to fluid intake during hot weather.
- If residents cannot drink unaided, offer fluids frequently and assist as needed.
- If a resident is on intake, record the amount of fluid consumed each time the resident drinks. If this is not possible, the amount of water left in a pitcher can be measured before the pitcher is refilled. The amount left is subtracted from the total amount of water in the pitcher originally.
- Fluid intake over 24 hours is usually consumed during the day and evening shifts (0700 to 2300). It is important for nursing assistants on these shifts to encourage residents to drink adequate fluid.

On the Job

Residents may still become dehydrated even if they eat well-prepared, balanced meals.

- Provide alternatives for residents who do not like water. Check dietary card for beverage preferences. Check if resident prefers and is allowed ice in beverages
- Serve water as well as other beverages at mealtime

The procedure for changing water is outlined in the facility procedure manual. Be sure you know the requirements for changing water, especially the steps to prevent the spread of infection. For example, if pitchers are taken to a central area to be refilled, be sure each resident receives her own pitcher and not one belonging to another resident. Pitchers must be covered before being taken back to the residents' rooms and should remain covered in the room.

KEY POINTS

- Vital signs tell you how well the body's vital organs are working.
- Body temperature can be measured orally, rectally, axillary, or at the tympanic membrane.
- The site used most often for taking the pulse is the radial artery.
- Because respirations are under voluntary control, the resident should not know when you are counting them.
- The systolic blood pressure is the first sound heard when the heart is contracting.
- The diastolic blood pressure is the last sound heard when the heart is resting.
- Abnormal vital signs must be reported to the nurse immediately.
- Accuracy is very important when taking and recording vital signs.
- The nursing assistant is responsible for obtaining and accurately recording the resident's height and weight.
- Accurate measuring & recording of intake and output.

REVIEW

A. Multiple Choice

Select the one best answer.

1. The nurse assigns you to take vital signs on Mr. Vasquez. You know this means you will take the
   a. TPR.
   b. B/P.
   c. TPR and B/P.
   d. B/P and mmHg.
2. The aural (tympanic) temperature is taken
   a. in the ear.
   b. rectally.
   c. under the arm.
   d. in the mouth.
3. The normal rectal temperature is
   a. 97.6°F.
   b. 98.6°F.
   c. 99.6°F.
   d. 100.6°F.
4. The normal oral temperature is
   a. 97.6°F.
   b. 98.6°F.
   c. 99.6°F.
   d. 100.6°F.
5. The normal axillary temperature is
   a. 97.6°F.
   b. 98.6°F.
   c. 99.6°F.
   d. 100.6°F.
6. You are assigned to take Mr. Washington's temperature rectally with a glass thermometer. After lubricating the thermometer, you will insert it into the anus
   a. ¼ inch.
   b. ½ inch.
   c. 1 inch.
   d. 2 inches.

7. The oral thermometer is marked with a
   a. blue dot.
   b. red dot.
   c. green dot.
   d. yellow dot.

8. The rectal thermometer is marked with a
   a. blue dot.
   b. red dot.
   c. green dot.
   d. yellow dot.

9. When taking an axillary temperature, you should use a/an
   a. green probe.
   b. red probe.
   c. rectal thermometer.
   d. oral thermometer.

10. Before taking a temperature with a glass thermometer, shake the thermometer down to
    a. 96°F.
    b. 97°F.
    c. 98°F.
    d. 99°F.

11. The most commonly used site for taking the pulse in adults is the
    a. temporal artery.
    b. apex of the heart.
    c. brachial artery.
    d. radial artery.

12. When palpating the pulse, always use your
    a. thumb.
    b. stethoscope.
    c. first three fingers.
    d. third and fourth fingers.

13. Which of the following pulse rates should you report to the nurse?
    a. 60
    b. 72
    c. 96
    d. 112

14. A pulse rate that is abnormally slow is called
    a. tachycardia.
    b. hypotension.
    c. bradycardia.
    d. pulse pressure.

15. The normal respiratory rate in adults is
    a. 14 to 20.
    b. 16 to 24.
    c. 10 to 20.
    d. 20 to 30.

16. You are assigned to take vital signs on Team A. Which of the following would you report to the nurse?
    a. 98.4°F (O)-80-18
    b. 97.6°F (Ax)-64-16
    c. 100.2°F (R)-110-24
    d. 99.2°F (O)-96-20

17. Which artery is used for taking blood pressure?
    a. carotid
    b. brachial
    c. radial
    d. femoral

18. Hypertension is blood pressure
    a. under 140/90.
    b. over 140/90.
    c. under 100/60.
    d. over 120/80.

19. Hypotension is blood pressure
    a. under 140/90.
    b. over 140/90.
    c. under 100/60.
    d. over 120/80.

20. The instrument used to take a blood pressure is the
    a. sphygmomanometer.
    b. thermometer.
    c. aneroid dial.
    d. mercury probe.

21. When weighing a resident on the balance scale, you know that each marking on the large bar represents
    a. 1 pound.
    b. 5 pounds.
    c. 25 pounds.
    d. 50 pounds.

22. Oral temperatures should not be taken on residents
    a. over the age of 80.
    b. with colostomies.
    c. with seizure disorders.
    d. who are alert.

23. Rectal temperatures should not be taken on residents
    a. with respiratory disease.
    b. with fecal impaction.
    c. using oxygen.
    d. who are confused.

24. The normal pulse rate in adults is
    a. 40–60.
    b. 20–80.
    c. 60–100.
    d. 70–90.

25. Which of the following is the *least accurate* method of taking the temperature?
    a. 1 pound.
    b. rectal
    c. tympanic
    d. oral
    e. axillary

B. Clinical Applications

Answer the following questions.

You are assigned to take vital signs on the north hallway. Your facility uses glass thermometers that are covered with disposable sheaths.

26. You obtained Mrs. White's TPR, but cannot hear her blood pressure. What should you do?

27. Mr. Camp is a new admission. He is using oxygen by mask at six liters per minute. Mr. Camp has an old, well-established colostomy. What method should you use to take his temperature? What type of personal protective equipment should you wear when taking a temperature using this method?

28. You have taken Mr. Camp's temperature. It is 103.2°F. You still have to take vital signs on four more residents. What action should you take?

29. You are assigned to do monthly weights on east wing. After obtaining the weights, you go to the nurses' station to document them. Mr. Lyer weighed 154 pounds last month. Today's weight is 138 pounds. What action should you take?

30. Mrs. Roosevelt is a new admission who has a doctor's order for bed rest. As part of the admission process, you must obtain her height and weight. Mrs. Roosevelt is an obese resident. Her left leg has been amputated above the knee. How will you obtain her height and weight?

C. Determine the resident's intake using the chart on the following page. The resident has consumed:

	mL
31. $^2/_3$ of a drinking glass of water	___
32. $^3/_4$ of a small glass of orange juice	___
33. $^2/_3$ of a small glass of apple juice	___
34. ½ of a water pitcher	___
35. $^3/_4$ of a water pitcher	___
36. $^1/_3$ of a cup of coffee	___
37. ¼ of a carton of milk	___
38. $^3/_4$ of a dish of gelatin	___
Total intake	___

D. On the chart provided, on the following page, make a record of the resident's intake and output for an 8-hour period.

39.

Time	Item	Amount
0730	urine	300 mL
0800	orange juice	90 mL
	coffee	120 mL
0930	water	60 mL
1130	tea	120 mL
	soup	120 mL
1300	urine	400 mL
1315	water	80 mL
1500	cranberry juice	100 mL
1515	vomitus	120 mL
1620	tea	120 mL
	sherbet	120 mL
1730	urine	300 mL
1800	water	150 mL
2100	ginger ale	100 mL
2130	urine	300 mL
2200	water	90 mL

E. Match the metric amounts with their approximate equivalents.

a. 500 mL
b. 0.06 mL
c. 30 mL
d. 3,840 mL
e. 1,000 mL

40. ________ 1 minim
41. ________ 1 quart
42. ________ 1 gallon

43. _______ 1 pint

44. _______ 1 ounce

F. Show your understanding of fractions by completing the following problems.

45. $\frac{1}{2} + \frac{1}{2} =$ ____________

46. $\frac{2}{3} + \frac{1}{3} =$ ____________

47. $\frac{1}{4} + \frac{1}{4} =$ ____________

48. $\frac{3}{4} + \frac{1}{4} =$ ____________

49. Your resident drinks 2/3 of her juice. The glass held 120 mL. How much juice did she drink? Show how you determined your answer.

50. You picked up an empty coffee cup when your resident finished eating. How much did he drink if the cup held 150 mL and you filled it twice? Show how you determined your answer.

51. Your resident consumed a bowl of soup that contained 300 mL. How many ounces of soup did your resident consume? Show how you determined your answer.

INTAKE AND OUTPUT

Room: Name: Date:

Instructions:

Intake	Output	Intake	Output	Intake	Output
Total		Total		Total	

Drinking Glass.........200 mL	Full Water Pitcher....950 mL	Milk Carton..............236 mL	Jello...........................90 mL
Styrofoam Cup........200 mL	Coffee or Teapot.....300 mL	Soup Bowl...............250 mL	Ice Cream Cup..........90 mL
Juice Glass (small)..100 mL	Coffee Cup.............150 mL	Soup Bowl (small)...100 mL	Creamer....................50 mL
Juice Glass (large)..250 mL			

FOLEY CATHETER DRAINAGE: (Circle the following when applicable)

Color: Yellow Amber Brown Red

Appearance: Cloudy Clear Sediment Mucous Bloody

Abdomen Distended Catheter Irrigated Catheter Changed

24 hour INTAKE___________

24 hour OUTPUT___________

UNIT 11

Resident Care Procedures

OBJECTIVES

After reading this unit, you will be able to:

- Spell and define key terms.
- Describe the purpose of the urinary system.
- Identify the common problems with urinary elimination associated with aging, trauma, and disease.
- List the responsibilities of the nursing assistant in assisting residents with urinary elimination.
- Describe the purpose of the urinary catheter.
- Describe the ability to accurately measure urinary output.
- Describe the purpose of collecting urine and stool specimens and demonstrate the procedure.
- Identify the common problems with bowel elimination and list the responsibilities of the nursing assistant in assisting residents with bowel elimination.
- Demonstrate procedures related to elimination.

OBSERVATIONS TO MAKE AND REPORT RELATED TO ELIMINATION

Sores or ulcers inside the mouth
Difficulty chewing or swallowing food
Unusual or abnormal appearance of feces
Blood, mucus, parasites, or other unusual substances in stool
Unusual color of feces
Hard stool, difficulty passing stool
Extremely small or extremely large stool
Loose, watery stool
Complaints of pain, constipation, diarrhea, bleeding
Frequent belching
Changes in appetite
Excessive thirst
Fruity smell to breath
Complaints of indigestion
Excessive gas (flatus)
Nausea, vomiting
Choking
Abdominal pain
Abdominal distention (swelling)
Oral or rectal bleeding
Vomitus, stool, or drainage from a nasogastric tube that looks like coffee grounds
Urinary output too low when compared with oral intake
Urinary output greatly exceeds fluid intake
Fluid intake and output not reasonably balanced on your shift
Resident not drinking sufficient fluids
Resident on fluid restriction drinking excessive fluids, exceeding limitations

Abnormal appearance of urine: dark, concentrated, red, cloudy
Unusual substances in urine: blood, pus, particles, sediment
Complaints of difficulty urinating
Foul-smelling urine
Complaints of pain, burning, urgency, frequency, pain in lower back
Urinating frequently in small amounts
Sudden-onset urinary incontinence
Dribbling of urine
Edema; obvious fluid in tissues, particularly face, fingers, legs, ankles, feet
Sudden weight loss or gain
Respiratory distress
Changes in mental status
Resident complains of inability to empty bladder, or cannot empty bladder completely
Signs of dehydration, including low fluid intake; low output of dark urine with strong odor; weight loss; dry skin; dry mucous membranes of the lips, mouth, tongue, eyes; drowsiness; confusion; poor skin turgor

A: Elimination/Specimen Collection

Urinary System

The urinary system removes waste products and regulates water in the body. The parts of the urinary system are shown in Figure 11.1. The urinary system consists of the **kidneys**, **ureters**, **bladder**, and **urethra**. The kidneys are organs that filter and remove waste products from the blood, forming urine. The ureters are two hollow tubes leading from the kidneys to the bladder. Urine passes from the kidneys through the ureters to the bladder. The bladder is a hollow muscle that stores urine until it is eliminated from the body. When urine is eliminated, it leaves the bladder through a hollow tube called the urethra and passes to the outside of the body. Several medical terms are used to describe the elimination of urine from the body. These are **urination**, **voiding**, and **micturition**. Most people feel the urge to urinate when the bladder contains 100 to 200 mL.

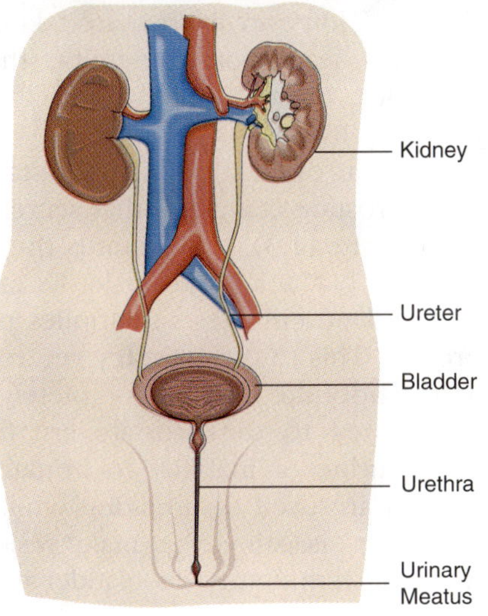

FIGURE 11-1 The urinary system

External Organs

The external organs associated with elimination in the female are the **urinary meatus**, **labia majora**, and **labia minora** (Figure 11.2A). The urinary meatus is the external opening of the urethra to the outside of the body. The labia majora are two large, hair-covered structures on the external female genitalia. The labia minora are smaller, liplike structures on the inside of the labia majora. The external organs in the male are the **penis**, **urinary meatus**, and **foreskin** (Figure 11.2B). The penis is the external male sex organ used for sex and elimination. The foreskin is the loose tissue at the tip of the penis. If the resident has been circumcised, the loose skin has been removed.

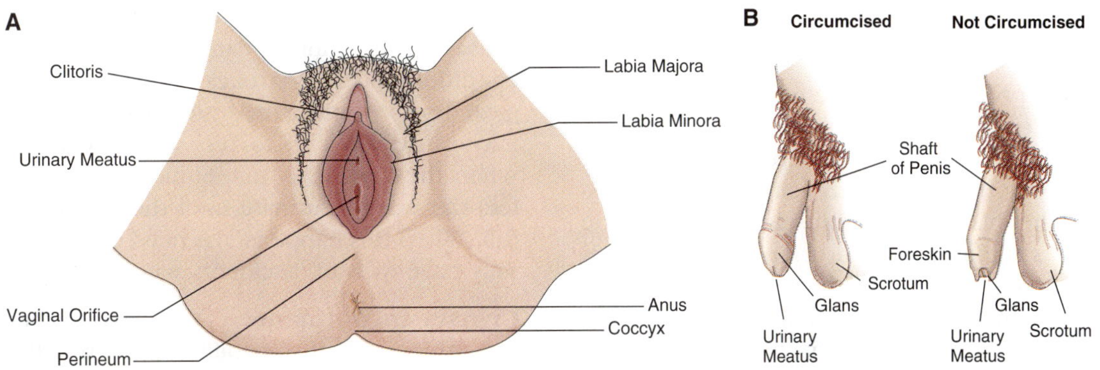

FIGURE 11-2 (A) The external female genitalia (B) The external male genitalia

Normal Elimination

You have learned that the normal fluid intake for most adults is 2000 to 3000 mL per day. The average adult eliminates about 1500 to 2000 mL of urine a day from the bladder. The remaining liquid is eliminated from the body in sweat (450 to 1050 mL), moisture in respiratory secretions (250 to 500 mL), and liquid in bowel elimination (50 to 200 mL). Many factors influence urine production. Some factors, such as disease, ingestion of salt, and certain medications, reduce urine production and cause the body to retain fluid. Drinking coffee, tea, or alcoholic beverages, and some medications increase urine production.

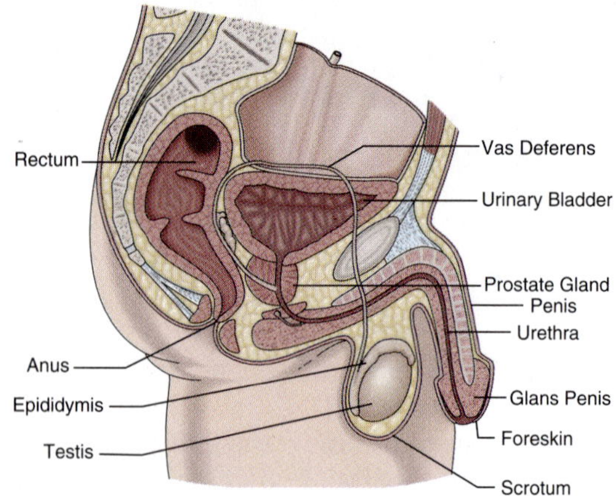

FIGURE 11-3 The prostate gland encircles the urethra. It enlarges in aging, causing partial or complete urinary obstruction.

Common Problems Related to the Urinary System

Problems with elimination have many causes. These are related to aging, medications, and many different diseases. Elimination is very private for most people, and even a change in routine can cause embarrassment. This is particularly true if someone else must assist with this very personal body function. Physical changes in elimination can have a major impact on the resident's self-esteem. Considering the resident's feelings when assisting with urinary elimination procedures is important. The care provider must be sensitive, understanding, and professional.

Incontinence is a medical problem. Health care workers often use underpads, incontinent pads, and briefs to contain urine, prevent skin breakdown, and avoid embarrassment to the resident. Select your words carefully and do not call these medical aids *diapers*, or other words that can be demeaning. Appropriate words to use include *adult brief, garment protector*, and *clothing protector*. Your facility may have specific names for the products you will be using.

Changes in Urinary Function Associated with Aging and Disease

The aging process affects the urinary system. The kidneys do not filter the blood as efficiently as they did previously, so less urine is produced. Muscle tone decreases with aging and some diseases. The bladder is a muscle. Although the bladder is still able to hold urine, the capacity is reduced, and it cannot hold as much as it once did. A common myth is that incontinence is a normal part of aging. This is not true. Incontinence usually indicates a physical problem. It can also occur in mentally confused residents because they cannot express the need to use the bathroom. However, if they are taken to the bathroom and seated on the toilet, they will usually urinate. Most do not forget this basic activity of daily living.

Elderly men often develop **prostate** problems. The prostate is a gland that secretes fluid in semen (Figure 11.3). It surrounds the urethra just below the bladder in the male. As men age, the prostate gland enlarges and applies pressure to the urethra. This causes **urinary retention**, or inability to empty the bladder completely. Other problems related to the prostate are frequent dribbling of urine or inability to urinate at all. Because men are used to urinating while standing, sometimes assisting the male resident to stand will help him empty his bladder more efficiently.

Many diseases also affect the urinary system. In heart disease, the blood is not circulated through the body efficiently, so less urine is produced. Edema often results. High blood pressure causes severe kidney damage over time. Other conditions, such as strokes, trauma, and neurological diseases, affect the resident's sensation. This may cause inability to feel the urge to urinate when the bladder is full. Some residents do not feel the need to urinate until the bladder is very full. When this happens, the need is immediate. If they have to wait, accidents will result.

Urinary Incontinence. You have learned that incontinence is the inability to control the passage of urine from the bladder. Incontinence can be temporary or permanent. In addition to the problems listed earlier, other common causes of incontinence are disease, trauma, surgery, infection, stress, anxiety, tumors, mental confusion, and loss of muscle control. **Constipation**, or passage of hard, dry stool from the lower bowel, may also contribute to incontinence. Some residents are unable to communicate the need to use the bathroom or are physically unable to get to the bathroom. These problems can also cause incontinence. When caring for residents who are incontinent, provide perineal care after each incontinent episode. Some facilities used premixed sprays for this purpose. Some are rinsed off with water. Others are no-rinse solutions or disposable wipes. Follow the directions for the type of product you are using, but apply the principles of peri-care when you perform the procedure. Notify the nurse of any signs of skin redness, irritation, or breakdown.

Types of Incontinence. Some residents have a condition called **stress incontinence**. This is a common problem in women, caused by weak muscles, having multiple children, and aging. In stress incontinence, the bladder leaks urine when the pelvic muscles are strained during activities such as laughing, coughing, sneezing, and lifting.

Urge incontinence is often caused by infection. Other causes of urge incontinence include tumors, neurological problems, reproductive problems, and constipation. Residents with this condition have little warning of the need to use the bathroom. When they feel the urge, the need is immediate. If the urine begins to escape, the resident may be unable to control it, and the bladder empties involuntarily.

Functional incontinence occurs when the resident is physically unable to get to the bathroom on time or is disoriented and unable to find the bathroom. It is easily treated by anticipating residents' needs in advance, answering call signals immediately, and meeting residents' needs responsively. If the resident is in a restraint, he or she will be unable to get to the bathroom without your help. Anticipate the need and offer to toilet the resident routinely.

Mixed incontinence is a combination of urge and stress incontinence. **Overflow incontinence** occurs when the bladder is very full. When it can hold no more, urine leaks out to ease the pressure. **Reflex incontinence** is loss of urine that occurs without awareness in residents who are paralyzed or have other neurologic problems.

Mental Confusion. Residents who are mentally confused present a special challenge. Most are able to urinate if they are taken to the toilet. Some residents who are mentally confused have behavior problems caused by the discomfort of needing to use the toilet. They are not able to express themselves verbally, so they yell, scream, hit, or cry. After they have eliminated, the behavior problems cease. Some confused residents become restless and will pull at or remove their clothing. Anticipate the need for toileting and take confused residents to the bathroom every two hours. Managing incontinence requires planning and effort on your part. However, preventing accidents makes your work easier. A wet bed is a warm, moist, dark environment, so it presents an ideal breeding ground for bacteria. The risk of skin and bladder infections is increased by incontinence. Preventing incontinence also prevents skin breakdown, discomfort, and other complications for the resident.

Urinary Tract Infections. Urinary tract infections (UTIs) are common in women. The urethra in the female is only 1½ to 2½ inches long (Figure 11.4). Because the urethra is so short, bacteria can easily enter it and travel to the bladder. This is why following the correct procedure for perineal care is so important. The urethra in the male is six to eight inches long. Bacteria can travel through the male urethra, but because of the length, the problem is less common than it is in women.

Urine is normally amber or straw colored and clear. There is no mucus or sediment. It has a faint odor. In a urinary tract infection, an unusual

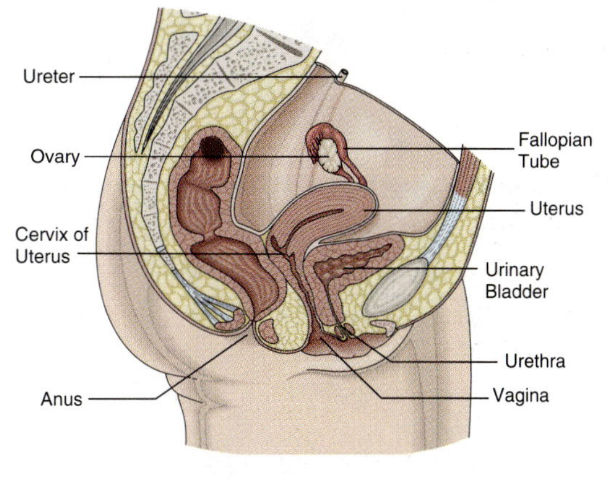

FIGURE 11-4 The female urethra is 1½ to 2½ inches long, providing easy access for invading pathogens to enter a sterile area.

GUIDELINES FOR

Assisting Residents with Urinary Elimination

- Provide adequate fluid intake. Many residents drink less because they believe they will urinate less. The opposite is true. If the resident does not drink enough fluids, the bladder capacity will shrink, and the resident will void more frequently.
- Answer call signals promptly. Take residents to the bathroom, or provide a **bedpan**, **urinal**, or bedside commode (Figure 11.5), if necessary. The bedpan is a device used for elimination in bed. A urinal is used by some male residents for urination.
- Assist residents to assume an upright position for urination. Emptying the bladder in the supine position is difficult.
- Provide privacy by closing the door, privacy curtain, and window curtain. Cover the resident with a bath blanket when using the bedpan or commode, even if alone in the room. Leave the resident alone if doing so is safe. Return immediately when the resident signals. Remain nearby if the resident is unable to safely be left alone.
- Never restrain a resident on the toilet or commode.
- Allow adequate time for the resident to empty the bladder. Leave toilet paper and the call signal nearby.
- If the resident has difficulty urinating, try running a slow, steady stream of water so the resident can hear it. Placing the hands in warm water, offering the resident a drink of water, or pouring warm water over the genital area may also be helpful.
- After the resident has voided, give perineal care if needed.
- Bedpans and urinals should always be covered when removing them from the bedside. Some agencies use covers designed for this purpose. Others use disposable underpads. Wear gloves when handling the bedpan or urinal. Avoid contaminating side rails, door knobs, and faucets with your gloves. Wearing a glove on one hand (Figure 11.6) is a good method of preventing environmental contamination. If removing a glove is not possible, use a paper towel under your gloved hand to avoid touching environmental surfaces.
- Before discarding the specimen, check to see if a urine specimen is needed or if the resident's urinary output must be measured.
- Follow your facility policy for discarding urine and disinfecting the bedpan or urinal after each use.
- Assist the resident to wash hands after emptying the bladder.

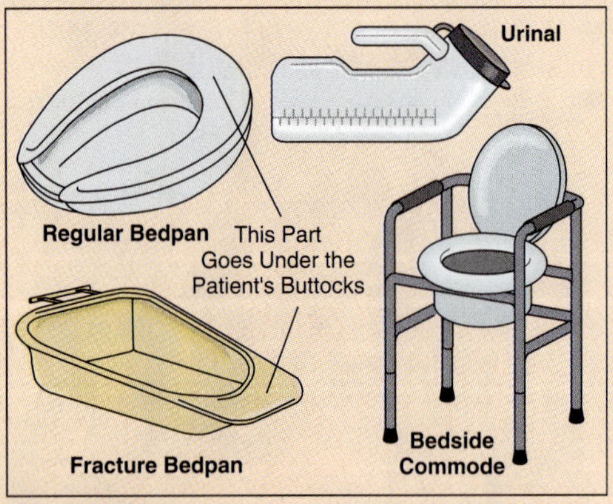

FIGURE 11-5 Devices used to assist residents with elimination

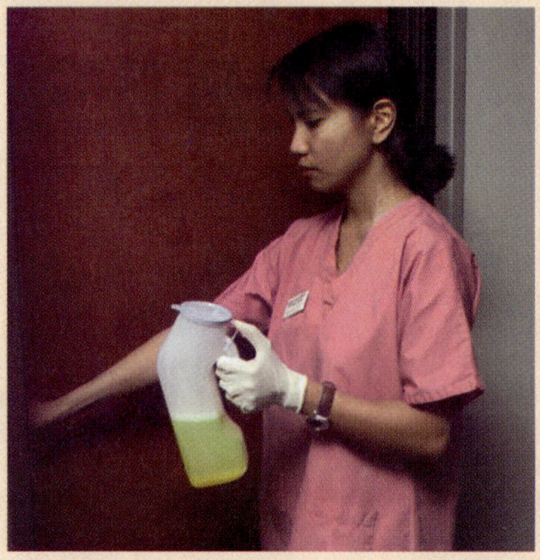

FIGURE 11-6 To avoid environmental contamination, open doors and turn on faucets with your ungloved hand.

color or odor, blood, mucus, or pus may be present in the urine. If you think the urine appears abnormal, save it for the nurse to observe. Pain in the **flank**, or the area of the back immediately above the waist, may indicate an infection. Other signs and symptoms include:

- Voiding frequently in small amounts
- Incontinence or dribbling
- Having an urgent need to void
- Getting up at night to urinate
- New onset of mental confusion
- Burning or pain on urination
- Feeling as if the bladder will not empty
- Being unable to urinate despite having an urge to do so
- Foul odor
- Change from clear to cloudy appearance

If you observe any of these signs in a resident, notify the nurse. If a resident normally has bladder control, and begins to have episodes of incon-

PROCEDURE 52 Assisting the Resident with a Bedpan

1. Perform your beginning procedure actions.
2. Gather supplies needed: gloves, bedpan, bedpan cover, two bed protectors, toilet tissue, basin of water, soap, washcloth, towel.
3. Cover the top linen with a bath blanket and remove the upper linen without exposing the resident, or fold the upper linen down to expose the buttocks.
4. Optional measures for comfort and convenience:
   a. You may run the bedpan under warm water before placing it, for resident comfort. Dry the outside of the bedpan before placing it under the resident.
   b. Dust the edges of the (dry) bedpan lightly with baby powder, then rub the powder around evenly with your gloved hand. This reduces friction, making the bedpan easier to insert and remove. The powder reduces inadvertent shearing on the resident's skin.
5. Ask the resident to flex the knees, resting weight on the heels, and lift the buttocks off the bed, if able.
6. Help the resident raise the buttocks by:
   a. Putting one hand under the small of the back and gently lifting while the resident pushes with the feet (Figure 11.7).
   b. With the other hand, insert the bed protector under the buttocks.
7. If the resident is unable to lift the buttocks:
   a. Assist the resident to turn on the side, with back facing you.
   b. Place the bed protector on the bed.

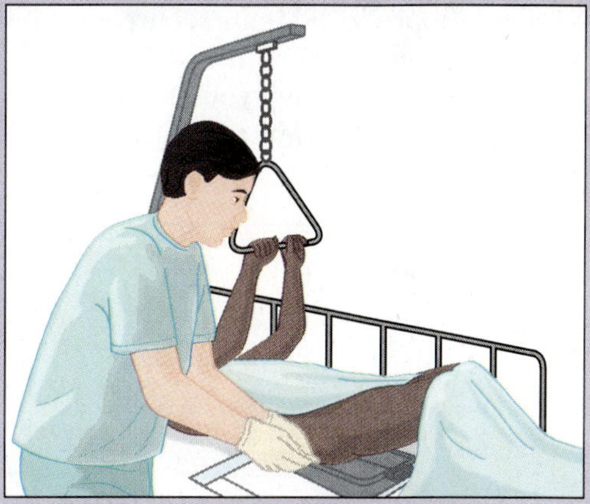

FIGURE 11-7 The resident pulls on the trapeze to lift her hips off the bed. The nursing assistant slides the bedpan under the buttocks.

PROCEDURE

52 Assisting the Resident with a Bedpan, *continued*

c. Place the bedpan flat against the buttocks (Figure 11.8).

d. Assist the resident to roll back while you hold the bedpan in place.

8. Cover the resident with the top sheet or bath blanket.
9. Raise the head of the bed up, for comfort.
10. Remove your gloves.
11. Raise the side rail.
12. Dispose of gloves according to facility policy.
13. Wash your hands.
14. Give the resident the call signal and toilet tissue and leave the room.
15. Return immediately when the resident signals.
16. Put on gloves.
17. Lower the side rail.
18. Remove the bedpan by asking the resident to raise his or her hips.
19. If the resident is unable to raise the hips, hold the bedpan securely while the resident rolls to the side with his or her back facing you. Remove the bedpan. Cover the pan with a bedpan cover or disposable underpad according to facility policy.
20. Place the bedpan on a bed protector on the chair in the room, or according to facility policy. It is usually not placed on the overbed table or bedside stand.
21. Remove one glove to avoid environmental contamination.
22. Fill the washbasin with water (105 °F). Help the resident to clean the perineal area. If you will be assisting with the procedure, wear two gloves. Follow the guidelines for perineal care.
23. Remove one glove and raise the side rail with the ungloved hand.
24. Take the covered bedpan to the bathroom. Empty and disinfect it according to facility policy. Use the ungloved hand to turn on faucets and flush the toilet. Store the bedpan in its proper location.
25. Assist the resident with handwashing.
26. Perform your procedure completion actions.
27. Report or record output. Note color, amount, or any abnormalities.

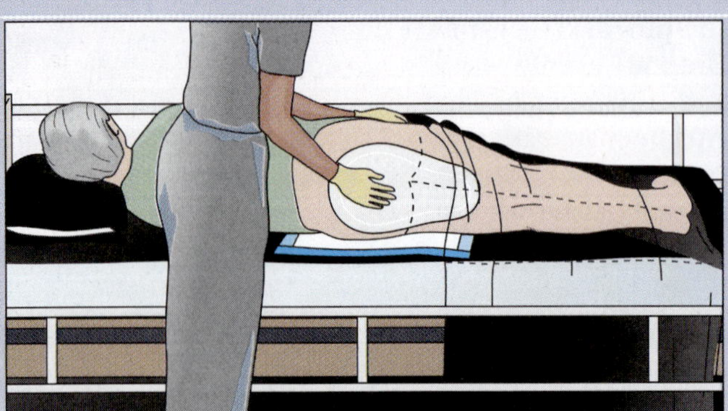

FIGURE 11-8 If the resident cannot lift his or her hips, the resident turns to the side. The nursing assistant places the bedpan against the buttocks, then holds it in place while the resident turns back.

tinence, this is also an important observation. If the resident has not voided at all on your shift, this could also indicate a problem. Notify the nurse of these findings.

Role of the Nursing Assistant in Assisting Residents with Urinary Elimination

The nursing assistant has a very important responsibility in assisting residents with elimination. Always apply the principles of standard precautions when assisting residents with elimination. The circumstances of elimination are highly personal. Use good judgment regarding when to apply and remove gloves. Avoid contaminating environmental surfaces with your gloves. Wear a gown, eye protection, and face mask if splashing is likely.

Assisting Residents with the Bedpan, Urinal, and Bedside Commode

Residents who are confined to bed must use the bedpan or urinal for elimination. The bedpans used in long-term care facilities are regular bedpans and fracture pans. Adjusting to using a bedpan in bed may be difficult for residents. The urinal is a container the male resident uses for urination. The urinal is a plastic or metal container with a handle and lid. It is usually marked on the side with measurements in milliliters. Male residents use the bedpan for bowel movements.

Assisting Residents with the Bedside Commode. The bedside commode is a raised seat placed over the regular toilet, or is used at the bedside with a bedpan or other container placed under the seat. It is used for residents who can get out of bed, but are unable to walk to the bathroom. Using the commode positions the resi-

PROCEDURE 53 Assisting the Male Resident with a Urinal

1. Perform your beginning procedure actions.
2. Gather supplies: gloves, urinal with cover, basin of water, soap, washcloth, towel.
3. Put on gloves.
4. Lift the top covers and hand the resident the urinal. If the resident is unable to take the urinal, place it between the resident's legs and insert the penis into the opening.
5. Remove your gloves and discard according to facility policy.
6. Raise the side rail.
7. Wash your hands.
8. Give the resident the call signal and leave the room.
9. Return immediately when called.
10. Put on one glove.
11. Ask the resident to hand you the urinal. Remove it if he is unable, using the gloved hand. Close the lid if needed.
12. Assist the resident with perineal care. Wear two gloves, if assisting.
13. Take the covered urinal to the bathroom and empty and disinfect it according to facility policy. Store the urinal in its proper location.
14. Remove the glove(s) and dispose according to facility policy.
15. Wash your hands.
16. Lower the side rail.
17. Help the resident to wash his hands.
18. Raise the side rail.
19. Perform your procedure completion actions.
20. Report or record output. Note color, amount, or any abnormalities.

dent in a natural position for elimination, and increases resident independence. The bedside commode is more secure for some residents to sit on because it has sturdy arms that help with sitting, rising, and positioning. Some commodes have wheels. If this is the case, they should be locked securely at all times. Most commodes have a cover over the container used for elimination. However, the commode should be emptied each time it is used. The cover is used when transporting the container to the designated area for emptying and disinfecting.

The procedure for transferring a resident to the commode is the same as the procedure used to transfer from bed to chair. Apply the principles of standard precautions when handling the container the resident uses for elimination.

URINARY CATHETERS

A **catheter** is a hollow tube inserted into the bladder to drain urine. This is a sterile procedure that is done by the nurse. Sometimes a catheter is called a *Foley*, which is a common brand name for **indwelling catheters**. It may also be called a *retention catheter* or *indwelling catheter*. Catheters are inserted through the urethra, and are held in place with a balloon inflated with saline solution or sterile water (Figure 11.9). The catheter remains in the body for a period of time. Sometimes the resident will complain of feeling the urge to urinate after the catheter is inserted. This is due to the pressure of the balloon on the internal sphincter of the urethra. The pressure feels the same as the sensation of urine pressing on the sphincter. If the resident with a catheter complains of feeling the urge to void, notify the nurse.

A **suprapubic catheter** (Figure 11.10) is inserted surgically through the abdominal wall directly into the bladder. A **condom catheter** (Figure 11.11) is an **external catheter** used in males. It is applied over the penis and attached to

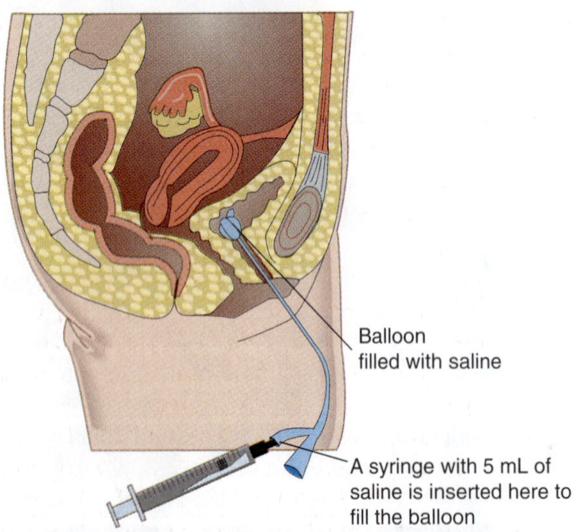

FIGURE 11-9 A small balloon filled with sterile saline solution holds the catheter in the bladder. Pressure from the balloon on the internal sphincter of the urethra may cause the resident to feel the urge to void.

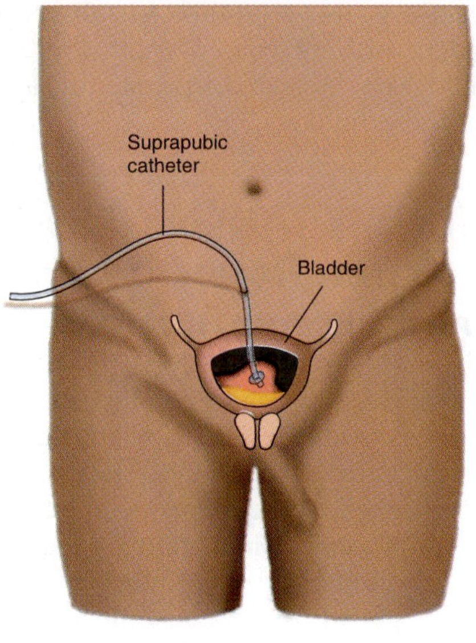

FIGURE 11-10 The suprapubic catheter is surgically inserted through the abdominal wall. The urethra is not functional.

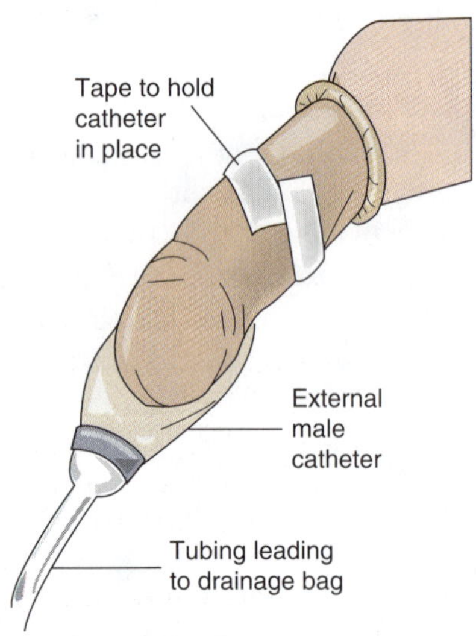

FIGURE 11-11 This male external catheter is secured with spiral-wrapped tape. Another type has a self-adhesive inner surface.

drainage tubing. It is sometimes called a *Texas catheter*. An **intermittent catheter** is inserted into the bladder for emptying the bladder or obtaining a urine specimen. After the bladder is emptied, the catheter is removed.

Purpose of Catheters

Catheters are used for many reasons. Some catheters are intermittent. Some are temporary and others are used permanently. Catheter use is avoided whenever possible because it presents a very high risk of infection. Because the catheter provides a direct opening into the bladder, pathogens can make their way up the tubing and cause serious problems. Residents who are elderly and those with weakened immune systems often become **septic** because of bladder infections. Sepsis is a very serious, sometimes fatal, systemic infection caused by bacteria.

Catheters are never used for staff convenience. Many residents with neurological problems or trauma are catheterized because the condition has affected sensation, and the resident cannot feel the urge to void. Some residents retain urine until the bladder is stretched beyond capacity. This is very painful. Catheters are used to empty the bladder in these cases. Catheters are also used after many surgical procedures. These catheters are used temporarily and are removed when the resident is able to use the toilet again. Residents with severe skin problems may also use catheters temporarily, allowing time for the skin to heal without the irritation of urine on the wound. Some residents routinely catheterize themselves to empty the bladder.

Drainage Systems

Catheters must be ordered by a physician and are inserted by licensed personnel. They must always be secured to the resident's body with a special strap (Figure 11.12). Securing the catheter prevents accidental pulling during movement. Pulling can cause damage to the bladder and urethra, and is very uncomfortable for the resident. After the catheter is inserted, it is connected to a **closed drainage system**. (Figure 11.13). The system is connected to the catheter with a long tubing that empties urine into a **drainage bag** (Figure 11.14), where urine is collected. As long as the system is not opened, it remains **sterile**, or free from all microbes. Each time the system is opened, the risk of infection increases. Opening a closed urinary drainage system is usually a licensed nursing responsibility. Do not open a closed system unless you have been taught the proper techniques and are permitted to do so in your facility.

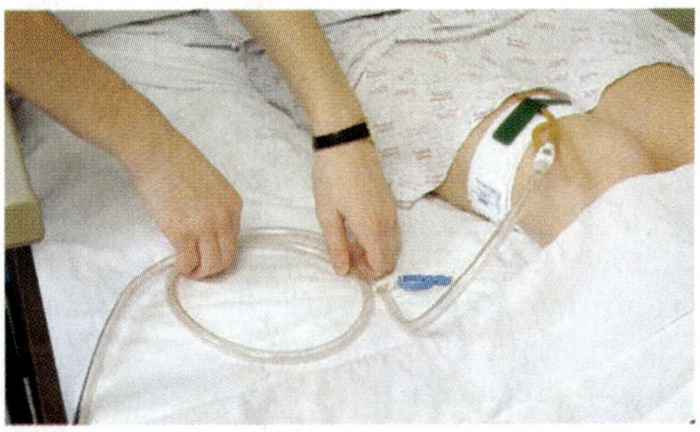

FIGURE 11-12 The catheter is secured with a Velcro strap to prevent pulling and damage to the bladder and urethra. For a male resident, the catheter may be taped to the abdomen.

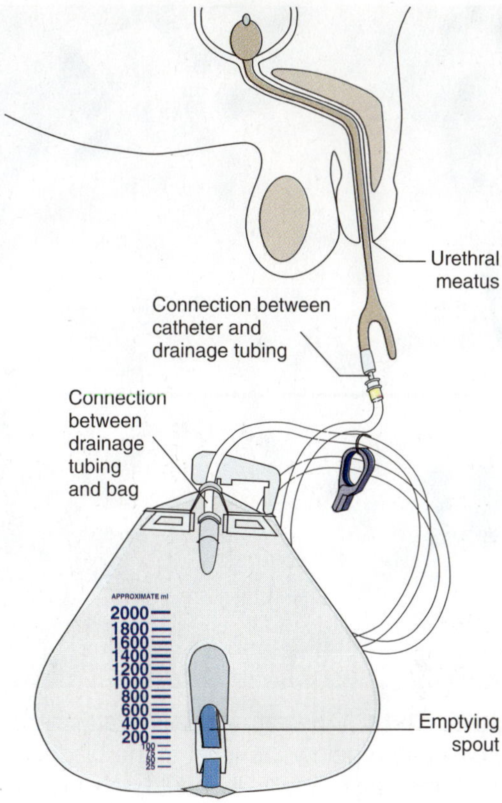

FIGURE 11-13 Handle the closed drainage system carefully to avoid accidental contamination of these areas.

Some facilities use **leg drainage bags** (Figure 11.15) on both indwelling catheters and condom catheters. These are used for ambulatory residents who are up and about during the day. The bag is attached to the leg with elastic straps or Velcro bands. The leg bag holds a smaller amount of urine than a normal drainage bag, and must be emptied more often. Use of the leg bag is avoided whenever possible, because it requires frequent

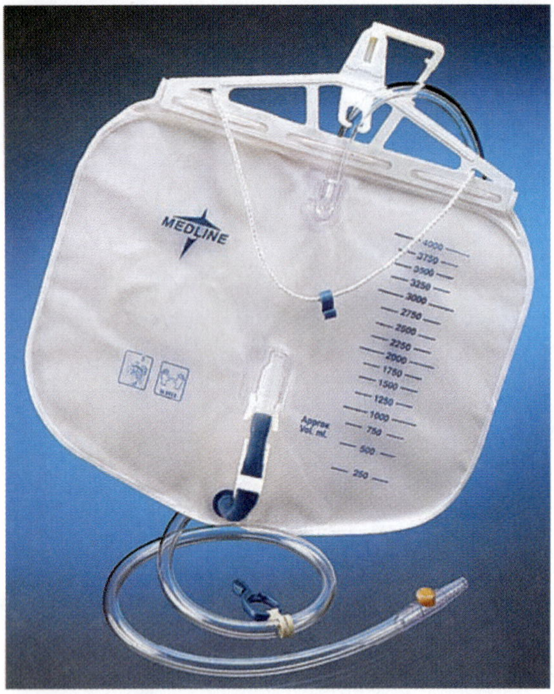

FIGURE 11-14 The catheter bag is attached to the bed frame below the level of the bladder. Handle the bag carefully. It should never be positioned so that urine flows back into the bladder. Note the numbers on the bag. These are approximations only, and are used for monitoring purposes. Do not use these numbers for intake and output measurements. *(Courtesy of Medline Industries, Inc. 1-800-MEDLINE)*

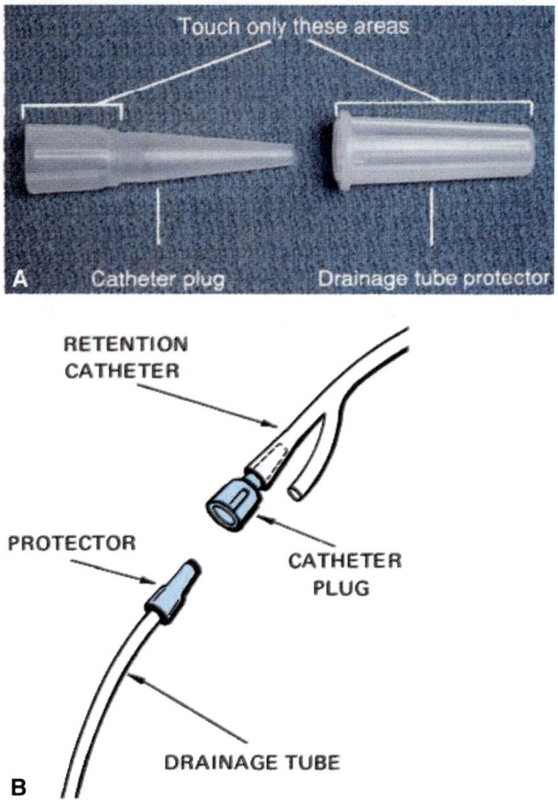

FIGURE 11-16A, B The sterile plug and drainage tube protector are used to maintain sterility of the closed catheter system. Never touch the inside of the cap or patient end of the plug with your fingers.

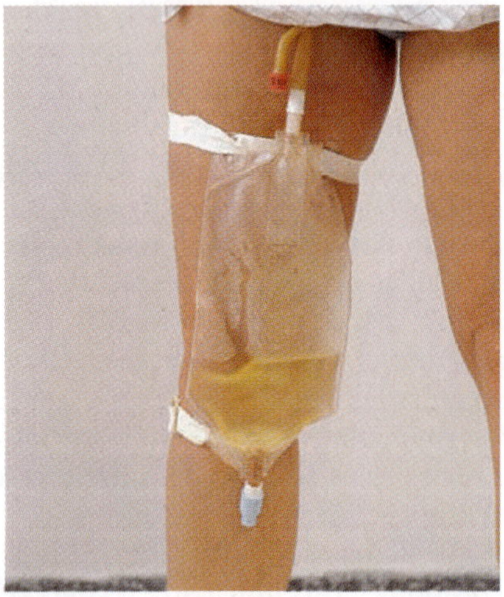

FIGURE 11-15 The leg bag is held in place by adjustable straps. The bag is smaller than a bed collection bag and must be emptied more often. Carefully connect the catheter to the leg bag. Avoid touching anything against the end of the catheter. The drainage tubing on the bed bag is covered with a sterile cap that is left in place until it is reconnected to the catheter.

manipulation and opening of the closed system and increases the chance of infection. Some facilities have policies and procedures for disinfecting and reusing them; others use a new bag each day. Know and follow your facility policy. Residents who use the leg bag are connected to the normal catheter drainage bag when they are in bed. Never put a resident to bed with a leg bag in place. Follow your facility policy for use of the leg bag.

If you are responsible for applying a leg bag or opening a closed system, use aseptic technique. Insert a catheter plug into the end of the catheter (Figure 11.16A). Cover the end of the drainage tube with the sterile cap (Figure 11.16B).

Caring for a Catheter

The nursing assistant is usually responsible for maintaining the closed drainage system. The tubing may be secured to the bed linen with a rubber band and clip. Maintaining the sterility of this system is an important responsibility. Apply the principles of standard precautions, and use the correct personal protective equipment when working with catheters.

GUIDELINES FOR

Maintaining a Closed Drainage System

- Always wash your hands and apply gloves before handling the catheter and closed drainage system. Avoid contaminating the environment with your gloves.
- Wear a face shield, mask, and gown if you are performing a procedure in which splashing is likely, such as emptying a very full drainage bag.
- The catheter, bag, and tubing are never disconnected unless sterile technique is used.
- When the resident is in bed, the closed drainage bag is attached to the frame of the bed, never the side rail.
- The urinary drainage bag must never touch the floor, as this contaminates the system.
- When the resident is in a chair or wheelchair, the closed drainage bag is attached to the frame of the chair.
- Many facilities use cloth catheter bags for privacy. The cloth bag is connected to the bed or chair frame, and the urinary drainage bag is placed in it. The cloth bag should not touch the floor.
- Avoid elevating the urinary drainage bag and tubing above the level of the bladder. This causes a back-flow of urine into the bladder, greatly increasing the risk of infection.
- When the resident is ambulating, the tubing and drainage bag are carried below the level of the bladder.
- Secure the catheter with a strap. Some facilities secure the catheter to the leg in women, and the abdomen, using tape, in men. When securing the catheter to the leg, it is positioned on the top side. Avoid placing the catheter under the leg, as this placement may pinch and obstruct the flow of urine. Know and follow your facility policy.
- Attach the tubing to the bed with a rubber band and plastic clip. The tubing should not hang below the drainage bag.
- Make sure the urine is draining freely through the system and that there are no kinks or obstructions in the tubing.
- Never disconnect the tubing, unless you are trained in this procedure.
- Use care when lifting, moving, and transferring residents with catheters, to avoid accidentally dislodging the catheter by pulling on the tubing.
- When the resident is positioned on his or her back, the catheter should be on top of the leg. The drainage bag is positioned on the bed frame on the same side of the bed as the catheter. (If the catheter is on the left leg, the bag is on the left side of the bed.)
- If the resident is positioned on his or her side, the catheter is positioned between the legs. Make sure the urine flow is not obstructed. The bag is placed on the bed frame on the side the resident is facing (if the resident faces right, the bag hangs on the right side of the bed).
- When transferring the resident to a chair or wheelchair, move the bag first, then the resident. Take care to avoid stepping on the tubing during the transfer.
- Monitor the level of urine in the drainage bag. Most people excrete about 50 to 80 mL of urine each hour. If the level of urine in the bag does not change, if the catheter is leaking, if no urine is present in the bag, or if the urine has an abnormal color, odor, or appearance, inform the nurse.
- Notify the nurse if redness, irritation, drainage, crusting, or open areas are present at the catheter insertion site.
- Notify the nurse if the resident complains of pain, burning, or tenderness, or has other signs or symptoms of urinary tract infection.
- Most facilities routinely measure intake and output on residents who are using a urinary catheter. Follow your facility policy.

You may be assigned to care for a resident who has recently had a catheter removed. Sometimes residents have difficulty urinating after the catheter is removed, or the bladder does not empty completely. After the catheter is removed, monitor the resident and record the time and amount of each voiding for the rest of your shift. If the resident has not voided by the end of your shift, notify the nurse. Monitoring of the resident's urination will continue for at least 24 hours after the catheter has been removed.

Providing Catheter Care

The nursing assistant is responsible for providing catheter care to residents who use catheters. Always apply the principles of standard precautions when caring for the catheter. Use **aseptic technique** when caring for the catheter or the drainage system. Aseptic technique means you will perform the procedure correctly so you do not introduce microbes to the area. The perineum should be as clean as possible, so perform perineal care before caring for the catheter.

Some facilities use specially packaged catheter care kits, but most use soap and water when providing perineal and catheter care. The supplies for performing this procedure will vary depending on which method you use, but the principles of care are the same.

Caring for the External Catheter

The risk of infection is not as great when using an external catheter. However, the catheter must be cared for correctly because infection can occur. Other complications, such as irritation and circulatory problems, can also occur. The external catheter is applied over the penis. It is usually attached with an adhesive strip. The strip should always be wrapped in a spiral. If it completely encircles the penis, severe injury can result. Some external catheters have a self-adhesive film on the inside, making the adhesive strip on the outside unnecessary. About one inch of the catheter should extend beyond the tip of the penis and attach to the drainage tubing. Always apply the principles of standard precautions when caring for an external catheter.

Emptying the Urinary Drainage Bag

The nursing assistant is responsible for emptying the urinary drainage bag at the end of the shift, and more often if the bag becomes full. The output is measured and recorded. Apply the principles of standard precautions when performing

GUIDELINES FOR

Opening a Closed Drainage System

Note: In some states, nursing assistants are not permitted to perform this procedure. Additionally, the policies of some facilities state that only licensed nurses may open a closed urinary drainage system. Perform this procedure only if you are permitted to do so by state law and facility policies.

- Always wash your hands and apply gloves before handling the catheter and closed drainage system. Avoid contaminating the environment with your gloves. Use sterile technique.
- Position an underpad under the connection between the catheter and drainage tube.
- Open the sterile package containing the catheter plug and cap. Leave it open on the table, but avoid touching it. Disconnect the catheter and tubing. Hold both ends in your hand. Do not set them down. Insert the catheter plug into the end of the catheter. Avoid touching the tip of the plug. Place the sterile cap over the end of the drainage tube. After covering, both items may be put down.
- If accidental contamination occurs, wipe the ends well with an antiseptic wipe before placing the cap or inserting the plug.
- Empty the drainage bag, if necessary. Secure the tubing to the bed so it does not touch the floor.
- Reverse these steps to reconnect the catheter. If you find an unconnected, disconnected catheter, do not reconnect it. Inform the nurse at once.

GUIDELINES FOR

Applying a Urinary Leg Bag

Note: In some states, nursing assistants are not permitted to perform this procedure. Additionally, the policies of some facilities state that only licensed nurses may open a closed urinary drainage system. Perform this procedure only if you are permitted to do so by state law and facility policies.

- Always wash your hands and apply gloves before handling the catheter and closed drainage system. Avoid contaminating the environment with your gloves. Use sterile technique.
- Position an underpad under the connection between the catheter and drainage tube.
- Open the sterile package containing the leg bag. Leave it open on the table, but avoid touching it.
- Open the sterile package containing the catheter plug and cap. Leave it open on the table, but avoid touching it. Disconnect the catheter and tubing. Hold both ends in your hand. Do not set them down. Insert the catheter plug into the end of the catheter. Avoid touching the tip of the plug. Place the sterile cap over the end of the drainage tube. After covering, both items may be put down.
- If accidental contamination occurs, wipe the ends well with an antiseptic wipe before placing the cap or inserting the plug.
- Secure the tubing to the bed so it does not fall on the floor.
- Remove the catheter plug. Place it on the open, sterile package.
- Insert the upper connector of the leg bag into the catheter.
- Fasten the leg bag to the resident's leg with the Velcro or vinyl straps. Make sure the catheter is straight and able to drain freely. Check for leaks.
- Empty the drainage bag, if necessary.
- Reverse these steps to reconnect the catheter. If you find an unconnected, disconnected catheter, do not reconnect it. Inform the nurse at once.

PROCEDURE 54

Providing Indwelling Catheter Care

Note: The guidelines and sequence for this procedure vary slightly from state to state. Your instructor will inform you if the sequence in your state differs from the procedure listed here. Know and follow the required sequence for your state.

1. Perform your beginning procedure actions.
2. Gather supplies needed: catheter care kit or basin, soap, two washcloths, towels, clean gown or clothing, bath blanket, bed protector, hamper or plastic laundry bag, gloves.
3. Place the equipment on the overbed table. Follow your facility policy for covering the overbed table with a barrier.
4. Perform perineal care.
5. Using a clean washcloth, wash the catheter for three to four inches from the insertion site into the body. Begin washing at the urinary meatus and wash downward. Avoid rubbing back and forth on the tubing.
6. Thoroughly rinse and dry the tubing.
7. Secure the tubing to the leg.
8. Perform your procedure completion actions.

GUIDELINES FOR

Caring for an External Catheter

- Wear gloves and apply the principles of standard precautions when caring for an external catheter and drainage system. Avoid contaminating the environment with your gloves.
- Provide perineal care before applying the external catheter.
- Dry the penis well before applying the catheter. Report redness, irritation, discharge, or signs of infection to the nurse.
- Roll the tip of the condom catheter over the tip of the penis and up the shaft. Leave one inch of space at the end.
- Wrap the adhesive strip in a spiral.
- Attach the connecting tube of the catheter to the drainage tubing and urinary drainage bag.
- Change the catheter daily. Discard the external catheter and apply a new one each day, and more often if necessary. Never reuse a catheter after it has been removed.
- To change the catheter, remove the adhesive strip and roll the condom down over the tip of the penis. Discard it in the biohazardous waste, according to facility policy.
- Observe the skin on the penis for redness, irritation, swelling, and open areas. If noted, report your observations to the nurse before applying a new external catheter.
- After the catheter has been removed, perineal care must be done before a new catheter is applied.

PROCEDURE 55

Emptying the Urinary Drainage Bag

Note: The guidelines and sequence for this procedure vary slightly from state to state. Your instructor will inform you if the sequence in your state differs from the procedure listed here. Know and follow the required sequence for your state.

1. Perform your beginning procedure actions.
2. Gather supplies needed: gloves; mask and eye protection, if necessary; graduated pitcher; paper towel; alcohol sponge.
3. Place the paper towel on the floor and place the graduated pitcher on it (Figure 11.17A).
4. Apply gloves.
5. Remove the drainage spout from the bag and center it over the graduate. Avoid touching the tip of the drainage spout with your hands or the side of the graduate.
6. Open the clamp on the drainage spout and drain the urine into the graduate (Figure 11.17B).
7. After the urine has drained into the graduate, wipe the spout with the alcohol sponge, if this is your facility policy. Some facilities do not wipe the tip of the spout unless it has contacted your hands or the graduate.
8. Replace the drainage spout into the holder on the side of the catheter bag. Pick up the graduate and dispose of the paper towel.

9. Note the amount, color, and character of urine.
10. Discard urine and disinfect the graduate according to facility policy. Store the graduate in its proper location.
11. Report or record output. Note color, amount, or any abnormalities.
12. Perform your procedure completion actions.

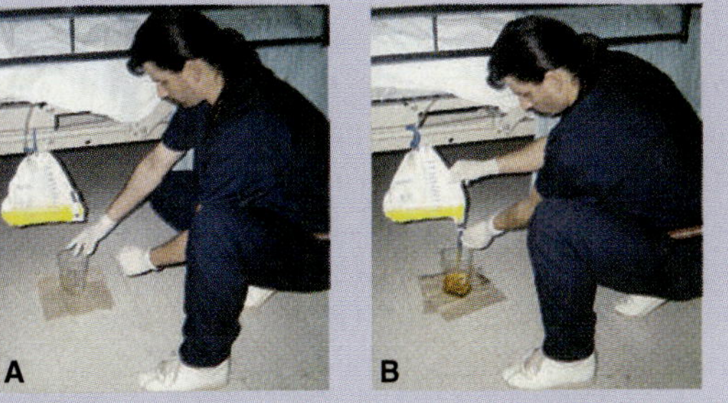

FIGURE 11-17 (A) Place a paper towel on the floor under the graduate. (B) Center the drain spout over the graduate to avoid accidental contamination.

this procedure. All facilities require you to wear gloves. Some also require the use of a face mask and eye protection, because of the risk of splashing if the drainage bag is full. Know and follow your facility policy.

MEASURING URINARY OUTPUT

You have learned that most people eliminate about 1500 mL of urine each day and the reasons for recording intake and output. If the

PROCEDURE 56 Measuring Urinary Output

1. Perform your beginning procedure actions.
2. Gather supplies needed: graduate, intake and output work sheet, gloves.
3. After the resident has voided, apply gloves.
4. Empty the urine into the graduate. Measure the amount of urine in the container at eye level (Figure 11.18).
5. Empty the graduate into the toilet, and rinse and disinfect the container.
6. Rinse, disinfect, dry, and replace the bedpan, urinal, or commode container.
7. Perform your procedure completion actions.
8. Record the output on the intake and output work sheet, or according to facility policy.

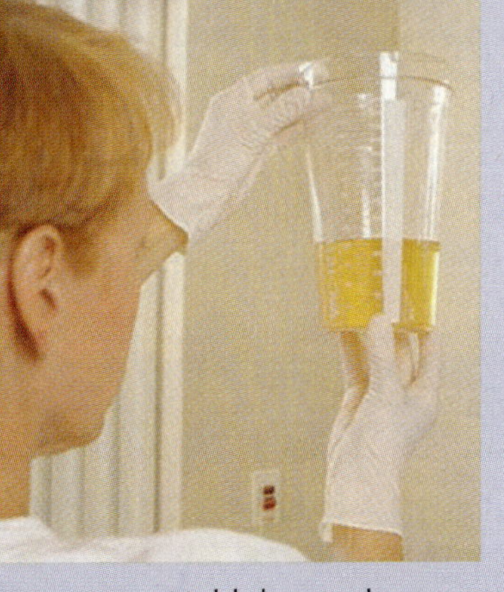

FIGURE 11-18 Hold the graduate at eye level or place it on the counter and view at eye level to measure the output accurately.

resident is incontinent, follow your facility procedure for recording fluid output. Some facilities count the number of episodes of incontinence. Others measure the size of the urine puddle or weigh the underpad. The dry weight of the pad is subtracted from the total weight, and an estimation of the amount of urine eliminated is made. A scale that measures weight in grams is usually used. The most common formula is 1 gram of weight is equivalent to 1 mL of urine.

A **graduate** is a container used for measuring liquids in the health care facility. The graduate is marked on the side in ounces and milliliters (or cubic centimeters). Measuring the urine in a graduate is more accurate than using the markings on a catheter bag or estimating the output.

If you will be measuring urinary output, remind the resident not to drop toilet tissue into the container holding the urine. The toilet tissue is discarded into a plastic bag, or according to facility policy. Apply the principles of standard precautions when measuring urinary output.

Collecting a Urine Specimen

The nursing assistant is responsible for collecting routine urine specimens for analysis by the laboratory. The physician will use the information gathered to aid in diagnosis and treatment of the resident. A **laboratory requisition** is completed and attached to each specimen. The requisition contains identifying resident information and specifies the type of test to be performed on the specimen.

Urine is collected in a clean bedpan, urinal, or specimen collection container in the toilet. This container may be called a specimen collection "hat," or "nun's hat" (Figure 11.19). The specimen is poured into a closed urine specimen container with a lid. A routine urine specimen is collected using clean technique. The specimen does not have to be sterile, but must be free from outside contamination.

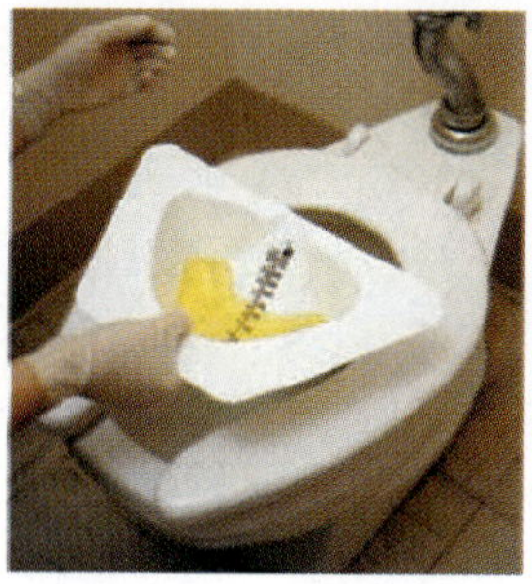

FIGURE 11-19 The specimen collection container may be called a specimen "hat" or "nun's hat."

A **midstream (clean-catch) specimen** is collected from the middle of the urinary stream and is as sterile as possible. The specimen cup is sterile. Urine in the bladder is normally sterile. Precautions are taken when obtaining the specimen to avoid contamination. The perineum is washed before collecting the specimen, to eliminate microbes on the skin. The resident starts to void into the toilet or other container, and stops the flow of urine partway through. The sterile specimen cup is placed under the urethra, and the resident voids into the container until an adequate amount of urine is obtained. The resident stops voiding again, the cup is removed, and the resident finishes the elimination in the toilet.

Catheterized Urine Specimen. When a urine specimen is needed that is free of contamination from organisms found in areas near the urinary meatus (opening), the specimen may be collected by inserting a sterile tube (**catheter**). The nurse will perform this procedure.

GUIDELINES FOR
Collecting a Urine Specimen

- Apply the principles of standard precautions. Avoid contaminating the environment with your gloves.
- *The lid to the specimen container is always placed topside down on the table, so the clean inner side faces up.*
- *Avoid touching the inside of the container or lid with your hands.*
- The specimen container is always labeled with the resident's name and other identifying information. Follow your facility policy for labeling the container.

- Ask the resident not to discard toilet tissue into the specimen. The toilet tissue is discarded into a plastic bag, or according to facility policy.
- Pour the specimen into the specimen collection container. If you will be placing the container on a counter or other flat surface, place a paper towel under it.
- After you have collected the specimen, put the lid on the container and place it in a sealed **transport bag** labeled with a biohazardous waste label (Figure 11.20). The transport bag is a plastic bag that can be sealed tightly to prevent leaking.
- If the urine specimen cannot be transported to the lab immediately, it can be stored in a designated refrigerator or cooler for lab specimens.

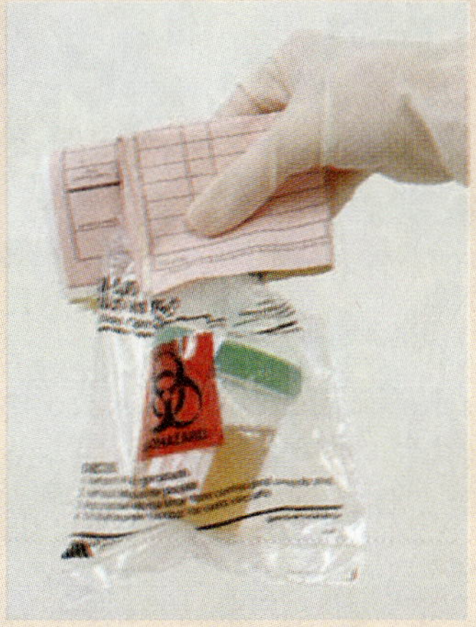

FIGURE 11-20 Specimens are transported to the laboratory in a sealed plastic transport bag with a biohazard label.

Twenty-Four-Hour Specimen. If a 24-hour urine specimen is ordered, all urine excreted by the patient in a 24-hour period is collected and saved. A 24-hour urine specimen requires that the patient start the 24-hour time period with an empty bladder. For this reason, the first specimen is discarded.

- All urine is saved in a large, carefully labeled container that is supplied by the laboratory and may contain a preservative.
- The container is usually surrounded by ice. If the patient has an indwelling catheter, place the catheter bag in a container surrounded by ice. Empty the bag into the container supplied by the laboratory.

PROCEDURE 57 Collecting a Routine Urine Specimen

1. Perform your beginning procedure actions.
2. Gather supplies needed: specimen collection container, label, transport bag, bedpan, urinal, commode or specimen collection device, plastic bag for waste disposal, gloves.
3. Complete the label and put it on the container.
4. Ask the resident to urinate into the collection device. Instruct the resident not to place toilet tissue into the specimen. Provide a plastic bag for this purpose.
5. Provide privacy and make sure the call signal and toilet tissue are within reach.
6. Return immediately when the resident signals.
7. Open the specimen collection container and place the lid on the counter, with the top side down.

PROCEDURE 57 Collecting a Routine Urine Specimen, *continued*

8. Apply gloves.
9. Take the container of urine to the toilet and raise the seat.
10. Measure the urine if the resident is on intake and output.
11. Hold the specimen collection container over the toilet. Pour the urine into the collection container. The container should be about three-quarters full. Discard the rest of the urine into the toilet.
12. Put the lid on the specimen container. Place it on a paper towel on the counter (Figure 11.21).

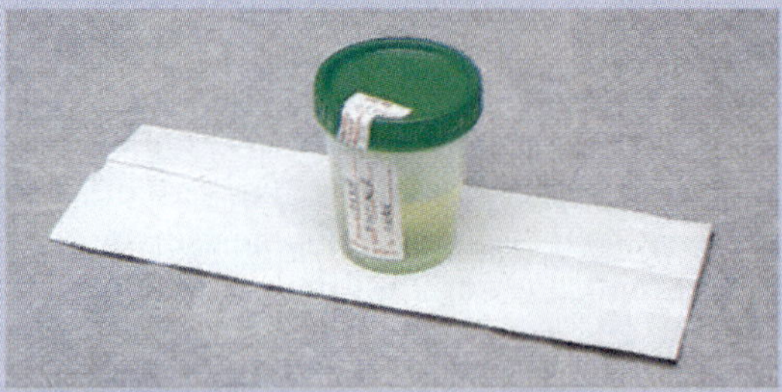

FIGURE 11-21 To prevent environmental contamination, place the specimen collection cup on a paper towel.

13. Rinse and disinfect the bedpan or other container according to facility policy.
14. Remove one glove and place the specimen into the transport bag with your gloved hand. Avoid touching the outside of the bag with your glove. Handle the transport bag with your ungloved hand.
15. Remove the other glove and discard according to facility policy. (Gloves can be discarded in the plastic bag with toilet tissue.)
16. Wash your hands.
17. Record output, if the resident is on intake and output.
18. Perform your procedure completion actions.
19. Discard the plastic bag containing the waste in the biohazardous waste container.
20. Take the specimen to the designated location.
21. Report that the specimen was collected, and report any abnormalities to the nurse.

PROCEDURE 58 Collecting the Midstream (Clean-Catch) Urine Specimen

Note: The guidelines and sequence for this procedure vary slightly from state to state. Your instructor will inform you if the sequence in your state differs from the procedure listed here. Know and follow the required sequence for your state.

1. Perform your beginning procedure actions.
2. Gather supplies needed: midstream specimen kit, or other equipment used by your facility; bedpan; urinal or com-

mode; transport bag; plastic bag for waste disposal; gloves.

3. Open the specimen collection kit. Remove the specimen collection container. Apply gloves.
4. Remove the towelettes or swabs from the collection kit.
5. Clean the penis or female perineal area with the swabs or towelettes. Use each swab or towelette once, then discard in a plastic bag. Do not place the used swabs near the clean kit. Discard in a plastic bag after use.
6. In a female resident, keep the labia separated until the specimen has been collected. In an uncircumcised male resident, keep the foreskin retracted until the specimen is collected.
7. Explain the procedure to the resident and ask him or her to begin urinating into the toilet or other container. Ask the resident to stop the stream. Hold the collection cup under the urethra without touching the body, and collect the specimen. Ask the resident to stop urinating, and remove the container. Instruct the resident to finish urinating in the toilet. Assist the resident to use toilet tissue, if necessary.
8. Put the lid on the specimen container. Place it on a paper towel on the counter.
9. Remove gloves and discard according to facility policy.
10. Wash your hands.
11. Assist the resident to wash his or her hands and return to bed, if necessary.
12. Wash your hands and apply clean gloves.
13. Rinse and disinfect the bedpan or other container, if used, according to facility policy.
14. Remove one glove and place the specimen into the transport bag with your gloved hand. Avoid touching the outside of the bag with your glove. Handle the transport bag with your ungloved hand.
15. Remove the other glove and discard according to facility policy.
16. Wash your hands.
17. Record output, if the resident is on intake and output.
18. Perform your procedure completion actions.
19. Discard the plastic bag containing the waste in the biohazardous waste container.
20. Take the specimen to the designated location.
21. Report that the specimen was collected, and report any abnormalities to the nurse.

- The patient is asked to void. This first urine is discarded so that the bladder is empty at the time the test begins.
- All other urine is saved, including that voided as the test time finishes.
- No toilet tissue should be allowed to enter the container.
- If you or the patient forget to save a specimen during the test period, report it immediately to the nurse. The test must be discontinued and started again for another 24 hours.

Remember to put on disposable gloves and remove and dispose of them properly each time you collect a specimen.

Gastrointestinal System

Excretion of wastes from the gastrointestinal system (Figure 11.23) is called *bowel elimination*. A process called **peristalsis** moves the food from the upper end of the gastrointestinal system to the lower end. Peristalsis is caused by the contraction and relaxation of the muscles in the intestines. As the muscles contract, the food is propelled downward in the system. Food and fluids are taken in orally and partially digested by the stomach. They are mixed with digestive juices, then move from the stomach to the small intestine, where nutrients are

PROCEDURE

59 Collecting a 24-Hour Urine Specimen

1. Carry out beginning procedure actions.
2. Assemble equipment:
   - disposable gloves
   - 24-hour specimen container (supplied by health care facility)
   - label
   - bedpan, urinal, or commode, or specimen collector for toilet
   - plastic bag
   - sign for patient's bed
   - biohazard bag
3. Label the container with:
   - patient's name
   - room number
   - test ordered
   - type of specimen
   - time started
   - time ended
   - date
   - physician's name
4. Emphasize to the patient the necessity of saving all urine passed.
5. Place the specimen collection container in the bathroom in a pan of ice (Figures 11.22A and 11.22B). The ice will keep the specimen cool for 24 hours.
6. Put on disposable gloves.
7. Allow the patient to void.
   a. Assist with the bedpan or urinal as needed.
   b. Discard the urine specimen.
   c. Measure the amount of urine passed if the patient's I/O is being monitored.
   d. Note the date and time of voiding. This time will mark the start of the 24-hour collection.

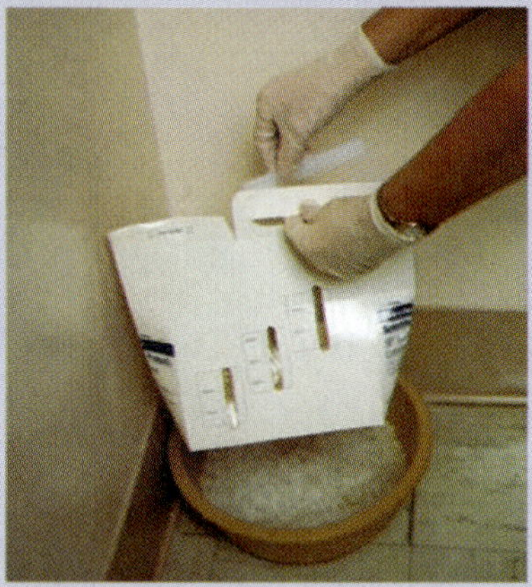

FIGURE 11-22A Close the container with the plastic fastener. Place the 24-hour specimen container in the patient's bathroom in a pan of ice.

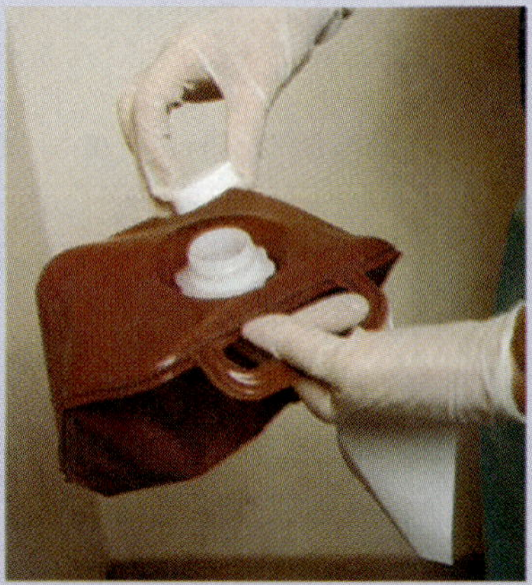

FIGURE 11-22B Some facilities use plastic containers for collecting a 24-hour specimen.

8. Place a sign on the patient's bed to alert other health care team members that a 24-hour urine specimen is being collected. (The sign may read: *Save all urine-24-hour specimen.*)
9. From this time on, for a period of 24 hours, all urine voided is added to the specimen container (Figure 11.22C). The container is kept on ice when not in use. Check facility policy regarding handling of the specimen container.

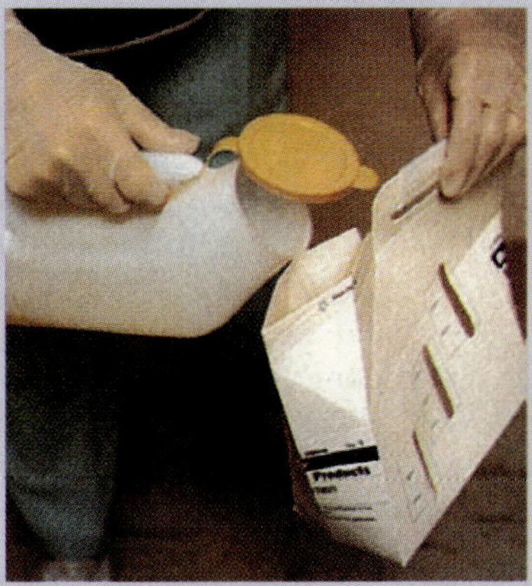

FIGURE 11-22C Open the mouth of the container wide to avoid spilling the specimen.

10. Instruct the patient not to discard toilet tissue into the specimen collection container. Provide small plastic bags for this purpose.
11. At the end of the 24-hour period:
    a. Put on disposable gloves.
    b. Ask the patient to void one last time.
    c. Add this urine to the specimen container.
12. Remove the sign from the patient's bed. Check the container label for accuracy and completeness. Attach the appropriate requisition slip.
13. Remove and dispose of gloves according to facility policy.
14. Place the specimen in a protective biohazard bag for transport.
15. Carry out procedure completion actions.
16. Clean and replace all equipment used, according to facility policy.
17. Follow facility policy for transporting the specimen to the laboratory.

absorbed and more digestion takes place. The food mass passes to the large intestine, where extra water is absorbed. After the liquid is absorbed, the solid food mass is called **feces**. The feces moves from the large intestine to the rectum, where it is stored until it is excreted through the **anus**. Additional water is absorbed from the stool in the rectum. The waste mate-

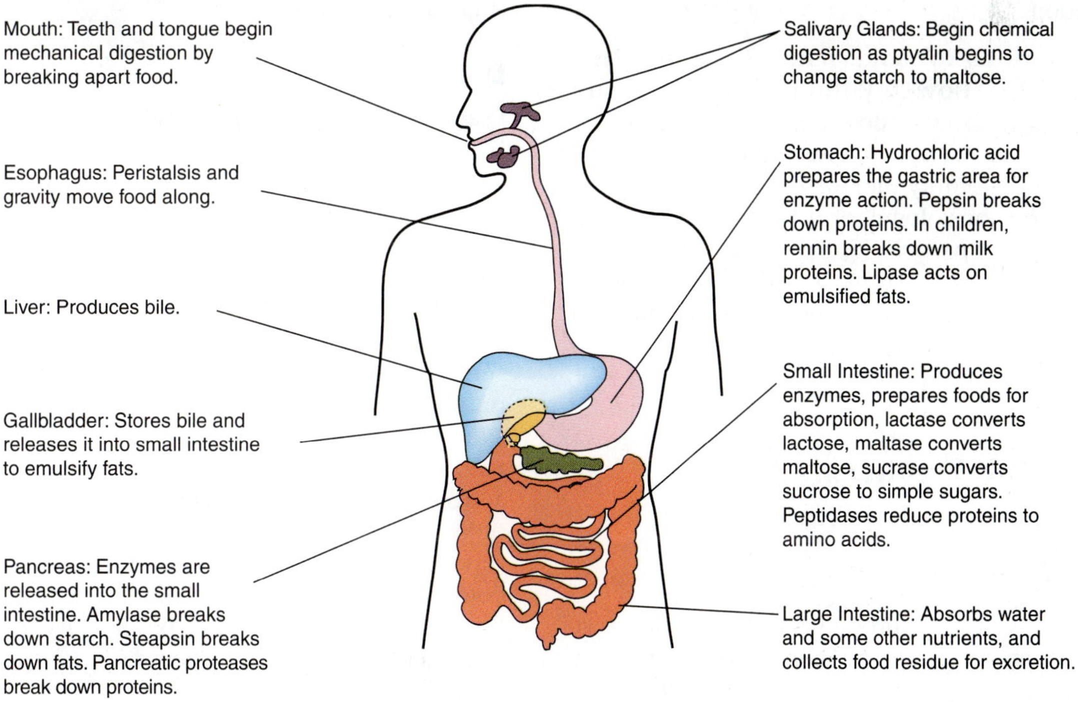

FIGURE 11-23 The gastrointestinal system.

rial excreted may be called feces, **fecal material**, **stool**, or **bowel movement (BM)**. The process of eliminating the waste from the anus is called **defecation**.

Bowel Elimination

The frequency of bowel movements varies with the individual. Some people have more than one bowel movement a day. Others have a bowel movement every two or three days. Fecal material is usually brown, but this color can be affected by certain foods, medications, and diseases. The bowel movement is normally soft and formed. If it passes through the colon too quickly, the stool is loose and watery. Passage of frequent liquid stools is called **diarrhea**. If it passes through too slowly, the fecal material becomes hard, dry, or sticky and pasty in consistency. This is called constipation. Certain foods, medications, infections, and diseases can cause constipation and diarrhea.

Flatus is intestinal gas. As foods move through the gastrointestinal tract by peristalsis, gas is formed. When the gas is expelled from the body, it is called "passing flatus," or flatulence. If the gas is not passed, it accumulates in the abdomen. The abdomen will enlarge and appear bloated. This is called **abdominal distention**, and is an important observation to report to the nurse. Abdominal distention may also be caused by constipation and urinary retention.

Observations to Make when Assisting Residents with Bowel Elimination. You must observe the color, odor, character, and consistency of the resident's bowel movement before discarding it. Notify the nurse if it has an unusual color, odor, or volume, or if blood, mucus, parasites, or food particles are present (except corn and raisins) in the stool. If you think a stool is abnormal, save the specimen for the nurse to assess.

Common Problems Related to the Gastrointestinal System

The most common problems in the gastrointestinal system are related to constipation, diarrhea, and excessive flatulence. Other problems are caused by cancer, diseases, and trauma.

Constipation and Fecal Impaction

Report problems with constipation to the nurse. If the resident has not had a bowel movement in more than three days, must strain to pass stool, or passes hard, marble-like stools, this is an indication of constipation. **Fecal impaction** (Figure 11.24) is the most serious form of constipation. This is caused by retention of stool in the rectum. Water is absorbed in the rectum, causing the fecal mass to become hard and dry. The resident may be unable to pass it. The resident may complain of abdominal or rectal pain, nausea, or lack of appetite. Sometimes fecal impaction will cause mental confusion and fever. Other signs and symptoms of fecal impaction are passing excessive flatus, bloating, frequent urination, inability to empty the bladder, or leaking around the catheter. Residents may complain of feeling the need to have a bowel movement, but being unable to do so. Eventually, liquid stool begins to seep from the rectum. This is easily mistaken for diarrhea. It occurs because liquid feces pass through the colon to the rectum, but are obstructed by the hard fecal mass. The rectum becomes so full that the fluid escapes around the impaction and is eliminated from the body. Fecal impaction is a very serious condition that is usually treated by manual removal of the mass by the nurse. Laxatives and enemas are also used to treat fecal impaction. The best thing to do is observe the resident's bowel elimination carefully and prevent fecal impaction from occurring.

Diarrhea

Diarrhea occurs when peristalsis in the intestines is very rapid. The need to defecate may be very urgent if the resident has diarrhea. The resident may also complain of abdominal pain and cramping. Some residents may become incontinent because of the force with which the fecal material moves through the intestines.

Diarrhea can cause dehydration and other serious medical problems if undetected or untreated. Most health care facilities do not consider one loose stool to be diarrhea. Diarrhea is usually defined as three or more loose stools in a designated period of time. Remember to be objective in reporting your observations. When reporting loose stools to the nurse, report the color, odor, consistency, character, amount, and frequency of stools. Also report any resident complaints of pain or other discomfort. If the resident is on intake and output, you may be asked to record the output from diarrhea. Use

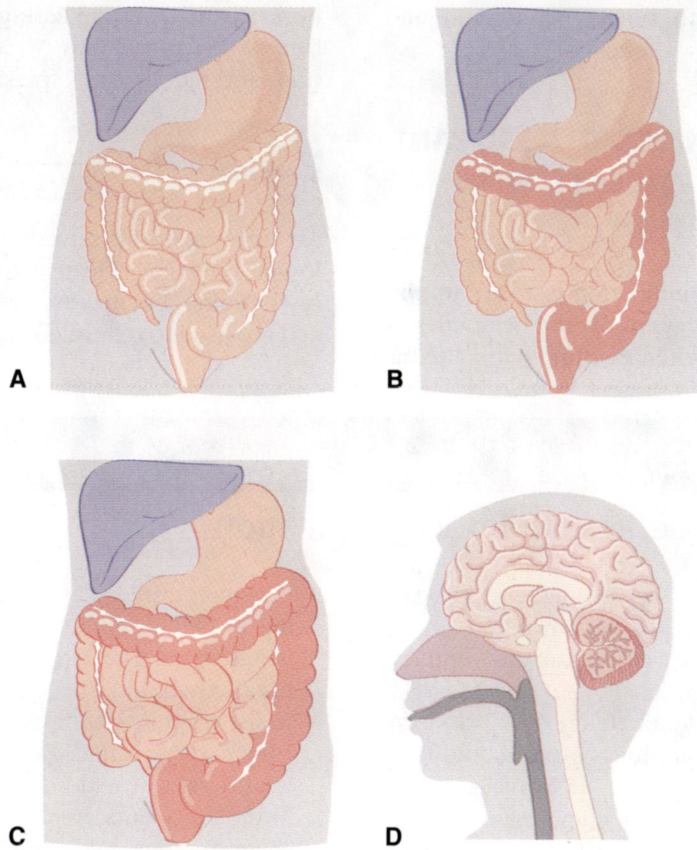

FIGURE 11-24 Progression of a fecal impaction, a life-threatening condition: **A.** A fecal impaction blocks the rectum. The rectum and sigmoid colon become enlarged. **B.** The colon continues to enlarge. **C.** Fecal material fills the colon. Digested and undigested food back up into the small intestines and stomach. The resident has signs and symptoms of acute illness, including lethargy, distention, constipation, and pain that is dull and cramping. **D.** The entire system is full, and the resident vomits fecal material. The feces are commonly aspirated into the lungs. At this point, the condition is life-threatening.

a specimen collection hat or graduate. Select PPE appropriate to the task. Avoid showing disgust for the procedure. Maintain a professional demeanor.

Changes in Function of the Gastrointestinal System Associated with Aging and Disease

Change in bowel function may be caused by aging, disease, surgery, diet, and medications. Lack of privacy may also affect the resident's ability to have a bowel movement. In aging, movement in the colon is decreased. Food absorption is slowed, and fewer digestive juices are produced. Constipation is a common problem. Other factors that affect bowel function are:

- Bed rest
- Inactivity
- Inadequate exercise
- Inability to chew foods properly
- Loose or missing teeth
- Inadequate fluid intake
- Stress
- Change in environment
- Change in diet

A diet that does not contain enough fiber, fruits, or vegetables may cause constipation and other nutritional problems.

Bowel Incontinence

Bowel incontinence is involuntary passage of fecal material from the anus. It has many causes, including trauma, neurological diseases, inability to reach the toilet quickly, and mental confusion. Fecal material is very irritating to the skin, so the resident must be cleansed well after each episode of incontinence. Skin exposed to fecal material will break down quickly. Bowel incontinence may lower the resident's self-esteem. Be professional, compassionate, and understanding when assisting residents with bowel elimination and incontinence.

Role of the Nursing Assistant in Assisting Residents with Bowel Elimination

Assisting with bowel elimination is a very important responsibility. Always apply the principles of standard precautions when assisting with elimination. Avoid contaminating environmental surfaces with your gloves. Wear a gown, eye protection, and face mask if splashing is likely.

Enemas

An **enema** is the introduction of fluid into the lower bowel to cleanse the anus, rectum, and lower colon. Enemas are ordered by the physician and are used to relieve constipation and empty the

GUIDELINES FOR

Assisting Residents with Bowel Elimination

- Apply the principles of standard precautions when assisting with bowel elimination. Avoid contaminating the environment with your gloves.
- Encourage residents to consume an adequate amount of fluid. Maintaining fluid intake is as important for bowel elimination as it is for urinary elimination.
- Encourage residents to eat a well-balanced diet.
- Allow adequate time for residents to eat meals.
- Encourage residents to chew food well. Cut food into small pieces if necessary. Report chewing problems to the nurse for further assessment.
- If you observe that a resident has not eaten fiber foods, fruits, or vegetables, offer a substitute. The dietitian may have to visit the resident to discuss likes and dislikes and assure that the resident will eat the foods served.
- Encourage exercise and activity as allowed and as tolerated.
- Assist residents with toileting at regular intervals and provide privacy.
- Position residents in a sitting position, if allowed, for bowel elimination.
- Use a bath blanket to cover residents when using the bedpan or commode, for privacy and warmth.
- Leave the call signal and toilet tissue within reach and respond to the call signal immediately.
- Allow adequate time for defecation.
- Provide perineal care as needed, or according to facility policy. Fecal material is very irritating to the skin and promotes skin breakdown and infection.
- Assist residents with cleaning the anal area (this may be called the rectal area by some health care providers).
- Assist residents with handwashing and other personal hygiene after bowel elimination.
- Monitor bowel elimination and report irregularities.
- Record bowel movements on the flow sheet or other designated location. If a resident is independent with bowel elimination, ask if he or she has had a bowel movement each day. In some facilities, the size of the bowel elimination is documented. The most common measurements used are small, medium, large, and extra large. Your facility will have guidelines for these amounts. In general, small is a 3-inch elimination, medium is a 6-inch elimination, large is a 9-inch elimination, and extra large is a 12-inch elimination.
- Report frequent stools, absence of stools, pain, cramping, excessive flatulence, abnormal color or consistency of stool, extremely small amounts of stool, hard, dry stool, or enlargement of the abdomen to the nurse.
- Specific abnormalities in stools to report are presence of blood, pus, mucus, black or other unusual color, undigested food (except corn and raisins), or presence of parasites in the stool.

colon before some tests and surgeries. Occasionally, enemas are given to relieve excessive flatulence. The physician always specifies the type of enema to give and the solution to use. The nursing assistant is responsible for administering enemas in many health care facilities. Always apply the principles of standard precautions when you are performing this procedure. Avoid contaminating environmental surfaces with your gloves.

A **cleansing enema** removes fecal material from the rectum and lower bowel. It also stimulates peristalsis and softens stool. A water-based solution is used in a cleansing enema. The cleansing enema is administered through a special enema bag or other container.

A **retention enema** may be given for constipation or fecal impaction. An oil-based solution, packaged in a small, commercial container, is used for the retention enema. The purpose of this enema is to soften hard stool and gently stimulate evacuation. The enema lubricates the rectum, making it easier to pass the stool.

Commercially prepared enemas (Figure 11.25) are administered in small, premeasured containers. Commercially prepared enemas are available with either cleansing or retention enema solutions.

The **Sims' position** (Figure 11.26) is a side-lying position used for giving enemas, rectal examinations, and other rectal treatments. This position promotes evacuation of the bowel. To assist a resident into the Sims' position, turn

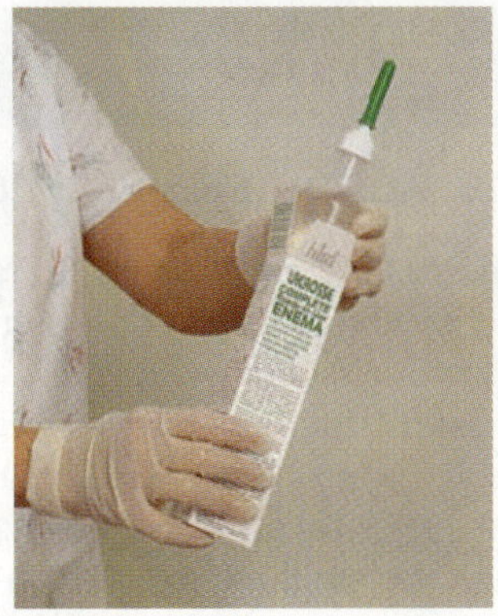

FIGURE 11-25 A commercially prepared enema

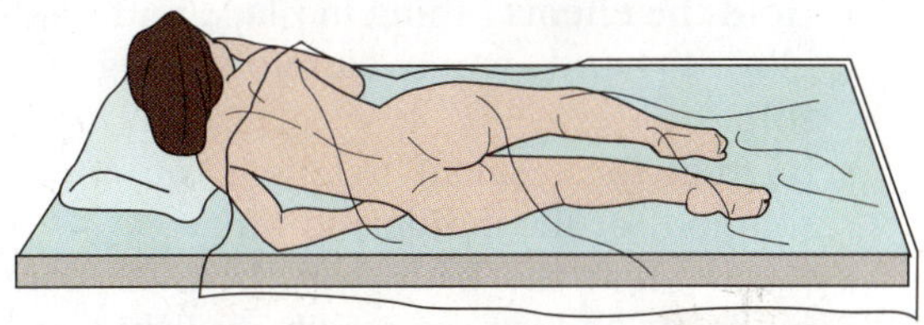

FIGURE 11-26 The Sims' position is used for enema administration and rectal treatments.

GUIDELINES FOR

Enema Administration

- Apply the principles of standard precautions. Avoid contaminating the environment with your gloves.
- Administer an enema only upon the direction of a licensed nurse.
- Avoid giving an enema within an hour after a meal, because the increased peristalsis makes it difficult for the resident to retain the solution. Avoid administering an enema to a resident who is in a sitting position, such as on the toilet. The solution will not flow high into the colon when administered to a resident who is seated. It will cause the rectum to enlarge, causing rapid expulsion of the fluid.
- Consult the care plan or nurse for the amount and type of solution to use and any special instructions.
- Provide privacy. Cover the resident with a bath blanket.
- Check the temperature of a water-based solution with a bath thermometer. The solution temperature should be 105 °F.
- Commercially prepared enemas can be administered at room temperature, or warmed by placing the container in a basin of warm water.
- Lubricate the tip of the enema tubing well with a water-based lubricant before inserting it into the rectum. Most disposable units are prelubricated. However, if the tip appears dry, apply additional lubricant before inserting it into the rectum.
- Insert the enema tube gently into the rectum. The tube should be inserted two to four inches. If you meet resistance, do not force the tube. Remove it and consult the nurse.

GUIDELINES FOR

Enema Administration, *continued*

- An enema in a bag should be raised 12 to 16 inches above the rectum (Figure 11.27). Follow your facility policy.
- Administer the enema solution slowly. Instruct the resident to inhale and breathe in slowly through the nose and exhale through the mouth. If the resident complains of pain, stop the solution briefly before proceeding. If the pain is severe or persistent, stop the solution and notify the nurse.
- Hold the enema tubing in place with your gloved hand when administering the solution.
- Instruct the resident to retain the enema solution for the designated time.
- Ensure that the bathroom, bedside commode, or bedpan are readily available.
- Assist the resident to a sitting position on the bedpan, commode, or toilet, if possible, to expel the enema.
- Leave the resident alone to expel the enema solution, if doing so is safe. Place the signal light and toilet tissue within reach.
- Respond promptly when the resident signals.
- Save the enema results for the nurse to observe before discarding.
- Assist the resident to cleanse the perineal area and wash hands after the enema has been expelled.

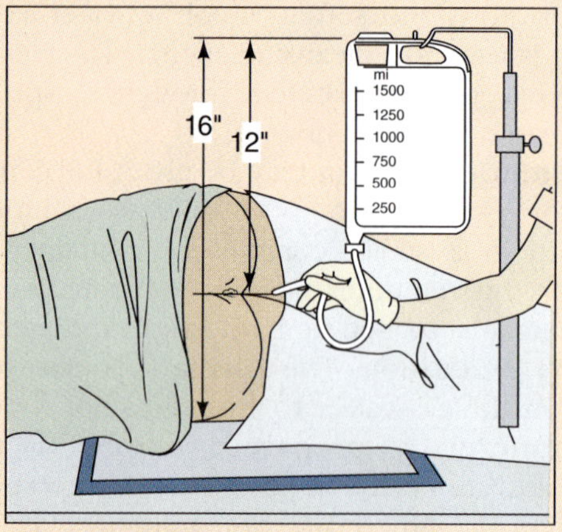

FIGURE 11-27 Hang the enema bag 12 to 16 inches above the rectum.

PROCEDURE 60

Administering a Cleansing Enema

Note: In some states, nursing assistants are not permitted to perform this procedure. Additionally, the policies of some facilities state that only licensed nurses may perform rectal treatments, including enemas. Perform this procedure only if you are permitted to do so by state law and facility policies.

1. Perform your beginning procedure actions.
2. Gather supplies needed: assembled enema kit, prescribed solution, water-soluble lubricant, bath blanket, bath thermometer, bed protector, bedpan, toilet tissue, washcloth, towel, washbasin, paper towel, plastic bag, gloves.
3. Close the clamp on the enema container.
4. Prepare the enema solution in the bathroom or utility room, according to facility policy. Fill the enema container with water in the specified amount. This usually varies from 500 to 1500 mL, but more or less solution can be used. Follow the nurse's instructions. Check the water temperature with a bath thermometer. It should be 105 °F.
5. If you are instructed to administer a soapsuds enema, empty the contents of the soap packet into the container *after* the water has been added. Squeeze and agitate the bag slightly to mix the solution.

6. Open the clamp on the tubing and allow the solution to flow through the tubing to the tip, to prevent the injection of air into the body. Close the clamp when the solution begins to flow through the tip.
7. Take the solution to the bedside. Squeeze some water-soluble lubricant onto a paper towel or gauze sponge.
8. Place the bed protector under the buttocks. Cover the upper bedding with a bath blanket, then remove the linen from under the blanket without exposing the resident.
9. Assist the resident into the Sims' position and ensure that he or she is comfortable.
10. Apply gloves.
11. Expose the rectal area.
12. Remove the cap from the end of the tubing, and lubricate the tube if it is not prelubricated. If the tip appears dry, apply extra lubricant.
13. Separate the buttocks to expose the anal area.
14. Tell the resident you are going to insert the tube and ask him or her to take a deep breath and then exhale.
15. Gently insert the enema tubing two to four inches while the resident exhales.
16. Hold the solution 12 to 16 inches above the rectum, or according to facility policy.
17. Unclamp the tubing and allow the solution to flow into the rectum. Instruct the resident to try to relax and retain the solution.
18. Allow the desired amount of solution to flow into the rectum. When the fluid level reaches the bottom of the bag, clamp the tubing to avoid injecting air into the rectum.
19. Remove the tubing and insert the tip into the enema administration container.
20. Instruct the resident to retain the solution for the designated amount of time.
21. Place the enema container in a plastic bag.
22. Remove your gloves and place them in the plastic bag.
23. Assist the resident to the bathroom or commode, or place the bedpan. Instruct the resident not to flush the toilet after expelling the enema.
24. Make sure the resident is safe, warm, and comfortable. Leave the signal light and toilet tissue within reach.
25. Wash your hands.
26. Leave the room if doing so is safe. Take the plastic bag containing the enema container and gloves and discard it in the biohazardous waste.
27. Return immediately when the resident signals.
28. Apply gloves and assist the resident with cleansing and perineal care.
29. Remove one glove or use a paper towel to turn on the faucet, and assist the resident with hand-washing.
30. Remove the bed protector with the gloved hand, and discard according to facility policy.
31. Remove the other glove and discard according to facility policy.
32. Wash your hands.
33. Assist the resident back to bed, or position the resident in bed for comfort and safety.
34. Observe the results of the enema and save them for the nurse, or discard according to facility policy.
35. Perform your procedure completion actions.
36. Observe and report to the nurse:
    - Type of enema and amount of solution
    - Results of the enema, estimated amount of solution returned, amount and consistency of stool
    - Unusual observations (if noted, save the returns for the nurse to assess)
    - Presence of blood, mucus, undigested food (except corn and raisins), or parasites in stool
    - Resident's response to the procedure

PROCEDURE

61 Administering a Commercially Prepared Enema

Note: In some states, nursing assistants are not permitted to perform this procedure. Additionally, the policies of some facilities state that only licensed nurses may perform rectal treatments, including enemas. Perform this procedure only if you are permitted to do so by state law and facility policies.

1. Perform your beginning procedure actions.
2. Gather supplies needed: commercial enema, water-soluble lubricant, bath blanket, bed protector, bedpan, toilet tissue, washcloth, towel, washbasin, plastic bag, paper towel, gloves.
3. Warm the container of enema solution in a basin of warm water, if this is your facility policy. Dry the outside of the container.
4. Take the solution to the bedside.
5. Place the bed protector under the buttocks. Cover the upper bedding with a bath blanket, then remove the linen from under the blanket without exposing the resident.
6. Assist the resident into the Sims' position and ensure that he or she is comfortable.
7. Apply gloves.
8. Expose the rectal area.
9. Remove the cap from the end of the container and lubricate the tip, if it is not prelubricated.
10. Separate the buttocks to expose the anal area.
11. Tell the resident you are going to insert the tube and ask him or her to take a deep breath and then exhale.
12. Gently insert the tip of the container while the resident exhales.
13. Gently squeeze and roll the container until the desired quantity of solution is administered. A small amount of solution will remain in the container. Avoid releasing pressure on the container, or the solution will return.
14. Instruct the resident to hold his or her breath, then gently remove the tip of the container.
15. Place the enema container in a plastic bag to avoid contamination.
16. Remove your gloves and place them in the plastic bag.
17. Assist the resident to the bathroom or commode, or place the bedpan. Instruct the resident not to flush the toilet after expelling the enema.
18. Make sure the resident is safe, warm, and comfortable. Leave the signal light and toilet tissue within reach.
19. Wash your hands.
20. Leave the room if doing so is safe. Take the plastic bag containing the enema container and gloves, and discard it in the biohazardous waste.
21. Return immediately when the resident signals.
22. Apply gloves and assist the resident with cleansing and perineal care.
23. Remove one glove or use a paper towel to turn on the faucet, and assist the resident with handwashing.
24. Remove the bed protector with the gloved hand and discard it according to facility policy.
25. Remove the other glove and discard it according to facility policy.
26. Wash your hands.

27. Assist the resident back to bed, or position the resident in bed for comfort and safety.
28. Observe the results of the enema and save for the nurse, or discard according to facility policy.
29. Perform your procedure completion actions.
30. Observe and report to the nurse:
    - Type of enema and amount of solution
    - Results of the enema, estimated amount of solution returned, and amount and consistency of stool
    - Unusual observations (if noted, save the returns for the nurse to assess)
    - Presence of blood, mucus, undigested food (except corn and raisins), or parasites in stool
    - Resident's response to the procedure

him or her onto the left side. Position the shoulder, arm, and hip for comfort. Bend the right leg at the knee and flex the leg forward slightly.

Collecting a Stool Specimen

Stool specimens are collected and analyzed by the laboratory for presence of blood, parasites, fat, bacteria, and other abnormalities. Analysis of the stool assists the physician with diagnosis and treatment. The resident is instructed to defecate in a specimen collection device, commode, or bedpan. The stool is then transferred into the specimen collection container and packaged according to facility policy prior to transport to the laboratory. The resident should be instructed not to urinate into the stool specimen. Follow the general guidelines for collecting a urine specimen when collecting a stool specimen. Apply the principles of standard precautions. Some stool specimens must be analyzed while warm, so they must be transported to the laboratory immediately. Check with the care plan or nurse for special directions for the type of specimen you are collecting.

Caring For Residents With Ostomies

An **ostomy** is a surgically created opening into the body. There are many types of ostomies (Figure 11.28). Some are performed for bowel elimination. These are usually done because of cancer, bowel disease, and trauma. The opening to the outside of the body is called a **stoma**. An ostomy may be temporary or permanent. The location of the ostomy is determined by the part of the colon that is injured or diseased.

In most facilities, a licensed nurse will care for a newly created ostomy. However, in residents with well-established ostomies, the nursing assistant is usually responsible for caring for the area. Know and follow your facility policy.

Colostomies

The **colostomy** is the most common type of ostomy. This ostomy is located between the colon and the abdomen. The intestines are brought to the outside of the body to create the stoma. A bag is attached to the stoma to collect fecal material. When the ostomy is first performed, the stool is loose and watery, but becomes soft and formed over time. The amount of liquid in the stool is also determined by how much of the colon remains after surgery. If a large amount of colon is left, the colon will absorb water and the stools will be formed. If most of the colon has been removed, the body will be unable to absorb the water in the stool, so the stools in the ostomy are more liquid. Flatus is also passed through the stoma.

Many people live successfully for years with an ostomy, but this type of surgery is very difficult for the resident to adjust to psychologically. Residents are often upset by this change in normal function. They worry about the appliance showing under their clothing. They also worry about odors and sounds that are offensive. The resident may have to adjust the diet to avoid gasforming foods. Adjusting a dietary pattern that a person has established over a lifetime may be difficult. The resident with an ostomy requires you to be very professional, tactful, patient, and understanding.

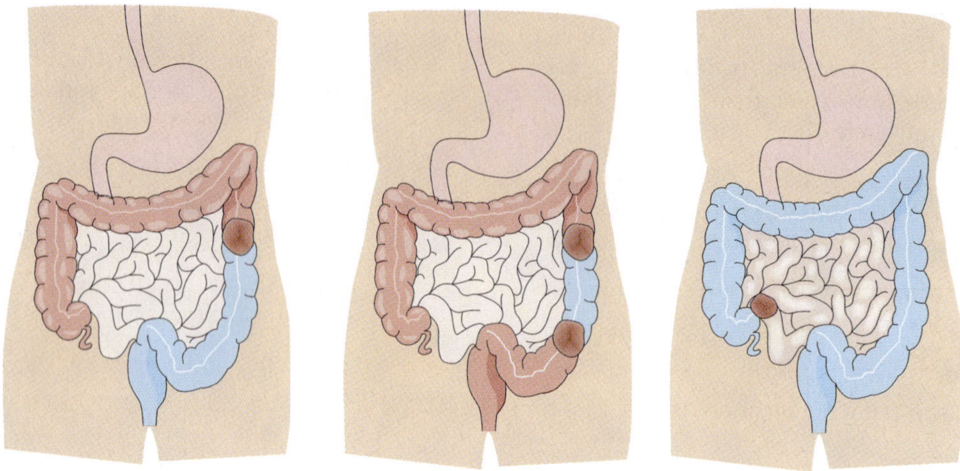

FIGURE 11-28 The location of the ostomy determines the amount of water in the stool. The double-barrel colostomy is usually temporary. After the digestive system rests, the intestines are surgically reconnected.

PROCEDURE 62 Collecting a Stool Specimen

1. Perform your beginning procedure actions.
2. Gather needed supplies: bedpan and cover, commode, or specimen collection pan; specimen container with lid; transport bag; tongue blade; toilet tissue; plastic bag; gloves.
3. Complete the label and put it on the container.
4. Ask the resident to defecate into the designated collection device. Instruct him or her not to discard toilet tissue into the collection device. Provide a plastic bag for this purpose.
5. Provide privacy and make sure the call signal and toilet tissue are within reach.
6. Return immediately when the resident signals.
7. Apply gloves and remove the stool specimen collection container.
8. Provide a clean container or bedpan for urination, if necessary. Allow the resident to urinate. Provide privacy.
9. Cover the specimen collection container and assist the resident with cleansing, returning to bed, or positioning. Wear gloves and apply the principles of standard precautions if appropriate to the activity.
10. Take the collection device to the bathroom or other designated location according to facility policy.
11. Open the specimen collection cup and place the lid on the counter, with the top side down.
12. Apply gloves.
13. Uncover the container. Use the tongue blade to remove the feces from the collection device and place it in the specimen container. About two tablespoons of stool are necessary. Taking a small sample from each part of the stool is best. Discard the tongue blade in the plastic bag.
14. Put the lid on the specimen container. Place the container on a paper towel on the counter.

15. Rinse and disinfect the bedpan or collection container according to facility policy.
16. Remove one glove and place the specimen into the transport bag with your gloved hand. Avoid touching the outside of the bag with your glove. Handle the transport bag with your ungloved hand.
17. Remove the other glove and discard according to facility policy.
18. Wash your hands.
19. Perform your procedure completion actions.
20. Discard the plastic bag containing the waste in the biohazardous waste container.
21. Take the specimen to the designated location.
22. Report that the specimen was collected, and report any abnormalities to the nurse.

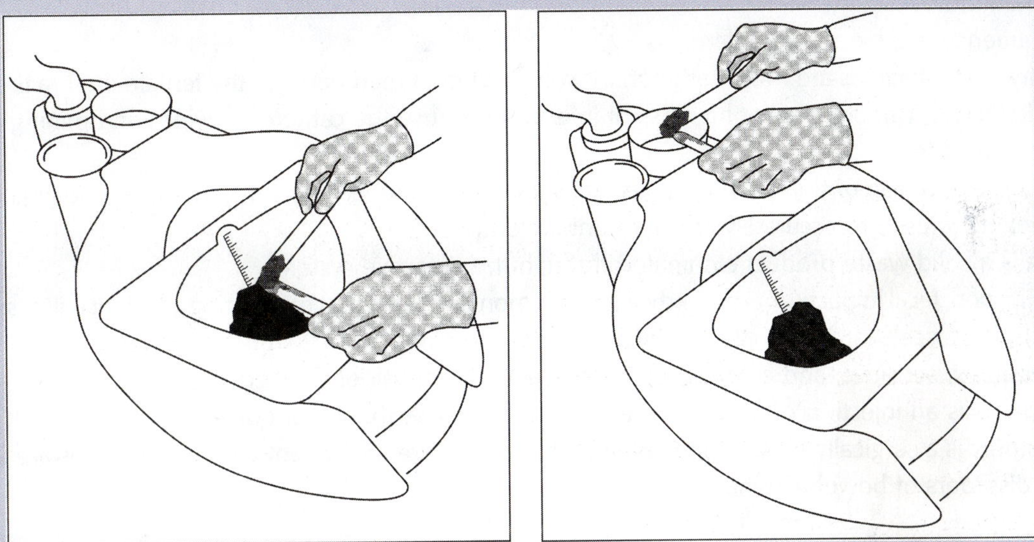

FIGURE 11-29 Use tongue blades to transfer the specimen from the collection device to the specimen cup.

The Ostomy Appliance. The ostomy **appliance** (Figure 11.30) is the plastic container into which the contents of the bowel are emptied. It is fastened to the body with a belt or a self-adhesive seal around the bag. Remember that fecal material is very irritating to the skin. A new ostomy is sore and tender. The fecal material, particularly liquid stool, causes additional irritation. Even established ostomies become irritated from the combination of fecal material and adhesive on the skin. The care plan will guide you in caring for the ostomy. Report redness or skin irritation to the nurse. Always apply the principles of standard precautions when caring for the ostomy appliance.

Odors from ostomies are a particular problem. Good personal hygiene is essential. The skin around the stoma is washed and dried well each time the bag is removed. A special skin

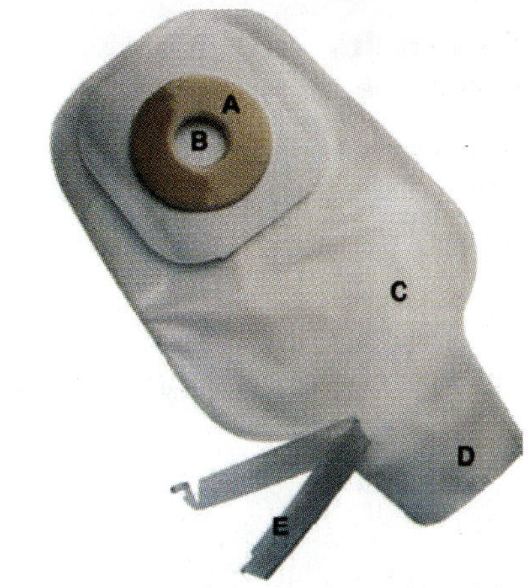

A. Adhesive ring seals around stoma to prevent leakage
B. Opening placed over stoma
C. Collection bag
D. Drainage end of bag
E. Secures drainage end of bag to prevent leakage

FIGURE 11-30 A disposable ostomy appliance.

barrier product may also be used. The used bag is discarded in the biohazardous waste. Various deodorizing products are available to place inside the bag to reduce or eliminate odors. Only nurses or nursing assistant II may apply new ostomy appliance.

KEY POINTS

- The urinary system regulates water in the body and filters waste products from the blood and eliminates them from the body.
- The average adult eliminates 1500 mL of urine from the body each day. Additional fluid is lost in respiration, perspiration, and bowel elimination.
- The nursing assistant must be professional, sensitive, and understanding when assisting residents with elimination needs.
- Incontinence is a medical problem.
- Urinary tract infections are more common in women than in men because the female urethra is shorter.
- Residents with catheters are at high risk of infection because the catheter provides an opening directly into the bladder.
- Maintaining sterility of the catheter by using aseptic technique is a very important responsibility.
- A graduate is used to accurately measure urinary output.
- Feces is a solid waste product eliminated through the digestive system.
- Constipation, fecal impaction, and diarrhea are common problems that the nursing assistant will assist with.
- The resident's self-esteem is affected by problems with elimination, and the nursing assistant must be professional, sensitive, and compassionate in meeting the resident's needs.
- An enema is an injection of fluid into the rectum to cleanse the lower bowel.
- An ostomy is a surgically created opening into the body. Several different types of ostomies are used to treat disorders of bowel elimination.

REVIEW

A. Multiple Choice

Select the one best answer.

1. The urinary system
   a. removes solid waste from the digestive tract.
   b. removes waste from the blood and regulates water in the body.
   c. recirculates waste products through the system.
   d. removes waste from the pancreas and intestines.

2. The average adult eliminates
   a. 500 mL of urine per day.
   b. 1000 mL of urine per day.
   c. 1500 mL of urine per day.
   d. 4500 mL of urine per day.

3. Which of the following affect urinary elimination?
   a. starches
   b. salt
   c. sugars
   d. high-fiber foods

4. Incontinence
   a. occurs naturally in aging.
   b. is always a psychological problem.
   c. is a medical problem.
   d. always occurs when residents are confused.

5. Aging and disease may affect
   a. length of the urethra.
   b. the kidney's ability to filter efficiently.
   c. color of urine.
   d. clarity of urine.

6. A common cause of urge incontinence is
   a. infection.
   b. multiple childbirths.
   c. physical inability to get to the bathroom.
   d. lifting heavy objects.
7. Which of the following are signs or symptoms of urinary tract infection?
   a. diarrhea
   b. voiding frequently in small amounts
   c. vomiting
   d. profuse sweating
8. A container that the male resident uses for urination in bed is the
   a. urinal.
   b. regular bedpan.
   c. fracture bedpan.
   d. indwelling catheter.
9. A catheter is used
   a. for staff convenience.
   b. to drain urine from the bladder.
   c. to obstruct the bladder so urine cannot escape.
   d. only for diagnostic tests.
10. The inside of the unopened closed drainage system is
    a. clean.
    b. contaminated.
    c. septic.
    d. sterile.
11. When a resident is in bed, the catheter drainage bag should be positioned
    a. above the level of the bladder.
    b. on the bed frame above the floor.
    c. on the side rail above the floor.
    d. on the floor.
12. When caring for a catheter, you should practice
    a. contact precautions.
    b. airborne precautions.
    c. medical asepsis.
    d. isolation technique.
13. The catheter should always be
    a. secured to the resident's body.
    b. opened and cleaned twice a day.
    c. washed from bottom to top with alcohol.
    d. drained every two hours.
14. The adhesive strip that secures the external catheter to the penis should be wrapped
    a. in a circle.
    b. diagonally.
    c. in a spiral.
    d. very tightly.
15. Condom catheters should be disposed of in the
    a. trash can in the resident's room.
    b. biohazardous waste.
    c. puncture-resistant container.
    d. sanitary sewer.
16. You are assigned to measure urinary output on Mr. Davis, a resident with an indwelling catheter. To obtain an accurate measurement, you should
    a. record the level of urine according to the markings on the catheter bag.
    b. empty the catheter bag into a bedpan.
    c. withdraw the urine with a syringe.
    d. empty the catheter bag into a graduate.
17. When preparing to collect a midstream urine specimen from a female resident, you should wipe the labia
    a. from front to back.
    b. from back to front.
    c. back and forth.
    d. from side to side.
18. Water is absorbed from fecal material in the
    a. stomach.
    b. small intestine.
    c. large intestine.
    d. liver.
19. The medical term for passing gas is
    a. impaction.
    b. distention.
    c. flatulence.
    d. obstruction.
20. The most serious form of constipation is
    a. flatulence.
    b. impaction.
    c. distention.
    d. diarrhea.
21. Which of the following affect normal bowel elimination?
    a. sugar in food
    b. inadequate fluid intake

c. confusion
d. skin breakdown

22. The enema tubing is inserted into the rectum

a. 1 to 2 inches.
b. 2 to 4 inches.
c. 4 to 6 inches.
d. 6 to 8 inches.

23. The opening of a colostomy to the outside of the body is called the

a. rectum.
b. insertion site.
c. stoma.
d. appliance.

24. Fecal material is

a. very irritating to the skin.
b. normally liquid.
c. excreted through the urethra.
d. hard and pasty.

25. The ostomy appliance is

a. an irrigating device.
b. similar to a catheter.
c. difficult to apply.
d. a plastic bag.

B. Clinical Applications

Answer the following questions.

26. Mr. Hoover is a 76-year-old confused resident. He ambulates in his room and is normally pleasant and talkative, even though he does not always make sense. He recognizes you as his primary caregiver. Mr. Hoover uses the urinal for elimination. When you enter his room to give AM care, you find him sleeping in the chair, which is unusual. His skin is hot to the touch and he is lethargic. He does not speak or answer your questions. You notice his urinal on the floor next to his chair. The urine in the urinal is reddish in color with mucus threads in it. What should you do?

27. Mrs. Sanders tells you that she has burning on urination. You notice that she is voiding every 30 to 45 minutes in small amounts. What do you think is wrong? What should you do?

28. Miss Gonzalez has just started eating her breakfast. The nurse instructs you to give the resident an enema this morning. What should you do?

29. Mr. Deck has a colostomy. You change the bag and care for the stoma each day. When you remove the self-adhesive bag, Mr. Deck flinches as if in pain. The area around the stoma is very red. What should you do?

30. You are assigned to collect a stat midstream urine specimen from Mrs. King. The resident accidentally contaminates the specimen with BM. What should you do?

B: Applying Warm or Cold Applications

OBJECTIVES

After reading this unit, you will be able to:

- Spell and define terms.
- List the physical conditions requiring the use of heat and cold.
- Name types of heat and cold applications.
- Describe the effects of local cold applications.
- Describe the effects of local heat applications.
- List safety concerns related to application of heat and cold.
- Demonstrate the following procedures:
  - Applying an Ice Bag
  - Applying a Disposable Cold Pack
  - Applying an Aquamatic K-Pad®
  - Performing a Warm Soak
  - Applying a Warm Moist Compress
  - Assisting with Application of a Hypothermia Blanket

INTRODUCTION

Heat and cold applications are used only on written orders from the physician or nurse, and only for a specific length of time. Some facilities allow only professional personnel to apply heat and cold. **Some states have laws against nursing assistants applying heat or cold in a home health setting**. In other facilities, nursing assistants who have been specially trained are permitted to carry out these procedures under the supervision of the nurse. Be sure you know and follow the policy of your facility and are adequately prepared and *supervised*.

THERAPY WITH HEAT AND COLD

The physician orders the use of heat or cold applications to:

- relieve pain.
- combat local infection, swelling, or inflammation.
- control bleeding **(hemorrhage)**.
- reduce body temperature.

Local applications of heat and cold are made with:

- Ice bags.
- Electronically operated Aquamatic K-Pads®. K-Pads® come in many shapes and sizes. They can be used to apply dry heat. By using an attachment, they can also be used for cooling.
- Prepackaged, single-use units for the application of hot and cold. A single hit on the surface activates the contents, providing a controlled temperature.
- Gel packs that can be cooled or heated as needed.

General treatments of heat and cold consist of thermal mattresses known as **hypothermia-hyperthermia blankets**. These are widely used to:

- lower body temperature when there is fever.
- elevate body temperature in cases of hypothermia.

Applications of warm and cold may be either dry or moist. Moisture makes both heat and cold more penetrating. Therefore, moist heat or moist cold is more likely to cause injury. Extra care must be taken to protect the patient when moist treatments are used. Be sure you know:

- Exact method to be used
- Correct temperature and placement
- Proper length of time the warm or cold application is to be performed
- How often the area being treated is to be checked

Table 11.1 summarizes types of warm and cold applications.

TABLE 11-1 Warm and Cold Applications

Dry Warm Applications	Dry Cold Applications
Aquamatic K-Pad®	Ice cap
Disposable warm pack	Ice bag
Electric heating pads	Disposable cold pack
Aquathermia blanket	Aquamatic K-Pad®
	Hypothermia blanket
Moist Warm Applications	**Moist Cold Applications**
Warm soaks	Compresses
Compresses	Soaks
Tub baths	Packs
Sitz baths	

Commercial Preparations

Easy-to-use commercial warm and cold packs are available for dry applications. For one type of pack, a single hit or blow to the pack before application activates it. The pack is discarded after one use. Reusable packs are also available, but infection control issues make them less desirable.

Use of Cold Applications

Applications of cold are given only with a physician's order. The application of cold:

- Constricts or decreases the size of blood vessels (**vasoconstriction**) and reduces swelling
- Decreases sensitivity to pain
- Reduces temperature
- Slows inflammation
- Reduces itching

GUIDELINES FOR

Warm and Cold Treatments

You must be very watchful when applying cold or warm treatments. When assigned to this task, keep in mind the following:

- The age and condition of the patient. Give extra care to:
  - Young children
  - The aged
  - Patients with cognitive impairment
  - Patients who are uncooperative
  - Patients who are unconscious
  - Patients who are paralyzed
  - Patients with tissue damage
  - Patients with poor circulation
- Apply the principles of standard precautions if your hands will contact blood, moist body fluids (except sweat), secretions, excretions, nonintact skin, or mucous membranes.
- If the patient has a dressing covering the area to be treated, consult the nurse for directions.
- Check the temperature of the solution with a thermometer. You may need to add more liquid during the treatment to maintain the temperature. Avoid pouring hot or cold liquid directly over the patient.
- Remove all metal jewelry, buttons, or zippers that could conduct heat or cold and thereby injure the skin.
- Avoid using heat treatments with temperatures over 110°F. Temperatures greater than this can cause burns, particularly in infants and the elderly.
- Avoid using heat in the first 48 hours after an injury.
- Follow all safety rules to prevent spills and falls.
- An electric heating pad must not be used with moist dressings unless a rubber cover is placed over the pad. If the wires become damp, a short circuit may result. The patient must not lie on the pad, because severe burns can result. Sensitivity to heat varies, so patients receiving heat treatments must be checked frequently. Although heating pads are not used in health care facilities, they are used by individuals in homes.
- Heat is not applied to the head because it could make blood vessels in the area dilate, causing headache.
- Heat should not be applied to the abdomen if there is any chance that the

patient has appendicitis, because it would increase the chance of the appendix rupturing.

- Check the skin under the application every 10 minutes, or according to facility policy. If the skin under a heat application appears red, or a dark area appears, stop the treatment. Notify the nurse immediately. Stop a cold application and notify your supervisor if the patient's skin appears cyanotic, pale, white, or bright red; if the patient complains of numbness; or if the patient is shivering. Cover the patient with a blanket.
- Rubber or plastic should never touch the patient's skin. Be sure all appliances are covered with cloth.
- Heat and cold applications are usually not left in place longer than 20 minutes, according to the purpose and type of treatment. Follow the care plan and the nurse's instructions.
- After the treatment, pat the skin dry. Make the patient comfortable. Clean and store used equipment. Remove gloves, if worn, and dispose of them according to facility policy. Wash your hands. Report to your supervisor that the procedure was completed and the patient's reaction to the treatment.

Cautions

Remember, moisture intensifies the effect of cold just as it does heat. Caution must be used in the application of moist cold.

- Excessive cold can damage body tissues.
- Report color changes such as *blanching* (turning white) or *cyanosis* (becoming bluish).
- Report feelings of numbness or discomfort experienced by the patient.
- Stop the cold treatment if the patient starts to shiver. Cover the patient with a blanket and report immediately to the nurse.

Dry Cold Applications

There are several methods for applying therapeutic cold. Careful attention to the application is needed to prevent injury.

- Disposable *cold pack*—This single-use commercial pack can be stored until needed. Reusable commercial packs are also available (for both warm and cold applications). The pack remains effective for approximately 15 to 30 minutes. If the cold pack must be activated, follow the manufacturer's instructions exactly. When activating the pack, do not hold it in front of your face. If the pack leaks or bursts, the chemicals inside the pack may splash. Check the area being treated every 10 minutes. Discard the chemical cold pack after one use, or when the pack warms. Do not attempt to refreeze it.
- **Ice bag**—This reusable, waterproof, canvas or rubber container can be filled with ice to provide temporary local cold. An ice bag is never placed directly on the affected area because the weight of the bag will cause the patient discomfort.

SAFETY *Alert*

Cold therapy should not be used for patients with:

- Deep vein thrombosis
- Peripheral vascular disease
- Open wound(s)
- Skin sensation impairment
- Severe cognitive impairment
- Cold intolerance, cold allergy
- Some medical conditions such as rheumatoid arthritis and Reynaud's phenomenon.

If a patient has any of these conditions, check with the nurse before applying a cold application.

- *Thermal blanket*—This is a large, fluid-filled blanket that is placed over or around the patient. The temperature of the fluid in the blanket may be raised or lowered. The blanket is used to lower or raise the patient's body temperature. However, it is most often used in care facilities to lower the body temperature. This process is called inducing **hypothermia**. A licensed professional usually monitors the use of this type of blanket.

Note: Paper or styrofoam cups of ice are sometimes used to gently massage an injured area. To apply cold this way, hold the cup and make small, overlapping circles on the affected area for 20 minutes. An examination glove filled with ice and secured with a rubber band is also sometimes used as an alternate ice application.

Moist Cold Applications

- **Wet compresses** are moistened with a solution and placed on the affected area.
- A syringe may be used to add water to the compresses to keep them moist.
- The compresses can be kept cold by placing a covered ice bag against the affected area. Make sure the patient can tolerate the weight of the ice bag without increased pain.
- Each time the pad is removed and replaced, be careful to reposition the protective covering.

Follow facility policy for:

- method of applying the treatment.
- length of time the treatment is to be applied.
- how often the patient is to be checked for condition of the skin in the treatment area and general response to the treatment.
- signs that treatment should be discontinued.

PROCEDURE 63 Applying an Ice Bag

1. Assemble equipment:
   - ice bag
   - cover (usually cotton, such as a towel, or cover specified by your facility)
   - paper towels
   - spoon or similar utensil
   - ice cubes or crushed ice
2. Prepare the ice bag as follows:
   a. Fill the ice bag with cold water and check for leaks.
   b. Empty the bag.
   c. If ice cubes are used, rinse them in water to remove sharp edges. The use of crushed ice makes the bag more flexible and is more comfortable for the patient.
   d. Fill the ice bag half full, using an ice scooper, paper cup, or large spoon (Figure 11.31). Avoid making ice bags too heavy. Do not allow the scoop to touch the ice bag.
   e. To remove air from the ice bag:
      - Rest the ice bag flat on a paper towel on a flat surface.
      - Put the top in place, but do not screw it on.

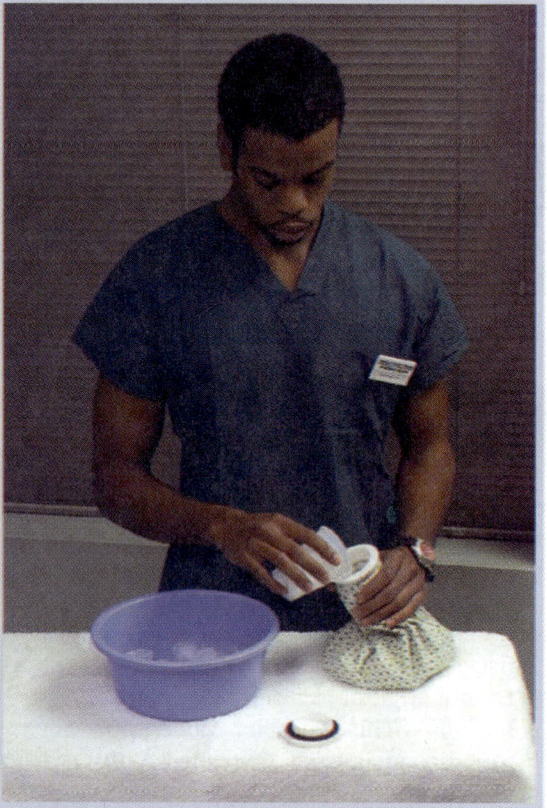

FIGURE 11-31 Fill the ice bag half full.

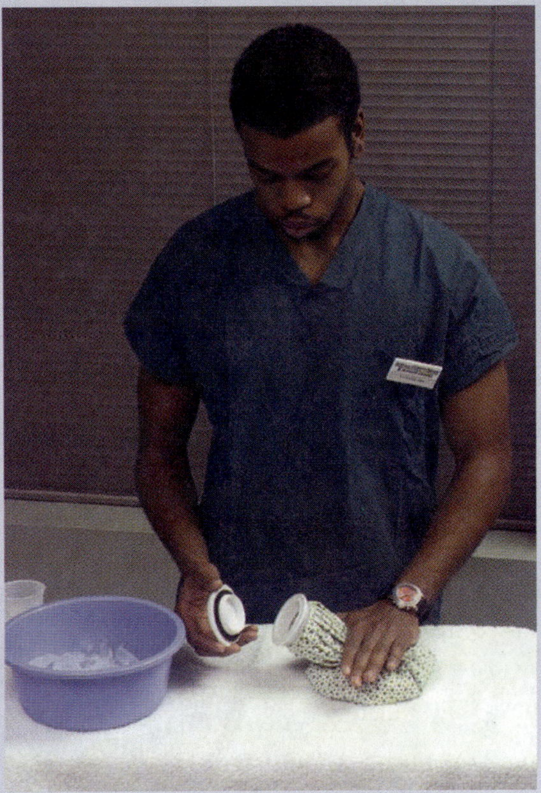

FIGURE 11-32 Place the ice bag on a flat surface, then press firmly to remove the air.

- Press the bag until the air is removed (Figure 11.32).

f. Fasten the top securely.

g. Test for leakage.

h. Wipe the ice bag dry with paper towels. Place it in a cloth cover.

Note: As an alternative, a gel pack stored in the freezer can be used for cold applications. These packs can be refrozen and reused if this is facility policy.

3. Take the equipment to the bedside on a tray. Carry out beginning procedure actions.
4. Apply the ice bag to the affected part.
5. Refill the ice bag before all the ice has melted.
6. Check the skin area under the ice bag every 10 minutes. Report to supervising nurse immediately if skin is discolored or white or if the patient reports that the skin is numb.
7. Continue the cold application for the amount of time specified by your supervisor. If the patient feels cold, cover with a blanket, but do not cover the area being treated.
8. Carry out procedure completion actions.
9. When the treatment is complete, wash the bag with soap and water. Rinse and dry it completely, and then screw the top on. Wipe the bag with a disinfectant if this is your facility policy. Leave air in the ice bag to prevent the sides from sticking together.
10. If a reusable cold pack is used, wash it thoroughly with soap and water or wipe with a disinfectant, according to facility policy. Return the pack to the refrigerator. Discard a disposable pack.

Use of Warm Applications

Warm applications are ordered to:

- relieve muscle spasms.
- reduce pain.
- reduce inflammation.
- promote healing.
- combat local infection.
- increase circulation.
- improve mobility before exercise periods.
- soothe the patient.

The value of heat treatments (**diathermy**) is that heat dilates or increases the size of blood vessels (**vasodilation**). This brings more blood to the area to promote healing. Warmth is very soothing when there is pain.

There must be a specific order for a warm application. Some groups of people require extra care when they receive warm applications.

Cautions

Follow these cautions when working with patients:

- Constant warmth must be carefully monitored.
- Moisture intensifies the effect of warmth. Use extra caution.

PROCEDURE

64 Applying a Disposable Cold Pack

1. Carry out beginning procedure actions.
2. Assemble equipment:
   - disposable commercial cold pack
   - cloth covering (towel, warm water bag cover, or other cover specified by the facility)
   - tape or rolls of gauze
3. Expose the area to be treated. Note the condition of the area.
4. Place the cold pack in a cloth covering (Figure 11.33).
5. Strike or squeeze the cold pack to activate chemicals. (Follow manufacturer's instructions.)
6. Place the covered cold pack on the proper area and cover it with a towel (Figure 11.34). Note time of application.
7. Secure the cover with tape or gauze, if necessary, to hold it in place.
8. Leave the patient in a comfortable position, with the signal cord within easy reach.
9. Return to the bedside every 10 minutes. Check the area being treated for discoloration or numbness. If these signs and symptoms occur, discontinue treatment and report them to your supervisor.
10. If no adverse symptoms occur, remove the pack after 30 minutes, or after the amount of time given in your instructions. Note the condition of the area. Continuous treatment requires application of a fresh pack.
11. Remove the pack from the cover and discard according to facility policy. Return unused gauze and tape.
12. Put the cover in a laundry hamper.
13. Carry out procedure completion actions.

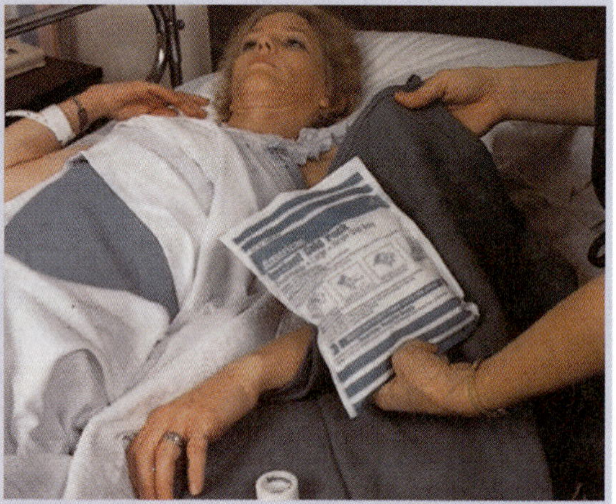

FIGURE 11-33 Cover the disposable cold pack with a cover before applying it to the patient.

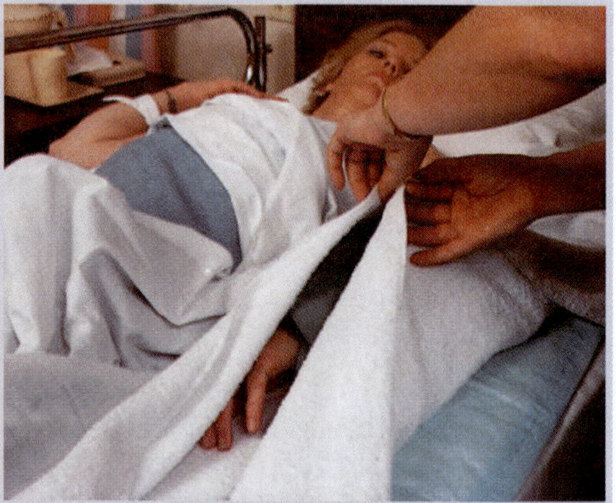

FIGURE 11-34 After positioning the cold pack, cover the application with a towel.

SAFETY *Alert*

The heat application should feel comfortably warm to the patient, not uncomfortably hot. If you will be applying a pack or pad, touch the device to your forearm to check the temperature before applying it. If the patient complains of burning, remove the application and consult the nurse.

- Hot packs are contraindicated for paralyzed areas or areas without sensation, acute edema or inflammation, infection, and hemophilia. They must be used with caution for patients with many medical conditions, including impaired circulation, sensory impairment, cancer, rashes, and open skin conditions. Take extra care with hot packs for very young and very old patients.

SAFETY *Alert*

Heat therapy should not be used for patients with:

- Acute inflammation
- Dermatitis
- Deep vein thrombosis
- Peripheral vascular disease
- Open wound(s)
- Recent soft tissue injuries in which swelling or bleeding would be increased by heat
- Skin sensation impairment
- Severe cognitive impairment

Some physicians also recommend avoiding heat use with children and women during pregnancy. If a patient has any of these conditions, check with the nurse before applying a heat application.

- Never allow a patient to lie on a constant heat unit, because heat may be trapped and build up to dangerous levels.
- Temperature of a constant heat unit should be between 95° and 100°F.
- Always use a bath thermometer to check solution temperatures.
- Always remove the body part being soaked before adding warm solution.
- Always stay with the patient during the treatment.
- Protect areas not being treated from excessive exposure.
- Warmth is not applied to the head because it could cause blood vessels in the area to dilate, resulting in headache.
- Rubber or plastic should never touch the patient's skin. Be sure all appliances are covered with cloth.

Dry Warm Applications

The **Aquamatic K-Pad®** is commonly used to provide dry warmth. It consists of a plastic pad with fluid-filled coils and a control unit that maintains a constant temperature of the fluid.

The fluid in the pad is distilled water that is supplied from a reservoir in the control unit. The control unit is placed on the bedside stand and is plugged into an electrical outlet. In most facilities, the temperature is preset by the central supply department. The temperature is usually set at 95° to 100°F.

Note: When setting up the K-Pad® for the first time, check the pad for leaks. Tip it back and forth several times to eliminate air pockets, which cause hot spots. Place the control unit on the bedside stand so it is higher than the patient, so that water will run into the pad by gravity. Make sure the tubing is free of kinks.

Moist Warm Applications

SAFETY *Alert*

Moisture intensifies heat and you must use extra care.

For each of the warm treatments, follow facility policy for:

- method of applying the treatment.
- length of time the treatment is to be applied.
- how often the patient is to be checked for condition of the skin in the treatment area and general response to the treatment.
- signs that treatment should be discontinued.

Moist warm treatments include:

- **Warm soaks**—The patient, or the part of the patient's body that is being treated, is immersed in a tub filled with water at a specific temperature, usually 105°.
- **Wet compresses**—The same cautions apply to warm compresses as to cold compresses. They may be kept wet with a syringe and warm by covering them with an Aquamatic K-Pad®

PROCEDURE 65 Applying an Aquamatic K-PAD®

1. Carry out beginning procedure actions.
2. Assemble equipment:
   - K-Pad® and control unit
   - distilled water
   - covering for pad
3. Check the cord for frayed or damaged insulation. Also check that the tubing between the control unit and the pad is intact.
4. Place the control unit on the bedside stand (Figure 11.35).

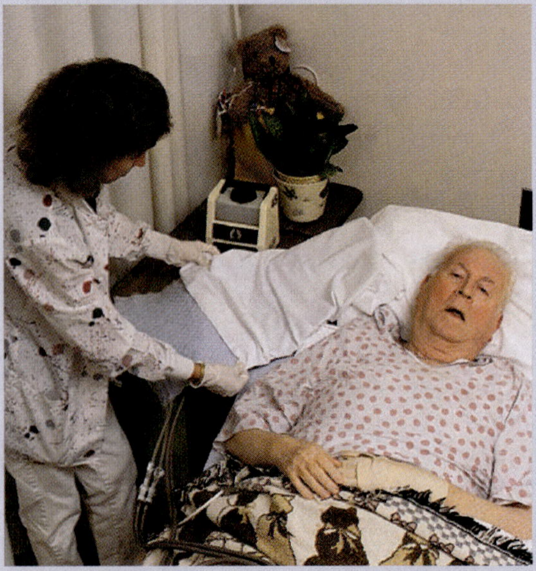

FIGURE 11-35 The control unit for the aquathermia pad maintains a constant temperature.

5. Remove the cover of the control unit and check the level of the distilled water. If it is low, fill the unit two-thirds full or to the fill line using distilled water. Tilt the unit back and forth gently to clear the tubing of air.
6. Screw the cover in place and loosen it one-quarter turn.
7. If the temperature was not preset, check with the nurse for the proper setting before turning on the unit. Remove the key after setting the temperature.
8. Plug in the unit.
9. Cover the pad with an appropriate cover, according to facility policy or as specified by the manufacturer of the unit. Do not use pins to hold the cover in place.
10. Expose the area on the patient to be treated. Place the covered pad on the patient and note the time.
    - Be sure the tubing between the control unit and the pad does not hang over the side of the bed. It should be coiled on the bed to promote the flow of liquid.
11. Following facility policy, periodically check the skin under the pad.
12. Check the level of the water in the control unit. Refill if necessary to the fill line.
13. Remove the pad after the prescribed amount of time.
14. Carry out procedure completion actions.

PROCEDURE

66 Performing a Warm Soak

1. Carry out beginning procedure actions.
2. Assemble equipment:
   - bath thermometer
   - soak basin
   - pitcher
   - large plastic sheet
   - bath towel
   - bath blanket
3. Bring equipment to the bedside.
4. Cover the patient with a bath blanket.
5. Fanfold bedding to the foot of the bed.
6. Expose the limb to be soaked.
7. Position the patient for comfort on the far side of the bed (opposite the part to be soaked). Be sure the side rail is up and secure.
8. Cover the bed with a plastic sheet and towel.
9. Fill the soak basin half full with water at the prescribed temperature (usually 105 °F). Check the temperature with a bath thermometer.
10. Take the soak basin from the overbed table and position it on the bed protector.
11. Assist the patient to gradually place the limb in the basin (Figure 11.36). Cover the basin with a towel to help maintain temperature.
12. Check the temperature every 5 minutes. Use a pitcher to get additional water and add to the soak basin to maintain temperature. Remember to remove the patient's limb before adding water to the container.

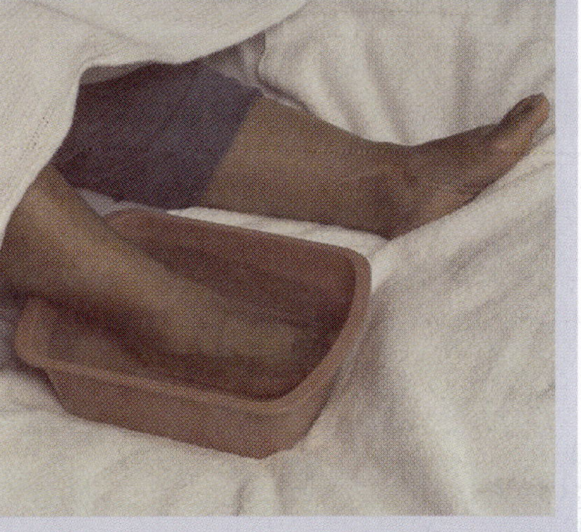

FIGURE 11-36 The patient is receiving warm soak therapy.

13. Discontinue the procedure at the end of the prescribed time.
    a. Lift the patient's limb out of the basin.
    b. Slip the basin forward and allow the limb to rest on the bath towel.
    c. Place the basin on the overbed table. Gently pat the limb dry with a towel.
14. Remove the plastic sheet and towel.
15. Adjust bedding and remove the bath blanket. If the treatment is to be repeated, fold the bath blanket and place it in the bedside stand. Leave the unit tidy and the call bell within reach.
16. Lower the head of the bed and make the patient comfortable.
17. Take equipment to the utility room. Clean and store it according to facility policy.
18. Carry out procedure completion actions.

PROCEDURE

67 Applying a Warm Moist Compress

1. Carry out beginning procedure actions.
2. Assemble equipment:
   - disposable gloves
   - syringe
   - bed protector
   - compresses
   - bath thermometer
   - binder or towel
   - pins or bandage
   - basin with prescribed solution at temperature ordered
3. Bring equipment to the bedside.
4. Expose only the area to be treated.
5. Protect the bed and the patient's clothing with a bed protector (Figure 11.37A).
6. Put on disposable gloves.
7. Check the temperature of the solution. Moisten the compresses; remove excess liquid (Figure 11.37B). Apply to treatment area (Figure 11.37C).
8. Secure the compresses with a bandage or binder. The compress must be in contact with the patient's skin.
9. Help the patient to maintain a comfortable position throughout the treatment.
10. Unscreen the unit. Leave the unit neat and tidy, with the signal cord within easy reach.
11. Maintain proper temperature and moisture.
    - If the compresses are to be kept warm, a K-Pad® may be applied.
    - If the compresses are to be kept cool, an ice bag may be applied.
    - A syringe may be used to apply more solution to keep the compresses wet.
12. Remove the compresses when ordered. Change as ordered or once in 24 hours. Check skin several times each day.
13. Discard the compresses.
14. Remove and dispose of gloves according to facility policy.
15. Carry out procedure completion actions.

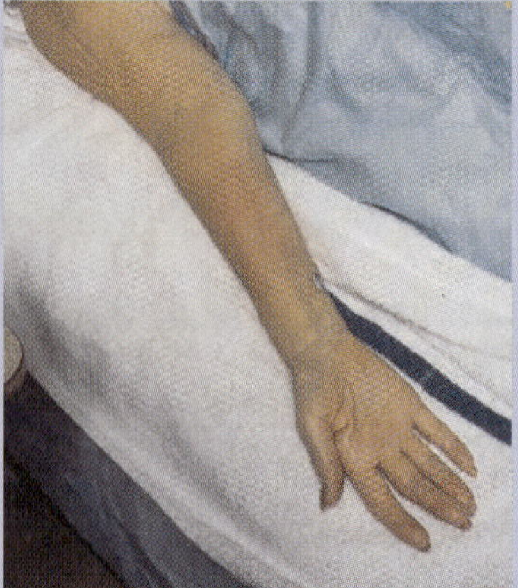

FIGURE 11-37A Protect the bed with a towel or underpad.

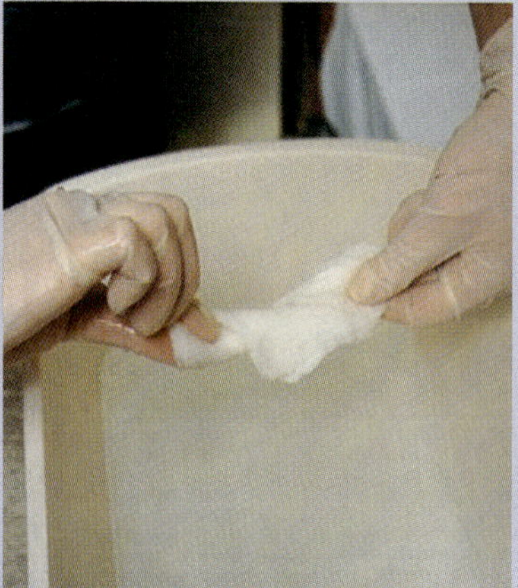

FIGURE 11-37B Dip the compress into a basin of warm (105 °F) water. Grasp the edges, then squeeze out excess liquid.

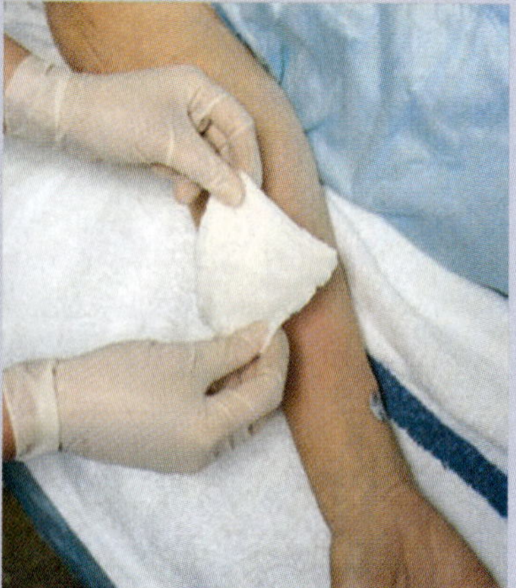

FIGURE 11-37C Open the compress and apply it to the inflamed area.

Temperature Control Measures

Excessively high or low body temperatures are treated in acute care facilities by placing hypothermia-hyperthermia blankets (Figure 11.38) over and under the patient. These blankets are units filled with water. The blankets may be called **aquathermia blankets**. "Aqua" is the Latin term for *water*. The temperature of the water can be adjusted higher or lower depending on whether the patient's body temperature is to be raised or lowered.

Using the Aquathermia Blanket

The aquathermia blanket is operated either manually or automatically. For manual operation, the licensed nurse will set the blanket to a predetermined temperature, which is ordered by the physician. The blanket maintains this temperature regardless of changes in the patient's body temperature. When the unit is set for automatic operation, it monitors the patient's temperature through a rectal, skin, or esophageal probe. The probe is secured to the body with tape to prevent injury. The blanket temperature changes according to the patient's temperature. The goal is to maintain the patient's body temperature. An alarm will sound for abnormal temperature variations. Before using the blanket, check it for cracks, tears, or leaks in the system. Do not use it if there are cracks or an electrical malfunction.

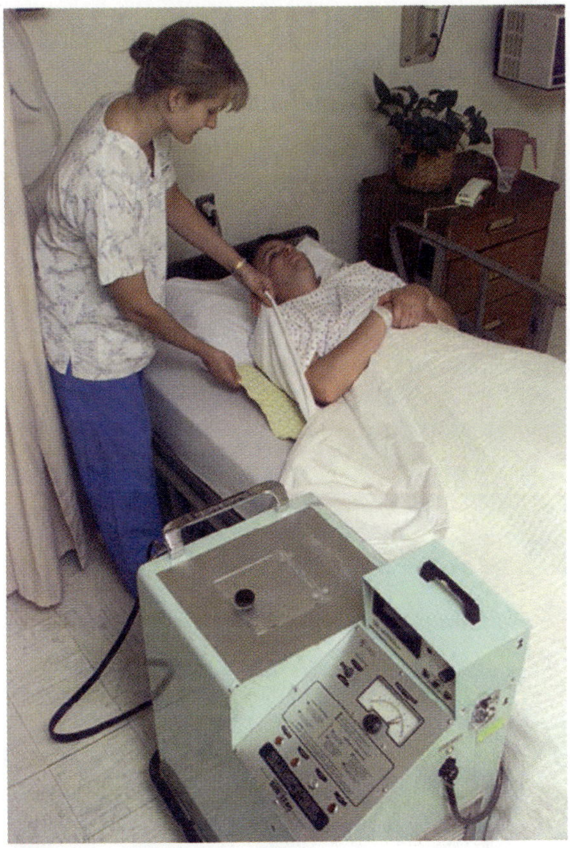

FIGURE 11-38 Hypothermia-hyperthermia blanket.

The patient should wear a hospital gown when the aquathermia blanket is used. Use a gown with tie closures. Snaps, pins, or other metal may cause injury to the skin. Before beginning the procedure, check and record the patient's baseline vital signs as a basis for comparison.

One or two aquathermia blankets may be used. The nurse may instruct you to place one under the patient, and to cover him or her with the other. The blankets must be covered with a disposable cover, sheet, or bath blanket to absorb perspiration and prevent complications. Avoid using pins to cover the blanket. These can puncture the unit or injure the patient's skin by creating hot or cold spots. Use tape or Velcro® fasteners, if necessary, to cover the unit.

The blanket should be set up and preheated or precooled before it is applied to the patient. Connect the blanket to the control unit by plugging in the tubing. The nurse will set the blanket for automatic or manual operation. He or she will also set the desired body temperature or blanket temperature and instruct you as to what temperature values are being used. Turn the device on, then add distilled water to the reservoir. Position the controls at the foot of the bed. After the blanket has reached the designated temperature, apply it to the patient. If the patient will be lying on a blanket, place a pillow or folded bath blanket under the patient's head.

The patient's head should not contact the blanket directly. The combination of heat or cold and the surface of the blanket promotes skin breakdown on the back of the head. The nurse may instruct you to apply lanolin or another designated product to the skin in exposed areas that contact the blanket directly. You may wrap the patient's hands and feet to prevent chilling, if desired.

Complications. Immediately notify the nurse if you observe any of these complications:

- Changes in skin color
- Cyanosis of the lips or nail beds
- Sudden changes in body temperature
- marked changes in pulse, respirations, and blood pressure

- respiratory distress
- pain
- changes in sensation
- edema
- shivering and chills
- urinary output below 50 mL/hour

Discontinuing Blanket Use. The nurse will inform you when to discontinue use of the blanket. Follow the manufacturer's directions for the type of blanket you are using. Turn the unit off. (Some types must remain plugged in for 30 to 60 minutes to dry condensation inside the unit.) Dry the patient's skin and assist him or her into a dry gown. Position the patient in a comfortable position. Remove the aquathermia blanket from the bed after the designated time. Continue checking vital signs and intake and output every 30 minutes for the first 2 hours, then hourly or as directed by the nurse.

Hypothermia

Hypothermia is a drop in core body temperature below 95 °F (35 °C) rectally. This can occur:

- when people are exposed to cold without adequate protection.
- in the elderly, when a person is exposed to external temperatures as warm as 60 °F.
- when deliberately induced before surgery to slow body metabolism.

SAFETY Alert

The nurse will instruct you on the frequency for monitoring vital signs when an aquathermia blanket is being used. The patient's temperature and the blanket temperature are usually monitored and documented every 15 to 30 minutes. Inform the nurse immediately if the patient's temperature drops more than one degree in 15 minutes. Continued temperature monitoring is necessary after the blanket is removed because the patient's temperature can continue to drop as much as 5 degrees after the procedure ends.

Indications of hypothermia to report include:

- Drop in body temperature
- Poor coordination and confusion
- Slurred speech
- Decreased respiratory and heart rates

Nursing Assistant Actions

- Report observations to the supervisor.
- Check the environmental temperature and adjust it.
- Provide external warmth with a sweater or blanket.
- Reduce drafts with screens or curtains.
- If permitted, give something warm to drink.
- Check vital signs.

Hyperthermia

Hyperthermia is an elevation of core body temperature to 104 °F (40 °C) rectally or higher. This can occur:

- when a person is exposed to high external temperature.
- with serious injuries such as burns.
- when there is damage to the temperature control center in the brain.
- with infections.

Indications of hyperthermia to report include:

- Elevated body temperature
- Hot, flushed skin
- Faintness
- Headache
- Nausea
- Convulsions

Fever or *pyrexia* occurs when core body temperature rises to at least 101 °F (rectally). Fever is often associated with infections, injury, surgery,

AGE-APPROPRIATE CARE Alert

In children, temperatures tend to rise higher than in adults. This puts children at greater risk for seizures.

and serious trauma. Indications of fever are the same as those for general hyperthermia.

Nursing Assistant Actions

- Report observations to the supervisor.
- Check environment temperature and adjust it.
- Reduce external warmth. Cover the patient only with a gown or sheet.
- If permitted, give cooling drink.
- Carry out cooling procedures as ordered. For example, give cooling baths or enemas.
- Check vital signs frequently.

PROCEDURE 68 Assisting With Application of a Hypothermia Blanket

Applying a hypothermia blanket and monitoring a patient who is receiving a hypothermia treatment is a professional nursing responsibility. The nurse will supervise the procedure and monitor the patient throughout the treatment. The nurse will check the specific gravity of the patient's urine, vital signs, and nervous system response. The nursing assistant may be asked to assist in setting up equipment, positioning the patient and the thermal blanket, observing the patient during the treatment, and keeping the patient comfortable. In addition, the nursing assistant may be asked to transport equipment to and from the central supply service.

1. Wash your hands, collect equipment, and take equipment to the bedside.
2. Assemble equipment:
   - disposable gloves
   - hypothermia-hyperthermia control unit
   - fluid for control unit
   - thermometer probes (rectal or skin)
   - adhesive tape
   - sphygmomanometer
   - stethoscope
   - hypothermia-hyperthermia blanket (disposable or reusable), one or two as ordered
   - bath blanket or sheet, one or two as ordered
   - lanolin-based skin cream
3. Follow manufacturer's directions for setting up equipment. Check equipment for safety. Be sure the control unit is grounded.
4. Connect the blanket(s) to the control unit and set the control.
5. Turn on the control unit and add liquid.
6. Allow the blanket(s) to precool as you prepare the patient.
7. Carry out beginning procedure actions.
8. Place the patient in a hospital-type gown with ties.
9. Measure vital signs and record.
10. Place the hypothermia-hyperthermia blanket on the bed and cover it with a sheet. Position the patient on the sheet-covered thermal blanket in the recumbent position, with the head on a pillow that does not touch the blanket.
11. Wash your hands. Put on gloves.
12. Insert a rectal thermometer probe into the patient's rectum (unless contraindicated) and tape it in place. (Alternatively, place a skin probe into an axilla and tape it in place.)
13. Plug the end of the probe into the proper jack on the control panel.
14. Place a second sheet over the patient and place a second thermal blanket over the sheet, if ordered.

15. Apply lanolin-based cream to the patient's skin where it contacts the blanket.
16. Remove gloves. Discard according to facility policy. Wash your hands.
17. Monitor vital signs, neurologic response, and intake and output every 5 minutes until the desired body temperature is reached, and then every 15 minutes, or as ordered.
18. Report color changes in skin or excessive shivering.
19. The blanket's texture increases the risk of skin breakdown. The patient should be repositioned every 30 minutes to 1 hour. Reapply skin cream as necessary. Change the gown and top sheet as often as necessary if the patient is actively perspiring. Put on gloves each time you care for patient. At the end of care, remove gloves, discard according to facility policy, and wash your hands.
20. At completion of the treatment, follow manufacturer's instructions for turning off the unit, disconnecting the blanket(s), and returning them to storage.
21. Put on gloves. Continue to monitor the patient as you remove the equipment.
22. Replace any damp bedding or garments and cover the patient. Continue to monitor the patient every 30 minutes until he or she has been stable for 2 hours.
23. Clean the thermometer probe and store it according to facility policy.
24. Remove gloves and discard according to facility policy.
25. Carry out procedure completion actions.

REVIEW

A. True/False.

Mark the following true or false by circling T or F.

1. T F Heat and cold treatments should be supervised by the nurse.
2. T F If a patient has a possible diagnosis of appendicitis, heat should not be applied to the abdomen.
3. T F The temperature of a warm soak solution should be approximately 100 °F.
4. T F Special blankets used to alter the patient's temperature are called infrared blankets.
5. T F A patient who is unconscious must receive special attention during a heat treatment.
6. T F Hyperthermia is an elevation of core body temperature to below 95 °F.
7. T F Heat is frequently applied to the head.
8. T F When charting an application of cold, always include the length of time of the application.
9. T F Aquamatic K-Pads® are usually set at 115 °F.

B. Multiple Choice

Select the one best answer.

10. Heat affects the body by
    a. causing constriction.
    b. increasing blood supply to the area.
    c. reducing oxygen in tissues.
    d. increasing white blood cells.
11. Special care with heat and cold treatments must be taken when the patient is
    a. alert and oriented.
    b. very young.
    c. cooperative.
    d. ambulatory.

12. Dry cold is provided by
    a. compresses.
    b. a hyperthermia blanket.
    c. ice caps.
    d. soaks.
13. Cold affects the body by
    a. reducing pain sensations.
    b. stimulating life processes.
    c. promoting inflammation.
    d. promoting healing.
14. Moist cold is applied with
    a. ice bags.
    b. ice caps.
    c. ice collars.
    d. soaks.
15. When applying heat and cold treatments, the nursing assistant should
    a. always remain in the room for the duration of the treatment.
    b. check the temperature of the solution with an elbow.
    c. monitor the skin under the application every 30 minutes.
    d. remove jewelry, buttons, or zippers that may conduct heat or cold.
16. When caring for a patient who is using an aquathermia blanket, the nursing assistant should
    a. regulate blanket temperature at least every 15 minutes.
    b. give the patient plenty of iced liquids to drink to reduce fever.
    c. monitor the patient for cyanosis or changes in vital signs.
    d. turn the patient at least every 2 hours.

C. Matching

Choose the correct word from Column II to match each blank in Column I.

Column I	Column II
17. ____ excessive blood loss	a. diathermy
18. ____ increase in size of blood vessel	b. vasoconstriction
19. ___ heat treatment	c. vasodilation
20. ____ decrease in size of blood vessel	d. hypothermia blanket
21. ____ used to lower body temperature	e. hemorrhage
	f. infrared

D. Nursing Assistant Challenge

Peggy, 17 years of age, was admitted to your unit from the emergency room. She fractured an ankle and will require internal repair with screws and wire. You will care for her prior to surgery. The physician has ordered an ice bag for her ankle and her leg is to be elevated. Answer the following questions.

22. What are two reasons for applying the ice bag?
23. How full should the ice bag be filled?
24. Why should ice cubes be rinsed?
25. How should the metal cap be positioned when the ice bag is placed on the patient?
26. When should the ice bag be refilled?
27. How is the ice bag held in place?
28. What important observation should be reported immediately to the nurse?

C: Assisting with Coughing and Deep Breathing Exercises

OBJECTIVES

After reading this unit, you will be able to:

- Spell and define key terms.
- Describe the purpose of deep breathing and coughing.
- Demonstrate procedure for deep breathing and coughing.
- Demonstrate standard precautions when assisting with coughing and deep breathing procedure.

DEEP BREATHING AND COUGHING

Breathing Exercises

Residents can be taught breathing exercises that improve respiration and general respiratory muscle tone. Breathing exercises stress the expiration phase of respiration. The resident is first taught the basic breathing pattern, which is to:

- Breathe in through the nose to the count of one, allowing the abdomen to rise.
- Purse the lips to the count of two and three as the abdominal wall is contracted and air is forced out of the lungs.

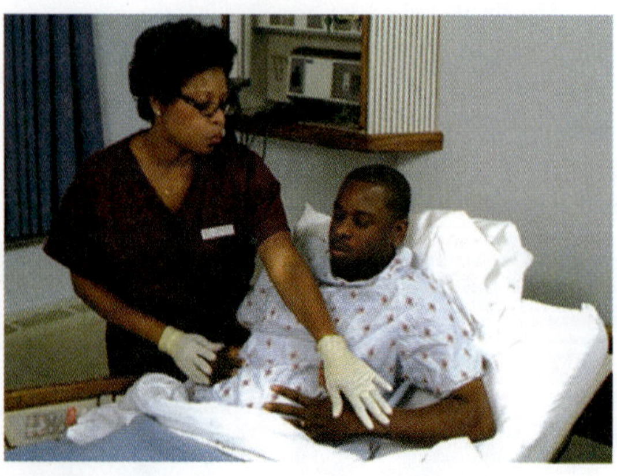

FIGURE 11-39 Encourage the patient to perform deep breathing exercises.

Deep breathing and coughing clear the air passages. This helps to prevent postoperative respiratory complications such as pneumonia and atelectasis, which is the collapse of the alveolar air sacs. This may be an uncomfortable task when the patient has a new incision and feels fatigued. You can best assist the patient by:

- Explaining the value of the exercise and carrying out the following procedure.

SAFETY *Alert*

Although we routinely encourage postoperative patients to cough and deep breathe, there are a few exceptions you must be aware of. Avoid this procedure with patients who have had eye, nose, or neurologic surgery. Coughing and deep breathing will increase pressure, causing complications in these patients. Check with the nurse if you are unsure of what action to take.

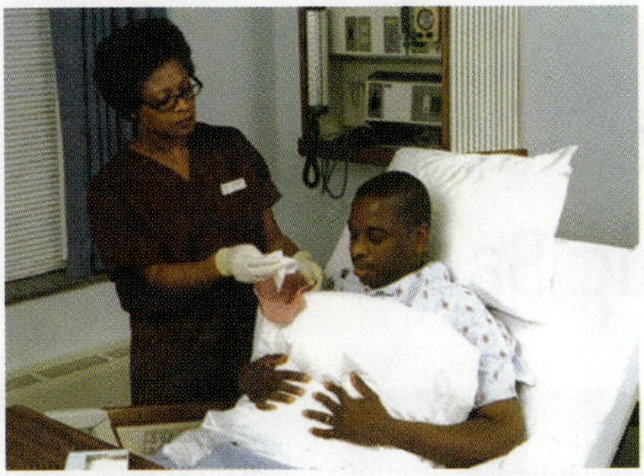

FIGURE 11-40 A pillow helps support the abdomen and splint the incision during coughing and deep breathing.

- Checking with the nurse to see if medication for pain is to be administered before the exercise. If so, wait for 45 minutes after the medication has been given before carrying out the exercise.
- Learning from the nurse how many deep breaths and coughs should be attempted. The usual number is 5 to 10 breaths and 2 to 3 coughs.
- Using a pillow or binder to support the incision during the procedure.

OSHA Alert

Apply the principles of standard precautions when assisting with coughing and deep breathing procedures. If the patient is expelling loose secretions, select and wear appropriate protective equipment, including gloves, gown, mask, and face shield. Show the patient how to contain secretions in a tissue. Assist him or her with handwashing after the activity.

REVIEW

A. Multiple Choice

Select the one best answer.

1. The purpose of deep breathing and coughing is to
   a. control pain
   b. prevent skin breakdown
   c. prevent pneumonia
   d. manage acid reflux
2. A post-operative respiratory complication is
   a. thrombophlebitis
   b. dermatitis
   c. atelectasis
   d. gastritis
3. If secretions are expelled following coughing and deep breathing exercises, the nursing assistant should
   a. maintain bedrest
   b. restrict fluids
   c. ask nurse to give cough medicine
   d. wear protective equipment
4. Patients who are exceptions to routine coughing and deep breathing exercises are patients
   a. on strict bedrest
   b. who have had eye, nose or neurologic surgery
   c. with continuous gastric tubing feeding
   d. with chronic obstructive pulmonary disease
5. The patient's body position used for coughing and deep breathing exercises
   a. Semi-Fowler's
   b. Supine
   c. Lateral
   d. Trendelenburg

D: Applying Elastic Stocking (TED Hose) and Elastic Bandages

OBJECTIVES

After reading this unit, you will be able to:

- Define key terms.
- List purposes that require anti-embolism hose
- State when to apply and remove anti-embolism hose
- Demonstrate the procedure for applying and removing anti-embolism hose
- List purposes for application of elastic bandages
- Observe circulation and report complaints of pain and numbness

OBSERVATIONS

TED stockings applied evenly and smoothly with no wrinkles
Appropriate type and size of anti-embolism hose
Edema
Tingling
Pain or discomfort
Cyanotic skin
Appropriate size bandage
Apply elastic bandage so that two skin surfaces do not rub together
Signs of skin breakdown
Elastic stockings removed and reapplied at least twice a day or as ordered

Elasticized Stockings

Elasticized stockings, called **TED hose** or **anti-embolism hose**, or Ace bandages that extend from the ankle or foot to calf or mid-thigh, are often applied during the preoperative and post-operative periods to support the veins of the legs. This reduces the incidence of **thrombophlebitis**, which is inflammation of the veins that can lead to blood clots. The stockings must be applied smoothly and evenly before the patient gets out of bed. They should be removed and reapplied at least every eight hours—more often if necessary or as ordered.

Several different types of anti-embolism hose are used. Some have closed toes, but most have an opening near the toe end. The hole is positioned

PROCEDURE 69 Applying Elasticized Stockings

1. Carry out beginning procedure actions.
2. Assemble equipment:
   - elasticized stockings of proper length and size
3. Always apply stockings with the patient lying down. Expose one leg at a time.
4. Grasp the stocking with both hands at the top and roll it toward the toe end (Figure 11.41A).
5. Adjust over the patient's toes, positioning the opening at the base of the toes (unless the toes are to be covered) (Figure 11.41B). Remember that the raised seams should be on the outside.

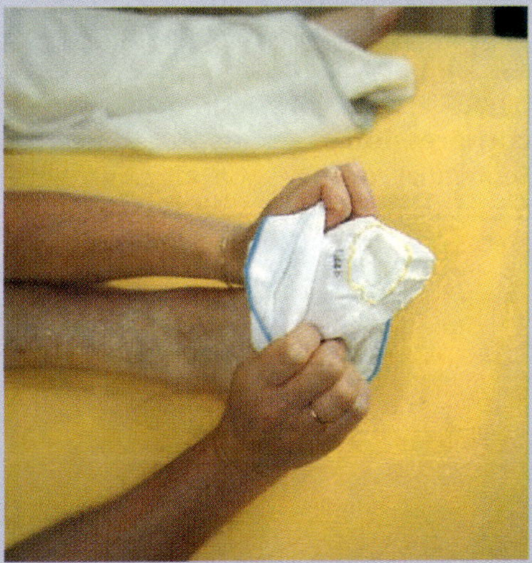

FIGURE 11-41A Gather the stocking and slip it over the patient's toes.

6. Apply the stocking to the leg by rolling it upward toward the body (Figure 11.41C).
7. Check to be sure the stocking is applied evenly and smoothly and that there are no wrinkles (Figure 11.41D).
8. Repeat the procedure on the opposite leg.
9. Carry out procedure completion actions.

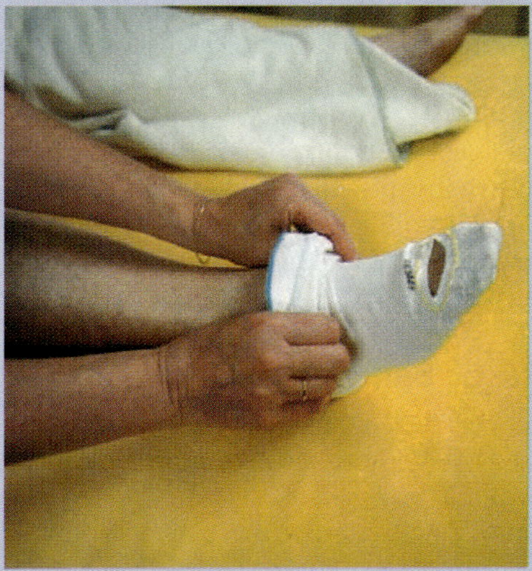

FIGURE 11-41B Position the opening on the top of the foot, at the base of the toes.

(continues)

PROCEDURE 69

Applying Elasticized Stockings, *continued*

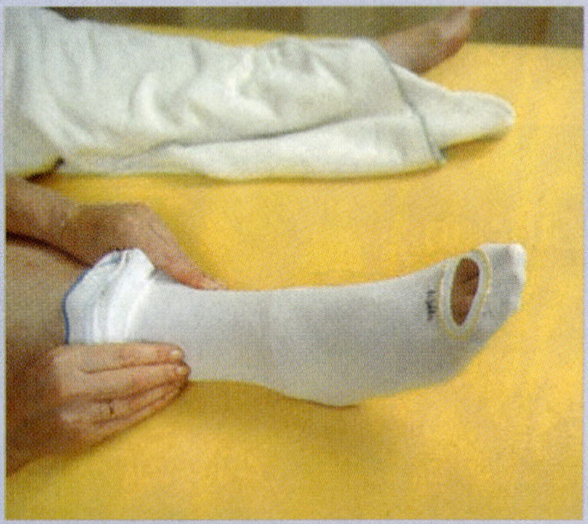

FIGURE 11-41C Draw the stocking smoothly up to the knee.

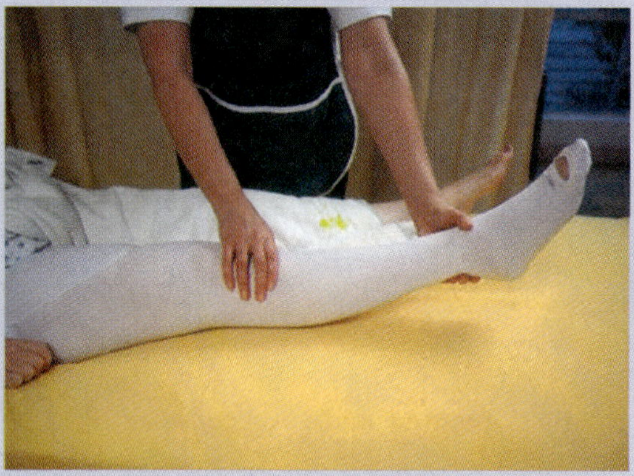

FIGURE 11-41D Check to make sure the stocking is free of wrinkles.

on the top or the bottom of the foot, just proximal to the toes. Check the heel placement on the stocking. By using the heel as a landmark, you will see where to position the hole in the stocking.

Make sure the legs are dry before attempting to apply the hose. Elastic hosiery fit tightly. An apparatus is used in some facilities to make them easier to apply. If this is not available, the nurse may permit you to dust the legs lightly with baby powder, making the hose easier to apply. Avoid using powders if the patient has respiratory difficulty, a rash, or dressings on the legs.

Elastic Bandage

An elasticized bandage (Ace bandage) may be used to keep dressings in place, especially on an extremity or on the head. You may need to remove and reapply the bandage once or twice on your shift. Elastic bandages are also used on nonsurgical patients, to promote venous blood flow in the legs, and for injuries of the musculoskeletal system, to reduce swelling. Elastic bandages come in 2-inch to 6-inch widths and in 4-foot and 6-foot lengths (Figure 11.42). Check with the nurse for the appropriate size bandage.

Sequential Compression Therapy

Deep vein thrombosis and **pulmonary embolism** (blood clot in the lungs) are serious postoperative complications. Approximately 10% of all patients with DVT die from pulmonary embolism. Most have no symptoms until they develop the pulmonary embolus. The femoral vein, the large blood vessel in the groin, is particularly susceptible to clot formation. Because of the high risk and serious consequences associated with blood clots, the physician may order **sequential compression therapy** to reduce the risk. Sequential compression therapy massages the legs using a milking, wavelike motion.

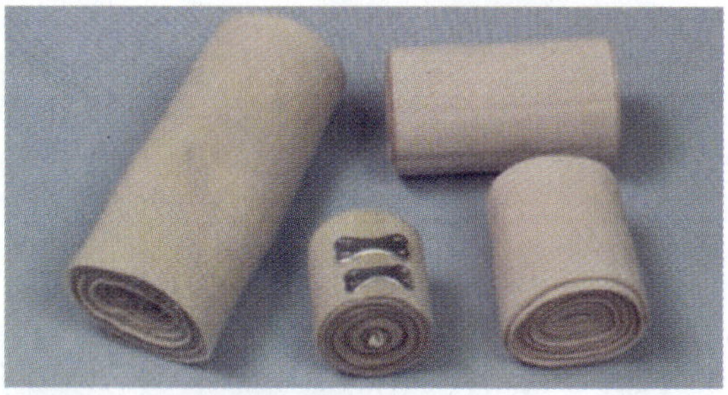

FIGURE 11-42 Elastic bandages are available in a variety of widths.

PROCEDURE

70 Applying Elastic Bandage

1. Carry out beginning procedure actions.
2. Assemble equipment:
   - appropriate size bandage (check for cleanliness)
   - tape, pins, or self-closures that come with bandage
3. Check the area to be bandaged.
   a. If there are lesions or signs of skin breakdown, report to the nurse before bandaging.
   b. If there are dressings underneath the bandage, the nurse may want to check them before you reapply the bandage.
   c. If an arm or leg is to be bandaged, elevate it for 15 to 30 minutes before application to promote venous blood flow.
   d. Apply the bandage so that two skin surfaces do not rub together (toes, fingers, under breasts and arms). Place gauze or cotton to prevent friction (Figure 11.43A).

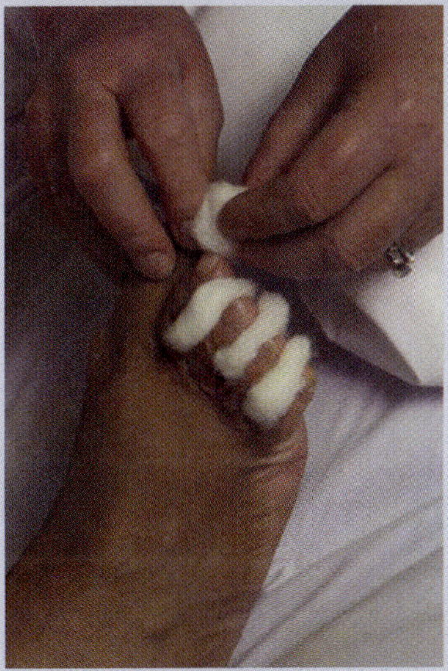

FIGURE 11-43A Pad the toes with cotton to keep them from rubbing together.

4. Hold the bandage with the roll facing upward in one hand and the free end of the bandage in your other hand (Figure 11.43B).
   a. Hold the roll close to the part being bandaged so that pressure is even.
   b. When bandaging an extremity, always wrap from the distal (far) area to the proximal (near) area (Figure 11.43C).
   c. Unroll the bandage as you wrap the body part. Never unroll the entire bandage at once.
5. Use appropriate bandaging technique (Figure 11.43D). Overlap each layer of bandage by one-half the width of the strip.
6. When finished rolling, secure the bandage with pins, tape, or self-closures. Avoid using the clips that may come with the bandage, if possible. They tend to come loose and could injure the patient's skin. The bandage should be smooth and wrinkle-free.

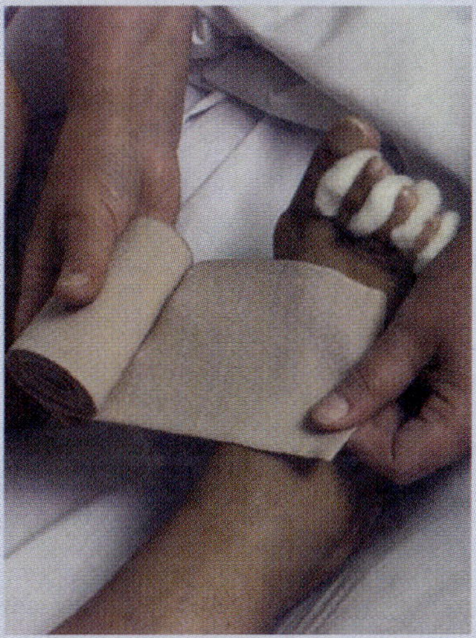

FIGURE 11-43B Hold the bandage with the roll facing upward in one hand and the free end of the bandage in your other hand.

(continues)

PROCEDURE 70 Applying Elastic Bandage, *continued*

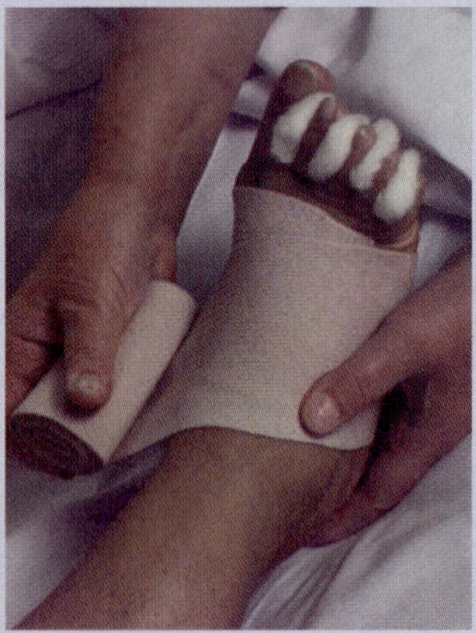

FIGURE 11-43C Always wrap from distal to proximal.

7. Check distal circulation just after the bandage has been applied and once or twice every 8 hours thereafter (check the skin under the bandage for color and temperature; note patient complaints of burning, tingling, or other discomfort).
8. Remove and reapply the bandage every shift, or more often if needed. The patient should have two bandages so that they can be laundered daily. Ask the nurse whether the bandage is to be worn continuously or only at specified times.
9. Carry out procedure completion actions.

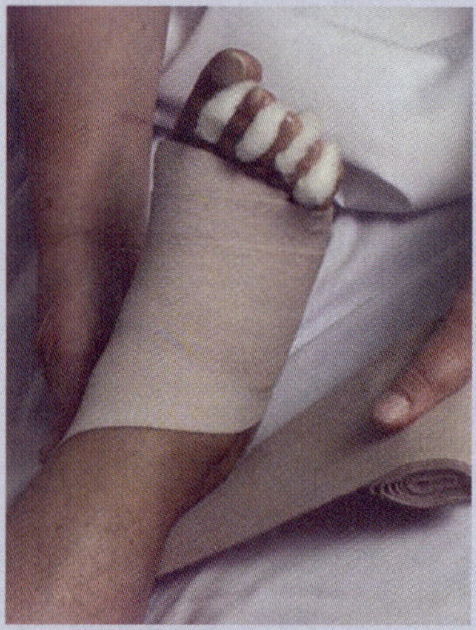

FIGURE 11-43D Use the correct bandaging technique. Overlap each layer of bandage by one-half the width of the strip. The finished bandage should be smooth and wrinkle-free.

Pneumatic hosiery (Figure 11.44) are also called *sequential compression hosiery*. This device prevents blood clots by massaging the legs mechanically. Pneumatic hosiery inflate and deflate rhythmically to produce the milking, wavelike massaging motion. The device should not be used on patients with lower leg ulcers, blood clots, massive edema, deformities, infected or broken skin, or arterial disease. Shiny, hairless skin is an indication of arterial problems. If you observe any hard nodules, red areas, or warm areas on the patient's lower legs, inform the nurse before applying the hosiery.

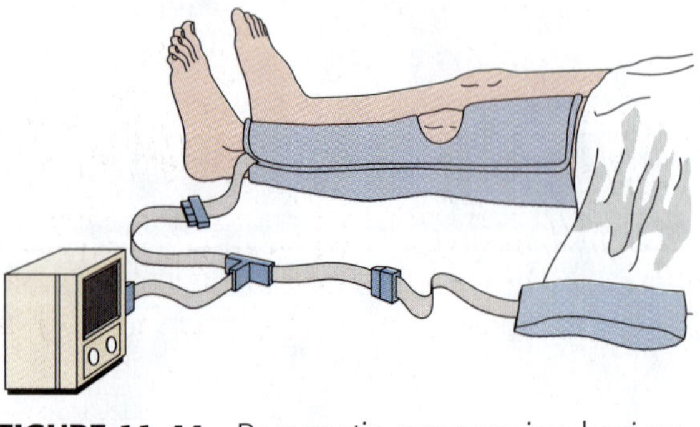

FIGURE 11-44 Pneumatic compression hosiery is used to prevent blood clots.

Measuring and Connecting the Hosiery. Before beginning this procedure, you must determine the proper size hosiery for the patient. Do this by measuring the circumference of the patient's upper thigh with a tape measure when she is in bed. Hold the measure snugly against the leg and note the circumference. Compare the measurement with the sizing chart, and select the proper size hosiery.

Familiarize yourself with the hosiery and compression controller if you have not used them before. Open the package and lay the hose on a flat surface. Open them completely, with the cotton lining facing up. Inside you will notice markings for the ankle and knee. When you apply the garment to the patient's leg, line it up exactly with these landmarks. Next, familiarize yourself with the compression controller. The device may have a cooling adjustment. This is used to cool the patient. It is turned off during routine use. Follow your facility policy and the nurse's instructions for activating this feature. The controller also has arrows to adjust the pressure inside the hose. It should be set at 35 mm Hg to 55 mm Hg. The unit may automatically set at 45 mm Hg, the midway point. The nurse will set the unit or instruct you on the setting to use.

Both hosiery must be connected to the controller for the unit to operate. Position the arrows on the hose opposite the arrows on the tubing. Push the ends together firmly until you hear a clicking sound. If the patient will be using only one sleeve, such as when she has a cast on one leg, leave the unused sleeve in the sealed plastic bag. Cut a small hole in the bag and connect the tubing.

Applying Pneumatic Hosiery. Before applying the hosiery, palpate the pedal (Figure 11.45A) and posterior tibial pulses (Figure 11.45B). In most facilities, staff mark the location of these pulses with a marker, making a small "X" on the patient's skin. Compare the movement, sensation, and color in both feet. If abnormalities are noted, consult the nurse before continuing. The nurse will assess the patient's legs and check for contraindications. Follow the nurse's instructions

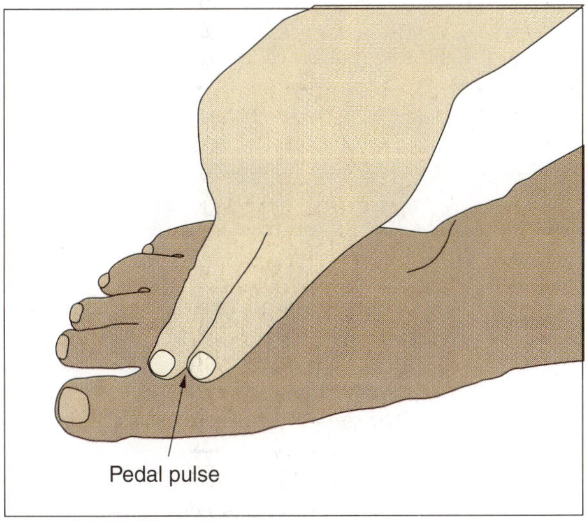

FIGURE 11-45A The pedal (dorsalis pedis) pulse.

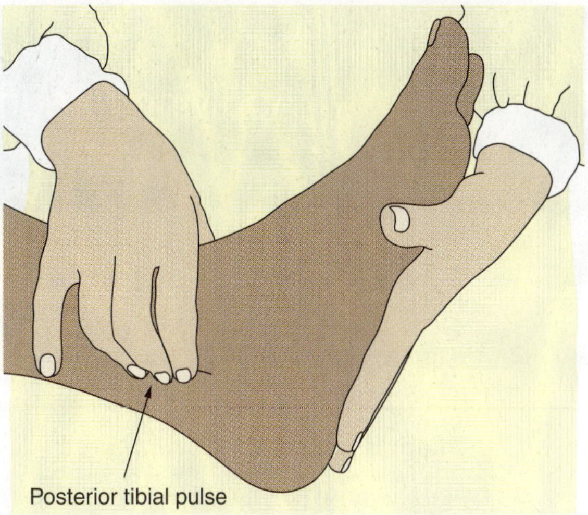

FIGURE 11-45B The posterior tibial pulse.

Pneumatic hosiery may be applied over antiembolism hose, but both the sleeves and the antiembolism hose must be smooth and wrinkle-free to reduce the risk of skin breakdown. The device is used 24 hours a day, when the patient is lying down, until the patient is completely ambulatory. It may be removed for bathing and ambulation, then reapplied immediately. The nurse may instruct the patient to perform certain leg exercises while the device is being used.

Caring for the Patient with Pneumatic Hosiery. The compression controller has a visual display that notes which chamber is inflated. When the chambers decompress, the unit will say "vent." Make sure the audible alarm is turned on, and check that the key has been removed. If the alarm sounds, the panel will display a message code. A card in a slot in the top of the unit will display the numerical message code with the nature of the problem. Follow the directions on the card to correct the problem, or notify the nurse, according to facility policy. The hose deflates automatically when the alarm sounds.

Turn the power off and remove the hose every 4 hours. Disconnect the sleeves from the tubing by releasing the latches on each side of the connectors, then pulling the connectors apart. Observe the skin under the device, and provide skin care as ordered. Avoid massaging the legs.

PROCEDURE 71 Applying Pneumatic Compression Hosiery

1. Carry out beginning procedure actions.
2. Assemble equipment:
   - hosiery of proper size
   - compression controller
3. Open the hose, laying them flat on the bed with the markings opposite the knee and ankle.
4. Lift the patient's leg, and slide the hose under it. Begin on the side of the leg opposite the plastic tubing. Wrap the sleeve smoothly around the leg with the opening in front, over the knee. Make sure there are no dents, folds, or creases in the garment.
5. Beginning at the ankle, fasten the Velcro fasteners securely. Next, secure the ankle and calf, then the thigh.
6. Check the fit by inserting two fingers between the sleeve and the patient's leg. The fit should feel snug and secure, but not tight.
7. Wrap the other leg in the same manner, beginning on the side opposite the plastic tubing. After wrapping the leg, check the fit.
8. Attach the plastic tubing on each leg to the compression controller by lining up the arrows on the tubing.
9. Plug the controller in and turn on the power.
10. Remain with the patient for one complete cycle (usually 60 to 90 seconds) to ensure that she tolerates the procedure.
11. Carry out procedure completion actions.

Massage may dislodge a blood clot, which will quickly migrate to the lungs. Inform the nurse when you will be removing the device so that he or she can assess the patient's legs.

Use of the hose will be discontinued when the patient is fully ambulatory. The unit is not disposable. Clean and store the device according to facility policy after use, or return it to central supply.

Documentation. Follow your facility policy for documenting use of the pneumatic compression device. You may be asked to document the procedure, pulse checks in the feet, skin color, the patient's response, and the settings, including use of the alarm and cooling settings.

REVIEW

A. Multiple Choice

Select the one best answer.

1. Anti-embolism hose reduce the incidence of
   a. Arthritis
   b. Thrombophlebitis
   c. Gastritis
   d. Dermatitis
2. Prior to applying an elastic bandage, elevate the arm or leg
   a. 24 hours
   b. 12 hours
   c. 1–2 hours
   d. 15 to 30 minutes

3. The best time to apply TED's is

    a. while the resident is sleeping
    b. while the resident is sitting in a chair
    c. before the resident gets out of bed in the morning
    d. while the resident's skin is moist with lotion

4. Pneumatic hosiery also called sequential compression hosiery prevent blood clots by:

    a. promoting immobility
    b. massaging the legs mechanically
    c. promoting mobility
    d. warming the legs

5. Thirty minutes after applying anti-embolic, resident complains of numbness and tingling in both feet. Which pulses may be checked for circulation?

    a. brachial
    b. posterior tibia
    c. right temporal
    d. anterior carotid

E: Non-sterile Dressing and Bandages

OBJECTIVES

After reading this unit, you will be able to:

- Spell and define key terms.
- State the purposes of clean dressings and bandages
- Define clean dressing and bandages
- List dressing supplies
- Demonstrate application of non-sterile dressing following the RN's directions

OBSERVATIONS

Observe and report color, size, drainage, or odor

Report resident's response to procedure

Clean Dressings and Bandages

Caring for surgical wounds, injuries, and ulcers is very important. **Dressings** are gauze, film, or other synthetic substances that cover a wound, ulcer, or injury. Some dressings have an adhesive backing. Some are affixed with tape. Many different types of tapes are available in the health care facility. Some patients need special **hypoallergenic tape**, which reduces the incidence of a skin reaction in patients who are allergic to the adhesive backing. **Bandages** are sometimes used to hold dressings in place. These are fabric, gauze, net, or elasticized materials used to cover the dressing and keep it securely in place. Bandages are available in different sizes and shapes. Gauze bandages are commonly used to cover dressings. Elastic bandages are used to reduce edema and support injured body parts. When wrapping bandages, avoid wrapping them so tightly that they restrict circulation.

Occasionally, **Montgomery straps** (Figure 11.46) are used to hold dressings in place. These are long strips of adhesive attached to the skin on either side of the wound. They are less traumatic to the skin because the adhesive is not removed with each dressing change unless the straps are soiled.

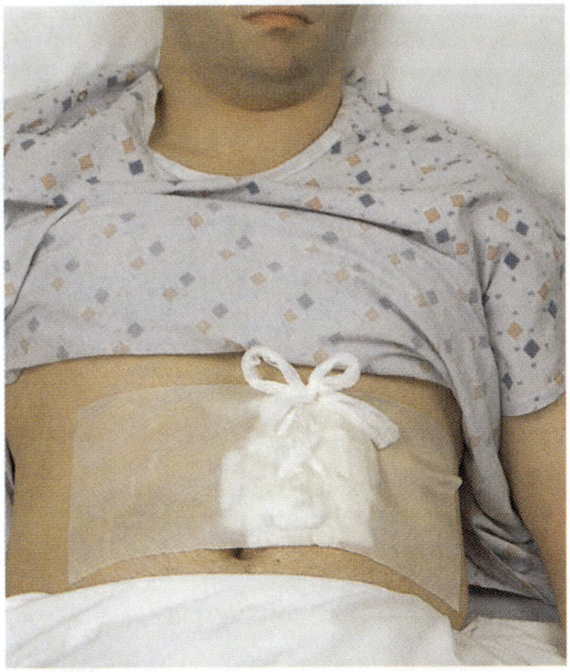

FIGURE 11-46 Montgomery straps hold dressings securely in place so they can be observed, changed, and reinforced without tape. This is much less traumatic for the patient.

After the dressing is in place, the straps are tied to hold the dressing securely. **Binders** (Figure 11.47) may also be used to hold dressings in place.

Clean Technique

Any break in the skin increases the risk of infection. Wounds are most susceptible to infection during the first four days, although infection can begin at any time. Dressings protect the wound, preventing contamination. They also increase comfort and prevent further injury. Some dressings are used to apply pressure to the wound to control bleeding. Always apply the principles of standard precautions when caring for wounds. **NA I may not do sterile dressings.**

Clean technique may be used for superficial pressure ulcers and other minor wounds. Clean dressing supplies may be used in an emergency to stop bleeding in any wound.

Applying a Dressing

Before applying the dressing, receive direction from RN. Gather your supplies. Select a dressing that will extend at least one inch beyond the borders of the wound. If gauze dressings are used, several layers may be necessary to protect the wound and collect drainage. Wounds with heavy drainage may need additional composite dressings over the gauze. Extra dressings may be applied to some wounds for protective padding. This prevents discomfort and trauma to the wound.

It may be necessary to reposition the patient for the procedure. Place the patient in a position that he or she can maintain for the entire procedure without discomfort.

After you have applied the dressing and the wound is covered, you can remove your gloves, if necessary, so tape does not stick to them. (Do not remove your gloves if the wound is draining.) Secure the dressing with tape, bandage, or binder. Discard the used gloves, dressings, and supplies in a plastic bag, according to facility policy. Assist the patient to a comfortable position.

Changing A Clean Dressing

Clean dressings are used on minor, uninfected wounds. You will handle only the corners of the dressings. Avoid touching the center, which contacts the wound.

PROCEDURE

72 Changing a Clean Dressing

Supplies needed:

- 2 pairs clean, disposable exam gloves
- Cleansing solution
- Plastic bag for used supplies
- Clean or sterile gauze pads or other dressing, as ordered, and according to facility policy
- Tape or bandage material

1. Perform your beginning procedure actions.
2. Holding gentle traction on the skin, loosen the tape by pulling the ends toward the wound, and then remove the dressing. Discard in the plastic bag.
3. Cleanse and rinse the wound as ordered. If the wound appears abnormal or infected, notify your supervisor.
4. Remove the gloves and discard in the plastic bag.
5. Wash your hands.
6. Set up your dressing supplies and open packages.
7. Apply clean exam gloves.
8. Pick up the gauze dressing, holding it only by the corners.
9. Center the dressing over the wound.
10. Tape the dressing securely in place, or cover with a bandage as instructed.
11. Perform your procedure completion actions.

PROCEDURE

73 Applying a Bandage

1. After applying the dressing, apply the bandage. Most bandaging materials are conforming, self-adhering gauze. Brand name products, such as Kling® and Kerlix®, or generic products, such as conforming gauze, are commonly used in health care facilities.
2. The bandage must cover the dressing completely. Begin by holding the bandage in your dominant hand. Hold the bandage against the skin with your nondominant thumb, approximately one inch below the dressing.
3. Wrap the bandage around the extremity two or three times to hold it securely in place.
4. Wrap the bandage from distal to proximal, in overlapping spiral turns (Figure 11.47). Each turn should overlap 1\2 to 3\4 of the previous turn. The bandage should be snug so it does not fall off. However, it must not be so tight that it restricts blood flow.
5. Wrap the bandage at least one inch above the top of the dressing. Wrap it completely around the extremity twice, then cut the end. Tape the end to the bandage, not the skin.
6. Assess the circulation distal to the bandage to ensure that the circulation is adequate.
7. Perform your procedure completion actions.

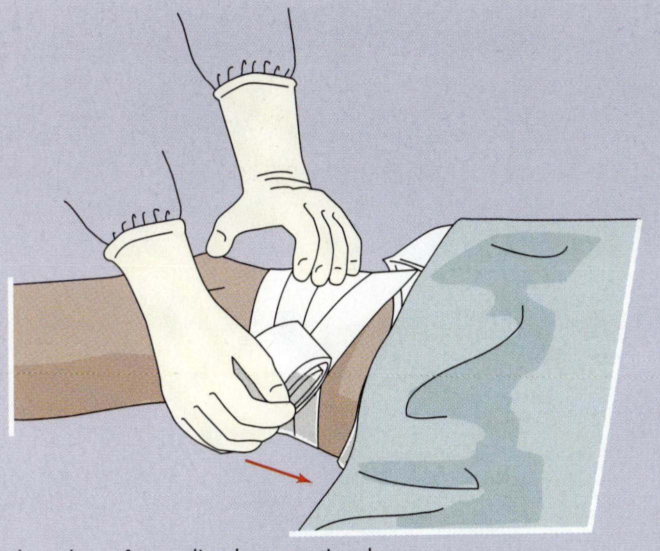

FIGURE 11-47 Wrap bandage from distal to proximal.

REVIEW

1. Why must dressings be secure over wounds?
2. Name two methods of securing dressings in place.
3. Why might a Nurse Aide choose paper tape over adhesive tape?

A. Multiple Choice

Select the one best answer.

4. A purpose of the non-sterile bandage is to:
   a. decrease dehydration
   b. absorb heavy bleeding
   c. hold dressings in place
   d. cover fresh open surgical wound
5. The scope of practice allows the Nursing Assistant I to:
   a. clean surgical wounds
   b. apply dressings using clean technique
   c. apply dressings using sterile technique
   d. apply sterile gloves for dressing change
6. After transferring Mrs. Green to the shower chair, you observe an inch-long skin tear above her right ankle. The Nurse Assistant should:
   a. Apply an elastic bandage to the wound
   b. report and receive directions from the nurse
   c. apply a bandage, shower the resident, and then report to your nurse
   d. wash the tear and leave open to air

B. Matching

Choose the correct word from Column II to match each blank in Column I.

	Column I	Column II
______	Used to reduce edema and support body parts	1. Elastic bandages
______	Holds dressings in place	2. Skin tears
______	Numbness, cyanosis, tingling	3. Montgomery straps
______	Minor breaks in the skin	4. Gauze bandages
______	Less traumatic to the skin than tape	5. Signs of poor circulation

UNIT 12

Death and Dying

OBJECTIVES

After reading this unit, you will be able to:

- Spell and define key terms.
- Examine your personal feelings about death, dying, and terminal illness.
- List the five steps in the grieving process and describe what happens in each.
- List 14 signs and symptoms of impending death.
- Describe the care of a dying resident.
- Explain why standard precautions are used when providing postmortem care.
- Demonstrate the procedure related to death and dying.

OBSERVATIONS TO MAKE AND REPORT RELATED TO DEATH AND DYING

Decreasing level of responsiveness
Decreasing movement, muscle tone, and sensation
Relaxation of lower jaw
Mouth falls open
Skin pale, moist, cool to touch; progresses to cold to touch
Skin progresses to blue, gray, or dusky appearance, beginning in the lower extremities and moving upward
Lips, fingernails, and mucous membranes become dusky, gray, or blue
Pulse becomes rapid, weak, or thready
Respirations become slow, labored, irregular, or noisy
Cheyne-Stokes respirations
Blood pressure decreases; blood pressure can no longer be heard at the brachial artery, but the resident remains alive
Mucus collects in the throat, may rattle during respirations
Resident becomes incontinent of urine and feces
Eyes stare and pupils do not respond to light

Introduction

Health care professionals deal with life and death daily. Caring for residents who are dying and caring for the body after death will probably be part of your responsibility. Death is expected in some residents. Others die suddenly, without warning. The nursing assistant plays an important role in the care of the dying resident. Although you can do nothing to prolong the resident's life, you will take comfort in the fact that you did all you could to make the resident's last moments on earth as comfortable as possible.

All staff members must be aware of what the resident has been told about his or her condition. In some situations residents are not told of their impending death. This is a medical decision made by the physician. If this is the case, you must respect this decision and abide by it whether you agree or not. In other cases residents are told they are dying and may wish to discuss it. Your listening and communication skills are especially important when caring for the dying resident (Figure 12.1).

Resuscitation Orders

Resuscitation is performed on all residents unless the physician has written a **do not resuscitate (DNR) order.** Residents with DNR orders are usually terminally ill and have signed an advance directive indicating that they do not want life-sustaining procedures performed in the event of death. If the resident has a DNR order, no CPR will be performed if the resident's heart stops beating. In the absence of a DNR order, cardiopulmonary resuscitation is performed if a resident shows signs of clinical death. In many facilities, the nursing assistant is trained to perform CPR and may initiate and assist with this procedure.

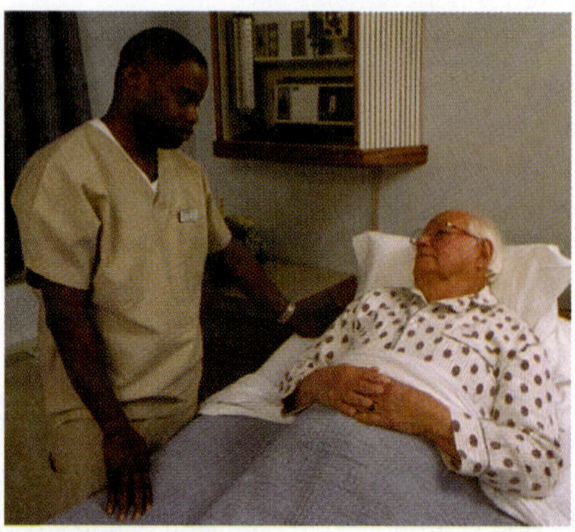

FIGURE 12-1 Active listening is an important communication skill.

Each facility has an emergency code designated for resuscitation. Many agencies use the term **code blue** to signify a **cardiac arrest.** A cardiac arrest occurs when the resident's heart and breathing have stopped. Announcing a resuscitation event (or code blue) on the public address system will alert the emergency response team to respond to the unit. CPR and other aggressive measures will be performed to save the resident's life. The ambulance will be called to transport the resident to the hospital. When paramedics arrive, they will use drugs and advanced life support devices to try to save the resident's life.

Examining Your Feelings About Death and Dying

As a whole, society in the United States avoids meaningful discussions about death and dying. As a result, we may be very uncomfortable speaking about this subject. Some people avoid making wills because it reminds them of their own mortality. For some, speaking about death and dying is painful because it reminds them of personal experiences with friends and loved ones. The AIDS epidemic of the 1980s and 1990s has evoked strong feelings about death and dying. Most victims of AIDS were young and in the prime of their lives. Approximately 11% of all new AIDS cases reported to the CDC are in people over age 50. State reporting requirements vary, so people who are HIV positive but have not yet developed AIDS are not necessarily included in this number. Many individuals have not been diagnosed, so the statistics do not accurately reflect the prevalence of HIV disease and AIDS. The incidence of HIV infection and AIDS is increasing. Unfortunately, this age group may not be tested for HIV because they are perceived to have few risk factors. The scientific community is beginning to view AIDS in a new light. We are beginning to see it as a chronic, manageable disease. However, many people are fearful of the disease and continue to see it as a **terminal illness.** A terminal illness is a condition from which the resident is not expected to recover. Young people tend to see themselves as invincible, and receiving a terminal diagnosis is traumatic and painful. A nurse who died of AIDS summed up her feelings about the disease and about dying. She explained that before she developed AIDS, she felt it was a disease for "them." After she became ill, it was difficult for her to accept care given to her by other nurses. As a nurse, she felt she should be giving care, not receiving it. It was embarrassing to lose control of her body functions. She said that the disease caused her to realize that "them is us." There is a great deal of wisdom and insight in this statement. The "them is us" philosophy can be applied to many different diseases in addition to AIDS.

Factors That Influence Your Feelings about Death and Dying

As a nursing assistant, you will care for both young and old residents who are dying. It is never your responsibility to inform them that they are dying. However, once the information has been delivered, you must be prepared to assist the dying resident to meet physical, emotional, psychological, social, and spiritual needs. In some cases, you will also be a source of strength and support for the family.

You may feel that death in infants, children, and young adults is unfair. Health care workers often have different views of death and dying in the elderly, who have lived long lives. Your body begins to age as soon as you are born. Death is a natural extension of life. Your feelings and beliefs about death and dying will affect the care you give. In order to care for dying residents effectively, you must examine and understand your own feelings about death. Sometimes we feel that we have failed in our job if the resident dies. As long as you have done all you can for the dying resident, you have succeeded in your responsibilities. Learn to take comfort in that.

Your age, culture, experiences, religion, values, and personal losses all influence your feelings about death and dying. Sometimes your attitude about death changes because of your personal experiences. As we age, we also may view death differently. Many elderly residents see death as a relief from pain and suffering. Some people fear death. It is a journey into the unknown. They are afraid that it will be lonely and painful. Studies of people who have had near-death experiences have shown that death is not unpleasant or frightening. Residents may also worry about dying alone. Many people worry about unfinished personal business and what will happen to family members and pets after their death.

Hospice. There is no cure for some diseases. Sometimes trauma and injuries to the body are so severe that the resident cannot recover. Some residents do not respond to medical treatment. Some die soon after receiving a terminal diagnosis. Others live for extended periods of time. We cannot predict when death will occur.

A **hospice** is an agency that cares for residents who are dying. Hospice workers are members of an interdisciplinary team who work to meet the resident's and family's physical, emotional, psychological, social, and spiritual needs. Hospice care is delivered in many different settings. Sometimes care is given in a hospital or nursing home. Many individuals use hospice services in their own home. Hospice care is not designed to be aggressive or to prolong life. It is designed to make the resident and family as comfortable as possible as death approaches. The quality of care given is as good as the care given to all other residents. Family members may participate in resident care if they wish. Hospice care is designed to ensure that the resident dies in comfort, with dignity and respect.

Coping Mechanisms. Coping mechanisms are responses to stress that people use to protect their self-esteem. An understanding of some of the coping mechanisms that people use to deal with losses and stress in life will help you understand resident and family reactions to dealing with terminal illness. Coping mechanisms develop throughout a person's life. Success or failure in developing coping skills depends on how well the developmental tasks of earlier life have been mastered. When a person's ability to cope is inadequate, the following reactions may be seen:

- Chronic complaining
- Anger
- Irritability
- Crying and tearfulness
- Agitation
- Restlessness
- Sleep disturbances
- Muscle tension and headaches
- Depression
- Withdrawal
- Weight loss or gain

Residents may criticize and blame you for things that are not your fault. Do not take their comments personally. These residents usually need emotional support. Your understanding of basic human needs, normal developmental tasks, and coping mechanisms will help you provide quality care. The following are other ways you can provide this support:

- Offer choices over routines and as much control as possible.
- Realize that angry outbursts may be the result of feelings of hopelessness, loss, and unmet needs.
- Direct the resident's emotional energy in positive ways.
- Avoid responding to the resident in a negative manner.
- Report any change in the resident's behavior to the nurse.

GRIEVING PROCESS

When we anticipate or experience a loss, we go through a series of emotional changes and behaviors called the **grieving process.** This process was first described by Dr. Elisabeth Kübler-Ross. Loss of someone or something you love is very difficult. The resident, family, friends, and care providers each go through the grieving process, which involves five steps. The grieving process varies with each of us, so all persons do not experience each step. The steps are not always obvious to others. Sometimes we recognize the steps in other people, but fail to recognize them in ourselves. Some people move from one stage to another and back again. It may take a long time to complete all the steps in the grieving process. The resident may die before completing the process. Throughout the grieving process, the nursing assistant must offer honesty, reassurance, understanding, caring, and empathy. Helping a resident die in comfort and dignity is very important. Table 12.1 gives examples of typical resident reactions and appropriate nursing assistant responses in each stage of the grieving process.

Denial

The first stage in the grieving process is **denial.** This occurs when a person first learns of a terminal diagnosis. The resident may feel that the diagnosis is incorrect. He or she may exhibit false hope, tell untrue stories, and spend a tremendous amount of energy keeping denial alive. The resident may refuse to participate in his or her care, and may not follow the directions of the physician and other staff. The resident and family need strong emotional support in order to move through this stage. Allow them to express their feelings, but do not provide false hope. Conversations should be based in reality. Spend time with the resident to show that he or she will not be

TABLE 12-1 Stages of grief

Stages of Grief	Response of the Nursing Assistant
Denial	Reflect the resident's statements, but try not to confirm or deny the fact that the resident is dying. *Example: "The lab tests can't be right. I don't have cancer."* *"It must have been difficult for you to learn the results of your tests."*
Anger	Understand the source of the resident's anger. Provide understanding and support. Listen. Try to meet reasonable needs and demands quickly. *Example: "This food is terrible–not fit to eat."* *"Let me see if I can find something that would appeal to you more."*
Bargaining	If it is possible to meet the resident's requests, do so. Listen attentively. *Example: "If only God will spare me this, I'll go to church every week."* *"Would you like a visit from your clergy person?"*
Depression	Avoid clichés that dismiss the resident's depression ("It could be worse. You could be in more pain"). Be caring and supporting. Let the resident know that it is okay to be depressed. *Example: "There just isn't any sense in going on."* *"I understand you are feeling very depressed."*
Acceptance	Do not assume that, because the resident has accepted death, she or he is unafraid, or that she or he does not need emotional support. Listen attentively and be supportive and caring. *Example: "I feel so alone."* *"I am here with you. Would you like to talk?"*

left alone. Later in the denial stage, the resident may isolate himself or herself from others.

Anger

The second stage of the grieving process is **anger.** The resident feels angry with himself or herself, family, staff, the doctor, and God. He or she may use abusive language and refuse care and nutrition. Recognize that the resident is not angry with you personally. Practice empathy and let the resident know you understand how he or she feels.

Bargaining

The third stage of the grieving process is **bargaining.** The resident hopes he or she can live to see a certain event, such as a graduation or birth of a grandchild. Sometimes the resident bargains with God and makes promises, such as attending church every Sunday in return for more time. Bargaining is an attempt to postpone the inevitable. This stage is usually short. Realize that the resident still needs time to accept his or her impending death. Spend as much time as you can with the resident to show that you sincerely care.

Depression

Depression (Figure 12.2) is the fourth stage in the grieving process. The resident is dealing with the loss of everything that he or she has. The resident's physical ability may decline. He or she is losing his or her home, possessions, loved ones, hopes, and dreams. The resident may also be feeling regrets for things he or she has said or done throughout life. The resident may experience **apathy**, decreased ability to concentrate, insomnia, fatigue, constant crying, poor appetite, and lack of interest in people and the environment. In this stage, the resident is beginning to separate himself or herself from life. Do not attempt to humor or cheer the resident. Allow him or her to express feelings, and be available to sit quietly and provide support.

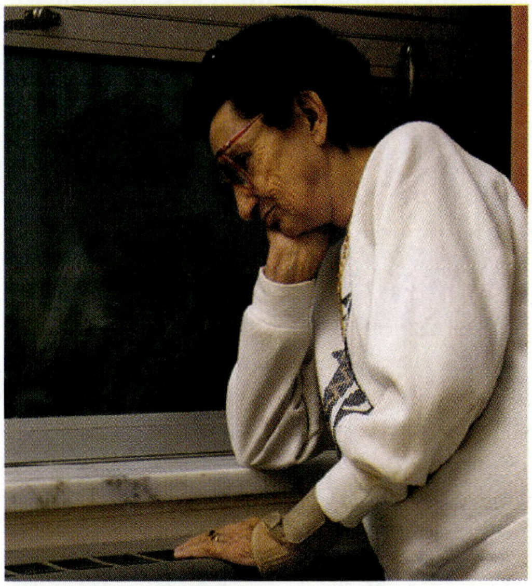

FIGURE 12-2 The depressed resident is beginning to separate herself from life.

Acceptance

The final stage in the grieving process is **acceptance.** The resident may feel empty and peaceful. This stage usually brings less emotional pain and discomfort, and the resident calmly waits for the end. The resident may not want to be alone during this stage. If the resident does not object, allow others with whom he or she is comfortable to assist with care. Allow the resident to express needs in his or her own time and way. Communication may be limited in this stage.

Signs of Approaching Death

Signs of death may occur slowly or rapidly. Always report changes in the resident's condition to the nurse. Some residents are alert until the moment of death. Others have a period of unconsciousness first. After the resident dies, the physician will examine the resident and pronounce death. In some states, registered nurses may pronounce death. This is never the responsibility of the nursing assistant. The nurse or physician is also responsible for notifying the family after death has been established.

Signs of approaching death are:

- Decreasing level of responsiveness.
- Movement, muscle tone, and sensation decrease until they are eventually lost.
- The lower jaw relaxes and the mouth falls open.
- The skin appears pale and is moist and cool to touch.
- The lips, fingernails, and mucous membranes take on a dusky, gray, or blue color.
- The pulse becomes rapid, weak, or thready.
- Respirations become slow, labored, irregular, or noisy. Cheyne-Stokes respirations may be present. Mucus collects in the throat. This is sometimes called a "death rattle."
- Blood pressure decreases. Sometimes blood pressure can no longer be heard at the brachial artery, but the resident remains alive.
- The resident may become incontinent of urine and feces.

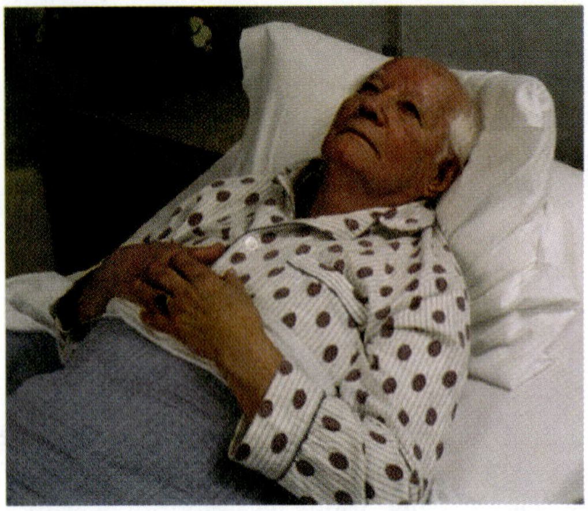

FIGURE 12-3 As death approaches, the eyes stare and the pupils do not respond to light. The resident can still hear, however.

- The eyes stare and pupils do not respond to light (Figure 12.3).
- The skin takes on a blue or dusky appearance beginning in the lower extremities, and moving upward. The skin feels cool or cold to touch.

Care of the Dying Resident

Some facilities are now setting aside private rooms for residents who are dying and their families. These rooms may be called *hospice rooms*, even though true hospice care is not being provided. This provides a place for the resident and family to spend their last moments together and say their goodbyes without disturbing a roommate. It also avoids upsetting a roommate at the time of the resident's death.

Care of the dying resident is a continuation of care that shows support, dignity, and respect. The Dying Person's Bill of Rights (Figure 12.4) provides guidelines and should be used as a basis for care.

The Dying Person's Bill of Rights

- I have the right to be treated as a living human being until I die.
- I have the right to maintain a sense of hopefulness, however changing its focus may be.
- I have the right to be cared for by those who can maintain a sense of hopefulness, however changing this may be.
- I have the right to express my feelings and emotions about my approaching death in my own way.
- I have the right to participate in decisions concerning my care.
- I have the right to expect continuing medical and nursing attention even though "cure" goals must be changed to "comfort" goals.
- I have the right not to die alone.
- I have the right to be free from pain.
- I have the right to have my questions answered honestly.
- I have the right not to be deceived.
- I have the right to have help from and for my family accepting my death.
- I have the right to die in peace and dignity.
- I have the right to retain my individuality and not be judged for my decisions, which may be contrary to the beliefs of others.
- I have the right to discuss and enlarge my religious and/or spiritual experiences, regardless of what they may mean to others.
- I have the right to expect that the sanctity of the human body will be respected after death.
- I have the right to be cared for by caring, sensitive, knowledgeable people who will attempt to understand my needs and will be able to gain some satisfaction in helping me face my death.

FIGURE 12-4 The dying person's bill of rights. *(From Barbus, A. J.: American Journal of Nursing 75(1):99, 1975)*

Postmortem Care

Your facility will have a policy and procedure for physical care of the body after death. This is called **postmortem care**, and in most cases, the nursing assistant delivers this care. Some facilities have a morgue to which the body is taken. In most facilities the body will be left in the room until it can be transferred to a mortuary. Within two to four hours after death, a condition called **rigor mortis** develops. In this condition, the muscles and limbs of the body become rigid and stiff. Position the body in good alignment before this condition occurs. When circulation stops, the body begins to pull blood into the lowest areas of the body. This process can begin within 20 minutes of death. Over time, this will result in a stained appearance on the back of the body (if the resident is in the supine position). To reduce the risk of staining about the head and neck, elevate the head of the bed 30 degrees, in the semi-Fowler's position. Some facilities do not use ties in the morgue pack to position the body. Follow your facility policies. If used, tie them loosely. If the ties are too tight, they will also cause permanent marks on the body.

Always use standard precautions when providing postmortem care. The body can be infectious after death. Handle the body very gently. Show the same respect and provide the same privacy that you would if the resident were alive. Respect the religious beliefs of the deceased. Spiritual beliefs vary, and people of some faiths have special religious requirements for preparation of the body. Table 12.2 describes some common religious and cultural beliefs.

TABLE 12-2 Cultural/religious beliefs affecting care at the time of death

Culture/Religion	Religious Belief
Adventist (Seventh Day, Church of God)	Some believe in divine healing, anointing with oil, and prayer.
American Indian	There are many different tribes, and beliefs vary with each. Some believe an owl is an omen of death. Some tribes have family members prepare the body for burial. Some tribes will not touch the dead person's belongings after death. Some tribes believe the dead are happy in the spirit world. Others believe the body is an empty shell. Some have extensive preparation of the body and visitation of the deceased. If a member of some tribes dies at home, the house is abandoned forever or may be burned.
Armenian Church	Holy Communion may be given as a form of last rites; laying-on of hands is practiced.
Baptist	Pastor, resident, and family counsel and pray. Resident may be given Communion. Some practice healing and laying-on of hands.
Black/African American	The deceased is highly respected. Health care providers usually prepare the body. Cremation is usually avoided. May have concerns about organ donation.
Black Muslim	Practices for washing the body, applying the shroud, and funeral rites are carefully prescribed.
Brethren	Anointing with oil is done for physical healing and spiritual guidance.
Buddhist Churches of America	The priest is contacted to provide Last Rites. Chanting may be done at the bedside after death.
Cambodian (Khmer)	Monks recite prayers. Family wants to be present at time of death and may want to care for the resident. Incense may be burned. Death is accepted in a quiet, passive manner. Family and monks may wish to prepare the body. A white cloth is used as a shroud, and mourners wear white.
Central American	Catholics may want a priest to administer Sacrament of the Sick. Candles may be used if oxygen is not in use in room. Family members may wish to prepare the body.
Chinese American	Family may prefer resident not be told of impending death, or may prefer to inform the resident themselves. May not want to talk about the terminal illness with anyone. Some believe that dying at home is bad luck. Others believe that the spirit gets lost if the resident dies in the hospital. Family members may place special cloths and amulets on the body. Some prefer to bathe their own family members after death.
Christian Scientist	A Christian Science practitioner may be called for spiritual support. Have concerns about organ donation.
Church of God	Believe in divine healing through prayer. Speaking in tongues may be used.
Church of Jesus Christ of Latter Day Saints (LDS or Mormon)	Body is dressed in white temple clothing before viewing by family members. Cremation is discouraged. Believe in baptism for others who have died and preaching to deceased.

(continues)

TABLE 12-2 *(continued)*

Culture/Religion	Religious Belief
Colombian	Catholic prayer and anointing of the sick common. Family may practice Catholic prayer at bedside. Family members may cry loudly or become hysterical. All family members may want to see the body before it is taken to the morgue. In Colombia, the decreased are usually buried within 24 to 36 hours. The nurse may need to inform them that in the United States the body may not be buried this quickly.
Cuban	Family may not want resident told of impending death. This varies according to Cuban culture. Family members may stay with resident 24 hours a day during terminal phase of illness.
Eastern Orthodox	Last rites are given. Anointing of the sick is performed as a form of healing with prayer. Cremation is discouraged.
Episcopal	Last Rites are available, but not mandatory. May practice prayer, Communion, and confession.
Ethiopian	Friends are told of death before family so they can be present when family is informed. Female family members are never told first. Great displays of feelings are encouraged at death. They may cry loudly and hysterically. Women may tear their clothing and beat their chests. Men may cry out loud. Some families may want to say goodbye to the decreased before the body is removed from the room.
Filipino	Head of family is informed away from resident's room. Catholic priest is called to deliver Sacrament of the Sick. DNR decisions may be made by the entire family. Religious objects may be placed around the resident. Family may pray at the bedside when resident is dying. After death, they may cry loudly and hysterically. Family may wish to wash the body. Death is considered a very spiritual event. All family members may say goodbye before body is removed from the room.
Friends (Quaker)	Do not believe in life after death (spiritual afterlife).
Greek Orthodox	The priest should be called while the resident is still conscious. Practice Last Rites and administration of Communion. Believe that life should be preserved until terminated by God.
Gypsy	In general, discussion of death is avoided in this culture. Eldest in authority is informed of death first. A priest may be present for body purification. Family may want the window open at the time of death and afterward so the spirit can leave the room. May ask for special personal items in room at the time of death. An older female relative may remain at the window to keep spirits out of room. The moment of death and the resident's last words are very significant. The body after death may represent a source of spiritual danger to the family. Family may want body embalmed immediately after death to remove blood. They may sit with the body around the clock after death, and will eat and drink at this location.
Haitian	Elaborate rituals after death. When death is imminent, family will cry hysterically and uncontrollably. Family members may bring religious symbols and medallions. They have a deep respect for the dead. Family members may wish to wash the body and participate in postmortem care.

Hindu	Specially prescribed rites. Priest may tie a thread around wrist or neck and place water in mouth. The family washes and dresses the body, and only certain persons may touch the dead. May prefer cremation to burial.
Hmong	Important to wear fine traditional Hmong clothing at the time of death. Family may put amulets on body, which should not be removed. The family usually prepares the body at the funeral home. The body cannot be buried with hard objects, buttons, or zippers against the body.
Iranian	Death is seen as the beginning of a spiritual relationship with God, not the end of life. Family may wish to be present at all times when resident is dying, and may cry and pray at bedside. Families may wish to wash the body.
Islam (Muslim)	Begging forgiveness and confession of sins must be done in presence of family members before death. There are five steps to preparing the body for burial. The first step involves washing of the body by a Muslim of the same gender. May offer special prayers at bedside to ease pain and suffering. Some have spiritual leader give resident holy water to drink prior to death to purify body. After death, arms and legs are straightened and the toes tied together with a bandage. May be opposed to autopsy.
Japanese	Resident and family may be aware of impending death, but will not speak about it. Family may wish to remain at bedside during terminal stage of illness. Cleanliness and dignity of the body are very important.
Jehovah's Witness	Practice baptism and Communion. May be opposed to autopsy.
Judaism (Orthodox and Conservative)	Jews believe in the sanctity of life. Medical care is generally expected, and there are no medication restrictions. Most surgical procedures are permitted, but body parts that have been removed are traditionally saved for later burial. For most Jews, medical treatment cannot be stopped once it has been started, but members are not required to use extraordinary measures to prolong life. May be opposed to prolonging life if resident has irreversible brain damage. However, active euthanasia is forbidden. Traditional Jews use a burial society to care for the body after death. Society members may or may not be members of the deceased's congregation. They usually prefer no autopsy, but this is permitted if legally required. Embalming is generally discouraged. The resident is buried as soon after death as possible. Cremation is discouraged. For traditional Jews, mourning begins with a seven-day period called *shiva*, in which men do not shave, and family and close friends do not read the newspaper or watch television. Mourning extends over a year. Jewish practices and beliefs can be very different from family to family. Asking the resident or family members about their practices is probably best. Asking is not offensive, and shows that you care about and respect the resident's and family's wishes.
Korean	Chanting, incense, and praying may be used. Family crying and mourning may be extreme. Family may want to spend time alone with the resident after death. Some may wish to wash the body.
Lutheran	Practice prayer. Last Rites optional; the resident may request anointing of the sick.

(continues)

TABLE 12-2 *(continued)*

Culture/Religion	Religious Belief
Methodist	May request donation of body or body parts to medical science.
Mexican American	Entire family may be obligated to visit the sick and dying. Pregnant women may be prohibited from visiting. Spiritual items may be important. May want to die at home because of the fear that the spirit will get lost in the hospital. Crying loudly and wailing is culturally accepted and a sign of respect. A Catholic priest is called for the Sacrament of the Sick. A family member may wish to assist with postmortem care. Family will want time alone with the body before it is removed from the room.
Orthodox Presbyterian	Scripture reading and prayer. Full forgiveness is granted for any illness connected with a sin.
Puerto Rican	If death is imminent, family may stay around the clock. Some believe that all immediate family members must be present at the time of death. Believe that the body must be treated with great respect.
Roman Catholic	Prayer and the rite for anointing of the sick is desired. Resident or family may request anointing if prognosis is poor.
Russian	Family may not want the resident to know of a terminal diagnosis. Depending on religion, family may wish to wash the body and dress it in special clothes.
Russian Orthodox	Practice prayer, Communion, and Last Rites by priest. Many wear a cross necklace, which should not be removed if at all possible. After death the arms are crossed, and fingers set in the form of a cross. Clothing must be a natural fiber so the body changes to ashes sooner. May be opposed to autopsy, embalming, or cremation.
Samoan	Resident and family prefer to be told of terminal diagnosis as early as possible. Family would prefer to care for resident at home, if possible. Family members usually prefer to prepare the body.
Sikh	Believe that the soul remains alive after death. Family washes the body and dresses deceased member in new clothing.
Unitarian Universalist	Cremation may be preferred to burial.
Vietnamese	DNR decisions are made by entire family. For Catholic families, religious items are kept close to resident. For Buddhist families, incense is burned. Families prefer time alone with the deceased before body is moved. The body is highly respected, and the family may prefer to wash it. Some may prefer the body left as it is.
West Indian	When death is near, close family and friends wish to remain at the bedside to pray. Family members may wish to view the body exactly as the resident was at the time of death. Most wish to be alone with the deceased

GUIDELINES IN

Caring for the Dying Resident

- Practice empathy for the resident, friends, and family.
- Check the care plan for special care instructions.
- Consider and respect the religious beliefs of the resident and family even if they are different from your own.
- Provide privacy when clergy visit (Figure 12.5).
- Learn the resident's cultural and religious practices regarding death.
- Keep the resident clean and comfortable.
- Keep the lips and mouth moist and give frequent oral care.
- Turn the resident every two hours or more. Position with props and pillows for comfort.
- Keep the skin clean. Apply lotion as needed.
- Change the linen immediately if it is wet or soiled. Provide blankets for warmth.
- Provide perineal care after each episode of incontinence.
- The room should be well lighted and as comfortable and pleasant as possible.
- Allow privacy if the family is present, but check on the resident frequently.
- Touch and continue to talk to the resident as you normally would.
- Avoid saying things that you do not want the resident to hear. Explain all procedures before doing them. The resident may appear unconscious, but the sense of hearing may be present. During the dying process, hearing is the last sensation to be lost.
- Support family members. Allow them to be involved in care, if appropriate.
- Make the family as comfortable as possible by providing coffee, pillows, blankets, or other needed items.

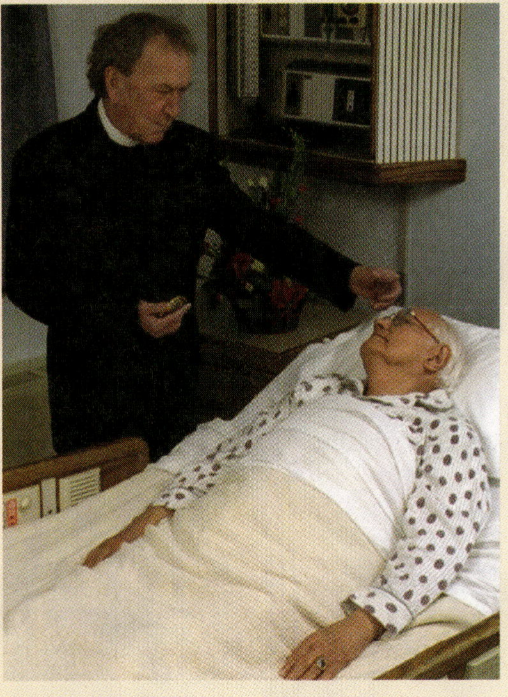

FIGURE 12-5 Respect the resident's religious beliefs. Assist him in preparations for a clergy visit, and provide privacy when religious workers are visiting.

PROCEDURE

74 Postmortem Care

1. Perform your beginning procedure actions.
2. Gather supplies needed: shroud kit or morgue pack (Figure 12.6) with gown and identification tags, a basin of warm water, soap, washcloth, towels, swabs for oral care, linen, gloves.

PROCEDURE

74 Postmortem Care, *continued*

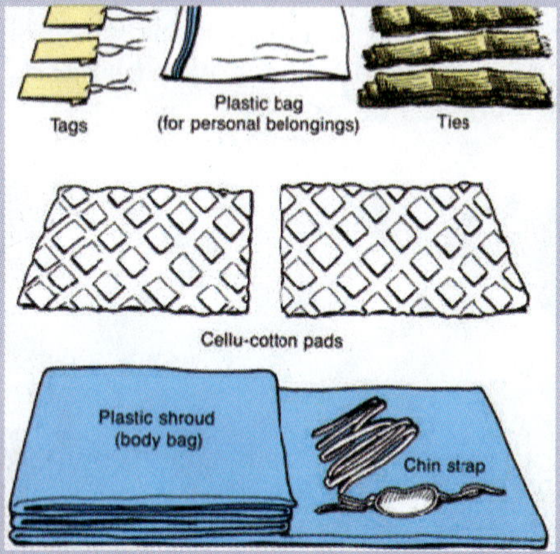

FIGURE 12-6 Standard morgue pack

3. Apply gloves.
4. Position the resident on the back with a pillow below the head and shoulders. Elevate the head of the bed 30 degrees.
5. Close the eyes by gently pulling the eyelids down (Figure 12.7).
6. Provide mouth care using moistened oral care swabs or sponges.
7. Close the mouth. A rolled-up washcloth may be placed under the chin to keep the jaw closed.
8. Follow your facility policy for removal of tubing from the body. In most facilities, the nurse will remove tubing. If the death is considered reportable to your coroner's office, the tubing should not be removed.
9. Bathe the body, straighten the arms and legs, and comb the hair.
10. Apply clean dressings to wounds, if necessary. Check with the nurse if dressings are soiled.
11. Place a bed protector or underpad under the buttocks. Urine and stool may continue to seep out after death.

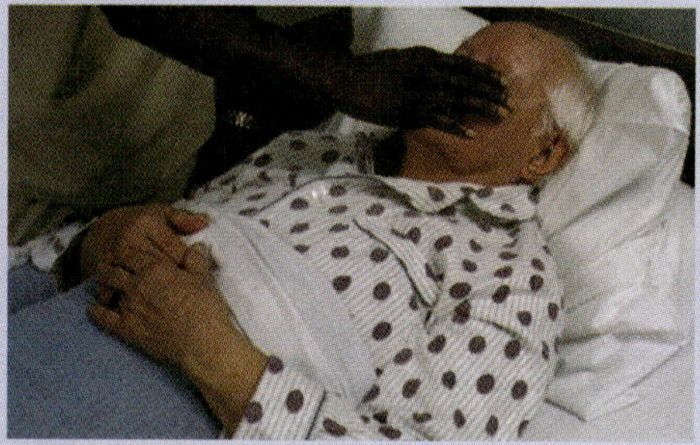

FIGURE 12-7 Gently close the resident's eyes.

12. Put a gown on the body.
13. Attach identification tags to the body according to facility policy.
14. Replace soiled linen and cover the body to the shoulders with a sheet.
15. Remove gloves and discard according to facility policy.
16. Wash your hands.
17. Straighten the room and remove unnecessary equipment.
18. Wash your hands.
19. Provide privacy and allow family members to be alone with the body.
20. Clean the resident's dentures, and place them in a denture cup. Make sure they are sent to the funeral home with the body.
21. Collect the resident's personal belongings, place them in a bag, and label them correctly. Usually these are given to the family. If no family members are present, follow facility policy. Complete and sign the inventory sheet according to your facility policy.
22. After the family leaves, wash your hands and put the **shroud** on the

body, if used in your facility. (The shroud is a cloth, paper, or plastic covering used to wrap the body after death.) Wear gloves if contact with blood or body fluid is likely.

23. Remove gloves and discard according to facility policy. Wash your hands.
24. Follow facility policy: either take the body to the morgue or close the door until representatives from the funeral home arrive.
25. Notify the nurse when representatives from the funeral home arrive.
26. Assist the funeral home representatives to move the body if necessary.
27. Strip and clean the unit according to your facility policy after the body has been removed.

KEY POINTS

- The nursing assistant is expected to provide care to residents who are dying and to care for the body after death.
- When caring for residents who are dying, the nursing assistant will assist residents and families to meet physical, emotional, psychological, social, and spiritual needs.
- Residents with terminal illness are not expected to recover, but the exact time of death cannot be predicted.
- The nursing assistant's personal beliefs about death and dying will affect the care given to the resident.
- A hospice is an agency that cares for dying residents.
- Hospice care focuses on keeping residents comfortable and allowing them to die with dignity and respect.
- Coping mechanisms are responses to stress and loss that are used to protect self-esteem.
- The five steps in the grieving process are denial, anger, bargaining, depression, and acceptance.
- The resident and family's cultural and religious beliefs about death and dying must be respected.
- Standard precautions are used when caring for the deceased, because the body can be infectious after death.

REVIEW

A. Multiple Choice

Select the one best answer.

1. Our feelings about death and dying are influenced by
   a. residents.
   b. the nurse.
   c. experiences.
   d. doctor's orders.
2. Hospice care is designed to
   a. treat the resident aggressively.
   b. keep the resident comfortable.
   c. prolong life.
   d. care only for the family.
3. Coping mechanisms are
   a. signs of grief.
   b. used to protect self-esteem.
   c. religious rituals.
   d. signs of approaching death.
4. In the first stage of the grieving process, the resident shows signs of
   a. denial.
   b. bargaining.

c. depression.
d. acceptance.

5. The resident is trying to separate himself or herself from life during the
   a. denial stage.
   b. anger stage.
   c. depression stage.
   d. bargaining stage.

6. Signs of approaching death include
   a. cooling of the skin, beginning with the lower extremities.
   b. constricted pupils.
   c. steady, slow pulse.
   d. elevated pulse and blood pressure.

7. When caring for the dying resident,
   a. be as quiet as possible and do not speak when providing care.
   b. always explain procedures before doing them.
   c. do not move the resident in bed, as this is painful and disturbing.
   d. keep the room very dark and warm.

8. Which of the following is a true statement about providing postmortem care?
   a. There is no need to provide privacy.
   b. The dentures are always removed from the mouth and given to the family to take home.
   c. Standard precautions are used because the body can be infectious.
   d. The nursing assistant removes all tubes and dressings.

9. The condition in which the muscles become stiff and rigid is
   a. algor mortis.
   b. liver mortis.
   c. muscle mortis.
   d. rigor mortis.

10. When a resident is dying, the room should be
    a. dark and cold.
    b. well lighted and ventilated.
    c. dark and hot.
    d. well lighted and cold.

B. Clinical Applications

Answer the following questions.

11. Mrs. Long has a history of severe depression. She attempted suicide years ago. Mrs. Long's husband has been told that the resident has terminal cancer. Her husband is the resident's legal guardian. He does not want her to know of her terminal diagnosis because he is afraid she will become depressed and attempt suicide again. When you are giving Mrs. Long a bed bath, she asks you if she is dying. How will you respond?

12. You are assigned to care for Mr. Street, a terminally ill resident who is not conscious. The family is in the room. They are discussing how bad the resident looks. What should you do?

13. Mr. Street's daughter tells you that she wants to help you turn the resident on his side. She would like to put lotion on her father's back. What will you do?

14. Mrs. Miles has a terminal diagnosis. When you enter her room to remove her supper tray, you find that she has thrown the food onto the wall. She yells that she is angry with you for giving her poor care. What do you think the problem is? How will you respond?

15. Miss Gantz is an 84-year-old resident who is dying. She tells you she is comfortable because she knows she is going home to be with the Lord. The resident's religious beliefs are not the same as your own. What will you do?

UNIT 13

Basic Restorative Services

A: Restorative Care

OBJECTIVES

After reading this unit, you will be able to:

- Spell and define key terms.
- Describe restorative care and the restorative environment.
- Describe restorative care for at least 10 common conditions seen in long-term care facilities.
- Explain why promoting independence is important in restorative care.
- List and describe common restorative programs.
- List three types of range-of-motion exercises and describe how each is different.
- Describe how a bowel and bladder management program is established and list the nursing assistant's responsibilities.
- Describe the nursing assistant's role in using restorative equipment.
- Demonstrate the procedures related to restorative care.
- List three prosthesis.

OBSERVATIONS TO MAKE AND REPORT RELATED TO RESTORATIVE CARE

Change in level of consciousness, orientation, awareness, or alertness
Feeling faint or lightheaded, losing consciousness
New-onset inability to recognize familiar persons or objects
New-onset disorientation; does not know person, place, time
Increasing memory loss or mental confusion, worsening confusion
Progressive lethargy
Loss of sensation
Numbness, tingling
Change in pupil size; unequal pupils
Abnormal or involuntary motor function
Spasticity (sudden, frequent, involuntary muscle contractions that impair function)
Loss of ability to move a body part
Incoordination (uncoordinated, irregular voluntary muscle movement)
Changes in speech
Changes in ability to swallow
Drooping of one side of the face
New-onset weakness or paralysis on one side of the body
Pain
Deformity
Edema

Immobility
Inability to move arms and legs
Inability to move one or more joints
Limited/abnormal range of motion
Shortening and external rotation of one leg in resident with history of fall
Sudden onset of falls, difficulty balancing
Jerking, tremors, shaky movements, muscle spasms
Weakness
Sensory changes
Changes in ability to sit, stand, move, or walk
Pain upon movement

Introduction to Restoration

Restorative care is given to assist the resident to attain and maintain the highest level of function possible in the resident's individual situation. A **restorative environment** is one in which the resident can function as independently as possible. The environment may require modification to meet the resident's need for independence. Being **dependent** on others has a negative effect on self-esteem. Dependence means you are unable to care for or do things for yourself, and that others must care for you. Disabled persons do not want to be treated differently than anyone else. They worked hard to become **independent**, or self-reliant and able to care for themselves. Most can do the same things you do, but they may do them differently. Their bodies work differently. Being independent is important for most people. This is especially true with personal care. Imagine how you would feel if someone had to bathe you and feed you. This would be very frustrating. Your self-esteem might suffer. Feeling helpless causes feelings of hopelessness.

The Restorative Team

Many departments assist in providing restorative care to residents (Figure 13.1). All members of the interdisciplinary team provide restorative care. The therapy departments usually take the lead role in resident restoration. **Rehabilitation** is a program designed by a therapist to help residents regain lost skills, or to teach new skills. Therapists teach residents, families, and staff members techniques for reinforcing and maintaining what the residents have learned. When you follow the restorative program established by the therapist to accompany the rehabilitation program, this reinforces what the therapists are teaching, and the resident masters the skill more quickly. This process is called **restoration**. Restorative nursing involves using basic measures to assist the resident to attain the highest degree of independence and self-care possible. Some facilities use the terms *rehabilitation* and *restoration* interchangeably, but rehabilitation really refers to a higher level of care provided by licensed therapy personnel. Restoration is delivered by both unlicensed and licensed caregivers in many departments. A restorative nurse may also develop restorative programs. The interdisciplinary approach provides continuity of care, because all staff members are working on the same goals 24 hours a day to benefit the resident.

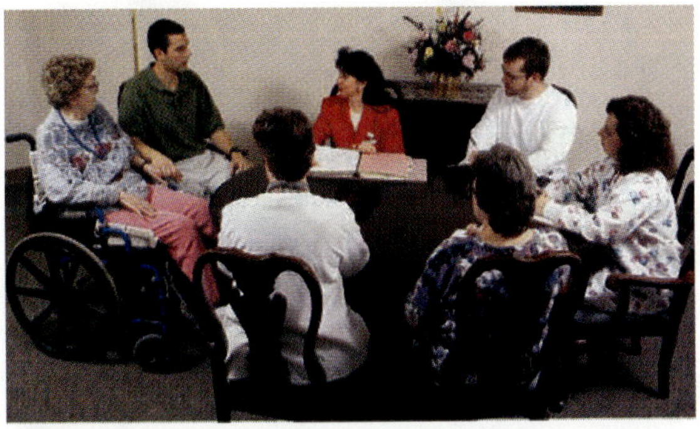

FIGURE 13-1 The interdisciplinary team meets to find out which skills are most important to the resident and develop a plan to assist her.

Complications of Bed Rest

Years ago, people who were sick stayed in bed for long periods. After childbirth, women were kept on bed rest for at least seven days. We now know that early activity is best for the resident. Rest is essential to the treatment of many illnesses. Nevertheless, the physician and other members of the interdisciplinary team will assess the resident and determine how much activity the resident can tolerate. This assessment forms the basis for the restorative program. Like the nursing process, the resident's response to the program is continuously evaluated, and the program modified to meet the resident's individual needs. Remember, **bed rest, inactivity**, and **immobility** affect every system in the body. Bed rest is a medically prescribed treatment in which the resident cannot get out of bed. A resident who is inactive is quiet and still. Immobility means the resident is motionless and unable to move. A summary of the major complications of immobility on each body system is found in Table 13.1.

Common Conditions

Some chronic conditions are commonly seen in the long-term care facility. Residents with these conditions usually receive restorative care to maintain independence, prevent declines, and prevent injuries.

Arthritis

Arthritis is a common condition in long-term care facility residents. There are many different types of arthritis. The most common are osteoarthritis, rheumatoid arthritis, and gout, or gouty

TABLE 13-1 Major complications of immobility

System	Complication
Respiratory	The resident has more difficulty expanding the lungs. Fluid and secretions collect in the lungs. This increases the risk of pneumonia and other lung infections.
Circulatory	Blood clots are caused by pooling of blood and pressure on the legs. Edema may be caused by lack of movement. The heart must work harder to pump blood through the body. Changes in the blood vessels may cause dizziness and fainting when the resident is placed in an upright position.
Integumentary (skin)	Pressure sores may develop in a short time from lack of oxygen to the tissues. Pressure ulcers may worsen quickly and be difficult or impossible to reverse.
Muscular	Weakness and atrophy develop from lack of use. Contractures (deformities) develop because of the resident's position. Contractures may be painful and are difficult or impossible to reverse. Contractures also promote pressure ulcer development, and make treating pressure ulcers more difficult. The contractures cause reduced capillary blood flow to bony prominences, and estimates are that up to 60% of all pressure ulcers involve some sort of unattended contracture. Voluntary movement of the contracted joint becomes difficult or impossible as the contracture worsens.
Skeletal	Calcium drains from the bones when they are inactive. This contributes to fractures, non-healing, osteoporosis, and other complications.
Genitourinary	The extra calcium in the system from the bones promotes the development of kidney stones. Retention of urine is common, and is often caused by the resident's position in bed. Overflow of a full bladder leads to incontinence. The resident is at high risk of urinary tract infection.
Gastrointestinal	Indigestion and heartburn may result if the resident is not positioned properly for meals. The resident is at risk for choking unless positioned upright during and after meals. Loss of appetite may occur from lack of activity, illness, and boredom. Constipation and fecal impaction result from immobility.
Nervous	Weakness and limited mobility develop. Insomnia may result from sleeping too much during the day, then being unable to sleep at night.
Mental changes	Irritability, boredom, lethargy, and depression result from the resident's frustration and feelings of helplessness.

arthritis. The most common symptom of arthritis is pain. Arthritis can cause mild discomfort to severe deformities and disability (Figure 13.2). The pain is usually described as a deep, aching pain that occurs after exercise, weight bearing, or exertion. It is often relieved by rest. Changes in the weather may also cause pain. Other symptoms include limited ability to move and stiffness, particularly upon arising in the morning. This also may occur after strenuous exercise or physical over activity. In some individuals, an audible grating sound can be heard in the joints during movement. Arthritis may cause redness and swelling in the joints. Conditions such as obesity and stress aggravate the symptoms.

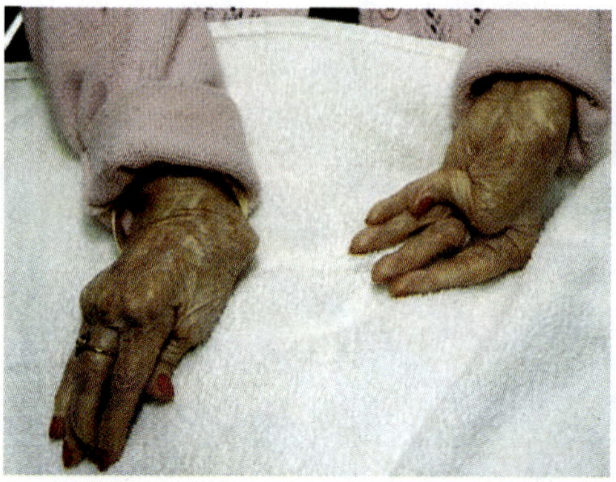

FIGURE 13-2 Signs and symptoms of arthritis can range from mild discomfort to severe deformity, making joint movement difficult or impossible.

Residents with arthritis are at high risk of contractures. The care plan may instruct you to place residents with this condition in the prone position periodically. This reduces the risk of contractures of the hips and knees. Avoid placing pillows under the knees or elevating the knee area of the bed. Using a small, flat pillow under the head and neck is best. A large pillow pushes the neck into a position of flexion. You will perform range of motion procedures on residents with arthritis. Be very gentle. Avoid moving joints past the point of resistance.

Osteoporosis

Osteoporosis is a metabolic disorder of the bones. It is most common in elderly females. Bone mass is lost, causing the bones to become porous and spongy (Figure 13.3). Bones affected are at very high risk of fracture. Fractures can occur spontaneously, such as when the resident is walking. They can also occur when the resident is turned in bed or during transfers.

The cause of osteoporosis is unknown. It is thought to result from years of inadequate calcium intake. Other potential causes are declining adrenal function, faulty protein metabolism, estrogen deficiency, and lack of exercise or activity. The first sign of osteoporosis is usually a fracture. Commonly, the resident moves or lifts something. He or she hears a "pop" or snapping sound in a bone. This frequently occurs in the lower back or hip. Sometimes the resident is walking and falls because of a fracture. (In most falls, the opposite is true.) After the initial incident, the area is very painful, particularly upon movement.

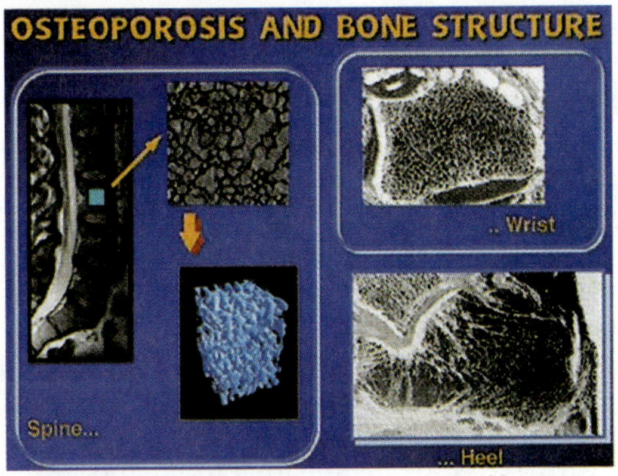

FIGURE 13-3 Bone loss from osteoporosis causes painful, disabling fractures in both genders. About 40% percent of women and 13% of men will suffer a bone fracture in their lifetime due to osteoporosis.Sharmila Majumdar, Ph.D., Professor, University of California, San Francisco)

Sometimes the onset of osteoporosis begins with a curvature of the spine and loss of height. The back progressively weakens, straining the neck, hips, and low back. Spontaneous fractures may occur on movement or as a result of a minor injury. The care plan may instruct you to use a turning sheet and two assistants for moving the resident in bed. Handle the resident gently.

Hip Surgery

Hip fractures are the most common type of fracture in the elderly. The most common cause of hip fractures is falls, but they may also occur because of osteoporosis. The term "hip fracture" really is not accurate. This term refers to a fracture anywhere in the upper third or head of the femur.

Caring for the Resident Who Has Had Hip Surgery. Hip fracture is almost always treated with surgery. Depending on the condition of the bone, the fracture may be repaired, or the hip completely replaced. Hip replacement surgery may also be done when the joint is painful and damaged, but not fractured. When the resident is admitted or readmitted to the long-term care facility following hip surgery, the following general hip precautions will be ordered:

- A trapeze is attached to the bed to assist with movement. The resident is instructed not to press down on the foot of the affected leg when using the trapeze.
- Antiembolism stockings are applied.
- A fracture bedpan or urinal is used initially for elimination. When the resident is able to use the toilet, an elevated toilet seat is used.
- The head of the bed is not elevated more than 45 degrees.
- Acute flexion of the hip and legs is avoided. The therapist will give directions for positioning and the degree of flexion permitted. Generally, the resident should never flex the hip more than 90 degrees.
- A special pillow, called an **abduction pillow**, will be used to keep the legs apart (Figure 13.4) after the resident has had hip replacement surgery. This is particularly important when the resident is turned on the side.
- The resident will be instructed to avoid crossing the legs, which can cause a dislocation.
- The affected leg should not be internally or externally rotated. Maintain good alignment without internal or external rotation.

The physician will specify how long the resident must avoid weight bearing after surgery. The

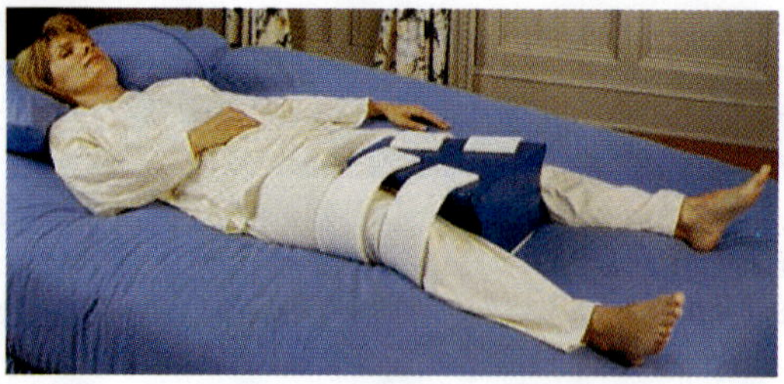

FIGURE 13-4 An abduction pillow is commonly used after hip surgery to keep the legs from adducting or crossing at the ankles.(Photo courtesy of Sammons Preston)

physical therapist will work with the resident to restore mobility. Some residents are able to ambulate soon after surgery. A walker is commonly used for a period of time after surgery. Some physicians do not permit full weight bearing for as long as four to six weeks. Initially, you will assist with procedures to prevent the complications of immobility. Restorative care of a resident who has had hip surgery will include:

- Range-of-motion exercises on the unaffected extremities
- Turning and repositioning
- Coughing and deep breathing exercises if the resident is bedfast
- Pressure ulcer prevention

Residents with hip surgery are at very high risk of developing heel pressure ulcers. Follow the care plan and get specific instructions from the nurse for positions and techniques to use for turning and repositioning the resident. Relieve pressure from the heels and check the resident's skin carefully each day for signs of red or open areas.

Cerebrovascular Accident

Cerebrovascular accident (CVA) is a common condition in the long-term care facility. A CVA may also be called a *stroke*. A newer term is *brain attack*. A CVA is caused by a sudden interruption of blood to the brain. This can be caused by a blood clot, which blocks a small vessel. Sometimes a vessel bursts, causing blood to spill out into the brain cavity. Both conditions decrease blood supply and often cause permanent damage (Figure 13.5).

CVA is the third leading cause of death in the United States, affecting about 500,000 people annually. About half of these die. About half of the survivors develop a permanent disability. Survivors often experience a recurrence some time later in life. This could be days or weeks later. It could also be many years after the initial CVA. The resident is usually hospitalized for aggressive treat-

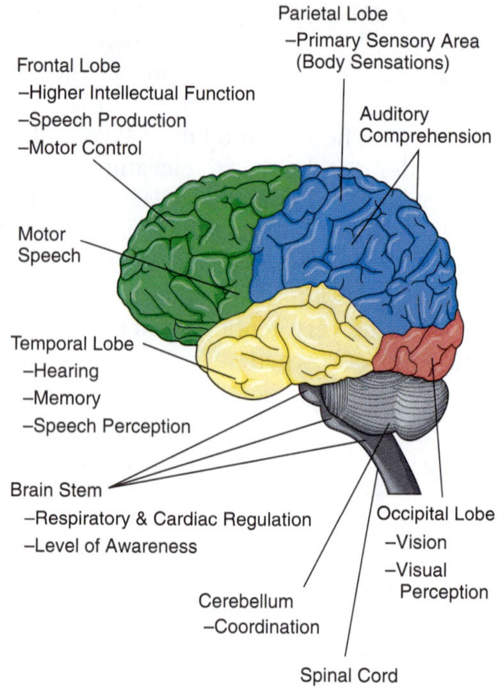

FIGURE 13-5 A stroke or head injury in the areas of the brain shown will result in loss of ability.

ment as soon as the signs and symptoms of CVA are recognized. Some treatments will reverse the damage from the CVA. However, the treatment must be given within the first four hours.

When a resident has a stroke, one side of the body becomes weak or paralyzed. These conditions may be temporary or permanent. **Hemiparesis** is weakness on one side of the body. **Hemiplegia** is paralysis on one side of the body. The ability to speak or understand the spoken word may be affected, depending on the location of the attack in the brain. The resident may develop loss of half of a visual field. Recognizing the effects of a CVA on vision is important.

Some residents lose the ability to differentiate right from left, or up from down. Some residents have a condition that causes them to ignore the affected side of the body. Stroke may also affect emotions. The resident may cry, laugh, or become angry for no apparent reason. This is very embarrassing for the resident. He or she is aware of the behavior but cannot control it.

Restorative Care. Rehabilitation and restorative nursing are started soon after admission or readmission to the facility. The resident will usually require physical, occupational, and speech therapy. The goals of care are to:

- Maintain or improve the resident's condition
- Prevent contractures and deformities

- Restore as much self-care ability as possible
- Prevent injury
- Prevent complications of immobility

Rehabilitation and restoration programs focus on activities such as ADLs and bowel and bladder control. Restoration of residents with CVA takes a long time. It is a great deal of work for the resident. Several restorative programs may be ordered for residents with CVA. Allow the resident to rest between treatments. Fatigue is a common problem.

The care plan usually list these approaches:

- Monitor the position of affected extremities during positioning, transfers, and ambulation, to prevent injury.
- Use a transfer belt for transfers and ambulation.
- Position the resident in good alignment to prevent contractures and deformities, using pillows and props if necessary.
- Use pressure ulcer prevention measures, including special mattresses, turning, repositioning, props, and skin care.

Care of a resident who has had a stroke is highly individual, depending on the area of the brain affected. Residents who have had a CVA on either side of the brain may have memory and behavior problems. These may interfere with the restorative program. Remember that the problems are beyond the resident's control. If the resident ignores one side of the body, the care plan will direct you to approach the resident from the affected side. You will encourage the resident to look at the affected side so he or she knows where it is. Touch the extremity gently, but firmly, periodically. Residents with CVA often have an impaired sense of balance. Assist the resident to develop an awareness of good posture and balance.

Residents with hemiplegia may complain of pain in the affected arm and shoulder. This occurs because the force of gravity pulls it downward. Avoid pulling on the arm or shoulder during transfers. A sling may be ordered to help support the arm. Other devices, such as a lap board or table, may also be used to provide support and relieve pressure on the shoulder joint.

Transient Ischemic Attack

A **transient ischemic attack (TIA)** is a temporary period of diminished blood flow to the brain. The attack occurs suddenly and may last from 2 to 15 minutes. Rarely, an attack will last as long as 24 hours. Signs and symptoms are similar to those of a stroke, but are reversible and temporary. Persons who experience TIAs are at high risk for eventually suffering a stroke.

Parkinson's Disease

Parkinson's disease (PD) is a neurological disease. Symptoms usually begin between the ages of 40 and 60. Occasionally they begin as early as the late teens or early twenties. About 1% of individuals over age 50 have the disease. Self-care in the home becomes difficult or impossible because the disease increases the risk of injury. Residents with Parkinson's disease have many restorative care needs.

In the early stages of the disease, the individual is slow when completing ADLs. He or she will also experience:

- Muscle stiffness
- Mild pain
- Tremors of the upper extremities
- Difficulty walking

The tremors are very embarrassing for some residents. The disease is progressive and symptoms gradually worsen with age. As symptoms progress, voluntary movement becomes difficult (Figure 13.6). As the condition worsens, the resident develops:

- Pill-rolling motions in the fingers (in this condition, the fingers move involuntarily in a circular motion as though the resident were rolling a pill between the thumb and fingers)
- Stooped posture
- Shuffling gait; falls are common
- Mask-like expression
- Low-pitched, monotonous speech
- Difficulty controlling oral secretions
- Dementia (only in some individuals)

The effects of the disease can be controlled to a degree with drug therapy. There is no known treatment for Parkinson's dementia.

Restorative Care. Licensed nurses will administer medication to control the tremors. Restorative nursing care includes:

- Range-of-motion exercises and other activities to prevent contractures
- Safety measures to prevent falls and injuries
- Using a gait belt and/or walker for ambulation
- Encouraging the resident to maintain good posture when walking
- Avoiding flexion of the neck and shoulders
- Using assistive devices for ADLs
- Being very patient; the tremors cause the resident to be very slow with ADLs and movement
- Allowing adequate time for residents to complete tasks independently

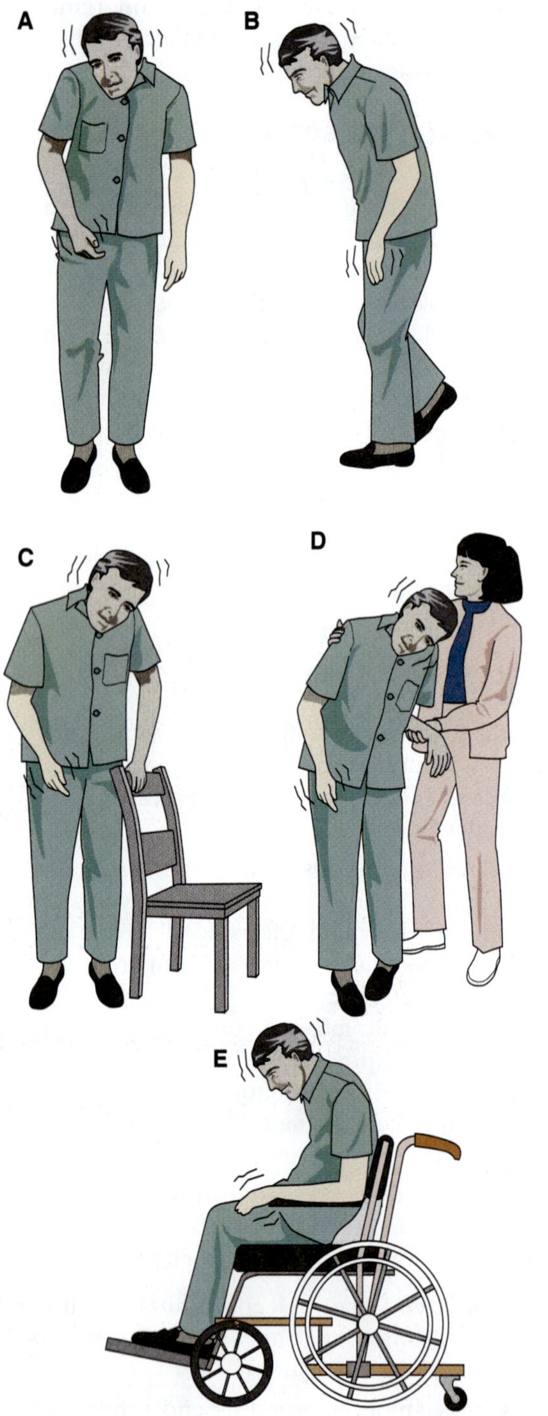

FIGURE 13-6 Progression of Parkinson's disease. (A) The resident leans slightly forward and develops flexion of the affected arm. (B) The resident stoops forward slightly and walks with a shuffling gait. (C) As the disease progresses, the resident needs support to prevent falling. The resident tends to shuffle faster and faster, leaning farther forward until he falls on his face. (D) The disease progresses to the point of needing assistance for ambulation. (E) The resident has profound weakness and severe tremors. Ambulation becomes impossible.

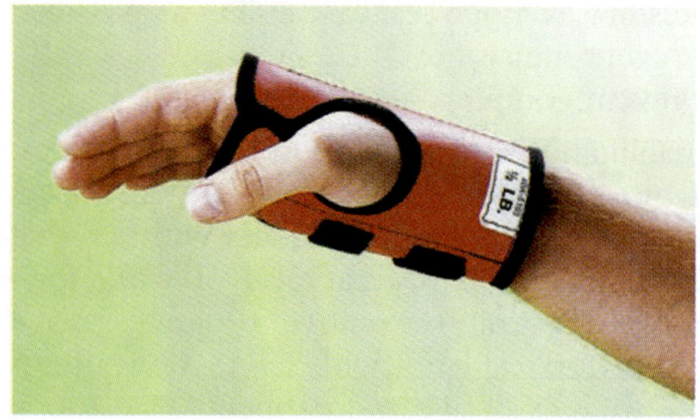

FIGURE 13-7 Various weights are available to reduce tremors of the hands and arms, enabling the resident to maintain greater independence.(Photo courtesy of Sammons Preston)

Some residents with Parkinson's disease have difficulty feeding themselves. The tremors may be so severe that the food spills before it gets to the mouth. In this situation, the therapist may evaluate the resident and establish a restorative program. Weights are often used to control the tremors (Figure 13.7). Some therapists prescribe weights to the backs of the hands. Others use weighted silverware. You will assist the resident to become proficient in eating while using the weights or weighted utensils. Special cups with lids are also used to prevent spilling. Feeding the resident is not desirable, if it can be avoided. However, the resident's weight must be monitored closely. The tremors of Parkinson's consume extra calories. The resident is at very high risk for weight loss. This is because of the extra caloric need, combined with problems such as spilling. Residents are often given nutritional supplements or nourishing snacks to help maintain their weight.

Huntington's Disease

Huntington's disease (HD) is also called *Huntington's chorea*. This is a hereditary disease. In recent years, a genetic test has become available to show if individuals with a family history of the disorder have the Huntington's gene. If the gene is present, development of the disease is inevitable.

Clinical signs of the disease usually begin when individuals are in their 40s or 50s. In some individuals, symptoms of the disease first appear in childhood or young adulthood. The disease is progressive and there is no cure. Disability and death occur within 15 to 20 years. Abnormal movements, called **chorea**, are the primary sign of Huntington's disease. The movements are subtle early in the course of the illness. The individual will appear anxious or restless. He or she appears to move frequently. Most people are aware of this movement. The resident may try to disguise the activity with voluntary movements, such as scratching the head or crossing the legs. As the disease progresses, rapid, jerking choreiform movements develop. These movements involve the entire body. The individual eventually loses voluntary control of all movement. He or she also loses control of the bowel and bladder. The **spasticity** (involuntary movement) increases with stress and attempts to control the choreiform motions. The resident becomes totally dependent on others. The risk of skin breakdown is high in the later stages. Individuals with Huntington's disease develop mental changes that progress to dementia.

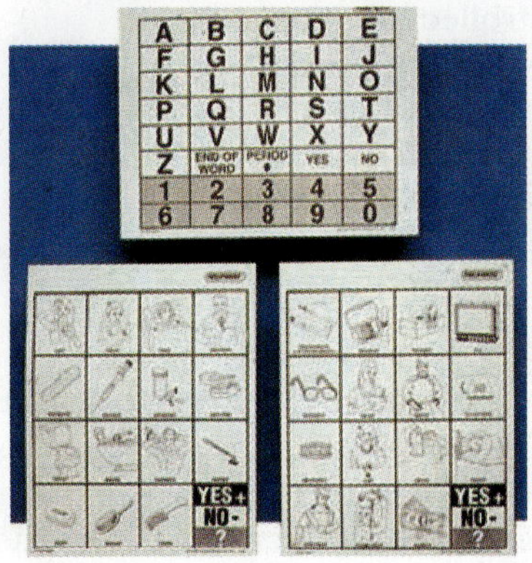

FIGURE 13-8 Alternate methods of communication may be used by residents who have difficulty speaking.(Permission given for reprint/reproduction courtesy of Maddak, Inc.)

Restorative Care. Residents with Huntington's disease are commonly admitted to the long-term care facility because they cannot function safely at home. There is no known treatment or cure. Care is designed to:

- Keep the resident as independent as possible for as long as possible
- Prevent injury
- Maintain nutrition and prevent weight loss

The rapid movements consume many extra calories. The resident is at very high risk for weight loss. Extra nutrition and hydration will be ordered. Restorative nursing programs for residents with chorea usually involve ambulation with a gait belt. Some residents can walk independently by pushing an empty wheelchair.

Residents with HD will develop difficulty swallowing and are at very high risk for choking. When residents with Huntington's disease are eating, they must sit completely upright to prevent choking. The care plan will specify other special feeding techniques.

Poor muscular control makes communication difficult. The speech-language pathologist will assess the resident and establish a communication program. The resident will be taught to use either hand signals, cards (Figure 13.8), or a communication board. Give the resident feedback when he or she speaks. Repeating what the resident says is a good way to show that the communication was successful.

Multiple Sclerosis

Multiple sclerosis (MS) is another neurological disorder commonly seen in long-term care. Sadly, many young adults are affected (Figure 13.9). This progressive disease causes a degeneration of the nervous system that interferes with conduction of nerve impulses. The exact cause is not known. It is thought to be an **autoimmune disorder**. In this type of condition, the individual makes antibodies that work against his or her own body. Recent research suggests that a virus may cause MS. The signs and symptoms of MS vary widely. They include:

- Weakness
- Numbness and tingling in one or more extremities, with eventual progression to complete loss of sensation
- Visual disturbances
- **Incoordination** (uncoordinated, irregular voluntary muscle movement)
- Poor muscular control, muscle spasms, and tremors
- Paralysis

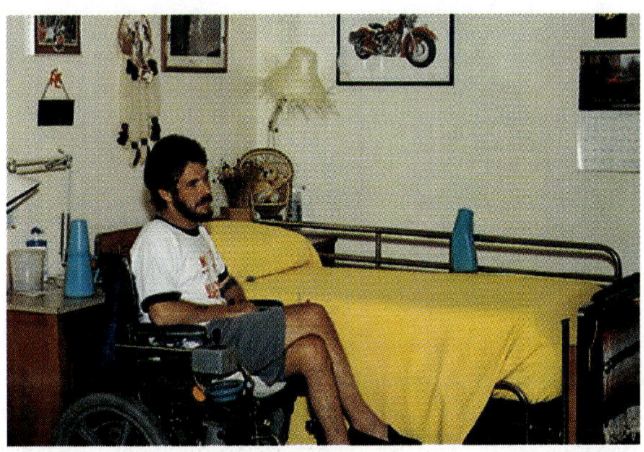

FIGURE 13-9 Multiple sclerosis often affects young adults. This resident is independent with ambulation because he uses a motorized wheelchair.

- Uncontrolled emotions
- Slow, scanning speech
- Short attention span
- Incontinence
- Urinary retention
- Fatigue that worsens as the day progresses
- Seizures
- Depression

Residents with MS often develop a **neurogenic bladder**. In this condition, the resident cannot feel the sensation of urine in the bladder. The bladder will become very full, retaining urine. The resident may have to be catheterized to relieve the problem.

Multiple sclerosis is a condition in which there are **exacerbations** and **remissions**. During an exacerbation, signs and symptoms worsen. Stress, infection, and injury are risk factors for exacerbations. Some residents are relatively stable for long periods of time. Others deteriorate rapidly. They quickly become dependent on staff for care. Residents in remission appear stable and relatively symptom-free.

Restorative Care. Preventive skin care is important for the resident with MS. Residents with this condition are at high risk for breakdown. MS causes impairment in the resident's sensation. He or she may not notice the discomfort of an early pressure ulcer. Pressure-relieving mattresses and other preventive devices are used routinely. The care plan will also list measures to prevent contractures and maintain independence.

Post Polio Syndrome (PPS)

Polio is a very serious neurological disease caused by a virus. It has been with us since at least 1350 BC. The virus attacks the motor neurons in the brain and spinal cord. Muscles affected by these neurons no longer function properly. Some individuals had respiratory paralysis and required a special ventilator to breathe. Others had speech and swallowing problems. Most had paralysis and weakness in the arms and legs. Many people died as a result of polio. Most of those who survived learned to overcome their disabilities and lead productive lives.

Post polio syndrome (PPS) is a neurologic condition marked by increased weakness and abnormal muscle fatigue in persons who had polio many years earlier (Figure 13.10). Estimates are that 30% to 70% of all polio survivors will develop this condition. There are several theories about the cause of PPS. The most common involves the motor neurons. Most polio survivors have about half as many motor neurons as others who were not affected by polio. It is believed that motor neurons that were not destroyed by the initial polio infection compensated by sprouting new connections. Some of the new neurons adapted to innervate areas that are five to seven times larger than normal. These neurons may be slowly dying, perhaps because of years of overuse. As the neurons die, they lose their muscle connections, and muscles stop responding when a nerve signals them.

Signs and symptoms of PPS range from annoying to debilitating. Onset may be sudden, following trauma, infection, surgery, a fall, or a stressful event. The new injury stresses the remaining motor neurons, causing new reduction in function and increased pain and fatigue. Signs and symptoms of PPS include:

- Fatigue that may be debilitating and worsens as the day progresses
- New joint and muscle pain
- New weakness in muscles affected by polio; unaffected muscles are also affected. (The new weakness may be more prominent on one side of the body).
- New dyspnea and other respiratory problems
- Severe cold intolerance, even with mild cold exposure. This causes the muscle weakness to worsen, the arms or legs to become pale or cyanotic, and the extremities to feel cold to touch. The resident may say," It's so cold it hurts."
- Muscle spasms and cramps that are sometimes severe and painful
- Difficulty swallowing and increased risk of choking
- Difficulty falling asleep and waking frequently during the night
- Anxiety, anger, frustration, and emotional outbursts due to loss of ability
- Disturbed sleep, sleep apnea

Post Polio Syndrome Diagnostic Criteria

Prior episode of polio with residual motor neuron loss.
A period of neurologic recovery followed by neurologic and functional stability (usually lasts 15 years or more).
Gradual or abrupt onset of new weakness and/or abnormal muscle fatigue.
May also have generalized fatigue, muscle atrophy, pain.
Exclusion of other conditions that may cause symptoms similar to post polio syndrome.

FIGURE 13-10 Post polio syndrome is diagnosed in persons who had polio many years previously, based on identification of new signs and symptoms. Many other conditions are ruled out before this diagnosis is made.

Restorative Care. Most polio survivors are fiercely independent, making them difficult to care for. PPS residents fear becoming dependent on others. Coping with the new problems from PPS is often very difficult for the resident. Residents may not complain because most were taught that they had to appear normal as part of their recovery. They have spent their lives trying to appear normal. Asking for and accepting help is very difficult. Because of this, pay attention if the resident says he or she cannot do something. Anticipate the resident's needs, and ask if assistance is needed. Even if the resident refuses your help, stand by to see if he or she can perform the task safely. Adapt the environment, whenever possible, for independent function. You may do this by moving furniture, or bringing a bedside commode, for example. Goals of restorative care are designed to:

- Maintain maximum independence
- Prevent falls and injury
- Prevent pain, pressure ulcers, and deformities
- Conserve energy

Residents with PPS have serious problems with cold because the nerves that control blood vessel size were destroyed by the virus. The legs and feet are commonly affected. One theory is that people with PPS function as if it were 20 degrees colder than the actual temperature. Their legs and feet turn bright red following a hot bath. When the resident stands to get up, she may become dizzy or faint as blood pools in the legs, causing her blood pressure to drop. If the resident complains of cold, assist her with socks or extra blankets. You may be instructed to soak the feet in warm water, or assist with a warm bath. Caution the resident to call for help before getting out of the tub.

Brain Damage

Some individuals are admitted to the long-term care facility because of head injuries. These usually result from trauma, falls, or automobile accidents. The injury often results in severe, permanent brain damage. Many young adults are admitted to long-term care facilities with this condition.

Signs and symptoms of brain damage vary widely. Most residents admitted to the nursing facility show signs and symptoms of severe damage. They are often dependent on staff for care. Common signs and symptoms of severe brain damage are:

- Ability to open eyes, but unaware or minimally aware of the surroundings
- Inability to follow commands, make decisions, or participate in care
- Loss of bowel and bladder control
- Inability to speak or communicate
- Paralysis of the extremities
- Lack of safety awareness
- Impaired sensation

Restorative Care. The goal of restorative care is to prevent complications. The care plan will list measures to:

- Prevent skin breakdown
- Prevent contractures, which are common
- Prevent deformities
- Prevent injuries

Spinal Cord Injuries

Some residents are admitted to the facility because of injuries or other conditions of the spinal cord resulting in paralysis. Paralysis affects sensation and voluntary movement below the level of injury (Figure 13.11). The most common cause is trauma, but medical problems and birth defects can also cause paralysis.

Restorative Care. Restorative nursing depends on the level of injury. Overall, treatment is directed at:

- Preventing pressure ulcers and other complications of immobility
- Preventing contractures and deformities
- Restoring the resident to the highest degree of independence possible

Promoting Independence

Promoting independence is part of restorative care. Independence is relative to the resident. No one is 100% independent. We all depend on others for some things. Independence for the resident, then, means being as self-sufficient as possible. Preventing total dependence on others is important both physically and psychologically. It is better for the resident to complete part of a task than it is for you to perform the task. Allowing the resident to do what he or she is able makes the resident feel useful and worth-while. It may take longer for the resident to complete a task than it takes you (Figure 13.12). However, maintaining the resident's ability to perform the skill and the effect of personal independence on the resident's self-esteem are worth the investment of your time.

Some residents have medical problems that cause physical dependence. For example, a resident who suffered a neck injury in an accident may be paralyzed from the neck down. This resident is physically dependent. However, if the

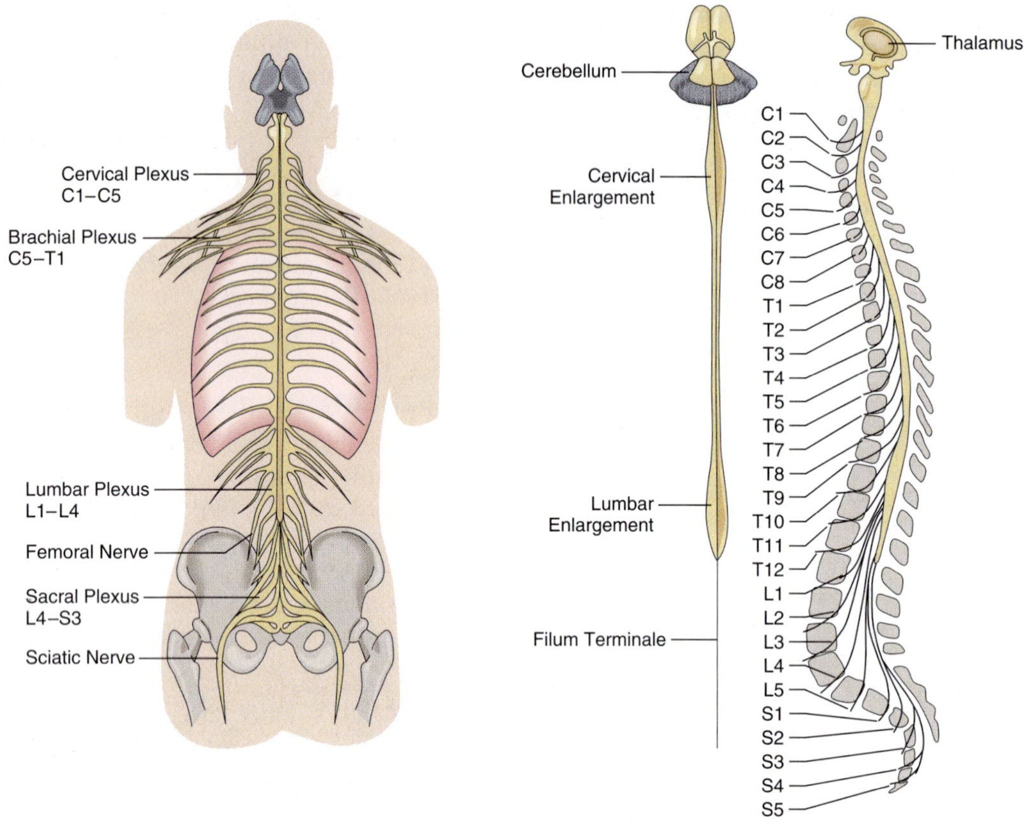

FIGURE 13-11 The type of paralysis is determined by the level of injury to the spinal cord.

resident is allowed to set the care routine, and tell you what he or she wants, the resident is psychologically independent. Psychological independence is also very important.

Principles of Restoration

The principles of restoration and rehabilitation are the same, and apply to all residents:

- *Begin treatment early*. If restorative care is started early in the resident's disease, the outcome will be better.
- *Activity strengthens and inactivity weakens*. The goal should be to keep the resident as active as possible, considering the medical condition. The resident should do an activity whenever possible. For example, passive range-of-motion exercises given by the nursing assistant will prevent deformity and complications. However, active range-of-motion exercises done by the resident will prevent deformity and strengthen muscles.
- *Prevent further disability*. Follow the care plan to prevent injury and deformity. Practice safety.
- *Stress what the resident can do*. Minimize what the resident cannot do. Emphasizing what the resident can do is better than telling the resident he or she can't do something.
- *Treat the whole person*. Restorative care works on the principle that residents are complex individuals. Each individual has many strengths and needs. You cannot isolate the medical pro-

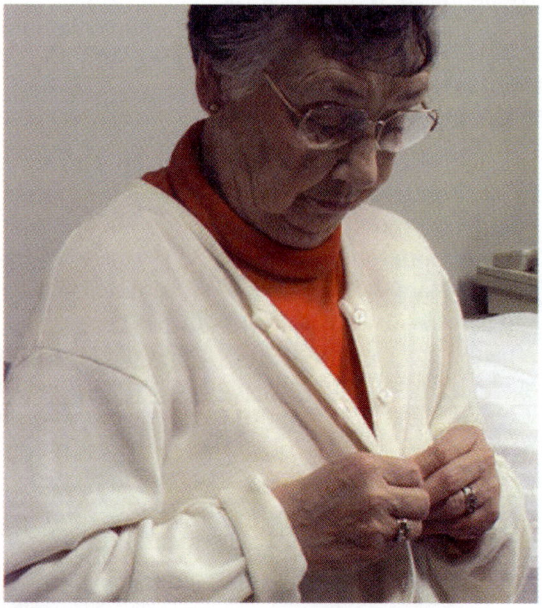

FIGURE 13-12 Although it may take a long time for the resident to button her buttons, you are helping her by encouraging independence.

blem from the rest of the person. Consider all of the resident's strengths and needs when delivering restorative care. Use and build on the resident's strengths to overcome the needs. The program must be individualized for the resident. The care plan will guide you in the approaches to use. If you discover something that works for the resident, share this information with the nurse and other team members so it can be included on the care plan.

Providing Restorative Care

When providing restorative care, always follow the care plan. The amount and type of activity allowed are ordered by the physician. The care is supervised by the licensed nurse. The care plan will guide you in the type of restorative care to deliver.

Providing restorative care takes a great deal of patience. We did not learn to care for ourselves overnight. Think about how long it takes a small child to learn to take a bath and get dressed. When adults lose the ability for self-care, it takes time to restore. The process can be frustrating for both the resident and the nursing assistant. Being patient, positive, and supportive is the best approach.

Monitoring the Resident's Response to Restorative Care

It is important to observe how the restorative program affects the resident. This is particularly true in the early stages of illness. The resident may become easily frustrated. Allow the resident to struggle, but intervene before he or she reaches the point of frustration. Encourage the resident and remind him or her that learning takes time. Practice empathy. Tell the resident you understand how frustrated he or she feels. Be aware of the resident's fears. Sometimes fear of falling or spilling will prevent the resident from participating in the restorative program.

Early in the restorative program, the resident may also have a physical response. Bed rest, even for a short period, can have a negative effect on the body. Any movement or exertion may cause a change in the resident's physical condition. Monitor for signs of fatigue. Be alert for changes, and report them to the nurse. A good practice is to take the resident's pulse before you begin restorative care. Then perform the activity. Monitor the pulse every five minutes during the activity. Normally, the pulse will increase. If the rate is more than 100, or if the resident shows signs of other problems, such as pain, shortness of breath, nausea, or perspiration, stop the activity and notify the nurse. After you complete the activity, check the pulse again. It should return to within 10 beats of the resting pulse rate within 5 minutes.

Maintaining a Restorative Attitude

Your attitude affects the resident and has a major effect on the care you deliver. You must believe that restorative care works and that it is good for the resident. Do not judge the value of restorative care by the results you see tomorrow. It takes a long time for the effects to become evident. Restorative care should be viewed as a positive process that is best for the resident, but results are usually slow in coming. Understanding this in advance will help you to avoid discouragement. Be patient, sincere, tactful, sensitive, and empathetic. Explain the importance of the program to the resident and provide encouragement. Good communication is part of restorative care.

Applying the Principles of Restorative Care to Activities of Daily Living

Most of the restorative care you provide will be done when you assist residents with activities of daily living. Observe the resident carefully. Learn which activity of daily living the resident is most interested in accomplishing. Share this information with the nurse. The information you contribute to the interdisciplinary team based on your observations of the resident is very important.

Role of the Nursing Assistant in Assisting with Restorative Programs

Many residents have nursing diagnoses listed on the care plans that include the words **self-care deficit**. A self-care deficit is an inability to perform an activity of daily living. The care plan will guide you in implementing restorative programs. Each program is designed specifically by the therapist or restorative nurse to meet the resident's needs. You must develop a sensitivity to the resident's abilities. Provide what the resident needs, but do not do more than necessary. Be available to assist, but do not help until you are certain the resident cannot accomplish the task. This may be difficult, but the only way the resident will relearn the skill is by doing it.

Bathing and Personal Hygiene Programs. Residents with many different illnesses lose the ability to bathe themselves and perform routine

GUIDELINES FOR

Restorative Care

- Practice good body mechanics for yourself and the resident.
- Provide restorative care at the usual time of day for the activity.
- Remember that all ADLs have many steps. If the resident cannot complete one step, he or she will not be able to do the activity.
- Do not rush the resident.
- Give verbal **cues**, if necessary. Cues are brief verbal hints that indicate what you want the resident to do. Make your directions as clear and simple as possible. If the resident does not understand, demonstrate.
- If the resident does not respond to verbal cues, use hand-over-hand technique (Figure 13.13) by placing your hand on top of the resident's hand and performing the activity.
- Practice safety and teach the resident safety measures.
- Allow the resident to do as much self-care as possible. Show the resident that you are confident in his or her ability.
- Use adaptive devices, if necessary.
- Apply **orthotic** and **prosthetic** devices as ordered by the therapist and described on the care plan. Orthotic devices improve function and prevent deformities. Prosthetic devices are replacements for body parts, such as the eye, breast, hand, leg, or foot.
- Modify the environment to promote independence, if necessary.
- If the resident cannot complete an ADL, praise his or her accomplishment and complete the task for the resident.

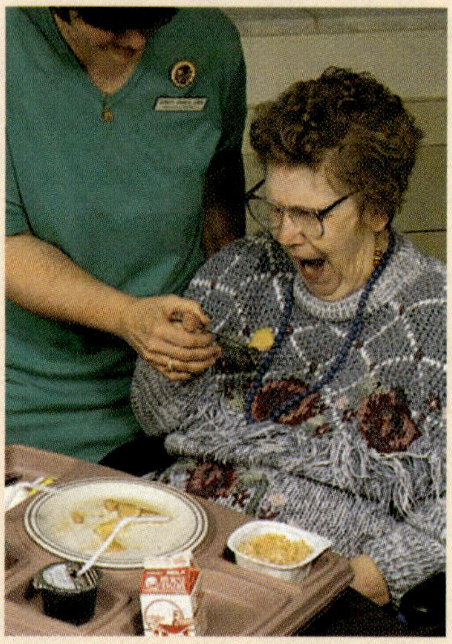

FIGURE 13-13 Use hand-over-hand technique if the resident does not respond to verbal cues.

hygienic measures. This is very difficult and frustrating for the resident. The occupational therapist often develops restorative programs to assist in this area. The care plan will provide directions for each program. The therapist does a **task analysis**, Table 13.2 of the steps in each procedure. The task analysis analyzes a procedure to determine which steps the resident can do independently. For example, part of the task analysis for brushing your teeth includes turning on the faucet, wetting the toothbrush, removing the cap from the toothpaste, and squeezing the toothpaste onto the brush. If the resident cannot do any of these steps, he or she will be unable to brush his or her teeth. The therapist will assess the resident to determine which steps he or she can do, then instruct you to work on the next step. After the resident accomplishes this step, the therapist will instruct you to add another step until the resident can accomplish the entire task. As you can see from the number of steps involved, this takes time, but is a very worthwhile process.

Common hygiene and grooming ADL programs include bathing and dressing skills, applying makeup, styling hair, and shaving. You will assist the resident to perform small parts of a skill, then build on his or her accomplishments. For example, a resident may be unable to wash his or her face. You will assist the resident to wash one cheek. When he or she accomplishes this, assist the resident to wash the other cheek. Build on this ability until the resident is able to wash his or her entire face. All ADL skills start with small tasks. Like building blocks, each new step is built on mastery of the previous step.

Feeding Programs. Eating is a social activity. Residents who eat alone may not eat as well as those who eat with others. Being spoon-fed also takes some of the pleasure out of eating. The resident

TABLE 13-2 Toothbrushing task analysis

Key: 1 = Resident can complete task
0 = Resident cannot complete task
N/A = Not applicable

Date	Key	Initial	Step
			1. Identifies equipment for toothbrushing.
			2. Gathers equipment.
			3. Removes cap from toothpaste.
			4. Turns on cold water.
			5. Wets toothbrush.
			6. Squeezes tube slowly and applies toothpaste to toothbrush.
			7. Places cap on toothpaste.
			8. Fills a cup with water for rinsing mouth.
			9. Turns off water.
			10. Grasps toothbrush handle.
			11. Turns bristles upward and brushes chewing surface of upper teeth.
			12. Brushes upper teeth beginning at one side, moving across front teeth, and ending on opposite side.
			13. Turns toothbrush and brushes inside of upper teeth.
			14. Brushes lower teeth beginning at one side, moving across front teeth, and ending on opposite side.
			15. Turns toothbrush and brushes inside of lower teeth.
			16. Brushes tongue.
			17. Turns bristles upward and gently brushes roof of mouth.
			18. Takes a sip of water from the cup.
			19. Rinses mouth.
			20. Spits water from mouth.
			21. Turns on cold water.
			22. Rinses toothbrush.
			23. Turns water off.
			24. Dries face with towel.
			25. Returns toothbrushing supplies to storage area.

may be able to eat finger foods, but will need to be spoon-fed the remainder of the meal. Restorative feeding programs frequently involve teaching the resident to use adaptive feeding equipment. The goal of restorative feeding is to assist the resident to be as independent as possible with meals. Your responsibility is to set up the tray by uncovering containers, opening milk cartons, buttering bread, cutting meat, or seasoning foods. Do only what the resident needs. If the resident is able to do some of these things for himself or herself, allow the resident to do so. You will also help the resident use adaptive dishes, silverware, and cups.

Restorative Mobility Programs. **Mobility** means the ability to move about. The restorative program may start out by teaching the resident how to move about independently in bed. The program then progresses to transfers from bed to wheelchair. Eventually, the program will progress to ambulation, if the resident is able.

Restorative mobility programs are prescribed for many residents. You may be asked to assist residents to move themselves in bed by using the side rails, trapeze, or other equipment. Teaching a resident to use a wheelchair is also a mobility program. Residents in wheelchairs may be taught to lean over, shift their weight, or do pushups in the chair to relieve pressure and prevent skin breakdown.

Restorative Ambulation Programs. These programs are designed for residents who have completed an intensive therapy rehabilitation program. Restorative ambulation further strengthens the resident and ensures that he or she will maintain the ability to ambulate. In most cases, you will support the resident by using a gait belt. You may also assist with the use of a cane, crutches, or walker.

Range of Motion

Maintaining a resident's **range of motion** is a very important part of restorative care. Range of motion is the normal movement of the joints. Joint motion is affected by age, body size, genetics, and the presence or absence of disease. We do range of motion many times each day during our normal activities of daily living, and at work.

Reasons for Range-of-Motion Exercises

People who are ill or who have been confined to bed do not move as actively, so the joints are not exercised normally. Weakness occurs quickly. Weakness and muscle wasting from lack of use is called **atrophy**. Over time, the muscles become rigid, and the joints do not move as freely as they once did. Joint movement may become painful because the muscles have become short from lack of use. When the joint is moved, the muscle is stretched, and this is uncomfortable or painful. **Contractures** and **deformities** develop (Figure 13.14). Contractures are usually permanent distortions of the body, caused by muscle shortening from lack of use. Contractures cause deformities, or disfigurement. These are serious complications of inactivity, and are painful for the resident. They make bathing, dressing, and caring for the resident more difficult. Every muscle has an antagonist that works in the opposite direction. If a muscle group is not moved for a period of time, or if the resident is not positioned in good body alignment, the stronger muscles will control the weaker ones, causing contractures. Residents with existing contractures are at high risk of developing additional contractures. Contractures can begin to develop in as little as four days of immobility and inactivity. After 15 days, the resident will lose range of motion.

Doing range-of-motion exercises stimulates circulation and improves the resident's sense of wellbeing. Residents' joints must be moved regularly to prevent complications. If residents cannot move independently, the nursing assistant is responsible for exercising the joints several times each day.

If you are assigned to assist residents with range-of-motion exercises, take this responsibility very seriously. Sometimes the physical or occupational therapist will prescribe a special routine. The care plan will describe your responsibilities. All residents, including those with no potential for rehabilitation, should be exercised regularly to prevent deformities. Like pressure ulcers, contractures and deformities are much easier to prevent than to reverse. Sometimes, contractures become permanent and cannot be reversed. Your facility will have a policy for how often to perform range-of-motion exercises on residents. Most facilities exercise residents two to three times a day. Each joint is taken through its normal range of motion three to five times. Know and follow your facility policy.

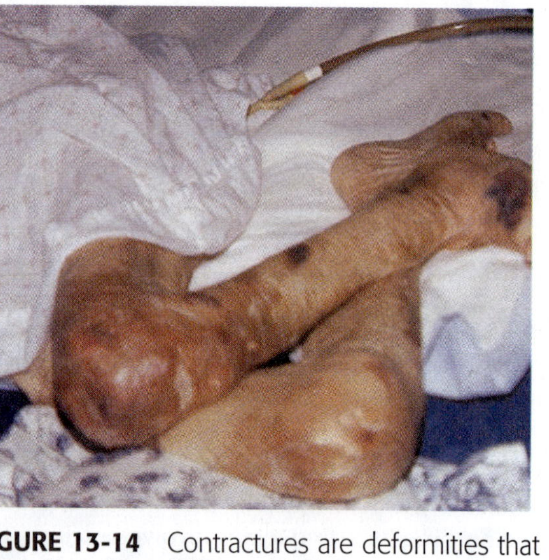

FIGURE 13-14 Contractures are deformities that result from immobility and lack of exercise.

Precautions and Special Situations

Residents with certain conditions require special care and handling. Avoid exercising extremities with fractures or dislocations. Residents with osteoporosis or bone cancer have bones that break very easily. Osteoporosis is a condition in which bone mass decreases, leading to fractures with little or no trauma. Check with the nurse and care plan before proceeding. If the resident has a wound or open area on the joint you are exercising, check with the nurse to see if exercise will be harmful to the healing tissue. If a resident is combative or resists exercise, try to explain why it is important and coax him or her into participating. However, do not force the resident. Notify the nurse if the resident continues to refuse.

Active Range of Motion

Active range-of-motion exercises are done by the resident each day during movement and ADLs. Some residents cannot move all of their joints independently. However, they may be able to use a strong extremity to exercise a weaker extremity. For example, a resident who has had a stroke has a strong right arm and a weak left arm. The resident can be taught to move the weak arm with the stronger right arm (Figure 13.15). Active range of motion maintains movement, prevents deformity, and strengthens muscles.

Active Assistive Range of Motion

Active assistive range-of-motion exercises are either started or completed by the resident. The nursing assistant assists with the exercise. Sometimes a piece of equipment, such as a pulley, is used to exercise the joint. This is another form of active assistive range of motion.

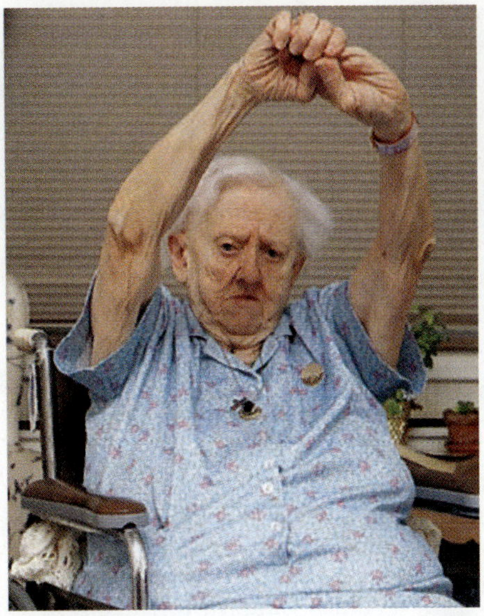

FIGURE 13-15 The resident's left arm is paralyzed from a stroke. She uses her right arm to exercise it several times each day, preventing contractures and deformities.

Passive Range of Motion

Passive range-of-motion exercises are performed by the nursing assistant. The joint is taken through the normal range of movement. Passive range-of-motion exercises maintain movement and prevent deformities, but do not strengthen the muscles.

Range-of-Motion Terminology

Range of motion involves taking the joint through its normal movements. Some important terms describing common joint movements are listed in Table 13.3.

PROCEDURE 75

Passive Range-of-Motion Exercises

1. Position the resident in good alignment in the supine position.
2. Exercise each extremity as indicated on the care plan, supporting the extremity above and below the joint. Repeat each motion 5 times.

A. Head and neck (if this is your facility policy or if you have a physician's order)

1. Tip the head forward, bringing the chin to the chest.

(continues)

PROCEDURE

75 Passive Range-of-Motion Exercises, *continued*

2. Tip the head backward, with the chin up.
3. Move the head from side to side.
4. Move the head back and forth in a circular motion.

B. Shoulders, arms, and elbows

1. Raise the arm over the head, then return the arm to the side.
2. Move the arm from side to side, as far away from the body as possible, then return to the side.
3. Move the arm across the chest until the fingers touch the opposite shoulder. Return the arm to the side.
4. With the arm straight out at the side, bend at the elbow and rotate the shoulder. Return the arm to the side.
5. Bend at the elbow and bring the hand to the chin or shoulder. Return the arm to the side.

C. Wrists, fingers, and forearms

1. Support the elbow.
2. Grasp the hand as in a handshake. Turn the palm up, then down.
3. Bend the hand backward at the wrist, then return to the neutral position.
4. Bend the hand forward at the wrist, then return to the neutral position.
5. Move the hand from side to side, first toward the thumb, then outward.
6. Move the hand in a circle.
7. Clench the fingers and thumb as if making a fist.
8. Extend the fingers and thumb.
9. Move fingers and thumb together and then apart.
10. Flex and extend joints in the thumb and fingers.
11. Move the thumb in a circular motion.

D. Legs, hips, and knees

1. Keeping the knee straight, raise the leg up and down.
2. Bend and straighten the knee.
3. With the leg resting on the bed, roll it inward and outward.
4. Stretch the leg out from the body. Return the leg to touch the other leg.

E. Ankles, foot, and toes

1. With the leg straight on the bed, push the foot and toes toward the knee, then back down.
2. Push the foot and toes out straight, pointing toward the foot of the bed.
3. With the leg straight, turn the foot and ankle from side to side.
4. Bend the toes downward and upward.
5. Spread each toe apart, then back together again.

GUIDELINES FOR

Assisting Residents with Range-of-Motion Exercises

- Check the care plan for limitations and guidelines for each resident.
- In many facilities, the neck is not exercised without a physician's order. Know and follow your facility policy.
- Perform each joint motion three to five times, or according to facility policy.
- Make sure you have enough space for full movement of the extremities.
- Use good body mechanics and position the resident on the back, in good body alignment, before beginning.
- Expose only the part of the body you are exercising.
- Work systematically from the top of the body to the bottom.
- Never push the resident past the point of joint resistance. Move each joint as far as it will comfortably go.
- Stop the exercise and report to the nurse if the resident complains of pain. Watch the resident's face for an indication of pain or discomfort.
- Support each joint while you exercise it by placing one hand above and one hand below the joint.
- Move each joint slowly and consistently. Stop briefly at the end of each motion before repeating it again.
- Be alert for any changes in the resident's condition during the activity. If you feel that the activity is harming the resident, stop the exercise and notify the nurse. Changes that indicate a potential problem are pain, shortness of breath, sweating, and change in color.
- Help the resident relax during exercise.
- Use the time spent during range-of-motion exercises as quality time to communicate with the resident.
- For residents who are stiff or combative, performing range-of-motion exercises in the bathtub or whirlpool may be helpful. Check with the nurse.

TABLE 13-3 Range-of-motion terminology

- **Abduction** (Figure 13.16) is moving an extremity *away from* the body.

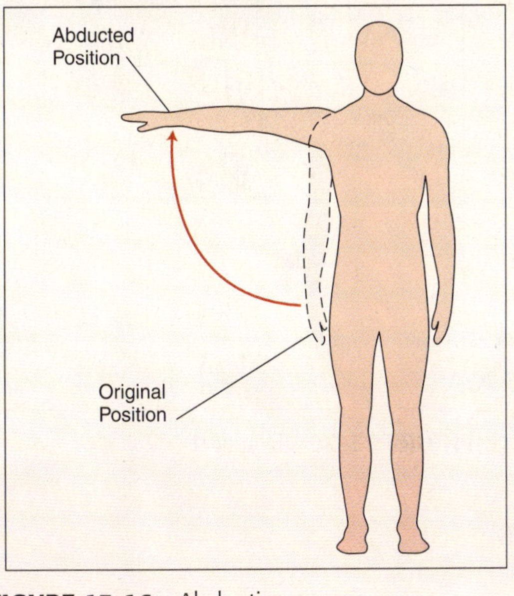

FIGURE 13-16 Abduction

- **Adduction** (Figure 13.17) is moving an extremity *toward* the body.

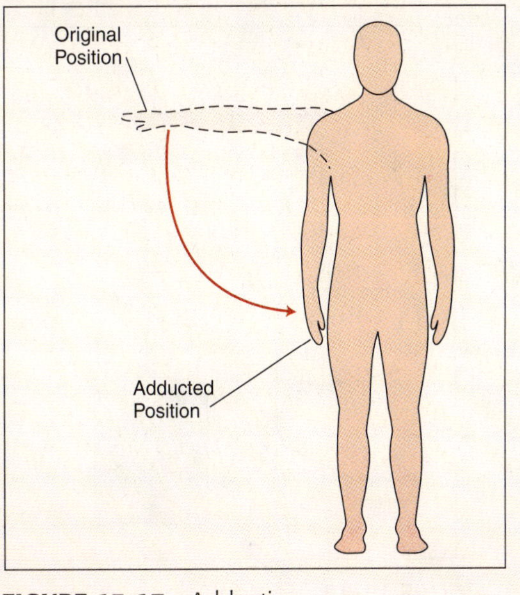

FIGURE 13-17 Adduction

TABLE 13-3 *(continued)*

- **Circumduction** is a circular movement of a joint, such as the thumb or wrist.
- **Dorsal flexion**, or **dorsiflexion**, is pulling the foot upward toward the head.
- **Eversion** is turning a joint outward.
- **Extension** (Figure 13.18) is straightening a joint.

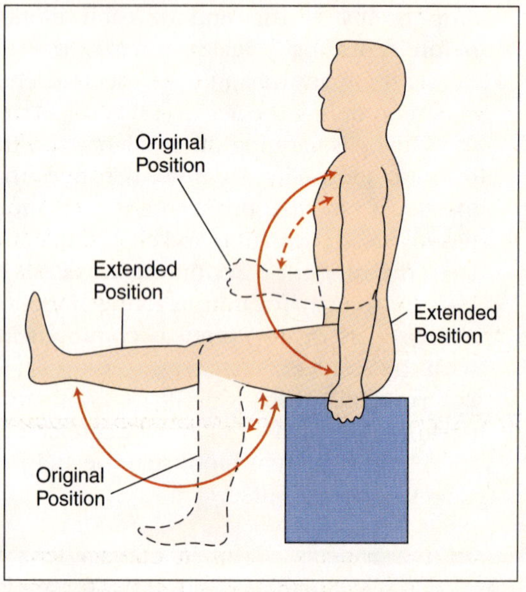

FIGURE 13-18 Extension

- **External rotation** is turning a joint outward away from the median line.
- **Flexion** (Figure 13.19) is bending a joint.

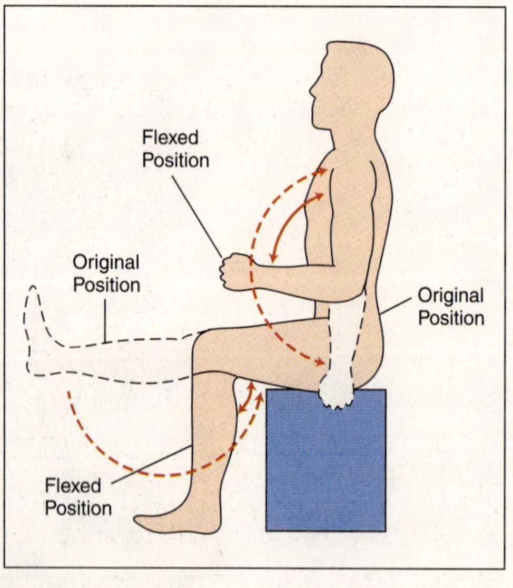

FIGURE 13-19 Flexion

- **Hyperextension** is gentle, excessive extension of a joint, slightly past the point of resistance.
- **Internal rotation** is turning a joint inward toward the median line.
- **Inversion** is turning a joint inward.
- **Medial** pertains to or is situated toward the midline of the body.
- **Median** means situated in the median plane or in the midline of the body.
- **Opposition** is touching each of the fingers against the thumb.
- **Palmar flexion** is the act of bending the hand down toward the palm.
- **Plantar flexion** is bending the foot downward, away from the body.
- **Pronation** is moving a joint to face downward.
- **Radial deviation** is turning the wrist inward, toward the radius.
- **Retraction** is drawing back, away from the body.
- **Rotation** (Figure 13.20) means moving a joint in, out, and around.
- **Supination** is moving a joint so it faces upward.
- **Ulnar deviation** is turning the wrist outward, toward the ulna.

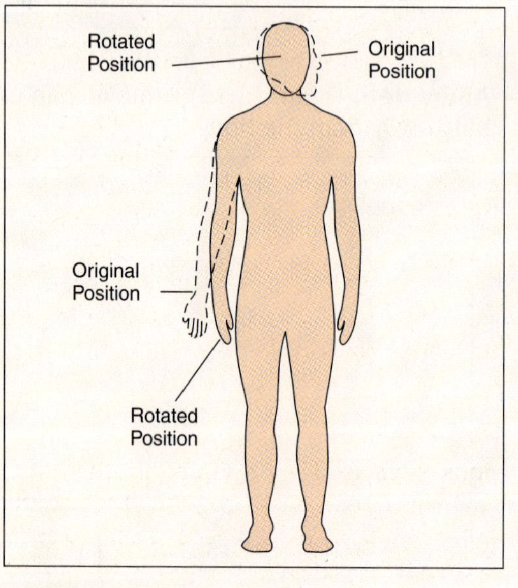

FIGURE 13-20 Rotation

GUIDELINES FOR

Caring for a Resident Who Has a Prosthesis

- Always check the care plan for special instructions regarding applying, removing, and caring for the prosthesis.
- The prosthesis and the skin under the prosthesis must be kept clean and dry.
- Check the skin under the prosthesis. Notify the nurse of any redness, irritation, dark spots, open areas, or blisters.
- Follow the directions on the care plan for covering the extremity under the prosthesis. A **stump sock** is a garment used to protect the extremity from irritation caused by rubbing against the prosthesis and is usually worn under artificial limbs.
- For residents with lower extremity amputation, position the remaining joints in extension (as straight as possible). Residents with leg amputation are at risk for contracture development. Follow the positioning instructions on the care plan. Avoid elevating the stump on pillows.
- Report to the nurse if you feel that the prosthesis needs repair. Do not attempt to fix it yourself.
- An artificial eye is usually cared for by the nurse or resident. If you will be caring for residents with artificial eyes, make sure you are properly trained. Follow facility policy. Handle the eye carefully. The eye socket and the artificial eye must be cleaned as indicated on the care plan. Apply the principles of standard precautions when inserting, removing, and cleaning the eye.

Prosthesis Care

Some residents use a prosthesis to replace a body part. Many types of prostheses are used. A resident may have an artificial eye or breast. Others have artificial arms, hands, legs, or feet. The prosthesis helps the resident function as normally as possible. Remember, the prosthesis is part of the resident's body and should be treated with care. You will be responsible for keeping the prosthesis clean. This usually involves washing with mild soap, rinsing, and drying. Follow the instructions on the care plan or check with the nurse.

Artificial Eye

Situations such as severe injury to the eye or untreatable cancer may require the surgical removal of an eye. An eye prosthesis (artificial eye) is usually inserted after the surgery. The care plan should provide information if the patient has an artificial eye.

Some patients remove the artificial eye at night. Others prefer not to remove the eye at all. You may be responsible for removing the eye. If the eye is to remain out of the socket, store it in a marked cup in contact lens disinfectant solution (Figure 13.21). The socket is usually cleansed and irrigated when the eye is removed. Irrigation of the socket may be a licensed nursing procedure in your facility. Know and follow your facility policy. Apply the principles of standard precautions when caring for the artificial eye and mucous membranes in the eye socket.

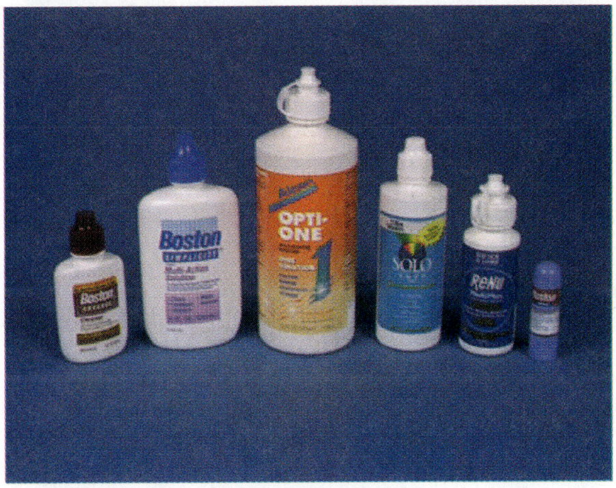

FIGURE 13-21 Many different disinfectant solutions are used to clean the artificial eye.

PROCEDURE 76 Caring for the Eye Socket and Artificial Eye

1. Carry out beginning procedure actions.
2. Assemble equipment:
   - eye cup or clean denture cup
   - prescribed solution, if ordered
   - small plastic bag
   - 4 to 6 cotton balls
   - 24 × 4 gauze pads
   - emesis basin with lukewarm water
   - disposable gloves
   - towel
3. Place the patient in supine position, if tolerated. Place a towel across the patient's chest.
4. Put on disposable gloves.
5. Moisten cotton balls in lukewarm water in the emesis basin.
   a. Ask the patient to close his eyes.
   b. Wipe the upper lid of the affected eye from the inner corner of the eye to the outer edge. Repeat with a clean cotton ball until the area is clean and free of mucus.
6. Dispose of the used cotton balls in a plastic bag.
7. Place a 4 × 4 gauze pad in the bottom of the eye cup or denture cup.
8. Remove the artificial eye:
   a. Gently pull down the lower eyelid with your thumb (Figure 13.22A). Open the upper lid with your index finger.
   b. Grasp the artificial eye as it comes out of the eye socket and place it on the gauze in the cup.
   c. Some patients use a small suction cup to remove the eye. Gently hold the eye open with the fingers of one hand. Depress the suction cup between your thumb and index finger (Figure 13.22B). Place the suction cup in the center of the artificial eye. Release the pressure. Gently pull the eye from the socket (Figure 13.22C).

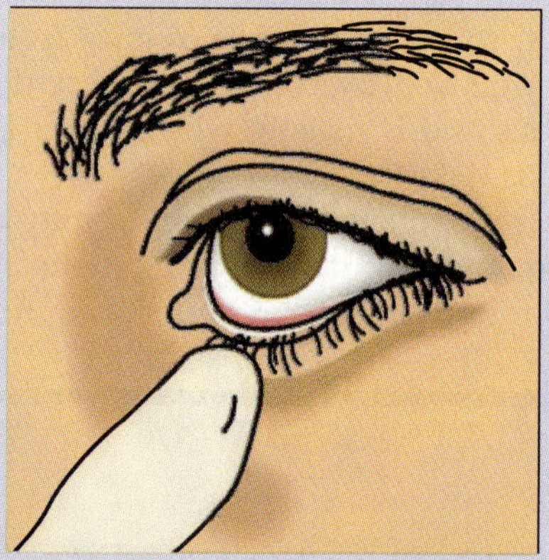

FIGURE 13-22A To loosen the eye, pull the lower lid down, then push back up slightly.

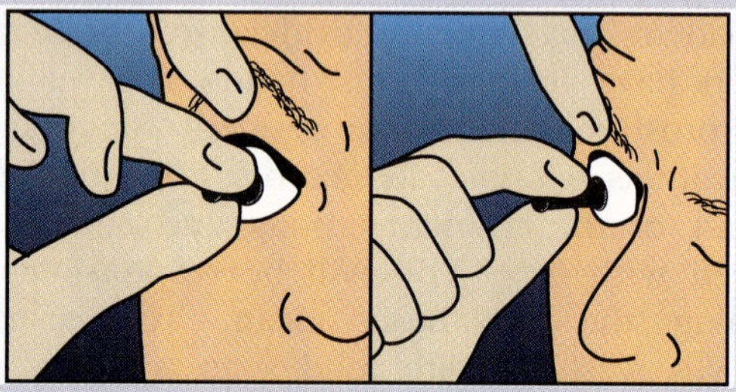

FIGURE 13-22B Squeeze the cup, place it against the eye, then release the suction.

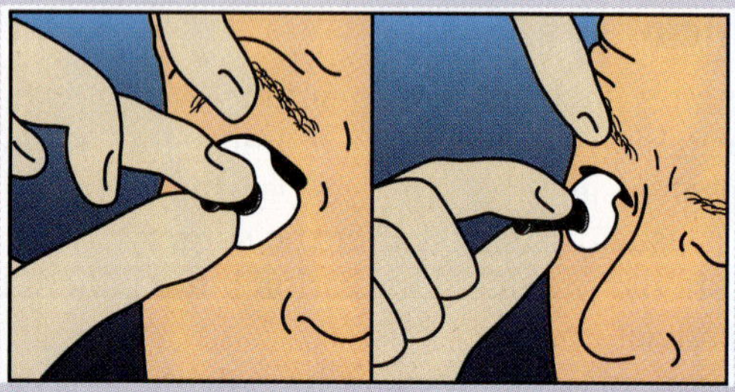

FIGURE 13-22C Pull the eye down gently from the socket.

9. Use clean cotton balls moistened with water or solution as ordered and clean the empty eye socket. Dry gently with clean, dry cotton balls. Use a new cotton ball for each wipe. Pat the patient's face dry, as needed.
10. Carry the cup with the artificial eye to the sink. Fill the sink one-third full with lukewarm water.
11. Wash the eye under lukewarm running water, or use the prescribed solution. Use gauze if necessary to loosen and remove any accumulation from the eye.
12. Rinse the eye and place it on a dry 4 × 4 gauze pad, or store the eye in sterile water or the prescribed solution, according to the care plan. (Do not dry an artificial eye.)
13. Discard the water or solution in the eye cup and rinse the cup.
14. Remove your gloves. Wash your hands. Carry the artificial eye to the patient's bedside.
15. Explain to the patient what you are going to do.
16. Insert the artificial eye into the eye socket:
    a. Carry out beginning procedure actions.
    b. Put on disposable gloves.
    c. Clean and rinse the artificial eye with the prescribed solution, if you have not already done so.
    d. Position the notched edge of the eye toward the patient's nose (Figure 13.22D).
    e. Gently open the upper eyelid. Bring the prosthesis up past the lower lid and under the upper lid. Set it flush once it is past the lower lid and touching the upper tissues (Figure 13.22E).
    f. Place your index finger on the prosthesis and slip it up under the upper lid (Figure 13.22F).

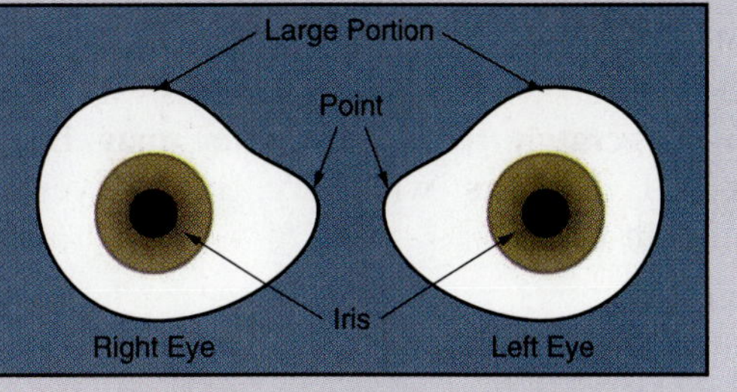

FIGURE 13-22D The notched part of the eye is positioned next to the patient's nose.

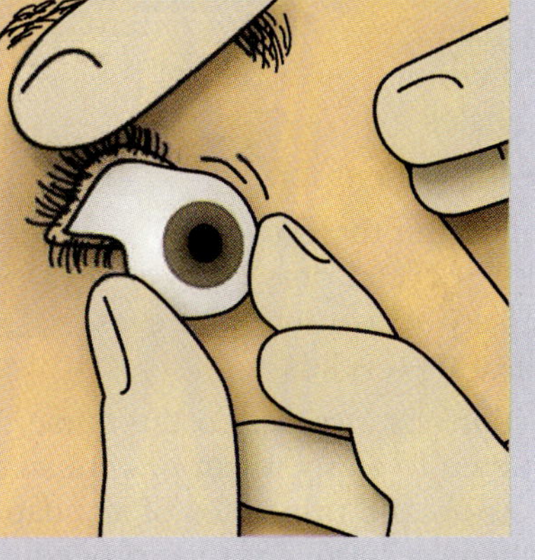

FIGURE 13-22E Gently move the artificial eye up past the lower lid.

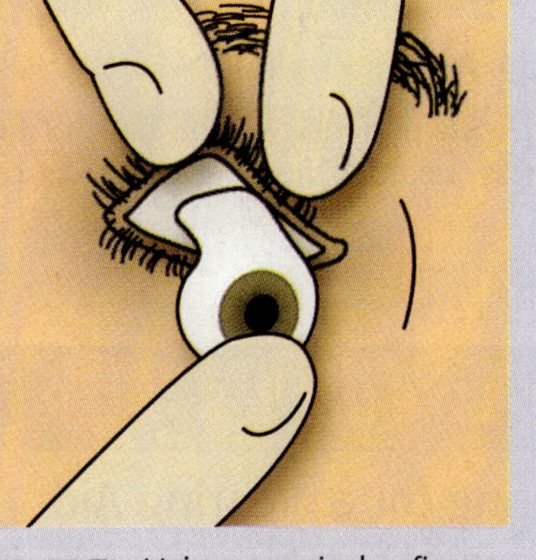

FIGURE 13-22F Using your index finger, push the eye the rest of the way up and under the upper lid.

    g. Release the upper lid.
    h. Draw the edge of the lower lid forward, covering the lower edge of the eye. Press down lightly.
17. Carry out procedure completion actions.

Warm and Cool Eye Compresses

Many elderly patients have dry, itchy eyes. This may be caused by allergies, irritants, squinting, rubbing, or blinking the eyes. The eyes may appear red, with swollen eyelids. If patients rub or scratch their eyes, they may become infected. Patients with dry, itchy eyes may complain of:

- burning
- scratchy feeling
- itching
- light sensitivity
- difficulty moving eyes
- excess mucus production
- severe pain
- blurred vision
- seeing halos

Observe the patient for:

- drainage from the eyes
- redness of eyelid rims
- scaly, flaky skin around the eyes
- edema of the eyelids

Report your observations to the nurse. You may be instructed to apply warm or cool soaks to the eyelids. Apply the principles of standard precautions when performing this procedure. If an infection is suspected, use separate equipment for each eye. This will prevent the infection from spreading.

Hearing Aids

Some of your patients will be hard of hearing or completely deaf. A hearing aid (Figure 13.23A and 13.23B) will sometimes improve the patient's level of hearing and comprehension. Lip reading or sign language may be needed to communicate.

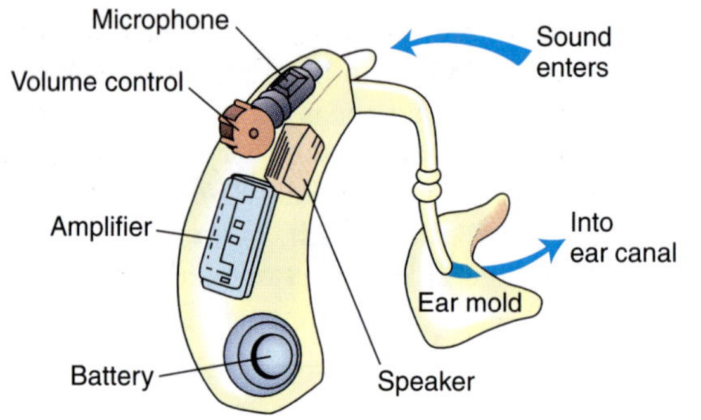

FIGURE 13-23A Parts of a behind-the-ear hearing aid. The ear mold is placed in the ear canal. The rest of the hearing aid is worn outside and over the top of the ear.

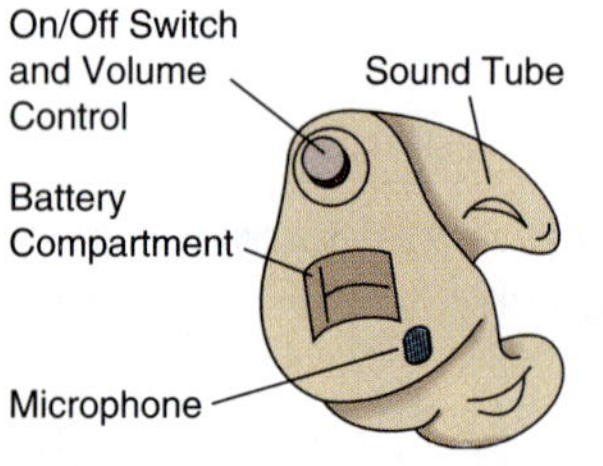

FIGURE 13-23B This hearing aid is worn inside the outer ear canal.

GUIDELINES FOR

Caring for a Hearing Aid

- Store hearing aids at room temperature when they are not being worn. Temperature extremes can damage hearing aids. They should not be worn for more than a few minutes in very cold weather. Avoid exposing them to hair dryers.
- Keep hearing aids dry. If an aid is worn accidentally in the shower, ask the nurse how to dry it. Never try to dry the aid with a hair dryer.
- Store extra batteries in a cool, dry place. Remove the batteries from the hearing aid at night or open the battery compartment. This allows any moisture to evaporate.
- Keep hearing aids safe. They break easily if dropped on a hard surface.

- Remove the hearing aid if hair spray is being used, as the spray may cause damage.
- Turn the hearing aid off when it is not in use. Turn the aid off before removing it.
- Wipe in-the-ear aids daily with a dry tissue.
- Check regularly to make sure the opening of the aid or ear mold is free of wax. In-the-ear types come with a cleaning tool. This should be used only by someone who has been instructed how to use it. Never use a toothpick, paper clip, or other sharp object to clean the hearing aid.
- Insert the hearing aid properly. Sometimes the shape of the ear changes with aging and the hearing aid may have to be refitted. If the patient complains of pain or the aid is difficult to insert, this may be the problem. Advise the nurse if this occurs.
- When communicating with the patient, follow the same guidelines that you use when communicating with a patient who has hearing impairment.
- Check bed linen carefully before placing it in the soiled linen hamper. A hearing aid is small, expensive, and easily lost. It will not survive a trip through the washer and dryer!

GUIDELINES FOR

Troubleshooting Hearing Aids

If the aid is not producing sound, before inserting it in the patient's ear:

- Check to make sure the "+" (positive) side of the battery is next to the "+" inside the hearing aid battery case or compartment.
- Try a new battery–the old one may be dead. Hold the hearing aid in the palm of your hand. Turn the volume all the way up. Cup the aid between your hands. You should hear a loud whistle. A weak or absent sound indicates that the battery is low.
- Before changing the battery, check the position of the old battery so you can put the new one in the same way. When inserting a new battery, place it in the unit gently. If you meet resistance, do not force it. Consult the nurse.
- Check the ear mold to see if it is plugged with wax.
- Make sure the hearing aid is set on "M" (microphone), not "T" (telephone switch).
- If the hearing aid works intermittently or makes a scratchy sound, check for dirt under and around the battery. Also check the volume control and connections. If the hearing aid has a connecting wire, make sure it is plugged in tightly and is not cracked or bent.

If the hearing aid is making squealing sounds:

- If the hearing aid is in the patient's ear and makes a loud, whistling sound, check the position. The aid should be securely in the ear. Make sure that hair, ear wax, or clothing are not interfering with the position. Check the tubing for cracks. Whistling usually indicates an air leak.
- Determine if the ear mold fits properly. It should be completely in the ear. If it does not fit well, report it to the nurse.
- Check the volume on the aid. If it is too high, turn it down until the squealing stops.
- Check the plastic tubing on a behind-the-ear aid. If it is cracked or split, it must be replaced.

PROCEDURE 77 Applying a Behind-the-Ear Hearing Aid

1. Carry out beginning procedure actions.
2. Assemble equipment:
   - hearing aid
3. Check the appliance to be sure the batteries are working and the tubing is not cracked (Figure 13.24).
4. Check to make sure the hearing aid is off or the volume is turned to its lowest level.
5. Check the patient's ear for wax buildup or any abnormalities.

   Note: *If the patient complains that the hearing aid hurts or does not fit properly, it may have to be refitted; the ear structure changes with age. Report this to the nurse.*
6. Handle the aid carefully.
   - Do not drop it.
   - Do not allow it to get wet.
   - Store it carefully with the switch in the off position when it is not in use. Some aids should have batteries removed when being stored.
7. Hand the aid to the patient so that you support the appliance as the patient inserts the ear mold into the ear canal.

Alternate Actions:

8. Place the hearing aid over the patient's ear, allowing the ear mold to hang free.
9. Adjust the hearing aid behind the patient's ear.
10. Grasp the ear mold and gently insert the tapered end into the ear canal.
11. Gently twist the ear mold into the curve of the ear, pushing upward and inward on the bottom of the ear mold while pulling on the ear lobe with the other hand.
12. Turn on the control switch and adjust the volume to a comfortable level.
13. Carry out procedure completion actions.

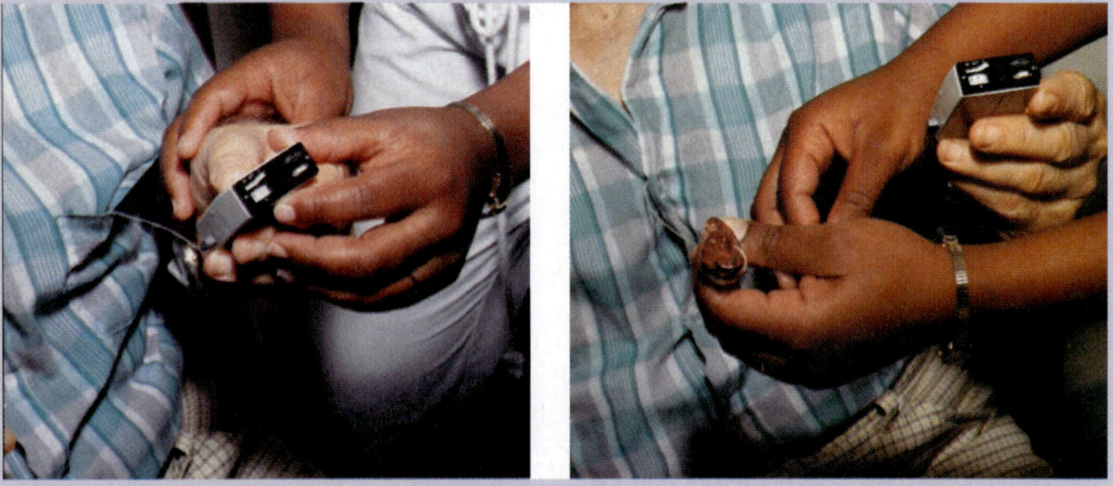

FIGURE 13-24 Check the appliance to make sure the batteries are working and the tubing is not cracked.

PROCEDURE 78 Removing a Behind-the-Ear Hearing Aid

1. Carry out beginning procedure actions.
2. Explain to the patient what you plan to do.
3. Turn off the hearing aid.
4. Loosen the outer portion of the ear mold by gently pulling on the upper part of the ear.
5. Lift the ear mold upward and outward.
6. Make sure the on-off switch is in the off position. Store the hearing aid in a safe area.
7. Carry out procedure completion actions.

PROCEDURE 79 Applying and Removing an In-the-Ear Hearing Aid

Applying the Hearing Aid

1. Carry out beginning procedure actions.
2. Assist the patient into a comfortable position, with head turned so that the ear needing the hearing aid is closest to you.
3. Turn the hearing aid off and turn the volume down.
4. Make sure you insert the aid in the correct ear.
   a. Grasp the ear mold and gently insert the tapered end into the ear canal (Figure 13.25).
   b. Gently twist the ear mold into the curve of the ear while gently pulling on the ear lobe with the other hand. The hearing aid should fit snugly but comfortably, flush with the ear.
5. Turn on the control switch. To adjust the volume, talk to the patient as you increase the volume. Stop when the patient can hear you.

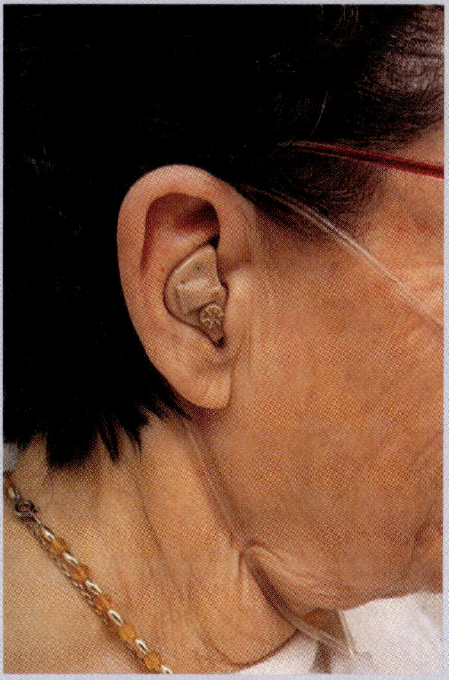

FIGURE 13-25 Gently insert the tapered end of the in-the-ear hearing aid into the ear canal.

(continues)

PROCEDURE 79 Applying and Removing an In-the-Ear Hearing Aid, *continued*

Removing the Hearing Aid

1. Wash your hands and explain to the patient what you plan to do.
2. Turn off the hearing aid.
3. Loosen the outer portion of the ear mold by gently pulling on the upper part of the ear.
4. Lift the ear mold upward and outward.
5. Store the aid in a safe area. Either remove the batteries and store them in a safe place, or open the battery compartment.
6. Carry out procedure completion actions.

Caring for Hearing Aids

A hearing aid is a delicate and expensive prosthesis. It requires safe handling and regular care.

Bowel and Bladder Management

The OBRA legislation specifically requires the prevention of declines. Incontinence is a decline. Acute illness and deterioration in mental status may cause a loss of bowel or bladder control. Remember, incontinence is not a normal consequence of aging. Incontinence should be prevented and treated aggressively. Managing incontinence is difficult and unpleasant for the nursing assistant and affects the resident's self-esteem. Incontinence greatly increases the risk for skin breakdown. Apply the principles of standard precautions when assisting residents with incontinence and bowel and bladder management programs.

Incontinence Management Programs

Incontinence management programs are not active restorative programs. These programs are designed for residents who are mentally confused and unable to communicate the need to use the toilet. However, if the resident is placed on the toilet he or she will use it correctly. The resident is taken to the bathroom at regular intervals, typically every two hours. This prevents incontinence most of the time. A trial of incontinence management should be used on all mentally confused residents who are physically able to use a toilet or commode. Although the resident is not actually "trained" to use the toilet, a successful incontinence management program benefits the resident and facility staff in many ways.

Bowel and Bladder Retraining Programs

Bowel and bladder retraining programs are individually designed for residents who have become incontinent due to acute illness, trauma, infection, medications, and other factors. Residents do not have to be mentally alert to participate. However, they must have some ability to follow directions and cooperate with the program. For the best results, bowel and bladder programs should be developed as early in the illness as possible. Members of the interdisciplinary team assess the resident's physical condition, mental status, and ability to participate. An environmental assessment is also completed to determine access and distance to the toilet, whether the resident can get out of the bed or chair independently, and so forth. The nursing assistant contributes important information to this assessment. After all data are collected, an individual program is developed to meet the resident's specific needs.

GUIDELINES FOR

Assisting Residents with Bowel and Bladder Retraining Programs

- Follow the care plan exactly.
- Answer the call signal promptly.
- Do not rush the resident when toileting.
- Provide privacy by closing the door and privacy curtain. Close the bathroom door even if you must remain in the bathroom with the resident for safety.
- Avoid scolding the resident for accidents. Tell the resident that he or she can try again next time. Praise the resident for using the toilet and for staying dry.
- If the resident cannot physically use the toilet, assist with the bedpan, urinal, or commode.
- Keep the path to the bathroom well lit and free from obstacles.
- If used, keep the wheelchair, walker, or cane close to the bed.
- Keep the resident's skin clean and dry.

Part of the bowel and bladder assessment involves identifying factors that contribute to or cause incontinence. After these factors are identified, the nurse will develop a plan to eliminate them. The nurse will take a history of the resident's previous bowel and bladder habits. A detailed analysis of the resident's incontinent episodes over a period of 7 to 14 days will be completed. The nursing assistant is usually responsible for checking the resident hourly and recording information about incontinence or resident requests to use the toilet (Figure 13.26). Accurate completion of this analysis is very important, because the resident's individual toileting schedule will be developed based largely on this information. Because you are more aware of the resident's habits and patterns than many other care providers, notify the nurse if you believe the resident shows a pattern of urge incontinence, stress incontinence, or overflow incontinence.

Following the initial assessment period, the nurse will analyze all the information collected and develop a plan for the resident. The plan is based on the resident's previous routines and habits and information about times when the resident was incontinent during the assessment. The nurse will write a specific schedule with times to toilet the resident. There may or may not be a pattern to this schedule. It is based on the resident's individual needs. Some people can wait for six hours before urinating. Others urinate every hour or two. The resident's medical condition, specific habits, and needs are considered when the schedule is written. Some environmental modification may be necessary. The schedule will be implemented and reassessed by the nurse every few days. During this time, you will continue to record each time the resident eliminates. The nurse will review the information and readjust the schedule as necessary until success is achieved. Treat the resident with dignity at all times. Flexibility in your schedule, consistency, and punctuality in being available at the scheduled toileting times will help guarantee success. In addition, believe that the program will succeed and maintain your motivation to help the resident.

Scheduled Toileting. **Scheduled toileting** is used for residents who require physical assistance to get to the bathroom. You will be assigned to assist the resident to the bathroom according to a fixed schedule, usually every two to four hours.

Prompted Voiding. Some residents know that their bladders are full, but do not communicate the need to use the toilet. The nurse may instruct you to use **prompted voiding** for these residents. In a prompted voiding program, you will check the resident frequently to determine if he or she is wet or dry. Each time you are in the room, you will ask the resident if he or she needs to use the toilet. Assist the resident to the bathroom or to use the commode, bedpan, or urinal. Praise the resident for remaining dry and for trying to use the toilet. Inform the resident when you will return to take him or her to the bathroom again.

Habit Training. **Habit training** is done for residents who are mentally confused and urinate at fairly predictable times. The resident is taken

ASSESSMENT FOR BOWEL & BLADDER TRAINING

PATIENT: Frank Martin ROOM NO: 629C

	DAY 1	DAY 2	DAY 3	DAY 4	DAY 5	DAY 6	DAY 7
DATE	10/2/XX	10/3/XX	10/4/XX	10/5/XX	10/6/XX	10/7/XX	10/8/XX
7 AM	D	IU	IU	D			
8 AM	IU	D	D	D			
9 AM	D	IU	D	IU			
10 AM	D	D	D	D			
11 AM	D	D	IU	IU			
12 AM	IU	D	D	D			
1 PM	IU	IU	IU	IU			
2 PM	D	D	D	D			
3 PM	D	D	D	D			
4 PM	IBM	D	D	IU			
5 PM	IU	IBM	D	IBM			
6 PM	D	IU	IU	D			
7 PM	D	D	D	IU			
8 PM	IU	IU	IU	D			
9 PM	D	D	D	D			
10 PM	D	D	D	IU			
11 PM	D	IU	IU	D			
12 AM	D	D	D	D			
1 AM	IU	D	D	D			
2 AM	D	IU	IU	IU			
3 AM	IU	D	D	IU			
4 AM	D	D	D	D			
5 AM	D	D	IU	D			
6 AM	IU	IU	D	D			
CODE:	D = DRY IBM = INCONTINENT BM IU = INCONTINENT URINE		TBM = TOILET BM TU = TOILET URINE				

FIGURE 13-26 The resident is checked hourly, but no retraining is done. If the resident asks to use the bathroom, honor the request. At the end of the assessment period, the nurse will develop an individualized toileting schedule based on this information.

to the toilet at those times. Praise the resident for being dry and for using the toilet.

Special Situations. Some residents are placed on bladder retraining programs because they have an indwelling catheter. Facilities manage these programs differently. Some facilities completely remove the catheter and begin the retraining assessment. Other facilities clamp and unclamp the catheter at intervals so the resident gets used to the sensation of urine in the bladder. You may be asked to clamp and unclamp the catheter during the retraining process. This does not involve opening the closed system. While the catheter is clamped, urine remains in the bladder. Report resident complaints of pain or discomfort to the nurse. Be punctual in the scheduled times to unclamp the catheter to prevent discomfort from the bladder overfilling.

Kegel Exercises. Some residents must do exercises to make the bladder muscles stronger. These exercises are called **Kegel exercises**. Restorative nurses work with these residents initially. Later in the program, you may be instructed to assist and remind the resident to perform the Kegel exercises. Kegel exercises are helpful in preventing incontinence. Over time, they strengthen the muscles of the pelvic floor and the muscles surrounding the urethra and vagina. These muscles contribute to the closing of the urethra and support the pelvic structures. The resident is taught to draw in, or lift up, the muscles surrounding the vagina and anus. This is the same as the action used for controlling urination and defecation. Residents are instructed to contract the muscles, then hold the contraction for at least 10 seconds, then release for 10 seconds. The exercises are done regularly, many times a day, for at least eight weeks. They may have to be continued indefinitely. More time may be required in the elderly before results are seen. Over time, the exercises condition the muscles to contract when abdominal pressure increases. Residents are reminded to contract the pelvic muscles in situations when leakage may occur.

Intake and Output. You may also be asked to record the resident's intake and output during the retraining period. The overall fluid intake for the resident may be increased during retraining. In some facilities, fluids are limited during the evening and night hours. The retraining program may take several months. You must be empathetic, patient, and supportive, and encourage the resident's success.

Restorative Equipment

Special restorative equipment is used for many residents to prevent contractures and deformities. These can develop very quickly as a result of immobility. Follow the care plan and use common sense in using restorative equipment. The nursing assistant is usually responsible for placing and applying the equipment. Some items, such as splints, are worn according to a schedule. Other equipment, such as handrolls, are used at all times. If the equipment is fastened to the resident's body, you are responsible for keeping the skin clean and dry under the device. Usually, the equipment is removed when range-of-motion exercises are being performed, then replaced. Follow the care plan and your facility policy.

Handrolls

Handrolls are used to prevent the fingers from contracting into a tight fist. Although some devices can be fashioned from common items in the health care facility, using commercially manufactured handrolls is best. Years ago, rolled wash-cloths were used for handrolls. We now know that the softness and texture of a rolled washcloth promotes squeezing and actually worsens contractures! Handrolls should be used by all dependent residents. Soft handrolls (Figure 13.27A) are the most comfortable and commonly used. Most commercial varieties have a Velcro® strip attached that is fastened to the hand. Semi-rigid, cone-shaped handrolls (Figure 13.27B) are also available. These are used by residents who may have early contractures and those whose fingers are rigid. The cones are fastened to the hand with the large end by the little finger.

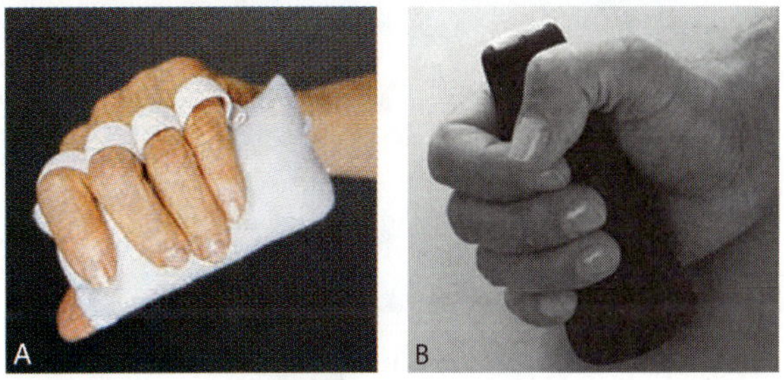

FIGURE 13-27 (A) The soft handroll is comfortable and prevents deformity. (B) The small end of the cone is placed on the thumb side of the hand. The nursing assistant is responsible for keeping the hands clean and the nails trimmed.Skil-Care Corporation, Yonkers, NY (800) 431-2972)

Splints

Splints (Figure 13.28) are rigid devices used on the hands, arms, legs, and feet. They are used to maintain good alignment, prevent and reverse early contractures, and maintain the extremity in a fixed position. Sometimes splints are used to maintain good alignment of a fracture until the area is casted or an operation is performed. The physical or occupational therapist usually fabricates splints or orders splints for a specific medical purpose. The care plan will describe the reason for the splint and provide instructions for applying and removing the splint. Splints used to support broken bones are not removed by the nursing assistant. Splints used to prevent or reverse contractures are worn according to a schedule. For example, the splint may be worn during the day and removed at night. Keeping the extremity under the splint clean and dry is very important. The splint must be removed at least once each 24 hours for bathing. Check the area under the splint for signs of redness, irritation, and breakdown. Report your observations to the nurse.

Trochanter Rolls

The **trochanter roll** (Figure 13.29) is used to prevent external rotation of the hip. Trochanter rolls should be used routinely for bedfast residents to prevent deformities. Unless the resident has a specific medical condition, such as a hip fracture, no special order is necessary. To hold the trochanter roll in place, roll it away from the resident's body. Rolling the trochanter roll toward the body will cause it to slip, making it ineffective.

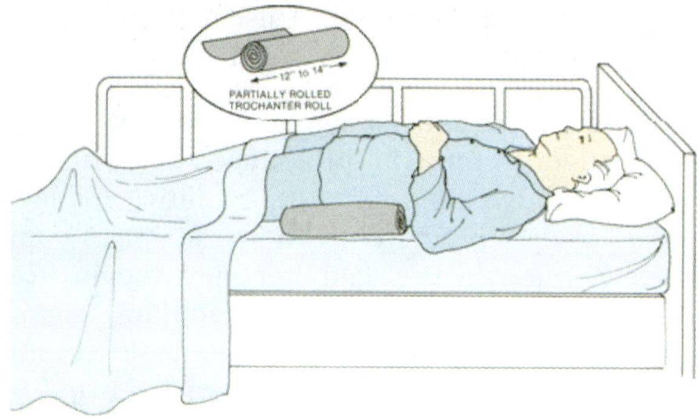

FIGURE 13-29 The trochanter roll is used to prevent the hips from contracting in a position of external rotation.

Foot Boards

Foot boards (Figure 13.30A) are used to prevent foot drop (Figure 13.30B). Foot drop is a severe contracture that is difficult or impossible to reverse. It occurs quickly in residents who are confined to bed. The toes of a resident with foot drop point downward, similar to the position of a woman's foot in high heels. The muscles in the foot become stiff and rigid, and the resident is unable to pull the ball of the foot and toes toward the body. This prevents the resident from standing normally on the foot with the heel flat on the floor. Residents with

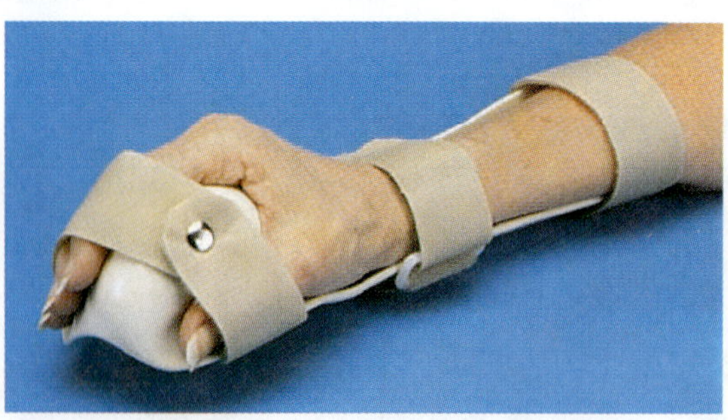

FIGURE 13-28 Apply the splint according to the individual use schedule on the care plan. The nursing assistant is responsible for keeping the resident's hand clean under the splint. Inform the nurse if the splint does not fit correctly. *(Neutral Position wrist/hand orthosis is provided by Sammons Preston, Inc., a Bissell® HealthCare Company. Reprinted with permission.)*

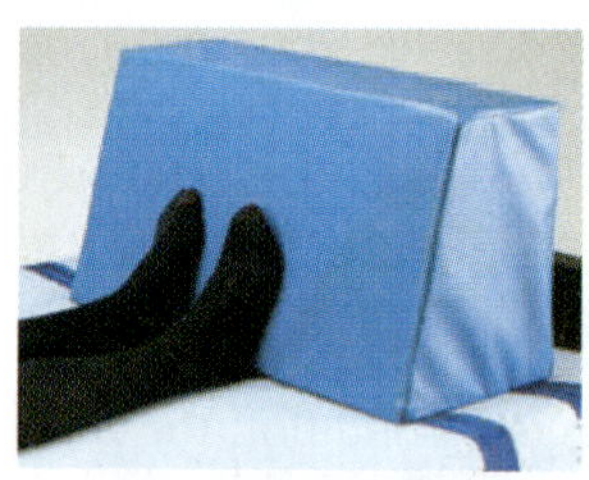

FIGURE 13-30A Foot boards are used to prevent foot drop, a severe contracture of the feet.Skil-Care Corporation, Yonkers, NY (800) 431-2972)

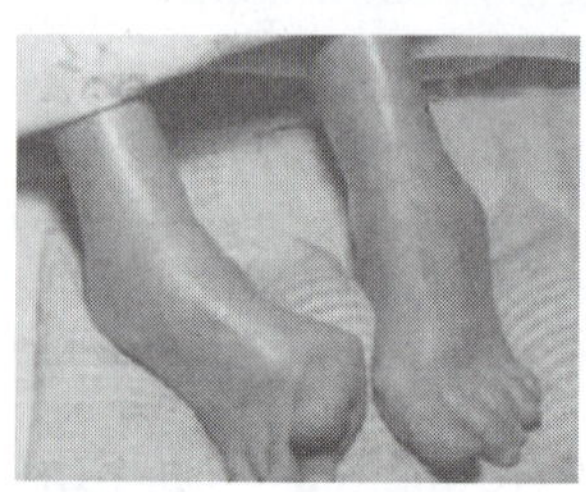

FIGURE 13-30B Foot drop is a serious contracture deformity that prevents the resident from standing or ambulating. Foot drop may be released surgically in some residents, but may become severe and irreversible.

PROCEDURE

80 Making a Trochanter Roll

1. Perform your beginning procedure actions.
2. Gather your equipment: bath blanket, gloves if contact with blood or body fluids is likely.
3. Place the bath blanket on a flat surface. Fold it in thirds lengthwise.
4. Place the blanket on the bed, extending from the waist to the mid-thigh area.
5. Position the resident in the center of the blanket.
6. Roll the center of the blanket outward (away from the resident) until it is firmly against the femur area.
7. Tuck the roll inward to maintain position.
8. Perform your procedure completion actions.

contractures of the feet and ankles are unable to walk.

Some foot boards are positioned at the end of the mattress. The heels hang over the end of the mattress so there is no pressure on them. The ball and sole of the foot are positioned flat against the foot board to prevent the toes from pointing downward. An alternative is to position the foot board on the bed and then to place a pillow in front of the foot board for the feet to rest against. A small pillow under the ankles keeps the heels off the mattress.

No matter which position is used, monitor the resident's heels frequently, relieve pressure as much as possible, and alert the nurse to signs and symptoms of skin irritation or breakdown. Heel breakdown often begins with an area that appears black, brown, purple, or bruised under the skin. It may look like a large blood blister. The heels are a high-pressure area, and the skin may be thinner than on other areas of the body. The risk of heel breakdown is very high, and because of the anatomy, heel ulcers will develop quickly and worsen rapidly, invading underlying structures. Many elderly individuals have diabetes and other conditions that cause reduced circulation to the feet. Because of decreased blood flow, the risk of complications and amputation from heel ulcers is very high.

Other commercial devices that fasten to the foot may be used as substitutes for the foot board (Figure 13.31). Preventing contractures of the feet is an important responsibility.

Other Positioning Devices

Sometimes it is hard to differentiate positioning devices from restraint alternatives. Many devices are used for both purposes. Restraints are commonly used because the resident has a particular positioning problem. When trying to decide how to meet the resident's positioning needs, consider restraint alternatives mentioned in Unit 15. The devices listed can be used for support and to keep residents positioned comfortably in good body alignment.

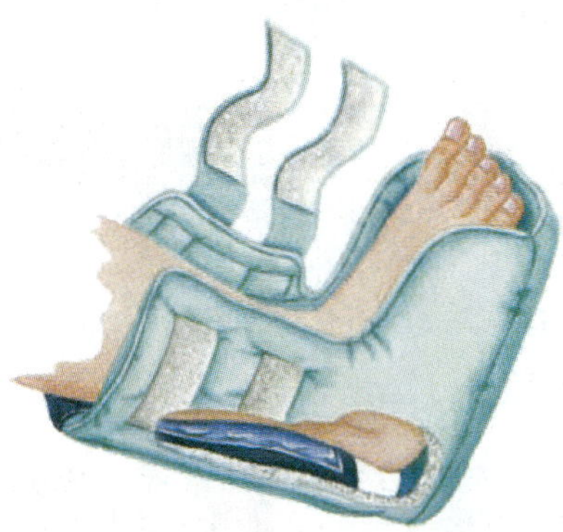

FIGURE 13-31 This heel float boot reduces pressure to the heel, and also keeps the sole of the foot in good alignment to prevent foot drop.Skil-Care Corporation, Yonkers, NY (800) 431-2972)

Adaptive Devices

Adaptive devices are pieces of equipment used to perform everyday tasks (Figure 18.32). A person with a disability may be unable to perform activities of daily living. Sometimes adding a device that changes the way the task is done will enable the resident to perform it independently. Adaptive devices are usually prescribed by the occupational therapist or restorative nurse based on an evaluation of the resident's individual needs. The resident is taught how to use the device for everyday tasks. Your role as a nursing assistant is to make sure the device is clean, available, and used by the resident. The care plan will provide instructions in the types of devices used by residents.

Adaptive Devices for Eating. The most common adaptive devices are used to enable residents to feed themselves. Many individual devices are available to meet residents' needs. The most common devices are adaptive silverware (Figure 13.33A and B), plates (Figure 13.33C), plate guards, and cups (Figure 13.33D). Other items, such as straw holders (Figure 13.33E), may also be necessary.

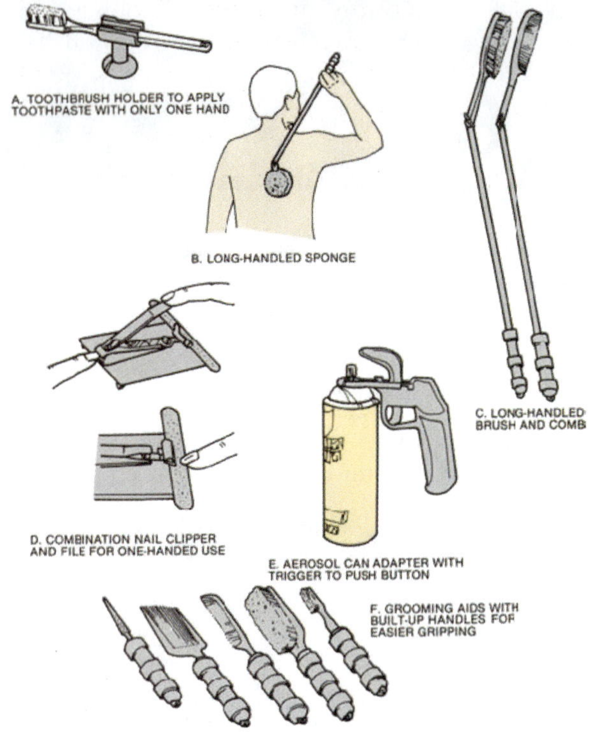

FIGURE 13-32 Adaptive devices enable residents to be independent.

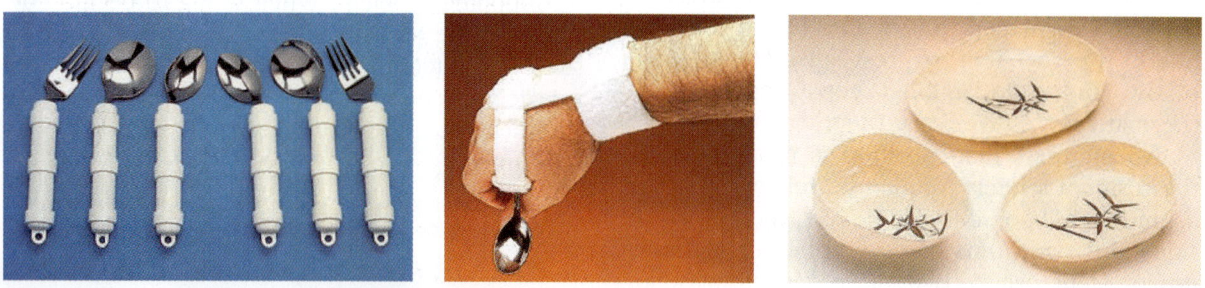

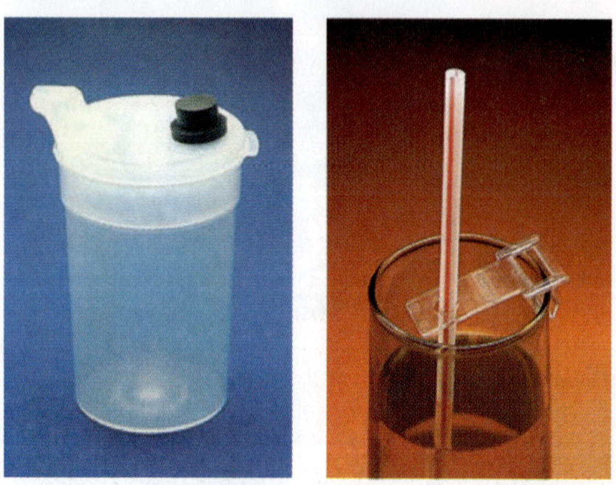

FIGURE 13-33 (A) Many types of adaptive utensils are available to meet individual needs and enable residents to feed themselves. (B) The wrist cuff enables the resident to hold silverware and eat independently. (C) Adaptive plates and bowls have raised edges so residents can scoop food easily. (D) An adaptive cup. (E) The straw holder centers the straw and holds it in place. Maddak, Inc.)

Adaptive Devices for Dressing. Dressing aids are also commonly used (Figure 13.34A and B). These devices make it easier for residents to dress themselves. Using these adaptive devices may appear awkward to you, but for the resident, being able to dress himself or herself is important for self-esteem.

Adaptive Devices for Grooming and Hygiene. Bathing and grooming are important skills. Each person has a personal hygienic routine. Grooming and hygiene are very private activities. Using adaptive devices permits the resident to perform these skills and increases self-esteem and comfort.

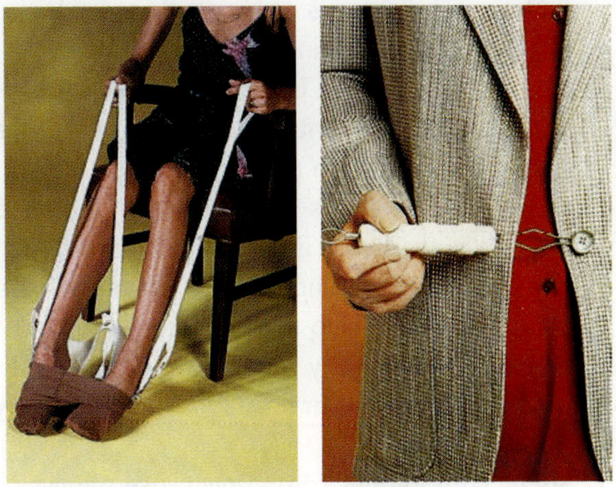

FIGURE 13-34 (A) Various adaptive devices are used by residents to put on socks and hosiery. (B) The hook is threaded through the button hole. The resident grabs the button and pulls it through the hole.Maddak, Inc.)

KEY POINTS

- Restorative care is given to assist residents to attain and maintain their highest level of function.
- Promoting independence is part of restorative care.
- Restorative care is most effective if it is started early in the resident's illness.
- Activity strengthens residents and inactivity weakens.
- When providing restorative care, stress what the resident can do.
- When providing restorative care, the nursing assistant should look at the entire person and not just the illness.
- Many restorative programs involve assisting residents to relearn ADL skills.
- Range of motion is normal movement of joints.
- If a resident's joints do not move through the normal range of motion each day, contractures and deformities may develop.
- Contractures promote pressure ulcer development, and make treating pressure ulcers more difficult.
- Residents with existing contractures are at high risk of developing additional contractures. Contractures can begin to develop in as little as four days of immobility and inactivity. After 15 days, the resident will lose range of motion.
- Arthritis can cause mild discomfort to severe deformities and disability; the most common symptom is pain.
- Osteoporosis is a metabolic disorder in which bone mass is lost, causing bones to become porous and spongy. Residents with this condition are at very high risk for fracture.
- Hip fracture is the most common fracture in the elderly. The term "hip fracture" refers to a fracture anywhere in the upper third or head of the femur.
- A cerebrovascular accident is caused by a sudden interruption of blood to the brain. Residents with this condition will experience weakness or paralysis on one side of the body; other complications such as speech and vision problems may also occur.
- A transient ischemic attack is a temporary period of diminished blood flow to the brain that occurs suddenly and usually lasts from 2 to 15 minutes. Residents with this condition are at risk of stroke.

- Parkinson's disease is an incurable neurological disease that causes tremors and shuffling gait, and increases the risk of injury.
- Huntington's disease is an incurable neurologic disease that is hereditary. The resident develops choreiform movements, loss of voluntary movement, and dementia.
- Multiple sclerosis is a progressive neurological disorder that causes a degeneration of the nervous system and interferes with conduction of nerve impulses.
- Post polio syndrome is a neurologic condition marked by increased weakness and abnormal muscle fatigue in persons who had polio many years earlier. Estimates are that 30% to 70% of all polio survivors will develop this condition.
- Head injuries usually result from trauma, falls, or automobile accidents. The injury often causes severe, permanent brain damage. Residents with brain injury are often totally dependent on staff for care.
- Spinal cord injuries commonly cause paralysis that affects sensation and voluntary movement below the level of injury.
- A self-care deficit is an inability to perform an activity of daily living.
- Bowel and bladder retraining programs are individualized to the resident's needs based on an assessment.
- Kegel exercises strengthen pelvic floor muscles, and the muscles surrounding the urethra and vagina; they are helpful in preventing incontinence.
- The nursing assistant is responsible for applying and removing many types of restorative equipment.
- Trochanter rolls should be used routinely for bedfast residents to prevent deformities caused by external rotation of the hip.

REVIEW

A. Multiple Choice

Select the one best answer.

1. Being dependent on others may cause feelings of
   a. security.
   b. helplessness.
   c. self-esteem.
   d. hopefulness.

2. Restorative care is
   a. highly skilled.
   b. designed to maintain and improve residents.
   c. always given by licensed personnel.
   d. very technical and complex.

3. Continuity of care involves
   a. being assigned to different residents each day.
   b. providing total care to all residents.
   c. all caregivers using the same approaches.
   d. working independently.

4. Which of the following is true?
   a. Bed rest, immobility, and inactivity affect every system of the body.
   b. All sick residents should remain on bed rest.
   c. The cardiopulmonary system is not affected by bed rest.
   d. Most elderly residents need bed rest.

5. You are assigned to care for an alert resident who is paralyzed and cannot perform self-care. You should
   a. perform total care as quietly as possible.
   b. allow the resident to determine the care routine.
   c. provide the care you think is best.
   d. ask the resident's family what to do.

6. Principles of restoration include
   a. beginning treatment early.
   b. inactivity strengthens the resident.
   c. stress what the resident cannot do.
   d. do as much as possible to help the resident.

7. You are assisting a resident with a restorative ADL program. The resident is struggling to squeeze the water out of the washcloth. You should
   a. allow the resident to struggle for a few seconds.
   b. intervene immediately.
   c. complete the procedure for the resident.
   d. get the nurse right away.
8. The therapist who develops bathing, hygiene, and grooming programs is the
   a. physical therapist.
   b. occupational therapist.
   c. speech-language pathologist.
   d. respiratory care practitioner.
9. The weakness and muscle wasting caused by immobility are called
   a. range of motion.
   b. edema.
   c. atrophy.
   d. adduction.
10. Contractures are
   a. extensions of the joints.
   b. pressure ulcers.
   c. blood clots.
   d. painful deformities.
11. You are assigned to do passive range-of-motion exercises on Mr. King. He had knee surgery yesterday and his left knee is bandaged. You should
   a. consult the nurse before performing range of motion on the left knee.
   b. not do the range-of-motion exercises because of the surgery.
   c. exercise all of Mr. King's joints.
   d. perform only flexion and extension exercises on the left knee.
12. When performing range-of-motion exercises, you should
   a. stretch all joints as far as you can.
   b. move each joint as far as it comfortably will go.
   c. ask the resident to tolerate discomfort.
   d. exercise extremities with fractures only.
13. An incontinence management program
   a. is an individual bladder retraining program.
   b. is an assessment of the resident's ability to void.
   c. involves toileting residents on a fixed schedule.
   d. involves using diapers to prevent skin problems.
14. You will assist with the assessment for a bowel and bladder retraining program by
   a. taking the resident to the bathroom every two hours.
   b. writing down the times the resident is incontinent.
   c. administering suppositories and enemas daily.
   d. telling the nurse when the resident requests toileting.
15. Handrolls are used to
   a. prevent contractures of the hands.
   b. promote squeezing.
   c. increase strength.
   d. improve range of motion.

B. Matching

Choose the correct word from Column II to match the phrases in Column I. Write the letter of the matching term in the appropriate blank.

	Column I	Column II
16. ——	60% of all pressure ulcers involve some type of this problem	a. post polio syndrome
17. ——	the most common symptom of arthritis	b. hip fracture
18. ——	metabolic condition in which bones become porous and spongy	c. Parkinson's disease
19. ——	avoid elevating head of bed more than 45 degrees	d. Kegel

20.	—— interruption of blood to the brain	e. neurogenic bladder
21.	—— choreiform movements	f. remission
22.	—— fracture anywhere in the upper third or head of the femur	g. brain damage
23.	—— cannot feel sensation of urine	h. Huntington's disease
24.	—— worsening of symptoms	i. self-care deficit
25.	—— symptoms are stable	j. paralysis
26.	—— tremors, shuffling gait	k. hip precautions
27.	—— degeneration that interferes with conduction of nerve impulses	l. trochanter roll
28.	—— unaware or minimally aware of the surroundings	m. contracture
29.	—— increased weakness, abnormal muscle fatigue, cold intolerance	n. cerebrovascular accident
30.	—— affects sensation and voluntary movement below level of injury	o. osteoporosis
31.	—— inability to perform an activity of daily living	p. exacerbation
32.	—— exercises to help prevent incontinence	q. pain
33.	—— prevents external rotation of hips	r. multiple sclerosis

C. Short-Answer

Answer the following questions.

34–37. List the principles of rehabilitation.

34. ________ 35. ________
36. ________ 37. ________

D. Clinical Applications

Answer the following questions.

38. Mrs. Lincoln is on a restorative ambulation program. Her goal is to walk from her room to the dining room. Before beginning the walk, you check the resident's pulse. The rate is 64. You ambulate Mrs. Lincoln to the dining room and assist her to sit in a chair. You return to check her pulse 5 minutes later and discover that her pulse is 74. What does this indicate? What action should you take?
39. Mr. Lee is a newly admitted resident. He seems to understand what you say to him, but has aphasia and cannot speak. As part of your routine care, the care plan instructs you to perform passive range-of-motion exercises, five repetitions for each joint. Mr. Lee's joints seem stiff. He makes a face and grimaces when you abduct his right shoulder. You ask him if he is in pain and he looks at you with a blank expression on his face. What should you do?

The restorative nurse is conducting an assessment for bowel and bladder retraining on Miss Rogers. You know that the resident has a bowel movement daily about 30 minutes after eating lunch. You also know that the resident has increased motor activity shortly before she is incontinent of urine. The resident does not appear restless at any other time. She does not urinate often. When she does void, it is usually a large quantity.

40. Is any of this information important to the bladder retraining assessment? Which information is important?
41. List each observation you will share with the nurse and explain why it is important.
42. What are the nursing assistant's responsibilities during the assessment phase of the retraining program? Why is it important to conscientiously fulfill these responsibilities?

B: Assisting Residents with Mobility

OBJECTIVES

After reading this unit, you will be able to:

- Demonstrate how to lift and move residents from one location to another using the rules of good body mechanics.
- Describe how to check the wheelchair to ensure it fits the resident properly.
- List at least eight guidelines for positioning residents in a chair or wheelchair.
- Describe how to prevent pressure ulcers in residents who are chairfast.
- List at least twelve guidelines for safe use of a wheelchair.
- Discuss how to transport a resident by wheelchair and by stretcher.
- Demonstrate how to assist residents with ambulation.
- Demonstrate procedures related to assisting residents with mobility.
- Demonstrate procedure to support cast with palms of hands.

OBSERVATIONS TO MAKE AND REPORT RELATED TO ASSISTING RESIDENTS WITH MOBILITY

Pain
Deformity
Edema
Immobility
Inability to move arms and legs
Inability to move one or more joints
Limited/abnormal range of motion
Shortening and external rotation of one leg in a resident with a history of fall
Sudden onset of falls, difficulty balancing
Jerking, tremors, shaky movements, muscle spasms
Weakness
Sensory changes, dizziness
Changes in ability to sit, stand, move, or walk
Pain upon movement
Changes in ability to assist with procedure

Assisting Residents With Mobility

The nursing assistant frequently helps **transfer** residents. A transfer is done to move a resident from one location to another. The procedures in this section involve helping residents to get out of bed. Make sure that your uniform fits loosely enough to allow you to lift and move residents without tearing or binding. As with the other procedures, use of good body mechanics and helping residents maintain proper body alignment in both bed and chair are very important.

Assisting Residents to Sit on the Side of the Bed

Sitting on the side of the bed with the legs over the edge of the mattress is called **dangling**. This is the first step to getting out of bed. Sitting on the side of the bed helps residents who have been lying down to balance before getting up. The resident may become dizzy after lying down for a long time. Dangling helps to equalize the system before the resident is transferred to the chair or begins to walk. The resident should sit in this position for a few minutes before getting up. This helps prevent fainting and loss of balance. Stay with the resident while dangling. Monitor the skin for perspiration or pale color. If these changes occur, return the resident to the supine position and notify the nurse.

Assisting Residents Out of Bed

If the resident tolerates dangling without difficulty, the next step is to assist the resident out of bed. The nursing assistant should evaluate the resident and check the care plan before moving the resident. Follow the directions for transfer on the care plan. If the resident is larger than you are, cannot follow directions, or is otherwise unable to help you with the transfer, ask another nursing assistant to help you.

Before beginning, explain the procedure to the resident. Tell him or her what is expected. Get feedback to make sure the resident understands. Use simple commands or counts to time your movements. For example, tell the resident, "We will move when I count to three," or, "We will move when I say lift."

PROCEDURE 81 Assisting the Resident to Sit Up on the Side of the Bed

1. Perform your beginning procedure actions.
2. Place the bed in the lowest horizontal position.
3. Elevate the head of the bed.
4. Assist the resident to move to the side of the bed closest to you.
5. Place your arm closest to the head under the resident's shoulders, palm side up.
6. Place your other arm under the resident's knees, palm side up.
7. Lift the back and knees up and pivot the resident so the legs are hanging over the side of the bed and the back is straight.
8. Help the resident maintain balance, if necessary.
9. If the resident will be getting out of bed, assist him or her to put on a robe and footwear appropriate to the floor surface.
10. Stay with the resident and observe for changes in color and moisture of the skin.
11. To return the resident to bed, reverse the procedure and pivot the resident back to the supine position.
12. Perform your procedure completion actions.

GUIDELINES FOR

Assisting Residents with Mobility

- Wear a back support belt if this is your preference or facility policy.
- Refer to the care plan or nurse for specific instructions.
- Explain the procedure to the resident. Before beginning the move, make sure the resident understands what is to be done and what is expected.
- Always use a transfer belt (unless contra-indicated) to prevent injury to yourself and the resident.
- Adjust the bed to the lowest horizontal position. Elevate the head of the bed 90 degrees to make it easier for the resident to get up.
- Lock the brakes on beds, wheelchairs, lifts, stretchers, or other equipment before beginning the move.
- Use lifting devices, if needed.
- Make sure that mechanical lifts and other moving devices are in good working condition.
- When transferring a resident with a weak or paralyzed side, move toward the stronger side.
- Support the resident's weaker side during transfers.
- Be alert to catheters and other tubes so they are not accidentally pulled or removed.
- Have the resident wear footwear appropriate to the floor surface if standing during the transfer.
- Apply artificial limbs and braces correctly before transferring the resident.
- Make sure the resident's feet are firmly on the floor before standing.
- Avoid lifting the resident under the arms. This can cause pain, dislocation, and other injuries.
- The resident should never place hands or arms around your neck during the transfer.
- When ambulating residents, look for hazards on the floor and approach corners slowly, watching for approaching traffic.
- Check the tips of canes, crutches, and walkers. If they are worn through, do not use them.
- If you will be transferring the resident into a wheelchair, check the position of the small front wheels. The large part of the small wheels should be facing forward before you begin the transfer.

Moving simultaneously with the resident is important. This helps prevent injury to you and the resident.

Transferring the Resident into a Wheelchair

If you will be transferring the resident into a wheelchair, you must position the chair and lock the brakes before beginning the transfer. The footrests should be removed or pushed up and out of the way during the transfer. (If you remove the leg rests, make sure to replace them immediately upon completion of the procedure.) Before beginning the transfer, position the wheelchair at a 45° to 60° angle to the surface from which you are transferring. If the resident has a strong side, position the chair so the strongest leg moves toward the chair. Pay close attention to the small, front caster wheels of the wheelchair. These wheels provide the ability to move in all directions. The large part of the wheel faces back when the chair is moving. During transfers, position the large part of the small front wheels to face forward (Figure 13.35). This changes the center of gravity of the chair and reduces the risk of tipping. To reposition the wheels, back the chair up, then move forward until the wheels are in good alignment, then lock the brakes.

The resident must be able to move to the side of the bed or front edge of the chair before standing, and for most transfers. Sitting in this position moves the resident's center of

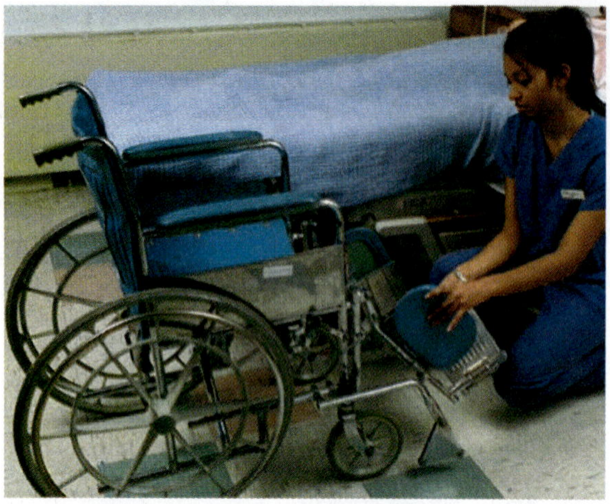

FIGURE 13-35 Prepare for the transfer by positioning the chair correctly at a 45° to 60° angle. Position the large part of the small front wheels facing forward. Lock the brakes. Move the footrests back or up and out of the way.

gravity over the base of support in the feet, making standing easier and safer. Several methods can be used for moving the resident forward. If he or she cannot scoot forward independently, the care plan will list the method to use.

The Transfer Belt

The transfer belt is a heavy canvas belt. In some facilities, each resident is given a belt that is used only for that resident. Other facilities require the nursing assistant to wear the belt and use it to transfer all residents. Use of the transfer belt is safer for both you and the resident. It prevents pulling and tugging on the resident's skin. The belt makes it easier for you to move the resident and gives you control if the resident starts to slip or fall. The belt should be used for most routine transfers. Never use the belt on a pair of pants in place of a transfer belt.

Contraindications for use of the transfer belt

The transfer belt may be contraindicated in residents with some conditions. Facilities have different policies for use of the transfer belt. Know and follow your facility policy. Check with the nurse or the resident's care plan for specific instructions. In general, contraindications to use of the transfer belt are:

- A **colostomy**, a surgical procedure in which the colon is attached to the outside of the body and waste is eliminated into a plastic bag attached to the skin
- A **gastrostomy** tube, or feeding tube that is surgically inserted into the resident's stomach with the end extending through the side of the abdomen
- Recent abdominal surgery or a fresh surgical **incision** (cut in the skin made with a knife)
- Severe cardiac and respiratory disease
- Fractured ribs or vertebrae
- Pregnancy
- An abdominal **pacemaker**. This is a surgically implanted device that regulates the rate of the heartbeat. Most commonly, the pacemaker is implanted in the chest, but occasionally it is placed in the abdomen. You will see the shape of the device beneath the skin surface.

GUIDELINES FOR

Using the Transfer (Gait) Belt

- The resident should be dressed before the belt is applied. Do not apply it over bare skin.
- Make sure the resident is wearing footwear appropriate to the surface of the floor. If you are unsure, check with the care plan or nurse. As a rule, nonslip soles are used in facilities with tile floors. Leather or plastic soles may be used on carpeting. The physical therapist will evaluate the resident to determine what type of sole is safest for the resident.
- The belt is placed around the waist and buckled in front.
- For a female resident, be sure the breasts are not under the belt.

- Thread the belt through the teeth side, then back through the opening on the other side so that it is double-locked (Figure 13.36).
- Check the fit of the belt by placing three fingers under it. The belt should be snug, but there should be enough space for your fingers to fit comfortably.
- Before attempting to move the resident, be sure his or her feet are flat on the floor.

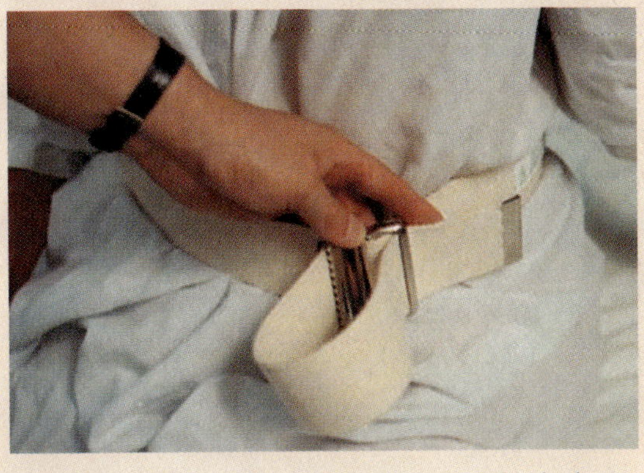

FIGURE 13-36 Threading the transfer belt through the teeth ensures that the belt will not slip during the transfer.

If they are not, use the belt to assist the resident to the edge of the bed until the feet are resting firmly on the floor.
- If you are transferring a resident into or out of a wheelchair, the footrests should be out of the way during the transfer. After the resident is seated, the legs should not dangle. The feet are supported on the floor or on the wheelchair footrests.
- Teach the resident to assist by pushing off the bed with the hands when you count to three.
- Always hold the belt with an underhand grasp. For transfers, one hand should be on each side of the buckle in front.
- When the resident is standing, pivot to transfer.
- The chair should be close enough so the resident can feel the back of the chair with the hands after you pivot.
- The belt is removed after the resident is seated.
- Keep your belt clean. Wash it at least weekly, and whenever it becomes soiled.

- Implanted medication pumps. Some residents have implanted medication pumps under the skin of the abdomen. These are not always visible, although an incision will be present over the implant. The care plan, nurse, or resident will inform you if such a device is present. If the surgical site is well healed, it is probably safe to use the gait belt. However, you should always follow the care plan or check with the nurse before using a gait belt to move a resident with any type of implanted device.
- Abdominal **aneurysm**. An aneurysm is a ballooning of the wall of an artery due to a structural weakness. If the aneurysm ruptures, the resident will die.

Moving the Resident with a Mechanical Lift

Several types of mechanical lifts are available. Some are hydraulic. Others are electric. The most commonly used lift is the hydraulic lift. It is used when a resident is heavy, unable to assist, or unbalanced, or has an amputation or other condition that makes transfer with a belt difficult or impossible. For safety reasons, the hydraulic lift should be operated by two or more nursing assistants. Never attempt to operate it alone. Some electric and battery-operated lifts can safely be used by one person. Know and follow your facility policy for use of the mechanical lift.

Because the mechanical lift is a hydraulic unit, check the floor by the lift each time you use it. If you see an oily substance on the floor, do not use the lift until it has been checked and repaired. The fluid may be hydraulic fluid. If hydraulic fluid is leaking, the lift may slip, causing injury to both the resident and the nursing assistant. Check the sling, release mechanisms, attachment straps, and chains for safety before using the lift. If anything is in need of repair, do not use the lift. Follow your facility policy for tagging the lift out of service. Obtain safe equipment before attempting to move the resident.

PROCEDURE

82

Assisting the Resident to Transfer to Chair or Wheelchair, One Person, with Transfer Belt

1. Perform your beginning procedure actions.
2. Assist the resident to dress and put on footwear appropriate to the floor.
3. Apply the transfer belt snugly around the resident's waist and check it with three fingers for tightness.
4. Stand in front of the resident. Keep your feet apart, knees bent, and back straight. Place one hand under each side of the transfer belt, using an underhand grasp (Figure 13.37A).
5. Move the resident so the feet are touching the floor. The resident's knees should be separated to provide a wide base of support.
6. Instruct the resident on the count of three to lean forward and push up from the bed with the hands while you lift up on the belt. Support the resident's knees and feet by placing your knees and feet firmly against them (Figure 13.37B).
7. Assist the resident to pivot until the knees touch the back of the chair and the resident can reach the armrests with his or her hands.
8. Bend your knees and assist the resident to lower himself or herself into the chair.
9. Remove the transfer belt.
10. Adjust the wheelchair legs and footrests.
11. Perform your procedure completion actions.
12. Reverse the procedure to return the resident to bed.

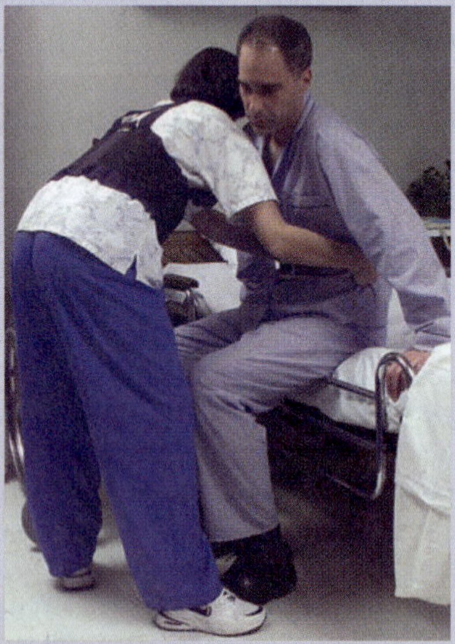

FIGURE 13-37A Always use an underhand grasp for transferring and ambulating residents.

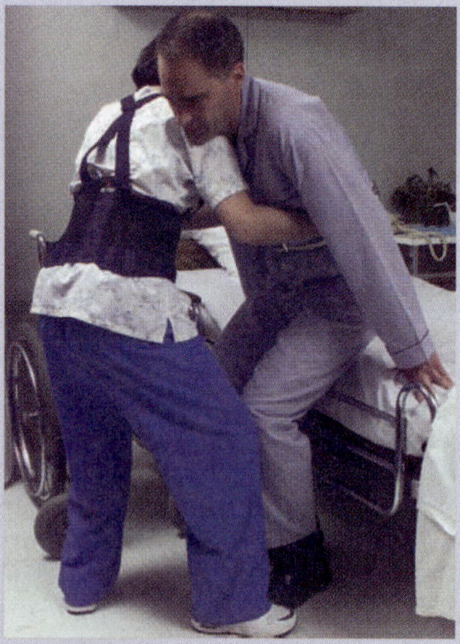

FIGURE 13-37B Supporting the resident with your knees and feet reduces the risk of slipping.

PROCEDURE 83 Assisting the Resident to Transfer to Chair or Wheelchair, Two Persons, with Transfer Belt

1. Perform your beginning procedure actions.
2. Assist the resident to dress and put on footwear appropriate to the floor.
3. Apply the transfer belt snugly around the resident's waist and check it with three fingers for tightness.
4. Stand in front of the resident. Keep your feet apart, knees bent, and back straight. Each nursing assistant places one hand under the front of the belt and one hand under the back of the belt, using an underhand grasp (Figure 13.38).
5. Move the resident so the feet are touching the floor. The resident's knees should be separated to provide a wide base of support.

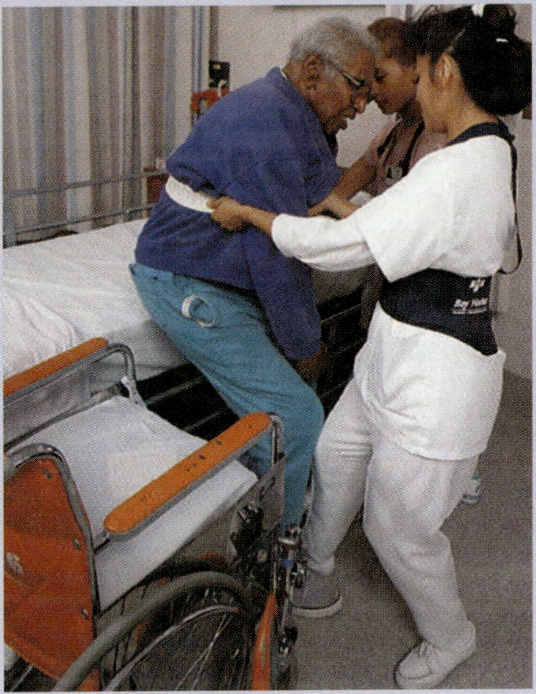

FIGURE 13-38 During a two-person transfer, each assistant places a hand on the front and back of the belt.

6. On the count of three, both nursing assistants move the resident at the same time. Coordination of movement is important.
7. The nursing assistant on the side closest to the chair stands in a position so that he or she can pivot and move away, allowing the resident unobstructed access to the chair. This nursing assistant should stand with one leg behind the other, so that he or she can step back quickly.
8. The other nursing assistant uses one knee to support the resident's weak leg. This nursing assistant's other leg is positioned further back.
9. Instruct the resident to lean forward and push off the bed, using the palms of the hands, on the count of three.
10. The resident's knees should be spread apart. Instruct the resident to put both feet down with the stronger foot behind the weaker foot.
11. Both nursing assistants bend their knees, squat slightly, and spread their feet to provide a wide base of support.
12. On the count of three, the resident is lifted to a standing position. The nursing assistants pivot slowly and smoothly by moving their feet, legs, and hips to the left side until the resident can feel the back of the wheelchair with his or her legs.
13. Instruct the resident to place his or her hands on the armrests of the chair and lean forward slightly.
14. Both nursing assistants bend their knees and lower the resident into the chair (Figure 13.39).

(continues)

PROCEDURE 83 Assisting the Resident to Transfer to Chair or Wheelchair, Two Persons, with Transfer Belt, *continued*

15. Remove the transfer belt.
16. Adjust the wheelchair legs and footrests.
17. Perform your procedure completion actions.
18. Reverse the procedure to return the resident to bed.

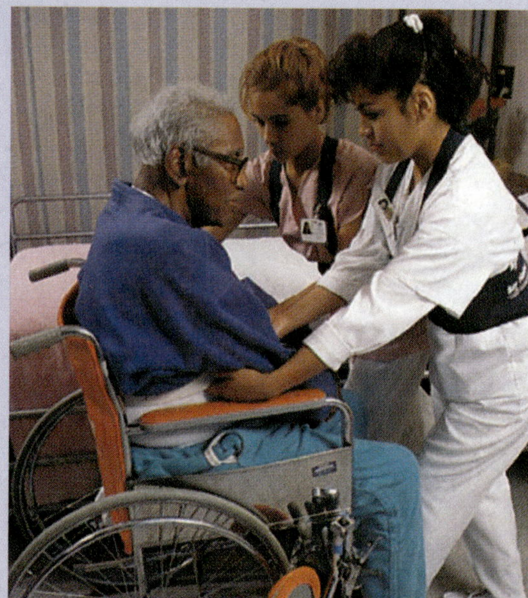

FIGURE 13-39 Bending from the knees and using good body mechanics, lower the resident into the chair.

PROCEDURE 84 Assisting the Resident to Transfer from Bed to Chair or Wheelchair, One Assistant

1. Perform your beginning procedure actions.
2. Assist the resident to dress and put on footwear appropriate to the floor.
3. Bring the resident to the edge of the bed so the feet touch the floor. The resident's knees should be separated to provide a wide base of support.
4. Place your hands under the resident's arms and around the back of the shoulders (Figure 13.40).
5. Brace the resident's knees and feet with your knees and feet.
6. On the count of three, pull the resident to a standing position. Avoid pulling upward under the arms.
7. Pivot the resident until the knees touch the back of the chair and the

resident can reach the armrests with his or her hands.

8. Bend your knees and assist the resident to lower himself or herself into the chair.
9. Adjust the wheelchair legs and footrests.
10. Perform your procedure completion actions.
11. Reverse the procedure to return the resident to bed.

Note: For the safety of both the nursing assistant and the resident, use this procedure only if use of the transfer belt is contraindicated.

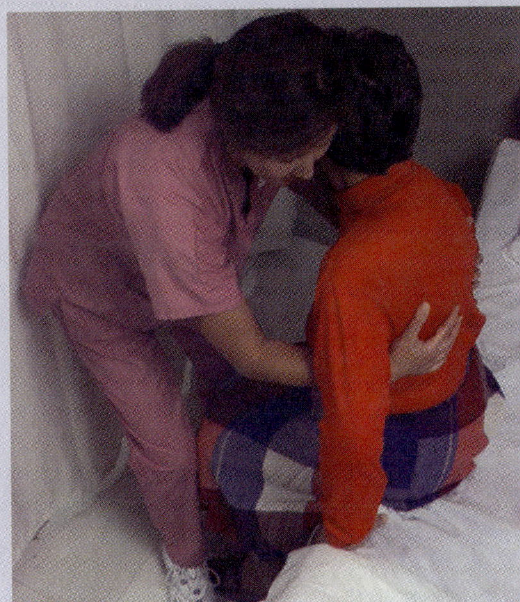

FIGURE 13-40 Place your arms around the resident to the back of the shoulders. Avoid pulling under the arms.

PROCEDURE 85

Transferring the Resident Using a Mechanical Lift

1. Perform your beginning procedure actions.
2. Place the chair at right angles to the foot of the bed, facing the head.
3. Lower the side rail on the side nearest you.
4. Roll the resident on the side.
5. Position the sling under the resident's body so that it supports the shoulders, buttocks, and thighs. Straighten the sling.
6. Roll the resident onto the sling and properly position it on the other side (Figure 13.41A).

(continues)

PROCEDURE

85 Transferring the Resident Using a Mechanical Lift, *continued*

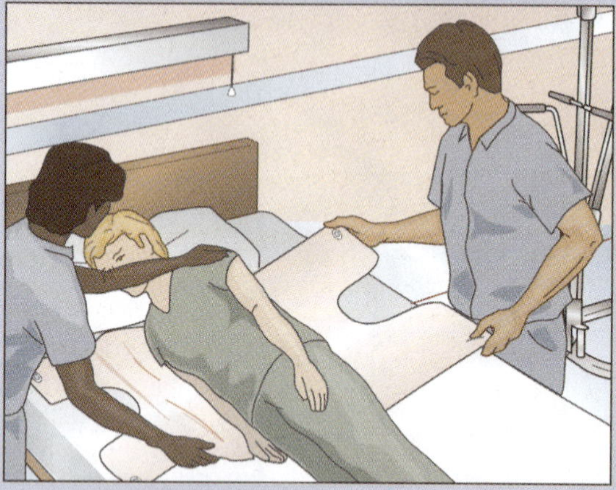

FIGURE 13-41A Position the sling between the shoulder blades and thighs.

7. Position the lift over the bed (Figure 13.41B). Spread the legs of the lift to the widest open position to maintain a broad base of support.
8. Attach the suspension straps or chains to the sling. The "S" hook should face away from the resident to prevent injury (Figure 13.41C).

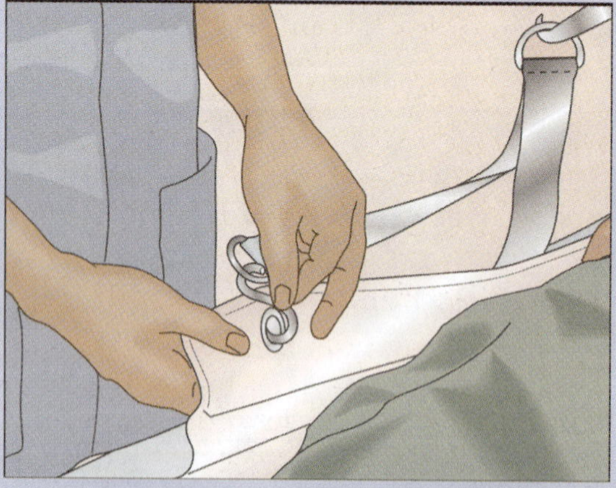

FIGURE 13-41B Center the lift over the resident.

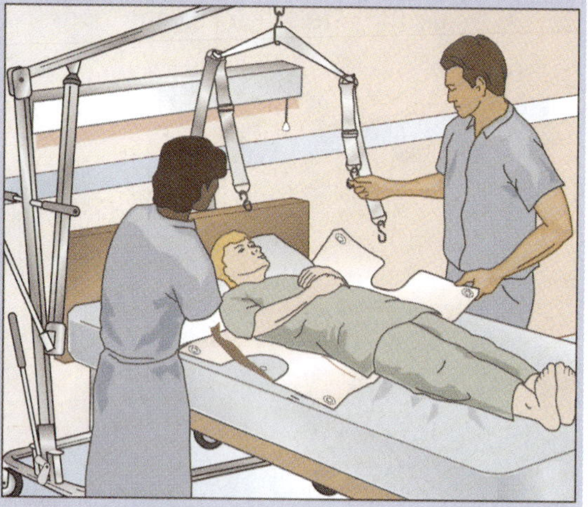

FIGURE 13-41C Fasten the straps with the "S" hooks facing outward, to prevent injury to the resident.

9. Position the resident's arms comfortably inside the sling.
10. Attach the straps or chains to the lift frame.
11. Reassure the resident, lock the hydraulic mechanism, and slowly raise the boom of the lift until the resident is suspended over the bed.
12. Slowly guide the lift away from the bed.
13. Position the lift above the chair.
14. The nursing assistant helping you holds the sling back and helps lower the resident slowly into the chair, keeping the hips back while you slowly release the hydraulic and lower the lift.
15. When lowering the lift, monitor the location of the resident's feet and arms to prevent injury (Figure 13.41D).

16. Unhook the straps or chains and remove the lift. The lift seat remains under the resident.
17. Position the footrests to support the feet.
18. Perform your procedure completion actions.
19. Reverse the procedure to return the resident to bed. When raising the resident from the chair, monitor the position of the "S" hooks, which sometimes catch under the arms of the chair.

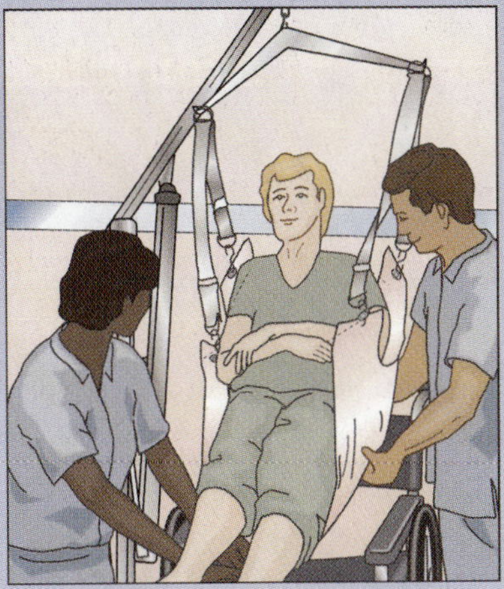

FIGURE 13-41D Slowly lower the lift while monitoring the resident's legs and arms and guiding the hips back into the chair.

Sliding Board Transfers

A sliding board (Figure 13.42) transfer is used for residents who have good upper body strength and sitting balance. This type of transfer is commonly used for residents with paraplegia. The procedure is performed by doing a series of pushups. The resident locks the elbows and pushes with the hands. To transfer, the resident must be able to lift the buttocks off the bed. After lifting the buttocks, he or she lowers onto the sliding board, then lifts and slides until the transfer is complete.

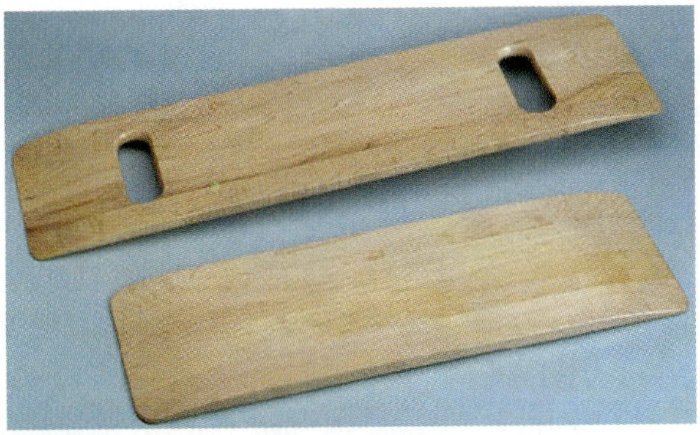

FIGURE 13-42 The sliding board is used when the wheelchair has removable arms and swing-away leg rests. Make sure the resident is wearing pants that will slide easily across the surface.(Photo courtesy of Briggs Corporation)

The wheelchair must have removable armrests when a sliding board is used. The resident must have clothing on the lower half of the body. Blue jeans do not slide well on the board. Cotton or synthetic slacks are best. If the resident has difficulty sliding on the board, draping a pillowcase across the board may be helpful. (Do not encase the board in the pillowcase as you would a pillow.) The board can also be waxed to maintain a slippery surface. Some residents perform this transfer independently, whereas others need help. If you will be assisting, always use a transfer belt.

Two assistants can move dependent residents by using a sliding board. One assistant stands in front and the other behind the resident. At the count of three, both assistants hold the belt and slide the resident across the board.

Toilet Transfers

A survey of long-term care facility workers revealed that toilet transfers were the most difficult. This is because the bathrooms in most facilities are small. Many meet the OSHA definition of "confined spaces." Working in a confined space increases the risk of injury. The wheelchair takes up a great deal of space. The toilet is close to the wall. There is little room for the assistant to move during the transfer. Follow all safety precautions carefully to prevent injury to the resident and yourself.

PROCEDURE

86 Sliding Board Transfer from Bed to Wheelchair

1. Perform your beginning procedure actions.
2. Remove the arm of the wheelchair closest to the bed. Remove the legs or fold them back.
3. Position the wheelchair parallel to the bed, or at a slight (about 35°) angle. Lock the brakes.
4. Apply a transfer belt. Check the fit with three fingers.
5. Assist the resident to move close to the edge of the bed.
6. Tell the resident to lean away from the wheelchair. Place the sliding board well under the buttocks, with the beveled side of the board facing up. Avoid pinching the resident's skin between the board and the bed.
7. Place the opposite end of the board well onto the seat of the wheelchair.
8. Instruct the resident to push up with the hands, lock the elbows, and move across the board. Repeat until the resident is seated in the chair with one buttock on the board.
9. Be prepared to assist by lifting the resident's buttocks during the sitting pushup. If the resident is having trouble balancing, place your hands on the shoulders for support.
10. Support and move the resident's legs with your hands, if necessary.
11. Instruct the resident to lean away from the bed. Remove the board.
12. Remove the transfer belt.
13. Position the legs on the leg rests, or as instructed. Replace the arm on the chair.
14. Perform your procedure completion actions.
15. Reverse the procedure to return the resident to bed.

Note: The resident may push on the opposite armrest of the wheelchair with one hand. This will help achieve greater height in the pushups. The resident may also push on the board. Caution the resident to avoid placing the fingers under the edges of the board.

PROCEDURE

87 Transferring the Resident from Wheelchair to Toilet

1. Perform your beginning procedure actions.
2. Position the wheelchair at a right angle to the toilet, if possible. Position the chair so that the toilet is on the resident's strong side, if possible.
3. Lock the brakes.
4. Remove the wheelchair legs or fold them back.
5. Apply the transfer belt.
6. Assist the resident to unfasten clothing.

7. Instruct the resident to place the hands on the wheelchair armrests and slide forward in the chair.
8. Tell the resident to pull the feet back under the body, placing them firmly on the floor.
9. Have the resident lean forward and push up, turning to the strong side (Figure 13.43) until he or she feels the toilet seat on the legs. Hold the transfer belt, but assist only to the degree necessary.
10. Instruct the resident to hold the grab rail and use the other hand to undress. Assist as needed.
11. Tell the resident to hold the rail and slowly lower his or her body to the toilet seat.
12. Remove the transfer belt, or leave it on according to resident preference and facility policy.
13. Provide privacy. Instruct the resident to call for assistance when done.
14. Perform your procedure completion actions.

Note: Reverse this procedure to return the resident to the chair. If possible, position the wheelchair on the resident's strong side. To rise from the toilet, the resident holds the rail. Tell the resident to slide forward slightly. Then remind the resident to pull the feet back and lean forward. He or she pushes up with the hands on the rails, or pulls up using the rail on the wall. Remind the resident to face forward, keeping the head over the feet. After the resident is seated in the chair, assist him or her to the sink. Provide supplies or assist with handwashing.

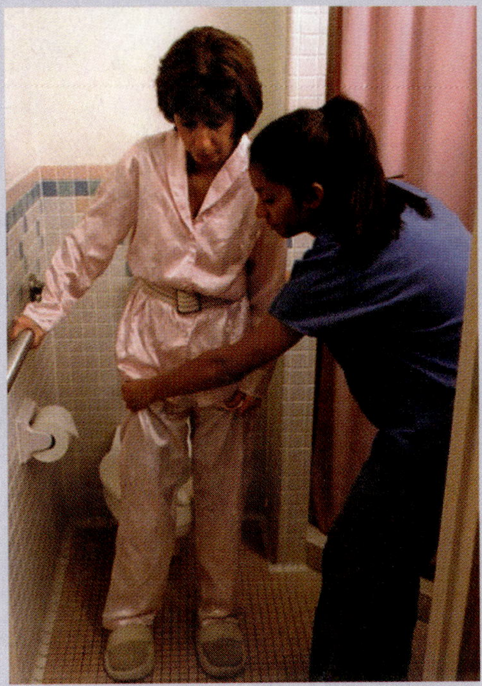

FIGURE 13-43 Assist the resident to pivot or back up until his legs touch the toilet. Hold the belt for support, if necessary, when adjusting the resident's clothes.

Transporting a Resident by Stretcher

Most long-term care facility residents are ambulatory or can be safely transported by wheelchair. Residents who are comatose or bedfast may need to be transported on a stretcher. A stretcher may also be needed for transporting residents in certain emergencies. Residents who must be transported in this manner are usually unable to assist in moving from the bed to the stretcher and back. Four or more staff members will be needed to safely move the resident. The **sliding technique** is used for transfers when the resident cannot bear weight. Use this technique for moving residents on a sheet, such as from bed to stretcher. Use your body weight to hold the two surfaces together during the transfer. This keeps them from separating. One or more caregivers stand on each side of the resident. The sheet is rolled close to the resident's body. On the count of three, lift the sheet, pulling and sliding the resident over to the stretcher.

Wheelchairs

The wheelchair is an important piece of equipment in the long-term care facility. Many residents use wheelchairs for mobility. Some will progress to ambulation. Others will always use the wheelchair to move about. Whenever possible, the facility should restore the resident's ability to ambulate.

PROCEDURE

88 Transferring the Resident from Bed to Stretcher

1. Perform your beginning procedure actions.
2. Gather your supplies:
   - Stretcher
   - Bath blanket
3. Ensure that three to four other staff members are available to assist in moving the resident.
4. Raise the bed to a horizontal position equal to the height of the stretcher. Lock the wheels. Lower the side rail on the side where you are working.
5. Cover the resident with the bath blanket.
6. Remove the linen by pulling it down from underneath the blanket. Avoid exposing the resident. Fanfold the linen at the foot of the bed or dispose of it according to facility policy.
7. Roll the turning sheet up against the resident's body on both sides. The turning sheet should be long enough to support the resident's torso from the knees to the shoulders. If no turning sheet is available, use the bottom bed sheet.
8. Move the stretcher in next to the bed. Lock the brakes.
9. Two or three people stand on the open side of the stretcher. One or two more go to the other side of the bed and lower the rail. The staff on this side should be prepared to get on their knees in the bed during the transfer, if necessary, to avoid back injury from lifting and reaching. If another assistant is available, he or she should stand at the head of the bed to support the resident's head.
10. All staff grasp the sheet using an overhand grasp.
    - The assistant(s) at the end of the bed grasps the lifting sheet by placing one hand on the lower leg area and one at the hip area.
    - The middle assistant(s) grasps the lifting sheet by placing one hand at the hip and one at the shoulder.
    - The assistant at the head (if present) grasps the sheet on either side of the resident's head.
11. On the count of three, all staff lift, push, and pull the sheet from the bed to the stretcher (Figure 13.44).
12. Center and position the resident in good body alignment, with a pillow for comfort.
13. Secure the safety straps.
14. Raise the side rails on the stretcher.
15. Transport the resident as directed. When complete, return to the unit to straighten the bed and prepare for the resident's return.
16. Perform your procedure completion actions.

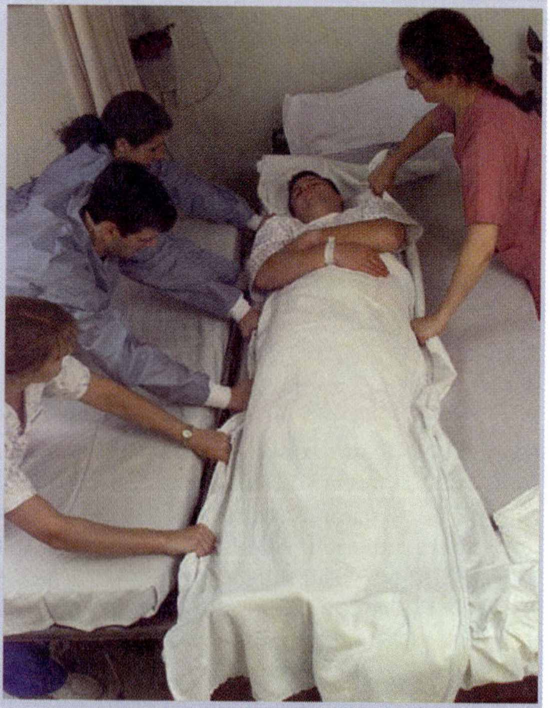

FIGURE 13-44 On signal, all staff move the sheet from the bed to the stretcher.

If the resident is unable to ambulate, it may be best to use the wheelchair to move from one location to another, then transfer into a regular chair. For example, the resident propels the wheelchair to the dining room. For pressure relief and mealtime positioning, transferring her into the dining room chair may be best. Follow your facility policies and the residents' care plans.

Because residents spend so much time in wheelchairs, careful attention to fitting the chair to the resident is very important for comfort and pressure ulcer prevention. Sometimes wheelchairs are ordered or modified to meet special resident needs. For example, some residents with hemiplegia can propel the wheelchair independently. They use the strong arm on the wheel and push the strong leg on the floor. The leg rest is removed on this side.

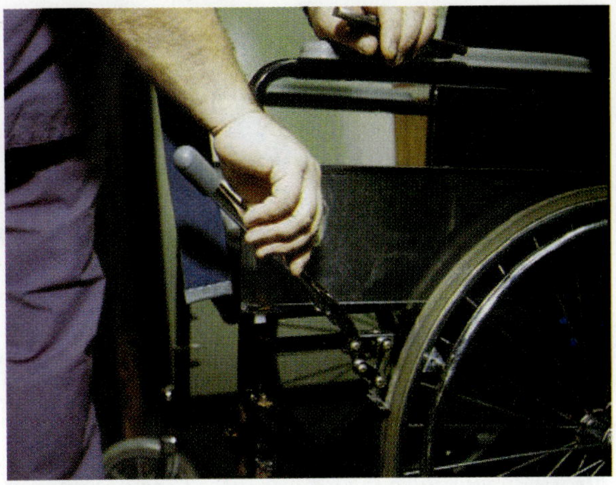

FIGURE 13-45 The brake extension is attached so the resident can reach it with the opposite arm, if necessary.

Wheelchair Size

For safety, the wheelchair must be used correctly and must fit the resident properly. There is no "one size fits all" wheelchair. Residents may not be able to propel a wheelchair that does not fit correctly. Fewer positioning aids are necessary if the chair fits the resident. A wheelchair that is the wrong size causes discomfort, contributes to skin breakdown, and increases the need for restraints. Positioning residents upright, in good body alignment, is difficult and further increases the risk of complications. As you can see, attention to chair size is very important.

The therapist or restorative nurse will evaluate the chair to determine whether it fits the resident. The type of chair selected is determined by:

- An assessment of the resident's physical condition
- The resident's special needs
- The needs of caregivers
- The environment in which the chair will be used

Brakes

The brakes are an important safety feature of the wheelchair. Several types of brakes are available. The most common type uses a lever system to lock the chair. The brakes must be secure during transfers. Set them when the wheelchair is parked. If the chair slips even slightly, the brakes are not working properly. Notify the nurse or the appropriate person in your facility if you believe the brakes are not working correctly. Do not transfer the resident into or out of the chair until the brakes have been repaired. If a transfer is essential, have another assistant immobilize the chair while you transfer the resident.

Some residents do not lock the brakes on the wheelchair because they cannot reach them. For example, a resident with hemiparesis may not be able to reach the brake on the affected side. Extensions are available to lengthen the brake handle (Figure 13.45). Some facilities create brake extensions by attaching PVC pipe.

Caster Wheels

The small, front caster wheels of the chair provide the ability to move in all directions. The large part of the wheel faces back when the chair is moving. Before beginning a transfer, and when parking the chair, position the large part of the front wheel facing forward. This will stabilize the chair by changing its center of gravity. Back the chair up, then move it forward until the wheels are properly positioned.

Drive Wheels

The large, rear wheels are the drive wheels. The most common type of wheel is made from solid rubber.

The outer rim of the drive wheels is used for pushing the chair. Propelling the wheelchair independently is better for the residents. It provides exercise, and permits them to move about the facility at will. This is much more satisfying than having to wait for someone to transport them.

Seat Depth

The depth of the seat is very important. The seat must be deep enough to support the pelvis and thighs correctly. A short seat can be very uncomfortable for residents with long legs. If the seat is too long, the resident's weight is shifted toward the sacrum. This causes discomfort and increases the risk of skin breakdown. A long seat also makes it more difficult for the resident to propel the chair. Some residents slide to the front edge of the wheelchair. A seat that is too long is often the problem. Facilities often look for restraints and alternatives to keep residents from sliding when a different wheelchair may be all that is necessary! Staff members may not recognize this problem. When the resident is seated properly in the chair, the hips should be near the back. The front edge of the seat should end two or three inches before the back of the knees.

Seat Width

Proper seat width is also important for comfort. It affects ease in moving the drive wheels and resting the arms on the armrests. A wheelchair that is too wide is difficult for residents to move. The resident may lean to one side. A seat that is too narrow increases pressure on the thighs, buttocks, and hips. If the seat width fits the resident correctly, there should be enough space to slide your hand in on either side between the resident's hips and the side of the wheelchair.

Back Height

The height of the chair back is determined by the resident's need for back support. The back should be supported from the hips to the bottom of the shoulder blades. If the resident uses a foam cushion in the wheelchair, the back must be the proper height with the cushion in place. Some wheelchairs have an extension piece that is elevated to provide head support, if needed.

Armrests

Armrests can be removable or nonremovable. Removable armrests are necessary for use of sliding boards, and for some other transfers. Armrest height is important for comfort and good sitting posture. If the armrests are too high, shorter residents will have problems propelling the chair.

Armrests are available in two lengths. The desk-length armrest is lower in the front than in the back. This enables the resident to get close to tables. The chair works well for residents who sit in wheelchairs at mealtime. The full-length armrest is most common and is comfortable when the resident is seated. However, getting close to tables may be a problem. Elevating the table height does not solve the problem. Raising the table allows the resident to move closer. However, most residents are too short to benefit from the increased table height. They may end up eating with their elbows in the air because the table is too high. This is very uncomfortable and causes shoulder strain. It may cause some residents to have problems eating. Attaching a lap tray to the armrests corrects the problem.

Leg Rests and Footrests

Many wheelchairs have removable leg rests. Remove the leg rests or fold the footrests up during transfers. If they fall down, notify the nurse. The footrest is easily tightened. If you remove the leg rests, make sure to replace them when you finish. Facilities have many different types of wheelchairs. If the parts become separated from the chair, matching them up may be difficult.

Some wheelchairs have swing-away or pivoting legs. A lever on the side releases the leg. These leg rests can be folded to the sides during transfers. When using wheelchairs with fixed legs, raise the footrests during transfers.

Some residents with edema or fractures need chairs with elevating legs. This type of leg rest may also be used for residents with contractures, or those who cannot flex the knees. A lock on the side holds the leg rest in place. For safety, support the leg with one hand while operating the lock with the other. Support the calf with a pad when the leg rests are elevated.

Residents' feet must be supported when the chair is being moved. Their feet should never dangle in the air or drag on the floor. The length of the chair legs can be adjusted to provide proper support. If the leg rest cannot be adjusted, a footrest elevator (Figure 13.46) may be used. Your maintenance department may make footrest elevators out of wood. When the wheelchair is parked, the resident's legs should be supported on the footrests or the floor. Allowing the legs to dangle is uncomfortable and increases the risk of blood clots. Advise residents to avoid leaning forward or picking up items from the floor. If the feet are on the footrests, the chair will tip. There should be at least two inches of clearance from the bottom of the footrest to the floor.

Reclining Chairs

Reclining-back wheelchairs (Figure 13.47A) and geriatric chairs (Figure 13.47B) should be used only for residents who cannot sit upright. The chair back supports the head and neck. Adjust the back for comfort and maximum functional ability. When adjusting the back, support the resident. Suddenly releasing the lock will cause him or her to fall back quickly, frightening

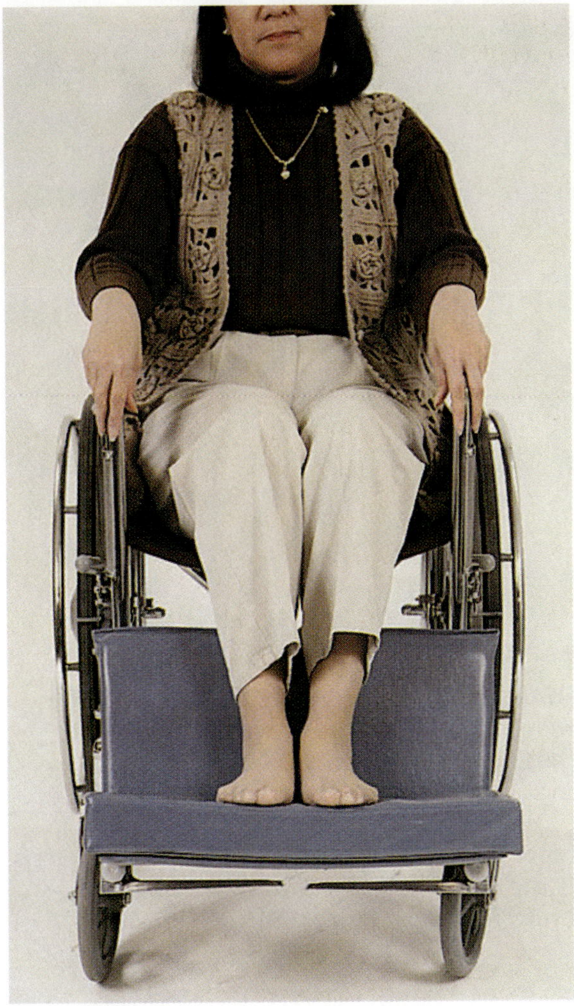

FIGURE 13-46 The feet must always be supported when the resident is seated. The foam footrest elevator may be used if the feet do not reach the footrests.Skil-Care Corporation, Yonkers, NY, (800) 431-2972)

the resident and causing pain and potential injury.

Avoid placing residents in reclining chairs unless such a chair is medically necessary. At first glance, using a recliner looks like a good way to position the resident comfortably in a chair without using restraints. However, placing a resident in a reclining chair unnecessarily can cause serious physical and mental declines. If a recliner must be used, avoid reclining the back farther than necessary. This often causes loss of orientation. The resident looks at the ceiling all day and cannot see people or activity in the room. He or she becomes more dependent because the resident cannot perform activities, such as feeding, in this position. Use of reclining chairs is discussed in greater detail in Unit 15.

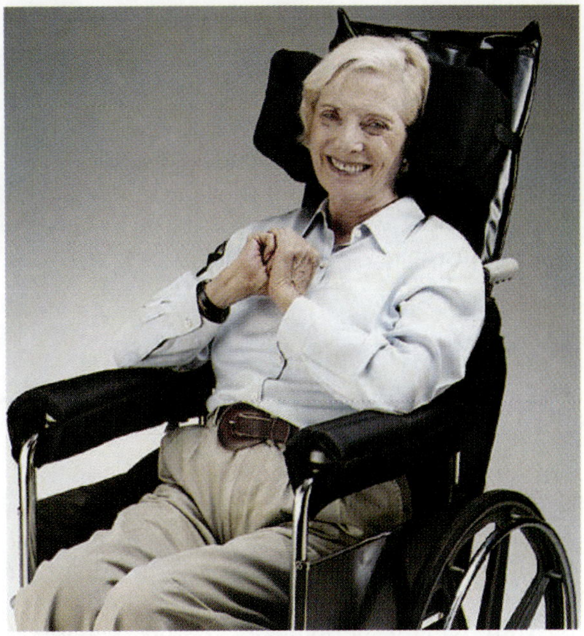

FIGURE 13-47A The reclining wheelchair may be used for residents who do not have trunk, head, or neck control. Keep the back as upright as possible to maintain orientation to the environment. Skil-Care Corporation, Yonkers, NY, (800) 431-2972)

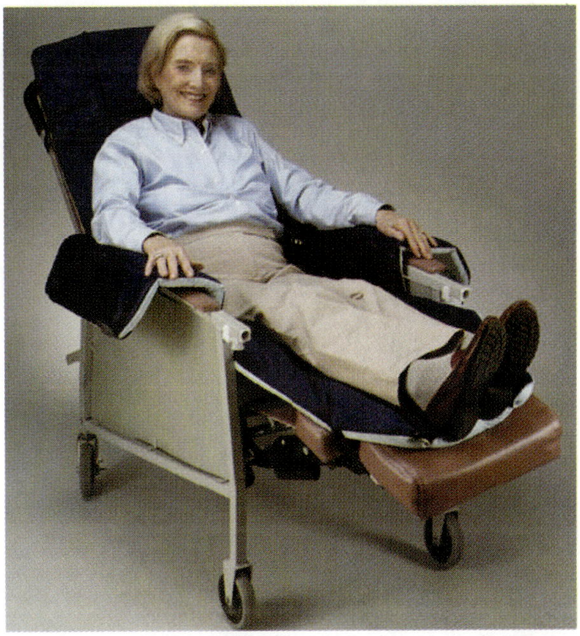

FIGURE 13-47B The reclining geriatric chair is a restraint if the resident cannot get out of it at will. Keep the chair as upright as possible so the resident can interact with the environment.Skil-Care Corporation, Yonkers, NY, (800) 431-2972)

Preventing Skin Tears

Torn armrests and seats on wheelchairs are a common cause of skin tears and resident injury. Surveyors will write up deficiencies if they observe worn wheelchairs. The armrests and seats should be replaced if they become cracked or torn. Notify your supervisor if you observe a chair in disrepair.

Positioning the Resident in a Chair or Wheelchair

Proper positioning is as important for residents who are sitting in chairs as it is for residents who are in bed. Use foam or padding on the chair seat if the resident will be sitting for long periods. Assist the resident to stand or shift weight periodically. Before leaving a resident seated in a chair, make sure that he or she is in good alignment (Figure 13.48). Good sitting posture begins with positioning the pelvis correctly. Position the resident upright in the center of the chair seat, with the hips to the back. The resident's hips and knees are positioned at a 90° angle. Make sure the weight is evenly distributed on the buttocks. You should be able to place a flat hand between the armrests and the resident's hips. If the resident leans to the side, use props to bring him or her to an upright position. Posi-

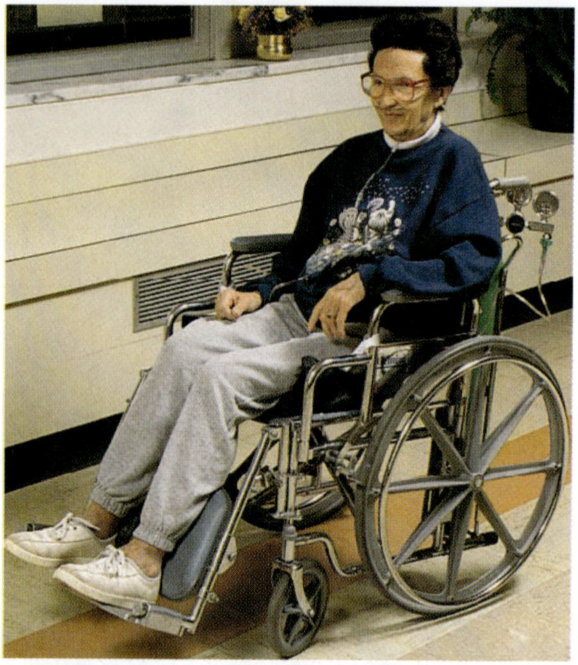

FIGURE 13-48 This resident is sitting in good body alignment and the chair fits her properly. These two factors improve her body function and ability to propel the chair.

PROCEDURE 89 Positioning the Resident in a Chair or Wheelchair

1. Perform your beginning procedure actions.
2. Make sure the brakes are locked and that the small, front caster wheels on the wheelchair are properly positioned before beginning.
3. Seat the resident upright so the head is erect and centered over the spine.
4. Position the resident's arms for comfort.
5. The back of the wheelchair should be at the lower level of the resident's shoulder blades.
6. The hips and back are positioned at a 90° angle.
7. The edge of the seat should be two to three inches from the back of the resident's knees. Position the legs at a 90° angle. If the knees touch the seat, place a cushion behind the back to move the resident forward.
8. Position the feet and ankles at 90° angles on the footrests or floor.
9. Perform your procedure completion actions.

tion the arms on the armrests. Check to make sure the shoulders are not pushed up. Check behind the knees. There should be three or four finger widths between the knees and the seat. Adjust the feet and legs so they are in line with the pelvis. Support the feet on the footrests so the legs do not dangle.

Pressure Relief in the Chair

Years ago, pressure ulcers were called decubitus ulcers. The term *decubitus* means lying down. Pressure ulcers can also develop while a person is sitting in a chair, so the name was changed to more accurately describe the cause of the problem. Residents who sit in chairs for long periods can develop skin breakdown. Anticipate this risk. If the resident is wearing a gown, cover the seat of the chair with a sheet or bath blanket. If a resident will be sitting in a chair for a prolonged period, make sure the seat is well padded. Follow the care plan for guidance as to which device to use. However, even with padding, pressure relief must be provided by assisting residents to move regularly to relieve pressure.

PROCEDURE 90 Assisting with Wheelchair Pushups

1. Perform your beginning procedure actions.
2. Position the small front wheels of the wheelchair facing forward. Lock the brakes.
3. Remove the leg rests or fold them back. Place the resident's feet on the floor.
4. Position yourself in front of the resident.
5. Instruct the resident to place both hands on the armrests, push the body up, lock the elbows, and lift the hips off the seat (Figure 13.49).
6. If the resident can use one or both legs, instruct him or her to push on the floor with the feet while pushing up with the hands.
7. Instruct the resident to unlock the elbows, slowly flex the knees, and lower gradually to the seat.
8. Repeat as instructed by the restorative nurse or therapist.
9. If the resident can perform the procedure independently, remind him or her to practice.
10. Assist the resident to return the leg rests and legs to a position of comfort.
11. Perform your procedure completion actions.

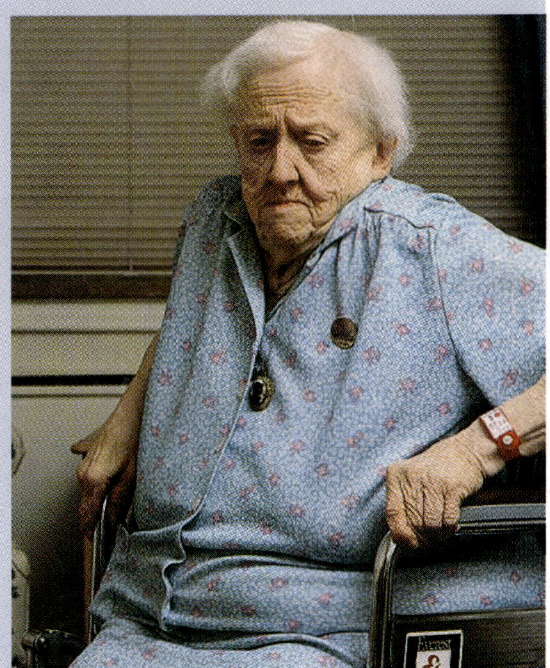

FIGURE 13-49 To perform wheelchair pushups, position the small front wheels facing forward. Elevate the footrests and place the resident's feet on the floor. Lock the brakes. Teach the resident to push on the armrests with the hands and raise the body off the seat.

PROCEDURE

91 Leaning to the Side for Pressure Relief

1. Perform your beginning procedure actions.
2. Position the small front wheels of the wheelchair facing forward. Lock the brakes. For extra security, back the wheelchair against a wall.
3. Remove the leg rests or fold them back. Place the resident's feet on the floor.
4. Position yourself in front of the resident.
5. Instruct the resident to lean forward slightly, then lean back.
6. Have the resident lean from side to side. Advise him or her to lift as much weight off the buttocks as possible. Repeat five times, or as stated in the care plan.
7. Assist the resident to return the leg rests and legs to a position of comfort.
8. Perform your procedure completion actions.

You will work with many residents who are **chairfast**, or confined to chairs. Assist and remind the residents to perform pressure-relieving activities. When the resident is learning pressure-relieving techniques, stay with him or her to give directions and encouragement. The therapist or restorative nurse will recommend a frequency for the pressure-relieving activities.

Wheelchair pushups

Wheelchair pushups are the best method of relieving pressure when the resident is seated. The resident places the palms on the armrests of the wheelchair. The feet are flat on the floor. Caution the resident against performing pushups with the feet on the footrests. Instruct the resident to push down with the hands, extend the elbows, and lift the buttocks from the chair. This should be done at least five times, or the frequency specified by the care plan.

Wheelchair pushups relieve pressure on the hips, buttocks, and coccyx. They are helpful to the resident who sits in a chair for long periods of time. Wheelchair pushups increase upper body strength. This helps prepare the resident for transfer procedures. The care plan will list directions.

Leaning to the Side for Pressure Relief
Some residents do not have the arm strength or trunk control to perform pushups. These residents can lean to the sides and front of the chair to relieve pressure. For more dependent residents, have the resident grab your hands. Instruct the resident to pull on your hands to shift the weight off the buttocks.

Wheelchair Mobility

The wheelchair is a mobility device, not a transportation device. Propelling the wheelchair independently is good exercise. It promotes communication, independence, confidence, and self-esteem. Wheelchair mobility provides opportunities for residents to make choices and decisions. They can decide where they will go and what activities to attend. A facility emphasis on efficiency may create problems with wheelchair mobility. Pushing the chairs is faster for staff, but it deprives residents of much-needed exercise and independence. Some residents do not propel their wheelchairs because of physical problems. However, adaptations may allow them to move independently. Some do not propel the chair because it does not fit correctly. Fitting wheelchairs and teaching residents to use them is best. The therapy and restorative nursing departments will work with the residents to teach them to move their wheelchairs independently. For example, a resident may propel the chair by pushing with the foot on one side. Assist and encourage residents with independence whenever possible.

GUIDELINES FOR

Wheelchair Safety

- Make sure the wheelchair fits the resident correctly and has all necessary parts, such as leg rests and brakes.
- Position the small front wheels in the forward position when transferring the resident into and out of the chair, and when the chair is parked.
- Keep the brakes locked during transfers and when the chair is parked.
- Position the resident in good body alignment; reposition as often as necessary.
- Support paralyzed body parts so they do not slip over the chair arm, drag the floor, or become entangled in the wheels.
- Cover the resident's lap with a lap blanket or bath blanket, as needed for modesty and warmth. This is especially important for a female resident who is wearing a skirt or dress. Make sure the blanket and the resident's clothing do not drag on the floor or become entangled in the wheels.
- Remind residents about wheelchair safety, including:
  - locking the brakes when the chair is parked.
  - parking the chair with the large part of the small front wheels facing forward.
  - holding the armrests and feeling the chair with the back of the legs before sitting.
  - not reaching down between the knees or bending over to pick up items from the floor.
- Push the wheelchair from behind by guiding it with the handgrips. Avoid walking too fast. Slow down and look before turning corners.
- Approach swinging doors with caution. Prop the door open before entering, if possible. If not, back the wheelchair through the doorway.
- Always back over the thresholds of doorways.
- Lock the elevator, turn the wheelchair around, and back in. When the elevator stops at your destination, lock it again, turn the chair around, and back out. (Remember to go back and unlock the elevator.)
- To transport a wheelchair up a ramp, instruct the resident to lean forward slightly. Push the resident up, from behind the chair.
- To move a wheelchair down a ramp, turn the chair around. Position yourself behind the chair and walk backward. Guide the chair by using the handgrips. Periodically look over your shoulder to make sure the path is clear. Walk slowly, using your body to guard the chair. Avoid very steep ramps, if possible.

GUIDELINES FOR

Transporting a Resident by Stretcher

- Make sure the side rails are up and all safety belts are fastened.
- Push the stretcher by standing at the resident's head.
- Approach corners slowly and look before you go around them.
- Slow down and look for oncoming traffic when approaching a swinging door. Prop the door open to propel the stretcher through the door. If this is not possible, back through swinging doors.
- When entering an elevator, push the stop button to lock the doors open. Back the stretcher into the elevator by walking backward and pulling the head end.

(continues)

GUIDELINES FOR

Transporting a Resident by Stretcher, *continued*

- Stand by the resident's head while an elevator is in motion. When the elevator stops, push the stop button to lock the door open. Push the stretcher out so the feet exit the elevator first. (Remember to go back and unlock the elevator.)

  If the elevator threshold is uneven, go to the foot end of the stretcher and pull it out of the elevator. After the stretcher is safely out of the elevator, unlock the door mechanism.
- When transporting a stretcher down a ramp or incline, walk backward, slowly guiding the stretcher from the head end. Periodically look over your shoulder to make sure the path is clear.
- When parking a stretcher, avoid blocking a doorway.
- Never leave a resident unattended and unsupervised on a stretcher.

Assisting Residents with Ambulation

Walking, or **ambulation**, is an excellent form of exercise. The body functions more efficiently in an upright position. Residents may have difficulty walking because of illness, injury, surgery, or weakness. In the initial stages of ambulation, the nursing assistant will assist residents until they regain strength and become more independent. Some residents may never become independent. However, walking them is important so that they do not lose the use of their legs. You will be assigned to walk residents a specified distance each day to help them maintain the ability to walk. If the resident is in a physical therapy or restorative nursing program, the care plan will contain specific instructions for you to follow during ambulation.

Make sure the resident's shoes are appropriate for the floor surface. Residents should not ambulate with bare feet or stocking feet. Ambulate residents on a tile floor whenever possible. Uneven surfaces make walking more difficult. They may also cause fatigue and loss of balance. Use good judgment when ambulating residents. Safety is always a primary concern. Check for hazards on the floor, such as spills, or objects that could cause the residents to fall.

Goal-Oriented Ambulation

The therapist or restorative nurse develops assessment-based ambulation goals for each resident (Figure 13.50). They try to consider goals that will be useful or purposeful for the resident. For example, going to the dining room is a functional skill. In this case, the care plan will state to ambulate the resident to and from the dining room for meals. Instead of ambulating in the hallway, walking to and from the dining room gives the activity a useful purpose. Other purposeful goals are ambulating residents:

- To and from activities programs
- To and from the bathroom
- To the nurses' station for medications

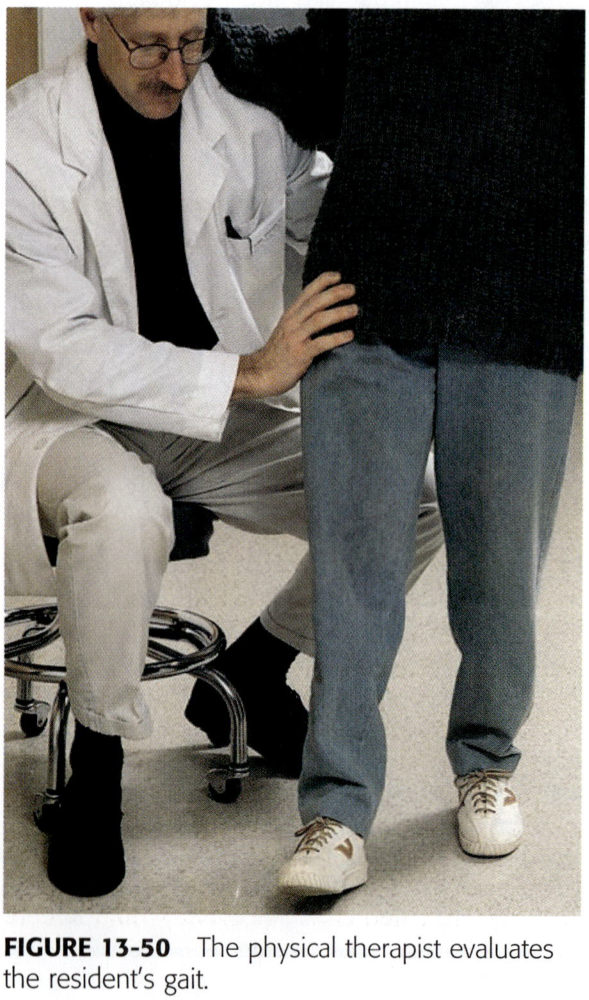

FIGURE 13-50 The physical therapist evaluates the resident's gait.

If the ambulation care plan involves walking back and forth in the hallway, residents may not see the functional purpose of the ambulation. Because of this, they view the activity as exercise, and will depend on their wheelchairs for mobility instead. The overall goals of ambulation are to:

- Maintain or improve the resident's ability to ambulate
- Ensure that the resident can ambulate safely
- Prevent the loss of independence
- Prevent **atrophy**, or muscular wasting from lack of use
- Provide a safe, consistent, purposeful ambulation activity for residents who otherwise would be unable or unwilling to ambulate regularly
- Increase residents' endurance for ambulation outside their rooms
- Increase residents' confidence and sense of well-being

Gait

The way a person walks is called the **gait**. Residents with certain musculoskeletal and neurologic problems have a gait that is peculiar to the illness. For example, residents with Parkinson's disease walk with a shuffling gait. This is because of muscle rigidity. Residents with some neurological problems walk with an **ataxic** gait. The residents appear uncoordinated. They keep their legs farther apart. This makes the residents more stable. Residents with an ataxic gait need a very wide base of support to prevent falls. Their movement is somewhat irregular. They may walk with jerking movements. Residents having pain may walk slowly. The resident's body language and facial expression may appear strained. The resident may move the painful area differently or abnormally.

Normal Gait

The normal gait pattern consists of two steps. The resident begins with the feet flat on the floor. He or she raises a leg, dorsiflexes the foot, and begins walking. The heel strikes the floor first. The resident rolls forward on the sole of the foot, and moves ahead. The arms swing back and forth, in the same direction as the opposite leg (Figure 13.51). The care plan will list special approaches to use for a resident with an abnormal gait, and special risk and safety factors.

Some residents may require more than one assistant for safe ambulation. The physical therapist or restorative nurse will determine if this is necessary. The therapist or restorative nurse will also decide whether the resident would benefit from use of an assistive device.

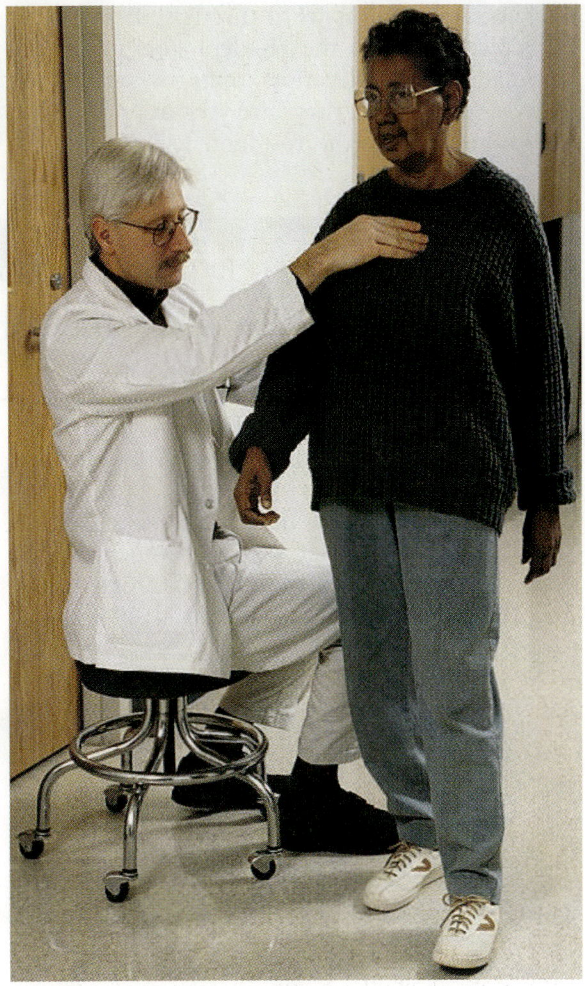

FIGURE 13-51 The arms swing in the same direction as the opposite leg.

When developing ambulation goals, the interdisciplinary team determines the distance that the resident can ambulate safely. Preventing increased pain, edema, shortness of breath, or weakness is important. If you observe these problems when you are walking a resident, stop the activity. Notify the nurse promptly.

Assisting the Resident to Walk with a Cane, Walker, or Crutches

Canes, crutches, and walkers are used to provide support during ambulation. They redistribute the balance of the resident's weight, shifting the center of gravity over a wider area. The device helps prevent loss of balance. Usually, the physical therapist will provide the device and teach the resident how to use it correctly. Use of these devices enables residents who are weak or unsteady to be independent with ambulation. Check the rubber tips before the resident ambulates. If the rubber is worn through, the tip must be replaced before the resident gets up. If the ambulation device has nuts, bolts, or pushbutton locks, make sure they are securely fastened before ambulating the resident. Each leg of the walker has a pushbutton lock. All four legs must be the same height before the resident uses the device. If you feel that a resident is not using the assistive devices correctly, notify the nurse, who will contact the therapy department.

GUIDELINES FOR

Assisting Residents with Ambulation

- Check the resident's shoes to make sure they are appropriate for the floor surface. Never ambulate a resident who has bare feet or is wearing only socks.
- Dress the resident in street clothes. If this is not possible, make sure the resident's body is covered. Avoid long pants, long robes, and slippers that could cause the resident to trip.
- Assist the resident to dangle, then stand at the bedside to balance before ambulating. If the resident feels weak, dizzy, or faint, return him or her to bed. Notify the nurse.
- Always use a gait belt, even if the resident is steady on his or her feet.
- If an assistive device is ordered, have the resident practice using it. The therapist or restorative nurse will determine the gait pattern to use. Ambulate the resident with the device for the distance and time ordered.
- If the care plan or your assignment is not specific, ask for clarification.
- Practice good body mechanics for both yourself and the resident.
- Teach and remind the resident to practice safety.
- Position your body so it moves with the resident's body. You should not interfere with the resident's movement. Match the resident's stride.
- Support the resident's weak side (if any). Stay close, slightly behind and to the resident's side. Hold the center back of the gait belt with an underhand grasp (Figure 13.52).
- Encourage the resident to stand upright and erect when walking. The head, shoulders, hips, knees, and feet should be aligned.
- Encourage the resident to take moderate, even steps. Make sure he or she maintains a wide base of support. The distance between the feet should be about equal to the resident's shoulder width.
- Allow adequate time for ambulation. Avoid making the resident feel rushed.
- Allow the resident time to rest, if necessary.
- Provide only the amount of assistance necessary.
- If the resident is not motivated, place a chair ahead of him or her. Tell the resident the goal is to walk to the chair.
- Have another assistant follow behind you with a wheelchair, if the resident's endurance is in doubt.
- Inform the nurse if you believe the resident is unsafe.
- Stop ambulation immediately if the resident shows signs of illness, pain, extreme fatigue, shortness of breath, dizziness, sweating, or anxiety. Notify the nurse.
- Never leave the resident standing unattended. When you are through, leave the resident safely sitting in a chair.

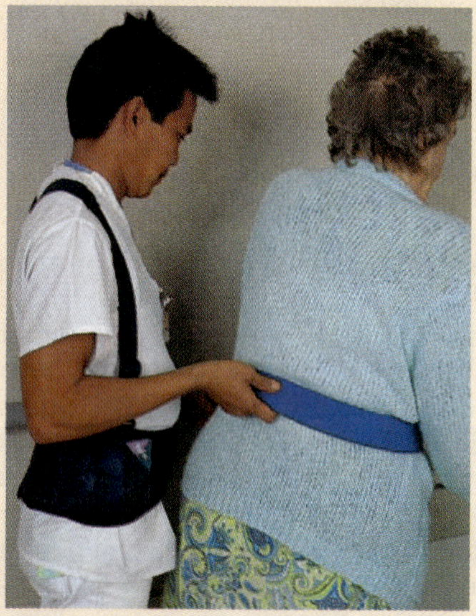

FIGURE 13-52 Stand behind and to the side of the resident, grasping the center of the belt with an underhand grasp.

PROCEDURE 92 Ambulating the Resident with a Gait Belt

1. Perform your beginning procedure actions.
2. Lower the bed to the lowest horizontal position.
3. Assist the resident to dangle.
4. Assist the resident to dress and put on footwear appropriate to the floor.
5. If the resident is not familiar with the gait belt, explain how and why it will be used.
6. Check the fit of the belt with three fingers.
7. Using an underhand grasp, place your hands under the belt on each side and bring the resident to a standing position.
8. Walk behind and slightly to one side of the resident. Maintain a firm, underhand grasp at the center back of the gait belt.
9. Encourage the resident to use the handrails in the hallway.
10. Walk the distance specified by the care plan, physical therapist, or nurse's instructions.
11. Monitor the resident for signs of fatigue. If fatigue occurs, assist the resident to sit in a chair.
12. If the resident starts to fall, pull him or her close to your body. Protect the resident's head. Using good body mechanics, hold the belt securely and ease the resident down your leg to the floor (Figure 13.53). Bend your knees as you lower the resident. Do not attempt to hold the resident up. This could cause injuries to the resident and nursing assistant. Use of the belt gives you control of the fall and helps prevent head injuries.
13. After the ambulation, return to the resident's room.
14. Assist the resident to sit in the chair or return to bed.
15. Remove the gait belt.
16. Perform your procedure completion actions.
17. Upon completion of this procedure, you may be asked to record the distance the resident walked and the resident's vital signs.

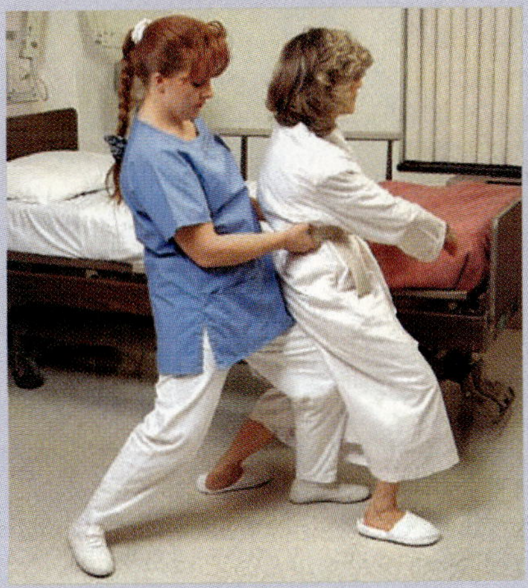

FIGURE 13-53 Keep your back straight and bend from the hips and knees. Guide the resident down your leg to the floor.

Canes

Canes are ordered for residents who have balance problems, pain, or weakness in the legs. One or two canes may be used. They are most commonly used when only one side of the body is weak. Many types of canes are available (Figure 13.54). The standard cane is shaped like an upside-down letter J. The **quad cane** has four feet. Of the canes available, it is the most stable. The resident can release the hand grip and it will

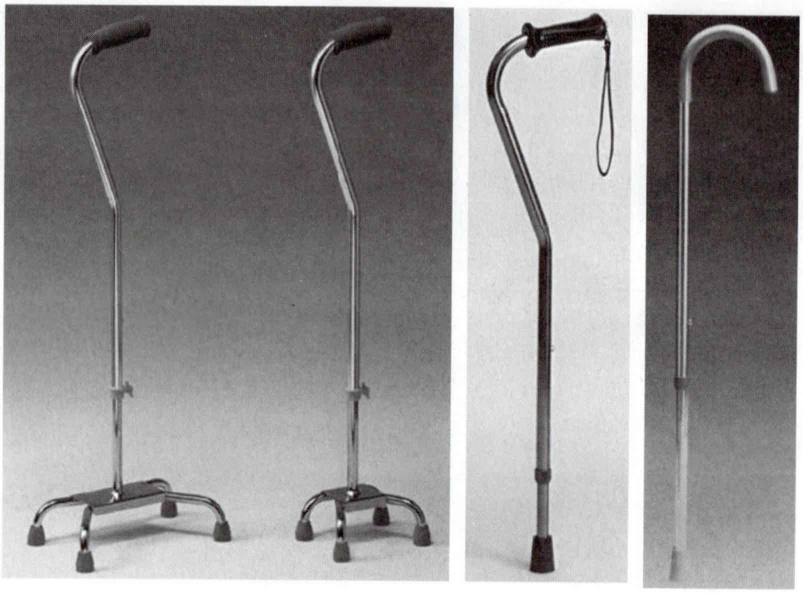

FIGURE 13-54 Various types of canes.Lumex Medical Products)

not fall to the floor. The base of the quad cane comes in two sizes, small and large. The large base provides the greatest stability. However, its size may make maneuvering in tight spaces difficult. Canes are available with many different types of hand grips. Some have an offset shaft, which changes the center of gravity. This shifts the weight over the tip of the J cane or the center of the base of the quad cane.

For safety, the cane must fit the resident. The hand grip of the cane should be at the panty-line level. If the cane is the correct height, the resident's shoulders will be even and not raised. Wooden canes can be adjusted only by cutting them. Metal canes are adjusted by releasing the pushbutton lock and moving the telescoping shaft.

The physical therapist will select the gait pattern to use, depending on the resident's problem. The most common gait pattern involves holding the cane in the hand opposite the weak leg. The cane and the weak leg move forward at the same time. This provides extra support and balance on the weak side.

Walkers

Walkers are commonly used for elderly residents. Indications for using a walker are:

- Debilitating conditions
- Generalized weakness in one or both legs
- Need to reduce weight bearing on one leg
- Poor coordination
- Injury to one leg
- Inability to use crutches
- Difficulty balancing without support

The walker provides a sturdy base of support. The resident propels the walker by using elbow extension and shoulder depression. Residents who are recovering from hip fractures often begin ambulation using a walker. Several different types of walkers are available (Figure 13.55). The therapist will select the type that meets the resident's needs. The walker is adjusted so that the handgrip is at panty-line height. If the shoulders are raised during ambulation, the walker is too high. Platforms may be attached to the walker to support the arms.

The therapist will measure the walker height to fit the resident. The walker is adjusted by turning the device upside down. Each leg has a pushbutton lock. Depress the lock and push or pull the telescoping leg to adjust the height. All four legs should be the same height before the resident uses the device.

The most common types of walkers are pictured in Figure 13.55. The aluminum walker with rubber tips on all four legs is used most often. Walkers are also available with two and four wheels. These are used for residents who cannot lift a walker, or who have weak hands. Some walkers have brakes on the wheels. The brakes lock automatically when weight is placed downward on the walker.

Safety Precautions for Ambulating Residents with a Walker

The therapist or restorative nurse will recommend a gait for the resident to use. The standard walker is picked up and placed a comfortable

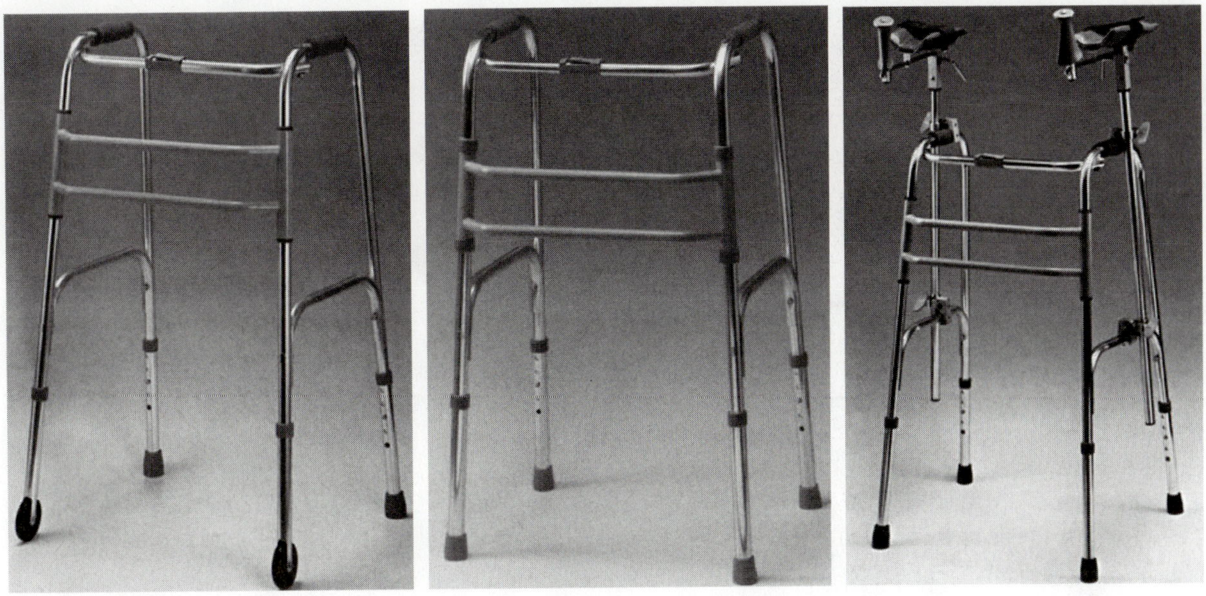

FIGURE 13-55 Various types of walkers.Lumex Medical Products)

distance ahead of the resident. Comfortable distance is important. If the resident must lean forward to reach the handles, the walker is too far away. If you are assisting, stand on the resident's weak side, holding the gait belt in the center back with an underhand grasp. All four legs of the walker should strike the floor at the same time. Some residents have a tendency to touch the back legs on the floor first, rocking the walker forward onto the front legs. This is an unsafe practice that causes falls. When all four legs are securely on the floor, the resident steps forward. He or she steps into the walker with the weak leg, then the strong leg. If the resident has visual or cognitive deficits, assist with steering. Place one hand on the gait belt and one hand on the walker, guiding the resident.

Some residents pick up the walkers and carry them. This also increases the risk of injury. If the resident can carry the walker, he or she probably does not need the device, or may do better with a different type of device. Consult the nurse.

Many residents want to use the walker as a transfer device. They may try to hold the walker while they get into or out of the chair. This is an unsafe practice, as the walker is not stable and may tip, resulting in a fall. The resident should be taught to push against the arms of the chair when sitting and rising.

Crutches

Crutches are used by residents who have only one leg, or have an injury to one leg. The correct height of the crutch is three finger-widths below the armpit. Several different gaits are used in crutch walking, depending on the resident's medical problem. The therapist will teach the resident the correct gait for his or her condition.

Crutches are not commonly used by elderly residents. Most do not have sufficient arm strength to lift the body. Balance and coordination may also be a problem.

Fractures/Cast Care

A **fracture** is any break in the continuity of a bone. Falls are the most common cause of fractures. If the bone breaks through the skin, the injury is called an *open compound fracture*. If the bones do not break through the skin, the fracture is known as *closed*.

Fractures (Figure 13.56) are classified by the type of break in the bone and whether or not the skin is broken:

- A **complete fracture** involves a break across the entire cross-section of the bone. It is often displaced, or improperly aligned, and must be reduced and straightened.
- An **incomplete fracture** involves only part of the cross-section of bone.
- A **closed** or **simple fracture** (Figure 13.56A) occurs when the skin is intact and not broken.
- An **open** or **compound fracture** (Figure 13.56B) occurs when the skin over the fracture is broken. The bone may or may not protrude.

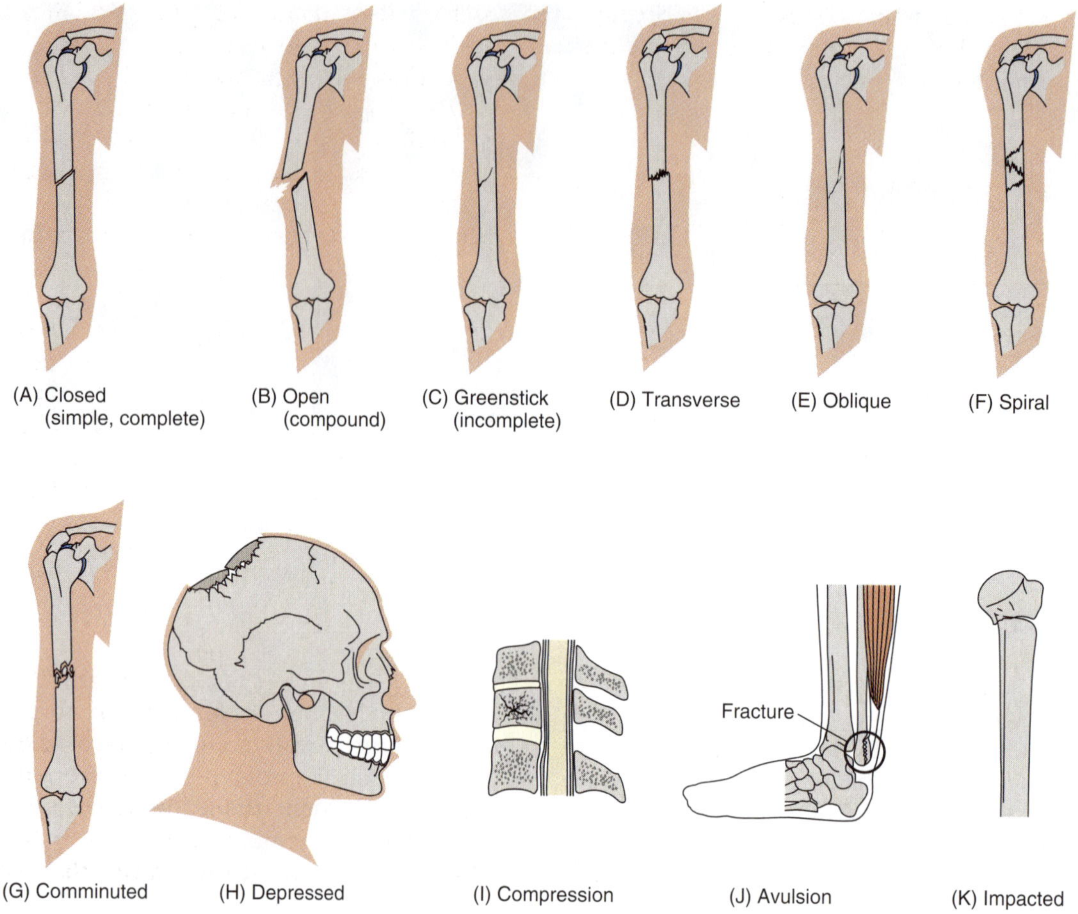

FIGURE 13-56 Types and patterns of fractures.

- A **pathologic fracture** is a fracture in a diseased bone.It occurs as a result of osteoporosis, a tumor, or cancer.

The pattern of a fracture describes the manner in which the bone is broken:

- A **greenstick fracture** (Figure 13.56C) occurs when only one side of the bone is broken and the other side is bent. This fracture is common in children, whose bone growth is incomplete. The bones tend to bend like young trees; hence the name "greenstick" fracture.
- A **transverse fracture** (Figure 13.56D), breaks completely across the bone.
- An **oblique fracture** ((Figure 13.56E) runs at an angle across the bone.
- A **spiral fracture** (Figure 13.56F) twists around the bone.
- A **comminuted fracture** (Figure 13.56G) involves shattering and splintering of the bone into more than three fragments.
- A **depressed fracture** (Figure 13.56H) is seen only in fractures of the skull and face. This type of fracture depresses the bone and drives fragments inward.
- A **compression fracture** (Figure 13.56I) is seen only in the vertebrae of the spine. This type of fracture collapses the bone inward.
- An **avulsion fracture** (Figure 13.56J) occurs when a bone fragment is pulled off at the point of ligament or tendon attachment.
- An **impacted fracture** (Figure 13.56K) occurs when the fragment from one bone is wedged into another bone.

Signs and Symptoms

Signs and symptoms of fractures will vary with the type of fracture and location. Fractures are painful conditions. Movement is limited, or the patient may be unable to move the injured area. The skin surrounding the fracture may appear deformed. Edema is common. **Ecchymosis**, or bruising, may occur. Some parts of the body, such as the area over the femur, are very **vascular**. Areas that are vascular contain many blood vessels.

They bleed readily under the skin. An ecchymosis the size of an adult's fist over the femur indicates loss of approximately one pint of blood.

Treatment

A new fracture is usually treated in the hospital emergency department. Admission for surgical correction of the fracture may be necessary. The immediate goals of care are to:

- control pain
- prevent complications of immobility
- prevent or reduce edema
- keep the fracture in good alignment
- keep the fractured extremity immobile

Fractures of any kind are treated by keeping the part that is injured immobilized in proper position until healing takes place. Injured bones take from several weeks to several months to heal. Immobilization is achieved through the use of:

- Pins (Figure 13.57)
- Screws
- Splints
- Bone plates
- Casting
- Traction

Special beds and attachments are used to make nursing care easier. The patient may be placed on a Stryker frame or the CircOlectric® bed.

Be sure you know how to operate each bed and attachment before attempting care. In many facilities, an RN must be present when the bed is turned. Know and follow the policy of your facility.

You will assist patients who have fractures with range-of-motion exercises several times each day. Check with the nurse or care plan for specific instructions. In most cases, you will not exercise the fractured extremity. You may be assigned to exercise the patient's joints above and below the cast to keep them mobile. For fractured arms and legs, you may be permitted to exercise fingers and toes. Exercising the rest of the patient's body is important. The exercise prevents complications related to immobility and inactivity.

You may also assist the patient with coughing and deep breathing exercises to prevent pneumonia. When working with patients with fractures, encourage adequate fluid intake. The increased fluid liquefies secretions that accumulate in the lungs. Coughing and deep breathing exercises are the same as those used in postoperative care. A **trapeze** (Figure 13.58) may be attached to the bed to assist the patient with movement. Your supervisor will teach you how to move and reposition the patient without interfering with the traction. The casted extremity is elevated on pillows if traction is not used.

Treatment for patients with fractures begins soon after admission. The type of treatment is determined by the location and type of fracture, and method of fracture reduction. Patients with fractures will be evaluated by the physical and occupational therapists. Therapists will design rehabilitation programs to meet the patients'

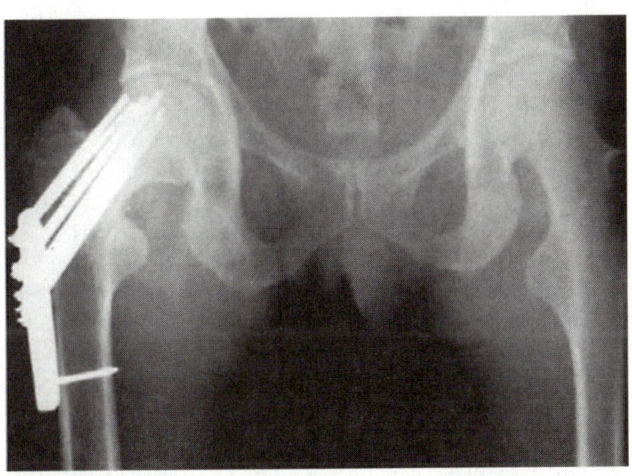

FIGURE 13-57 Certain fractures are repaired using plates, pins, or screws.

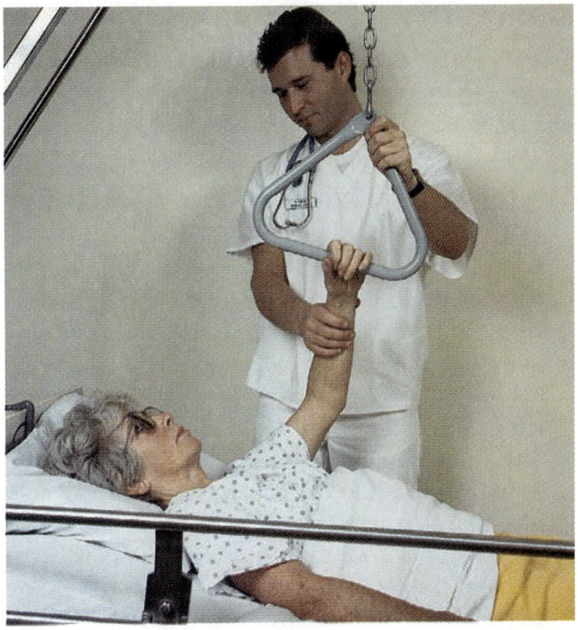

FIGURE 13-58 The overhead trapeze is a helpful adjunct that enables the patient to move in bed. The trapeze is not used for some patients with back injuries and back surgeries, because independent positioning can worsen the condition or cause further injuries.

SAFETY *Alert*

A fiberglass cast dries immediately. A plaster arm or leg cast will take 24 to 48 hours to dry completely. A plaster body or spica cast will take 48 to 72 hours to dry. Proper positioning of the cast is essential during the drying period to prevent depressions that can cause pressure and edema. Never use a table or hard object to support the cast during the drying period. Avoid rubber or plastic pillows, which increase heat under the cast. When the cast is dry, it will look white and shiny. It will not appear soft or damp.

needs and help them to regain as much mobility as possible.

Care of Patients with Casts

Two types of cast materials are commonly used:

1. Plaster of Paris, which can take up to 48 hours to dry completely
2. Fiberglass, which dries very rapidly

Cast material is wet when it is applied. During the drying period, the cast gives off heat. Special care for the newly casted patient includes:

- Supporting the cast and body in good alignment with pillows covered by cloth pillowcases, and keeping the cast uncovered.
- Elevating the casted extremity on a pillow as instructed. When positioning a patient with a leg cast, elevate the foot higher than the hip. The fingers should be higher than the elbow. Avoid placing the cast on a flat surface. Avoid placing anything plastic under a wet cast. Check the skin distal to the cast frequently for signs of poor circulation.
- Turning the patient frequently to permit air circulation to all parts of the cast. Maintain support. Use the palm of your hand, not your fingers, to support the wet cast.
- Not positioning the cast against the footboard or side rail. Leaving the cast open to air until it dries is best. If the patient is cold, cover the cast loosely with a sheet. Avoid tucking the sheet under the mattress. A bed cradle may be used, if necessary. The greatest area of heat loss is the head. Covering the upper body and back and top of the head with a blanket may help keep the patient warm.
- Closely observing the uncasted areas of the extremities, such as the fingers and toes, for signs of decreased circulation. Report coldness, cyanosis, swelling, increased pain, numbness, or tingling immediately.
- Closely observing skin areas around the cast edges for signs of irritation (Figure 13.59). Rough edges should be covered with adhesive strips to prevent skin irritation.

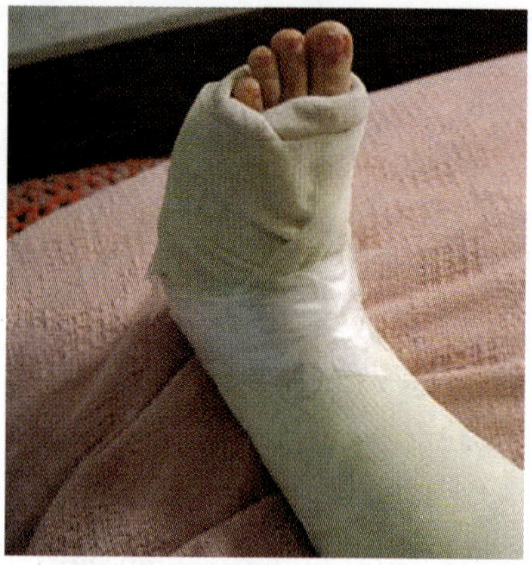

FIGURE 13-59 Check the skin around the edges of the cast regularly for signs of irritation. Check the circulation in the toes.

Recall the following key of reportables when checking the patient:

- C = color
- M = motion
- E = edema
- T = temperature

Special Care After Cast Is Dry

After the cast has completely dried:

- Turn the patient to the noncasted side. This is particularly important in moving a patient with a body cast (**spica cast**) (Figure 13.60) because turning to the casted side may crack the cast.
- Always support the cast when turning or moving a patient.
- Encourage use of a trapeze to assist the patient in helping herself.
- Tape edges of casts to prevent pressure and abrasive areas, if edges were not covered when the cast was applied.

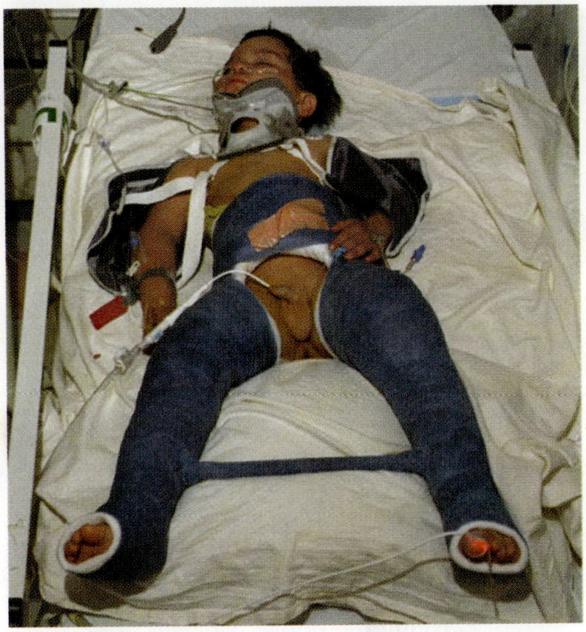

FIGURE 13-60 The spica cast is a full-body cast that is commonly used to treat hip fracture and after hip surgery in children.

- Use plastic to protect cast edges that are near the genitals and buttocks, to help prevent soiling during toileting.

After the cast dries, you may observe changes that indicate infection or ulceration under the cast:

- odor from the cast
- drainage through the cast

The care plan may instruct you to keep the casted extremity elevated to prevent edema. A sling may be used to elevate an arm cast when the patient is out of bed. A wheelchair with an elevated leg rest is used for patients with leg casts. Cover the cast with plastic during bathing. Keep small objects from getting inside the cast. The patient may complain of an itching sensation under the cast. Discourage him or her from placing objects down the cast to scratch. This could cause a skin injury and infection. Report complaints of itching to your supervisor.

KEY POINTS

- A transfer involves moving a resident from one location to another.
- Sitting on the side of the bed is called dangling; this is the first step in the transfer procedure if the resident has been bedfast.
- A transfer belt should always be used when moving residents, unless contraindicated.
- Lock the brakes on the bed and wheelchair before transferring the resident.
- Move the footrests out of the way if the resident is transferring into a wheelchair.
- A key to maintaining stability of a wheelchair is positioning the large part of the front caster wheels facing forward.
- Always lock the brakes during transfers into and out of a wheelchair, and when the chair is parked.
- Position the resident in the wheelchair in good body alignment.
- The resident's legs must be supported on the footrests or the floor when the resident is seated in a wheelchair.
- The mechanical lift is a two-person device.
- A resident with good upper body strength can use a sliding board to transfer from the bed to a wheelchair and back.
- The wheelchair must fit the resident properly for comfort, safety, and to reduce the use of restraints.
- Pressure ulcers can develop when a resident is seated in the wheelchair; pressure relief must be provided.
- The wheelchair is a mobility device, not a transportation device. The resident should propel the chair independently whenever possible.
- The care plan will list purposeful activities for maintaining residents' ambulation ability.
- Residents may need canes, walkers, or crutches for balance, stability, and support during ambulation.

REVIEW

A. Multiple Choice

Select the one best answer.

1. Sitting a resident on the side of the bed is called
   a. proning.
   b. supining.
   c. semisitting.
   d. dangling.
2. When transferring residents from one place to another, you should
   a. lock the brakes of the bed, wheelchair, or stretcher.
   b. adjust the bed to the highest horizontal height.
   c. use a transfer belt only if the resident has had a stroke.
   d. advise the resident not to help, for safety.
3. Contraindications for using the transfer belt include residents who have
   a. had a stroke.
   b. head injuries.
   c. a gastrostomy.
   d. confusion.
4. When moving a resident (by yourself) with a transfer belt,
   a. use an underhand grasp.
   b. use an overhand grasp.
   c. stand behind the resident.
   d. lift from the side.
5. When using the mechanical (hydraulic) lift,
   a. ask another nursing assistant to help you.
   b. apply a transfer belt to the resident.
   c. fasten the "S" hooks facing inward.
   d. unlock the brakes so the wheelchair can be moved.
6. You are assigned to ambulate Mr. Wells using a gait belt. You are in the middle of the hallway, and the resident starts to fall. You should
   a. let go of the belt.
   b. hold Mr. Wells up and call for help.
   c. ease the resident down your leg.
   d. tell the resident to grab the handrail.
7. The correct height for the hands on a walker or cane is at the
   a. waist level.
   b. panty-line level.
   c. mid-thigh level.
   d. wrist level.
8. When transferring the resident from the bed to the wheelchair, position the wheelchair
   a. facing the door.
   b. at a 90° angle.
   c. at a 45° to 60° angle.
   d. on the resident's weak side.
9. When a resident transfers using the sliding board, he or she should wear
   a. cotton pants.
   b. a hospital gown.
   c. blue jeans.
   d. underwear only.
10. When transferring a resident from the bed to a stretcher,
    a. lower the bed to the lowest horizontal height.
    b. ensure that three or four people are available to help.
    c. logroll the resident onto the stretcher.
    d. lift the resident from the head and feet.
11. For wheelchair safety, all of the following are correct *except*
    a. lock the brakes during transfers and when the chair is parked.
    b. the small part of the front wheel faces sideways during transfers.
    c. the resident's feet should be supported when seated in the chair.
    d. the wheelchair must fit the resident properly.
12. Pressure ulcers
    a. can develop in chairfast residents.
    b. are not a concern in elderly persons.

c. develop only when the resident is in bed.
d. occur if the resident is not moved every four hours.

13. When pushing a wheelchair or stretcher, you should
    a. always avoid ramps and inclines.
    b. make sure the resident faces forward to enter an elevator.
    c. not use belts or rails, to avoid restraining the resident.
    d. back over thresholds and uneven surfaces.
14. If the resident's hips slide forward in a wheelchair, you should
    a. apply a restraint.
    b. check the chair depth.
    c. get a larger chair.
    d. shorten the leg rests.
15. Ideally, the resident who is chairfast should
    a. relieve pressure every 15 minutes.
    b. be moved by staff every four hours.
    c. use a five-inch foam or eggcrate cushion.
    d. stand up at least once each hour.

B. Short-Answer

Answer the following questions.

16–20. List at least five contraindications for using the gait (transfer) belt.

16. ____________ 19. ____________
17. ____________ 20. ____________
18. ____________

21–30. List at least 10 guidelines for proper chair positioning.

21. ______________________________
22. ______________________________
23. ______________________________
24. ______________________________
25. ______________________________
26. ______________________________
27. ______________________________
28. ______________________________
29. ______________________________
30. ______________________________

C. Clinical Applications

Answer the following questions.

31. You must transfer Mr. Hall from the chair to his bed. The care plan states that a transfer belt should be used for moving Mr. Hall. You cannot find a transfer belt. Mr. Hall has a belt on the trousers he is wearing. What should you do?
32. You have never transferred Mrs. Livingston before. The resident is smaller than you are. The care plan states that she uses a one-person transfer, but the resident is confused, agitated, and seems fearful. She is not following your directions. What will you do?
33. Mrs. Tsai asks you to take her to the bathroom. Because of the design of the room, the toilet is on her paralyzed side. How will you safely transfer this resident to the toilet?
34. You enter Mr. Secrest's room to walk him to the dining room for lunch, as listed on the care plan. The resident tells you he has a headache and feels weak. What action will you take?
35. After getting Miss Hegle up in the wheelchair, you discover that one leg rest is missing. The resident is confused. You were instructed to transport her to the activities room for a church service. What will you do?

UNIT 14

Prevention of Pressure Ulcers

OBJECTIVES

After reading this unit, you will be able to:

- Spell and define key terms.
- Demonstrate good body mechanics when lifting and moving residents and other heavy objects.
- Describe why positioning residents in good body alignment is important.
- Define ergonomics and describe how cumulative trauma disorders occur.
- Demonstrate proper positioning in the supine, prone, lateral, Fowler's, semisupine, and semiprone positions.
- Describe the cause of pressure ulcers and list 10 methods of preventing pressure ulcer development.
- Demonstrate procedures related to body mechanics, moving and positioning residents.

OBSERVATIONS TO MAKE AND REPORT RELATED TO BODY MECHANICS, MOVING AND POSITIONING RESIDENTS

Rash
Redness
Redness in the skin that does not go away within 30 minutes after pressure is relieved from a bony prominence or pressure area
In dark- or yellow-skinned residents, spots or areas that are darker in appearance than normal skin tone
Pressure ulcers, blisters
Abrasions, skin tears, lacerations
Irritation
Bruises
Skin discoloration
Swelling
Lumps
Abnormal skin growths
Change in color of a wart or mole
Abnormal sweating
Excessive heat or coolness to touch
Open areas/skin breakdown
Drainage
Foul odor
Complaints such as numbness, burning, tingling, itching
Signs of infection
Unusual skin color, such as blue or gray color of the skin, lips, nail beds, roof of mouth, or mucous membranes
Skin growths
Poor skin turgor/Tenting of skin on forehead or over sternum
Sunken, dark eyes

Body Mechanics

The nursing assistant routinely lifts, moves, and positions residents and other heavy objects. Good **body mechanics** involves using your body correctly. Good body mechanics should always be used when performing lifting or moving procedures, transferring residents, picking up items from the floor, and bending and lifting. Proper body mechanics means using the largest, strongest muscles to do the job. Your strongest muscles are in your legs and arms. Your weakest muscles are in your back and abdomen.

Practice the principles of good body mechanics until they become a habit. They will make your job easier and prevent fatigue by making the best use of your strength and energy. Use of proper body mechanics helps prevent injury to the nursing assistant and resident.

Posture

Good posture is the foundation on which proper body mechanics is built. Good posture is the same whether you are standing, sitting, or lying down. Keep your back straight with your feet flat on the floor and your weight distributed evenly on both feet. The feet should be at least 12 inches apart to maintain a wide base of support. Your knees should be bent slightly and your arms should be at your sides (Figure 14.1).

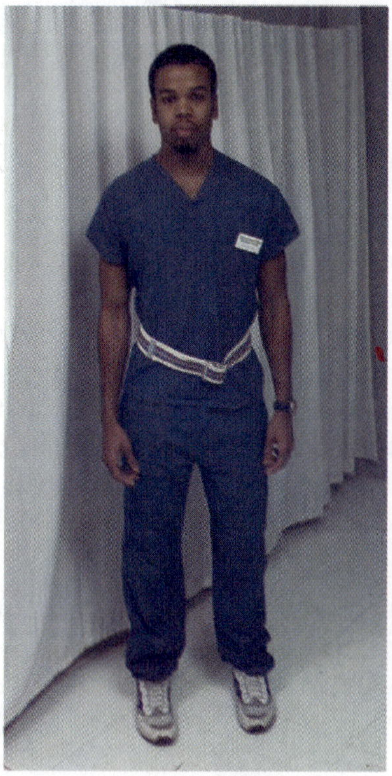

FIGURE 14-1 Good standing posture

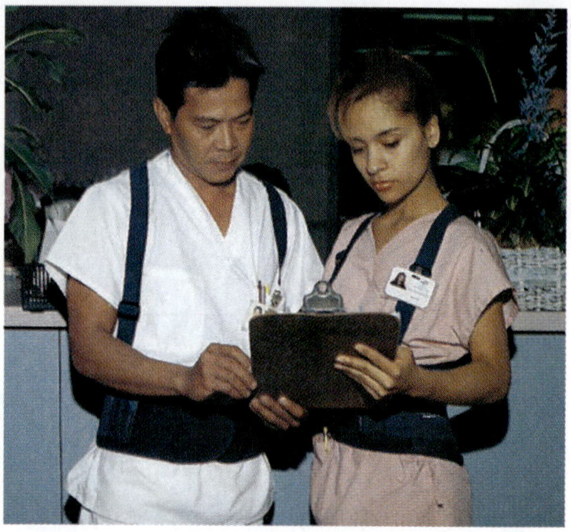

FIGURE 14-2 A back support belt reminds you to use good body mechanics. It does not make you stronger.

Back Support Belts. Use a back support belt (Figure 14.2) if this is your preference or the policy of your facility. Back injuries are very common in health care workers. Many nursing assistants feel better if they are wearing the belt for support. Several studies have shown that workers using the back support have fewer back injuries. Other studies have shown that there is no difference in the rate of injuries. The belt reminds you to keep your back straight and to use good body mechanics. Remember that wearing the back support belt does not make you stronger, and you should not lift more weight than you would if you were not wearing the belt. Using improper body mechanics when wearing the belt is difficult. For this reason alone, the belt may prove beneficial. You are less likely to become injured if you are using good body mechanics.

Ergonomics

Ergonomics is a method of fitting the job to the worker. When the job and the worker do not match, physical injuries can result. Ergonomic hazards are workplace conditions that place biomechanical stress on the worker. Examples of hazards are improper work methods, improper equipment, poor posture, force, repetition, and inadequate work-rest regimens.

Two types of injuries commonly affect the nursing assistant. **Instantaneous injuries** are injuries that occur suddenly and without warning,

GUIDELINES FOR

Using Good Body Mechanics

- Keep your back straight.
- Your feet should be at least 12 inches apart.
- Use the large muscles in your legs when lifting residents or heavy objects.
- Bend from the hips and knees, never from the waist.
- Face your work. Avoid twisting at the waist. If you must turn, pivot instead.
- If you must turn or change direction, take a few short steps. Turn your entire body instead of twisting your back or neck.
- Squat when lifting heavy objects from the floor.
- Keep heavy objects as close to your body as possible when lifting, moving, and carrying.
- Use both hands when lifting and moving heavy objects.
- Push, pull, or slide heavy objects instead of lifting them whenever possible. Use your body weight to help you.
- Use smooth, even movements instead of quick, jerking motions.
- Avoid unnecessary bending and reaching.
- Check the care plan before moving residents. The care plan often provides individualized instructions for moving, positioning, and transferring each resident.
- Always use a **transfer belt** for moving residents from one place to another, unless **contraindicated**. A transfer belt is a heavy canvas belt used for lifting and moving residents. The same belt is also called a **gait belt** when it is used for walking residents. Contraindicated means the belt should not be used for moving a resident because of a specific medical condition.
- Ask for help from others if you are not sure whether you can move a resident or lift an object.
- Use mechanical lifting devices for moving heavy residents.
- When giving bedside care, raise the height of the bed to a comfortable height for your body so you will not have to bend at the waist. When finished, remember to lower the bed to the lowest horizontal position.
- Avoid lifting heavy objects that are above your shoulder height.

such as in an accident. An example of an instantaneous injury is a fall. **Cumulative trauma disorders** are bodily injuries to nerves, tissues, tendons, and joints that occur from repeated stress and strain over a period of months to years. Cumulative trauma disorders are caused by performing repetitious tasks, using muscular force to perform a job, doing heavy lifting without assistance, poor posture, standing in awkward positions, and inadequate rest.

Back injuries are common in workers who lift and move residents frequently. Using the principles of body mechanics will help protect you from injury. Good posture is very important as well. Use mechanical lifting devices and transfer belts for moving residents whenever possible. If the resident is not able to assist with the transfer in any way, always ask another nursing assistant to help you. Raising the height of the bed to a comfortable working height when you are performing bedside procedures is an important method of protecting your back. Avoid placing stress on your body whenever possible. Use a cart to transport heavy objects instead of carrying them. Do a job at waist height instead of bending or reaching up and down. Pivot to reach an object instead of twisting from the waist. Squat instead of bending. Always use good body mechanics when standing, lifting, moving, and turning.

PRESSURE ULCERS

The skin is the largest organ of the body, and it performs many vital functions. The skin protects the body from infection and injury. If the skin is broken, pain results, and there is an increased risk of infection. The skin also removes waste products, water, and salt through sweat. At certain places the skin joins with mucous membranes that line openings into body cavities. Some of these areas are covered with hair. The hair is a natural defense of the body to trap

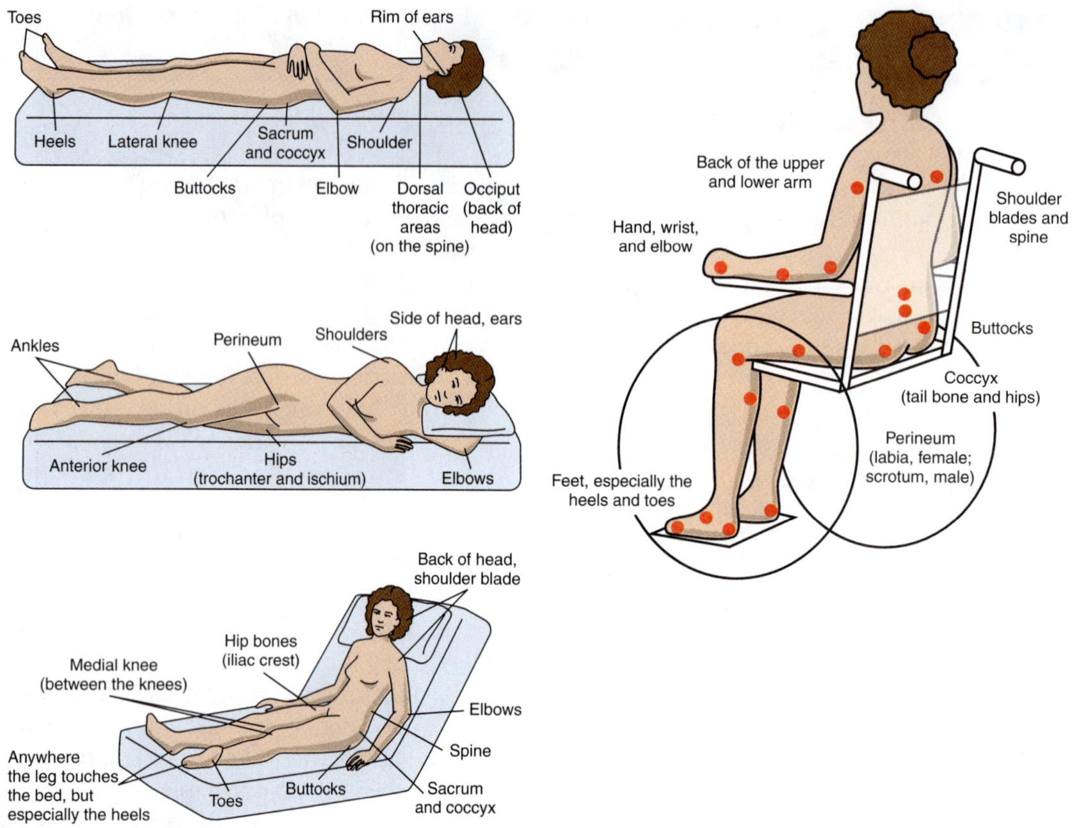

FIGURE 14-3 Common areas of pressure ulcer development in bed and chair

invading microbes and prevent them from entering. The hair and nails are considered part of the skin system.

One of the primary purposes of moving and positioning residents is to prevent **pressure ulcers**. Pressure ulcers may appear on the skin in areas where the skin is close to an underlying bone. They are the result of prolonged pressure, moisture, and other irritants. Older terms you may hear to refer to pressure ulcers are **pressure sores**, **bedsores**, **decubitus ulcers**, or **decubiti**. These areas usually develop as the result of pressure over **bony prominences**, or areas where the bone is close to the skin. Figure 14.3 shows common sites for pressure ulcer development. Pressure ulcers can also develop in other areas if tubing or clothing is constricting, pressing, or rubbing on the skin. Ulcers are the result of inadequate blood and oxygen flow to an area of the body. They can develop in a short time and will quickly cause tissue destruction. Residents can develop pressure ulcers while lying in bed or sitting in a chair. Pressure ulcers are painful and heal slowly. Infections and other complications may develop. They are much easier to prevent than they are to treat.

Risk Factors for Pressure Ulcers

Pressure ulcers are a very serious complication of immobility that should be prevented at all costs. Understanding the contributing causes and risk factors for pressure ulcers will help you prevent them. Many residents are identified as being at high risk of developing pressure ulcers by the minimum data set (MDS) and various assessments completed by nurses. A preventive care plan is always started when a resident is known to be at high risk. The presence of a risk factor does not make deterioration or development of a condition inevitable; rather, it is a "red flag" to staff that a serious complication or condition *may* develop. When one or more risk factors are present, staff is expected to plan and implement aggressive preventive care appropriate to the potential problem. Remember that OBRA requires facilities to maintain or improve residents' conditions whenever possible. Pressure ulcers are declines. If ulcers are present at the time of admission, the facility is expected to heal them. If the resident's skin is clear, it should remain clear. Pressure ulcers are considered unavoidable only when the resident has a medical condition that increases the risk of skin breakdown, and the:

- Resident has been accurately assessed.
- Risk of skin breakdown has been accurately assessed, and is adequately addressed in the care plan.
- Care plan is actually implemented.
- Interventions are evaluated periodically and modified according to the resident's responses to the plan of care.

When these factors are analyzed honestly, we find that most pressure ulcers are preventable.

Unfortunately, some residents slip through the cracks and their risks are not identified accurately or promptly, if at all. Serious skin breakdown can occur in a surprisingly brief period of time. Sometimes residents' conditions change quickly and breakdown occurs before the risk assessment is updated. Generally speaking, residents with low risk scores are at greater risk for developing pressure ulcers if they become ill, because no preventive plan of care is in place for them. If a resident who normally moves about independently suddenly becomes ill, he or she can develop a pressure ulcer rapidly. Thus, you must have a basic understanding of risk factors and take steps to prevent skin breakdown. Report to the nurse promptly if you feel there has been a change in a resident's condition. Tight and constricting clothing reduces oxygen and nutrients to the skin. Pressure does the same thing by reducing blood flow and nourishment. Tissues that are starved for oxygen become painful and begin to die. The full extent of the damage may not be immediately visible until the deep tissue ulcerates and sloughs off, leaving a large, deep crater in the resident's skin. An alert staff will recognize the potential danger and implement a preventive plan promptly.

Risk factors for pressure ulcer development are:

- Having a current pressure ulcer or a history of healed pressure ulcers
- Diabetes, peripheral vascular disease, edema of the feet and legs, or conditions such as stroke, in which extremities are paralyzed or sensation is impaired
- Being bedfast, chairfast, or unable to move and turn independently
- Weight loss, inadequate nutrition
- Poor fluid intake, dehydration
- Underweight (very thin) or overweight
- Skin that is dry, is thin, tears, or bleeds easily
- Confusion or coma
- Inability to communicate
- Bowel and/or bladder incontinence
- Contractures
- Restraint use

Exposure to moisture, powder, friction, shearing, chemicals, secretions, excretions, and other irritants also influences pressure ulcer development. Friction occurs when the skin rubs against another surface. Skin damage is worsened by rapid movement. Friction and shearing occur readily when residents are pulled up in a bed or chair. These minor injuries rapidly turn into pressure ulcers.

Stages of Pressure Ulcer Development

Pressure ulcers are staged according to their severity (Figure 14.4). If a pressure ulcer is detected in the early stages of development, it can be prevented from worsening.

- Stage I pressure ulcers (Figure 14.5) begin as red areas. The redness does not go away within 30 minutes after pressure has been relieved. In a dark-skinned person, a Stage I pressure ulcer begins as a dark blue or black area on the skin. The skin is not broken in a Stage I area.
- Stage II pressure ulcers (Figure 14.6) are blistered or open areas. They are shallow and involve part of the top layer of skin.
- Stage III pressure ulcers (Figure 14.7) are areas in which the entire layer of skin is lost and the subcutaneous fat and muscle are exposed.
- Stage IV pressure ulcers (Figure 14.8) involve destruction of the entire top layer of skin. Damage extends through the fat into the muscle, tendon, and bone.

Prevention of Pressure Ulcers

Keeping pressure off the skin over bony prominences is the best and most important way to prevent pressure ulcers. This is done by proper positioning, padding, and moving the resident frequently. Good nutrition and hydration play important roles in keeping the body healthy and preventing skin breakdown. Pressure ulcers are a leading cause of lawsuits against long-term care facilities. Pressure ulcers are declines that must be prevented. Remember that the nursing assistant has an important responsibility in the prevention of pressure ulcers. Take this responsibility seriously!

Observation and Reporting

In the early stages, pressure ulcers are quite painful because the nerve endings in the skin are

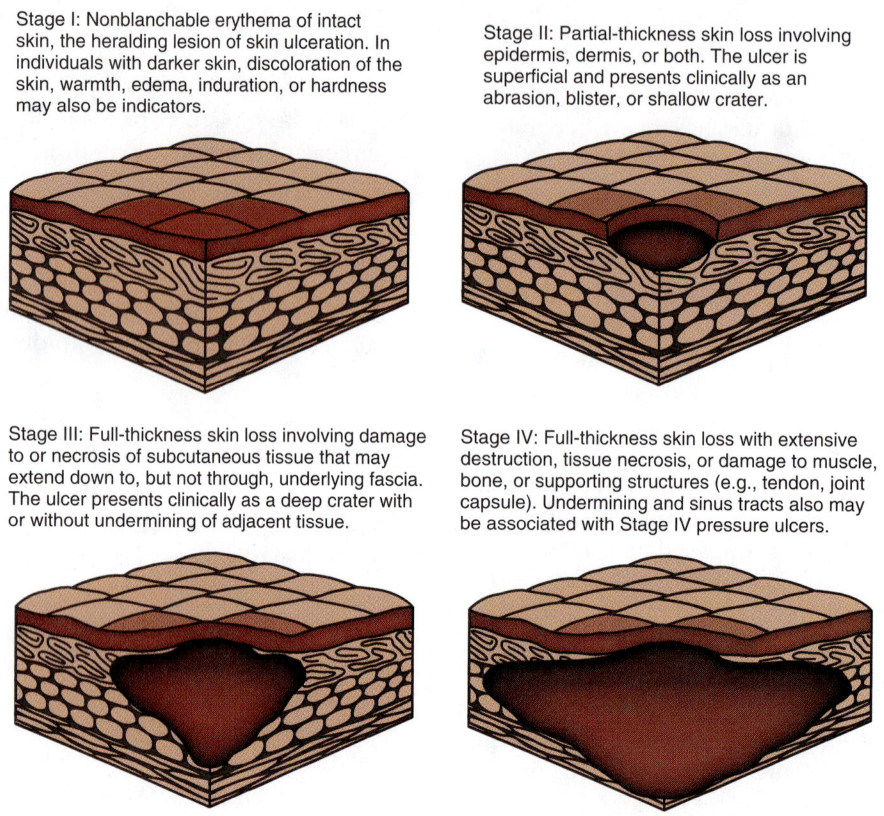

FIGURE 14-4 The pressure ulcer stages reflect the amount of tissue destruction.

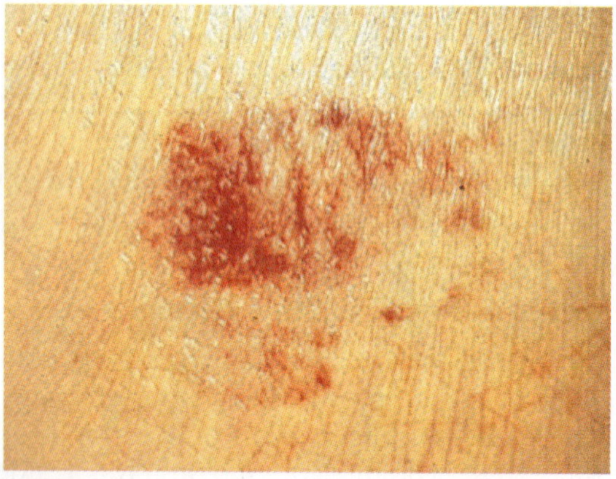

FIGURE 14-5 Stage I pressure ulcer. *(Permission to reproduce this copyrighted material has been granted by the owner, Hollister, Incorporated.)*

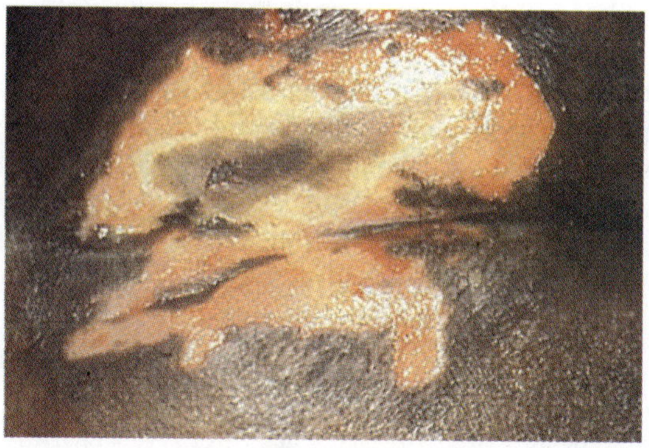

FIGURE 14-6 Stage II pressure ulcer. *(Permission to reproduce this copyrighted material has been granted by the owner, Hollister, Incorporated.)*

exposed. Early detection and treatment of pressure ulcers will prevent the areas from worsening. If the resident presently has, or has previously had, a pressure ulcer, consider this a high risk factor for further breakdown and use aggressive preventive measures. Immediately report to the nurse if you discover a red area that does not go away after the pressure has been removed for 30 minutes. Also report blisters, **abrasions** (scrapes that rub off the skin surface), open areas, bruises, areas of pain, or areas that appear discolored.

POSITIONING RESIDENTS

The nursing assistant positions residents frequently throughout the day. You will use good posture and good body mechanics when

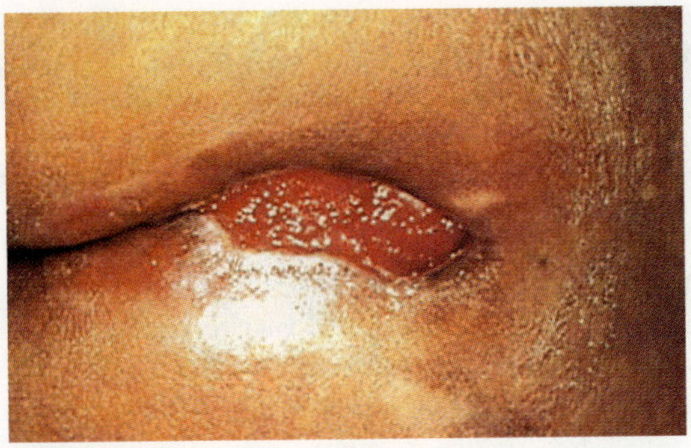

FIGURE 14-7 Stage III pressure ulcer. *(Permission to reproduce this copyrighted material has been granted by the owner, Hollister, Incorporated.)*

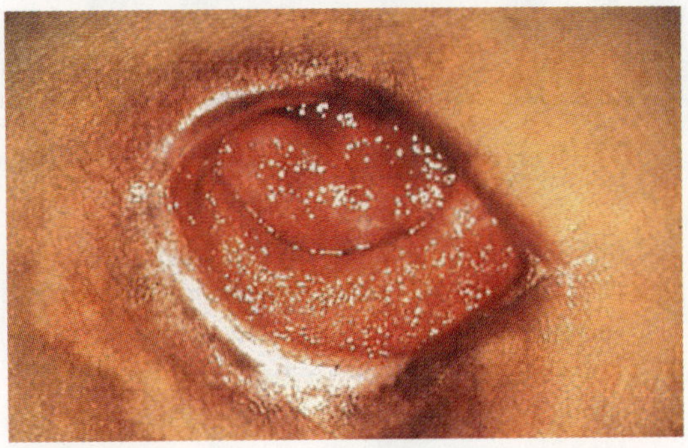

FIGURE 14-8 Stage IV pressure ulcer. *(Permission to reproduce this copyrighted material has been granted by the owner, Hollister, Incorporated.)*

GUIDELINES FOR

Prevention of Pressure Ulcers

- Turn the resident at least every two hours, and more often if necessary. Follow the care plan and the resident's individual turning schedule.
- Encourage residents who are able to move to reposition themselves frequently to relieve pressure.
- Teach residents who are seated in chairs to shift their weight every 15 minutes, if physically able, to relieve pressure.
- Residents who are sitting in chairs should also be moved and repositioned at least every two hours.
- Keep the skin clean and dry. Excessive moisture promotes skin breakdown.
- Avoid using very hot water to bathe residents.
- Use nonirritating soap to bathe residents.
- Rinse the skin well after using soap. Soap residue promotes irritation and skin breakdown.
- Avoid using powder and corn starch, which can be irritating to the skin.
- If the resident does not have control of bowel or bladder, wash the resident well with soap and water or a facility-approved cleansing agent after each episode of incontinence. Rinse the skin well. Urine and stool are very irritating to the skin.
- Use facility-approved moisturizing lotions on residents who have dry skin. Skin that is supple and well hydrated will not break as easily as dry skin.
- Keep bed linens crumb- and wrinkle-free. The pressure from wrinkles and crumbs can cause skin breakdown.
- Use lifting sheets to move residents in bed whenever possible, to avoid **friction** and **shearing**. Friction is rubbing the skin against another surface, such as bed linen. Excess friction in moving residents can cause abrasions, which can quickly worsen into pressure ulcers. Shearing (Figure 14.9)

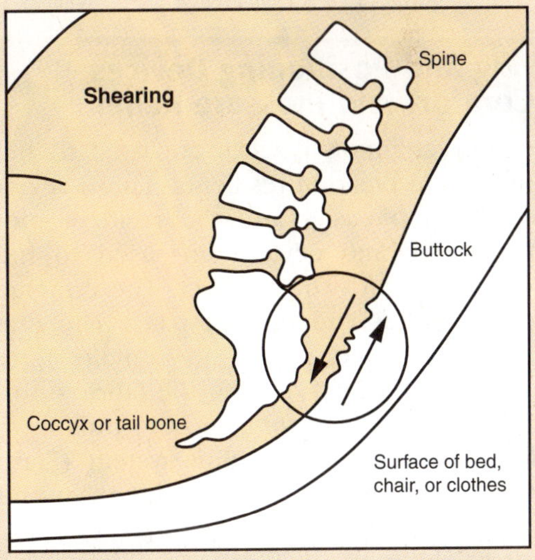

FIGURE 14-9 Shearing occurs when the skin is pulled in one direction while the underlying bone moves in the opposite direction. Many pressure ulcers develop because of shearing.

GUIDELINES FOR

Prevention of Pressure Ulcers, *Continued*

occurs when the skin moves in one direction while the underlying bones move in the opposite direction. The skin is stretched between the sheet (or other surface) on the outside and the bone on the inside.

- Use pressure-relieving pads in bed and chair.
- Pad areas of the resident's body where the skin or bones rub together.
- Use pillows, pads, and other props to maintain the resident's position.
- Inspect the resident's skin daily when bathing, dressing, and undressing. Report abnormal findings to the nurse.
- Check the skin folds under the breasts, abdomen, and groin for signs of redness or irritation. Dry these areas well after bathing.
- Follow the directions on the care plan for preventive skin care.
- Avoid elevating the head of the bed more than 45 degrees, to prevent shearing. If the head of the bed is elevated for any reason, help the resident change positions frequently to prevent pressure on the buttocks and hip area.
- Provide adequate nutrition to meet the resident's calorie and protein needs. Provide adequate fluids. Provide oral nourishments, supplements, and snacks as ordered.
- Wear gloves and apply the principles of standard precautions if contact with blood, moist body fluids (except sweat), secretions, excretions, mucous membranes, or nonintact skin is likely.

performing these procedures. In addition, positioning the resident in good alignment is very important. This means that the spine is straight and other parts of the body are in good position. When the resident is positioned correctly, function of the body systems is improved.

Moving and Positioning Devices for Comfort and Pressure Relief

Sometimes common devices are used to help you move and position residents. These devices make your job easier and the resident more comfortable. Some devices are used to help you physically turn the resident. These include the **draw sheet** and turning pads. The draw sheet is a half sheet placed horizontally across the center of the bed. Pulling the fabric on the sheet or pad is easier for you than pulling the resident. The bed positioning system (Figure 14.10) is similar to using a draw sheet. You pull the resident toward you, then place a long bolster to help maintain the position. Using these devices prevents accidental injury to the resident's skin and trauma to muscles, bones, and joints. The turning pad can be secured to the side rails after the move is completed to maintain the resident's position.

Foam wedges (Figure 14.11) are used to keep the resident in good alignment in bed. Sometimes residents will slip, move, or turn themselves after you have positioned them. Use of the foam wedge as a prop will help maintain the resident's position. They are also useful in preventing pressure ulcers.

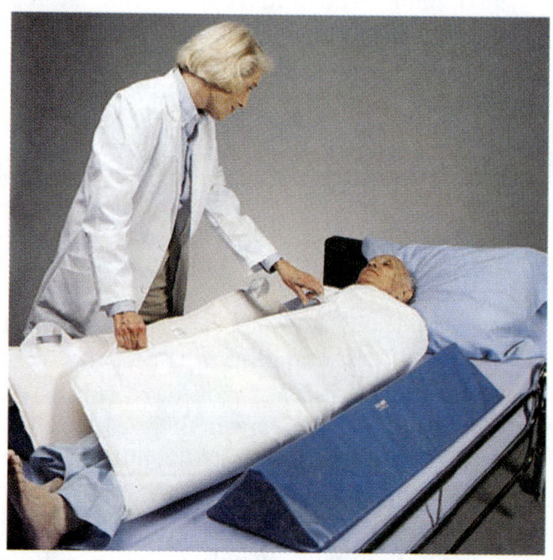

FIGURE 14-10 The bed positioning system is used for moving the resident. The positioning pad is inserted to maintain position, then Velcro fasteners are used to attach the pad to the bolster cushion. *(Courtesy of Skil-Care Corporation, Yonkers, NY (800) 431-2972)*

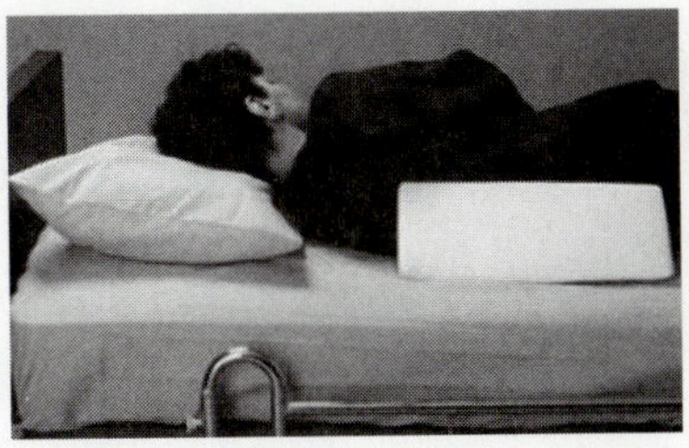

FIGURE 14-11 The foam wedge is used to support body parts and promote good alignment. *(Courtesy of Skil-Care Corporation, Yonkers, NY (800) 431-2972)*

Pillows may also be used to position residents. They are sometimes used when the resident is in a side-lying position, to prevent rolling over to the back. Small, flat pillows or a bath blanket may also be used as pads to prevent the knees and ankles from rubbing together when the resident is lying on his or her side. Commercial devices (Figure 14.12) are also available for this purpose. Pillows are also used to support the forearms and may be placed under the knees when the resident is lying on his or her back. Using pillows for positioning helps the resident feel more comfortable and secure. Sheepskins (Figure 14.13) are synthetic devices that can be used for padding bony areas. They may also be placed on the bed to promote resident comfort and prevent friction and shearing. Heel and elbow protectors (Figures 14.14A and 14.14B) also increase resident comfort and prevent friction and shearing. They do not relieve pressure.

A resident who is using a pressure-relieving pad or device still requires turning. Although some pressure is relieved, the devices do not remove it entirely, so further breakdown is possible. Commonly used pressure-relieving devices include:

- Foam heel elevators (Figure 14.15)
- Foam wedges, squares, and other foam pads
- Special foam, gel, air, and water mattresses, cushions, and overlays
- Low air loss and other therapeutic beds (Figure 14.16)
- Other devices used by your facility

Side rail pads (Figure 14.17) may be used for residents who are restless or have seizures, or diseases that cause involuntary movement of the

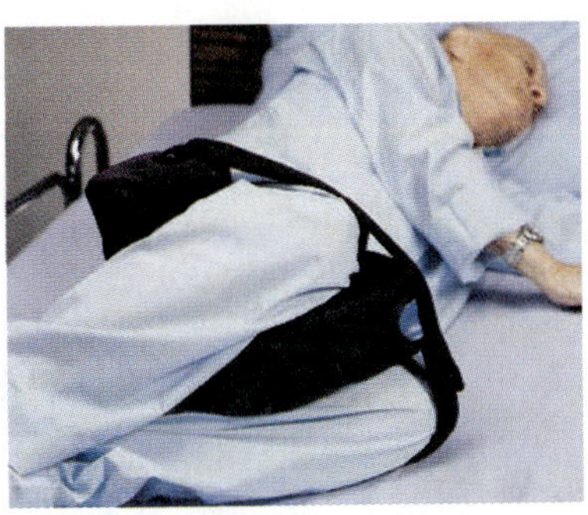

FIGURE 14-12 Keeping the legs apart will prevent pressure ulcers at the knees and ankles. The pad may also be used after some surgical procedures to position the legs. *(Courtesy of Skil-Care Corporation, Yonkers, NY (800) 431-2972)*

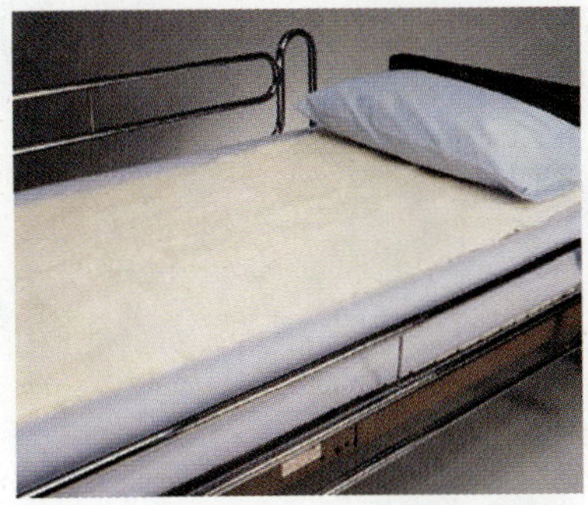

FIGURE 14-13 The sheepskin is used to prevent friction and shearing caused by skin surfaces rubbing against each other or against the sheet. It does not reduce pressure. *(Courtesy of Skil-Care Corporation, Yonkers, NY (800) 431-2972)*

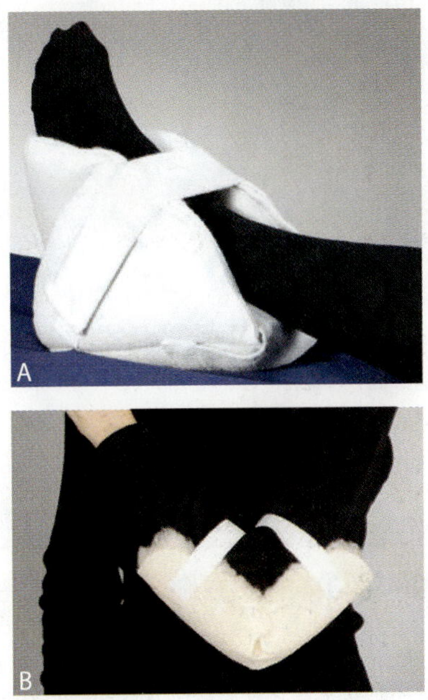

FIGURE 14-14 (A) Heel protectors and (B) elbow protectors are used to relieve pressure and prevent friction and shearing caused by rubbing against the linen. *(Courtesy of Skil-Care Corporation, Yonkers, NY (800) 431-2972)*

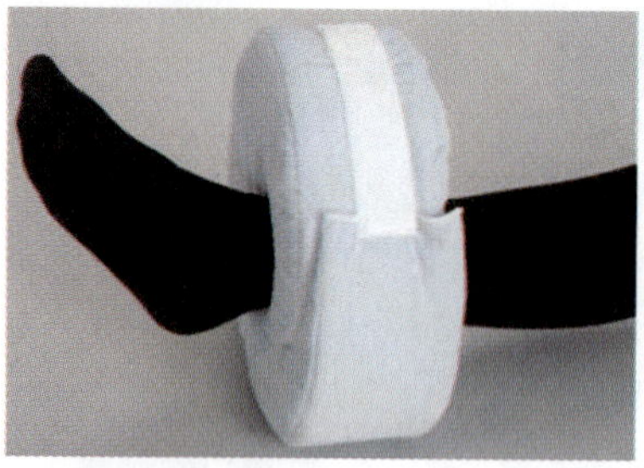

FIGURE 14-15 Foam heel elevators keep the heels off the surface of the bed, relieving all pressure. *(Courtesy of Skil-Care Corporation, Yonkers, NY (800) 431-2972)*

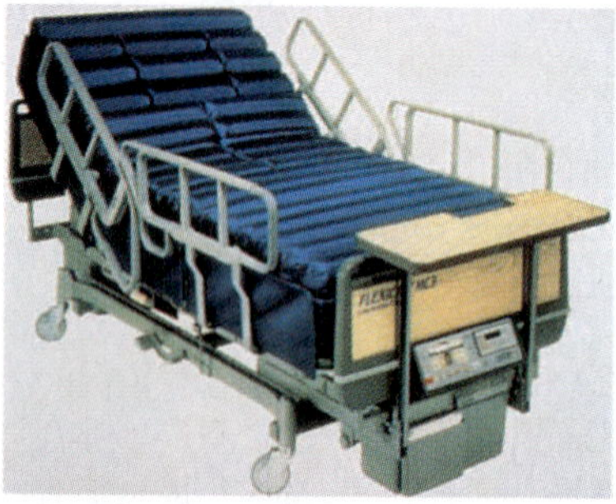

FIGURE 14-16 Low air loss and other therapeutic beds are used for residents with serious skin problems. *(Courtesy of Hill-Rom)*

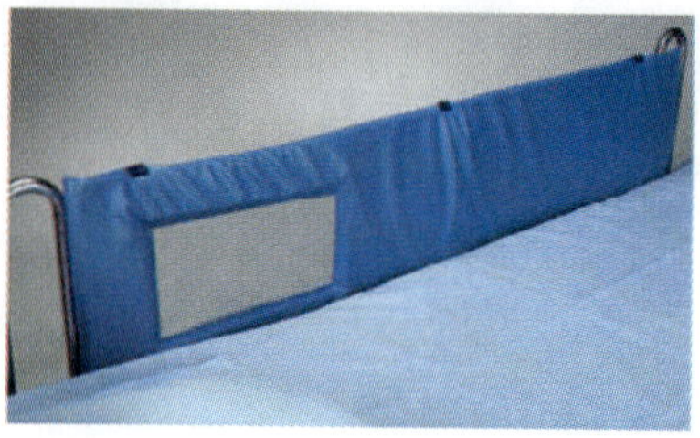

FIGURE 14-17 Side rail pads prevent serious injury. *(Courtesy of Skil-Care Corporation, Yonkers, NY (800) 431-2972)*

arms and legs. The pads prevent the resident from striking or slipping through the rails, causing injury.

The **bed cradle** is used to keep the weight of the bedding off the resident's skin. This device is made of metal or plastic and fastens to the bed to provide a frame. When the resident is in bed, the sheet and blanket are placed over the top of the cradle.

A wooden or plastic **foot board** may be used at the end of the mattress. A foot board is used to prevent pressure on the heels and to keep the feet upright so deformities do not develop. When a foot board is used, the heels

GUIDELINES FOR

Moving and Positioning Residents

- Evaluate the resident's ability to participate in the procedure. This involves the ability to follow directions and the ability to move, considering physical limitations.
- Ask another nursing assistant to help you if the resident is heavy, **combative** (hits or fights), unable to follow directions, unable to assist with the move, or larger than you are, or if you are unsure of your ability to move the resident alone.
- Know and follow your facility policies for positioning. In some facilities, a doctor's order is required to use certain positions.
- Consult the care plan or the nurse for specific turning and positioning instructions.
- Some facilities use "turn schedules," which specify designated positions at certain times for the resident. Follow the individual turn schedule for each resident.
- Use good body mechanics.
- Encourage residents to participate in care to the extent of their ability. Before beginning the procedure, make sure that residents understand what is expected and how to do it.
- Draw sheets, lifting sheets, and similar devices should be used whenever possible to avoid friction, shearing, and pulling on the resident's skin. Using a lift sheet to move residents helps prevent back strain for the nursing assistant as well.
- Use mechanical lifting devices, if needed.
- Use smooth, easy motions. Do not tug or jerk the resident over quickly.
- Avoid trauma and injury to the resident during the procedure.
- Use pillows, props, or other devices to maintain position, if necessary.

- Pad bony areas, such as between the knees and ankles, to prevent discomfort and skin breakdown caused by the skin surfaces rubbing together.
- Position the resident in good body alignment. The spine should be straight and supported. Sometimes residents curl up into a **fetal position** (turned on the side with the head tucked down and knees drawn up) to stay warm, or because they are in pain. If possible, identify the cause of the problem and correct it. Lying in this position for a prolonged period of time greatly increases the risk of complications. If you discover a method of positioning that reduces a resident's use of the fetal position, inform the nurse so the information can be added to the care plan.
- Support the arms, legs, or back with pillows, if needed for resident comfort. Special supportive devices may be listed on the care plan to maintain good body alignment. If so, make sure they are in place.
- Avoid tucking in the top linen too tightly. This pushes the feet downward, increasing the risk of deformities.
- If you are using a new position with a resident for the first time, check the resident frequently to be sure the position will be well tolerated.
- Monitor the location of catheters and tubing and avoid pulling them or accidentally dislodging them. After the move, position them correctly so they are not obstructed and do not put pressure on skin.
- Change the resident's position at least every two hours, and more often if indicated.
- Accurately document turning and repositioning on the flow sheet, or according to facility policy. Avoid documenting in advance. Do not document care that you did not provide. Documentation of turning and positioning residents is very important. Accurate documentation verifies that care was given as ordered, and according to the plan of care.

PROCEDURE 93 Moving the Resident to the Side of the Bed

1. Perform your beginning procedure actions.
2. Cross the resident's arms over the chest.
3. Place your upper hand, palm side up, under the resident's shoulders.
4. Place your lower hand, palm side up, under the mid back.
5. Lift the upper part of the body toward the near side of the bed.
6. Place your hands under the resident's waist and thighs.
7. Lift the middle section of the body toward the near side of the bed.
8. Place your hands under the thighs and lower legs and lift them toward you.
9. Perform your procedure completion actions.

hang over the end of the mattress and the sole of the foot rests against the board. Other devices are available that perform the same function as the foot board. These are applied directly to the resident's foot.

Basic Body Positions

Four basic body positions are used for positioning residents in bed. These are the **supine** (face up), **lateral** (side-lying), **Fowler's** (semisitting), and

PROCEDURE

94 Turning the Resident on the Side Toward You

1. Perform your beginning procedure actions.
2. Move the resident to the opposite side of the bed, if necessary.
3. Cross the resident's arms over the chest.
4. Cross the leg farthest away from you over the near leg.
5. Place your top hand behind the resident's far shoulder. Place your bottom hand on the resident's hip (Figure 14.18A).
6. Instruct the resident to assist with the move by pulling on the side rail with the far hand, according the plan of care, and as able. Keep your feet and knees separated to maintain a wide base of support. Brace your body against the side of the bed. Roll the resident toward you.
7. Raise the side rail and move to the opposite side of the bed.
8. Lower the side rail.
9. Place your hands under the resident's bottom shoulder and pull back slightly toward the center of the bed. The resident should not be lying directly on the shoulder. Repeat this action for the resident's hips (Figure 14.18B).

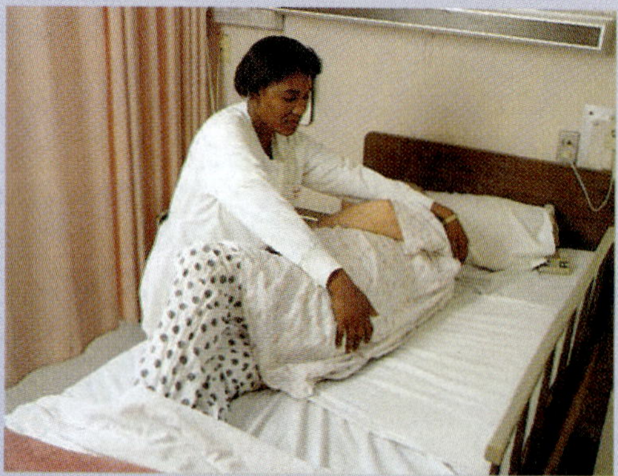

FIGURE 14-18A Place one hand on the shoulder and the other on the hip.

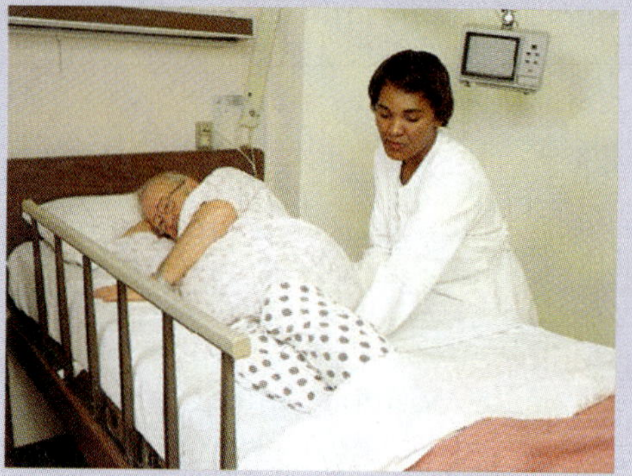

FIGURE 14-18B Pull the shoulder and hip back slightly so the resident is not lying directly on them.

10. Roll a pillow or place a positioning device behind the resident's back to maintain the position, if necessary.
11. Raise the side rail and return to the opposite side of the bed.
12. Lower the rail.
13. Bend the resident's knees slightly. The upper leg should be positioned slightly ahead of the lower leg. Place a pillow or folded bath blanket from the knees to the ankles to keep the legs from rubbing together (Figure 14.18C).

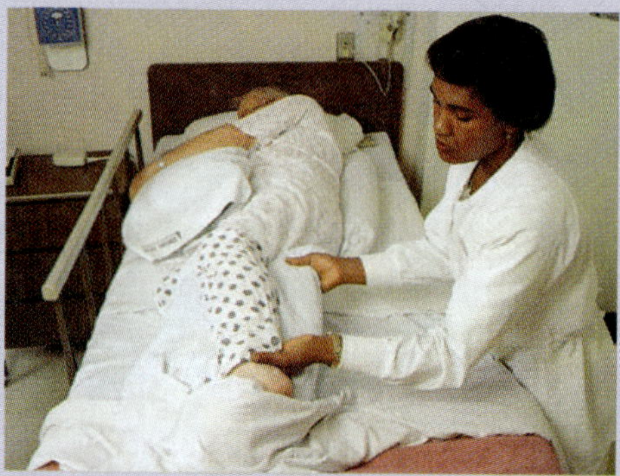

FIGURE 14-18C Place a pillow or pad between the legs for comfort and to prevent pressure.

14. Place a pillow under the resident's upper arm, if necessary, for support.

15. Check the lower arm to be sure it is not under the resident. If the resident is not able to move the arm, place it in a position of comfort at the side of the body or bent at the elbow with the hand by the head. Make sure the resident's body is in good alignment.

16. Perform your procedure completion actions.

PROCEDURE 95 Turning the Resident on the Side Toward you with a Lift Sheet

1. Arrange for another assistant to help you, as needed.
2. Perform your beginning procedure actions.
3. Make sure that a draw sheet or large pad is in place from the resident's shoulders to the knees. If not, turn the resident on the side facing you. Your assistant should put the draw sheet in position, then roll it in toward the resident's body.
4. Ask your assistant to turn the resident toward him or her. Pull the end of the lifting sheet to your side of the bed.
5. Coordinate the move with your assistant to prevent friction and shearing. Obtain additional help if necessary.
6. On a signal, use the sheet to move the resident to the far side of the bed, to provide enough space for the turn.
7. Cross the resident's arms over the chest.
8. Cross the leg farthest away from you over the near leg.
9. Roll the lifting sheet inward on the opposite side of the resident, so it is close to the body. Place your top hand on the sheet behind the resident's far shoulder. Place your bottom hand on the sheet near the resident's hip. Keep your feet and knees separated to maintain a wide base of support. Brace your body against the side of the bed.
10. Pull on the sheet to roll the resident toward you. *Note:* An alternate method is to position one hand on the resident's shoulder and the other on the hip. On a signal, turn the resident toward you while the other nursing assistant uses the lift sheet to roll the resident.
11. Raise the side rail and move to the opposite side of the bed. (If present, the second nursing assistant performs steps 13 and 14).
12. Lower the side rail.
13. Place your hands under the resident's bottom shoulder and pull back slightly toward the center of the bed. The resident should not be lying directly on the shoulder. Repeat this action for the resident's hips.
14. Grasp the draw sheet on the opposite side of the resident at the hips and shoulders. Hold the resident on the side facing you while the second nursing assistant rolls a pillow or places a positioning device behind the resident's back (under the draw sheet) to maintain the position, if necessary. Straighten the sheet to remove wrinkles.

PROCEDURE 95 Turning the Resident on the Side Toward you with a Lift Sheet, *continued*

15. Bend the resident's knees slightly. Position the upper leg slightly ahead of the lower leg. Place a small, flat pillow or folded bath blanket from the knees to the ankles to keep the legs from rubbing together.
16. Place a pillow under the resident's upper arm, if necessary, for support.
17. Check the lower arm to be sure it is not under the resident. If the resident is not able to move the arm, place it in a position of comfort at the side of the body, or bent at the elbow with the hand by the head.
18. Perform your procedure completion actions.

PROCEDURE 96 Turning the Resident on the Side Away from You

1. Perform your beginning procedure actions.
2. Move the resident to the side of the bed, if necessary.
3. Bend the resident's far arm at the elbow, so the hand is near the head. Cross the near arm over the chest.
4. Cross the near leg over the far leg.
5. Place your top hand on the resident's shoulder and your bottom hand on the hip. Turn the resident on the side facing away from you.
6. Roll a pillow or place a positioning device behind the resident's back to maintain the position, if necessary.
7. Raise the side rail and move to the opposite side of the bed.
8. Lower the side rail.
9. Bend the resident's knees slightly. The upper leg should be positioned slightly ahead of the lower leg. Place a pillow or folded bath blanket between the knees, calves, and ankles to keep them from rubbing together.
10. Place a pillow under the resident's upper arm, if necessary, for support.
11. Check the lower arm to be sure it is not under the resident.
12. Perform your procedure completion actions.

prone (lying on the abdomen) positions. The semi-prone and semisupine positions are variations of these positions and are excellent for relieving pressure and preventing pressure ulcers. Fowler's position also has several variations. Variations in Fowler's position are determined by the height of the head of the bed. Special positions may be used if the resident has

PROCEDURE 97 Assisting the Resident to Move to the Head of the Bed

1. Perform your beginning procedure actions.
2. Lower the head of the bed.
3. Remove the pillow and place it against the head-board.
4. Instruct the resident to bend the knees and place the feet flat on the bed. The arms should be at the sides with elbows bent.
5. Place your top arm under the shoulders.
6. Place your bottom arm under the hips.
7. On the count of three, instruct the resident to push up with the elbows and feet while you lift.
8. Replace the pillow and straighten the bed linen.
9. Perform your procedure completion actions.

PROCEDURE 98 Moving the Resident to the Head of the Bed with a Lifting (Draw) Sheet

1. Ask another nursing assistant to assist you.
2. Perform your beginning procedure actions.
3. Lower the head of the bed.
4. Lower the side rails.
5. Remove the pillow and place it against the headboard.
6. Roll the lift sheet inward until it touches the resident's body (Figure 14.19).
7. Grasp the lift sheet with your top hand at the level of the resident's shoulder and your bottom hand at the hip.
8. Face the head of the bed. On the count of three, shift your weight from the rear foot to the front foot and lift the resident toward the head of the bed.
9. Replace the pillow.
10. Straighten the lift sheet.
11. Perform your procedure completion actions.

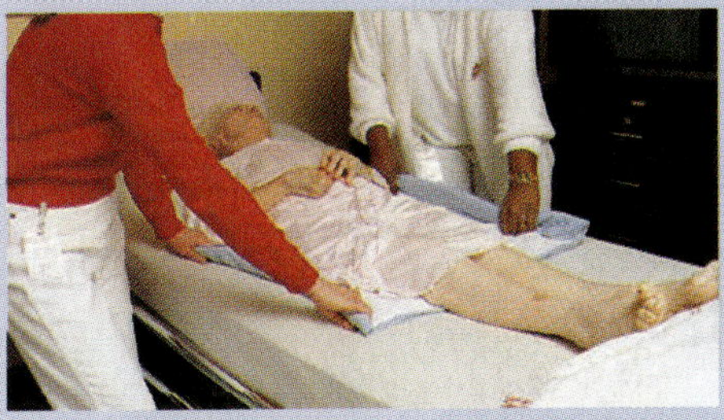

FIGURE 14-19 Roll the lift sheet inward until it touches the resident's body.

PROCEDURE 99 Moving the Resident Up in Bed with One Assistant

1. Ask another nursing assistant to help you.
2. Perform your beginning procedure actions.
3. Lower the head of the bed.
4. Lower the side rails.
5. Remove the pillow and place it against the headboard.
6. Place your top arm under the resident's shoulders and your bottom arm under the resident's hips. Your assistant should do the same.
7. Grasp arms with your assistant.
8. Face the head of the bed. On the count of three, shift your weight from the rear foot to the front foot and lift the resident toward the head of the bed.
9. Replace the pillow.
10. Perform your procedure completion actions.

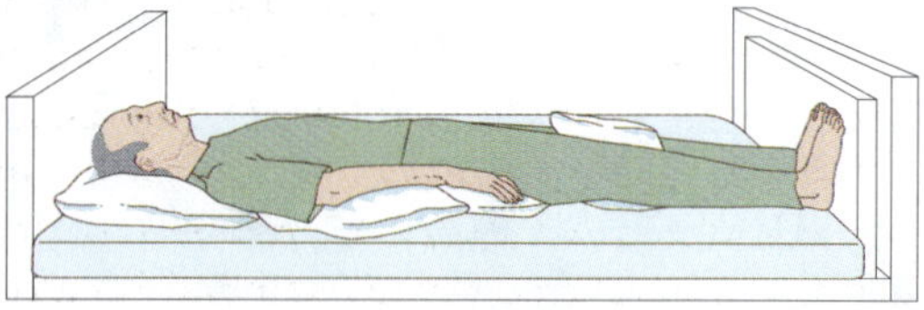

FIGURE 14-20 When the resident is in the supine

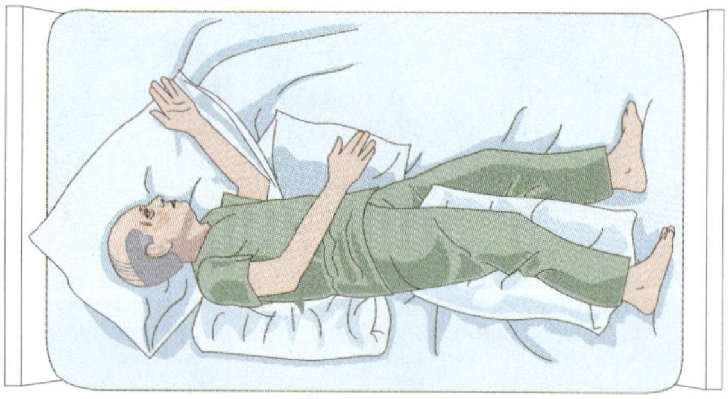

FIGURE 14-21 The semisupine position is a very comfortable position that relieves pressure from all major bony prominences.

special medical needs. The care plan and the nurse will provide specific instructions if special positioning is necessary.

Supine Position

The resident in the supine position (Figure 14.20) is lying on the back. This position may be preferred for sleeping. When the body is in good alignment, the resident's head and shoulders are supported on a pillow. The spine is straight. The arms are at the sides. They may be supported on pillows for comfort. The legs are straight. A pillow may be placed behind the knees for comfort. The feet are upright. A foot board or other supportive device may be used at the end of the bed.

Semisupine Position

The **semisupine position** (Figure 14.21) is also called the tilt position. It should not be confused with the lateral position. The resident in this position is not lying directly on the side. When correctly used, this position relieves pressure from all bony prominences. The spine is straight and the resident is positioned so that he or she is leaning against a pillow for support. Both legs are straight. The top leg is slightly behind the bottom leg. A pillow is placed under the top leg to keep it even with the hip joint. The lower shoulder is pulled slightly forward so that pressure is distributed over the back, not the shoulder joint. The arms can be at the sides or folded across the abdomen. Support the arms on pillows for comfort.

Prone Position

The resident in the prone position (Figure 14.22) is lying on the abdomen. Some elderly residents cannot tolerate this position. Some

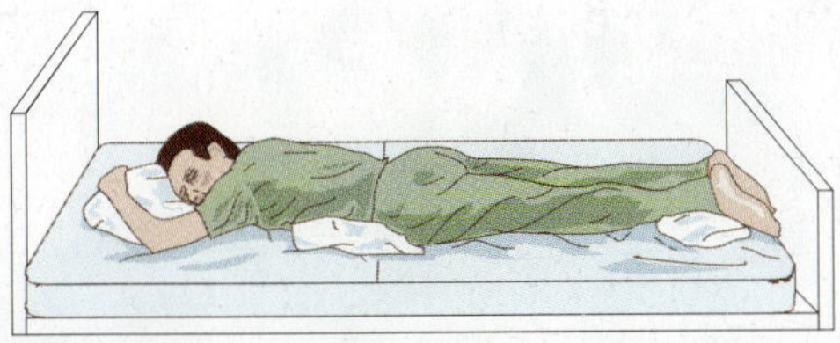

FIGURE 14-22 Check the resident frequently when using the prone position.

facilities do not use the prone position without a physician's order. Know and follow your facility policy. When using the position for the first time, remain in the room for the first 15 minutes to make sure the resident tolerates the position without distress. After this, routinely check every 15 minutes to be sure the resident continues to tolerate the position and is not having difficulty breathing. Make sure the call signal or a manual bell is close to the resident's dominant hand.

When positioning the resident in the prone position, turn the head to one side. A small, flat pillow may be used under the head. Additional padding may be used under the shoulders if they roll forward. The arms should be along the sides, or one arm bent so the hand is next to the head. Both arms should not be up, as this strains the shoulder muscles. Another flat pillow may be placed under the abdomen for comfort. The spine is straight. The legs are straight. The feet should be positioned so the toes are between the mattress and the end of the bed. A small pad may be used to keep pressure off the ankles.

The Semiprone Position (SIMS')

The **semiprone position** (Figure 14.23) is the opposite of the semisupine position. It is a very comfortable position for the resident. Like the semisupine position, it eliminates pressure on the major areas of pressure ulcer formation. To place the resident in the semiprone position, begin by placing the resident prone. Lift the resident's chest and shoulder closest to you and place a pillow under them.

If the resident has had a stroke, put the affected (paralyzed) side on top, if possible. Support the affected arm on a pillow, in a position of function with the elbow bent. Position the opposite arm behind the resident. Fold a second pillow in half and place it under the top leg. Check to make sure the legs and spine are straight, and the pelvis is not twisted. Check the hip to make sure the resident is not lying on it. Position a pillow lengthwise under the resident from the chest to the abdomen. Support the upper leg on a pillow. Turn the resident's head to either side and place it on a small, flat pillow. Avoid a large, fluffy pillow, which may inhibit the resident's breathing.

Follow your facility policies for using the semiprone position. Like the prone position, some facilities require a doctor's order for this position. When using this position for the first time, remain in the room for the first 15 minutes to be sure the resident tolerates the position without respiratory distress. After that, check the resident at least every 15 minutes to make sure he or she is not having trouble breathing. Position the call signal close to the resident's unaffected (good) hand.

Lateral Position

A resident in the lateral position (Figure 14.24) is lying on either side. The spine is straight. The bottom shoulder and hip are pulled slightly forward so that there is no pressure directly on the joint. A pillow may be rolled behind the back to hold the resident in this position. The arms can be positioned where they are most comfortable for the resident.

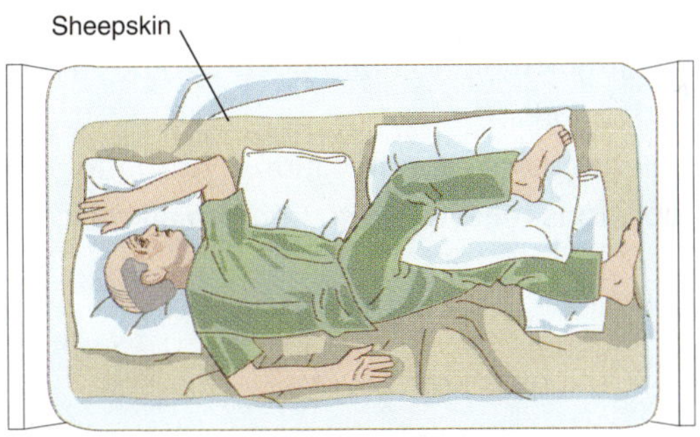

FIGURE 14-23 The semiprone position is very comfortable for the resident (SIMS').

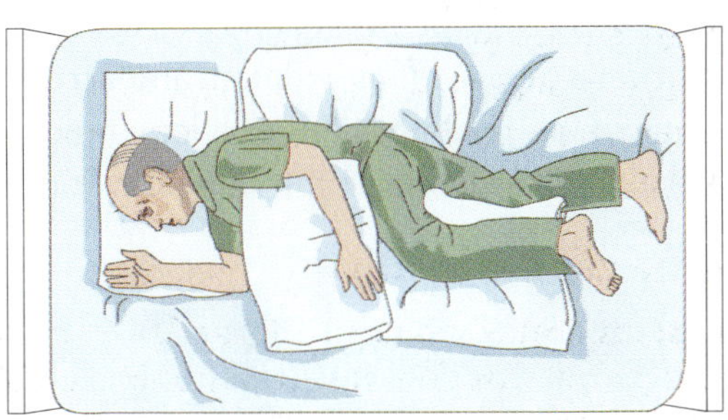

FIGURE 14-24 Use pillows to support the resident in the lateral position.

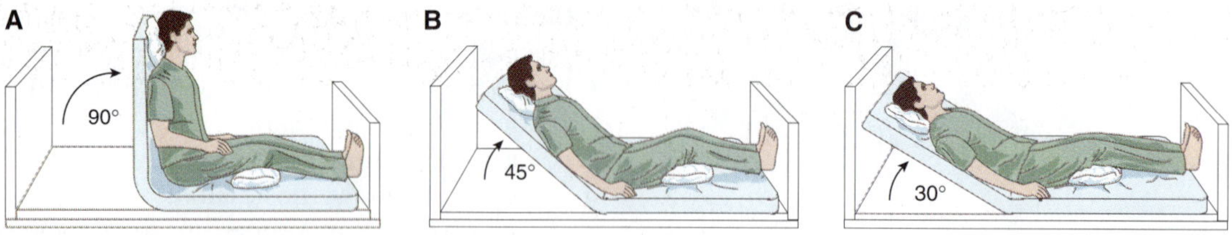

FIGURE 14-25 (A) High Fowler's position is used for meals and for residents who have difficulty breathing. (B) Fowler's position. (C) Semi-Fowler's position.

Usually, the elbow of the bottom arm is flexed and the hand placed near the head. The upper arm is folded across the abdomen and supported on a pillow. The upper leg is flexed and pulled slightly ahead of the bottom leg. A pillow is used to support the upper leg and keep the knees from rubbing together.

Fowler's Position

A resident in Fowler's position is lying on the back with the head elevated. This position is used for residents who are receiving tube feedings, or having difficulty breathing. The knee of the bed may also be elevated slightly for comfort. This position places extra pressure on the resident's buttocks and spine and increases the risk of pressure ulcer formation, so careful attention must be paid to skin care. You may be directed to position residents in three different Fowler's positions (Figure 14.25):

- High Fowler's position—the head of the bed is elevated 90 degrees
- Fowler's position—the head of the bed is elevated 45 degrees
- Low Fowler's position—the head of the bed is elevated 30 degrees

KEY POINTS

- Good body mechanics are used when lifting and moving residents and other heavy objects.
- Ergonomics is a method of fitting the job to the worker to prevent injuries.
- Residents must always be positioned in good body alignment.
- The primary cause of pressure ulcers is lack of oxygen and circulation to the skin, caused by pressure.
- Pressure ulcers are easier to prevent than to treat.
- Wearing a back support belt does not make you stronger; avoid lifting more weight than you would if you were not wearing the belt.
- Pressure ulcers are declines; most pressure ulcers are preventable.
- Residents with current pressure ulcers or a history of healed pressure ulcers are at high risk for additional skin breakdown.
- Documentation of turning and positioning residents is very important; accurate documentation verifies that care was given as ordered, and according to the plan of care.
- Lying in the fetal position for a long time greatly increases the risk of complications.
- Positioning residents in the semiprone and semisupine positions relieves pressure from all major bony prominences.

REVIEW

A. Multiple Choice

Select the one best answer.

1. Using your body correctly to do the job is good body
   a. maintenance.
   b. mechanisms.
   c. muscles.
   d. mechanics.
2. Your strongest muscles are in the
   a. back.
   b. abdomen.
   c. legs.
   d. shoulders.
3. Using your body correctly involves
   a. keeping your feet eight inches apart.
   b. using the strong muscles in your legs when lifting.
   c. lifting heavy objects instead of pushing them.
   d. bending from the waist and knees.
4. Which of the following is true about pressure ulcers?
   a. They are the result of inadequate blood and oxygen to the skin.
   b. Pressure ulcers take a long time to develop.
   c. Infections are not a consideration in preventing pressure ulcers.
   d. Pressure ulcers usually heal quickly.
5. A Stage II pressure ulcer may
   a. be a large, red area with intact skin.
   b. look like a blister or abrasion.
   c. involve the subcutaneous fat.
   d. involve muscle, tendon, and bone.
6. A Stage IV pressure ulcer
   a. is a large, red area with intact skin.
   b. looks like a blister or abrasion.
   c. involves only the top layer of skin.
   d. involves muscle, tendon, and bone.
7. A pressure ulcer in the early stages of development on a person with dark skin may appear
   a. black.
   b. pink.
   c. red.
   d. gray.
8. Which of the following measures prevents pressure ulcers?
   a. Turning the resident every four hours.
   b. Padding areas where bones and skin rub together.
   c. Using the Fowler's position.
   d. Positioning the resident on bony prominces.
9. When moving and positioning residents, the nursing assistant should *always*
   a. use the mechanical lift.
   b. use a gait belt.
   c. avoid friction and shearing.
   d. elevate the head of the bed.
10. Residents should be repositioned every
    a. two hours.
    b. three hours.
    c. four hours.
    d. shift.
11. Millie Davis is an obese, dependent resident. You are assigned to move her up in bed. Mrs. Davis has a pressure ulcer on her left hip. The best way to move her is to
    a. lift the resident by yourself.
    b. lift her on a draw sheet with one or more helpers.
    c. ask another assistant to lift the hips while you lift the feet.
    d. use a mechanical lift.
12. A resident in the supine position is lying
    a. face up.
    b. face down.
    c. on the abdomen.
    d. on the side.
13. A resident in the prone position is lying on the
    a. back.
    b. abdomen.
    c. left side.
    d. right side.

14. The nurse asks you to place Mr. Kay in Fowler's position while his tube feeding is running. You know the head of the bed should be elevated
    a. 15 degrees.
    b. 30 degrees.
    c. 45 degrees.
    d. 90 degrees.
15. The resident in the lateral position is lying
    a. face up.
    b. face down.
    c. with the head elevated.
    d. on the side.

B. Short-Answer

Answer the following questions.

16–20. List five methods the nursing assistant can use to prevent pressure ulcers.

16. ______________________
17. ______________________
18. ______________________
19. ______________________
20. ______________________

21–30. List 10 rules of good body mechanics.

21. ______________________
22. ______________________
23. ______________________
24. ______________________
25. ______________________
26. ______________________
27. ______________________
28. ______________________
29. ______________________
30. ______________________

C. Clinical Applications

Answer the following questions.

31. Martha Harris is an underweight, dependent resident. The care plan states that she is at high risk for skin breakdown and must be turned and repositioned every hour. It is very difficult to maintain Martha's position because she turns herself over onto her back as soon as you leave the room. You changed Martha's position at 9 a.m. When you left the room, she was on her right side. You got busy and forgot to return exactly at 10 a.m. When you returned at 10:30, Martha was lying on her back. When you turned her onto her left side, you noticed a very red area on her coccyx. What action should you take?
32. You must turn and reposition Mr. Taylor in bed. Mr. Taylor is very heavy and is more than six feet tall. He is unable to assist in the move. The care plan states to use a draw sheet to turn the resident, then place pillows behind his back for support. Mr. Taylor has slipped down in bed and needs to be moved up to the head of the bed before he is turned. What should you do?
33. You are assigned to position Mrs. Strong in the prone position. This position has never been used for the resident before. After you position the resident on her abdomen, what should you do next? How often should you check on her?
34. It is almost time to leave for the day when you discover that one of your assigned residents is wet and soiled. You change and clean the resident and discover a new open area that looks like a Stage II pressure ulcer. You did not notice the open area this morning. After cleaning the resident, you plan to report your observation to the nurse. The nurses are in report. Your ride is waiting outside. What action will you take?
35. You are assigned to give Mr. Walecki a shower. He has a loose dressing covering a pressure ulcer on his hip. The tape has fallen off two sides of the dressing. What action will you take?

UNIT 15

Restraints

OBJECTIVES

After reading this unit, you will be able to:

- Spell and define key terms.
- Define restraints and list six reasons for using restraints.
- Describe when and how restraints are used as enablers.
- List the guidelines for using restraints.
- List the complications of restraint use.
- Define restraint alternative and describe when to use an alternative device.
- Demonstrate procedures related to restraints and restraint alternatives.

OBSERVATIONS TO MAKE AND REPORT RELATED TO RESTRAINTS AND RESTRAINT ALTERNATIVES

Need for Restraints or Restraint Alternatives

Decreased ability to see or hear
Lack of connection to or awareness of environment
Use of corrective devices and aids
Lack of communication ability
Agitation
Situation-specific problem behaviors
Discomfort
Loneliness, isolation, boredom
Need for assistance in standing or ambulation
Falls

During Restraint Use

Decreased independence, increased dependence on staff
Impaired circulation, skin breakdown
Pressure ulcers
Weakness
Decreased range of motion
Muscle atrophy (wasting)
Contractures
Decreased ability to ambulate
Edema
Decreased appetite
Weight loss
Distended abdomen
Incontinence Constipation or fecal impaction
Increased or new-onset mental confusion
Lethargy
Restlessness
Crying, screaming, yelling
Depression
Irritability
Agitation, combativeness
Withdrawal
Forgetfulness
Ritualistic behavior

RESTRAINTS

Restraints are safety devices attached to or adjacent to the resident's body. Reasons for using restraints include:

- To prevent injury and falls.
- To prevent the resident from injuring himself or herself, or others.
- To prevent pulling on tubes, drains, wound coverings, or other forms of treatment.
- To maintain position when the resident is in bed or in a chair. Some residents are repositioned by staff, but quickly reposition themselves, causing complications or skin problems. Use of a restraint helps maintain position in some situations.
- To support the resident in good anatomical alignment to prevent discomfort and deformity.

Restraints are most commonly used to prevent falls and wandering, and to protect residents from injury. Some residents are unaware of hazards in the environment and unknowingly jeopardize their own safety as well as the safety of others.

Definition of Restraints

Restraints are physical, manual, or mechanical devices attached or adjacent to the resident's body. They cannot be removed easily by the resident and prevent access to the body. Restraints restrict freedom of movement. They are used to prevent injury to the resident and others, and allow medical treatment when the resident is confused and uncooperative. Restraints *may not* be used to force alert residents to accept specific treatments. Refusing a treatment is the resident's right, and a restraint is not used to administer treatment that an alert resident does not want. A physician's order is always needed for the use of restraints.

Physical restraints (Figure 15.1) are devices applied to the resident's body or chairs that prevent the resident from standing. Side rails are physical restraints. Many devices can be considered restraints, even those that are marketed as restraint alternatives. A device is considered a restraint if:

- It restricts access to the resident's body
- It restricts movement

  or
- The resident does not have the physical or mental ability to remove it easily

Examples of restraints, using this definition, are:

- Raising side rails to prevent a resident from voluntarily getting out of bed
- Tucking in or using Velcro to hold a sheet, fabric, lap blanket, or clothing tightly so that a resident's movement is restricted
- Using devices in conjunction with a chair, such as overbed tables, trays, tables, pads, bars, or belts, that the resident cannot remove easily and that prevent the resident from rising
- Placing a resident in a chair that prevents the resident from rising, such as a beanbag chair, reclining chair, or geriatric chair
- Placing a chair or bed so close to a wall that the wall prevents the resident from rising out of the chair or voluntarily getting out of bed

Chemical restraints are drugs used for discipline and staff convenience and not required to treat a resident's medical symptoms. Tranquilizers and mood-altering drugs are chemical restraints. In some residents these drugs have the opposite effect from that intended. Instead of calming the resident, they may cause agitation. They also may make the resident very lethargic. Side effects from long-term use of these drugs can be very serious. Licensed nurses and advanced care providers are responsible for medication administration. This chapter will focus on the use of physical restraints.

Enablers are devices that empower residents and assist them to function at their highest possible level. For example, a resident in a wheelchair is unable to sit up straight to feed himself or herself, so he or she is fed by staff. If a supportive device is applied to correct his or her posture and allow the resident to feed himself or herself, the device is an enabler. Devices used as enablers that maintain body position and alignment are commonly called **postural supports**. Used correctly, they give residents a higher degree of independence and enable them to perform tasks they were previously unable to do. In this case, using the restraint improves the resident's self-esteem.

The wheelchair lap tray (Figure 15.2) is a simple-to-use restraint alternative that is also used as an enabler. The tray is attached to the back of the wheelchair with Velcro straps. It can be used for residents to lean on, and it provides a surface

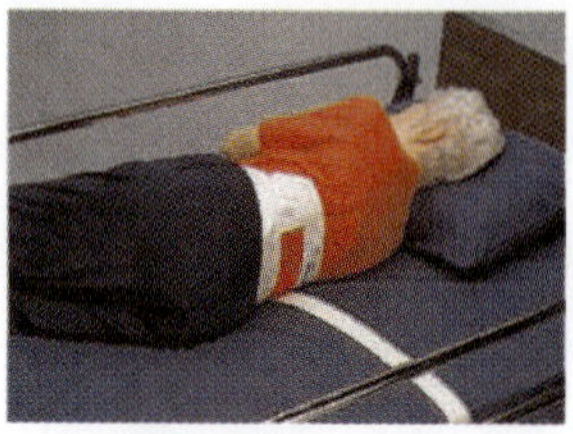

FIGURE 15-1 Physical restraints limit the resident's movement and access to her body. *(Courtesy of Skil-Care Corporation, Yonkers, NY (800) 431-2972)*

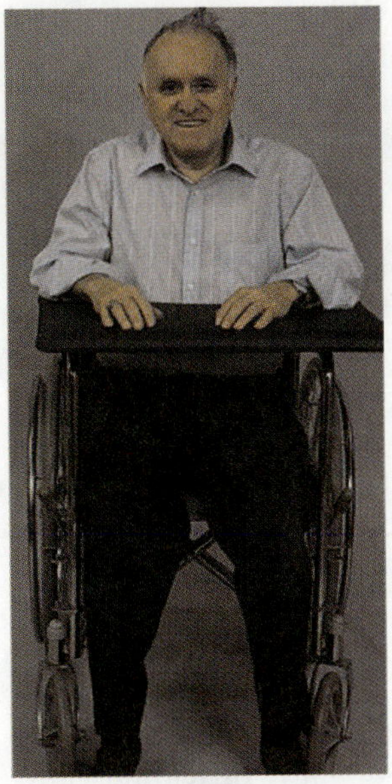

FIGURE 15-2 The Velcro lap tray is used as an enabler, restraint alternative, or restraint, depending on the resident's physical and mental ability. Some residents will push on the tray, releasing the Velcro straps. Because of this, using a lightweight tray is best. Heavy trays may cause injury to the legs and feet. *(Courtesy of Skil-Care Corporation, Yonkers, NY (800) 431-2972)*

to hold personal items and reading and writing supplies. A tray may enable the resident to feed himself or herself by moving the food closer so the resident can reach it. The tray serves as a reminder to the resident not to stand up. If the tray allows the resident to perform a task, it is an enabler. If it is used strictly to keep the resident in the chair, and the resident does not have the physical or mental ability to remove the tray, it is considered a restraint. If the tray can be removed by the resident, it is a restraint alternative.

Using Restraints

Unfortunately, most restraints are not used as enablers. They are commonly used to manage behavior problems, prevent wandering, and prevent falls. Several studies have shown that injuries related to falls are more severe in residents who are under restraint, compared with residents who are not restrained. Because residents tend to fight restraints, their behavior may be more aggressive than it was before the restraint was applied.

Before restraints are used, the staff must evaluate the resident's capabilities and the reasons for the restraint. If the reason for the resident's problem can be determined and corrected, the need for a restraint can be eliminated. For example, if use of restraints is being considered to prevent the resident from falling, all risk factors associated with falls are assessed. If some risk factors can be eliminated, this reduces the risk of falls, and restraint use may not be necessary. For example, the evaluation reveals that the resident rushes to the bathroom and loses his balance, falling along the way. A urinalysis reveals a urinary tract infection, which is treated. A care plan is developed based on the resident's needs and risk factors. The care plan states:

- The urinal must always be within reach
- Staff must check the resident hourly and offer to take him to the bathroom
- A second urinal must be placed in a cabinet next to the chair where the resident sits to watch television
- A hand bell must be placed by the resident's chair so he can call for help easily

Eliminating these risk factors reduces the risk of falls. Once the care plan is initiated, the resident stops trying to go to the bathroom by himself and the falls stop. The need for restraints has been eliminated by meeting the resident's individual needs. No single approach will be effective in eliminating the use of restraints for all residents. The answer lies in identifying and meeting each resident's needs.

If a resident is a danger to himself or herself, or to others, or requires emergency medical treatment, restraints may be appropriate. However, less restrictive alternatives to restraints must be considered first. Sometimes the environment can be modified to avoid restraint use. Many alternative devices are available for use instead of restraints. If a restraint is determined to be the best approach, it is applied. However, the factors necessitating use of the restraint are continuously reevaluated, and the interdisciplinary team works to reduce or eliminate the need for the restraint.

If the interdisciplinary team determines that restraints are needed, the least restrictive restraint required to keep the resident safe should be selected. The restraint should be used as infrequently as possible. Using restraints requires careful assessment, care planning, and monitoring by members of the interdisciplinary team. Studies have proven that it takes more time to care for residents in restraints compared with residents who are not restrained. The physician must agree to the use of restraints and write an order before they can be used. The care plan will specify the type of restraint to use, the time the restraint is to be applied, and other special information and instructions.

Although a physician's order is needed for the use of restraints, there must be a medical reason for their use. The decision to use restraints is a joint one made by facility staff, the resident (if alert), responsible family members, and the physician. Family members cannot demand that a facility use restraints unless the resident has a valid, documented medical problem that necessitates the restraint. Restraint assessment must be done except in an emergency. Dealing with family members' emotions and threats may take the skills of the entire interdisciplinary team. Restraint requests can present a very delicate situation for the facility. The outcome can be negative if this request is not handled correctly. If a family member asks you to apply a restraint to a resident, inform the nurse promptly.

Factors to Evaluate and Risk Factors to Eliminate

The nursing assistant makes a valuable contribution to the interdisciplinary team's restraint assessment. Because you have the most direct contact with the residents, you may be in the best position to know what does and doesn't work in managing the problem that creates the need for the restraint.

Many commercial devices are available to use in place of restraints. Sometimes clothing or other items can be used as restraint alternatives. For example, a male resident who pulls at his urinary catheter can be fitted with boxer shorts. A resident with a feeding tube can be covered with a t-shirt or abdominal binder. A resident with an intravenous infusion in the arm can wear a long-sleeved shirt or skin sleeve. Covering the medical device may be all that is necessary to keep the resident from pulling on it. Previously, wrist restraints would have been used routinely to keep the resident from dislodging tubes. Giving the resident something to hold, such as a Nerf ball, will occupy the hands and serve as a distraction. The nursing assistant plays an important role in knowing the residents' needs and making recommendations for restraint alternatives. Making sure the resident is in touch with his or her environment reduces agitation and confusion. Simply ensuring that the resident can see or hear well may improve mental orientation. Other observations that will help eliminate the need for restraints are:

- Does the resident see and hear well? Does the resident normally wear glasses? Is he or she wearing them now? Are they clean? Does the hearing aid work? Are the resident's ears plugged with wax? Sometimes behavior problems, balance problems, and other safety issues are caused because the resident is out of touch with the environment. Applying these simple corrective devices may eliminate the need for a restraint.
- Is the resident able to make his or her needs known? Unsafe behavior is often caused by fears or unmet needs. Discovering the unmet need and meeting it may help you avoid using a restraint.
- Does noise or confusion in the environment cause the resident to become agitated? Noise can be caused by other residents or staff, the public address system, radios, or television. Eliminating the noise may stop the behavior.
- Does the behavior occur during a certain time of day, during a certain activity, or when a specific person is providing care?
- Does the resident seem uncomfortable? Physical pain, hunger, thirst, or the need to use the bathroom can cause unsafe behavior.
- Does the resident seem lonely or isolated? Bored? Boredom, loneliness, or looking for a misplaced item can cause unsafe behavior.
- Does the resident try to get out of bed or the chair without help? Is the resident steady on his or her feet? Does the resident normally use a cane or walker? Is he or she using it now? Is the call signal available, and does the resident know how to use it? Would the resident benefit from the use of an alarm that sounds when he or she stands up? Would use of an alarm remind the resident to sit down, alert the staff, and eliminate the need for a restraint?

Complications of Restraints

Caution is used in making the decision to use restraints, because many complications and side effects are associated with their use. Residents have been severely injured and have died struggling to free themselves from restraints, so restraint use must be taken very seriously. Many burn injuries and burn-related deaths have occurred as a result of residents trying to burn off restraint straps to free themselves. In doing so, the residents themselves have caught on fire, sustaining serious burns. Several residents have died as a result of such injuries. Residents have also been injured by scissors, nail files, and other sharp objects that they used to try to cut restraint straps. If a resident is seriously injured or dies as the result of being restrained, the Safe Medical Device Reporting Act requires that the incident be reported to the government for investigation.

TABLE 15-1 Complications of restraints

Potential Physical Problems	***Potential Psychosocial Problems***
Decreased independence	Worsening of behavior problems
Increased dependence on staff	Withdrawal, loss of social contact
Pressure ulcers	Depression
Weakness	Forgetfulness
Decreased range of motion	Fear
Muscle wasting	Anger
Contractures (frozen, deformed joints)	Shame
Loss of ability to ambulate	Agitation
Edema of ankles, lower legs, feet, fingers	Mental confusion
Decreased appetite, weight loss	Combativeness
Dehydration	Restlessness
Acute mental confusion	Sense of abandonment
Distended abdomen	Loss of self-esteem
Urge to void frequently, dribbling	Crying
Incontinence	Screaming, yelling, calling out
Urinary tract infection	Loss of dignity
Constipation	Boredom
Fecal impaction	Feelings of hopelessness
Lethargy	Feelings of helplessness
Shortness of breath	Irritability
Pneumonia	Ritualistic behavior
Bruising, redness, cuts	
Falls	
Impaired circulation	
Blood clots	
Choking	
Death	

Accrediting and licensing organizations require health care facilities to reduce physical restraint use and track all restraint-related incidents. Complications related to the use of restraints are listed in Table 15.1

APPLYING RESTRAINTS

Despite the efforts of staff, restraints are sometimes necessary. The law is very clear regarding the use of restraints. It specifies that restraints

GUIDELINES FOR

Using Restraints

- Each facility has policies and procedures for the use and application of restraints. Know and follow your facility policies.
- Restraints are never used for staff convenience. They are used for the safety of the resident and others.
- Restraints are applied only with a physician's order and for a specific medical reason.
- The resident and family should clearly understand the purpose of the restraint. Emphasize safety; restraints are not used for punishment.
- The need for restraints is assessed by members of the interdisciplinary team, and alternatives are considered.
- The least restrictive type of restraint is used to keep the resident safe.
- The restraint is applied for the least time possible.
- Restraints are applied only according to manufacturers' directions.
- The proper size restraint must be used for the resident's weight and body size.
- Check the care plan for instructions on using restraints. The care plan will specify the type of restraint to use, the length of time it is to be applied, the reason for the restraint, when to release the restraint, and any special information.
- Check the restraint before using it. If it is worn, torn, cut, or frayed, discard it and obtain another restraint that is in good repair.
- Restraints used on the torso area of the body are always applied over clothing. They should not be applied directly against the skin. Extremity restraints are applied either over or under clothing on the arms and legs, but are padded to prevent restriction of circulation.
- The restraint straps should be smooth. Avoid twisting.
- When applying a restraint to a female resident, make sure the breasts are not under the strap to the restraint.
- After a restraint is applied, check the fit by slipping two or three fingers under the strap to be sure it is not too loose or too tight.
- The skin under the restraint is closely monitored to observe for signs of redness, irritation, or breakdown from the restraint.
- Check the skin above and below the restraint for signs of impaired circulation, such as blue or abnormal color and swelling.
- If the resident is restrained in the chair, the feet must be supported to prevent pain and circulatory problems.
- Restraints are tied in slipknots or bows so the health care provider can release them quickly in an emergency.
- The resident should be positioned using good body mechanics and good posture while in a restraint. Props and supports may also be necessary to keep the resident in good alignment.
- When the resident is restrained in a chair, the hips should be kept back. The purpose of the restraint is to keep the hips down. Restraint straps applied to the waist area instead of the hips may be incorrectly applied. Check the manufacturer's recommendations. The restraint should be at a 45° angle to keep the hips back.
- Most restraints are tied under the chair to the frame. Avoid tying them around the back of the chair, unless the manufacturer's directions clearly give this direction.
- When the resident is restrained in a wheelchair, the brakes should be locked when the chair is parked. The large part of the small front wheels of the chair should face forward. This changes the center of gravity of the chair, making the chair more stable and preventing tipping. The resident's feet should be supported.
- Facility policies vary on visual checks of residents in restraints, but a general rule is that the resident should be visually checked every 15 to 30 minutes while restrained.
- The resident should have the call signal, water, and other needed items within reach while restrained. Provide an alternative type of call signal, such as a manual bell, if the resident cannot use the regular call signal.
- The restraint is released every 2 hours for 10 full minutes. During this time the

resident is repositioned, exercised, ambulated, and taken to the bathroom.
- Report any changes in behavior or side effects from the restraint.
- Restraint use must be recorded on the medical record. A flow sheet is commonly used for this purpose.

must be applied according to manufacturers' directions. Each manufacturer determines the best way to apply its restraints. The directions for restraint application are sent to the government, which approves the instructions. There are many restraint manufacturers, so you must become familiar with the directions for applying the types of restraints used in your facility.

Consideration must also be given to the size of the restraints. Restraints come in different sizes. Each manufacturer lists weight and size guidelines for its restraints. Some restraints are color-coded so you can determine the size at a glance. Using a restraint that does not fit the resident correctly is dangerous. Applying the correct size is very important.

Restraint straps are tied where the resident is unable to reach them. This is usually under the frame of the chair or to the springs of a hospital bed. Many types of hospital beds are used in long-term care facilities. When applying a restraint to a resident who is in bed, fasten the straps to the moveable part of the bed frame, so that if the bed is repositioned the restraint moves with the resident. Tying the restraint to the stationary part of the bed frame can cause serious injury. Avoid tying restraints to the side rails. When applying restraints to a resident in a chair, the straps are usually inserted between the seat and the armrest. A common mistake is threading the straps *through the armrest*. Residents in wheelchairs frequently try to stand or slide their hips toward the front of the seat while restrained, causing injury. Threading the straps through the armrest places the restraint straps around the abdomen and fails to keep the hips down. If the resident attempts to stand or slides forward, the chair may tip or another injury may occur. Attention to manufacturer's directions for strap placement in the wheelchair is very important for preventing injuries.

Most restraints are tied in a slipknot. This allows for quick release in case of choking, fire, or other emergency.

After restraints have been applied, you must visually check the resident every 15 to 30 minutes, or according to your facility policy. The restraint must be completely released every 2 hours for 10 minutes. During this time, the resident should be repositioned, ambulated, offered fluids, taken to the bathroom, and exercised. The restraint may be reapplied after the 10-minute release.

Common Restraints

Although many types of restraints are available from different manufacturers, similar restraints are used in most health care facilities. They are all applied in a similar manner. The **vest restraint** (Figure 15.3) is applied to the upper body to prevent movement and sliding. The **belt restraint** (Figure 15.4)encircles the waist or hips and prevents rising. **Extremity restraints** encircle the arm or leg and prevent movement.

Vest Restraints. The vest restraint is a very secure restraint used for residents who are at high risk of injury. The restraint looks like a vest and crosses over in the front. Other similar restraints are pulled over the head (Figure 15.5). These are called by different names, such as jacket or poncho, but the principles of application are the same for all three devices. Years ago, health care providers were taught to cross the vest restraint over the resident's back. This is no longer acceptable and should never be done.

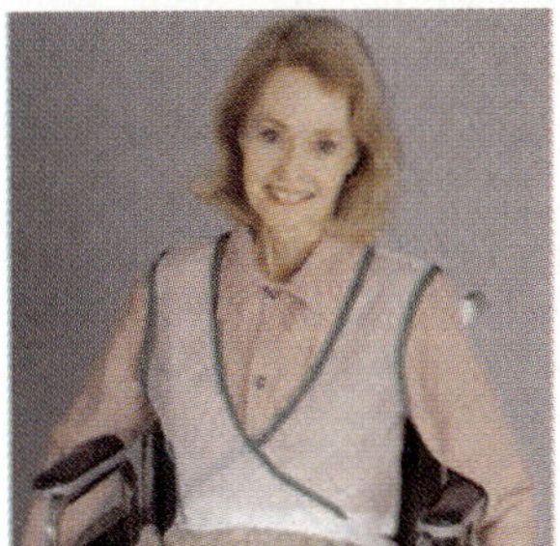

FIGURE 15-3 Vest restraints must be applied as pictured here, with the straps crossed over in front of the resident. Selecting the correct size is also very important. When the resident is in the chair, the straps should be positioned to keep the hips down. They should not encircle the waist. *(Courtesy of Skil-Care Corporation, Yonkers, NY (800) 431-2972)*

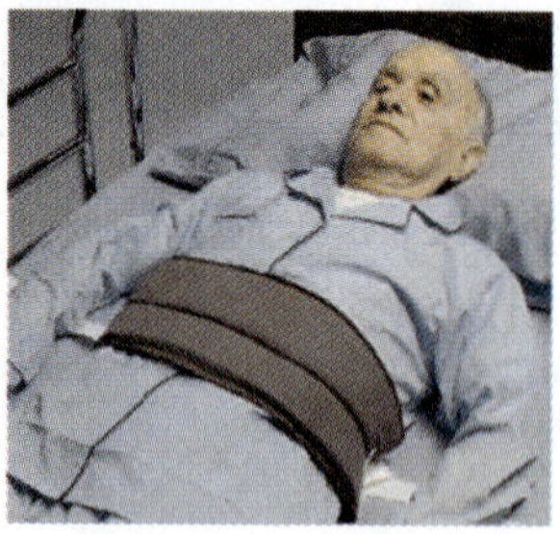

FIGURE 15-4 When the resident is in bed, the belt restraint permits him to turn from side to side. When the belt is used in the chair, it should be positioned to keep the hips down, preventing the resident from standing. *(Courtesy of Skil-Care Corporation, Yonkers, NY (800) 431-2972)*

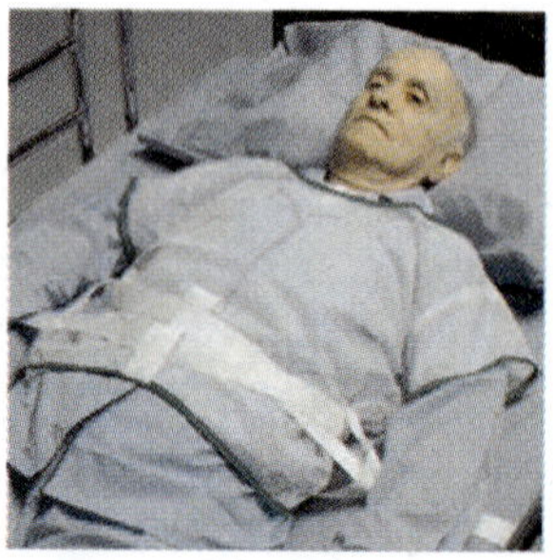

FIGURE 15-5 The jacket restraint is not interchangeable with the vest. This restraint is more secure than a vest, and requires a specific physician's order. *(Courtesy of Skil-Care Corporation, Yonkers, NY (800) 431-2972)*

Crossing the vest in the back can cause choking and other serious injury. A properly fitting vest restraint, crossed in front according to the manufacturer's directions and tied correctly out of reach, will safely and securely hold the resident.

The vest restraint is applied by placing the resident's arms through the sleeves, then crossing the vest over itself in the front. The straps thread through the vest on the side. The vest is pulled down as low as possible on the resident's torso. The straps are drawn behind the resident and fastened to the bed or chair frame.

Belt Restraints. A belt restraint may also be called a waist restraint or a soft tie. It is a wide, padded strap that encircles the resident's waist and attaches to the chair at a 45° angle to keep the hips down. Belts are usually used to remind the resident not to stand up.

Extremity Restraints. Extremity restraints (Figure 15.6) are used to hold the resident's arms and legs. They are usually used to prevent the resident from pulling at tubes or dressings, and to keep the resident still during a medical procedure. Many different extremity restraints are available. Most of these are padded with sheepskin or foam, so no additional padding is necessary. If your facility uses unpadded restraints, wrap a washcloth or other padding around the extremity before applying the restraint, to prevent circulatory problems. Some facilities require that hand rolls be placed in the resident's hands when wrist restraints are used. Commercial devices should be used. Do not use rolled washcloths as hand rolls, because they promote squeezing and can cause deformities. The resident's skin must be kept clean and dry under the hand roll.

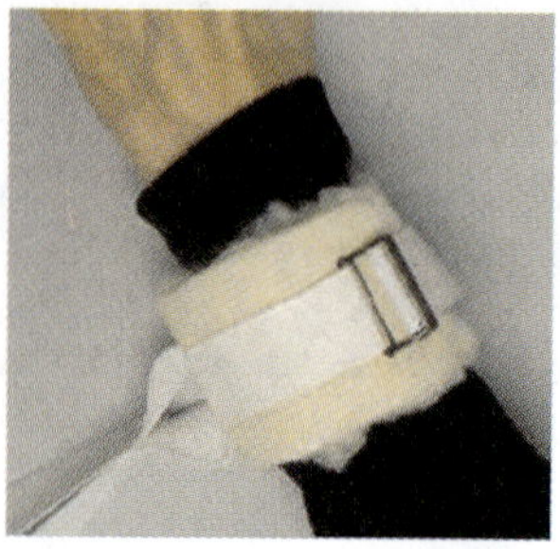

FIGURE 15-6 Extremity restraints are commonly used to keep the resident from pulling on tubes. Make sure the restraint is well padded. *(Courtesy of Skil-Care Corporation, Yonkers, NY (800) 431-2972)*

For residents who hit, scratch, or pull at tubes even if restrained, several types of mitten restraints are available. The fingers are inserted into the mitten (Figure 15.7). The bottom is padded to maintain alignment, prevent pulling at tubes, and prevent injury. Mittens with mesh on top are

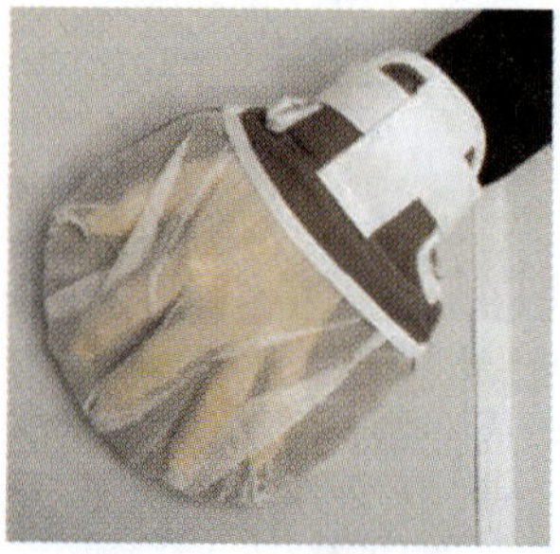

FIGURE 15-7 Mitten restraints are used to prevent self-injury from scratching, picking at the skin and hair, hitting, and pulling on tubes. They may be secured to the bed, like a wrist restraint, or the mitten may be worn alone, depending on the resident's needs. *(Courtesy of Skil-Care Corporation, Yonkers, NY (800) 431-2972)*

PROCEDURE 100 Applying a Vest Restraint

1. Perform your beginning procedure actions.
2. Get help from another nursing assistant if necessary.
3. Slip the resident's arms through the armholes of the vest.
4. Straighten the clothing to be sure it is not wrinkled under the vest.
5. Pull the vest down and smooth it over the clothing.
6. Cross the vest in the front and thread the straps through the slots on the sides.
7. Thread the straps *between* the seat and the armrest or *between* the back of the seat and back of the chair, according to the manufacturer's directions. If the resident is in bed, attach the straps to the moveable part of the bed frame.
8. Pull the straps securely and tie them in a slipknot under the chair or to the moveable part of the bed frame, according to the manufacturer's directions.
9. Insert three fingers under the restraint and check to be sure that it is not too tight.
10. Perform your procedure completion actions.

PROCEDURE 101 Applying a Belt Restraint

1. Perform your beginning procedure actions.
2. Get help from another nursing assistant, if necessary.
3. If the resident is in a wheelchair, lock the brakes, move the hips as far back as possible, and position the footrests to support the feet.
4. Place the belt around the waist. Cross the straps through the loops behind the resident.
5. After the straps are threaded through the loops, tighten the belt securely around the waist.
6. Insert three fingers under the restraint and check to be sure that it is not too tight.
7. Insert the straps between the seat and armrest, or between the seat and backrest, according to the manufacturer's recommendations for the type of restraint you are using.
8. Bring the straps down and tie them to the kick-spurs of the wheelchair, using a quick-release knot, according to the manufacturer's directions.
9. Perform your procedure completion actions.

PROCEDURE

102 Applying an Extremity Restraint

1. Perform your beginning procedure actions.
2. Get help from another nursing assistant if necessary.
3. Position the resident's extremity in good alignment. The joints should be bent slightly inward, in a state of **flexion**.
4. Pad the skin with a washcloth or other padding, if necessary.
5. Insert hand rolls into the hands.
6. Encircle the extremity with the restraint, and loop it over itself according to the manufacturer's directions.
7. Place two fingers under the restraint to check for tightness. Observe the toes or fingers farthest away from the center of the body, or **distal** to the restraint, to be sure circulation is adequate.
8. Tie the ends of the restraint to the bed frame or springs, according to facility policy.
9. Check the resident's circulation and pulse in the restrained extremity every 15 minutes.
10. Perform your procedure completion actions.

common and convenient because you can see through them to check the resident's circulation.

When caring for residents who are in wrist restraints, remember that the restraint renders the resident helpless. You must feed the resident and offer fluids frequently. The call signal should be positioned close to the dominant hand. If the resident cannot push the call signal because of a mitten, an alternative type of signal, such as a manually operated bell, should be provided.

Side Rails as Restraints. According to the definition of restraints at the beginning of the chapter, side rails are a restraint. They can also be an enabler. Many residents pull on them to position and turn themselves in bed. Some residents may feel more secure if the rails are up. Side rails must always be up when the resident who is in bed is restrained in a vest, belt, or extremity restraint.

Studies have shown that serious injuries can occur if residents attempt to climb over side rails and fall. This is a common cause of hip fractures in confused elderly residents. Leaving the rails down may be safer. Each resident's care plan will provide instructions regarding the use of side rails or alternative devices. Know and follow your facility policy.

When side rails are used, it is important to check the space between the rail and the mattress. Hospital beds are permanent pieces of equipment that are used for years. Mattresses wear out and are replaced. There have been cases of injury and death when residents became trapped between the mattress and side rails because the replacement mattress was not the same size as the original. Residents at high risk for entrapment include those with conditions such as confusion, restlessness, lack of muscle control, or a combination of these factors. *Make sure that the gap between the mattress and the side rail is not large enough to cause injury.* This is an important safety issue. Figure 15.8 shows potential areas of entrapment.

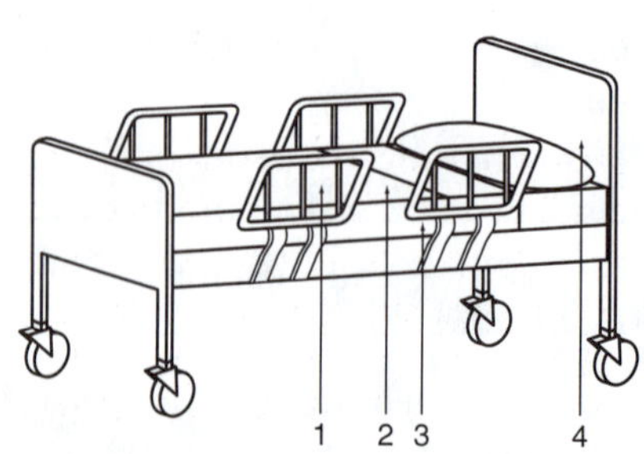

FIGURE 15-8 Entrapment occurs in one of the following ways: (numbered 1–4 in the diagram): (1) through the bars of an individual side rail; (2) through the space between split side rails; (3) between the side rail and mattress; or (4) between the headboard or footboard, side rail, and mattress.

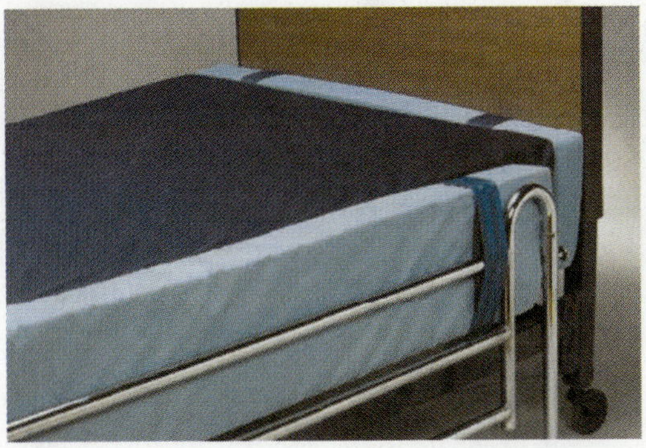

FIGURE 15-9 Various foam wedges and pads may be used to close the space between the side rails, bed frame, and mattress, reducing the risk of injury. *(Courtesy of Skil-Care Corporation, Yonkers, NY (800) 431-2972)*

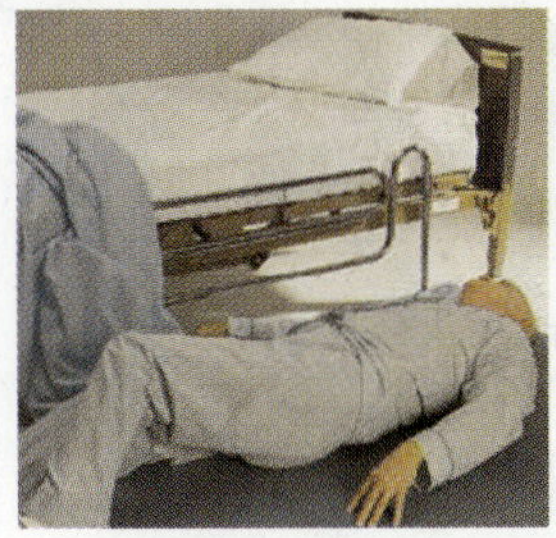

FIGURE 15-10 Placing foam mats on the floor reduces the risk of injury if the resident falls from the bed. *(Courtesy of Skil-Care Corporation, Yonkers, NY (800) 431-2972)*

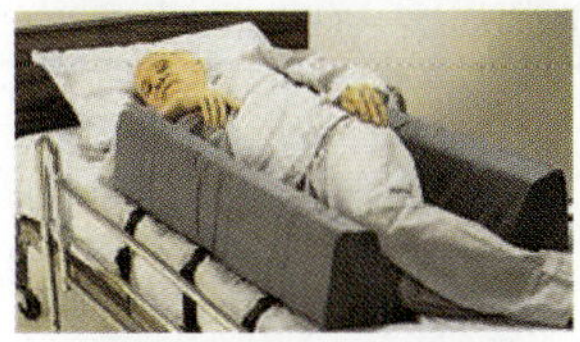

FIGURE 15-11 Bed control bolsters are a good option to use in place of side rails. *(Courtesy of Skil-Care Corporation, Yonkers, NY (800) 431-2972)*

Padded foam barriers may be used to close the space between the mattress, side rails, and bed frame (Figure 15.9) Limiting the space reduces the risk of choking, entrapment, and other injuries.

Facilities and commercial manufacturers have developed many excellent alternatives to the use of side rails. Each resident's care plan will provide instructions regarding the use of restraints, side rails, or alternative devices. Before applying restraints or raising the rails, ask yourself if the risks associated with their use presents less danger than other available options, including making the environment as safe and user-friendly as possible. Other possible alternatives to the use of side rails are:

- Keeping the bed in the lowest possible position with the wheels locked.
- Using a bed that can be raised and lowered close to the floor.
- Placing mats on the floor next to the bed (Figure 15.10) so that if a fall occurs, the resident will fall on a padded surface instead of the hard floor.
- Anticipating reasons the resident will use to get up, including need to use the bathroom, hunger, thirst, restlessness, and pain. Meet these needs promptly and provide calm interventions when you are in the room.
- Using side-rail bolster cushions (Figure 15.11) and side-rail pads (Figure 15.12).
- Using pressure-sensitive alarms that sound when a resident attempts to get up (Figure 15.13A–15.13C).

Each health care facility has policies addressing when side rails may be used. Know and follow your facility policies.

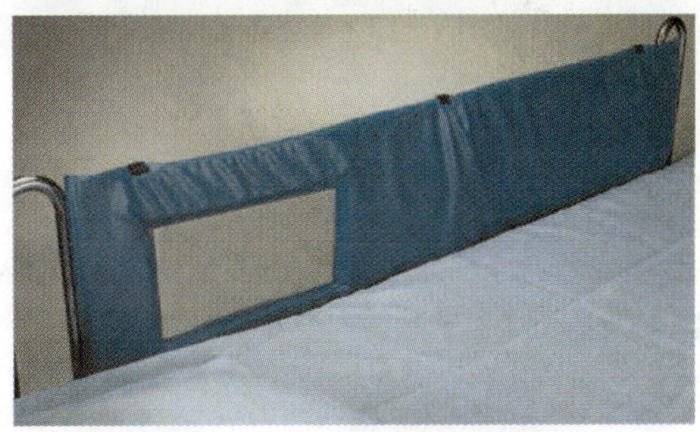

FIGURE 15-12 Side rail pads prevent injury and skin tears from contact with the side rails. They cover the side rail, eliminating the feeling that the resident is looking at the world through bars. *(Courtesy of Skil-Care Corporation, Yonkers, NY (800) 431-2972)*

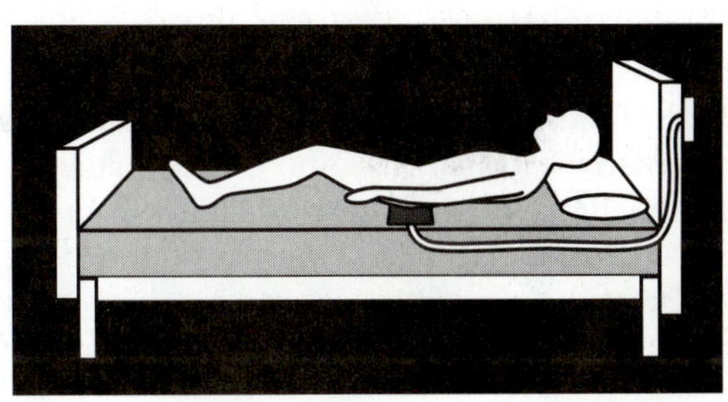

FIGURE 15-13A The pressure-sensitive pad is placed under the sheet. When the resident attempts to stand, an alarm sounds. The pad may also be used in a chair. *(Courtesy of RN + Systems/Tactilitics, Inc.)*

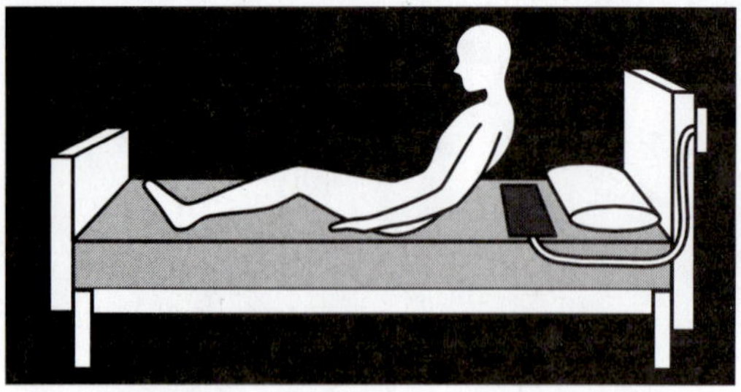

FIGURE 15-13B This pressure-sensitive pad is placed under the sheet beneath the resident's shoulders. When he lifts his upper body off the pad, the alarm will sound. *(Courtesy of RN + Systems/Tactilitics, Inc.)*

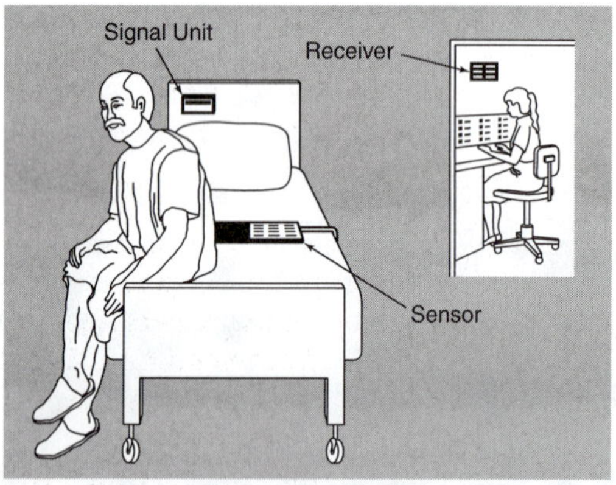

FIGURE 15-13C The pressure-sensitive pad is placed under the sheet. The sensor box is placed in the room. When the resident relieves pressure from the pad, a distinctive alarm sounds. The alarm may be set to sound only at the desk, at both the desk and the resident's room, or in the room only. *(Courtesy of RN + Systems/Tactilitics, Inc.)*

Alternatives To Restraints

Ideally, alternative devices will be used before the resident is placed in restraints. However, this does not always happen, because health care workers are not always aware of the wide variety of alternatives available. Some can be made from common items. Others are available from commercial manufacturers and are reasonably priced. If you know of a restraint alternative that you feel would be useful to a resident, inform the nurse.

Types of Restraint Alternatives

Lateral body supports (Figure 15.14) improve sitting posture for residents who lean to the side. They are commonly used for residents who have paralysis on one side of the body. The foam prevents leaning to the side and supports the resident's arm to prevent discomfort and swelling. Lateral stabilizer armrest bolsters are also used to correct leaning. These are commonly used for residents who have problems with motor control or balance.

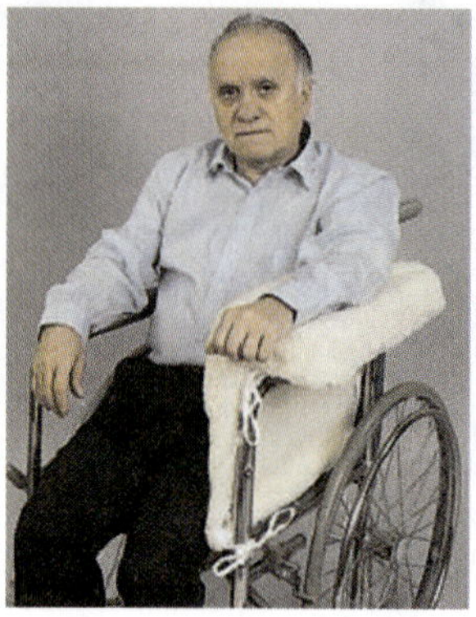

FIGURE 15-14 Some residents lean to the side, necessitating restraint to keep them upright in the chair. The lateral armrest supports and keeps the resident upright, making restraint unnecessary. *(Courtesy of Skil-Care Corporation, Yonkers, NY (800) 431-2972)*

The slide guard wedge (Figure 15.15) may also be called a pommel or saddle cushion. The wedge shifts the resident's weight to the back of the seat. The shape of the cushion and the pommel in the center prevent the resident from sliding. It is used for residents who slide forward on the seat of their chairs. Monitor the skin between the legs for redness and irritation.

The vinyl wedge cushion (Figure 15.16) is used for residents who slide forward in their chairs. The cushion also makes it more difficult for residents to stand, because the hips are lower than the knees. Wedges come in different sizes. The front of the wedge should be high enough to prevent the resident from rising, but should not raise the feet off the floor or footrests. When using a wedge cushion, make sure that the resident's legs are not dangling.

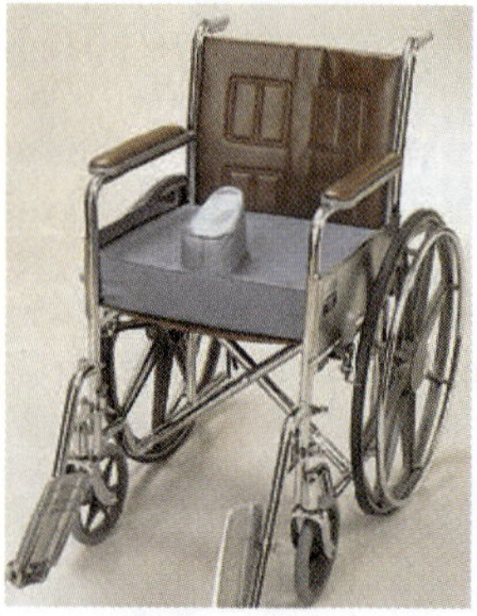

FIGURE 15-15 The pommel cushion keeps the resident from sliding and thrusting the hips forward. *Skil-Care Corporation, Yonkers, NY (800) 431-2972)*

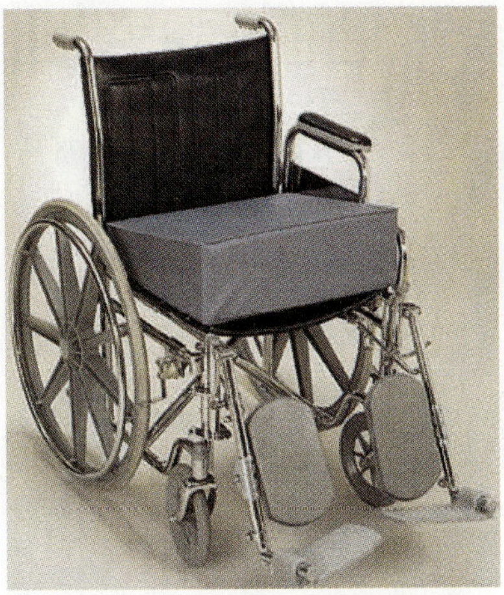

FIGURE 15-16 Some residents slide forward to the edge of the chair, and must be restrained to keep their hips back. The wedge cushion prevents sliding. A piece of gripper can be placed on top of and underneath the wedge for additional security. *(Courtesy of Skil-Care Corporation, Yonkers, NY (800) 431-2972)*

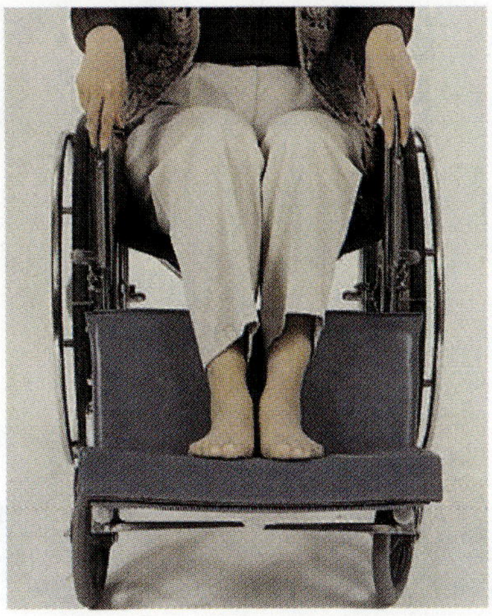

FIGURE 15-18 The resident's feet must be supported when she is sitting in a chair. The footrest elevator keeps the resident's legs from dangling and prevents sliding forward in the chair. *(Courtesy of Skil-Care Corporation, Yonkers, NY (800) 431-2972)*

Nonslip matting (Figure 15.17) is sometimes called "gripper" or Dycem. This is a useful restraint alternative. It can be used as a place mat to enable residents to feed themselves. Some residents scoop their food away from the body, causing the plate to slide. The matting prevents dishes from sliding away. It can be used alone on the seat of a wheelchair to prevent rising, or placed under a wedge cushion for extra security. Gripper comes on a roll, and you cut off a section of the correct size. It may be rinsed with water if it becomes soiled. Hang the matting to dry. The surface is slippery when wet, so do not use it until it is completely dry.

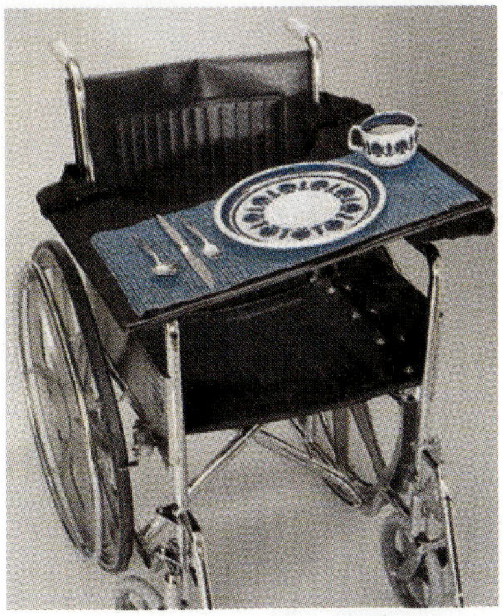

FIGURE 15-17 Gripper is a versatile product with many uses as an enabler and restraint alternative. It makes an excellent place mat, making cutting easier and preventing the dishes from sliding. Gripper may become slippery when wet. It may be rinsed if it becomes soiled, but should not be used until it is dry. *(Courtesy of Skil-Care Corporation, Yonkers, NY (800) 431-2972)*

Supporting the feet when the resident is seated in the chair is very important. Dangling the legs is painful and may allow complications such as blood clots to develop. The resident's legs may be too short to reach the floor or footrests of the chair. In this case, a footrest extender pad (Figure 15.18) is useful. The pad provides a firm base of support and makes it difficult to tip the chair.

Bed control bolsters (see Figure 15.11) are a good alternative to side rails. The bolsters can be used alone or in pairs. They protect the resident from rolling over the edge and serve as a reminder not to get up. The bolsters are half the length of the bed. They can also be used as a support to maintain good body alignment. They can be used for residents who are restless to prevent injury caused by striking or bumping the side rails.

Other Restraint Alternatives

- Magnetic sensor bracelets (Figure 15.19) set off alarms if the resident enters a dangerous area or tries to leave the premises. These work on the same principle as the magnetic detectors used in stores to prevent shoplifting. They are applied to the dominant hand to make them difficult to remove.

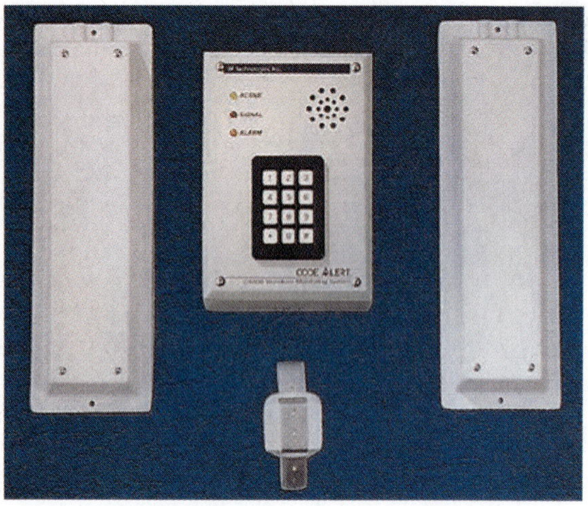

FIGURE 15-19 The magnetic sensor bracelet is used to allow cognitively impaired residents to wander within the unit. The door alarm will sound if the resident tries to exit. *(©1996, RF Technologies. Used by permission)*

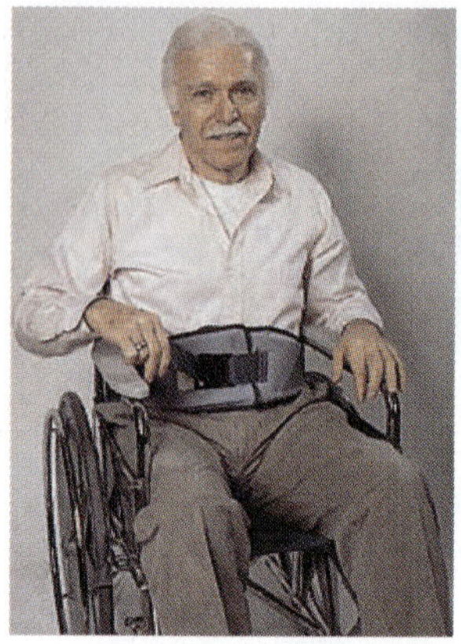

FIGURE 15-21 The self-release belt serves as a reminder to call for help before rising. It is not a restraint if the resident has the physical and mental ability to release the Velcro fastener. *(Courtesy of Skil-Care Corporation, Yonkers, NY (800) 431-2972)*

- Alarm cushions are available; these sound an alarm when the resident stands up or tries to get out of bed. Some facilities attach the signal cord to the resident's gown or clothing, so if the resident rises, it pulls the call signal. Various other personal alarms are also used, in which one end of the signal cord is attached to the resident's clothing. The alarm box is fastened to the bed or chair (Figure 15.20) When the resident stands, the signal cord pulls the alarm, sounding a very loud signal. These devices are used after careful resident evaluation. Some residents respond to the alarm by sitting down immediately. However, the noise from the alarm may startle some residents, increasing the risk of falls. In any event, you must respond to personal alarms immediately. Other personal alarms are used on doors for stairwells and other dangerous areas. There are many potential uses for this device.
- Self-releasing seat belts (Figure 15.21) are similar to the lap belts used in a car. Some belts have buckles and some have Velcro fasteners. Self-releasing devices are considered to be restraint alternatives only if the resident has the ability to remove them. If the resident does not know how to release them, they are restraints.
- "Lap buddies" (Figure 15.22), or foam cushions placed on the lap, keep the resident from rising.
- Special chairs are designed to make it more difficult for the resident to get up. Many chairs are available for residents with special positioning needs (Figure 15.23). Use caution, however. A common restraint alternative is a commercial reclining chair designed for health care facilities. Although some residents benefit from this device, it causes complications in others. Residents who stay in this type of chair for prolonged periods develop weakness in the neck muscles and lose the ability to hold their heads up. They are unable to feed themselves in the reclining position, so they are fed by staff. Eventually they lose the ability to feed themselves. Residents in reclining chairs look at the ceiling all day and may be out of touch with the environment because they cannot see it. Headrests are

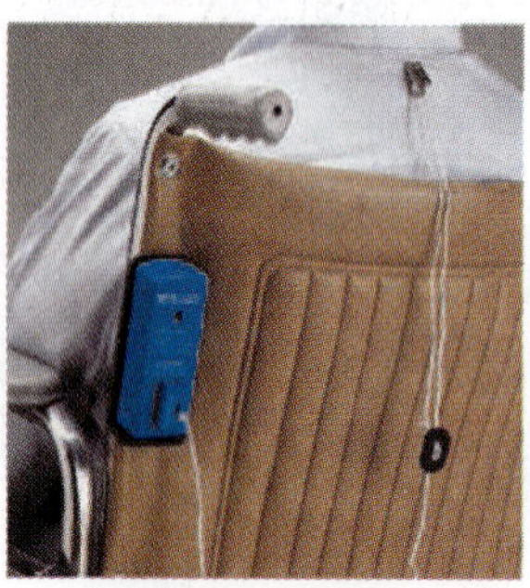

FIGURE 15-20 The personal alarm is a versatile restraint alternative that may be used in the bed or chair. *(Courtesy of Skil-Care Corporation, Yonkers, NY (800) 431-2972)*

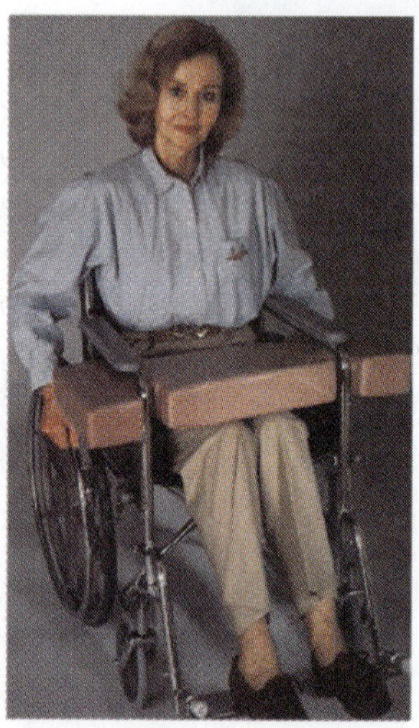

FIGURE 15-22 The lap buddy is foam covered with vinyl. It is lightweight and comfortable and may be used in place of a heavier tray. It is a restraint if the resident cannot remove it. *(Courtesy of Skil-Care Corporation, Yonkers, NY (800) 431-2972)*

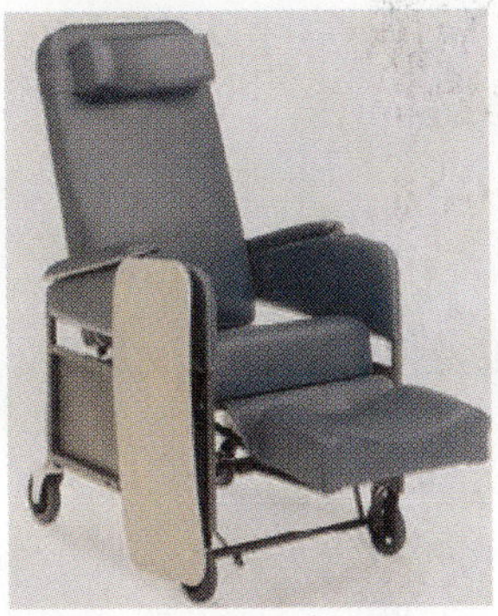

FIGURE 15-23 The geriatric chair can be used as a recliner for resident comfort. If the resident cannot stand, the chair is a restraint when in the reclining position. The tray is locked across the lap to prevent rising. It cannot be removed independently, and is considered a restraint. *(Photo courtesy of Hill-Rom Long Term Care Division)*

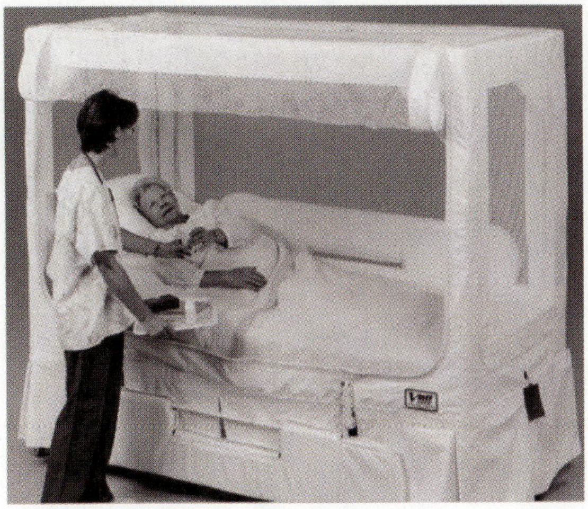

FIGURE 15-24 The Vail bed is a good alternative to physical restraints and side rails. *(Courtesy of Vail Products, Inc.)*

available to position the head forward and promote eye contact. Using these chairs as a restraint alternative must be considered cautiously, because although they solve one problem, they have the potential to create others.

- The **Vail bed** (Figure 15.24) is a useful alternative for confused adult residents who try to climb over the side rails. It is not used for mentally alert residents. This bed looks somewhat like a canopy bed or adult crib. The top and sides are surrounded by netting. From the inside, the netting seems to fade out and is not perceived as a barrier. The resident views the room as though looking through a screen door. The resident can move about in the bed without becoming entangled or falling out of bed. The netting protects the caregiver if the resident becomes aggressive. The bed is accessible from all sides through special zippers in the netting that open only from the outside. Residents should not be left unattended with the covers unzipped. Pediatric versions of this bed are also available for infant and child residents.

KEY POINTS

- Restraints are safety devices.
- Restraints can be dangerous if used incorrectly or inappropriately.
- The least amount of restraint required to keep the resident safe should be used.
- Restraints may be used as enablers to empower the resident and improve independence.
- Risk factors in the environment should be eliminated to reduce the need for restraints.
- The use of alternatives to restraints should be considered and continually reevaluated.

REVIEW

A. Multiple Choice

Select the one best answer.

1. Restraints are
   a. always used to prevent residents from wandering.
   b. enablers.
   c. devices that restrict freedom of movement.
   d. used when requested by the resident's family.

2. An enabler is
   a. a type of drug therapy.
   b. something that improves independent functioning.
   c. a mechanical device to manage behavior problems.
   d. a form of punishment.
3. Restraints may be used
   a. if the care provider feels they are needed.
   b. to punish the resident.
   c. with a physician's order.
   d. for convenience when the facility is short of staff.
4. Modifying the environment involves
   a. eliminating risk factors that contribute to the need for a restraint.
   b. assessing the resident for the proper size restraint.
   c. always restraining unsafe residents when out of bed.
   d. applying restraints correctly.
5. Which of the following will guide you in the type of restraint to use and the length of time the restraint should be applied?
   a. the resident
   b. the care plan
   c. the family
   d. the progress notes
6. Which of the following are complications of restraints?
   a. dehydration
   b. aphasia
   c. dysphagia
   d. independence
7. Which of the following should be considered when evaluating the resident for the need for restraints?
   a. age
   b. gender
   c. ability to see and hear
   d. staffing needs
8. Which of the following should be considered when obtaining a restraint from the linen closet to put on a resident?
   a. restraint size and condition
   b. the resident's age
   c. the resident's ability to ambulate
   d. the resident's mental status
9. Restraints should be released
   a. every 15 to 30 minutes.
   b. every 2 hours.
   c. every 4 hours.
   d. every shift.
10. When the resident is restrained in a chair, the hips should be
    a. as far forward as possible.
    b. flexed as much as possible.
    c. as far back as possible.
    d. extended as much as possible.
11. When applying a vest restraint to a resident
    a. apply the restraint directly against the resident's skin.
    b. cross the vest in the front.
    c. thread the straps through the armrests of the chair.
    d. cross the vest in the back.
12. Restraint alternatives are
    a. devices that hold residents very securely.
    b. devices to use instead of restraints.
    c. always postural supports.
    d. used only if the resident cannot remove the device.

B. Clinical Applications

Answer the following questions.

13. Mr. Black has an order for a vest restraint when he is up in the chair. He wears an extra-large vest. You are preparing to transfer him from the bed to the chair. When you go to the linen room, you find only one extra-large vest on the shelf. The vest is frayed around the edges. It appears that the straps have been cut. Both straps are very short. There are several size medium and large restraints on the shelf, all in good condition. What should you do?
14. Mr. Black has been restrained in the chair. You notice that when he is wearing a vest restraint, he yells, pulls at the restraint, and asks others for scissors to cut the straps. Sometimes he throws his food and water. When Mr. Black is unrestrained in bed, he does not behave this way. What do you think is the cause of the agitation? What can the nursing assistant do to help?

15. Mr. Long is a confused resident. He ambulates in the facility. Occasionally he goes into other residents' rooms and takes things. Mr. Long fell recently, but was not injured. Since the fall, he has been unsteady on his feet. Staff is concerned for his safety, and you know that restraints are being considered. The nurse has called a team conference and asked your opinion about how to keep the resident safe. David, your coworker, states that he thinks Mr. Long should be restrained. What suggestions do you have for nursing assistant measures to avoid the use of restraints?

16. Mrs. Stone uses a belt restraint when in bed to keep her from climbing over the side rails. You applied the restraint and correctly tied it to the moveable part of the bed frame. Mrs. Stone's daughters visited today. After they left, you noticed that the restraint straps were tied to the side rails. What action should you take?

17. Mrs. Decker is an alert resident with multiple sclerosis. She has poor motor control of her body. Mrs. Decker leans forward or to the side when she is seated in a chair. She is afraid of falling. What can the nursing assistant do to help her feel secure and prevent injury?

UNIT 16

Psychological Effects of Aging

OBJECTIVES

After reading this unit, you will be able to:

- Spell and define key terms.
- Identify common causes of behavior problems in alert and confused residents.
- Explain why physical and chemical restraints are not desirable in the management of behavior problems.
- Describe the effect of losses and unmet needs on residents' behavior.
- List the three steps in the ABC method of behavior management and explain how this method is used to eliminate undesirable behavior.
- Describe how to assist residents with specific behavior problems.
- Differentiate cognitive impairment from dementia and delirium.
- Describe methods of caring for and communicating with residents with cognitive impairment and dementia.
- List the three stages of Alzheimer's disease and describe signs and symptoms of each stage.
- List three groups of Maslow's Basic Needs
- Identify safety and security needs
- List four psychosocial needs

OBSERVATIONS TO MAKE AND REPORT RELATED TO SPECIAL BEHAVIORAL PROBLEMS

Change in consciousness, awareness, or alertness
Changes in mood, behavior, or emotional status
Changes in orientation to person, place, time, season
Change in communication
Changes in memory
Excessive drowsiness
Changes in ability to respond verbally or nonverbally
Sleepiness for no apparent reason
Sudden onset of mental confusion
Threats of suicide or harm to self or others
Signs or symptoms of illness or infection

Basic Human Needs

Basic human needs are the things and activities required by all persons to successfully and satisfactorily live their lives and realize their full potential as human beings. The needs are the same for all people at all ages, although individuals' abilities to meet these needs may vary widely.

Cultural backgrounds influence the way in which individuals fulfill these basic needs. *Culture* refers to those customs and practices that are common to groups of people, including beliefs, habits, health practices, expressions of spirituality, and ways of celebrating. These cultural patterns are part of the uniqueness of each individual and must be considered when providing for the person's care.

Abraham Maslow and Eric Erikson are two leaders in the field of human behavior. They helped us understand basic human needs and how people go about satisfying these needs.

Maslow's Hierarchy of Needs

Maslow originally proposed five steps in the continuum of needs: physical needs, safety and security needs, love and belonging needs, self-esteem needs, and self-actualization (accomplishment) needs. He later expanded the hierarchy to seven levels to include the growth needs of knowing, understanding, exploring, and appreciating symmetry, order, and beauty; and the ability to help others find self-fulfillment and realize their potential. This step he called *transcendence*.

The five original steps of the hierarchy help us understand the basic needs that must be met (Figure 16.1). Within the five original steps, Maslow described the basic needs as:

- Physical (physiological) needs
- Security and safety needs
- Psychosocial needs

Maslow believed that the order in which needs are satisfied is based on their importance to survival. Physical or physiological needs must be satisfied first. Safety and security needs are next in importance to survival. Only after these needs are satisfied can the psychosocial needs (emotional) be considered.

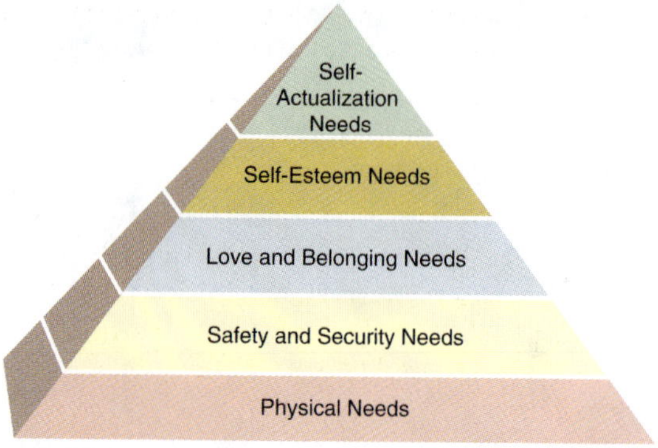

FIGURE 16-1 Maslow's Hierarchy of Needs. People meet needs in order of their importance to survival. Physical needs must be satisfied first.

Physical Needs (Physiological)

The most basic human needs relate to the physical functioning of our bodies. These needs must be met to maintain life:

- Oxygen
- Water
- Food
- Sleep/rest
- Activity
- Elimination
- Sexuality

Safety and Security Needs

Residents who do not feel safe will experience anxiety and fear. Living in a state of fear prevents an individual from achieving psychosocial well-being. You can help residents feel safe by:

- Being dependable and trustworthy
- Being kind and considerate
- Providing care promptly, gently, and safely
- Helping the residents maintain a life-style structured to their choice
- Protecting their possessions from theft
- Letting residents know that the facility is protected against fire and other disasters

Psychosocial Needs

The psychosocial needs of the elderly are the same as those at any age. There is a need to:

- Love and be loved
- Be treated with respect and dignity
- Feel needed
- Feel important as an individual
- Feel appreciated

On the Job

Health care workers often excel at giving physical care but neglect the psychosocial needs of residents.

When residents first enter a long-term care facility, they often feel depressed and frightened. They are in a strange environment and they fear that they will lose all privacy and control of their own lives.

Their self-esteem is threatened. Each person has in his or her own mind an idea of how they appear and wish to appear to others. This idea of self is referred to as **self-esteem** and must be protected. How residents respond to a threat to their self-esteem depends on how the resident has handled such threats previously and how those who are caring for the resident understand and respond to these feelings.

Some residents react to a threat of self-esteem with an aggressive response and complaints about all levels of care. Others may become quiet, withdrawn, and depressed. The nursing assistant must be aware of the residents' underlying feelings. Remain open and receptive and do not take personal offense at things the resident may say or do in frustration.

You can help residents meet their psychosocial needs if you:

- Treat each resident as an individual with specific characteristics and needs.
- Give the resident choices whenever possible (Figure 16.2).
- Honor the residents' identities. Call residents by the names they choose. Allow them to reflect their identity by the way they dress, the way they arrange their rooms, and the activities they choose.
- Allow residents to do as much as possible for themselves. Encourage their independence to the level their conditions permit.
- Respect the residents' rights.

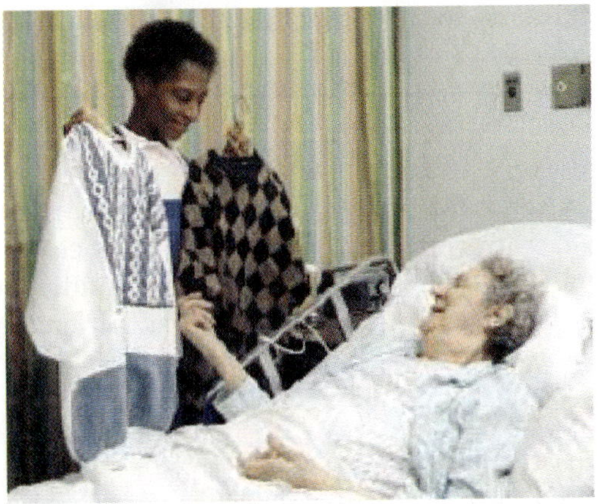

FIGURE 16-2 Assist the resident whenever necessary, but encourage her to make her own decisions.

Personality

The way each resident satisfies psychosocial needs depends on personality. **Personality** is the sum of the ways we react to the events in our lives. Personality is gradually formed through life experiences.

Erikson suggests that as we mature from infancy to old age, we pass through several developmental stages. During each stage, certain tasks must be accomplished. These are called **developmental tasks** (Figure 16.3).

The developmental tasks specific to older adults are just as important as those for younger people. They include the need to:

- Adjust to decreased abilities such as physical limitations caused by the aging process
- Integrate life experiences through reminiscing
- Accept the onset of chronic illness
- Accept one's place in the community structure
- Adapt to possible changes in social and financial security
- Recognize and accept that life is limited
- Act as a role model for others

Nursing assistants can play an important role in helping residents accomplish the developmental tasks by:

- Allowing residents to talk about their experiences and feelings
- Creating an atmosphere of acceptance where the residents are not judged

If these stages are interrupted and not completed because of illness, the individual may display behavior that is inappropriate for the age and the culture we live in.

Cultural Influences

The residents you care for may come from different cultures. More complete care is given if nursing assistants are sensitive to the cultural influences on a resident's behavior. People from the same culture usually share similar values, customs, clothing, and food preferences.

Even the cause of illness is influenced by cultural beliefs. Many European-Americans share in the belief that illness is punishment for sins and self-abuse. Many African Americans believe that illness is caused by spirits and demons and is punishment from God. Cultural values and customs are passed from generation to generation and are the foundation for accepted behavior. Cultural influences play an important role in how a person views and reacts to illness. For

Physical Stage	Year of Occurrence	Tasks to Be Mastered
Oral-sensory	Birth–1 year (infant)	To learn to trust (Trust)
Muscularanal	1–3 years (toddler)	To recognize self as an independent being from mother (Autonomy)
Locomotor	3–5 years (preschool years)	To recognize self as a family member (Initiative)
Latency	6–11 years (school-age years)	To demonstrate physical and mental skills/abilities (Industry)
Adolescence	12–18 years	To develop a sense of individuality as a sexual human being (Identity)
Young Adulthood	19–35 years	To establish intimate personal relationships with a mate (Intimacy)
Adulthood	35–50 years	To live a satisfying and productive life
Maturity	50+ years	To review life's events and examine how they have influenced the development of a unique individual (Ego integrity)

FIGURE 16-3 Erikson's tasks of personality development from infancy through old age

example, it is a common cultural practice in Asian American cultures to seek care from traditional healers. The healer reestablishes the balance between the negative (*yin*) energy that is believed to be the cause of illness and the positive (*yang*) energy of health.

Each culture may have its own belief system and religious faith. Belief systems influence choices in various cultures. For example, some Native American peoples create elaborate sand paintings to diagnose and treat illness. Hispanic Americans may treat illness with prayer, wearing of medals, and consumption of special food. An understanding of some of the major belief systems will help you assist your residents to meet their needs. Always remember that you are caring for an individual within a cultural framework. Within the framework of each belief system, there are individual differences in depth of belief and extent of practice.

Major Challenges to Adjustments

Each phase of life brings with it challenges to be met and adjustments to be made. The challenges that develop personality often come as the result of a major life crisis. Three crises older people are likely to experience are:

- Loss of a loved one (spouse or companion)
- Living with illness and disability
- Loss of independence

For many people, these events occur in close succession, and the stress can be overwhelming.

Loss of a Loved One

A person who loses a loved one faces major psychological adjustments. This is a time of great uncertainty at any age. It is particularly difficult when one is old, with failing health and limited resources. Many important decisions about the future must be made at a time when loneliness, confusion, and grief are at a peak.

When a spouse dies, the surviving spouse may sense a loss of identity or place in social situations. If able, he or she will eventually adjust to a new life alone. Although family and friends can help in the process, it is the individual who must face the loss and make the adjustment.

Sometimes a pet is a beloved member of the family to an elderly person. The loss of the pet through death can also require major psychological adjustments similar to those experienced when a human family member dies. Most facilities do not allow personal pets. The person who

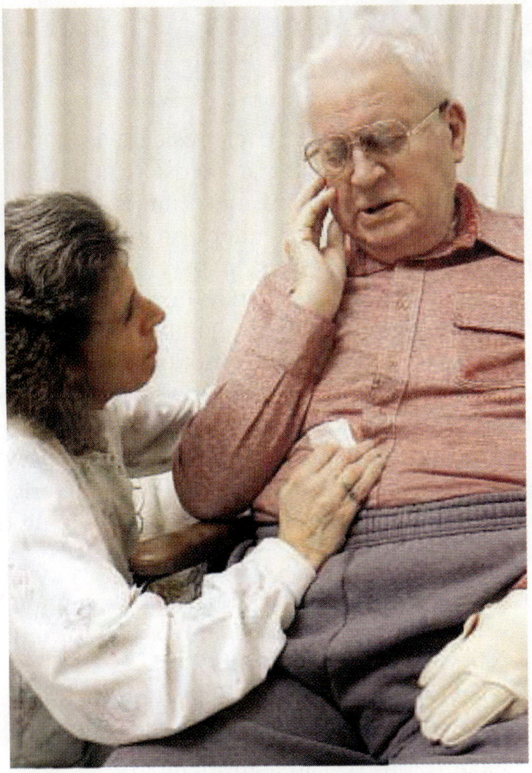

FIGURE 16-4 The nursing assistant can help residents work through a period of grieving.

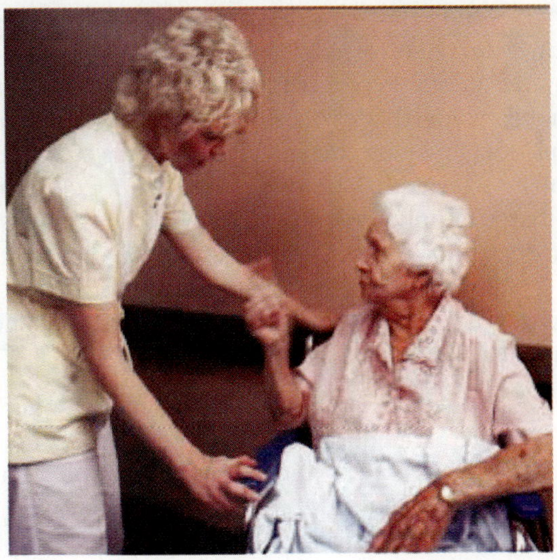

FIGURE 16-5 Residents may become frustrated with the changes occurring in their lives.

leaves a pet behind to enter a long-term care facility also feels a great sense of loss as well as guilt about leaving the pet. The separation is painful for the resident.

Having someone to confide in can help the elderly person work through the grief and adjustment period. The nursing assistant who has good **rapport** (sympathetic and understanding relationship) with the resident can help fill this role (Figure 16.4).

Giving the resident the opportunity to talk about lost loved ones helps to put feelings and memories into a proper perspective. Working through feelings gives the resident a sense of strength and better understanding of himself.

Chronic Illness

Many older people must adjust to the changes caused by aging and the problems associated with a chronic illness.

Some people try to deny these changes. They become angry when they realize they cannot control the changes going on in their bodies. Over time, most people adjust to and accept their limitations. Eventually they accept that life does not go on forever and that death is inevitable.

Loss of Independence

The third crisis involves the loss of independence that comes with the move to a long-term care facility. Dependency is natural for a child but not for a mature adult. The emotional distress before admission is high. Making the decision to enter a long-term care facility is never easy for the family or the person involved. It may require separation from loved ones, personal possessions, and pets. A person's sense of independence is threatened just by knowing that this type of care and support is necessary.

The anxiety and stress levels may be even higher once the person is admitted to the facility. New surroundings, new people, a room shared with another resident, and new procedures and rules now define the resident's world. Feelings of fear and frustration grow as the resident comes to know the degree to which independence is sacrificed (Figure 16.5). The calm manner, caring attitude, and patience of the nursing assistant are vital factors in helping the new resident adjust to life in the facility.

Using Defense (Coping) Mechanisms

Making positive psychological adjustments in later life depends to a large extent on how well the developmental tasks of earlier life periods were mastered and how the personality was formed. The ways of adjusting that a person used successfully through life become part of the person's **defense** (or coping) **mechanisms**.

Residents will react to situations using defense mechanisms that worked for them in the past. Residents may use defense mechanisms to protect their self-esteem. The use of defense mechanisms is harmful only when they become the major way of dealing with stressful situations. If this occurs, a mental health professional may counsel the resident. Here are some definitions for common defense mechanisms:

1. **Suppression**: refusing to recognize a painful thought, memory, feeling, or impulse. A person who has been abused, for example, may refuse to admit the memory of the abuse.
2. **Projection**: attributing one's own unacceptable feelings, thoughts, and actions to others. For example, a resident may tell you the bed is wet because you did not bring the bedpan on time. The resident is blaming you rather than admitting that she is incontinent.
3. **Denial**: pretending that a problem does not exist. For example, a resident is in denial when he or she talks about going home but there is little realistic chance that this will occur. This is different from similar expressions in dementia.
4. **Rationalization**: giving false but believable reasons for a situation. A resident may be rationalizing when he or she tells you that he or she must stay in bed all day because there was too much noise to sleep the night before.
5. **Compensation**: making up for a situation in some other way. A woman who received much satisfaction from caring for a husband and children may compensate for this loss by caring for and protecting other residents (Figure 16.6).

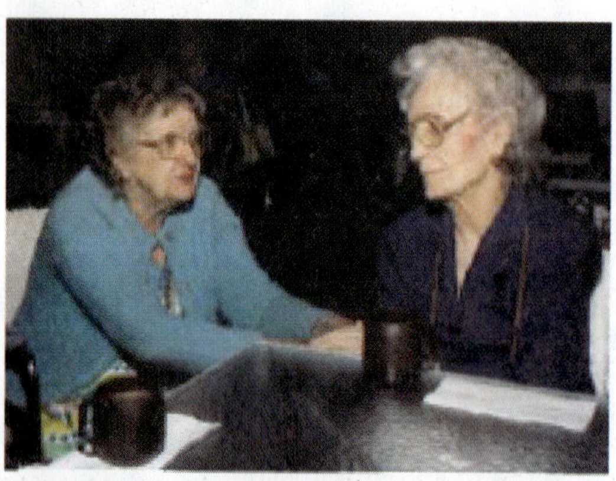

FIGURE 16-6 Treat relationships between residents with respect.

Meeting Residents' Psychosocial Needs

It is important to see each resident as a whole person. The psychological needs of each resident must be recognized and met. Unmet psychological needs have a great effect on physical needs and status. For example, if psychological needs go unmet, the resident may become depressed and refuse to cooperate in therapy. Such a refusal may start a physical and emotional decline that rules out any chance of the resident returning home and could lead to death.

Nursing assistants can do much to help the residents meet their needs. If the residents' rights are respected at all times, you will be helping the residents to fulfill their psychosocial needs.

1. Remember that emotional needs cannot be fulfilled unless the residents' physical and safety needs are first met.
2. New residents must adjust to living in the long-term care facility. Help them to:
   - Develop trust in staff members
   - Meet other residents
   - Adapt to the routine of the facility
   - Adjust to having less personal space. You must respect the space that is theirs
   - Adjust to the loss of a home and many personal belongings
   - Use their own personal possessions, such as clothing or books
   - Display family photos and mementos
   - Find activities that have meaning and contribute to the resident's sense of self-worth
3. Always give residents the opportunity to be as independent as possible. Allow choices whenever possible.
4. Attend to the residents' comfort. Report complaints of pain or signs of anxiety immediately.
5. Explain procedures and routines to residents; notify your supervisor if the resident does not understand procedures and routines.
6. Listen carefully to everything residents say.
7. Recognize that each resident is an individual with likes and dislikes.
8. Answer signal lights promptly.
9. Treat all residents as adults.
10. Help residents feel loved and accepted by:
    - Accepting each resident in a nonjudgmental manner
    - Using touch appropriately to indicate your acceptance of the person
11. Help residents feel positive self-esteem and respect from others by:

- Calling them by the names/titles of their choice
- Learning about them, their families, and their histories

12. Unless they choose not to, residents should have the opportunity to contribute to facility life. These activities must be voluntary and written into the care plan so no violation of the resident's rights occurs. Activities may include:
    - Visiting other residents who may have no family and few visitors
    - Sharing their knowledge of a hobby with other residents
    - Working on the facility newsletter
    - Creating items for a facility craft sale
    - Delivering mail to other residents
    - Stuffing envelopes for mailings
    - Caring for nursing home pets such as birds or fish
    - Serving on the Residents' Council
    - Playing the piano or leading singing groups
    - Leading current events groups

BEHAVIOR PROBLEMS

Behavior problems frequently have medical, social, or emotional causes that create great stress. Typical behavior problems include physical or verbal aggression, wandering, yelling or calling out, and other socially inappropriate behaviors. Some behavior problems are related to a decline in intellectual functioning called **cognitive impairment**. Problem behaviors may present a danger to the resident, staff, and other residents on the unit. Other behaviors may be annoying or distressing to the staff, but are harmless. Facility staff often have difficulty caring for residents who have behavior problems. Sometimes this results in overuse of physical restraints or sedation with chemical restraints. Both interventions may have serious consequences and do not always solve the underlying problem. They often worsen physical dependence, and may increase confusion and behavior problems. Although physical and chemical restraints are useful sometimes, other methods of dealing with the behavior should be tried first. If they are ineffective, treatments involving restraints are used as the last resort. Behavior management is a technique commonly used to modify the resident's behavior. Dealing with residents with behavior problems requires using patience, common sense, good communication skills, and a great deal of empathy. Health care professionals have taken positive steps, and the current trend is moving away from using physical and chemical restraints. Other methods of managing behavior have been found to be more effective and beneficial to residents.

The Effect of Losses on Behavior

When people are sick or injured, they suffer losses. The most obvious loss is their health. Loss of health causes loss of independence. Loss of health and independence causes loss of income and security. The loss of health, independence, income, and security may affect the resident's relationships with others. Family and friends may be lost. The resident may feel like a bother, unloved, or both. The resident may feel as if he or she has lost control. Changes in relationships and losses affect the resident's self-esteem. Although the losses may be only temporary, the resident may be afraid the loss will become permanent.

The resident in the long-term care facility has lost his or her home and the comfort of belongings. The loss may be temporary, but this is a difficult adjustment to make. When loss of home is combined with other losses, the resident may feel overwhelmed. Many people go through the grieving process when they suffer the types of losses described here. You will be caring for residents in various stages of the grieving process. Sadness and grief are normal when people suffer a loss. The resident may also be fearful and anxious. This is caused in part by fear of the unknown. The resident does not know what the outcome of the illness will be. He or she may fear a negative outcome. The resident may be afraid of treatments and procedures used to manage his or her illness. Over time, the resident begins to feel helpless and hopeless. He or she may feel frustrated and angry. The anger may be internal, or directed toward oneself. It is difficult to maintain your self-esteem when you are angry with yourself. The anger may also be external. The resident may direct anger toward family, friends, and caregivers. If anger is directed at you, try to understand that the real cause of the resident's anger is fear and anger at the situation. The resident is not mad at you personally.

Unmet Needs

Behavior problems usually develop in response to stress, loss, or unmet needs that exceed the resident's coping ability. Think about the needs in Maslow's hierarchy. Residents with behavior problems who are mentally alert are often responding to an unmet psychosocial need. They also may be responding to a feeling of lack of control over their bodies, their situations, or the environment. Get to know the resident and respect his or her uniqueness as a person. Offer the resident control and choices, showing that you respect him or her as a person. Promote and reward independence, decision making, and assertive behavior. If you are able to identify the resident's unmet needs, share the information with the nurse and other members of the interdisciplinary team. This will help in developing a care plan to meet the needs and minimize or eliminate the behavior problems.

Residents who are mentally confused often demonstrate problem behavior in response to fear, loneliness, boredom, too much stimulation in the environment, or an unmet physical need. The behavior may be the only way the resident has to express himself or herself. For example, a mentally confused resident screams frequently throughout the day. The resident is alone in bed in her room. This presents a challenge because there are so many potential reasons for the screaming. She may be hungry or thirsty, in pain, scared, lonely, bored, too hot, or too cold. She may need to use the bathroom, but is unable to tell you. There may be too much noise or stimulation in the environment, causing her to be agitated. The only way to find out why the resident is screaming is by using common sense and experimenting with different approaches. Offer her a drink or something to eat. Take her to the bathroom. Sit quietly with her and hold her hand. Rubbing lotion on the resident's hands and arms may have a calming effect. If you find an approach that calms her, share this information with other team members.

The Meaning of Behavior Problems. All behavior has a meaning. The meaning may not be apparent to you. The resident may not even realize that he or she is demonstrating a behavior that you consider abnormal. This is particularly true if the resident is from a different culture. Behavior that is acceptable in one culture may be considered abnormal by people from other cultures. Behavior patterns develop throughout a person's lifetime and are affected by heredity, culture, environment, and lifetime experiences.

Normal Coping and Defense Mechanisms. Residents react to losses by using methods they have learned over their lifetime. Residents use coping and defense mechanisms as tools to compensate for losses. Several defense mechanisms are commonly seen. These are:

- **Denial**, or refusing to admit there is a problem
- **Rationalization**, or providing an acceptable but untrue reason for the illness or behavior

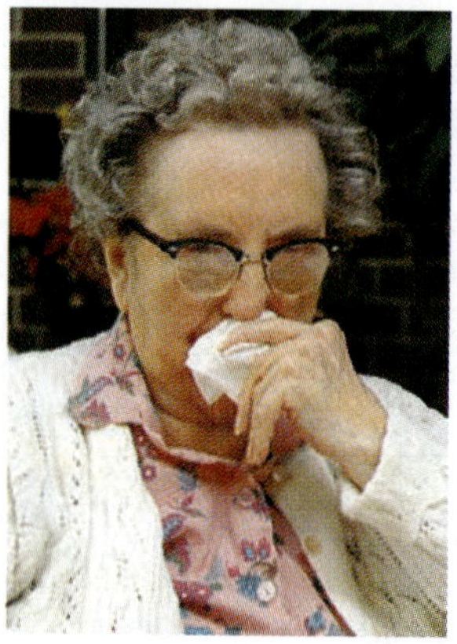

FIGURE 16-7 Residents entering the long-term care facility experience many losses.

- **Compensation**, or using strength and overachieving in one area to overcome a weakness in another area of life
- **Projection**, or placing the blame for the situation on someone or something else

The nursing assistant must use good communication and listening skills when dealing with residents who have suffered losses (Figure 16.7). Understand that residents are responding to stress when they use coping mechanisms. Do not take angry outbursts or other behavior personally. Although the resident may say he or she is angry with you, this is not always the case. The resident is usually angry because of his or her situation. You may need to modify your behavior. Monitor how the resident responds to you, and adjust your approach to achieve results. Practice empathy. Put yourself in the resident's shoes and try to understand what is happening.

THE ABCS OF BEHAVIOR MANAGEMENT

An effective technique of behavior management is the ABC plan (Table 16.1). This plan is useful with both alert and mentally confused residents. The theory behind this program is that if the **antecedent** or **consequences** of the behavior are eliminated or modified, the behavior will change or cease. The antecedent is the event that causes or triggers a behavior. The consequences are the outcome of the behavior.

The Three Steps of Behavior Management

There are three steps in the ABC method of behavior management:

TABLE 16-1 ABCs of behavior management

Identify the ABCs	Definition
A = Antecedent	The cause or trigger of the behavior
B = Behavior	The behavior itself
C = Consequences	The consequences, effect, or result of the behavior

Step 1: Attempt to determine the cause (trigger or antecedent) for the behavior. Does the behavior occur in specific environmental conditions, at a certain time of day, or during a certain activity? Does the presence or absence of other persons trigger the behavior?

Step 2: Eliminate the cause of the behavior. If the cause can be identified and eliminated, the behavior will cease or change.

Step 3: Examine the consequences of the behavior. They may also have to be eliminated or changed in order to change the behavior. Modifying the consequences of behavior requires practice. For example, a mentally confused resident yells and cries. You discover that if you sit and hold the resident's hand, the behavior stops. Sitting and holding her hand serves as a reward for the behavior. To modify the consequences, sit and hold the resident's hand *before* the yelling and crying start. Pay attention to the resident on a regular basis. In this case, modifying the consequences changes the behavior. If the resident's behavior has been rewarded for a long period of time, do not expect to see immediate results. All team members will have to practice the new approach consistently before results are apparent.

Using the ABC Method. Mentally alert residents who use the call signal frequently for minor requests can be distressing to staff. The resident may ask you to turn on the light, position the window blinds, or refill the water glass. Within minutes after you leave the room, the resident signals again. Residents who display this type of behavior are often lonely and scared. They may be using the call signal to get attention. An effective approach is to tell the resident what time you will return when you leave the room. Be sure to return at that time. Keeping your word shows the resident that you can be trusted. Stop in the room and check on the resident as often as you can. When the resident knows he or she can depend on you to check on him or her regularly, unnecessary use of the call signal will decrease.

This simple example shows how the ABCs of behavior management are used effectively. In this case:

A, or the antecedent, is the resident's loneliness and fear.

B, or the behavior, is using the call signal frequently for minor requests.

C, or the consequence, is attention and companionship when you are in the room.

By checking on the resident frequently and keeping your promise to return, you have changed the consequences. You are providing companionship and attention regularly. This eases the resident's loneliness and fear, so there is no reason to continue the behavior.

In these examples, the consequences were modified to change the behavior. Sometimes the antecedent must be changed. For example, a mentally confused resident is quiet all day. She begins to scream every night at bedtime after you have done HS care. You discover that she stops screaming when you enter the room and turn on the light. When you turn the light off, she screams again. The resident is frightened of the dark. Leaving a light on in the room or bathroom will cause the resident to stop screaming.

Role of the Nursing Assistant in Assisting with Behavior Management Programs. If a resident demonstrates a behavior problem, members of the interdisciplinary team will develop a care plan for all team members to use. If you identify a possible cause for the problem behavior, or know of an approach that is effective, inform the nurse. It is very important to include this information in the care plan. The plan will be based on the resident's individual strengths and needs. Behavior management is a form of restorative care, so the principles of restoration are used. The plan may have to be modified several times, depending on the resident's response. For the plan to be effective, all team members must be *consistent* in their approaches to the resident. For consistency, all care providers use exactly the same approaches in response to the resident.

Implementing the Behavior Management Plan. After the care plan has been developed, become familiar with it and implement the approaches listed. Your objective observations of the resident's response to the plan are important and should be reported to the nurse. The plan may call for you to modify your own behavior in response to the resident's behavior. Appropriate resident behavior is reinforced or rewarded. Residents tend to repeat behavior that is rewarded. Verbal praise, positive feedback, and other signs of approval are rewards. Nonverbal reinforcement such as a hug, smile, or pat on the back may also be used (Figure 16.8). Snacks and privileges are sometimes used as rewards.

The care plan will describe how to reduce the resident's inappropriate behavior. Sometimes this is done by ignoring the behavior, if this can safely be done. The care plan will specify other nonpunitive responses. The goal is not to punish the resident, but to show him or her a more positive way of directing energy.

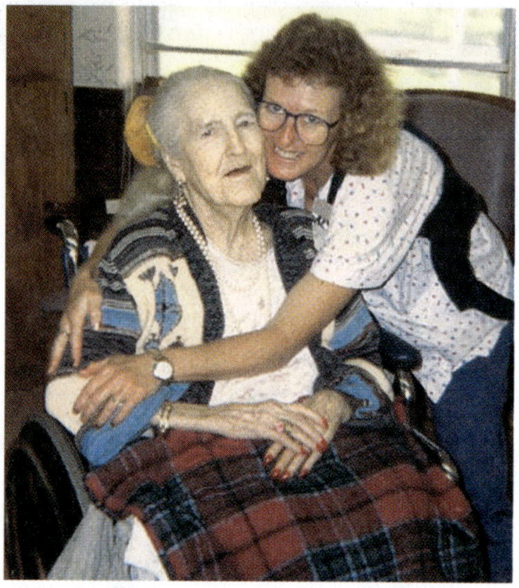

FIGURE 16-8 Residents respond warmly to touch and hugs.

Your Role in Assisting Residents with Specific Behavior Problems

Making generalizations about behavior management is difficult, because each person is a unique individual. However, certain common conditions are seen in residents in long-term care facilities. The general care you provide to residents with these conditions is similar. Always follow the care plan for specific resident information, goals, and approaches. Use common sense.

Depression. Feelings of despair or discouragement, called **depression**, may occur because of stress and loss. Sometimes depression occurs for unknown reasons. The signs and symptoms of depression vary widely. Decreased concentration, memory loss, fatigue, insomnia, sadness, crying,

GUIDELINES FOR

Assisting Residents Who Have Behavior Problems

- Follow the approaches listed on the care plan.
- Maintain control of your own responses and reactions.
- Remove the irritant, or cause of the behavior, if known.
- Protect the safety of the resident and others.
- If the care plan calls for you to respond when a resident demonstrates a specific behavior, implement the approaches as soon as the behavior starts. Do not wait for the resident to lose control.
- Use good communication and listening skills.
- Practice empathy.
- Attempt to learn the cause of the behavior, and communicate this information to other team members.
- Communicate effective approaches to other team members.
- Monitor the resident's response to your approaches. Adjust your approach if necessary.
- Discuss family, friends, or other pleasant information with residents. This provides a source of strength, comfort, and support.
- Make certain the resident's physical needs are met.
- Give alert residents as much control as possible. Offer choices in care and routines. Encourage residents to direct their own care.
- Be happy. Smile to communicate caring. Make sure your body language does not send a negative message. Positive behavior is contagious.

GUIDELINES FOR

Assisting the Resident Who Has Depression

- Be honest, supportive, and caring.
- Be a good listener (Figure 16.9). Encourage the resident to express feelings.
- Avoid passing judgment or criticizing what the resident feels. Avoid interrupting or changing the subject.
- Give positive feedback on the resident's strengths and successes.
- Acknowledge the resident's feelings.
- Do not make comments like "Cheer up. Things could be worse."
- Encourage physical activity to the extent possible. Exercise reduces stress.
- Encourage the resident to laugh regularly. Laughter is therapeutic and reduces stress. Turn on a funny television program or tell a joke.
- Monitor the resident's appetite and report overeating or undereating to the nurse.
- Report changes in behavior or talk of suicide to the nurse immediately.

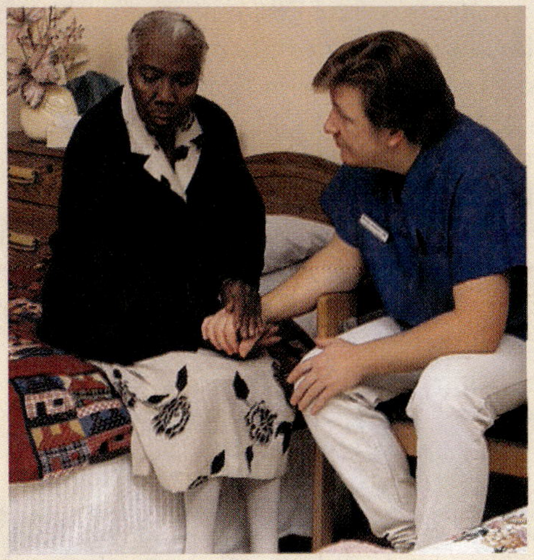

FIGURE 16-9 Allowing the resident to talk and express her feelings shows that you care.

GUIDELINES FOR

Assisting Residents Who Have Problems Sleeping

- Follow the resident's bedtime routine.
- Offer HS care by making the resident comfortable, giving a back rub, controlling room temperature, adjusting the lights, and eliminating noise in the environment.
- If the resident wakes up frightened during the night, provide support and reassurance. Make the resident comfortable.
- If the resident wakes up confused, provide orientation to person, place, and time. Assure the resident that he or she is safe and in the right place.
- If the resident wants to stay awake during the night, provide diversional activities and comfort measures that will not disturb others.
- Warm snacks may be helpful. Avoid beverages containing caffeine.

loss of appetite, overeating, apathy, and loss of self-esteem are all symptoms of depression.

Sleep Disturbances. Sleep problems may be related to physical, emotional, or environmental causes. Some residents complain of being unable to sleep. Others appear to sleep all the time. Look for causes of the sleep disturbance, such as excessive caffeine intake, pain, fear, anxiety, room temperature, or noise.

Complaining or Demanding Behavior. Listening to resident complaints requires a great deal of tact. Sometimes resident complaints are justified, but at times they are not. Listen objectively to what the resident says. Report the information to the

GUIDELINES FOR

Assisting the Resident Who Has Complaining or Demanding Behavior

- Reassure the resident that you understand the complaint or problem and will report it to the appropriate person.
- Use good listening skills and support the resident.
- If the complaints are about care given by others, remain neutral and do not criticize other workers. If complaints are about your care, listen, but do not argue or become defensive.
- Attempt to determine the cause of unjustified complaints and correct it if possible.
- Give the resident as much control over daily routines as possible.
- Offer choices to give the resident control, show respect for the resident as a person, and demonstrate that you value his or her opinion.

GUIDELINES FOR

Assisting the Resident Who Is Yelling or Calling Out

- Look for the cause of the behavior. If you can identify it, correct it.
- If the resident is alert, ask what the problem is. Use active listening skills and provide comfort.
- Realize that residents from some cultures scream with pain and grief. This is socially acceptable in the resident's culture.
- Offer the resident something to eat or drink.
- Monitor body language to see if the resident grimaces or shows other signs of pain.
- Try to distract the resident. Redirecting the behavior with a positive activity, such as a walk or looking at a picture album, may be helpful.
- Eliminate or minimize environmental stimulation. Try moving the resident to a quiet area.
- Provide physical comfort measures, such as turning, positioning, or a back rub.
- Take the resident to the bathroom. Some confused residents scream from the discomfort of a full bladder.

nurse objectively. If the complaint is something simple that you can correct, do so immediately.

Yelling and Screaming. Yelling and screaming may be the only way some residents can communicate or express displeasure. Most screaming behavior is seen in confused residents, but occasionally alert residents also yell and scream. Dealing with this type of behavior is usually done by trial and error. Remove the irritant, if known. Direct the resident's attention to another activity or try moving to another area, if possible.

Physical or Verbal Aggression. Physical aggression is hitting, scratching, kicking, biting, or fighting. This is called **combative behavior**. Verbal aggression is arguing, accusing, threatening, or swearing.

Sexual Behavior. All human beings need sexuality. Sexuality does not diminish with age (Figure 16.10). Sexual expression may be physical or psychological. Sexuality is a basic human need, according to Maslow. Always knock before entering a resident's room and wait for a response before entering.

Many health care workers feel that masturbation is inappropriate behavior. Masturbation is satisfying to the resident and is not harmful. It is an acceptable behavior as long as it is done in a private area. If you enter a resident's room and find the resident masturbating, provide privacy and leave the room.

If you enter a room and find two competent, consenting adults engaged in a sexual act, provide privacy and leave. Adults have a legal right to

GUIDELINES FOR

Assisting the Aggressive Resident

- Attempt to identify the cause of the behavior and eliminate it, if possible.
- Respect the resident's need for personal space.
- Do not back yourself into a room with no way to escape.
- Take physical threats seriously and keep your distance.
- Watch the resident's eyes. They will usually focus on the part of the body to be attacked.
- Remain calm.
- Speak in a soft, low, calm voice.
- Do not make the resident feel trapped or cornered.
- Do not turn your back on the resident.
- Avoid touching the resident, as this may cause further agitation.
- Show that you are interested in what the resident is saying.
- Empathize with the resident and acknowledge that you understand how he or she feels.
- Reassure the resident.
- Praise efforts at self-control.
- Do not argue or try to reason with the resident.
- Make sure your body language is not threatening.
- If aggressive behavior occurs in a public area, move the resident if it is safe to do so. If not, move others out of the way.
- Call for assistance from others, if necessary.

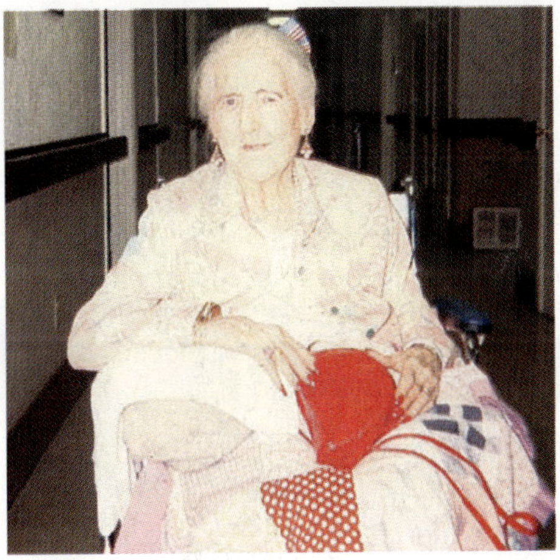

FIGURE 16-10 This resident's appearance is important to her. Assisting her to style her hair and apply makeup, nail polish, and jewelry help her feel attractive and promote a positive self-image.

do whatever is pleasing to them, as long as it is not medically contraindicated and both partners are mentally capable of consent. Do not pass judgment on the resident's choice of partner or methods of sexual expression.

Facility staff is responsible for protecting residents who are physically or mentally vulnerable to unwanted sexual contact. Sexual contact with unwilling, alert residents who are physically unable to defend themselves, or confused residents who cannot give full informed consent, is **sexual abuse**. Sexual abuse is a violation of resident rights and is illegal. No health care worker, visitor, or other resident is permitted to sexually abuse others. If sexual abuse occurs, the police are notified. Anyone who sexually harasses or abuses a resident or care provider should be reported to the nurse or other appropriate person according to your facility policy.

Sometimes residents may make unwanted sexual advances toward the nursing assistant. Humans have a normal need to express sexuality. The resident's desire for sexuality is normal, but the choice of person is not. If a resident makes sexual advances, do not ridicule or belittle him or her. Be patient and understanding, and speak to the resident in a matter-of-fact manner. Tactfully inform the resident that the behavior is not acceptable. Follow your facility policy for reporting sexual advances.

Table 16.2 lists types of inappropriate sexual behavior, potential triggers, and ways in which to manage the behavior. Table 16.3 lists observations to make of resident behaviors. Report your observations to the nurse.

COGNITIVE IMPAIRMENT

Cognitive impairment means damaged or impaired thinking. It is not a normal part of aging. It may be caused by disease, trauma, alcohol, street drugs, prescription medications, or anesthesia. Losses of

TABLE 16-2 Managing inappropriate sexual behavior

Behavior	Possible Trigger (Antecedent)	Approaches
Sexually suggestive comments, inappropriate sexual behavior (General Guidelines)	• Needs more affection, sense of belonging, need to be touched • As dementia progresses, the need for human contact is often expressed more physically • Environment reminds resident of sex • Fatigue, sensory overload, discomfort, boredom	• Focus on the person, not the behavior • *Remain calm, do not overreact* • *Inform the resident that the behavior is not appropriate* • Redirect the resident calmly and firmly • Involve the resident in an activities program • Do something the resident likes, such as listening to music, taking a walk, or having a snack • Give the resident something else to do • Leave and return later • Change your behavior • Change your physical position or approach • Touch the resident in an appropriate manner, such as by putting lotion on arms and hands • Find ways of incorporating appropriate touch into daily routine • Offer soothing objects to touch, fondle, and hold, such as stuffed animals or dolls • Assist in making the resident look good and feel physically attractive • If the behavior occurs at a certain time of day, keep the resident involved in a purposeful activity during this time • Do an environmental audit. Hot? Cold? Too much stimulation? Too little stimulation? • Offer to take the resident to the bathroom • Move the resident to another location • Encourage and reward appropriate behavior • Be aware of cues indicating unmet intimacy needs
Sexual gestures with staff or inappropriate touching during personal care or ADLs	• Misinterprets caregiver's intention • Resident misinterprets cues, perceives another's touch as sexual, such as touching or sitting next to the resident and touching his or her body with yours	• Distract during personal care • Avoid sending the resident mixed sexual messages, even in a joking manner • Ask a caregiver of the same gender (as the resident) to provide personal care

	• Environment reminds resident of sex • Mistakes caregiver for their partner	• *Remain calm, do not overreact* • *Inform the resident that the behavior is not appropriate* • Respond to the resident in a matter-of-fact manner • Be aware that the behavior is a symptom of the resident's illness • Be aware of your own behavior, body language, and the message you send • Decide ahead of time how you will react if a resident makes inappropriate sexual advances. Advance planning will help you react appropriately when confronted with the situation
Removing clothes Exposing self Undressing in public Wearing only a shirt	• Too hot in environment • Need to use the bathroom • Clothing uncomfortable • Memory loss, forgets to put on clothes • Unaware of environment; may think he is in his bedroom or getting ready to bathe • Tired, wants to go to bed • Does not remember rules of social behavior	• Check and modify room temperature • Take to bathroom • Make sure clothing fits properly, is comfortable and not too tight • Allow resident to rest in bed • Dress in clothing that opens in back or is difficult to remove (do not put clothing on inside out or backward, use clothing designed to open in back)
Public masturbation or fondling self	• Genital irritation • Reacts to what feels good • No longer has judgment, awareness of appropriate behavior	• Check for irritation at an appropriate time • Remove from public area and provide privacy • Give resident repetitive manual activities to do, such as folding towels
Inappropriate advances toward other residents Sexual behavior with another resident Touching someone else in an inappropriate way	• Other person may remind the resident of a former partner • Other resident may be giving cues that are perceived as sexual advances, such as a woman lifting her skirt • Mistakes other resident for a former partner	• Calmly and firmly inform resident that the behavior is not appropriate • Keep residents separated as much as possible • Monitor helpless residents carefully; protect helpless residents • Seat away from residents of the opposite gender • Have care provided by staff member of same gender as the resident

self-care ability are often the first sign of cognitive impairment. Over time, residents become unable to recognize familiar faces, objects, or surroundings. They lose the ability to learn and process new information. The most common symptoms are loss of ability to make decisions, memory loss, mental confusion, and poor judgment (Figure 16.11). In early stages of cognitive loss, the resident usually knows there is a problem. He or she may make up stories and spend a tremendous amount of energy trying to hide the memory loss. If the resident cannot remember something, he or she makes up a story. Avoid judging the resident. Avoid placing too many demands on the resident, which

TABLE 16-3 Behavior observations to make and report
Always report abnormal behavior to the nurse, even if you believe the behavior is "normal for the resident."
Who? Does the behavior involve another person or specific types of people? How are these individuals alike?
What? Describe the behavior. What were the circumstances in which the behavior occurred?
Where? Did the behavior occur in one specific location?
When? What is the time of day? Does the behavior occur at predictable times or in predictable situations, such as during bathing? When the resident is tired, when the resident awakens, or other times?
What were the environmental conditions? Was it light, dark, hot, cold, noisy, quiet?
How do others respond to the resident's behavior? Is there anyone who is never approached by the resident? If so, how does he or she manage or prevent the behavior?
Is there a pattern or clues to the behavior? Can you identify clues or signals that the behavior is about to begin?

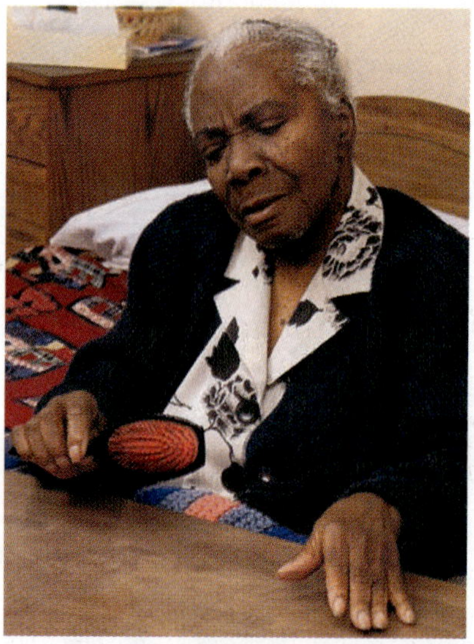

FIGURE 16-11 This resident with dementia has forgotten what the hairbrush is used for.

cause stress. Care of residents with cognitive impairment should maintain their quality of life, functional abilities, and dignity. Provide support. Monitor for safety in the environment.

Dementia

Dementia is a mental disorder that causes cognitive impairment. Dementia is not a disease. It can be acute or chronic, and occurs as the result of some diseases and conditions. Dementia is a set of symptoms affecting the resident's thinking, judgment, memory, and ability to reason. In persons with dementia, mental function declines over time. The rights of residents with dementia are the same as those of other residents, but the nursing assistant may need to help residents exercise their rights.

Delirium

Delirium is an acute confusional state. It indicates a treatable illness. There are many causes, including medications and drugs, fever, isolation, depression, use of restraints, recent relocation, and dehydration. The most common causes are infection, circulatory, respiratory, and metabolic disorders. Often two or three different causes contribute to the delirium. If one cause is eliminated, the delirium will remain until all causes have been discovered and are eliminated. Delirium is characterized by changing states of consciousness, disorganization, behavioral changes, and lack of awareness of the environment. The resident becomes **disoriented**, or loses awareness of person, place, or time. Delirium usually develops quickly, over several hours or several days. Rapid development of symptoms is a key indicator that there is an underlying medical problem. Dementia develops gradually over a much longer period of time. When the medical problem is treated properly, the resident's mental status clears. This may occur quickly, or take several weeks.

Sensory Losses

Sensory loss is difficulty seeing, hearing, smelling, or touching. Loss of sensation may produce signs of cognitive impairment. The problem is worsened if the resident has an existing dementia. If the resident cannot see, hear, feel, or otherwise communicate with others and the environment, he or she may appear cognitively impaired. Besides the inability to communicate with others, the resident may misinterpret noises, people, or other images. The resident may have self-care deficits because he or she cannot see what he or she is doing or hear your instructions. This may cause the resident to have behavior problems. Sometimes simple measures, such as having the eyes examined, putting the resident's glasses on, or using a hearing aid, are enough to improve the condition.

Observing the Resident

Careful assessment and observation by the interdisciplinary team are necessary to differentiate delirium from dementia. Sometimes delirium, medical problems, or sensory losses worsen existing dementia. Because the nursing assistants spend more time with the resident than other team members, their observational skills are very important. Small, seemingly minor changes may be important. Sometimes we think that certain behaviors are "normal for the resident." For example, each night when you give a resident HS care, the resident hits and fights. You accept this as normal for the resident, complete your care, and continue your assignment. Because you are the only person in the room with the resident, others may not know of this behavior. The behavior is not normal and may be important. Report your observations of the resident's physical and mental status to the nurse and be alert for changes. Some health care facilities keep a log of behaviors so they can study the time of day, type of behavior, and triggering events. This helps to determine if there is a pattern to the behavior.

Alzheimer's Disease

Alzheimer's disease is a disease that causes loss of mental abilities and judgment. It is the most common form of dementia. The cause is unknown, but it is believed that heredity plays a significant role in its development. Most cases of Alzheimer's disease occur in residents over the age of 65, but it can occur in middle-aged individuals. Alzheimer's disease causes physical and chemical changes in the brain. The brain atrophies. In muscles, atrophy is preventable, but this is not true with the brain. The disease progressively worsens and is eventually fatal. However, some individuals may live up to 20 years with the disease. Their physical health may be excellent in the early stages, but declines as the disease progresses. Some medications will improve the symptoms, but there is no cure. Residents with Alzheimer's disease are at high risk for dehydration. The resident may forget to drink, or may lose the sensation of thirst completely. Be aware of the risk and offer fluids frequently.

Three Stages of Alzheimer's Disease

Persons with Alzheimer's disease go through three stages. Physical and mental problems worsen in each stage. Eventually, all cognitive ability is lost. Initially, the resident can perform normal activities of daily living with verbal cues and reminders, but over time the resident becomes totally dependent on others.

Stage I: Mild Dementia. Residents in this stage of Alzheimer's appear normal and can function with minimum assistance and supervision. The changes in this stage are in memory and personality, and include:

- Short-term memory loss; long-term memory remains
- Indifference and apathy
- Resident is not outgoing and is not interested in life
- Decreased concentration and attention span
- Poor judgment
- Unaware of time
- Inability to calculate simple math problems, such as those needed to balance a checkbook
- May forget to eat and drink
- Moodiness
- Blames others for mistakes and problems
- Disorientation to location, inability to remember how to get home
- **Delusions of persecution**, or believing that others are attempting to cause personal harm
- Carelessness
- Unkempt appearance
- Anxiety, agitation, and depression

Stage II: Moderate Dementia. In this stage, short-term memory continues to decline. Long-term memory loss is apparent. All of the symptoms from the first stage continue. The person continues to be in good physical health. Other symptoms are:

- Loss of control over impulses and behavior
- Complete disorientation
- Unable to recognize danger
- Restlessness

GUIDELINES FOR

Caring for Residents Who Have Dementia

- Approach the resident from the front. Make sure the resident can see or hear you when you approach. Avoid startling the resident.
- Be calm, gentle, and flexible in your approach.
- Control your own body. Avoid sudden, abrupt movement.
- Stay in control of your own responses to the resident. Try to remain calm and soothing when responding to the resident.
- Be creative when responding to the resident. Modify your behavior according to how the resident responds and reacts to you.
- Be matter-of-fact and nondemanding.
- Speak in a "here and now" time frame.
- If the resident is not agitated, use touch to show you care.
- Speak slowly and clearly, using short, simple sentences and words.
- Offer simple choices, but do not overwhelm the resident with options. Best results are obtained if you ask the resident to select one of two choices.
- Break large tasks down into a series of smaller tasks.
- Give the resident familiar, orienting cues for performing ADLs.
- If a resident is combative or agitated, stand at the side when he or she is putting on shoes and socks, to avoid getting kicked.
- Follow the same routine each day.
- If the resident does not understand what you are trying to say, demonstrate. For example, put the brush in the resident's hand. Simulate brushing your hair and tell the resident to imitate you.
- Make eye contact when speaking. Try to be at the resident's eye level whenever possible.
- Make sure your body language matches your words (Figure 16.12).
- Keep your voice low and speak calmly.
- Use one-step commands. If the resident does not respond, count to five before repeating. After the resident completes one step, move to the next.
- Avoid rushing the resident. Allow adequate time to complete a task.
- Avoid words such as "don't" or "no" whenever possible. Instead, use words like "do" or "let's."
- Alternate periods of activity with rest.
- Monitor for signs of increasing frustration.
- Accept communication even if it does not make sense. Avoid arguing. For example, the resident tells you that her grandmother ate lunch with her. A good response is, "Are you thinking about your grandmother?"
- Concentrate on what the resident tells you, even if it does not make sense. Respond to what you think the resident is saying.
- Do not argue with the resident about fixed, false beliefs.
- Avoid situations that you know are upsetting to the resident.
- If the resident is upset or agitated, avoid turning your back. Keep your face protected or out of the resident's reach.
- Keep the environment simple and safe. Do not make changes in the environment.
- Provide activities at the time of day the activity would normally be done.
- Reduce excessive noise and stimulation in the environment.

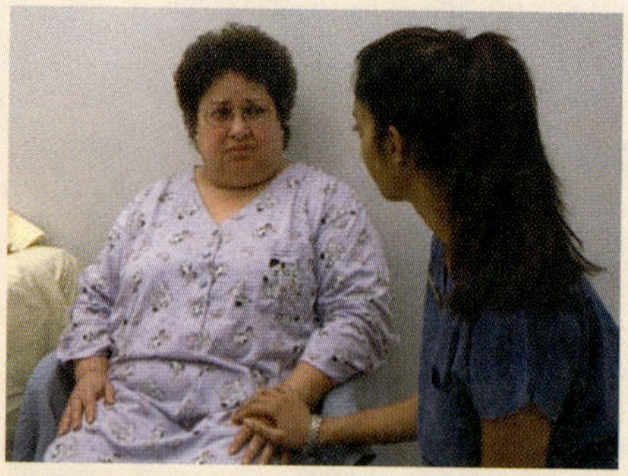

FIGURE 16-12 Your body language should send a caring message.

- Wandering and pacing
- **Sundowning**, or increased restlessness and wandering in the late afternoon, evening, and night
- Sensory and perceptual changes that cause the person to be unable to differentiate hot, cold, left, right, up, or down
- Loss of ability to recognize common items such as silverware or grooming items
- Loss of ability to perform motor skills, such as eating, dressing, and toileting
- Gradual loss of ability to follow directions
- **Perseveration**, or repetitious behavior, speech, movement, or action
- Difficulty speaking, reading, and writing
- Gradual loss of ability to understand others
- Walking and motor problems; development of a shuffling gait
- Incontinence of bowel and bladder
- **Hallucinations**, or seeing, hearing, smelling, or feeling something that is not real
- **Delusions**, or false beliefs
- **Catastrophic reactions**, or uncontrolled emotional outbursts in response to feeling completely overwhelmed

Stage III: Severe Dementia. The resident in stage III is totally dependent on others for care and develops severe physical problems. The ability to swallow is progressively lost, and the resident is at high risk for choking and aspiration. The resident becomes bedfast and unable to sit in the chair or walk. Seizures may be present. The resident progresses to coma and death. Other signs and symptoms of the third stage of Alzheimer's disease are:

- Complete mental disorientation to time, place, and person
- Loss of ability to communicate
- Inability to recognize family, friends, and facility staff
- Total dependence on others for all care
- Resistance to care
- Refusal to eat
- Sleep disturbances
- Lack of response to activity or environment

COMMUNICATION

Good communication skills are necessary when caring for residents with Alzheimer's disease and other dementias. Try to talk to the resident in an area that is free from distractions. These residents have lost the ability to screen out distractions and noises from the television, radio, or other conversations. Monitor your body language. Make sure it sends the proper message and does not communicate impatience or anger. Begin your conversation socially to win the resident's trust. One way of doing this is to sit and talk before beginning resident care. Always begin your conversation with orienting information. Call the resident by name and tell her who you are. After the resident is relaxed, explain what you are going to do. Make eye contact and be sure you have his or her attention before beginning to speak. Sit at the resident's eye level when you speak whenever possible. If the resident ignores you, wait a minute and try again. Gently touch the resident's arm to get his or her attention. However, avoid startling the resident, which can cause a catastrophic reaction. Speak slowly and clearly, using short, simple sentences. Ask questions that require a yes or no answer. Use concrete terms and familiar words. Keep your tone of voice low and speak in a calm, warm, pleasant manner.

You may have trouble understanding what the resident tells you. Listen actively and carefully. If you do not understand, apologize and ask the resident to repeat. Try to focus on a word or phrase that you understand. Repeat what you do understand and help the resident clarify it. Respond to the resident's emotion. For example, say, "You sound very angry." Remain calm and patient. If the resident repeats certain words, ask family members if they know the meaning. Sometimes people with Alzheimer's disease talk by using code words that close friends and family understand.

Residents with Alzheimer's disease lose the ability to reason. Avoid arguing, which makes the situation worse. Do not tell the resident what he or she can and cannot do. Instead, use distraction. The resident may say "I'm going home to cook dinner for my children." You know the children are grown and live in another state. Instead of arguing with the resident, ask what she likes to cook. Then distract her by asking her to sit with you and look at a magazine. Avoid asking the resident questions that require a good memory. People with dementia often recognize that they have memory loss and are humiliated and frustrated when they cannot remember. Do not talk about residents who have dementia in front of them. We do not know what they understand, and their understanding changes from one moment to the next.

Goals for Caregiving

Always keep in mind the following goals when caring for residents with Alzheimer's disease or other dementias:

1. Protect the resident from physical injury.
2. Maintain the resident's independence as long as possible.

3. Focus on what the resident is still able to do.
4. Provide physical and mental activities within the resident's capabilities.
5. Support the resident's dignity and self-esteem at all times.

To meet these goals:

1. The care must be consistent. Procedures should be carried out in the same way, all the time. All caregivers should use the same approach.
2. The routine of care should be structured but flexible to accommodate residents when they are more responsive or less responsive.
3. The care must be given in a peaceful, quiet environment that is simple, uncluttered, and unchanged.
4. Staff members must be educated to the needs of the residents with dementia and must learn how to meet these needs.

Alzheimer's Units

Many facilities have established special Alzheimer care units. These units differ from general units in several ways:

- There is a higher staff-to-resident ratio.
- The staff has received special training in Alzheimer's care.
- Cross-training of staff may be done. For example, nursing assistants may help with activities and activity staff or social service staff may help with meals.
- The unit is a "dedicated" unit. This means that the same staff work on the unit all the time. New staff are assigned to the unit only when there is an opening that has to be filled.

This type of staffing results in:

- Staff who have a special interest in Alzheimer's residents.
- Staff who know each resident, their strengths, and their weaknesses.
- Staff who better understand the need to facilitate an interdisciplinary support system.
- Staff who can provide valuable input for the plan of care.

The environment is specially designed to:

- Provide calmness and serenity through the use of color and design.
- Avoid disturbing noises. For example, there is no loudspeaker system, telephones do not ring, and televisions are turned on only when appropriate.
- Be secure, so that residents may wander at will without threat of danger.
- Most activities can take place on the unit. The dining room and activities areas are incorporated into the unit.
- Families are encouraged to take part in the care and activities if they wish.

Residents must meet certain pre-established criteria before being admitted to the special unit. This is to ensure that placement will benefit the resident and also the other residents.

Residents' Rights

Residents with dementia have the same rights as other residents. They may need assistance to ensure that these rights are protected. It is important to remember that:

- Making decisions and having choices is a resident's right. However, residents with dementia may be unable to make decisions and may become overwhelmed with too many choices. This can cause the resident to become very upset.
- Staff must protect residents with dementia. Do not allow them to be taken advantage of or abused by other people.
- The rights of residents with dementia do not have priority over the rights of other residents. For example, it is upsetting to other residents to have confused residents wandering into their rooms. The resident with dementia is not aware of this. It is the staff's responsibility to resolve these issues without infringing on the rights of either resident.
- Residents with dementia have the right to have possessions that give them pleasure as long as these do not impair the health or safety of the resident or other people. For example, if a resident receives pleasure from a doll or stuffed animal, do not take it away. Above all, do not tease or make fun of the situation. The resident deserves to be treated with dignity (Figure 16.13).

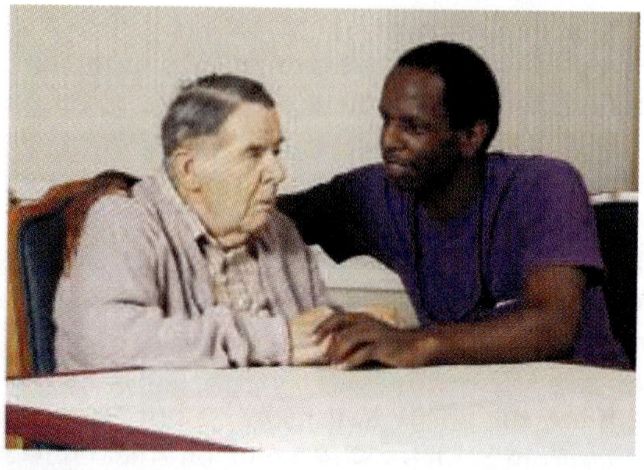

FIGURE 16-13 Always treat the resident with dignity.

Family Members

In most cases, family members have cared for the resident with a dementia for months or years prior to admission to the long-term care facility. By the time the decision is made to admit the individual, the family is often physically and emotionally drained. The admission is a traumatic experience. As you work with the residents with Alzheimer's or other dementias, remember:

1. The family remembers the resident as a vital family member. Acknowledge the family's presence.
2. The spouse of the resident may have no other support system. If they have children, they may be many miles away. It can be very upsetting not to be recognized by a spouse of many years. Some facilities have support groups for families.
3. Listen to the family's suggestions. They often know what will work and what will not be effective in caring for the new resident.
4. Allow the family to participate in the care, if they choose to and if it is appropriate. For example, many family members like to assist the resident at mealtime.

Special Problems

Alzheimer's disease is frustrating for the resident, family, and care provider. The resident is not responsible for the symptoms of the disease. Some residents say unkind things, hit, or act aggressively. The disease has triggered the problem. Because Alzheimer's disease also causes poor impulse control, the resident is powerless to do anything to correct the behavior. Caring for residents with Alzheimer's disease requires patience and understanding.

Catastrophic reactions occur as a result of being startled or in response to overwhelming stimulation. Anger and rage are signs that the resident is feeling loss of control. The resident cannot control the reaction. Catastrophic reactions are noted by increased agitation and physical activity. The resident may talk, yell, or mumble (Figure 16.14). Sometimes the behavior is violent. The best way to deal with catastrophic reactions is to anticipate and prevent them. Monitor the resident's behavior closely and watch for signs of increasing restlessness or agitation. Minimize noise and confusion in the environment. Make sure the resident's physical needs are met. If a catastrophic reaction occurs, avoid trying to reason with the resident. Avoid restraints and use of physical force. Approach the resident using a soft, calm, but firm voice. Touching the resident may make the reaction worse. Remove the resident from the stressful situation, if possible. Avoid responding with anger and hostility. Distraction may be effective. Reassure the resident by speaking gently. Make every effort to quiet the resident by speaking calmly and listening to what the resident says.

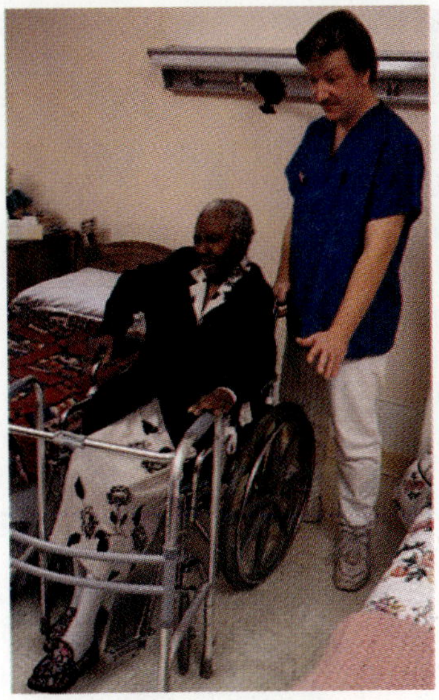

FIGURE 16-14 Recognize early signs of a catastrophic reaction and counteract them whenever possible.

If you feel that your physical safety is threatened during a catastrophic reaction, stand out of the resident's reach. Call for help. Avoid having many care providers approach the resident at one time. Avoid making the resident feel trapped or cornered. Watch the resident's eyes. Residents will usually stare at the person or body part that will be attacked. Protect yourself according to your facility policy.

Wandering

Wandering is a very serious concern for long-term care facilities. Residents who wander within the facility may become lost or injured. Residents who wander outside the facility are in danger of being hit by a car, overexposed to heat and cold, and placed in other situations that can be harmful or dangerous.

Residents in multi-story facilities often enter the elevator when wandering. Cover the buttons outside the elevator with fabric or duct tape. Staff and visitors will know that they can push the elevator buttons through the fabric, but a confused resident will not. Replace the tape or fabric when it shows signs of wear.

GUIDELINES FOR

Managing Wandering Behavior

- Consider physical causes for the behavior, including illness, the need to use the bathroom, hunger, thirst, and pain. By trial and error, eliminate each cause to see if it reduces the wandering.
- If the resident is wandering trying to find his or her room, place an identifying object on the door to the room. Direct the resident to find the object.
- Decrease noise and stimulation in the environment.
- Remove coats, purses, and other items that the resident associates with going outside.
- Check the resident daily to make sure the identification bracelet is in place.
- Always know what clothing the resident is wearing.
- Distract the resident with a magazine, conversation, activity, food, or drink.
- Give the wanderer a repetitious task, such as folding towels or sorting items.
- Provide a portable radio with a headset. Play the resident's favorite type of music. This simple distraction is often very effective.
- Remind and reassure the resident that he or she is safe and in the right place.
- Make sure that the wanderer gets adequate exercise.
- Avoid trying to reason with a wanderer who is determined to leave. Instead, provide distraction.
- Avoid telling a wanderer "Don't go outside." Thinking and understanding is a complex process. Instructing the resident not to leave will cause him or her to think about going outside. If someone tells you not to think of a green cat, you will think of it. Then you will have to unthink it. Saying "stay inside" is a more effective approach with a person who is cognitively impaired.
- Keep toxic substances, chemicals, matches, and other potentially harmful items in locked cupboards.
- Provide adequate lighting. Aging changes in vision make more light necessary to interpret the environment correctly.
- Monitor and respond to exit door alarms.
- Leave a night-light on in the room during the night.
- Make sure the resident is wearing eye glasses and hearing aids, if used. This helps to maintain contact with the environment.
- Post signs and labels on drawers, common rooms, and other items.
- Display familiar items and pictures in the resident's room.
- Consider seating the wanderer in a beanbag chair. They are comfortable but difficult to get out of.
- Know where a current picture of the wanderer is located in case he or she becomes lost.
- Apply a shirt or sweater to the resident and have him wear it for 6 to 8 hours. Remove the garment and place the *unwashed* item in a sealed plastic bag. Mark the resident's name on the bag and put it on the closet shelf. If the wanderer does become lost, the garment can be used by a tracking dog. In the event a tracking garment is not available, the dog may be able to pick up a scent from the pillow.

A key to understanding wandering behavior is to realize that there are different types of wanderers. If the type of wandering behavior can be identified, approaches can be planned to keep the resident safe. The types of wanderers are listed in Table 16.4.

Allowing residents to wander in a safe area is the best approach to take. Consider physical causes for the wandering, such as pain, thirst, hunger, or looking for the bathroom. Decrease noise levels in the environment. Approach the resident from the front, then walk with the resident by falling in step at her side. If the resident leaves the unit or goes outside, walk with her and circle back in. Distract the resident with food, drink, or activity. Monitor for signs of fatigue and encourage the resident to sit down and get adequate rest. There are many techniques to keep wanderers safe. Most important, wanderers require supervision and understanding. Restraints should be used only as a last resort.

TABLE 16-4 Wanderers

Type of Wanderer	Characteristics	Approaches
Exit seeker/ escapist wanderer	• Very high risk for leaving the facility. • The resident may not know where he or she is, but knows that he or she does not want to be there. • May be ambulatory or in a wheelchair. • Resident looks for opportunities to exit and leaves very quickly if presented with an opportunity. • Completely unaware of personal safety. • May not be properly dressed for the outside climate. • Uses very poor judgment. • Probably has a destination in mind.	• Try to determine the resident's intended location in advance. • Avoid arguing or using reality orientation, which agitate the resident. • Use distraction. • This wanderer is usually not looking for a physical location, but instead a state of mind. Try to provide it. If the resident says he or she must go to work, provide the state of mind by talking about the job, responsibilities, and so forth. • Make the resident feel good about himself or herself. • Remove hats, coats, coat rack, purses, shoes, and other items associated with going outside.
Critical/self-stimulation wanderer	• Completely disoriented. • Unaware of safety. • At very high risk of serious injury outside the facility. • Not deliberately trying to leave the facility. • If resident turns a doorknob or pushes the panic bar on the door for stimulation, he or she will exit.	• Close monitoring and supervision. • Diversional activity. • Exercise. • Walking in a small group inside the facility. • Responds well to repetition, structure, predictability, and familiar routines.
Akathisia wanderer	• Resident who has taken psychiatric drugs (chemical restraints) for many years. • Wandering is a side effect of years of drug therapy. • Very restless. • Wanders aimlessly with no apparent purpose. • May cross arms in front of the chest or abdomen when wandering. • Usually does not try to leave the facility.	• Close monitoring and supervision. • Diversional activity. • Exercise. • Walking in a small group inside the facility. • Responds well to repetition, structure, predictability, and familiar routines.
Purposeful wanderer	• Has a specific agenda, but is unable to communicate what it is. • May be looking for the bathroom. • May be bored. • May be overstimulated by noise and other factors in the environment. • May be in pain. • May be hungry or thirsty. • May be stressed and feeling overwhelmed. • May be dehydrated.	• Through trial and error, attempt to learn the resident's agenda and meet it.

TABLE 16-4 *(continued)*

Type of Wanderer	Characteristics	Approaches
Aimless wanderer	• Totally disoriented. May think he or she is in own residence. • Frequently wanders into others' rooms. • May rummage through others' belongings. • Will enter housekeeping closets and unlocked service areas. • Totally unaware of personal safety. • Usually very upsetting to other residents and stressful for facility staff.	• Place cloth shields over doorknobs to change the texture. • Tape paper streamers across doorways. • Post signs that say "Stop," "Do Not Enter," or "Construction Zone." • Provide a dresser or nightstand of items to rummage through in the hallways. • Give the resident a repetitious task, such as folding towels or sorting coins.
Modeling wanderer	• Wander in pairs, usually for stimulation and companionship. • If the first resident exits the facility, the second resident will follow. • Usually completely unaware of safety.	• Provide diversional activities. • Determine the leader's agenda and keep him or her in the facility. • Place dark tile or construction paper on the floor by the doorway. It appears to be a hole, and residents usually will not attempt to cross it.

Problems with ADLs

When performing ADL care, try to focus on familiar skills and tasks. Although the resident cannot learn new tasks, he or she may be able to do familiar ones. Give the resident control by offering one of two choices. Allow enough time for the resident to process the information. If the resident does not understand, repeat the instructions in exactly the same way. Break the task down into small, simple steps. Give only one direction at a time and allow the resident time to complete it before giving the next. Telling the resident to complete an entire task, such as bathing, may be overwhelming. Start by telling the resident to wash his or her face. After the face is washed, instruct the resident in the next step. Sincerely compliment the resident for success.

Problems with Bathing. Resistance to bathing is a common problem in residents with Alzheimer's disease. The resident may have forgotten the purpose of bathing. Residents may be uncomfortable and resist removing their clothing in front of you. Wrapping a towel around the shoulders and pinning it securely may help with modesty problems. Leave the towel in place during the bath. Some residents appear to be fearful of water or afraid of washing. Noises from running water, the whirlpool tub, and heaters in the shower room may frighten the resident. Sound tends to echo in some shower rooms, making the problem worse. Encouraging the resident to sing an old song or playing pleasant music may help. (You may also use a special battery-operated shower radio, or keep the radio plug away from sources of water.)

Because Alzheimer's disease causes problems with sensation, bathing may be uncomfortable. The resident may not be able to feel the water temperature. Bathing is a complex task involving many steps. Taking a bath may simply be too overwhelming for the resident. Residents with Alzheimer's disease may also be sensitive with an unfamiliar nursing assistant.

Maintain a flexible attitude when you are assigned to bathe a cognitively impaired resident. Avoid forcing the resident. If the resident becomes agitated and refuses to bathe, leave and try again later. Before bringing the resident to the tub or shower room, make sure the room is warm and private. Before beginning, ask the resident to feel the water. Say something like "This feels good." Explain what you are going to do and what you want the resident to do, one step at a time. Giving many directions at one time may be overwhelming and will trigger a catastrophic reaction. If you will be giving the resident a complete bath, giving the resident something to hold and occupy the hands may be helpful. Squeezing a sponge or washcloth may distract the resident. Washing the hair may also be frightening. Use the resident's responses to guide your actions.

Modify your behavior and care according to the resident's responses to the procedure. Be slow, calm, patient, and reassuring. If you are successful with bathing the resident, share the approaches you used with the nurse and other team members so that the approaches can be added to the care plan.

Dressing Problems. Some residents are resistive to dressing. Others remove their clothing after they are dressed. Keep the morning routine consistent and familiar. Once you start, avoid interruptions, which cause the resident to forget what he or she is supposed to be doing. Make sure the room is warm and private. Ask the resident to select the clothing, if this is not too overwhelming. The clothing should be color-coordinated and appropriate for the resident's age and the season. Lay out clothing in the order in which it will be put on. Break the task down into simple, manageable steps and give the resident easy instructions, one step at a time. Assist with dressing, if needed. Allow the resident to do as much for himself or herself as possible, but do not let the resident become overwhelmed or frustrated. Understand the resident's need for privacy and unwillingness to completely disrobe in front of you. Be sensitive to grooming issues and encourage residents to comb hair, shave, or wear cosmetics and jewelry. Praise the resident and compliment his or her appearance.

Other Helpful Techniques

The residents' care plans will list various methods for managing residents who have cognitive impairment or behavior problems. Some of the approaches you will see are described here.

Activities

The activities program has many important functions in the long-term care facility. The activities department plans social and therapeutic programs to meet residents' needs (Figure 16.15). Activities meet many resident needs, ranging from socialization to relief of boredom. Many activities meet residents' self-esteem needs. Some activities provide outlets for residents to express feelings. The activity department will post a schedule of daily activities and events. Schedule resident care around the activity programs the residents want to attend. Activities are available to meet the needs of both high-functioning and low-functioning residents. Activities such as parties are enjoyable to all residents.

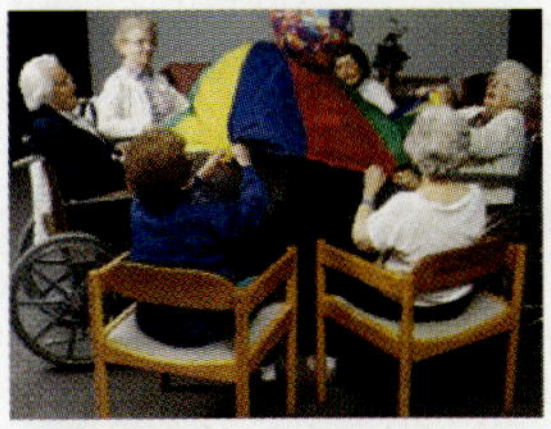

FIGURE 16-15 Activities serve many purposes. This parachute activity is enjoyable, but also provides excellent upper extremity exercise. *(Compliments of Briggs Corporation, Des Moines, IA [800] 247-2343)*

All residents, including those with behavior problems, will benefit from activities. Some residents will not be able to read the daily schedule. Plan your routine and offer to escort the residents to appropriate activities. The activity department will also provide activities to keep residents occupied on the nursing unit. They will do room visits for residents who are bedfast. They will obtain items such as talking books for residents who have sensory impairments. They plan trips and programs in the community. Special programs, such as music therapy and pet therapy, are enjoyable for many residents. The activity department can be a great source of assistance in the care of residents who have cognitive impairment and behavior problems. Find out what programs and resources are available in your facility, and use them to benefit the residents.

Validation Therapy

Validation therapy is a technique developed by Naomi Feil, who is a social worker, an actress, and a researcher. She describes the therapy as a way to communicate with persons over the age of 75. It is also used for persons with Alzheimer's disease and cognitive impairments (Figure 16.16). The program is based on the belief that developmental

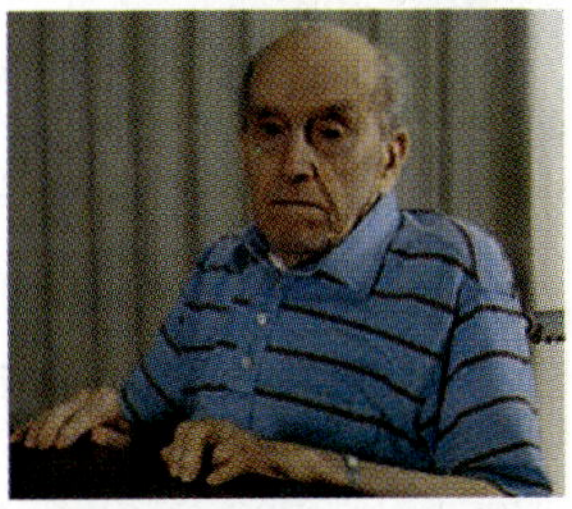

FIGURE 16-16 This cognitively impaired resident was once a child, then an adult. Use validation to reinforce his self-esteem and assist him to complete the developmental tasks of old age.

tasks from earlier years must be resolved. If they were not resolved, they will emerge in old age. The elderly person may display many emotions in trying to conclude them. Feil's research has shown that using validation reduces the need for restraints. It helps residents regain feelings of dignity and self-control. It also increases staff morale. Feil stresses the following concepts:

- Maintaining the identity and dignity of residents is important.
- People with dementia can feel good about themselves.
- All behavior has a purpose. Some disoriented behavior may be acting out of memories.
- The residents' memories and feelings should be acknowledged.
- Cognitively impaired residents have the right to express their feelings.
- Residents must resolve living in order to prepare for dying.
- The elderly have experienced many losses. Many have lost the ability to cope.
- Living in reality is not the only way to live.
- Disoriented residents are worthwhile. Staff can give them joy by allowing them to express their feelings.
- Each person was once a child, then an adult. Residents deserve to be cared for with dignity in their final years of life.

When using validation, allow residents to express their feelings. Reassure them that the feelings are worthwhile. Use a calm, nonthreatening manner. Speak in a loving tone of voice. When the resident describes an emotion, assure him or her that it is okay. A book, videotape, and training program are available for facilities that use this technique.

Reality Orientation

Reality orientation is a technique in which the residents are reoriented to time, place, person, and season. Some facilities do not use reality orientation because they believe it worsens agitation in some residents. The subject is controversial. It is most effective in orienting residents who are delirious. Memory loss in delirium is a temporary condition. After the resident recovers, the confusion clears. Newly admitted residents who are confused by the change in environment may also benefit. A large calendar is placed in the resident's room. Each day is marked off. Large clocks are placed throughout the facility. Signs with large letters label areas, equipment, and personal items (Figure 16.17). This enables the resident to find his or her way about the facility.

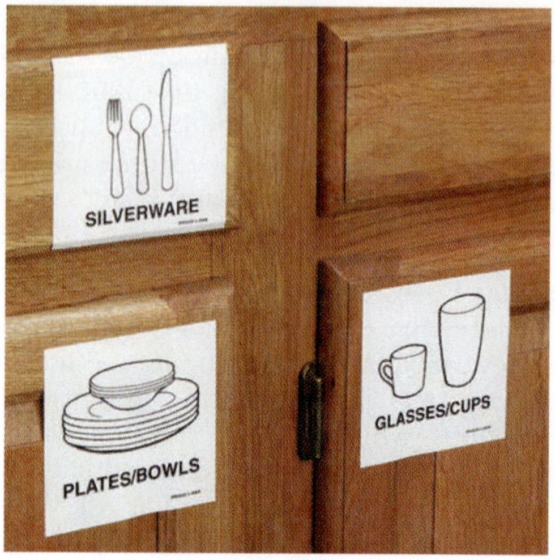

FIGURE 16-17 Using signs to label areas and personal items helps residents to function independently. *(Compliments of Briggs Corporation, Des Moines, IA [800] 247-2343)*

To be effective, reality orientation must be used by all staff during each resident contact. The goal is to give the resident a sense of identity in time and space. It may decrease anxiety in some residents. When approaching residents, call them by name. Tell them who you are. Do not expect them to remember you.

The principles of reality orientation are to:

- Treat residents as adults
- Treat residents with dignity
- Speak clearly and directly; avoid speaking loudly
- Use repetition; speak slowly if the resident does not understand
- Allow enough time for the resident to process thoughts and respond
- Keep instructions and responses simple and brief
- Maintain structure in routines
- Make sure residents are wearing hearing aids and glasses
- Promote resident independence
- Frequently provide orientation about the day, date, time, season, and weather
- Avoid making residents feel like you are putting them on the spot or criticizing them
- Answer questions honestly, but avoid information that is upsetting
- Avoid reinforcing the resident's confusion
- Avoid teasing the resident about his or her confusion
- Avoid arguing with residents who are delusional

Although reality orientation is effective in some residents, do not depend on it for keeping residents safe. For example, showing a confused resident how to use the call signal may be effective when you are in the room. Residents with cognitive impairment have short-term memory loss, and will probably forget how to use the call signal as soon as you leave the room. Do not depend on the resident's memory or safety awareness to prevent falls. Use other approaches, such as frequent monitoring or restraint alternatives, for safety.

Reminiscing

Reminiscing is the act of remembering the past (Figure 16.18A). It is a normal activity for all people. One of the developmental tasks of the elderly is a life review. Reminiscence helps residents complete this task. Studies have shown that reminiscence programs can improve cognitive function. A group of women studied had excellent results. Almost everyone enjoys this activity. Reminiscence is an effective one-to-one activity for residents with behavior problems and cognitive impairment. The resident discusses his or her past. You ask questions and make comments. If the resident expresses feelings and emotions, accept them. Reassure the resident that feeling this way is okay. The program can also be done as a group activity. Books, tapes, and kits are available for reminiscence programs (Figure 16.18B). Your activities department may have a formal reminiscence program, but you can also use this approach individually with the residents.

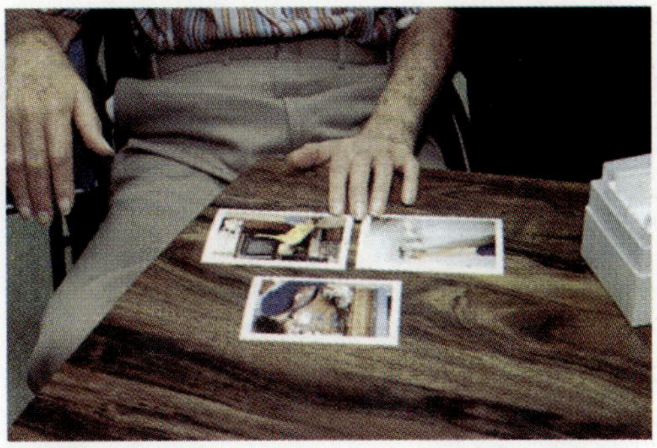

FIGURE 16-18A Discussing old photographs with residents is an excellent way of encouraging reminiscence.

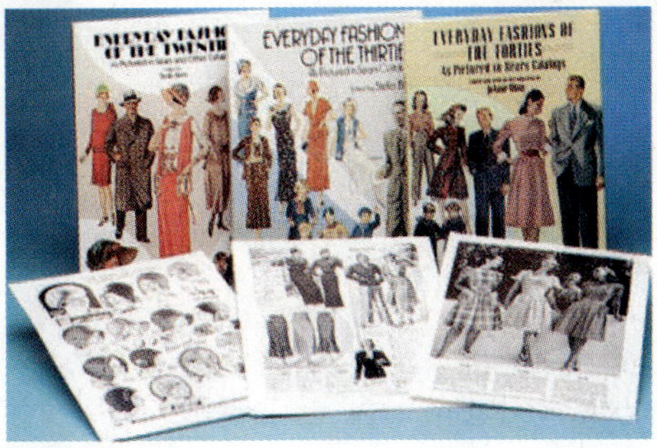

FIGURE 16-18B Looking at pictures of old clothing and furnishings brings back many fond memories. Seeing these items often stimulates residents to tell long-forgotten stories about their past. *(Compliments of Briggs Corporation, Des Moines, IA [800] 247-2343)*

KEY POINTS

- All behavior has meaning, even if the meaning is not evident to you.
- Losses and unmet needs affect residents' behavior.
- Physical and chemical restraints are the treatment of last resort in the management of behavior problems.
- When using the ABC method of behavior management, modifying the antecedent or consequences will change the behavior.
- Consistency is important to the success of a behavior management program.
- Cognitive impairment has many causes, and is not a normal part of aging.
- Safety is a primary concern when caring for residents who have cognitive impairment and dementia.
- Delirium is a reversible condition with medical causes.
- Sensory losses may mimic cognitive impairment or worsen existing dementia.
- Alzheimer's disease causes atrophy of the brain and progressive mental deterioration.
- Wandering is a serious problem in long-term care facilities. The nursing assistant plays an important role in preventing the wanderer from leaving or becoming injured.

REVIEW

A. Multiple Choice

Select the one best answer.

1. Cognitive impairment is
   a. a temporary, reversible condition.
   b. usually caused by infection.
   c. a means of validation.
   d. a decline in intellectual function.
2. A confused resident displays a behavior problem. She yells and screams loudly when she is in bed. A good first step in managing this behavior is
   a. applying a restraint.
   b. asking the nurse to give the resident a tranquilizer.
   c. attempting to learn the cause of the behavior.
   d. isolating the resident.
3. When an alert resident displays a behavior problem, it is most commonly in response to
   a. unmet psychosocial needs.
   b. cognitive impairment.
   c. dementia.
   d. delirium.
4. Defense mechanisms are
   a. means of defending yourself against physical assault.
   b. a response to stress, loss, or unmet needs.
   c. medical problems.
   d. techniques to use when residents are upset.
5. Projection is
   a. refusing to admit there is a problem.
   b. placing the blame for a problem on someone else.
   c. overachieving in one area to overcome a weakness.
   d. making excuses for a problem.
6. According to the ABC method of behavior management,
   a. *A* is an abbreviation for anger.
   b. *A* is an abbreviation for anxiety.
   c. *B* is an abbreviation for behavior.
   d. *C* is an abbreviation for control.
7. When caring for residents who have behavior problems,
   a. adjust your approach to the resident.
   b. leave until the resident calms down.
   c. implement the behavior care plan when the resident becomes upset.
   d. ask the nurse what to do.
8. Masturbation is
   a. acceptable if done in private.
   b. always inappropriate.
   c. harmful to the resident.
   d. an indication that the resident is homosexual.
9. Sexual abuse is
   a. acceptable if done by the resident's spouse.
   b. acceptable if a confused resident consents.
   c. unwanted sexual contact.
   d. appropriate in some situations.
10. Causes of stress and agitation in cognitively impaired residents include
    a. noise and confusion.
    b. validation therapy.
    c. consistent routines.
    d. having a caregiver of the same gender.
11. Dementia
    a. is a disease.
    b. has social causes.
    c. is usually reversible.
    d. is the resident's fault.
12. Delirium is
    a. a mental illness.
    b. caused by reversible medical problems.
    c. a sign of cognitive impairment.
    d. a normal part of aging.
13. Sundowning is
    a. agitation when the resident is put to bed.
    b. restlessness early in the morning.
    c. restlessness in the late afternoon and evening.
    d. a form of combative behavior.
14. Perceptual changes that occur in Alzheimer's disease include

a. inability to differentiate left from right.
b. loss of sense of smell.
c. deterioration in vision.
d. altered taste of food.

15. Activities are

a. only for fun and games.
b. for alert residents only.
c. planned social and therapeutic events.
d. always spontaneous and disorganized.

16. Validation is used to

a. orient confused residents to reality.
b. punish residents whose behavior is inappropriate.
c. reverse cognitive impairment.
d. help residents regain dignity and self-control.

17. Reality orientation works best in residents

a. with delirium.
b. with dementia.
c. who are alert.
d. who have good short-term memory.

18. Reminiscing is a program that helps

a. validate the residents' feelings.
b. the resident remember the past.
c. orient residents to time, place, person.
d. residents forget their past problems.

B. True/False Questions

Answer each statement true (T) or false (F).

19. _______ A person's job provides a sense of identity.
20. ________ Residents who are cognitively impaired may display abnormal behavior in response to too much stimulation in the environment.
21. _______Modifying the behavior changes the antecedent.
22. ________ When managing behavior problems, all care providers should use different approaches with the resident.
23. ________ Cognitive impairment is a normal part of aging.
24. _____ Safety is a primary concern when managing behavior problems and caring for residents who have cognitive impairment and dementia.
25. _______ When caring for residents who have dementia, assume they can do nothing for themselves and provide total care.
26. ____ Residents with Alzheimer's disease may be afraid of being bathed.
27. ________ Residents in the late stage of Alzheimer's disease may lose the ability to swallow.
28. ______ Wanderers should always be restrained for their own safety.
29. ____ Residents with Alzheimer's disease can easily remember something you told them an hour ago.

C. Clinical Application

Answer the following questions.

30. Mrs. Mallory is from a large family. She lived most of her life on a farm. Her husband was in the fields long hours. The resident ran the household and took care of the children. Mrs. Mallory has always been a very controlling person. She has been admitted to your facility for management of her diabetes. The resident is overweight and is unable to walk. The family can no longer care for her at home. Mrs. Mallory is angry with her children and tells you she resents being in the facility. She uses her call signal frequently. Her requests are minor. She asks you to turn the light on or off, add or remove a blanket, bring her ice, pour her a cup of water, and so forth. You are frustrated with her frequent requests. What do you think the cause of the demanding behavior is? How can you best assist this resident?
31. Mrs. Atkins is a confused resident. She wanders about in the facility, but has never attempted to leave. She comes to the nurses' station crying at least once each hour and asks for the location of her room. When she does this, a staff member takes her by the hand, leads her to her room, and gives her a hug. What are the consequences of the resident's behavior? Do you think that the staff is reinforcing the resident's behavior? What can be done to assist Mrs. Atkins?
32. Mr. Morrow sits in a chair in the lounge most of the day watching television. He frequently removes his clothing. What can you do to assist this resident?
33. Mr. Kosmanek immigrated from Poland after World War II. He has Alzheimer's disease and has been admitted to your facility. He sundowns in the evening. When he wakes up in the morning, he

routinely asks, "How many did they shoot last night?" You are working the 11 p.m. to 7 a.m. shift. Mr. Kosmanek has tried to leave the nursing home several times. He says, "I must hide so they can't find me." What can the nursing assistant do to keep the resident from leaving the facility and make him feel safe and secure?

34. Mr. Springer, a resident with Alzheimer's disease, frequently refuses to bathe. You are assigned to give him a shower today. The resident has a bad body odor. When you tell him it is time for his shower, he becomes agitated and tells you to leave him alone. He turns and walks rapidly down the hall. What can the nursing assistant do?

35. According to Maslow, which human needs must be met first?

    a. psychological needs
    b. social needs
    c. security needs
    d. physical needs

Glossary

abandonment leaving or walking off the premises before another worker has been assigned to care for your residents

abbreviation a shortened form of a word or term

abdominal distention enlargement of the abdomen due to excess gas, fecal matter, or urinary retention

abdominal pacemaker *See* pacemaker

abduction moving an extremity away from the body

abduction pillow a special pillow used to keep the legs apart for a resident who has had hip replacement surgery

abrasion a scrape or injury that rubs off the surface of the skin

abuse the willful infliction of injury, unreasonable confinement, intimidation, or punishment that results in physical harm, pain, or mental anguish

acceptance the final stage in the grieving process in which the resident calmly waits for death

accident an unexpected, undesirable event

accreditation a process in which health care facilities voluntarily participate to ensure that high standards of care are maintained

acquired immunodeficiency syndrome (AIDS) a progressively fatal disease caused by the HIV virus and spread by contact with blood or moist body fluids

active assistive range of motion exercises that are started or completed by the resident with some assistance from the care provider

active range of motion moving all joints through their normal movements independently

activities of daily living (ADLs) personal care activities people do each day to meet their human needs

acute illness illness that develops suddenly and last for a short time

adaptive devices pieces of equipment used to help a resident perform a task independently

adduction moving an extremity toward the body

ADLs *See* activities of daily living

admission the procedure for checking the resident into the health care facility and getting him or her settled

advance directive a document that designates the resident's wishes in the event that the resident is unable to speak for himself or herself

AED *See* automatic external defibrillator

afternoon care routine care that is given after lunch

AIDS *See* acquired immunodeficiency syndrome

airborne method of transmission in which very small germs suspended in dust and moisture in the air are inhaled by a susceptible host

airborne precautions practices that health care workers use to protect themselves from airborne pathogens

ALF *See* assisted living facility

AM care routine care given to prepare the resident for breakfast

ambulation the act of walking or moving from one place to another

analgesic pain-relieving medication

aneroid gauge a gauge that operates with a spring-loaded dial

aneurysm a ballooning of the wall of an artery due to a structural weakness

anger the second step in the grieving process, in which the resident is angry because of a terminal diagnosis

antecedent an event that causes or triggers a behavior

antecubital space the space in front of the elbow

antibiotics medications used to eliminate pathogens from the body

antiembolism stockings elastic hosiery used on some residents to relieve edema and prevent blood clots

antiseptic chemical agent designed to cleanse the skin

anus the outlet of the intestines at the rectum, from which waste products are eliminated

apathy indifference; lack of feeling or emotion

aphasia a condition in which the speech center in the brain has been damaged

apical pulse the pulse taken at the apex of the heart

apnea absence of respiration

appliance a plastic collection device used to contain the excretions from an ostomy

application the form on which employment information is written and a request for employment is made

arteries blood vessels that carry freshly oxygenated blood to body parts

arthritis a chronic condition that causes a range of problems from mild discomfort to severe joint pain, deformities, and disability

aseptic technique practices used that are free of all microbes

aspiration inhaling food, fluid, or other objects into the lungs

assess gather information and facts so as to identify the resident's problems and needs

assisted living facility (ALF) a senior housing option that provides housing and personal care support services in a residential setting

ataxic incoordinated; poorly or defectively coordinated

ataxic gait an uncoordinated gait caused by neurologic disease, in which the resident keeps the legs farther apart to maintain balance

atrophy weakness and muscle wasting from lack of use

attending behavior behaviors used to improve the transfer of verbal communication

attitude the outer reflection of feelings

aura a sensation, smell, or a bright light that precedes the onset of a seizure

aural temperature also called *tympanic temperature;* the temperature taken at the tympanic membrane inside the ear

autoimmune disorder a condition in which the individual makes antibodies that work against his or her own body

automatic external defibrillator (AED) a computerized device used when a resident is unresponsive, not breathing, and pulseless. When attached to the chest, the unit determines if an electrical shock is necessary to reestablish or regulate the heartbeat

axilla the area under the arm; the armpit

axillary temperature the temperature taken in the armpit

bacteria one-celled microorganisms that can cause disease

bargaining the third stage in the grieving process, in which the resident attempts to buy more time

barrier something that interferes with communication

bath blanket a soft cotton or flannel blanket used to protect resident privacy and provide warmth during procedures in which the body is exposed

bed bath the bathing procedure used for a resident who is unable to get out of bed

bed cradle a metal or plastic frame suspended over the hospital bed to keep the weight of the linen off the resident's body

bed rest a medically prescribed treatment in which the resident is not allowed out of bed

bedpan a device used for elimination in bed

bedside stand the nightstand used to store personal possessions, grooming, and hygiene items

bedsore *See* pressure ulcer

belt restraint a safety device that encircles the resident's waist and serves as a reminder to prevent rising

biohazardous waste disposable items that are contaminated with blood or body fluids

bioterrorism the use of biological agents, such as pathogenic organisms or agricultural pests, for terrorist purposes

bladder a hollow muscle in which urine is stored until it is eliminated from the body

bland diet a diet containing foods that are low in residue, with limited or no seasoning

blood pressure measurement of the force of the blood on the walls of the arteries

bloodborne pathogens microbes that cause diseases that are spread through contact with blood or body fluid

BM *See* bowel movement

body mechanics correct use of the body to lift or move heavy objects or residents

bony prominences places where the bones are close to the surface of the skin

bowel movement (BM) solid waste eliminated from the digestive system

brachial artery the artery in the antecubital space, in front of the elbow

bradycardia slow pulse rate, usually less than 60 beats per minute

bronchi the two large branches of the trachea through which air passes to the lungs

bruise injury to the skin caused by hitting or striking; the area turns black and blue

burnout complete physical, mental, or emotional fatigue or exhaustion

calorie-controlled diet a diet that restricts the total number of calories served to the resident; usually served to overweight residents

cannula a plastic or metal tube inserted into a tracheostomy to keep the stoma open

CAPD *See* continuous ambulatory peritoneal dialysis

carbohydrates foods that produce heat and energy in the body

cardiac arrest a condition that occurs when the heartbeat and respirations cease

care plan a plan developed by the interdisciplinary health care team that describes the goals and approaches to be used by all team members when caring for the resident

carrier a person who can give a disease to others; the person may not know of the infection

catastrophic reactions uncontrolled emotional outbursts in response to feeling completely overwhelmed or fearful; may include crying, sudden mood changes, anger, and combative behavior

catheter a hollow tube used to drain secretions from the body

causative agent a pathogen that causes disease

CDC *See* Centers for Disease Control and Prevention

Celsius (centigrade) scale a scale for measuring temperature in which the boiling point of water is 100

Centers for Disease Control and Prevention (CDC) a federal agency that studies diseases and makes recommendations on protective measures

Centers for Medicare and Medicaid Services (CMS) a governmental agency that sets policy and administers Medicare and Medicaid payments to health care facilities

centigrade scale *See* Celsius scale

cerebrovascular accident (CVA) also called a *stroke* or *brain attack*; a condition caused by a sudden interruption of blood to the brain, commonly a blood clot or breakage of a small blood vessel. May cause hemiparesis, hemiplegia, and/or speech, vision, emotional, and perception problems

certification an inspection process for facilities that accept state or federal funds as payment for health care

chain of command the lines of authority in each department

chain of infection a description of the factors necessary for an infection to spread

chairfast confined to a chair

chart the notebook or binder containing the resident's medical record

chemical restraint a medication or drug used to alter behavior for staff convenience, and not required to treat a resident's medical symptoms

chemicals substances that may be harmful if they touch the skin or mucous membranes, and are usually dangerous if swallowed

chemotherapy the treatment of cancer using specific chemical agents or drugs that destroy cancer cells

Cheyne-Stokes respirations periods of dyspnea alternating with periods of apnea

chorea abnormal, erratic, involuntary movements seen in Huntington's disease

chronic illness an illness or disease that lasts for a long time

circumduction circular movement of a joint, such as the thumb or wrist

citation a written notice that informs the health care agency or facility of alleged violations of OSHA rules and the time frame in which the conditions must be corrected

clean-catch (midstream) specimen a urine specimen collected from the middle of the urinary stream

cleansing enema introduction of fluid into the lower bowel to remove solid waste

clear-liquid diet a diet that is high in water and carbohydrates, with little nutritive value

clergy a minister of the gospel, a pastor, priest, or rabbi

client the person being cared for in the home

client care records documentation forms used for communication and reimbursement in home health care

closed drainage system a drainage bag and tubing connected to a catheter that is not opened

CMS *See* Centers for Medicare and Medicaid Services

coccyx the bone at the base of the spine

code blue an emergency designation to alert staff and summon help when a cardiac arrest occurs

cognitive impairment a decline in intellectual functioning

colostomy a surgical procedure in which the colon is attached to the outside of the body and waste is eliminated into a plastic bag attached to the skin

combative hitting or fighting the care provider

combative behavior physically aggressive behavior; hitting, kicking, scratching, biting

comfort a state of physical and emotional well-being in which the resident is calm and relaxed, and not in pain or upset

commercially prepared enema an enema solution prepackaged in a small dispenser

common vehicle food, water, or other items in which pathogens can live and multiply

compassionate kind and merciful

compensation using strength and overachieving in one area to overcome a weakness in another area of life

complete bath washing the entire body of a resident

condom catheter an external catheter applied to the penis of an incontinent male

confidentiality keeping personal information about the resident private; not revealing it to unauthorized persons

consent permission to perform care, treatments, and procedures

consequences the outcome of a behavior

consistent the same, uniform; describes approaches to care that used and performed the same by all care providers

constipation passage of hard, dry stool from the lower bowel

constrict to make smaller

contact precautions a category of transmission-based precautions used when caring for residents who have infections that can be spread by skin and wound drainage, secretions, excretions, blood, body fluids, or contact with mucous membranes

continuity of care all staff working on the same goals and providing the same approaches to the resident 24 hours a day

continuous ambulatory peritoneal dialysis (CAPD) a form of dialysis performed in subacute care centers that removes waste products from the resident's blood

contractures permanent shortening and deformity of muscles from lack of use

contraindicated not indicated, inappropriate

coping mechanisms responses to stress and loss that people use to protect feelings of self-esteem

cover letter a letter of introduction sent to a prospective employer with a resume

cubic centimeter (cc) a metric unit of measure used in health care facilities; equal to one milliliter (30 cc equal 1 ounce)

cues brief verbal hints to tell the resident what you want him or her to do

culture the pattern or lifestyle of an individual or group

cumulative trauma disorders injuries to nerves, tissues, tendons, and joints that occur over a period of months to years

CVA *See* cerebrovascular accident

cyanosis a dark bluish or purplish discoloration of the skin and mucous membranes caused by inadequate oxygen in the blood

dangling sitting on the side of the bed with the legs over the edge of the mattress

decline worsening or deterioration in the resident's physical or mental condition

decubiti more than one pressure ulcer

decubitus ulcer *See* pressure ulcer

defamation of character making false or damaging statements about another person

defecation elimination of solid waste from the lower bowel

defibrillation a method of treatment that uses an electric shock to reverse disorganized activity in the heart during cardiac arrest

deficiency a written notice of inadequate care or a substandard practice

deformity disfigurement of the body

degenerative changes deterioration of a body part or system due to age or disease

dehydration a serious condition resulting from inadequate water in the body

delirium an acute confusional state that is an indication of a treatable illness

delusions false beliefs

delusions of persecution thinking that others are trying to cause personal harm

dementia a set of symptoms affecting the resident's thinking, judgment, memory, and ability to reason

denial refusing to accept something as the truth; also, the first stage in the grieving process, in which the resident denies the terminal diagnosis

dentures artificial teeth

dependable being trustworthy and able to be relied on

dependent unable to care for oneself

depression feelings of despair and discouragement; also, the fourth stage in the grieving process, in which the resident is trying to deal with loss

dermis the thicker, inner layer of the skin

developmental disability a severe physical and/or mental impairment that is apparent before the age of 22 and is likely to continue indefinitely

developmental tasks intellectual, social, and emotional skills that a person must accomplish at a certain age level

diabetes a chronic disease caused by a disorder of carbohydrate metabolism

diabetic diet a diet calculated by the dietitian to meet the needs of a resident with diabetes mellitus; the diet limits free sugar and some other foods

diagnosis the term describing the resident's disease or condition; determination of what is wrong with the resident

dialysis a process of removing waste products from the blood; used for residents with kidney disease

diarrhea passage of loose, watery, liquid stools

diastolic blood pressure the last sound heard when taking the blood pressure; taken during the relaxation phase of the heart

dilate to become larger

direct contact the spread of infection by touching

disability inability to function normally because of a physical or mental problem

discharge the procedure by which the resident leaves the health care agency

discharge planner a social worker who is responsible for helping the resident make the transition between the long-term care facility and the community

disinfection a cleaning process that destroys most microorganisms; a chemical is usually used to disinfect reusable items

disoriented unaware of person, place, or time

distal situated farthest away from the center of the resident's body

distended enlarged

DNR *See* do not resuscitate order

do not resuscitate (DNR) order a physician's order indicating that no CPR or life-sustaining measures will be performed

dorsiflexion (dorsal flexion) pulling the foot upward toward the head

drainage bag a bag connected to a catheter to collect urine

draw sheet a small sheet placed horizontally across the center of the hospital bed

droplet method of transmission in which germs are spread by secretions produced during laughing, talking, singing, sneezing, or coughing; these germs are large and usually do not spread more than three feet in the air

droplet precautions the type of isolation used for infections that are transmitted in respiratory secretions; the pathogens that cause infections requiring droplet precautions are usually confined to an area within three feet of the resident

durable power of attorney for health care a document that designates another individual to make medical decisions on behalf of the resident

dysarthria a condition often caused by a head injury or stroke, in which the resident has weakness or paralysis of the lips, tongue, or throat

dysphagia difficulty swallowing food and liquids

dysrhythmia an abnormal heart rhythm

dyspnea difficulty breathing, labored respirations

E. coli 0157:H7 a strain of Escherichia coli that is found in the intestines of some cattle; it is most commonly transmitted to humans in undercooked ground meat. This dangerous strain can cause renal failure and death

ecchymosis a bruise; an injury caused by bleeding under the skin

edema swelling

emesis basin a kidney-shaped basin used for oral care procedures

empathetic able to understand how someone else feels

empathy understanding how someone else feels

EMS (emergency medical services) usually an ambulance or fire department

enabler a device that empowers residents and allows them to function independently

enema introduction of fluid into the lower bowel

entrance conference a meeting between surveyors and facility administration to discuss the purpose of a survey; the entrance conference is conducted at the beginning of a survey

environmental services department the housekeeping department; the department responsible for cleanliness and sanitation in most health care facilities

epidermis the thinner, outer layer of the skin

epiglottis a muscular flap that covers the trachea during swallowing

ergonomics adapting the job and the workplace to the worker's needs

Escherichia coli a type of bacteria that normally resides in the intestines

esophagus the tube through which food passes from the back of the throat to the stomach

evaluation the determination of how the resident's plan of care is working

eversion turning a joint outward

exacerbation a time in the course of a disease when signs and symptoms worsen

excretions human waste products eliminated from the body

exhalation breathing air out of the lungs

exit conference a meeting between surveyors and facility administration upon completion of a survey to discuss the surveyors' findings and the nature of any deficiencies

expiration breathing air out of the lungs

exposure control plan a written program that the employer is required to have that describes what to do if an employee contacts blood or body fluids

expressive aphasia a condition in which the speech center in the brain has been damaged; residents with this condition have difficulty saying what they want to say. They may also have trouble with gestures and writing

extended survey a survey that lasts longer than originally anticipated so surveyors can examine resident care and facility practices in greater detail

extension straightening a joint

external catheter a catheter applied to the outside of the penis of an incontinent male

external genitalia the reproductive organs on the outside of the body

external rotation turning a joint outward, away from the median line

extracurricular activities clubs, hobbies, volunteer work, and special interests

extremity restraint a safety device that encircles the arm or leg and prevents movement

factual something that you know to be true

Fahrenheit scale a scale commonly used for measuring temperature

false imprisonment holding or restraining a resident against his or her will

fats nutrients, found in food products such as butter and oil, that are used for heat and energy production in the body

fecal impaction a large, hard, dry mass of stool that the resident is unable to pass

fecal material solid waste eliminated from the digestive system

feces solid waste eliminated from the digestive system

fetal position a position in which the resident is turned on the side with the head tucked down and knees drawn up

fistula a method of suturing a vein to an artery for the purpose of performing hemodialysis

flammable combustible; burns readily

flank the area of the back immediately above the waist where the kidneys are located

flatus gas expelled from the digestive tract

flexion bending at a joint

flora microbes that inhabit the internal and external surfaces of healthy individuals

fluid restrictions limiting the total amount of fluid the resident can have in a 24-hour period

fomites linen, equipment, and other items contaminated with microbes

food pyramid a U.S. Department of Agriculture diagram that provides a guide to eating a well-balanced diet

foot board a piece of wood or plastic placed at the end of the hospital bed and used for positioning the resident's feet

force energy, strength, or power

force fluids an order to encourage the resident to drink as much liquid as possible

foreskin the loose tissue at the tip of the penis

Fowler's position a semi-sitting position in bed

fracture a broken bone

friction force created by rubbing the skin; for example, against bed linen

full-liquid diet a diet used for residents with digestive disorders; includes clear and milk-based liquids

functional incontinence inability to control the passage of urine due to physical inability to get to the toilet

gait the way a person walks

gait belt a heavy canvas belt used to assist the resident with ambulation

gastrostomy a surgical procedure in which a feeding tube is placed directly into the resident's stomach, with the end extending through the abdominal skin

gastrostomy tube also called *G-tube;* the feeding tube used in a resident who has had a gastrostomy

gatch handles handles at the foot of a bed that raise and lower the head, knee, and height of the bed

generalized spread throughout the entire body

generalized application applied to the resident's entire body

genital area the area of the body where the external reproductive organs are located

geriatrics care of the elderly

global aphasia inability to speak or understand

Good Samaritan laws laws that protect health care workers who provide emergency care outside the place of employment

graduate a measuring device with markings on the side

graft a method of connecting an artery and a vein with a tube for the purpose of performing hemodialysis

grievance a complaint

grieving process five steps that people go through when they anticipate or suffer a loss

habit training a type of bladder management program used for mentally confused residents who urinate at the same time each day

hallucination seeing, hearing, or feeling something that is not real

handroll prop that is placed in the hand to prevent contractures

hantavirus a virus that is spread by contact with rodents (rats and mice) or their excretions, including urine and feces

HD *See* Huntington's disease

head lice human parasites that feed on blood; they cannot be contracted from contact with pets or other animals

health care proxy an individual who has been legally designated to make medical decisions on behalf of the resident

Health Insurance Portability and Accountability Act (HIPAA) a law that applies to resident privacy, confidentiality, and medical records. The HIPAA regulations protect all individually identifiable health information in any form. The rules apply to paper, verbal, and electronic documentation, billing records, and clinical records. Staff members are provided with only the information needed to carry out their duties

health maintenance organization (HMO) a group of health care providers and hospitals paid by insurance companies to care for residents for a monthly fee

hemiparesis weakness on one side of the body

hemiplegia paralysis on one side of the body

hemodialysis removal of waste products from the body done by cleansing the resident's blood; this procedure must be performed at a special dialysis center

hemorrhage excessive bleeding

HEPA *See* high efficiency particulate air respirator

hepatitis B an infection of the liver caused by a virus; it can cause liver cancer and death

hepatitis C an infection of the liver caused by a virus; it can be spread through contact with blood or body fluids

herpes zoster *See* shingles

high efficiency particulate air (HEPA) respirator mask/respirator used to protect employees working in rooms of residents who have diseases spread by the airborne method of transmission

HIPAA *See* Health Insurance Portability and Accountability Act

HIV *See* human immunodeficiency virus disease

HMO *See* health maintenance organization

holistically focusing care on the whole person as an individual with many complex, interrelated strengths and needs

hormones chemical messengers of the body that originate in organs and glands of the body

hospice an organization that cares for dying residents

hospice care physical, psychological, and spiritual care provided to residents who have limited life expectancy and their families

hospital institution that cares for people with acute illnesses

host the place where a disease-causing germ can grow

HS care routine care given at bedtime to prepare the resident for sleep

human immunodeficiency virus (HIV) disease the disease caused by the human immunodeficiency virus that may progress to AIDS; it is spread by direct or indirect contact with blood and body fluids

humidifier a device that attaches to the oxygen supply to add moisture before oxygen is delivered to the resident

Huntington's disease (HD) a hereditary disease that causes choreiform movements, anxiety, and dementia

hygiene personal cleanliness

hyperalimentation a method of feeding a resident total nutrition intravenously, to allow the gastrointestinal system to rest and heal

hyperextension gentle, excessive extension of a joint, slightly past the point of resistance

hyperglycemia an abnormally high concentration of glucose (sugar) in the blood

hypertension high blood pressure, usually 140/90 or above

hypoglycemia an abnormally low concentration of glucose (sugar) in the blood

hypotension low blood pressure, usually 90/60 or below

hypothermia abnormally low body temperature (below 95°F)

I & O *See* intake and output

identification band a plastic bracelet, usually worn on the wrist or ankle, that contains the resident's name and other identifying information

immobility being motionless and unable to move

immobilize to support or restrain in a way that prevents movement

immune system part of the circulatory system that recognizes invading germs and works to eliminate them from the body

immunization administration of drugs that stimulate the immune system to protect against certain diseases

implementation the process of carrying out a plan

inactivity being still, quiet, sedentary, or immobile

incident an occurrence or event that interrupts normal procedures or causes a crisis

incident report a special form that is completed for each accident or unusual occurrence in a long-term care facility; the incident report describes what happened and contains other important information

incision a cut in the skin made with a knife

incontinence management programs a routine in which the resident is taken to the toilet at regular intervals

incontinent unable to control the passage of urine from the bladder, or stool from the bowel, or both

incoordination uncoordinated, irregular voluntary muscle movement

independent self reliant, able to care for self

indirect contact touching objects, equipment, or dishes contaminated with harmful microorganisms

indwelling catheter a hollow tube inserted into the bladder to remove urine; the catheter remains in the body for a period of time

infection a state of sickness or disease caused by pathogens in the body

infection control medical asepsis; methods used in health care facilities to prevent the spread of infection

infusion site the site where the intravenous needle is inserted into the body

inhalation breathing air into the lungs

inspiration breathing air into the lungs

instantaneous injuries injuries that occur suddenly and without warning, usually as a result of an accident

insulin a hormone secreted by the pancreas that regulates glucose metabolism

intake and output (I & O) an estimated measurement of all the liquid the resident takes in and all the fluid lost in a 24 hour period

interdisciplinary team a group of caregivers who work together for the good of the patient, resident, or client

intermittent catheter a catheter that is inserted into the bladder for the purpose of obtaining a specimen, or for emptying the bladder, and is then withdrawn

internal rotation turning a joint inward, toward the median line

interview a formal meeting in which the employer assesses the qualifications of an applicant and provides information about a job opening

intravenous (IV) feeding administering sterile liquid and nutrients into a vein with a needle

inversion turning a joint inward

involuntary seclusion isolating a resident as a form of punishment

isolation measures used when a resident has an infectious disease; it is used to prevent the spread of pathogens to others

IV standard a metal pole used to hang an IV bag, bottle, or pump above the infusion site

jaundice a yellow color of the skin seen in hepatitis and some other diseases

JCAHO *See* Joint Commission on Accreditation of Healthcare Organizations

job objective the section of your resume that lists the type of position you are seeking and states how your abilities and skills qualify you for this position

Joint Commission on Accreditation of Healthcare Organizations (JCAHO) an organization that inspects and accredits health care agencies that meet high quality standards

Kegel exercises exercises used to make the muscles around the bladder stronger

Kelly a special clamp used to close tubes quickly

kidneys the organs that filter waste products from the blood and produce urine

labia majora two large, hair covered structures on the external female genitalia

labia minora two small, liplike structures inside the labia majora on the external female genitalia

laboratory requisition a document with identifying resident information that specifies the type of lab test to be performed on a specimen

large intestine the lower part of the bowel

larynx the voice box

lateral position lying on the left or right side

leg drainage bag a bag attached to a catheter to collect urine; it is secured to the leg with an elastic or rubber strap

lethargy abnormal drowsiness or sleepiness

level of consciousness the degree of awareness or alertness, which ranges from fully awake and alert to confusion and unconsciousness

libel making false statements about another person in writing

license a state permit allowing the long-term care facility to operate

licensed practical nurse (LPN) a nurse who has completed one to two years of nursing school and passed a state licensing examination

licensed vocational nurse (LVN) a licensed practical nurse

living will a document that specifies the resident's wishes in the event that the resident is in a terminal condition

localized confined to a specific area of the body

localized application applied to a specific area of a resident's body

lockout-tagout placing a locking tag on a broken piece of equipment so that the equipment cannot be used

long-term care facility health care institutions that cares for residents with chronic diseases and personal care needs

low bed a bed in which the frame is four to six inches from the floor to the top of the frame deck; such beds reduce the risk of injury if the resident falls from the bed

low-cholesterol diet a diet that is low in fat and cholesterol; used for residents with heart, blood vessel, liver, and gallbladder disease

lowfat diet a diet that is low in fats; used for residents with heart, blood vessel, liver, and gallbladder disease

LPN *See* licensed practical nurse

LVN *See* licensed vocational nurse

malnutrition inadequate nutrition due to poor diet or inability to absorb nutrients

malpractice negligence that results in harm to the resident

Maslow's hierarchy of needs a chart based on a widely accepted theory of physical and psychological needs of all human beings

material safety data sheets (MSDS) information sheets on chemicals used in the workplace that list the health hazards, safe use, and emergency procedures for chemical exposure

MDS *See* Minimum Data Set 2.0

mechanical soft diet a diet that is finely ground or chopped; used for residents who have chewing or swallowing problems

mechanically altered diets a diet that is altered in texture to meet the needs of residents who have chewing, swallowing, or digestive problems

medial pertaining to or situated toward the midline of the body

median situated in the median plane or in the midline of the body

Medicaid a program funded by the state and federal governments that pays for health care for individuals with a low income

medical asepsis practices used in health care facilities to prevent the spread of infection

medical record a record of the resident's true condition and a record of progress and care

Medicare a program administered by the federal government that helps the elderly and disabled pay for care in a hospital, long-term care facility, and/or home health care setting

mentally retarded lower-than-average intellectual development; retardation ranges from mild to severe

metabolism rate the rate at which the body uses energy

methicillin-resistant Staphylococcus aureus (MRSA) a pathogen commonly seen in health care facilities that causes illness or infection; the pathogen resists treatment with most antibiotics

microorganisms living germs that cannot be seen with the naked eye

micturition the act of eliminating urine from the body

midstream (clean-catch) specimen a urine specimen collected from the middle of the urinary stream

milliliter (mL) a metric unit of measure used in health care facilities; 30 mL equal one ounce; one milliliter is the same as one cubic centimeter

minerals inorganic compounds in food used to build body tissues

Minimum Data Set 2.0 (MDS) the assessment tool upon which the care plan is based; completed upon admission and quarterly for all residents of long-term care facilities

misappropriation of property theft

mite a tiny parasite that cannot be seen with the naked eye

miter to tuck a sheet in by forming a 45° angle perpendicular to the mattress

mixed incontinence inability to control passage of both liquid and solid waste from the body

mobility the ability to move about

mode of transmission the way in which a disease-causing pathogen is spread

morning care routine care that is given after breakfast

MRSA *See* methicillin-resistant Staphylococcus aureus

MS *See* multiple sclerosis

MSDS *See* material safety data sheet

mucous membranes tissues of the body that secrete mucus; these areas open to the outside of the body

multiple sclerosis (MS) a progressive neurological disorder that causes a degeneration of the nervous system, which interferes with conduction of nerve impulses

multiskilled workers nursing assistants who have received additional education to enable them to perform additional tasks and procedures that are not taught in the original, basic NA program

musculoskeletal system the name commonly used to refer to the muscular and skeletal systems

myths commonly accepted beliefs that are not true

N95 respirator a mask with very small pores that may be worn when caring for residents in airborne precautions

nasogastric tube a tube inserted into the nose and threaded through the esophagus into the stomach; it can be used for feeding or medical procedures

negative pressure environment a description of the ventilation system used in an airborne precautions room; the room air is drawn upward into the ventilation system and is either specially filtered or exhausted directly to the outside of the building

neglect failing to provide services to residents to prevent physical harm or mental anguish

negligence failing to provide services to a resident in the same manner as a reasonably prudent person would do

network to communicate with people you know who have similar careers, goals, and interests

neurogenic bladder a condition in which the resident cannot feel the sensation of urine in the bladder, causing it to become very full and retain urine

NIC *See* Nursing Interventions Classification

nits the eggs left by lice; if untreated, the eggs will hatch into more lice

no concentrated sweets diet a regular diet that is not calorie restricted; however, free sugar, fruit in sugary syrup, and most regular desserts are not served on this diet

NOC *See* Nursing Outcomes Classification

nonintact skin skin that is broken, chapped, or cracked

nonrapid eye movement (NREM) sleep the part of the sleep cycle that begins when the resident first falls asleep. As he or she progresses through the cycle, arousal becomes more difficult and sleep becomes deeper

normal flora microorganisms that are healthful and necessary for the body to function correctly; they are not harmful in the area in which they reside, but can cause infection if spread to other parts of the body

nosocomial infection an infection acquired by a resident of a long-term care facility

Nursing Interventions Classification (NIC) a comprehensive, standardized language describing treatments that nursing personnel perform; this method was established by nurse researchers at the University of Iowa in 1987

Nursing Outcomes Classification (NOC) a method of measuring how well the resident is meeting care plan goals; this method was established by nurse researchers at the University of Iowa in 1991

nursing process the four-step process of assessment, planning, implementation, and evaluation of the resident and care provided to meet the resident's needs

nutrients chemical substances in food that are necessary for life

objective observations made by seeing, hearing, feeling, touching, and smelling

OBRA (Omnibus Budget Reconciliation Act of 1987) legislation that called for sweeping reforms of the long-term care industry; describes requirements for nursing assistant education

obstructed airway food or a foreign body blocking the trachea or windpipe, making it impossible to breathe

Occupational Safety and Health Administration (OSHA) a governmental agency responsible for developing and enforcing job safety and health standards to protect employees

occupied bedmaking procedure for making the bed with the resident in the bed

ombudsman a resident advocate; he or she can provide information on how to find a facility and get quality care, can help in solving problems, and can assist residents to file grievances, if requested

opposition touching each of the fingers against the thumb

oral temperature temperature taken by placing the thermometer in the resident's mouth

orthotic a device that restores or improves function and prevents deformity

OSHA *See* Occupational Safety and Health Administration

osteoporosis a decrease in bone mass that leads to fractures with minimal or no trauma

ostomy a surgically created opening into the body

ovaries glands in the female that produce eggs and are responsible for hormone production

overbed table a narrow table on wheels used to hold the resident's water, meal trays, and clean items

overflow incontinence the escape of urine that occurs when the bladder is very full and can hold no more urine

pacemaker a surgically implanted device that regulates the rate of the heartbeat. Most commonly, the pacemaker is implanted in the chest, but occasionally it is placed in the abdomen

pain a state of discomfort that is unpleasant for the resident; it is always a warning that something is wrong

palmar flexion the act of bending the hand down toward the palm

paraphrasing a method of restating the message communicated to you in clear, simple terms

paraplegic a person who has permanent loss of sensation and movement below the waist

parasites tiny animals that survive by feeding off another human or animal

Parkinson's disease (PD) a neurological disease that causes tremors, shuffling gait, and dementia

partial bath washing the face, hands, underarms, back, and genital area

passive range of motion joint exercises performed on the resident by the care provider

pathogen a microorganism that causes disease

patient a person who is cared for in a hospital

PD *See* Parkinson's disease

penis the external male organ used for sex and elimination

peri-care *See* perineal care

perineal care washing the genital and anal areas of the body

perineum the area between the anus and vagina in the female; the area between the anus and scrotum in the male

peripherally inserted central catheter (PICC) an intravenous line that is inserted in the arm and threaded through the venous system to the superior vena cava; used for long-term intravenous therapy and TPN

peristalsis muscular contractions of the digestive tract that move food and waste products through the intestines

peritoneal dialysis dialysis done by inserting solution through a cannula into the resident's abdominal cavity

perseveration repetitious behavior, movements, or actions

personal data the section of your resume that lists your name, address, phone number, and professional license or certification number

personal protective equipment (PPE) equipment worn to protect the health care worker and the resident from contact with disease-causing pathogens

personal space a comfortable distance in which to communicate with others

petechiae small purplish spots on the body surface, caused by minute hemorrhages

PFR95 respirator a mask with very small pores that may be worn when caring for residents in airborne precautions

pharynx the throat

physical restraints physical, manual, or mechanical devices attached or adjacent to the resident's body that the resident cannot remove easily and prevent access to the body

PICC *See* peripherally inserted central catheter

plan of correction a written plan submitted by the health care agency in response to deficient survey findings; the plan will list what corrections will be made, by whom, who will monitor the correction, and what will be done to prevent similar deficiencies in the future

planning deciding what to do with information gathered in an assessment

plantar flexion bending the foot downward, away from the body

plaque an acidic, decay-causing substance in the mouth

portal of entry the place where a pathogen enters the body

portal of exit the way pathogens leave the body. This may be in excretions, secretions, or body fluids, such as urine, feces, saliva, tears, drainage from open wounds, blood, mucus, or respiratory fluids

post polio syndrome (PPS) a neurologic condition marked by increased weakness and abnormal muscle fatigue in persons who had polio many years earlier

postmortem care physical care of the body after death

postoperative care care given to residents after surgical procedures

postural support a device that maintains good body alignment and posture

PPE *See* personal protective equipment

PPO *See* preferred provider organization

PPS *See* post polio syndrome

preferred provider organization (PPO) a list of physicians and health care facilities/agencies that contract with insurance companies to provide health care to insurance company subscribers

prefix the word element at the beginning of a word

prehypertension blood pressure between 120/80 and 139/89; persons with this condition are likely to develop high blood pressure in the future and should take steps to decrease their risk

pressure sore *See* pressure ulcer

pressure ulcer also called *bedsore, decubitus ulcer, pressure sore*; an ulcer that forms on the skin over a bony prominence as the result of pressure

priorities things that are very important that must be taken care of first

probe the attachment to an electronic thermometer used to measure temperature

probe cover the plastic, disposable cover or sheath used on the thermometer probe when taking a resident's temperature

professional a skilled practitioner who is capable, competent, and efficient

professional boundaries unspoken limits on physical and emotional relationships with residents; boundaries limit and define how a health care worker acts with residents

projection placing the blame for the illness or situation on someone or something else

prompted voiding a bladder management program used for residents who know that the bladder is full, but do not communicate the need to use the toilet

pronation moving a joint to face downward

prone position lying on the abdomen with the head turned to one side

prostate gland a gland in the male that encircles the urethra just below the bladder and secretes a fluid which forms part of the semen

prosthesis an artificial body part

prosthetic refers to a device that takes the place of a body part

protective isolation also called *reverse isolation*; used in some health care facilities to protect residents who have weakened immune systems from contacting pathogens in the environment

proteins nutrients in food that build and repair tissues

pseudomembranous colitis a very serious condition in which severe diarrhea is caused by a bacterium called Clostridium difficile (C. difficile); it develops in residents who have been on antibiotic therapy

pulse the expansion and contraction of an artery that can be felt on the outside surface of the body

pulse oximeter a device that measures the oxygen in the arterial blood

pulse points locations on the body where the pulse can be felt

pulse pressure the difference between the systolic and diastolic blood pressure

pulse rate the number of pulse beats per minute

pureed diet a diet blenderized to a smooth consistency

QA *See* quality assurance

quad cane a cane with four feet; the most stable type of cane

quality assurance (QA) an internal review made by facility staff to identify problems and find solutions for improvement

RACE System the steps that should be followed in case of fire

radial deviation turning the forearm toward the radius

radial pulse the pulse felt on the thumb side of the wrist

radiation therapy a type of cancer treatment in which the skin is exposed to high doses of radiation

range of motion normal joint movements

rapid eye movement (REM) sleep the part of the sleep cycle that restores mental function; the part of the sleep cycle in which dreams occur

rationalization providing an acceptable, but untrue reason for the illness or behavior

reality orientation a technique in which a resident is reoriented to time, place, person, and season

reasonable accommodation considering the resident's likes, dislikes, needs, and preferences when providing care and services

receptive aphasia a condition in which the speech center in the brain has been damaged; residents with this condition have trouble understanding spoken language, and may also have trouble reading and understanding gestures

rectal temperature the temperature taken by inserting the thermometer into the anus

rectum the last six to eight inches of the large intestine, where fecal material is stored until it is eliminated from the body through the anus

references individuals who know you will who will recommend you to the prospective employer for the job you are seeking

reflex incontinence a loss of urine that occurs without awareness in residents who are paralyzed or have other neurologic problems

reflexes unconscious or involuntary movements

registered nurse (RN) a nurse who has two to four years of nursing school and has passed a state licensure examination

regular diet a normal diet based on the five food groups in the food pyramid

rehabilitation program(s) designed by a therapist to help a resident regain lost skills or to teach new skills

reimburse to repay an institution for the cost of services provided

reminiscing the act of remembering the past

remission a time period when a chronic disease appears stable and relatively symptom-free

reprisal retaliation

reservoir host; the person who has an infection

resident the person who is cared for in a long-term care facility

Resident's Bill of Rights a legal document listing the rights of residents in long-term care facilities

resolved through, over, completed

respiration the act of breathing in and out

responsible behavior behavior that is dependable and trustworthy

rest a state of mental and physical comfort, calmness, and relaxation

restoration basic nursing care measures designed to maintain or improve a resident's function and assist the resident to return to self-care

restorative care nursing care designed to assist the resident to attain and maintain the highest level of function possible

restorative environment an environment that has been modified so the resident can function as independently as possible

restraints physical, manual, or mechanical devices attached or adjacent to the resident's body that the resident cannot remove easily and prevent access to the resident's body

resume a summary of your professional or work experience and qualifications

retention enema introduction of fluid into the lower bowel to soften, lubricate, and remove solid waste

retraction drawing back, away from the body

reverse chronological order the order in which your previous jobs are listed on your resume, beginning with most recent job first

reverse isolation *See* protective isolation

rhythm a recurring action or movement

rigor mortis a condition that occurs two to four hours after death, in which the muscles and limbs become stiff

risk factor condition that has the potential to cause the resident's health to worsen; condition indicating that a problem may develop or predisposing the resident to development of a problem

RN *See* registered nurse

root the element that gives meaning to a medical word

rotation moving a joint in, out, and around

scabies a skin condition caused by a mite; it causes a rash and severe itching and is highly contagious

scheduled toileting a bladder management program used for residents who cannot use the bathroom without physical help; the resident is taken to the bathroom on a fixed schedule developed by the nurse

scrotum the sac-like structure containing the testes on the male genitalia

secretions drainage, discharge, or seeping from the body

seizure a convulsion or condition characterized by severe shaking and jerking of the body

self-actualization the realization of one's full potential

self-care deficit inability to perform an activity of daily living

self-esteem your opinion of yourself

semiprone position a modified prone position in which the body is supported on pillows to relieve pressure from most of the bony prominences

semisupine position a modified side-lying position in which the body is supported on pillows to relieve pressure from most of the bony prominences

senile purpura dark purple bruises on the forearms and backs of hands in the elderly

sensory loss difficulty seeing, hearing, smelling, or touching

sepsis systemic poisoning of the body caused by bacteria; a serious infection

septic infected; poisoned

sexual abuse forcing a resident to perform a sexual act

shearing moving the resident so the skin is stretched between the bone inside and the surface (such as a sheet) outside, causing skin damage

sheath a cover for a probe or instrument

shingles (herpes zoster) a condition that occurs only in people who have had chickenpox. The resident develops blister-like lesions on the torso that follow the nerve pathways, and are extremely painful. The condition is infectious through the airborne and contact routes until all lesions crust over

shock the result of blood loss that causes inadequate blood flow to the vital organs

shroud a cloth, paper, or plastic covering used to wrap the body after death

shunt a passage between two blood vessels, commonly under the forearm skin in residents who are receiving hemodialysis

signs conditions of the resident that can be seen or observed by others

Sims' position a side-lying position in which the resident is placed on the left side with the right leg flexed and bent; used for rectal examinations and treatments

skin tears injuries in which the epidermis is torn

slander making false statements about another person

sleep a period of continuous or intermittent unconsciousness in which physical movements are decreased and allows the mind and body to rest.. Sleep is a basic need

sleep deprivation prolonged sleep loss (inadequate quality or quantity of REM or NREM sleep)

sliding technique a technique used for transfers when the resident cannot bear weight. The resident is moved on a sheet

small intestine the part of the digestive system that receives food from the stomach and completes digestion, absorbing nutrients from the food into the bloodstream

sodium-restricted diet a diet that is prepared with no sodium (salt) or limited sodium

soft diet a diet containing foods that are low in residue, with limited or no seasoning

source causative agent; a pathogen that causes disease

spasticity sudden, frequent, involuntary muscle contractions that impair function

sperm reproductive secretion from the testes in the male

sphygmomanometer the instrument used to measure blood pressure

splint a device used to maintain the position of an extremity or joint

standard precautions measures that health care workers use to prevent the spread of infection to themselves and others

standards of care common health care practices based on current information about health care and facility policies

stereotyping fixed images or beliefs that categorize an individual or group

sterile free from all pathogens

sterilization processes used to kill all germs

stethoscope the instrument used to listen to sounds inside the body

stoma the opening of an ostomy to the outside of the body

stool feces; solid waste eliminated from the digestive system

strain injury to a muscle or muscles from stretching or overuse

stress physical or emotional strain and tension

stress incontinence inability to control the passage of urine due to muscular weakness

strict I & O an accurate measurement of all the liquid the resident takes in and all the fluid the resident loses in a 24-hour period

stump sock a stocking that is placed over an amputated extremity before the prosthesis is applied

subacute a level of care for the resident who has complex care needs but is not critically ill

subcutaneous tissue the fatty layer below the epidermis

subjective describes observations based on what you think, or what the resident tells you; may or may not be factual

suffix the word element at the end of a word

sundowning increased restlessness and confusion in the late afternoon, evening, and night

supination moving a joint so it faces upward

supine position lying on the back; face up

supplemental feedings nourishments given to the resident in addition to meals, to meet special nutritional needs

suprapubic catheter a hollow tube surgically inserted into the bladder through the abdomen

survey a review and evaluation to ensure that a long-term care facility is maintaining acceptable standards of practice, quality of care, and quality of life for residents

surveyor a representative of a private or governmental agency who reviews long-term care facility policies, procedures, and practices for quality of care

susceptibility the ability of the body to resist disease

susceptible host a person who can become infected with a disease-causing pathogen

sympathy feeling very sorry for someone because of their physical condition or situation. Sympathy is not healthy for you or the resident; feeling sympathetic can cause you to cross professional boundaries and enter the relationship danger zone

symptoms an indication of a disease or disorder that is noticed by the resident, but cannot be observed by others

syncope fainting

systolic blood pressure the first sound heard when taking the blood pressure; taken during the contraction phase of the heart

tachycardia rapid pulse rate, usually more than 100 beats per minute

tact the ability to speak and act without offending others

tactful considerate, polite, and thoughtful

tagout *See* lockout-tagout

task analysis analyzing the steps of a procedure and determining which the steps the resident can complete independently

TB *See* tuberculosis

temperature measurement of heat within the body

tepid lukewarm

terminal illness an illness for which there is no cure

testes the egg-shaped reproductive glands located in the scrotum in the male

therapeutic diet a special or modified diet prepared to treat a resident's individual nutritional needs

thermal burn an injury to the skin caused by contact with flame, steam, hot water, or hot object

thermometer the instrument used to measure temperature

TIA *See* transient ischemic attack

time and travel records reports showing how the nursing assistant spent his or her time when working in home health care

toe pleat a fold in the top linen near the end of the bed that provides extra space and keeps the linen from pressing or pulling the feet downward

tornado warning a state of alert that occurs when a tornado is in the area

tornado watch a state of alert suggesting that conditions are right for a tornado to develop

total parenteral nutrition (TPN) a method of feeding a resident total nutrition intravenously, to allow the gastrointestinal system to rest and heal

TPN *See* total parenteral nutrition

trachea the upper windpipe extending from the larynx to the bronchus

tracheostomy an opening into the trachea through which the resident breathes

transfer moving the resident from one place, unit, or facility to another

transfer belt a heavy canvas belt used to move a resident from one location to another

transient ischemic attack (TIA) a period of temporarily diminished blood flow to the brain; occurs suddenly and commonly lasts from 2 to 15 minutes

transmission-based precautions isolation categories designed to interrupt the mode of transmission so the pathogen cannot spread

transport bag a sealed plastic bag labeled with a biohazard emblem; used to contain laboratory specimens during transport to the lab

tremors involuntary shaking

trochanter roll a rolled bath blanket used for bedfast residents to prevent external rotation of the hips

tuberculosis (TB) a contagious disease that is spread by airborne contact; it commonly affects the lungs, but can cause illness in other parts of the body

turgor elasticity of skin; skin that stretches and tents when pinched is an indication of dehydration

tympanic temperature also called *aural temperature*; the temperature taken at the tympanic membrane inside the ear

tympanic thermometer the thermometer used to measure temperature inside the ear

ulnar deviation turning the forearm toward the ulna

unit the resident's personal space in the facility; includes a bed, chair, overbed table, nightstand, dresser, wastebasket, and closet

universal choking sign one or both hands on the throat

ureters the tubes that carry urine from the kidneys to the bladder

urethra the hollow tube leading from the bladder to the outside of the body

urge incontinence inability to control the passage of urine in which the need to urinate is very strong and sudden, preventing the resident from getting to the toilet on time

urinal a container used for urinary elimination in the male resident

urinary meatus the external opening to the urethra where urine leaves the body

urinary retention inability to empty the bladder completely

urination the act of passing liquid waste to the outside of the body

uterus the internal organ in the female in which a baby develops and receives nourishment

vagina the canal in the female extending from the external genitalia to the uterus

validation therapy a technique that validates feelings, helps residents resolve developmental tasks, and enhances feelings of dignity and self-control

Vancomycin-resistant Enterococcus (VRE) a drug-resistant pathogen seen in health care facilities that commonly causes infections

vector an insect, rodent, or small animal that spreads disease

veins blood vessels that carry blood from the body parts back to the heart

ventilator a device used to assist or control breathing

vest restraint a safety device applied to the resident's upper body to limit movement and prevent rising

viruses tiny pathogens that cause disease; antibiotics will not eliminate them

vital signs temperature, pulse, respiration, and blood pressure

vitamins organic substances in food that are necessary for normal body function

voiding urination; the act of passing liquid waste to the outside of the body

VRE *See* Vancomycin-resistant Enterococcus

vulva the external genitalia in the female

waterless bathing a prepackaged bathing system in which a package of moistened washcloths is used instead of a water basin and soap

Index

(hemorrhage) 469
A 631
Abandonment 176
abbreviation 57
abdominal distention 260, 456
abduction pillow 299
Abrasions 310, 590
Abuse 174
acceptance 502
accidents 132
acquired immune deficiency syndrome (AIDS) 102
Activities of daily living 358
acute illnesses 2
ADLs 358
admission 81
advance directive 175
afternoon care 358
airborne 93
Airborne precautions 112
AM care 358
ambulation 572
analgesic 70
aneroid gauge 417
aneurysm 555
anger 503
antecedent 630
antecubital space 420
antibiotics 92
antiembolism stockings 389
antiseptic 92
anus 455
apathy 503
Aphasia 41, 274
apical pulse 412
apnea 414
appliance 463
Arteries 230
arthritis 290
aseptic technique 444
aspiration 157
assess 83
Assisted living facilities (ALFs) 5
Attending behavior 31
attitude 19
aura 151, 280
aural 400
Automatic external defibrillators (AEDs) 162
axilla 370
axillary temperature 400

B 631
Bacteria 92
bargaining 502
barrier 32
bath blanket 344
bed bath 366
bed cradle 594
bedpan 438
bedside stand 343
bedsores 588
belt restraint 612
biohazardous waste 109
Bioterrorism 125
bladder 435
bland diets 190
blood pressure 400
Bloodborne pathogens 101
body mechanics 586
bony prominences 588
bowel movement (BM) 456
brachial artery 417
bradycardia 413
bronchi 245
Bruises 157
Burnout 23

C 631
Calorie-controlled diets 191
Carbohydrates 185
cardiac arrest 500
care plan 10
carrier 94
Catastrophic reactions 641
catheter 442, 450
causative agent 94
Celsius 400
Centers for Disease Control and Prevention (CDC) 111
centigrade 400
cerebrovascular accident (CVA) 272
chain of command 10
chain of infection 94
chart 48
Chemical restraints 606
chemicals 135
Cheyne-Stokes respirations 414
chronic illnesses 2
cleansing enema 459
Clear-liquid diet 190
clergy 16
client 6
code blue 500
Colostomy 259, 463, 554
combative 594
combative behavior 634
Comfort 69
Commercially prepared enemas 459
common vehicle 93
compassionate 26
Compensation 628
complete bath 365
condom catheter 442
confidentiality 170
Consent 175
consequences 630
constipation 260, 437
constricts 139

Contact precautions 113
continuity of care 47
contraindicated 310, 587
Coping mechanisms 501
cubic centimeters (cc) 206
cultures 178
Cumulative trauma disorders 587
cyanosis 414

dangling 552
Declines 8
decubiti 588
decubitus ulcers 311, 588
Defamation of character 176
defecation 258, 456
defibrillation 162
Dehydration 204, 427
Delirium 638
Delusions 639
Delusions of persecution 639
Dementia 638
denial 132, 502, 628
Dentures 362
dependable 24
Depression 503, 632
dermis 307
developmental disability 3
developmental tasks 2, 625
diagnosis 54
dialysis 417
diarrhea 261, 456
diastolic blood pressure 415
dilate 139
direct contact 93
disability 3
discharge 81
discharge planner 87
disinfection 92
disoriented 638
distal 614
distended 119
do not resuscitate (DNR) order 500
drainage bag 443
draw sheet 592
droplet 93
Droplet precautions 113
durable power of attorney for health care 175
Dysarthria 41
Dyspnea 248, 414

E. coli 0157:H7 119
ecchymosis 157, 293, 578
edema 139, 425
emesis basin 361
empathetic 26
empathy 30
Enablers 606
enema 458
environmental services department 86
epidermis 307
epiglottis 157
Ergonomics 586
Escherichia coli 116
Evaluation 83
exacerbations 290
excretions 100
Exhalation 414
expiration 414
exposure control plan 105
expressive aphasia 41, 274
external catheter 442
Extremity restraints 612

factual 132
Fahrenheit scale 400
False imprisonment 176
Fats 185
Fecal impaction 260, 456
Fecal material 260, 456
feces 455
fetal position 595
flank 439
Flatus 258, 456
flexion 614
fluid restrictions 205
fomites 93
food pyramid 186
foot board 594
force 413
force fluids 205, 425
foreskin 435
Fowler's 595
fracture 156, 292, 577
Friction 311, 591
Full-liquid diet 190
Functional incontinence 437

gait belt 24, 587
gastrostomy 554
gastrostomy tube 201
gatch handles 344
generalized application 138
generalized 92
genital area 369
Geriatrics 3
Global aphasia 41, 274
Good Samaritan laws 177
graduate 425, 450
grieving process 502

Hallucinations 641
hantavirus 120
Head lice 122
health care proxy 175
Health Insurance Portability and Accountability Act (HIPAA) 51
health maintenance organization (HMO) 7
hemiplegia 272
Hemorrhage 157
Hepatitis B 102
hepatitis C 102
high efficiency particulate air (HEPA) respirator 112
holistically 213
hospice 6, 501
Hospice care 6
Hospitals 2
host 93
HS care 358
human immunodeficiency virus (HIV) disease 102
humidifier 140
hygiene 358
Hyperalimentation 203
Hyperglycemia 321
Hypertension 238, 416
Hypoglycemia 321
Hypotension 416
hypothermia 401, 469, 471

identification band 135
immune system 92
Immunizations 20
Implementation 83
incident 132
incision 554
incontinent 358
indirect contact 93
indwelling catheters 442
Infection 92
infection control 92
Inhalation 414
inspiration 414
Instantaneous injuries 586
Insulin 315
intake and output (I&O) 204, 425
interdisciplinary team 10
intermittent catheter 443
Intravenous feedings 203
Involuntary seclusion 176
Isolation 111
IV standard 81

jaundiced 102

Kidneys 252, 435

labia majora 323, 435
labia minora 323, 435
laboratory requisition 450
larynx 247
lateral 595
leg drainage bags 443
lethargy 204
level of consciousness 151
licensed practical nurses (LPN) 10
licensed vocational nurses (LVN) 10
living will 175
localized 92
localized application 138

lockout-tagout 135
Long-term care facilities 2
Low beds 345
low-cholesterol diets 191
Lowfat 191

Malnutrition 199
material safety data sheets (MSDS) 135
Mechanical soft diet 191
Mechanically altered diets 190
Medicaid 7
Medical asepsis 92
medical record 48
Medicare 7
mentally retarded 3
Methicillin-resistant Staphylococcus aureus (MRSA) 121
Microorganisms 92
micturition 435
midstream (clean-catch) specimen 450
milliliters (mL) 206
Minerals 186
Minimum Data Set 2.0 8
mite 124
Mixed incontinence 437
mode of transmission 94
morning care 358
mucous membranes 100
Multiple sclerosis (MS) 276
multiskilled workers 2

N95 respirator 113
nasogastric tube 201
nasogastric tube (NG tube) 259
negative pressure environment 112
Neglect 174
Negligence 176
nits 122
no concentrated sweets diet 191
nonintact skin 100
Nonrapid eye movement (NREM) sleep 74
Normal flora 92
Nosocomial infection 92
Nursing Interventions Classification (NIC) 10
Nursing Outcomes Classification (NOC) 10
nursing process 83
Nutrients 185

Objective 48
OBRA 7
Occupational Safety and Health Administration (OSHA) 146
occupied bedmaking 346
Oral temperature 400
Osteoporosis 291
ostomy 463
ovaries 315, 325
overbed table 343
Overflow incontinence 437

pacemaker 242, 554
Pain 69
Paraphrasing 31
paraplegic 36
parasites 122
Parkinson's disease 274
partial bath 365
Pathogen 92
patient 2
penis 435
peri-care 383
Perineal care 368
perineum 368
peristalsis 257, 453
Perseveration 641
personal protective equipment (PPE) 105
Personal space 178
petechiae 119
PFR95 respirator 113
pharynx 245
Physical restraints 606
Planning 83
plaque 360
portal of entry 94
portal of exit 94
Post polio syndrome (PPS) 277
postmortem care 504
postural supports 606
preferred provider organization (PPO) 7
prefix 57
Prehypertension 416
pressure sores 588
Pressure ulcers 311, 588
priorities 24
probe 404
probe cover 404
professional 19
professional boundaries 18
Projection 628
prostate 436
prosthesis 36
protective isolation. 111
Proteins 185
Pseudomembranous colitis 120
pulse 400
pulse points. 412
pulse pressure 417
pulse rate 413
Pureed diet 190

RACE System 143
radial pulse 412
Rapid eye movement (REM) sleep 74
Rationalization 628
Reality orientation 648
receptive aphasia 41, 274
Rectal temperature 400
Reflex incontinence 437
Reflexes 132
registered nurse (RN) 6
regular diet 190
rehabilitation 2
reimburses 7
Reminiscing 649
remissions 290
reservoir 94
resident 2
Residents' Bill of Rights 169
resolved 132
respiration 400
Responsible behavior 24
Rest 73
Restorative care 179
restorative care 2
Restraints 606
retention enema 459
rhythm 413
rigor mortis 504
Risk factors 8
root 57

Scabies 124
scale 400
scrotum 315
secretions. 93
seizure 151
self-esteem 14, 625
semiprone position 601
semisupine position 600
Senile purpura 310
Sensory loss 638
Septic 443
sexual abuse 635
shearing 591
sheaths 402
Shingles 121
Shock 157
Shroud 510–511
Shunt 417
Signs 48
Sims' position 459
Skin tears 308
Slander 176
Sleep 73
sleep deprivation 75
sodium-restricted diet 191
source 94
sperm 323
sphygmomanometer 417
standard precautions 105
Standards of care 177
Stereotyping 178
Sterile 443
Sterilization 92
Stethoscope 415
Stoma 463

Stool 258, 456
Strains 157
Stress 23
stress incontinence 437
strict I 203
stump sock 393
subacute 5
subcutaneous tissue 307
Subjective 48
Suffix 57
Sundowning 641
Supine 595
Supplemental feedings 192
Suppression 628
suprapubic catheter 442
Susceptibility 92
susceptible host 94
Sympathy 30
Symptoms 48
Syncope 149
systolic blood pressure 415

tachycardia 413
Tact 19
tactful 18
temperature 400
tepid 138, 310
terminal illness 500
testes 315
Therapeutic diets 191
Thermal burns 138
Thermometer 400
toe pleat 352
tornado warning 145
tornado watch 145
total parenteral nutrition (TPN) 203
Trachea 245
transfer 81, 552
transfer belt 587
Transient ischemic attack (TIA) 237, 272
transmission-based precautions. 111
transport bag 451
tremors 132, 274
Tuberculosis (TB) 121
Turgor 204
tympanic temperature 400
tympanic thermometer 404

unit 16, 343
universal choking sign 162
Ureters 252, 435
Urethra 252, 435
Urge incontinence 437
Urinal 438
urinary meatus 252, 324, 435
urinary retention 436
urination 435
Uterus 326

Vagina 326
Validation therapy 647
Vancomycin-resistant Enterococcus (VRE) 121
Vectors 93
Veins 230
vest restraint 611
Viruses 92
vital signs 149, 400
Vitamins 186
voiding 435
Vulva 323

Warm soaks 476
waterless bathing 368
Wet compresses 476